CONTENTS

UNIT 1: ASSESSMENT OF THE WHOLE PERSON

1 Evidence-Based Assessment, 1
2 Cultural Competence: Cultural Care, 11
3 The Interview, 29
4 The Complete Health History, 49
5 Mental Status Assessment, 71
6 Substance Use Assessment, 93
7 Domestic Violence Assessment, 103

UNIT 2: APPROACH TO THE CLINICAL SETTING

8 Assessment Techniques and the Clinical Setting, 115
9 General Survey, Measurement, Vital Signs, 127
10 Pain Assessment: The Fifth Vital Sign, 159
11 Nutritional Assessment, 175

UNIT 3: PHYSICAL EXAMINATION

12 Skin, Hair, and Nails, 203
13 Head, Face, and Neck, Including Regional Lymphatics, 251
14 Eyes, 279
15 Ears, 323
16 Nose, Mouth, and Throat, 351
17 Breasts and Regional Lymphatics, 383
18 Thorax and Lungs, 411
19 Heart and Neck Vessels, 455
20 Peripheral Vascular System and Lymphatic System, 499
21 Abdomen, 527
22 Musculoskeletal System, 565
23 Neurologic System, 621
24 Male Genitourinary System, 679
25 Anus, Rectum, and Prostate, 709
26 Female Genitourinary System, 725

UNIT 4: INTEGRATION OF THE HEALTH SYSTEM

27 The Complete Health Assessment: Putting It All Together, 763
28 Bedside Assessment of the Hospitalized Adult, 787
29 The Pregnant Woman, 795
30 Functional Assessment of the Older Adult, 829

Illustration Credits, 847

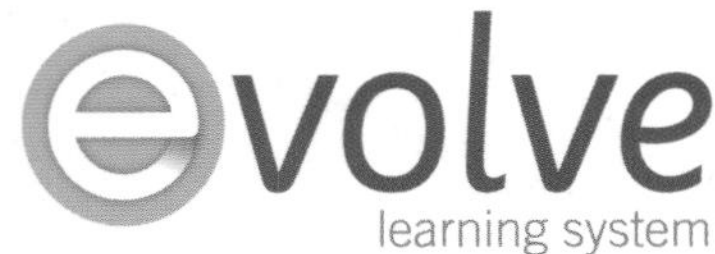

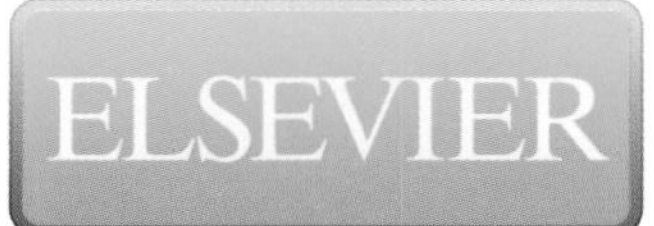

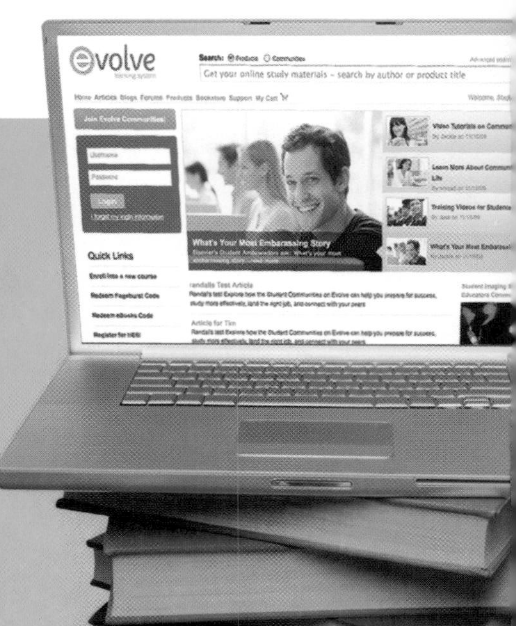

YOU'VE JUST PURCHASED MORE THAN A TEXTBOOK

ACTIVATE THE COMPLETE LEARNING EXPERIENCE THAT COMES WITH YOUR BOOK BY REGISTERING AT

http://evolve.elsevier.com/Jarvis

Once you register, you will have access to your FREE STUDY TOOLS:

- Abdomen, Heart, and Lung Sounds
- Animations
- Appendixes
- Assessment Videos
- Audio Key Points
- Bedside Assessment Summary Checklists
- Case Studies
- Complete Physical Examination Form
- Health Promotion Guides
- NCLEX® Review Questions
- Physical Examination Summary Checklists
- Quick Assessments for Common Conditions

REGISTER TODAY!

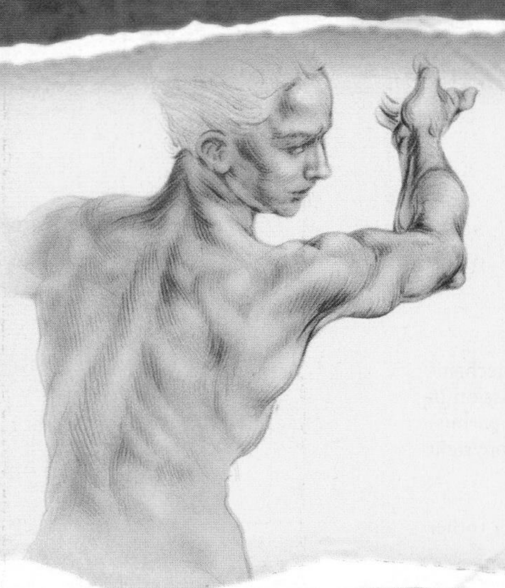

CAROLYN JARVIS, PhD, APN, CNP
Professor of Nursing
School of Nursing
Illinois Wesleyan University
Bloomington, Illinois
and
Family Nurse Practitioner
Bloomington, Illinois

Physical Examination & Health Assessment

6th Edition

Original Illustrations by Pat Thomas, CMI, FAMI
Oak Park, Illinois

Assessment Photographs by Kevin Strandberg
Professor of Art
Illinois Wesleyan University
Bloomington, Illinois

ELSEVIER
SAUNDERS

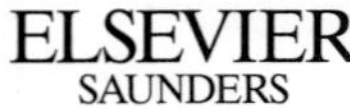

3251 Riverport Lane
St. Louis, Missouri 63043

PHYSICAL EXAMINATION AND HEALTH ASSESSMENT ISBN: 978-1-4377-0151-7

Notices

Knowledge and best practice in this field are constantly changing. As new research and experience broaden our understanding, changes in research methods, professional practices, or medical treatment may become necessary.

Practitioners and researchers must always rely on their own experience and knowledge in evaluating and using any information, methods, compounds, or experiments described herein. In using such information or methods they should be mindful of their own safety and the safety of others, including parties for whom they have a professional responsibility.

With respect to any drug or pharmaceutical products identified, readers are advised to check the most current information provided (i) on procedures featured or (ii) by the manufacturer of each product to be administered, to verify the recommended dose or formula, the method and duration of administration, and contraindications. It is the responsibility of practitioners, relying on their own experience and knowledge of their patients, to make diagnoses, to determine dosages and the best treatment for each individual patient, and to take all appropriate safety precautions.

To the fullest extent of the law, neither the Publisher nor the authors, contributors, or editors, assume any liability for any injury and/or damage to persons or property as a matter of products liability, negligence or otherwise, or from any use or operation of any methods, products, instructions, or ideas contained in the material herein.

ISBN: 978-1-4377-0151-7

Executive Editor: Robin Carter
Managing Editor: Laurie Gower
Publishing Services Manager: Deborah L. Vogel
Senior Project Manager: Jodi M. Willard
Design Direction: Teresa McBryan

Printed in the United States of America

Last digit is the print number: 9 8 7 6 5 4 3

To my mother, Frances,
With gratitude

ABOUT THE AUTHOR

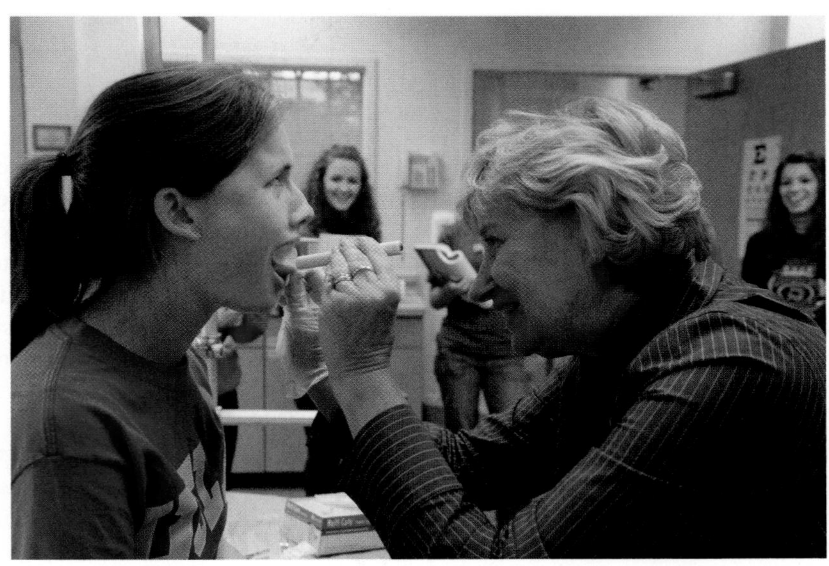

Carolyn Jarvis received her BSN cum laude from the University of Iowa, her MSN from Loyola University (Chicago), and her PhD from the University of Illinois at Chicago, with a research interest in the physiologic effect of alcohol on the cardiovascular system. She has taught physical assessment and critical care nursing at Rush University (Chicago), the University of Missouri (Columbia), and the University of Illinois (Urbana), and she has taught physical assessment, pharmacology, and pathophysiology at Illinois Wesleyan University (Bloomington).

Dr. Jarvis is a recipient of the University of Missouri's Superior Teaching Award; has taught physical assessment to thousands of baccalaureate students, graduate students, and nursing professionals; has held 150 continuing education seminars; and is the author of numerous articles and textbook contributions.

Dr. Jarvis has maintained a clinical practice in advanced practice roles—first as a cardiovascular clinical specialist in various critical care settings and as a certified family nurse practitioner in primary care. She is currently a Professor at Illinois Wesleyan University; is a nurse practitioner in Bloomington, Illinois; and is licensed as an advanced practice nurse in the state of Illinois. During the last 4 years, her enthusiasm has focused on learning Spanish to provide health care in rural Guatemala.

Martha Driessnack, PhD, PNP-BC, RN
The contributor for the health promotion content is a Pediatric Nurse Practitioner with more than 25 years of experience in teaching, practice, and research. She received her PhD from Oregon Health & Science University, completed a postdoctoral research fellowship in Clinical Genetics from the University of Iowa, and is an Assistant Professor in the College of Nursing at the University of Iowa.

Carla Graf, MS, RN, CNS-BC
The co-contributor for Chapter 30, Functional Assessment of the Older Adult, is a board certified Geriatric Clinical Nurse Specialist at the University of California, San Francisco (UCSF), and is an Assistant Clinical Professor at the UCSF School of Nursing. She is currently a doctoral student at UCSF, with a research focus on functional decline in hospitalized older adults.

Joyce K. Keithley, DNSc, RN, FAAN
The contributor for Chapter 11, Nutritional Assessment, is a Professor in the Department of Adult Health Nursing, Rush University College of Nursing and Rush University Medical Center in Chicago. Because she has worked in both clinical and instructional settings, she is an experienced and well-known practitioner, teacher, researcher, and author in the area of clinical nutrition.

Melissa A. Lee, MS, RN, CNS-BC
The co-contributor for Chapter 30, Functional Assessment of the Older Adult, is a Clinical Nurse Specialist at the University of California San Francisco Medical Center with experience in medical-surgical and telemetry nursing and education. She is certified in geriatrics by the American Nurses Credentialing Center.

Freda O'Bannon Lemmi, RN, MS, ANP-C, FNP
Images of normal and abnormal conditions are original photographs from patients in her clinical practice, students, relatives, and friends. She has been teaching physical assessment and curriculum of nurse practitioner programs as Professor of Nursing at California State University and at UCLA. She taught physical assessment classes in England to help prepare faculty to teach advanced nursing practice roles at the Royal Brompton Hospital in London in 1995 and at Oxford University in 1996. Carlos A.E. Lemmi, PhD, has taught microscopic anatomy to medical, dental, and graduate students at the UCLA school of medicine for over 15 years. His medical background and knowledge of computer graphics helped prepare the images for this book.

Shawna S. Mudd, MSN, CRNP
The co-contributor for Chapter 7, Domestic Violence Assessment, is a Pediatric Nurse Practitioner in the pediatric emergency department at the Johns Hopkins Hospital. She is also a member of the hospital's child protection team, which provides inpatient and outpatient consultation for cases of suspected child abuse and neglect. She is also faculty at the Johns Hopkins University School of Nursing.

Carolyn A. Nadeau, PhD
Dr. Nadeau contributed the Spanish terms at the back of this text. She is the Byron S. Tucci professor of Hispanic Studies at Illinois Wesleyan University, Bloomington, Illinois. She specializes in sixteenth-century and seventeenth-century Spanish literature and teaches the class, "Medical Spanish and Cultural Competency for Health Care."

Daniel J. Sheridan, PhD, RN, FAAN
The co-contributor for Chapter 7, Domestic Violence Assessment, is an Associate Professor in the Johns Hopkins University School of Nursing, where he coordinates forensic clinical nurse specialist graduate degree programs at the Masters, DNP, and PhD levels. Dr. Sheridan has 25 years of experience working with survivors of family abuse and sexual assault, and he lectures and consults nationally and internationally on these topics.

Rachel E. Spector, PhD, RN, CTN, FAAN
The contributor for Chapter 2, Cultural Competence: Cultural Care, has focused on culturally diverse health and illness beliefs and practices for more than 40 years. She retired from the Connell Boston College School of Nursing, Massachusetts. She was a Lady Davis Fellow in the Henrietta Zold-Hadassah Hebrew University School of Nursing in Jerusalem, Israel. The seventh edition of her text, *Cultural Diversity in Health and Illness,* was published in 2009. The Massachusetts Association of Registered Nurses honored her as a "Living Legend" in 2007, and in 2008 she received an Honorary Human Rights Award from the American Nurses' Association.

Deborah E. Swenson, MSN, ARNP, C-WHCNP
The contributor for Chapter 29, The Pregnant Woman, is a certified Women's Health Care Nurse Practitioner with Swedish Medical Center's Perinatal Medicine Clinic and OBSTETRIX Medical Group of Washington, Inc., P.S. in Seattle, Washington. She holds certification from the NCC as a Women's Health Care Nurse Practitioner. She is the author of *Telephone Triage for the Obstetric Patient: A Nursing Guide.*

INSTRUCTOR AND STUDENT ANCILLARIES

Health Assessment Online

Tim J. Bristol, PhD, RN, CNE
Faculty
Walden University
Waconia, Minnesota

Quick Assessments for Common Conditions

Ben Galatzan, MSN, RN
ADN Faculty
Southeast Community College
Lincoln, Nebraska

Health Promotion Guides

Nancy Haugen, PhD, RN
Associate Professor and ABSN Program Chair
School of Nursing
Samuel Merritt University
Oakland, California

Audience Response Questions, Instructor's Manual, Pre-Lecture Quizzes

Maria E. Lauer, MSN, RN, CNE
Nursing Instructor
School of Nursing and Allied Health Professions
Thomas Edison State College
Trenton, New Jersey

Case Studies, Student Laboratory Manual

Sharon R. Redding MN, RN, CNE
Nurse Educator
Alegent Bergan Mercy Medical Center
Omaha, Nebraska

Test Bank

Julie S. Snyder, MSN, RN-BC
Adjunct Faculty, School of Nursing
Old Dominion University
Norfolk, Virginia

Health Assessment Online

Lori Stephens, MN, RN
Nursing Faculty
Skagit Valley College
Mount Vernon, Washington

NCLEX® Review Questions

Jo A. Voss, PhD, RN, CNS
Associate Professor
South Dakota State University
Rapid City, South Dakota

Mary Anne Anderson, RN, BSN, MA, MS, CLC, LCCE
Professor, Nursing
Contra Costa College
San Pablo, California

Maureen Anthony, PhD, RN
Associate Professor
University of Detroit—Mercy
Detroit, Michigan

Susan Caplan, RN, MS
Assistant Professor, College of Nursing
University of Southern Maine
Portland, Maine

Patricia S. Conklin, MSN, RN
Assistant Professor of Nursing
Radford University
Radford, Virginia

Kristin H. Conrad, MSN, APRN, CNM
Instructor, School of Nursing
Radford University
Radford, Virginia

Paula Cox-North, MN, NP-C
Advanced Registered Nurse Practitioner
Harborview Medical Center
Seattle, Washington

Joseph T. DeRanieri, DM, MSN, RN, CPN, BCECR
Assistant Professor, Director of Health Services Administration Program
University of Delaware
Newark, Delaware

Sharon Forney, MSN, RN, MSHCA
Faculty, ADN Program
North Central Texas College
Gainesville, Texas

Jeannine Forrest, PhD, RN
Project Manager, Palliative Care for Advanced Dementia
Alzheimer's Association, Greater Illinois Chapter
Chicago, Illinois

Melissa Gutschall, PhD, RD
Assistant Professor, Department of Nutrition and Health Care Management
Appalachian State University
Boone, North Carolina

Mary Ann Jarmulowicz, RN, MSN, BC-GNP
Nursing Instructor
University of South Carolina Beaufort
Bluffton, South Carolina

Brenda Condusta Pavill, RN, CRNP, PhD
Associate Professor, School of Nursing
University of North Carolina at Wilmington
Wilmington, North Carolina

Demetrius James Porche, DNS, PhD, APRN, FNP, FAANP, FAAN
Dean and Professor, School of Nursing
Louisiana State University Health Sciences Center
New Orleans, Louisiana

Mary Shelkey, PhD, GNP-BC
Assistant Professor, College of Nursing
Seattle University
Seattle, Washington

Susan Shirato, RN, DNP, CCRN
Instructor, Jefferson School of Nursing
Thomas Jefferson University
Philadelphia, Pennsylvania

Beryl Stetson, RNBC, MSN
Assistant Professor, Nursing
Raritan Valley Community College
Somerville, New Jersey;
Nursing Education Specialist
Robert Wood Johnson University Hospital
New Brunswick, New Jersey

Donna Walls, MS, RN
Associate Clinical Professor, College of Nursing
Texas Woman's University
Dallas, Texas

Tami Wright, RN, MSN
Clinical Instructor, College of Nursing
The University of Texas at Arlington
Arlington, Texas

Joanne M. Yastik, PhDc, RN
Assistant Professor, McAuley School of Nursing
University of Detroit—Mercy
Detroit, Michigan

This book is for those who still carefully examine their patients and for those of you who wish to learn how to do so. You develop and practice, and then learn to trust, your health history and physical examination skills. In this book, I give you the tools to do that. Learn to listen to the patient—most often he or she will tell you what is wrong (and right) and what you can do to meet his or her health care needs. Then learn to inspect, examine, and listen to the person's body. The data are all there and are accessible to you by using just a few extra tools. High-tech machinery is a smart and sophisticated adjunct, but it cannot replace your own bedside assessment of your patient. Whether you are a beginning examiner or an advanced-practice student, this book holds the content you need to develop and refine your clinical skills.

Thank you for your enthusiastic response to the earlier editions of *Physical Examination & Health Assessment.* I am also grateful for your encouragement and for your suggestions, which are incorporated wherever possible. This revision of *Physical Examination & Health Assessment* presents a comprehensive textbook of health history–taking methods, physical examination skills, health promotion techniques, and clinical assessment tools.

NEW TO THE SIXTH EDITION

The sixth edition retains the strengths of the first five editions: a clear, approachable writing style; an attractive and user-friendly format; integrated developmental variations across the life span with age-specific content on the infant, child, adolescent, pregnant woman, and older adult; cultural competencies in both a separate chapter and throughout the book; hundreds of meticulously prepared full-color illustrations; sample charting of normal findings and sample clinical case studies; integration of the complete health assessment in a photo essay at the end of the book where all key steps of a complete head-to-toe examination of the adult and child are summarized; and a photo essay highlighting a condensed head-to-toe assessment for each daily shift of nursing care.

A new chapter and several new content features are presented in this sixth edition.

New Chapter 6, **Substance Use Assessment**, covers pertinent alcohol and drug abuse topics in the context of the health history/physical examination.

Chapter 1, **Evidence-Based Assessment,** is reoriented to reflect a focus on conducting the most effective, qualitative exams based on data showing their usefulness in patient assessment. Throughout the text, examination techniques are retained or dropped with explanation, depending on the **evidence.**

All chapters have current research citing new content on **genetics** and racial variations in disease incidence and response to treatment. The Jarvis text has the richest amount of cultural-racial-genetic content available in any assessment text.

New content on **obesity** is added to numerous chapters to address the important role we health care providers have in assessing and addressing obesity in adults and children.

Three new **Promoting a Healthy Lifestyle** boxes are presented and 15 others are thoroughly updated. These boxes describe an important teaching topic related to the body system discussed in each chapter—a teaching topic you can use to enhance patient health.

The **Abnormal Findings** tables located at the end of the chapters are revised and updated with many new clinical photos. These are still divided into two sections. The Abnormal Findings tables present frequently encountered conditions that every clinician should recognize, and the Abnormal Findings for Advanced Practice tables isolate the detailed illustrated atlas of conditions encountered in advanced practice roles.

All chapters are **revised and updated,** with expanded coverage in anatomy and physiology, physical examination, and assessment tools.

Growth and development content is integrated and thoroughly updated. **Developmental Competence** sections provide expected growth and development information, and the Examination section of each body system chapter details **exam techniques and clinical findings for infants, children, adolescents, and aging adults**. The Student Laboratory Manual accompanying the sixth edition text also includes appendixes that provide summaries of infant, toddler, preschooler, school-age, and adolescent growth, development, and health maintenance competencies.

Culture and Genetics data have been revised and updated in each chapter. Together with a revised Chapter 2 on cultural competence, these data highlight the importance of diversity and cultural awareness.

Full-color art includes over 200 new illustrations, including 100 new step-by-step images on examining the eye, mouth, throat, heart, neck, and peripheral vascular system; 50 newly drawn figures; and 50 new photos of abnormal findings.

New **audio reviews** with key points for every chapter are now provided so students can review content in a portable audio format.

Chapter bibliographies are up-to-date and meant to be used. They include the best of clinical practice readings as well as basic science research and nursing research, with an emphasis on scholarship from the last 5 years.

DUAL FOCUS AS TEXT AND REFERENCE

Physical Examination & Health Assessment is a **text for beginning students** of physical examination as well as a **text and**

reference for advanced practitioners. The chapter progression and format permit this scope without sacrificing one use for the other.

Chapters 1 through 7 focus on **health assessment of the whole person,** including health promotion for all age-groups, cultural environment and assessment, interviewing and complete health history gathering, the social environment of mental status, and the changes to the whole person on the occasions of substance use or domestic violence.

Chapters 8 through 11 begin the approach to the **clinical care setting,** describing physical data-gathering techniques, how to set up the examination site, body measurement and vital signs, pain assessment, and nutritional assessment.

Chapters 12 through 26 focus on the **physical examination and related health history** in a body systems approach. This is the most efficient method of performing the examination and is the most logical method for student learning and retrieval of data. **Each chapter has five major sections:** Structure and Function, Subjective Data (history), Objective Data (examination skills and findings), Documentation and Critical Thinking, and Abnormal Findings. The novice practitioner can review anatomy and physiology and learn the skills, expected findings, and common variations for generally healthy people and selected abnormal findings in the Objective Data sections.

Chapters 27 through 30 **integrate the complete health assessment.** Chapters 27 and 28 present the choreography of the head-to-toe exam for a complete screening examination in various age-groups and for the focused exam in this **unique chapter on a hospitalized adult.** Chapters 29 and 30 present special populations—the health assessment of the pregnant woman and the functional assessment of the older adult, including assessment tools, caregiver assessment, environmental assessment, and elder mistreatment.

Students will use this text in sequenced courses throughout their education and into advanced practice. As each course demands more advanced skills and techniques, students review the detailed presentation and the additional techniques in the Objective Data sections as well as variations for different age levels. Students can also study the extensive pathology illustrations and detailed text in the Abnormal Findings sections.

This text is valuable to both advanced practice students and experienced clinicians because of its comprehensive approach. *Physical Examination & Health Assessment* can help clinicians learn the skills for advanced practice, refresh their memory, review a specific examination technique when confronted with an unfamiliar clinical situation, and compare and label a diagnostic finding.

CONCEPTUAL APPROACH

Physical Examination & Health Assessment is committed to:

- **Holism,** the individual as a whole, both in wellness needs and illness needs
- **Health promotion,** in the health history questions that elicit self-care behaviors, the Promoting a Healthy Lifestyle boxes, nutrition information, and the self-examination teaching presented for skin, breast, and testicles
- Contracting with the person as an **active participant in health care** by discussing what the person currently is doing to promote health and by engaging the person to participate in self-care
- **Cultural competencies** that take into account this global society in which culturally diverse people seek health care
- Individuals **across the life cycle,** supporting the belief that a person's state of health must be considered in light of developmental stage. All chapters integrate relevant developmental content. Developmental anatomy, modifications of examination technique, and expected findings are given for infants and children, adolescents, pregnant females, and aging adults

FEATURES FROM EARLIER EDITIONS

Physical Examination & Health Assessment is built on the strengths of the previous edition and is designed to engage students and enhance learning:

1. **Method of examination** (Objective Data section) is clear, orderly, and easy to follow. Hundreds of original examination illustrations are placed directly with the text to demonstrate the physical examination in a step-by-step format.
2. **Two-column format** begins in the Subjective Data section, where the running column highlights the rationales for asking history questions. In the Objective Data section, the running column highlights selected abnormal findings to show a clear relationship between normal and abnormal findings.
3. **Abnormal Findings tables** organize and expand on material in the examination section. The atlas format of these extensive collections of pathology and original illustrations helps students recognize, sort, and describe abnormal findings. When applicable, the text under a table entry is presented in a Subjective Data–Objective Data format.
4. **Developmental approach** in each chapter presents prototypical content on the adult, then age-specific content for the infant, child, adolescent, pregnant female, and aging adult so that students can learn common variations for all age-groups.
5. **Cultural competencies** are extensive throughout and present the expected variations for culturally diverse people. Chapter 2 keynotes the cultural content, including customs to consider when planning the interview, cultural variations to consider when reviewing examination findings, and a Heritage Assessment Guide.
6. **Stunning full-color art** shows detailed human anatomy, physiology, examination techniques, and abnormal findings.
7. **Health history** (Subjective Data) appears in two places: (1) in Chapter 4, The Complete Health History, and (2) in pertinent history questions that are repeated and expanded in each regional examination chapter, including history questions that highlight health promotion

and self-care. This presentation helps students understand the relationship between subjective and objective data. Considering the history and examination data together, as you do in the clinical setting, means that each chapter can stand on its own if a person has a specific problem related to that body system.

Chapter 3, The Interview, has the most complete discussion available on the process of communication, interviewing skills, techniques and traps, and cultural considerations (for example, how nonverbal behavior varies cross-culturally and the use of an interpreter).

8. **Summary checklists** at the end of each chapter provide a quick review of examination steps to help develop a mental checklist.
9. **Sample recordings** of normal findings show the written language you should use so that charting, whether written or electronic, is complete yet succinct.
10. **Focused assessment/clinical case studies** of frequently encountered situations show the application of assessment techniques to patients of varying ages and clinical situations. These case histories, in SOAP format ending in diagnosis, are presented in the language actually used in recording. Diagnoses are derived from assessment data and show the relationship between medical and nursing diagnoses. Further nursing diagnoses are presented online on the Evolve website at http://evolve.elsevier.com/Jarvis/.
11. **Integration of the complete health assessment** for the adult, infant, and child is presented as an illustrated essay in Chapter 27. This approach integrates all the steps into a choreographed whole. Included is a complete write-up of a health history and physical examination.
12. **User-friendly design** makes the book easy to use. Frequent subheadings and instructional headings assist in easy retrieval of material.
13. **Spanish-language translations** highlight important phrases for communication during the physical examination and appear on the inside back cover.

SUPPLEMENTS

- The ***Pocket Companion for Physical Examination & Health Assessment*** continues to be a handy and current clinical reference that provides pertinent material in full color, with over 150 illustrations from the textbook.
- The ***Student Laboratory Manual*** with physical examination forms is a workbook that includes for each chapter a student study guide, glossary of key terms, clinical objectives, regional write-up forms, and review questions. The pages are perforated so that students can use the regional write-up forms in the skills laboratory or in the clinical setting and turn them in to the instructor. The Student Laboratory Manual also includes appendixes that provide summaries of infant, toddler, preschooler, school-age, and adolescent growth, development, and health maintenance competencies.
- The new revised ***Health Assessment Online*** is an innovative and dynamic teaching and learning tool with over **8000 electronic assets**, including video clips, anatomic overlays, animations, audio clips, interactive exercises, laboratory/diagnostic tests, review questions, and new **electronic charting activities.** Comprehensive **Self-Paced Learning Modules** offer increased flexibility to faculty who wish to provide students with tutorial learning modules and in-depth capstone case studies for each body system chapter in the text. The **Capstone Case Studies** now include **Quality and Safety Challenge** activities. Additional **Advance Practice Case Studies** put the student in the exam room and test history taking and documentation skills. The comprehensive **video clip library** shows exam procedures across the life span and is expanded to now include clips on the pregnant woman. Animations, sounds, images, interactive activities, and video clips are embedded in the learning modules and cases to provide a dynamic, multimodal learning environment for today's learners.
- ***Physical Examination*** & ***Health Assessment Video Series*** is an 18-video package developed in conjunction with this text. There are 12 body system videos and 6 head-to-toe videos, with the latter containing complete examinations of the neonate, child, adult, older adult, pregnant woman, and the bedside examination of a hospitalized adult. This series is available in DVD or streaming online formats. There are over 5 hours of video footage with highlighted Cross-Cultural Care Considerations, Developmental Considerations, and Health Promotion Tips, as well as Instructor Booklets with video overviews, outlines, learning objectives, discussion topics, and questions with answers.
- The companion ***EVOLVE Website*** (http://evolve.elsevier.com/Jarvis/) contains learning objectives, more than 300 multiple-choice review questions, system-by-system exam summaries, bedside exam summaries, and key points from the chapter that are downloadable into audio CD or MP3 player files, a comprehensive physical exam form for the adult, and numerous reference appendixes from previous editions that have been updated and moved online, including immunization schedules, Standard Precautions, growth charts, and blood pressure levels. **Case studies**—including a variety of developmental and cultural variables—help students apply health assessment skills and knowledge. These include 25 in-depth case studies with critical thinking questions and answer guidelines, as well as printable health promotion handouts. Also included is a complete Head-to-Toe Video examination of the adult that can be viewed in its entirety or by systems, as well as a new printable section on Quick Assessments for Common Conditions.
- ***Simulation Learning System.*** The new *Simulation Learning System* (SLS) is an online toolkit that incorporates medium- to high-fidelity simulation with scenarios that enhance the clinical decision-making skills of students. The SLS offers a comprehensive package of resources, including leveled patient scenarios, detailed instructions for preparation and implementation of the simulation experience, debriefing questions that encourage critical

thinking, and learning resources to reinforce student comprehension.

- For instructors, the Evolve website presents an Instructor's Manual and PowerPoint slides, a comprehensive Image Collection, Audience Response Questions for iClicker and other systems, and a Test Bank. The **Instructor's Manual** provides annotated learning objectives, key terms, teaching strategies for the classroom in a revised section with strategies for both clinical and simulation lab use and a focus on QSEN competencies, critical thinking exercises, websites, and performance checklists. The **PowerPoint** slides include 2000 slides with integrated images. **Audience Response Questions** provide 90 questions for in-class student participation. A separate 1200-illustration **Image Collection** is featured and, finally, the ExamView **Test Bank** has over 1000 multiple-choice questions with coded answers and rationales.

IN CONCLUSION

Throughout all stages of manuscript preparation and production, every effort has been made to develop a book that is readable, informative, instructive, and vital. Your comments and suggestions have been important to this task and continue to be welcome for this edition.

Carolyn Jarvis
c/o Nursing Editorial
Elsevier
3251 Riverport Lane
Maryland Heights, MO 63043

ACKNOWLEDGMENTS

It is my pleasure to recognize the many wonderful friends and colleagues who helped make the revision of this textbook possible. For their help and support I send my gratitude:

To my artistic colleagues, who made this book the vibrant visual display it is. Pat Thomas, medical illustrator, is a gifted artist with an eye for detail and clarity. Kevin Strandberg is a clever and careful photographer who has endless patience for capturing the images of children and adults in just the right moment of the examination. It is wonderful to collaborate with these two professionals. Our team has worked together for six editions, providing an artistic unity and clarity to this latest textbook. We are joined in this edition by Ronnie Lemmi, who contributed many photos of abnormal conditions, gathered through her clinical practice.

To my research assistants, whose tireless help enabled me to survive and proceed through manuscript preparation and revision. Erin Kugler and Abby Hoekstra searched for and retrieved countless articles. Abby read and reread endless copies of galleys and page proofs, making suggestions and finding errors.

To the faculty and students who took the time to write letters of encouragement and suggestions—your comments are gratefully received and are very helpful. To the reviewers who spent considerable time reading the chapter manuscript and filling out response questionnaires—your suggestions and ideas are very important for this sixth edition.

Thank you to the remarkable professional team at Elsevier. I am grateful to Sally Schrefer, Managing Director, Nursing and Health Professions, for her guidance and support for the book and its ancillaries. Sally knows the text well and has been personally involved in its advancement and promotion. Robin Carter, Executive Editor, has been a beacon of support for me and for the book. Robin always has sound suggestions for new ideas for the book and is everlastingly prompt and positive.

Many people worked very hard to guide this book through production. I am grateful to Debbie Vogel, Publishing Services Manager, for supervising the schedule for book production and making all the contacts to keep everyone on schedule. My thanks go especially to Jodi Willard, Senior Project Manager, who has been so organized and positive in our day-to-day production schedule. Her messages are always welcome. I know readers will share my pleasure in the striking colors and design of the sixth edition. I am grateful to Teresa McBryan, Design Manager, for coordinating the beautiful interior design. The design draws the reader into the book and guides one through all of the subsections. The dramatic illustration on the cover is the work of Max Fischer. The individual page layout is the wonderful work of Leslie Foster, Illustrator/Designer. Leslie crafts every page, always planning how the page can be made even better. Finally, I am so fortunate to have the support of Laurie Gower, Managing Editor. Laurie is so prompt and efficient and cheerful in directing the countless details of moving along the manuscript. It is always my pleasure to work with Deanna Dedeke, Developmental Editor. Deanna has been an instrumental part of the team for many editions. Deanna has worked tirelessly and efficiently to guide the instructor ancillaries, the Pocket Companion, and the Student Laboratory Manual. I am very grateful to Laurie and Deanna.

Most important are the members of my wonderful family for their help, love, and complete support. Their constant belief in me and their encouragement have kept me going throughout this process.

Carolyn Jarvis

UNIT 1: ASSESSMENT OF THE WHOLE PERSON

1 Evidence-Based Assessment, 1
2 Cultural Competence: Cultural Care, 11
3 The Interview, 29
4 The Complete Health History, 49
5 Mental Status Assessment, 71
6 Substance Use Assessment, 93
7 Domestic Violence Assessment, 103

UNIT 2: APPROACH TO THE CLINICAL SETTING

8 Assessment Techniques and the Clinical Setting, 115
9 General Survey, Measurement, Vital Signs, 127
10 Pain Assessment: The Fifth Vital Sign, 159
11 Nutritional Assessment, 175

UNIT 3: PHYSICAL EXAMINATION

12 Skin, Hair, and Nails, 203
13 Head, Face, and Neck, Including Regional Lymphatics, 251
14 Eyes, 279
15 Ears, 323
16 Nose, Mouth, and Throat, 351
17 Breasts and Regional Lymphatics, 383
18 Thorax and Lungs, 411
19 Heart and Neck Vessels, 455
20 Peripheral Vascular System and Lymphatic System, 499
21 Abdomen, 527
22 Musculoskeletal System, 565
23 Neurologic System, 621
24 Male Genitourinary System, 679
25 Anus, Rectum, and Prostate, 709
26 Female Genitourinary System, 725

UNIT 4: INTEGRATION OF THE HEALTH SYSTEM

27 The Complete Health Assessment: Putting It All Together, 763
28 Bedside Assessment of the Hospitalized Adult, 787
29 The Pregnant Woman, 795
30 Functional Assessment of the Older Adult, 829

Illustration Credits, 847

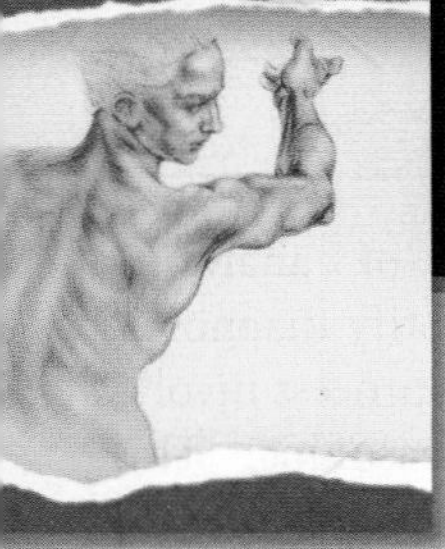

CHAPTER 1

Evidence-Based Assessment

evolve WEBSITE

http://evolve.elsevier.com/Jarvis/

- Audio Key Points
- NCLEX Review Questions

Ellen K. is a 23-year-old, white, unemployed woman who entered a substance abuse treatment program because of numerous drug-related driving offenses (Fig. 1-1).

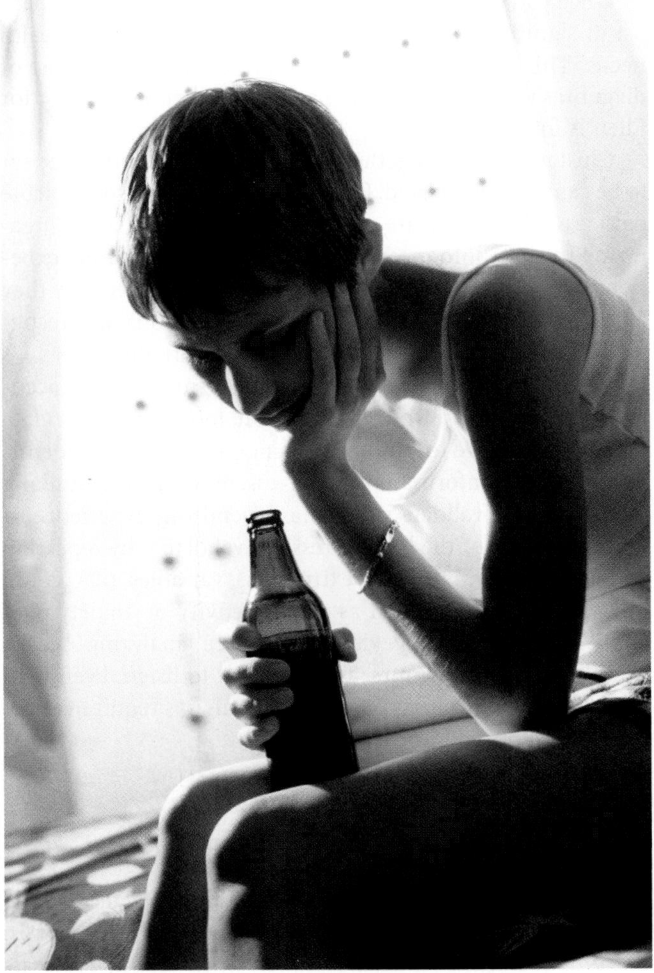

1-1

After Ellen's admission, the examiner collected a health history and performed a complete physical examination. The actual preliminary list of significant findings looked like this:

- High school academic record strong (A–/B+) in first 3 years, grades fell senior year but did graduate
- Alcohol abuse, started age 16, heavy daily usage × 3 years prior to admission (PTA), last drink 4 days PTA
- Smoked 2 packs per day (PPD) × 2 years, prior use 1 PPD × 4 years
- Elevated blood pressure (BP); 142/100 mm Hg at end of examination today
- Diminished breath sounds, with moderate expiratory wheeze and scattered rhonchi at both bases
- Grade II/VI systolic heart murmur, left lower sternal border
- Resolving hematoma, 2 to 3 cm, right (R) infraorbital ridge
- Missing R lower first molar, gums receding on lower incisors, multiple dark spots on all teeth
- Well-healed scar, 28 cm long × 2 cm wide, R lower leg, with R leg 3 cm shorter than left (L), sequela of auto accident age 12
- Altered nutrition—omits breakfast, daily intake has no fruits, no vegetables, eats meals at fast-food restaurants most days
- Oral contraceptives for birth control × 3 years, last pelvic examination 1 year PTA
- Unemployed × 6 months, previous work as cashier, bartender
- History of physically abusive relationship with boyfriend, today has orbital hematoma as a result of being hit; states, "It's OK, I probably deserved it."
- History of sexual abuse by father when Ellen was 12 to 16 years of age
- Relationships—estranged from parents, no close women friends, only significant relationship is with boyfriend of 2 years whom Ellen describes as physically abusive and alcoholic

The examiner analyzed and interpreted all the data; clustered the information, sorting out which data to refer and which to treat; and identified the diagnoses. It is interesting to note how many significant findings are derived from data the examiner collected. Not only physical data but also cognitive, psychosocial, and behavioral data are significant for an analysis of Ellen's health state. Also, the findings are interesting when considered from a life-cycle perspective; that is, Ellen is a young adult who normally should be concerned with the developmental tasks of emancipation from parents, building an independent lifestyle, establishing a vocation, making friends, forming an intimate bond with another, and establishing a social group.

A body of clinical **evidence** has validated the importance of using the assessment techniques in Ellen's case. For example, measuring BP screens for hypertension and early intervention here wards off heart attack and stroke. Listening to breath sounds screens (in Ellen's case) for asthma, which is compounded by her smoking. Listening to heart sounds yields Ellen's heart murmur, which could be "innocent" or a sign of a structural abnormality in a heart valve—further examination will tell. The physical examination is not just a rote formality. Its parts are determined by the best clinical evidence available and documented in the professional literature.

ASSESSMENT—POINT OF ENTRY IN AN ONGOING PROCESS

Assessment is the collection of data about the individual's health state. Throughout this text, you will be studying the techniques of collecting and analyzing **subjective data** (i.e., what the person *says* about himself or herself during history taking) and **objective data** (i.e., what you as the health professional *observe* by inspecting, percussing, palpating, and auscultating during the physical examination). Together with the patient's record and laboratory studies, these elements form the **database.**

From the database, you make a clinical judgment or diagnosis about the individual's health state or response to actual or risk health problems and life processes, as well as diagnoses about higher levels of wellness. Thus the purpose of assessment is to make a judgment or diagnosis.

An organized assessment is the starting point of diagnostic reasoning. Because all health care diagnoses, decisions, and treatments are based on the data you gather during assessment, it is paramount that your assessment be factual and complete.

Diagnostic Reasoning

The step from data collection to diagnosis can be a difficult one. Most beginning examiners perform well in gathering the data, given adequate practice, but then treat all the data as being equally important. This makes decision making slow and labored.

Diagnostic reasoning is the process of analyzing health data and drawing conclusions to identify diagnoses. Novice examiners most often use a diagnostic process involving hypothesis forming and deductive reasoning. This hypothetico-deductive process has four major components: (1) attending to initially available cues; (2) formulating diagnostic hypotheses; (3) gathering data relative to the tentative hypotheses; and (4) evaluating each hypothesis with the new data collected, thus arriving at a final diagnosis. A *cue* is a piece of information, a sign or symptom, or a piece of laboratory data. A *hypothesis* is a tentative explanation for a cue or a set of cues that can be used as a basis for further investigation.

For example, consider Ellen K., the case study presented at the beginning of this chapter. Ellen presents with a number of initial cues, one of which is the resolving hematoma under her eye. (1) You can recognize this cue even before history taking begins. Is it significant? (2) Ellen says she ran into a door, although she mumbles as she speaks and avoids eye contact. At this point, you formulate a hypothesis of trauma. (3) During the history and physical examination, you gather data to support or reject the tentative hypothesis. (4) You synthesize the new data collected, which support the hypothesis of trauma but eliminate the accidental cause. The final diagnoses are resolving right orbital contusion and risk for trauma.

Once you complete data collection, develop a preliminary list of significant signs and symptoms and all patient health needs. This is less formal in structure than your final list of diagnoses will be and is in no particular order. (Such a list for Ellen is found on p. 1.)

Cluster or group together the assessment data that appear to be causal or associated. For example, with a person in acute pain, associated data are rapid heart rate and anxiety. Organizing the data into meaningful clusters is slow at first; experienced examiners cluster data more rapidly because they recall proven results of earlier patient situations and recognize the same patterns in the new clinical situation.[9]

Validate the data you collect to make sure they are accurate. As you validate your information, look for gaps in data collection. Be sure to find the missing pieces, because identifying missing information is an essential critical-thinking skill. How you validate your data depends on experience. If you are unsure of the blood pressure, validate it by repeating it yourself. Eliminate any extraneous variables that could influence BP results, such as recent activity or anxiety over admission. If you have less experience analyzing breath sounds or heart murmurs, ask an expert to listen. Even with years of clinical experience, some signs always require validation (e.g., a breast lump).

Critical Thinking and the Diagnostic Process

The standards of practice in nursing, traditionally termed the **nursing process**, include six phases: assessment, diagnosis, outcome identification, planning, implementation, and evaluation.[2] This is a dynamic, interactive process; in today's complex clinical setting, practitioners move back and forth within the steps (Fig. 1-2).

Although the nursing process is a problem-solving approach, the way in which we apply the process depends on our level and time of experience. The *novice* has no experience with a specified patient population and uses rules to guide performance. It takes time, perhaps 2 to 3 years in similar clinical situations to achieve *competency,* in which you see actions in the context of arching goals or daily plans for patients. With more time and experience, the *proficient* nurse understands a patient situation as a whole rather than as a list of tasks. At this level, you can see long-term goals for the patient and how today's interventions apply to the point you want the patient to be in, say, 6 weeks. Finally, it seems that *expert* nurses vault over the steps and arrive at a clinical judgment in one leap. The expert has an intuitive grasp of a clinical situation and zeroes in on the accurate solution.[4]

Functioning at the level of expert in clinical judgment includes using intuition—that is, knowledge received as a whole. Intuition is characterized by immediate recognition of patterns—expert practitioners learn to attend to a pattern of assessment data and act without consciously labeling it. Whereas the beginner operates more from a set of defined, structured rules, the expert practitioner uses intuitive links, has the ability to see salient issues in a patient situation, and knows instant therapeutic responses.[5] The expert has a storehouse of experience about which interventions have been successful in the past.

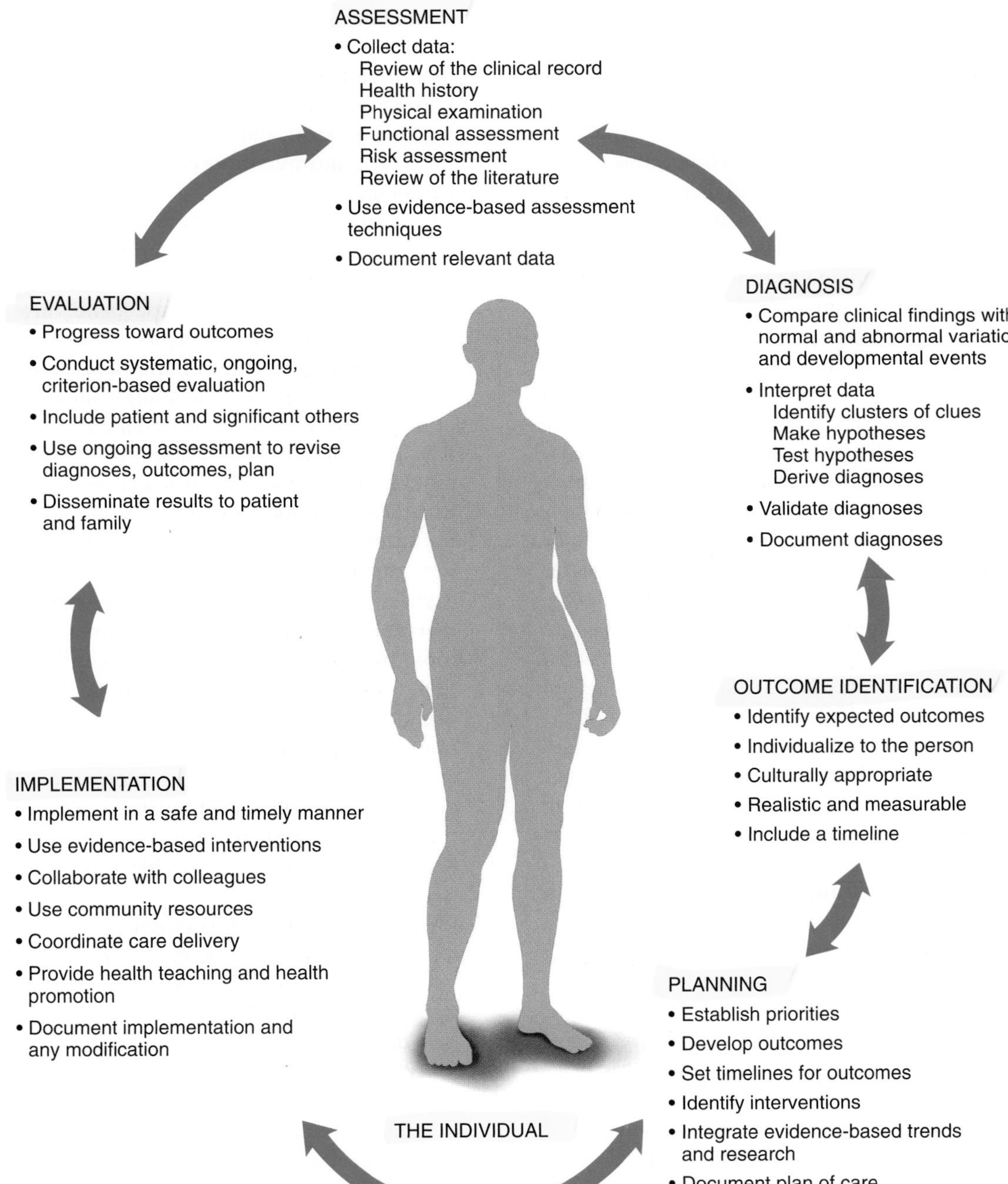
ASSESSMENT
• Collect data:
Review of the clinical record
Health history
Physical examination
Functional assessment
Risk assessment
Review of the literature
• Use evidence-based assessment techniques
• Document relevant data
DIAGNOSIS
• Compare clinical findings with normal and abnormal variation and developmental events
• Interpret data
Identify clusters of clues
Make hypotheses
Test hypotheses
Derive diagnoses
• Validate diagnoses
• Document diagnoses
OUTCOME IDENTIFICATION
• Identify expected outcomes
• Individualize to the person
• Culturally appropriate
• Realistic and measurable
• Include a timeline
PLANNING
• Establish priorities
• Develop outcomes
• Set timelines for outcomes
• Identify interventions
• Integrate evidence-based trends and research
• Document plan of care
THE INDIVIDUAL
IMPLEMENTATION
• Implement in a safe and timely manner
• Use evidence-based interventions
• Collaborate with colleagues
• Use community resources
• Coordinate care delivery
• Provide health teaching and health promotion
• Document implementation and any modification
EVALUATION
• Progress toward outcomes
• Conduct systematic, ongoing, criterion-based evaluation
• Include patient and significant others
• Use ongoing assessment to revise diagnoses, outcomes, plan
• Disseminate results to patient and family

1-2

For example, compare the actions of the nonexpert and the expert nurse in the following situation of a young man with *Pneumocystis jiroveci (P. carinii)* pneumonia:

> *He was banging the siderails, making sounds, and pointing to his endotracheal tube. He was diaphoretic, gasping, and frantic. The nurse put her hand on his arm and tried to ascertain whether he had a sore throat from the tube. While she was away from the bedside retrieving an analgesic, the expert nurse strolled by, hesitated, listened, went to the man's bedside, re-inflated the endotracheal cuff, and accepted the patient's look of gratitude because he was able to breathe again. The nonexpert nurse was distressed that she had misread the situation. The expert reviewed the signs of a leaky cuff with the nonexpert and pointed out that banging the siderails and panic help differentiate acute respiratory distress from pain.*[11]

The method of moving from novice to becoming an expert practitioner is through the use of critical thinking. We all start as novices, when we need the familiarity of clear-cut rules to guide actions. Critical thinking is the means by which we learn to assess and modify, if indicated, before acting.

Critical thinking is required for sound diagnostic reasoning and clinical judgment. During your career, you will need to sort through vast amounts of data and information in order to make the sound judgments to manage patient care. These data will be dynamic, unpredictable, and ever changing. There will not be any one protocol you can memorize that will apply to every situation.

The following critical-thinking skills are organized in a logical progression of the ways the skills might be used in the nursing process.[1] Although each skill here is described separately, they are not used that way in the clinical area. Rather than a step-by-step linear process, critical thinking is a multidimensional thinking process. With experience, you will be able to apply these skills in a rapid, dynamic, and interactive way. For now, follow Ellen's case study through the steps.

1. **Identifying assumptions.** That is, recognize that you could take information for granted or see it as fact when actually there is no evidence for it. Ask yourself, What am I taking for granted here? For example, in Ellen's situation, you might have assumptions of a "typical profile" of a person with alcohol abuse, based on your past experience or exposure to media coverage. However, drug abuse affects people of all ages and from all walks of life; the facts of Ellen's situation are unique.
2. **Identifying an organized and comprehensive approach** to assessment. This depends on the patient's priority needs and your personal or institutional preference. Ellen has many problems, but at her time of admission, she is not acutely physically ill. Thus you may use any organized format for assessment that is feasible for you: a head-to-toe approach, a body systems approach (e.g., cardiovascular, gastrointestinal), a regional area (e.g., pelvic examination), or the use of a preprinted assessment form developed by the hospital or clinic.
3. **Validation**, or checking the accuracy and reliability of data. For example, in addictions treatment, a clinician will corroborate data with a family member in order to verify the accuracy of Ellen's history. In Ellen's particular case, her significant others are absent or nonsupportive and the corroborative interview may need to be with a social worker.
4. **Distinguishing normal from abnormal** when identifying signs and symptoms. Spotting abnormal signs and symptoms leads to problem identification. At first it is difficult to discriminate abnormal signs and symptoms versus what is expected for the patient's age, gender, culture, and lifestyle. However, your ease will grow with study, practice, and experience. Increased BP, wheezing, and heart murmur are among the many abnormal findings in Ellen's case.
5. **Making inferences** or hypotheses. This involves interpreting the data and deriving a correct conclusion about the health status. This presents a challenge for the beginning examiner, because it needs a baseline amount of knowledge and experience. Is Ellen's increased BP caused by the stress of admission or a chronic condition? Is the heart murmur innocent or caused by heart valve pathology?
6. **Clustering related cues,** which will help you see relationships among the data. For example, heavy alcohol use, social consequences of alcohol use, academic consequences, and occupational consequences are a clustering of cues that suggest a maladaptive pattern of alcohol use.
7. **Distinguishing relevant from irrelevant.** A complete history and physical examination furnish a vast amount of data. Look at the clusters of data, and consider which data are important for a health problem or a health promotion need. This skill is also a challenge for beginning examiners and one area where a clinical mentor can be invaluable.
8. **Recognizing inconsistencies.** When Ellen gives the explanation that she ran into a door (subjective data), it is at odds with the location of the infraorbital hematoma (objective data). With this kind of conflicting information, you can investigate and further clarify the situation.
9. **Identifying patterns.** This helps fill in the whole picture and discover missing pieces of information. You need to know usual function of the heart, characteristics of innocent murmurs, and risk factors for abnormal or pathologic murmurs in order to decide if the systolic murmur is a problem for Ellen.
10. **Identifying missing information,** gaps in data, or a need for more data to make a diagnosis. Ellen will need more interviewing regarding any increasing tolerance to alcohol, any withdrawal signs or symptoms, and laboratory data regarding liver enzymes and blood count in order to name a diagnosis.
11. **Promoting health** by identifying risk factors. This applies to generally healthy people and concerns disease prevention and health promotion. To accomplish this skill, you need to identify and manage known risk factors for the individual's age-group and cultural status. This will drive

your wellness diagnosis. For example, counseling for injury prevention is an important intervention for Ellen because motor vehicle and other unintentional injuries are a leading cause of death for this age-group.

12. **Diagnosing actual and potential (risk) problems** from the assessment data. A full list of diagnoses (both medical and nursing) is derived from Ellen K.'s health history and physical examination and is found in Chapter 27. The biomedical focus is the diagnosis and treatment of the specific agents or pathogens that cause disease. Assessment factors are a list of biophysical symptoms and signs. The person is certified as healthy when these symptoms and signs have been eliminated. When disease does exist, medical diagnoses are worded to identify and explain the cause of disease.

    Nursing diagnoses are clinical judgments about a person's response to an actual or potential health state. The most recently approved North American Nursing Diagnosis Association (NANDA) 2009-2011 list includes (1) *actual diagnoses,* existing problems that are amenable to independent nursing interventions; (2) *risk diagnoses,* potential problems that an individual does not currently have but is particularly vulnerable to developing; and (3) *wellness diagnoses,* which focus on strengths and reflect an individual's transition to a higher level of wellness. Throughout this book, appropriate diagnoses from this list are presented and developed as they pertain to related content in each chapter. In Chapter 27, "The Complete Health Assessment," the list of findings for Ellen K. is analyzed and rewritten as diagnoses.

    Regarding Ellen's case study, the medical diagnosis is used to evaluate the etiology (cause) of disease. The nursing diagnosis is used to evaluate the response of the whole person to actual or potential health problems. For example, both the admitting nurse and later the physician auscultate Ellen's lung sounds and determine that they are diminished and that wheezing is present. This is both a medical and a nursing clinical problem. The physician listens to diagnose the cause of the abnormal sounds (in this case, asthma) and to order specific drug treatment. The nurse listens to detect abnormal sounds early, to monitor Ellen's response to treatment, and to initiate supportive measures and teaching; for example, the nurse may teach Ellen which behavioral measures may help her quit smoking and may recommend that Ellen initiate a walking program.

    The medical and nursing diagnoses should not be seen as isolated from each other. It makes sense that the medical diagnosis of asthma be reflected in the nursing diagnoses, as interpreted by the nurse's knowledge of the person's response to asthma. In this book, common nursing diagnoses are presented along with medical diagnoses to illustrate common abnormalities. Please observe how these two types of diagnoses are interrelated.

13. **Setting priorities** when there is more than one diagnosis. In the hospitalized, acute care setting, the initial problems are usually related to the reason for admission. However, the acuity of illness often determines the order of priorities of the person's problems (Table 1-1).

    For example, **first-level priority problems** are those that are emergent, life threatening, and immediate, such as establishing an airway or supporting breathing.

    Second-level priority problems are those that are next in urgency—those requiring your prompt intervention to forestall further deterioration, for example, mental status change, acute pain, acute urinary elimination problems, untreated medical problems, abnormal laboratory values, risks of infection, or risk to safety or security. Ellen has abnormal physical signs that fit in the category of untreated medical problems. For example, Ellen's adventitious breath sounds are a cue to further

TABLE 1-1 Identifying Immediate Priorities

PRINCIPLES OF SETTING PRIORITIES

1. **Make a complete list of current medications, medical problems, allergies, and reasons for seeking care. Refer to them frequently because they may affect how you set priorities.**
2. **Determine the *relationships* among the problems:** If problem Y causes problem Z, problem Y takes priority over problem Z. **Example:** If pain is causing immobility, *pain management* is a high priority.

Setting priorities is a dynamic, changing process; at times, the order of priority changes, depending on the seriousness and relationship of the problems. **Example:** If abnormal laboratory values are at life-threatening levels, they become a higher priority; if the patient is having trouble breathing because of acute rib pain, managing the pain may be a higher priority than dealing with a rapid pulse (first-level priority, listed below).

STEPS TO SETTING PRIORITIES

1. Assign high priority to *First-level* priority problems (immediate priorities): Remember the "ABCs plus V":
    - **A**irway problems
    - **B**reathing problems
    - **C**ardiac/circulation problems
    - **V**ital sign concerns (e.g., high fever)

Exception: With cardiopulmonary resuscitation (CPR) for cardiac arrest, begin chest compressions immediately. Go online to www.americanheart.org for the most current CPR guidelines.

2. Next, attend to *Second-level* priority problems:
    - Mental status change (e.g., confusion, decreased alertness)
    - Untreated medical problems requiring immediate attention (e.g., a diabetic who has not had insulin)
    - Acute pain
    - Acute urinary elimination problems
    - Abnormal laboratory values
    - Risks of infection, safety, or security (for the patient or for others)
3. Address *Third-level* priority problems (later priorities):
    - Health problems that do not fit into the above categories (e.g., problems with lack of knowledge, activity, rest, family coping)

Adapted from Alfaro-LeFevre, R. (2009). *Critical thinking and clinical judgment: a practical approach* (4th ed.). St. Louis: Saunders.

assess respiratory status to determine the final diagnosis. Ellen's mildly elevated blood pressure needs monitoring also.

Third-level priority problems are those that are important to the patient's health but can be addressed after more urgent health problems are addressed. In Ellen's case, the data indicating diagnoses of Deficient Knowledge, Dysfunctional Family Processes, and Chronic Low Self-Esteem fit in this category. Interventions to treat these problems are more long-term, and the response to treatment is expected to take more time.

Collaborative problems are those in which the approach to treatment involves multiple disciplines. Collaborative problems are certain physiologic complications in which nurses have the primary responsibility to diagnose the onset and monitor the changes in status.[7] For example, the data regarding alcohol abuse represent a collaborative problem. With this problem, the sudden withdrawal of alcohol has profound implications on the central nervous and cardiovascular systems. During detoxification, Ellen's response to the rebound effects of these systems is managed.

14. **Identifying patient-centered expected outcomes.** What specific, measurable results will you expect that will show an improvement in the person's problem after treatment? The outcome statement should include a specific time frame. For example: *After 5 days, Ellen will demonstrate how to manage balanced nutrition by keeping a food diary and by stating which food groups are present/absent in her diet.*
15. **Determining specific interventions** that will achieve your outcomes. These interventions aim to prevent, manage, or resolve health problems. This is the health care plan. For specific interventions, state who should perform the intervention, when and how often, and the method used.
16. **Evaluating and correcting thinking.** Look at the expected outcomes, and apply them for evaluation. Do the stated outcomes match the individual's actual progress? Then, analyze whether your interventions were successful or not. Continually think, "What could I be doing differently or better?"
17. **Determining a comprehensive plan** and evaluating and updating the plan. Record the revised plan of care and keep it up-to-date. Communicate the plan to the multidisciplinary team. Be aware that this is a legal document and that accurate recording is important for evaluation, insurance reimbursement, and research.

EVIDENCE-BASED ASSESSMENT

Does honey help burn wounds heal more quickly? Is St. John's wort effective in relieving the symptoms of major depression? Does male circumcision reduce the risk of transmitting human immunodeficiency virus (HIV) in heterosexual men? Can magnesium sulfate reduce cerebral palsy risk in premature infants? Can infusing hearts with stem cells help heal tissue damage after a heart attack?

Health care is a rapidly changing field. The amount of medical and nursing information available today has skyrocketed. Current efforts of cost containment result in a hospital population composed of people who have increased acuity and an earlier discharge than in the past. Clinical research studies are continuously pushing the field forward. Keeping up with these advances and translating them into practice are very challenging. Budget cuts, staff shortages, and increasing patient acuity mean that the clinician has little time to grab a lunch break, let alone browse the most recent journal articles for advances in a clinical specialty.

However, all patients deserve to be treated with the most current best-practice techniques. It is this conviction that led to the development of evidence-based practice (EBP). In 1972, a British epidemiologist and early proponent of EBP, Archie Cochrane, identified a pressing need for systematic reviews of randomized clinical trials. In a landmark case, Dr. Cochrane noted multiple clinical trials published between 1972 and 1981 showing that the use of corticosteroids to treat women in premature labor reduced the incidence of infant mortality. A short course of corticosteroid stimulates fetal lung development, thus preventing respiratory distress syndrome, a serious and common complication of premature birth. Yet these findings had not been implemented into daily practice and thousands of low-birth-weight premature infants were needlessly dying. Following a systematic review of the evidence in 1989, obstetricians were finally aware that the corticosteroid treatment was so effective. Corticosteroid treatment has since been shown to reduce the risk of infant mortality by 30% to 50%.[8]

EBP is more than the use of best-practice techniques to treat patients. "EBP is a systematic approach to practice that emphasizes the use of best evidence in combination with the clinician's experience, as well as the patient preferences and values, to make decisions about care and treatment"[13] (Fig. 1-3). This definition is comprehensive and holistic. Note how

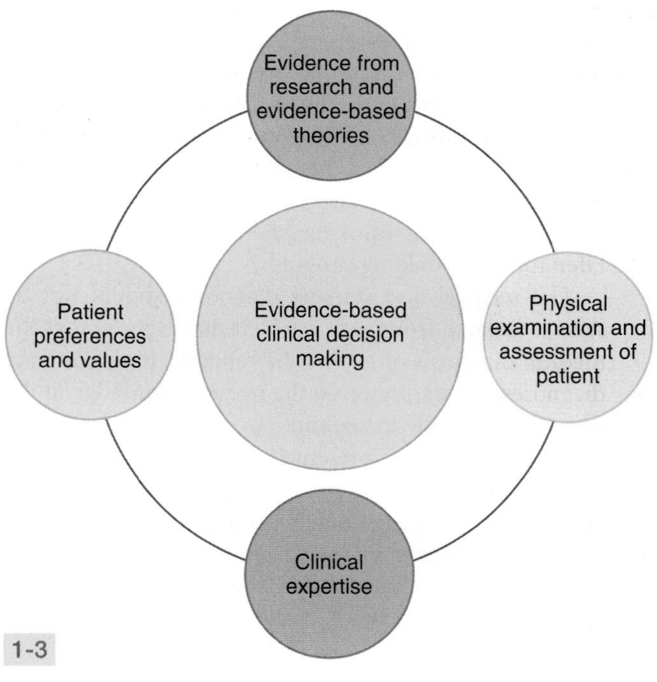

1-3

clinical decision making depends on all four factors: the best evidence from a critical review of research literature; the patient's own preferences; the clinician's own experience and expertise; and finally, physical examination and assessment. Assessment skills must be practiced with hands-on experience and refined to a high level.

Although assessment skills are foundational to EBP, it is important to question tradition when no compelling research evidence exists to support it. Some time-honored assessment techniques have dropped out of the examination repertoire because clinical evidence has shown them to be less than useful. For example, the traditional practice of auscultating bowel sounds was found to not be the best indicator of returning gastrointestinal (GI) motility in patients having abdominal surgery.[14] This research team first reviewed earlier studies suggesting that early postoperative bowel sounds probably do not represent the return of normal GI motility and therefore listening to the abdomen is not useful in this situation. Research did show the primary markers for returning GI motility after abdominal surgery to be the return of flatus and the first postoperative bowel movement. The Madsen team instituted a new practice protocol and monitored patient outcomes to check if discontinuing the auscultation of bowel sounds was detrimental to abdominal surgery patients. Detrimental outcomes did not occur; the new practice guideline was shown to be safe for patients' recovery and a better allocation of staff time.

Despite the advantages to patients who receive care based on EBP, it often takes up to 17 years for research findings to be implemented into practice.[3] This troubling gap has led researchers to examine closely the barriers to EBP, both as individual practitioners and as organizations. As individuals, nurses lack research skills in evaluating quality of research studies, are isolated from other colleagues knowledgeable in research, and lack confidence to implement change.[10] More significant barriers are the organizational characteristics of health care settings. Nurses lack time to go to the library to read research; health care institutions have inadequate library research holdings; and organizational support for EBP is lacking when nurses wish to implement changes in patient care.[10] Fostering a culture of EBP at the undergraduate and graduate levels is one way in which health care educators are attempting to make evidence-based care the "gold standard" of practice. Students of medicine and nursing are now taught how to filter through the wealth of scientific data and critique their findings. They are learning to discern which interventions would best serve their individual patients. Facilitating support for EBP at the organizational level includes time to go to the library; teaching to conduct electronic searches; journal club meetings; establishing nursing research committees; linking staff with university researchers; and ensuring adequate research journals and preprocessed evidence resources available in the library.[10] *"Without the ability to deliver EBP within a context of caring that embraces compassion, cultural sensitivity, and respect for patients and their families, healthcare would fall painfully short of its ultimate goal of providing safe, effective, and holistic care that meets the bio/psycho/social needs of its consumers."*[16]

COLLECTING FOUR TYPES OF DATA

Every examiner needs to establish four different types of databases depending on the clinical situation: complete, focused or problem-centered, follow-up, and emergency.

1. Complete (Total Health) Database

This includes a complete health history and a full physical examination. It describes the current and past health state and forms a baseline against which all future changes can be measured. It yields the first diagnoses.

In primary care, the complete database is collected in a primary care setting, such as a pediatric or family practice clinic, independent or group private practice, college health service, women's health care agency, visiting nurse agency, or community health agency. When you work in these settings, you are the first health professional to see the patient and have primary responsibility for monitoring the person's health care. This is the opportunity to build and strengthen your relationship with the patient. For the well person, this database must describe the person's health state, perception of health, strengths or assets such as health maintenance behaviors, individual coping patterns, support systems, current developmental tasks, and any risk factors or lifestyle changes. For the ill person, the database also includes a description of the person's health problems, perception of illness, and response to the problems.

For well and ill people, the complete database must screen for pathology as well as determine the ways people respond to that pathology or to any health problem. You must screen for pathology because you are the first, and often the only, health professional to see the patient. You will screen for pathology in order to refer the patient to another professional, to help the patient make decisions, and to perform appropriate treatments. But this database also notes the human responses to health problems. This factor is important because it provides additional information about the person that leads to nursing diagnoses.

In acute hospital care, the complete database also is gathered after admission to the hospital. In the hospital, data related specifically to pathology may be collected by the admitting physician. You will collect additional information on the patient's perception of illness, functional ability or patterns of living, activities of daily living, health maintenance behaviors, response to health problems, coping patterns, interaction patterns, and health goals. This approach completes the database from which the nursing diagnoses are made.

2. Focused or Problem-Centered Database

This is for a limited or short-term problem. Here, you collect a "mini" database, smaller in scope and more targeted than the complete database. It concerns mainly one problem, one cue complex, or one body system. It is used in all settings—hospital, primary care, or long-term care. For example, 2 days after surgery, a hospitalized person suddenly has a congested cough, shortness of breath, and fatigue. The history and examination focus primarily on the respiratory and cardiovascular systems. Or, in an outpatient clinic, a person presents with a rash. The history and examination follow the direction of this presenting concern, such as whether the rash had an acute or chronic onset, was associated with a fever, and was localized or generalized. History and examination must include a clear description of the rash.

3. Follow-Up Database

The status of any identified problems should be evaluated at regular and appropriate intervals. What change has occurred? Is the problem getting better or worse? What coping strategies are used? This type of database is used in all settings to follow up short-term or chronic health problems.

4. Emergency Database

This calls for a rapid collection of the data, often compiled concurrently with lifesaving measures. Diagnosis must be swift and sure. For example, in a hospital emergency department, a person is brought in with suspected substance overdose. The first history questions are "What did you take?," "How much did you take?," and "When?" The person is questioned simultaneously while his or her airway, breathing, circulation, level of consciousness, and disability are being assessed. Clearly, the emergency database requires more rapid collection of data than the episodic database.

EXPANDING THE CONCEPT OF HEALTH

Assessment is the collection of data about an individual's health state. A clear idea of health is important because this determines which assessment data should be collected. In general, the list of data that must be collected has lengthened as our concept of health has broadened.

Consideration of the whole person is the essence of **holistic health.** Holistic health views the mind, body, and spirit as interdependent and functioning as a whole within the environment. Health depends on all these factors working together. The basis of disease is multifaceted, originating both from within the person and from the external environment. Thus the treatment of disease requires the services of numerous providers. Nursing includes many aspects of the holistic model—the interaction of the mind and body, the oneness and unity of the individual. Both the individual human and the external environment are open systems, dynamic and continually changing and adapting to each other. Each person is responsible for his or her own personal health state and an active participant in health care. Health promotion and disease prevention form the core of nursing practice.

In a holistic model, assessment factors are expanded to include such things as culture and values, family and social roles, self-care behaviors, job-related stress, developmental tasks, and failures and frustrations of life. All are significant to health.

Health promotion and disease prevention now round out our concept of health. Guidelines to prevention emphasize the link between health and personal behavior. The report of the U.S. Preventive Services Task Force[19] asserts that the great majority of deaths among Americans younger than 65 years are preventable. Prevention can be achieved through counseling from primary care providers designed to change people's unhealthy behaviors related to smoking, alcohol and other drug use, lack of exercise, poor nutrition, injuries, and sexually transmitted infections. This is a wider, more dynamic concept of health. Health promotion is a set of positive acts we can take. In this model, the focus of the health professional is on teaching and helping the consumer choose a healthier lifestyle.

The frequency interval of assessment varies with the person's illness and wellness needs. Most ill people seek care because of pain or some abnormal signs and symptoms they have noticed. This prompts an assessment—gathering a complete, a focused, or an emergency database (Fig. 1-4). In addition, risk assessment and preventive services can be delivered in this context, once the presenting concerns are addressed

But for the well person, opinions are inconsistent about assessment intervals. The term *annual checkup* is vague. What does it constitute? Is it necessary or cost-effective? How can primary care clinicians deliver preventive services to persons with no signs and symptoms of illness? Routine health

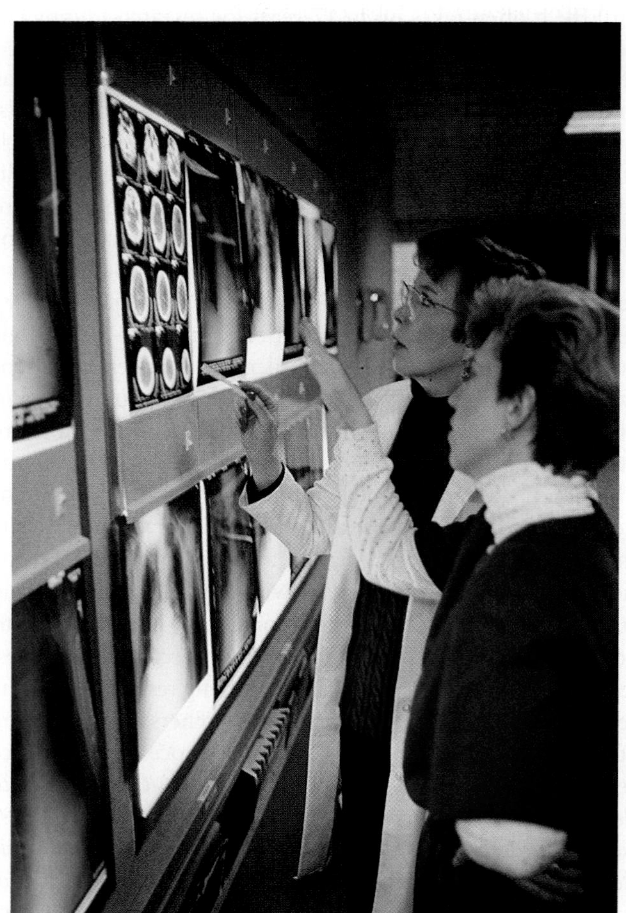

1-4

checkups are an excellent opportunity to deliver preventive services. Although routine health checkups could induce unnecessary costs and promote non-recommended services, advocates justify well-person visits because of delivery of some recommended preventive services and reduction of patient worry.[6]

The *Guide to Clinical Preventive Services* is a positive approach to health assessment and risk reduction.[19] The *Guide* is updated annually and is accessible online or in print. It presents evidence-based, gold standard recommendations on screening, counseling, and preventive topics and includes clinical considerations for each topic. These services include screening factors to gather during the history, age-specific items for physical examination and laboratory procedures, counseling topics, and immunizations. This approach moves away from an annual physical ritual and toward rational and varying periodicity. Health education and counseling are highlighted as the means to deliver health promotion and disease prevention.

For example, the guide to examination for Ellen K. (23-year-old female, nonpregnant, sexually active, tobacco user) would be recommended to include the following services for preventive health care:

1. **Screening history** for dietary intake, physical activity, tobacco/alcohol/drug use, and sexual practices
2. **Physical examination** for height and weight, blood pressure, and screening for cervical cancer, chlamydia, HIV, and other sexually transmitted infections
3. **Counseling** for tobacco use and interventions and for alcohol misuse and behavioral intervention
4. **Depression** screening
5. **Healthy diet** counseling including lipid disorder screening and obesity screening
6. **Chemoprophylaxis** to include multivitamin with folic acid (females capable of or planning pregnancy)
7. **Type 2 diabetes mellitus** screening for those with sustained BP over 135/80 mm Hg

Obviously, Ellen's individual health problems demand immediate intervention and preclude a strict adherence to this preventive list. Indeed, many of Ellen's findings are seen as "red flags" based on predictable risk factors from this list. Ellen will need a complete history, physical examination, and laboratory studies.

CULTURE AND GENETICS

In a holistic model of health care, assessment factors must include culture. An introduction to cross-cultural concepts follows in Chapter 2. These concepts are developed throughout the text as they relate to specific chapters.

Metaphors such as *melting pot, mosaic,* and *salad bowl* have been used to describe the cultural diversity that characterizes the United States. According to the U.S. Census Bureau, close to 50% of the population of the United States will consist of people from diverse racial, ethnic, and cultural groups by the year 2050. *Emerging minority* is a term that has been used to classify the populations that are rapidly becoming a combined numerical majority.[17]

The population of the United States surpassed 310 million people in the autumn of 2010; about 1 in 8 people was an immigrant, and about 1 in 3 U.S. residents was part of a group other than single-race non-Hispanic white according to national estimates by race, Hispanic origin, and age released by the Census Bureau. The nation's emerging majority population totaled 98 million, or 33%, of the country's total population. Hispanics are the largest and fastest growing group.

If current demographic trends continue, the following population diversity is expected in the United States in the twenty-first century: Hispanics, 24.3%; Blacks, 13.2%; Asian/Pacific Islander, 8.9%; and American Indian, 0.8%.[18] Hispanic and Asian populations are expected to double between now and 2050. It is expected that by 2040, the white, European majority will be a numerical minority population.

In the beginning of the twenty-first century, there is a steady flow of immigrants and refugees into the United States. Because the United States is sometimes perceived as the center of advanced health care and technology, foreign nationals who return home after treatment have been inflating the census reports at many U.S. hospitals, with the more popular types of U.S. interventions being cardiovascular, neurologic, and cancer treatments. For example, 35% of kidney transplant recipients at some U.S. hospitals have come from other countries. At the same time, U.S. health care providers go abroad to work in a wide variety of health care settings in the international community. Medical and nursing teams volunteer to provide free medical and surgical care in developing countries (Fig. 1-5). International interchanges are increasing among nurses and physicians, making attention to the cultural aspects of health and illness an even greater priority.

During your professional career, you may be expected to assess short-term foreign visitors, international university faculty, students from abroad studying in U.S. high schools and universities, family members of foreign diplomats, immigrants, refugees, members of more than 106 different ethnic

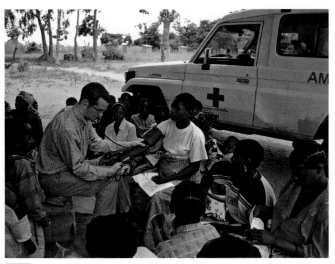

1-5

groups, and American Indians from 510 federally recognized tribes. A serious conceptual problem exists in that nurses and physicians are expected to know, understand, and meet the health needs of people from culturally diverse backgrounds without any formal preparation for doing so.

The inclusion of CULTURE in health assessment is important to gather data that are accurate and meaningful and to intervene with culturally sensitive and appropriate care. Members of some cultural groups are demanding culturally relevant health care that incorporates their specific beliefs and practices. An increasing expectation exists among members of certain cultural groups that health care providers will respect their "cultural health rights," an expectation that frequently conflicts with the unicultural Western biomedical world view taught in U.S. educational programs that prepare nurses and other health care providers. "Cultural malpractice" may soon become a recognized phenomenon.

Given the multicultural composition of the United States and the projected increase in the number of individuals from diverse cultural backgrounds anticipated in the future, a concern for the cultural beliefs and practices of people is becoming increasingly important.

BIBLIOGRAPHY

1. Alfaro-LeFevre, R. (2009). *Critical thinking and clinical judgment: a practical approach* (4th ed.). St. Louis: Saunders.
2. American Nurses Association. (2004). *Nursing scope and standards of performance and standards of clinical practice*. Washington, DC: American Nurses Publishing.
3. Balas, E. A., & Boren, S. A. (2000). Managing clinical knowledge for health care improvements. In J. Bemmel & A. T. McCray (Eds.), *Yearbook of medical informatics 2000*. Stuttgart, Germany: Schattauer.
4. Benner, P., Tanner, C. A., & Chesla, C. A. (1996). *Expertise in nursing practice*. New York: Springer.
5. Benner, P., Tanner, C. A., & Chesla, C. A. (1997). Becoming an expert nurse. *American Journal of Nursing, 97*(6), 16BBB-16DDD.
6. Boulware, L. E., Marinopoulos, S., & Phillips, K. A. (2007). Systematic review: The value of the periodic health evaluation. *Annals Internal Medicine, 146*(4), 289-300.
7. Carpenito-Moyet, L. (2004). *Nursing diagnosis: application to clinical practice* (10th ed.). Philadelphia: Lippincott Williams & Wilkins.
8. Cochrane Collaboration. (2009). Accessed May 10, 2009, from www.cochrane.org.
9. Coderre, S., Mandin, H., Harasym, P. H., et al. (2003). Diagnostic reasoning strategies and diagnostic success. *Medical Education, 37*(8), 695-703.
10. DiCenso, A., Guyatt, G., & Ciliska, D. (2005). *Evidence-based nursing: A guide to clinical practice*. St. Louis: Mosby.
11. Hanneman, S. K. (1996). Advancing nursing practice with a unit-based clinical expert. *Image, 28*(4), 331-337.
12. Hunter, A., Denman-Vitale, S., & Garzon, L. (2007). Global infections: Recognition, management and prevention. *Nurse Practitioner, 32*(2), 34-41.
13. Leufer, T. C. (2009). Evidence-based practice: Improving patient outcomes. *Nursing Standard, 23*(32), 35-39.
14. Madsen, D., Sebolt, T., Cullen, L., et al. (2005). Listening to bowel sounds: An evidence-based practice project. *American Journal of Nursing, 105*(12), 40-50.
15. McKenna, H. P., Ashton, S., & Keeney, S. (2004). Barriers to evidence-based practice in primary care. *Journal of Advanced Nursing, 45*(2), 178-189.
16. Melnyk, B. M., & Fineout-Overholt, E. (2005). *Evidence-based practice in nursing & healthcare*. Philadelphia: Lippincott Williams & Wilkins.

16a. Melnyk, B. M., Fineout-Overholt, E., Stillwell, S. B., et al. (2010). The seven steps of evidence-based practice. *American Journal of Nursing, 110*(1), 51-53.

17. Spector, R. E. (2004). *Cultural diversity in health and illness*. Upper Saddle River, NJ: Prentice Hall.

17a. Stillwell, S. B., Fineout-Overholt, E., Melnyk, B. M., et al. (2010). Asking the clinical question: A key step in evidence-based practice. *American Journal of Nursing, 110*(3), 58-61.

17b. Throckmorton, T., & Windle, P. E. (2009). Evidence-based case management practice. Part 1: The systemic review. *Professional Case Management, 14*(2), 76-81.

18. U.S. Bureau of the Census. (2000). *General population characteristics*. Washington, DC: U.S. Government Printing Office. Website: www.census.gov.
19. U.S. Preventive Services Task Force (USPSTF). (2009). *Guide to clinical preventive services, 2009*. Accessed August 17, 2010, from www.ahrq.gov/clinic/prevenix.htm.

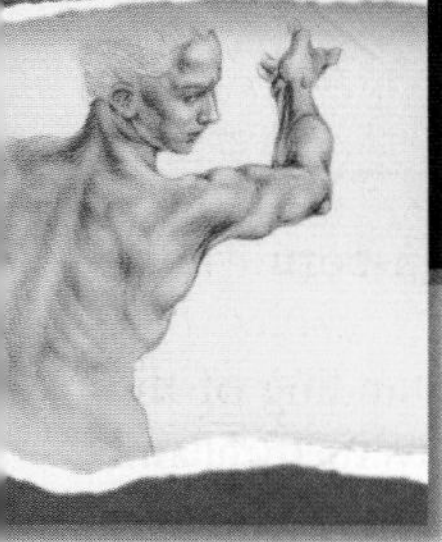

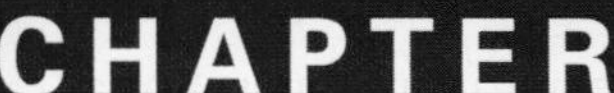

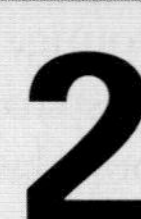

CHAPTER 2

Cultural Competence: CULTURAL CARE

evolve WEBSITE

http://evolve.elsevier.com/Jarvis/

- Audio Key Points
- NCLEX Review Questions
- Quick Assessment for Common Conditions
  Sickle Cell Anemia

Who am I? Where do I come from? What is my heritage—my cultural background—my ethnicity and religion? What is my primary language? Do I understand, speak, and read a language other than English? What are my HEALTH* and ILLNESS* beliefs and practices? You must also ask, WHO is the person whom I am meeting for the first time? Where does he or she come from? What is the person's heritage? What is the person's cultural background—his or her ethnicity and religion? Does the person understand, speak, and read English? What language does the person understand, speak, and read? What are the person's HEALTH and ILLNESS beliefs and practices?

Over the course of your professional education, you will study the physical examination and health promotion across the life span and learn to conduct numerous assessments, such as a complete health history, a mental health assessment, a domestic violence assessment, a nutritional assessment, a pain assessment, and a physical examination, on a patient. However, depending on the heritage of the person, there may be wide variations in the information you gather in the assessments and in the findings of the physical examination. Therefore a Heritage Assessment must be an integral component of a complete physical and health assessment.

The purpose of this chapter is:

1. To discuss the demographic profile of the United States
2. To describe the National Standards for Culturally and Linguistically Appropriate Services in Health Care
3. To discuss the background of the heritage assessment
4. To describe the methods for conducting the heritage assessment
5. To provide examples of traditional HEALTH and ILLNESS beliefs and practices
6. To describe the parameters of CULTURAL CARE
7. To discuss the steps to CULTURAL COMPETENCY

DEMOGRAPHIC PROFILE OF THE UNITED STATES

The population of the United States approached 310 million people in the summer of 2010.[22] About 1 in 8 people was an immigrant, and about 1 in 3 U.S. residents was part of a group other than single-race non-Hispanic white. The nation's minority, actually *emerging majority*, population totaled 102.5 million people, or 34% of the country's total population, in 2007. Of these, Hispanics, 15.1%, are the largest and fastest growing population. The second largest population is Asians, followed by Blacks, American Indians and Alaska natives, and Native Hawaiians and other Pacific Islanders. The findings from estimates of the U.S. population illustrate the increasing diversity in the population and contribute to the rationale for learning about the cultural aspects of health and illness from the point of view of the person seeking health care.[3]

The median age of the total population in 2007 was 36.6 years, and one fourth of these were younger than 18 years. Some population groups were younger than the total population as a whole. The median ages of those younger groups were Hispanics (27.6 years), Blacks (31.1 years), American Indians and Alaskan Natives (30.3 years), and Native Hawaiian/Pacific Islanders (30.2 years). These younger

*HEALTH: "The **balance** of the person, both within one's being—physical, mental, and/or spiritual—and in the outside world—natural, communal, and/or metaphysical, is a complex, interrelated phenomenon."[20]

*ILLNESS: "The loss of the person's **balance**, both within one's being—physical, mental, and/or spiritual—and in the outside world—natural, communal, and/or metaphysical."[20]

population groups also had close to one third of their members younger than 18 years of age. On the other hand, the non-Hispanic single-race white population was older than the population as a whole: the respective median ages were 40.8 and 36.6 years. About 21% of the population of this group were younger than 18 years, compared with 25% of the total population.[3]

IMMIGRATION

The 21st century began with the country in the midst of the greatest wave of immigration in its history.[5] The largest numbers of people ever to enter this nation happened during the 1990s, and the numbers of immigrants have more than tripled since the 1990s. The growth in immigration has been driven in part by legislative increases in legal admissions in 1965, 1976, and 1990 when refugees were admitted from Southeast Asia and other war-torn nations. The question "Can we accommodate this number of people?" is not much different from questions raised during other large waves of immigration. Other critical questions to ask are "What will be the impact on health care delivery and nursing practice?" and "How do the health care system and nursing meet the health care needs of people from diverse backgrounds?"

Immigrants are people who were not U.S. citizens at birth. In March 2003, the population in the United States included 33.5 million foreign-born people, representing 11.7% of the U.S. population. In 2008, a total of 1,107,126 people became legal permanent residents of this country. Among the foreign born, 44.4% were born in Central and South America, 34.6% in Asia, 10.8% in Europe, and the remaining 10.2% in other regions of the world.[17] The foreign-born population from Central America and Mexico accounted for more than two thirds of the foreign born from Latin America and more than one third of the total foreign born. It was estimated in January 2008 that there are also 11.6 million people who were foreign born and living here without legal documents. The sociopolitical questions that are constantly raised about the undocumented segment of the overall population relate to issues such as rights to health care and education.[9]

There are several terms and categories of immigrant populations that are of interest to health care providers[10]:

- **Legal Resident**—All persons who were granted lawful permanent residence
- **Naturalization**—The conferring, by any means, of citizenship upon a person after birth
- **Non-immigrant**—An alien who seeks temporary entry to the United States for a specific purpose
- **Parolee**—An alien, appearing to be inadmissible to the inspecting officer, allowed into the United States for urgent humanitarian reasons or when that alien's entry is determined to be for significant public benefit
- **Permanent Resident Alien**—An alien admitted to the United States as a lawful permanent resident
- **Refugee**—Any person who is outside his or her country of nationality who is unable or unwilling to return to that country because of persecution or a well-founded fear of persecution
- **Unauthorized Residents**—All foreign-born non-citizens who are not legal residents

Many new immigrants have minimal understanding of the modern health care delivery system and modern medical and nursing practices, and they speak and understand minimal or no English. Yet, it is imperative that your care be tailored to meet these immigrants' perceived needs.

NEW NATIONAL STANDARDS

In response to the demographic change and with knowledge that immigration was going to remain at high levels, the Office of Minority Health, an office with the Cabinet of Health and Human Services, published the *National Standards for Culturally and Linguistically Appropriate Services in Health Care* in 2001. The first and landmark standard states: "Health care organizations should ensure that patients receive from all staff members effective, understandable, and respectful care that is provided in a manner compatible with their cultural health beliefs and practices and preferred language"[14] (Table 2-1).

- EFFECTIVE CARE results in positive outcomes and satisfaction for the patient.
- RESPECTFUL CARE takes into consideration the values, preferences, and expressed needs of the patient.
- CULTURAL AND LINGUISTIC COMPETENCE is a set of congruent behaviors, attitudes, and policies that come together in a system among professionals that enables work in cross-cultural situations (Fig. 2-1).

Linguistic Competence

Under the provisions of Title VI of the Civil Rights Act of 1964, when people with limited English proficiency (LEP) seek health care in health care settings such as hospitals, nursing homes, clinics, daycare centers, and mental health centers, services cannot be denied to them. There are many

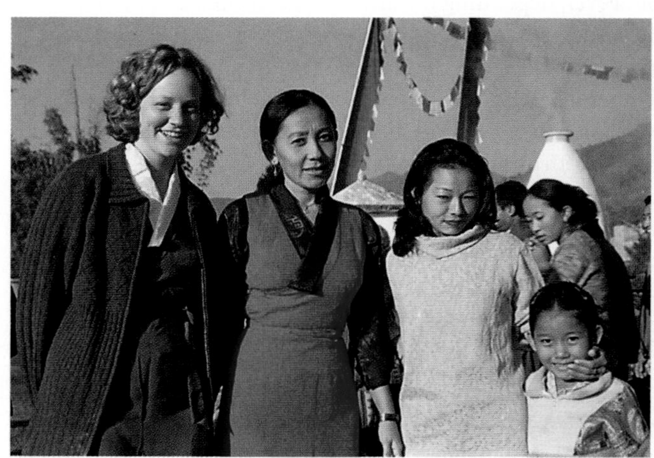

2-1

TABLE 2-1 National Standards for Culturally and Linguistically Appropriate Services in Health Care

1. Promote and support the attitudes, behaviors, knowledge, and skills necessary for staff to work respectfully and effectively with patients and each other in a culturally diverse work environment.
2. Have a comprehensive management strategy to address culturally and linguistically appropriate services, including strategic goals, plans, policies, procedures, and designated staff responsible for implementation.
3. Use formal mechanisms for community and consumer involvement in the design and execution of service delivery, including planning, policy making, operations, evaluation, training, and, as appropriate, treatment planning.
4. Develop and implement a strategy to recruit, retain, and promote qualified, diverse, and culturally competent administrative, clinical, and support staff who are trained and qualified to address the needs of the racial and ethnic communities being served.
5. Require and arrange for continuing education and training for administrative, clinical, and support staff in culturally and linguistically competent service delivery.
6. Provide all clients with limited English proficiency access to bilingual staff or interpretation services.
7. Provide oral and written notices, including translated signage at key points of contact, to clients in their primary languages informing them of their right to receive interpreter services free of charge.
8. Translate and make available signage and commonly used written patient educational material and other materials for members of the predominant language groups in service areas.
9. Ensure that interpreters and bilingual staff can demonstrate bilingual proficiency and receive training that includes the skills and ethics of interpreting and knowledge in both languages of the terms and concepts relevant to clinical or nonclinical encounters. Family or friends are not considered adequate substitutes because they usually lack these abilities.
10. Ensure that the clients' primary spoken language and self-identified race/ethnicity are included in the health care organization's management information system and in any patient records used by provider staff.
11. Use a variety of methods to collect and make use of accurate demographic, cultural, epidemiologic, and clinical outcome data for racial and ethnic groups in the service area, and become informed about the ethnic/cultural needs, resources, and assets of the surrounding community.
12. Undertake continuing organizational self-assessments of cultural and linguistic competency, and integrate measures of access, satisfaction, quality, and outcomes for CLAS (culturally linguistically appropriate services) into other organizational internal audits and performance improvement programs.
13. Develop structures and procedures to address cross-cultural ethical and legal conflicts in health care delivery and complaints or grievances by patients and staff about unfair, culturally insensitive or discriminatory treatment; difficulty in accessing services; or denial of services.
14. Prepare an annual progress report documenting the organizations' progress with implementing CLAS standards, including information on programs, staffing, and resources.

forms of illegal discrimination based on race or national origin that frequently limit the opportunities of people to gain equal access to health care services. It is said that "language barriers have a deleterious effect on health care, patients are less likely to have a usual source of health care, and have an increased risk of nonadherence to medication regimens."[6]

The United States is home to millions of people from different national origins. English is the predominant language of the United States. However, 12% of the people living in the United States from 2005 to 2007 were foreign born. Among people at least 5 years old living in the United States from 2005 to 2007, 20% spoke a language other than English at home. Of those speaking a language other than English at home, 62% spoke Spanish and 38% spoke some other language; 44% reported that they did not speak English "very well." The most common non-English languages spoken by people older than 5 years at home are Spanish, Chinese, French, German, and Tagalog (2.6%). Vietnamese, Italian, Korean, and Russian and Polish are next among the top 10 languages.[21]

People who are limited in their ability to speak, read, write, and understand the English language encounter countless language barriers that can result in limiting their access to critical public health, hospital, and other medical and social services to which they are legally entitled. Many health and social service programs provide information about their services in English only. When LEP persons seek health care at hospitals or medical clinics, they are frequently faced with receptionists, nurses, and physicians who speak English only. The language barrier faced by LEP persons in need of medical care or social services severely limits the ability to gain access to these services and to participate in these programs. In addition, the language barrier often results in the denial of medical care or social services, delays in the receipt of such care and services, or the provision of care and services on the basis of inaccurate or incomplete information. Services denied, delayed, or provided under such circumstances could have serious consequences for a LEP person as well as for a provider of medical care. Some states (e.g., California, Massachusetts, New York) recognize the seriousness of the problem and require providers to offer language assistance to patients in health care settings.

Chapter 3 describes in more detail how to communicate with people who do not understand English, how to interact with interpreters, and what services are available when no interpreter is available. It is vital that interpreters be present who not only serve to verbally translate the conversation but who also can describe to you the cultural aspects and meanings of the person's situation.

Health Disparities

A *health disparity* is the unusual and disproportionate frequency of a given health problem (e.g., diabetes, hypertension, certain cancers) within a population when compared with other populations. Disparities occur in a broader social and economic context. The factors that contribute to this phenomenon are multilevel and complex and include the health care system, health care providers, health care managers, and patients/families/communities. It is expected that, over time, this major problem in the delivery of health care in the United States will be overcome with the increasing knowledge and research necessary for the provision of culturally competent health care.[8]

Cultural Competence and CULTURAL CARE

One response to the government mandates for cultural competency is the development of CULTURAL CARE, a concept that describes professional health care that is culturally sensitive, appropriate, and competent. There is a discrete body of knowledge relevant to this, and much of the content is introduced in this chapter.

- *Culturally sensitive* implies that caregivers possess some basic knowledge of and constructive attitudes toward the diverse cultural populations found in the setting in which they are practicing.
- *Culturally appropriate* implies that the caregivers apply the underlying background knowledge that must be possessed to provide a given person with the best possible HEALTH CARE.
- *Culturally competent* implies that the caregivers understand and attend to the total context of the individual's situation, including awareness of immigration status, stress factors, other social factors, and cultural similarities and differences.[20]

CULTURAL CARE is critical to meeting the complex nursing care needs of a given person, family, and community. It is the provision of health care across cultural boundaries and takes into account the context in which the patient lives as well as the situations in which the patient's health problems arise.[20] Each chapter in this text will include information necessary for delivery of CULTURAL CARE.

More and more institutions are mandating that those who practice must be culturally competent; there are countless ways by which this can be achieved. However, it is NOT a one-lesson program but, rather, a lifetime journey of study and learning. Given the changes in the demographic profile of the United States and the enormous impact that immigration is having in this situation, it becomes imperative that a body of knowledge must be developed to meet this challenge. There are several discrete areas in which you must have knowledge:

1. Your own personal heritage
2. The heritage of the nursing profession
3. The heritage of the health care system
4. The heritage of the patient

HERITAGE

A given person's heritage is predicated on the concept of heritage consistency. **Heritage consistency** is a concept that describes "the degree to which one's lifestyle reflects his or her respective American Indian tribal culture."[4] The theory has been expanded in an attempt to study the degree to which a person's lifestyle reflects his or her traditional heritage, whether it is American Indian, European, Asian, African, or Hispanic. The values indicating heritage consistency exist on a continuum, and a person can possess value characteristics of both a heritage consistent (**traditional**—that is, living within the norms of the traditional culture) and a heritage inconsistent (**modern**—that is, acculturated to the norms of the dominant society). The concept of **heritage consistency** includes a determination of a person's cultural, ethnic, and religious background and **socialization** experiences.[20]

Culture

There is no single definition of culture, and too often, definitions tend to omit salient aspects of culture or are too general to have any real meaning. One example of a definition of culture is that it is the thoughts, communications, actions, beliefs, values, and institutions of racial, ethnic, religious, or social groups. Culture is a complex whole in which each part is related to every other part. It is learned, and the capacity to learn culture is genetic, but the subject matter is not genetic and must be learned by each person in his or her family and social community. Culture also depends on an underlying social matrix, and included in this social matrix are knowledge, belief, art, law, morals, and customs. Culture is also a web of communication, and much of culture is transmitted nonverbally.[20]

In addition, culture has four basic characteristics in that it is (1) *learned* from birth through the processes of language acquisition and socialization, (2) *shared* by all members of the same cultural group, (3) *adapted* to specific conditions related to environmental and technical factors and to the availability of natural resources, and (4) *dynamic* and ever changing.

Culture is a universal phenomenon without which no person exists. Yet the culture that develops in any given society is always specific and distinctive, encompassing all the knowledge, beliefs, customs, and skills acquired by members of that society. Within cultures, groups of people share different beliefs, values, and attitudes. Differences occur because of ethnicity, religion, education, occupation, age, and gender. When such groups function within a large culture, they are referred to as *subcultural groups.*

Ethnicity

Cultural background is a fundamental component of your **ethnic** background. Ethnicity pertains to a social group within the social system that claims to possess variable traits such as a common geographic origin, migratory status, religion, race, language, shared values, traditions, or symbols, and food preferences.

The term *ethnic* has aroused strongly negative feelings and often is rejected by the general population. In a nation as large as the United States and comprising as many different peoples as it does—with the American Indians being the only true native population—we find ourselves still reluctant to speak of ethnicity and ethnic differences. This stance stems from the fact that most foreign groups that came to this land often shed the ways of the "old country" and quickly attempt to assimilate themselves into the mainstream, or the so-called *melting pot.*[15] There are at least 106 ethnic groups and more than 500 American Indian nations in the United States. People from every nation on earth are now residing in this country[20] (Fig. 2-2).

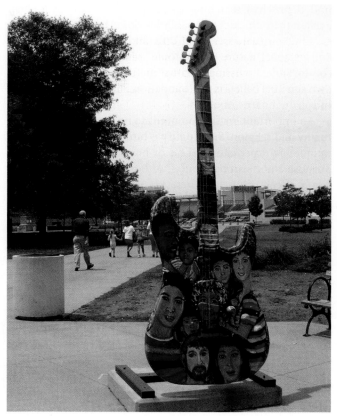

2-2

Religion

The third major component of a person's heritage is **religion.** Religion is the belief in a divine or superhuman power or powers to be obeyed and worshipped as the creator(s) and ruler(s) of the universe. A system of beliefs, practices, and ethical values is a major reason for the development of ethnicity.[1] Religion may be seen as a shared experience of spirituality or as the values, beliefs, and practices that people are either born into or may adopt to meet their personal spiritual needs through communal actions such as religious affiliation; attendance and participation in a religious institution, prayer, or meditation; and religious practices.

On the other hand, spirituality may be seen as focusing more on the self and includes belief systems other than religion.[18] The practice of religion is revealed in numerous cults, sects, denominations, and churches. Ethnicity and religion are clearly related, and religion quite often is the determinant of ethnic group. Religion gives a person a frame of reference and a perspective with which to organize information. Religious teachings vis-á-vis health help present a meaningful philosophy and system of practices within a system of social controls having specific values, norms, and ethics. These are related to health in that adherence to a religious code is conducive to spiritual harmony and health. Illness is sometimes seen as the punishment for the violation of religious codes and morals.

Religion plays a most significant role in the ways people practice their health care. Too often, this aspect of the person is ignored, and in many settings, the question "What is your religious preference?" is not asked. This may be to protect against discrimination based on religion. Yet, religion is seen as the domain of life beyond the body and mind.[12] The following are examples of how religion influences the health practices of countless people:

1. Religious affiliation and membership benefit health by promoting health behavior and lifestyles.
2. Regular religious fellowship benefits health by offering social support that buffers and affects stress and isolation.
3. Faith benefits health by leading to thoughts of hope, optimism, and positive expectation.

There are countless health-related behaviors promoted by nearly all religions. The following list presents selected examples. Not every religion speaks to each point: meditating, exercising and maintaining physical fitness, getting enough sleep, being vaccinated, being willing to have the body examined, undertaking a pilgrimage for HEALTH reasons, telling the truth about how you feel, maintaining family viability, hoping for recovery, coping with stress, undergoing genetic screening and counseling, being able to live with a handicap, and caring for children.[12]

As an integral component of the person's culture, religious beliefs may influence the person's explanation of the cause(s) of illness, perception of its severity, and choice of healer(s). In times of crisis, such as serious illness and impending death, religion may be a source of consolation for the person and for his or her family. Religious dogma and spiritual leaders may exert considerable influence on the person's decision making concerning acceptable medical and surgical treatment, choice of healer(s), and other aspects of the illness.

Spirituality and Religion

Religious concerns evolve from and respond to the mysteries of life and death, good and evil, and pain and suffering. In health care settings, you frequently encounter people who find themselves searching for a spiritual meaning to help explain their illnesses or disabilities. Some health care providers find spiritual assessment difficult because of the abstract and personal nature of the topic, whereas others feel quite comfortable discussing spiritual matters. Comfort with your own spiritual beliefs is the foundation for effective assessment of spiritual needs in others.

An important distinction needs to be made between spirituality and religion. **Spirituality** is borne out of each person's unique life experience and his or her personal effort to find purpose and meaning in life.[18] Although the religions of the world offer various interpretations to many of life's mysteries, most people seek a personal understanding and interpretation at some time in their lives. Ultimately, this personal search becomes a pursuit to discover a supreme being (called by names such as Allah, God, Yahweh, and Jehovah) or some unifying truth that will render meaning, purpose, and integrity to existence.

Religion, on the other hand, refers to an organized system of beliefs concerning the cause, nature, and purpose of the universe, especially belief in or the worship of God or gods. An extensive new survey by the Pew Forum on Religion and Public Life details statistics on religion in America.[16] The study found that religious affiliation in the United States is both very diverse and extremely fluid. The number of people who say they are unaffiliated with any particular faith is now 16.1%. Those reporting religious affiliation with a Christian church number 78.4%. The Christian denominations include Roman Catholic (23.9%); Protestant (51.3%), which includes Mainline Protestant (18.1%), Evangelical Churches (26.3%), and Historical Black Churches (6.9%); Mormon or Church of Jesus Christ of Latter-Day Saints (1.3%); Jehovah's Witness (0.7%); and others. Those belonging to non-Christian and other religions total 4.7% of the U.S. population; of these, the largest group is Jewish (1.7%), followed by Buddhist (0.7%), Muslim (0.6%), and Hindu (0.4%).

The Landscape Survey also found that among the foreign-born adult population, Catholics outnumbered Protestants by nearly a two-to-one margin (46% Catholic vs. 24% Protestant) and that immigrants are also disproportionately represented among several world religions in the United States, including Islam, Hinduism, and Buddhism.[16] Religious identification among people from different racial and ethnic groups is important because religion and culture are interconnected and play a critical role in HEALTH beliefs and practices.

There are many examples of how spirituality and religion are apparent in daily life and frequently play a role in one's HEALTH. Shrines are an essential component of this. There are countless shrines, both secular and from a religious tradition, where people visit to remember and/or to pray for favors or healing. Fig. 2-3, *A* is an image of the Vietnam Memorial Wall in Washington, DC, an example of a secular/spiritual shrine where people go to remember loved ones who died in the Vietnam War. Fig. 2-3, *B* is a statue of Saint Peregrine, the patron saint of people with cancer. This statue is in the chapel in the Mission San Juan Capistrano in California. Fig. 2-3, *C* is the Thai Spirit House, in Los Angeles, California. The shrine is on a public street and visited by believers; offerings such as flowers and food are frequently left at the base. Fig. 2-3, *D* is an example of a sacred Buddhist shrine that can be found in a store or in a home.

Just as the trends in immigration have influenced our newest citizens, there has been a growing interest in the religious preferences of the oldest group, the American Indians. The religious profile of American Indians is similar to that of non-Hispanic whites: 20% identified themselves as Baptist, 17% as Catholic, and 17% indicated no religious preference. Only 3% indicated their primary religious identification as a tribal Indian religion, perhaps a reflection of the growing number of native people who reside in non-reservation urban centers.[1a]

Socialization

Socialization is the process of being raised within a culture and acquiring the characteristics of that group. Education—be it elementary school, high school, college, or professional school—is a form of socialization. For many people who have been socialized within the boundaries of a "traditional culture" or a non-modern culture (usually associated with the East or with developing nations), modern "American," or Western, first-world culture becomes a second cultural identity. Those who immigrate here (legally or illegally) from non-Western or non-modern countries may find socialization into the American culture, whether in schools or in society, to be an extremely difficult and painful process. As time passes, many people experience biculturalism, which is a dual pattern of identification and often of divided loyalty.[11] In addition, many people who have been socialized in cultures in which traditional health care resources are used may prefer to use this type of care even when residing in a modern cultural setting with modern health care resources available.

It is not possible to isolate the aspects of culture, religion, ethnicity, and socialization that shape a person's worldview. Each is part of the other, and all are united within the person. When we write of religion, we cannot eliminate culture or ethnicity but descriptions and comparisons can be made.

There are several other terms related to socialization:

- **Acculturation**—the process of adapting to and acquiring another culture
- **Assimilation**—the process by which a person develops a new cultural identity and becomes like the members of the dominant culture
- **Biculturalism**—dual pattern of identification and often of divided loyalty

Not only is it vital that you develop the skills for conducting heritage assessments, but also it is equally important that, as you learn these concepts, you understand that the first step in developing CULTURAL COMPETENCY is to know yourself. Thus, as you examine the factors related to heritage consistency and the assessment questions used in a heritage assessment, ask these questions of yourself and your family.

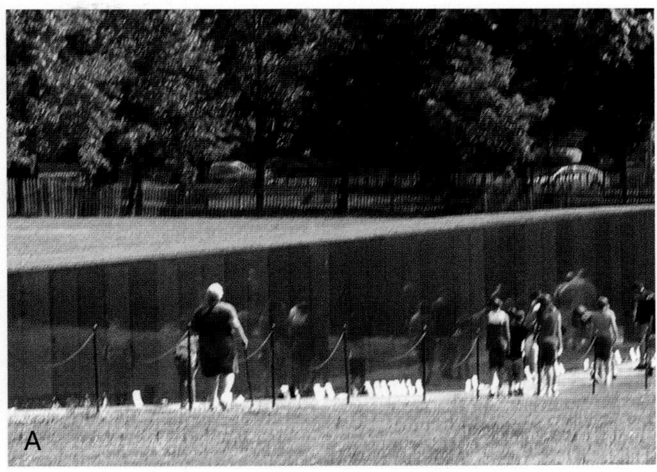

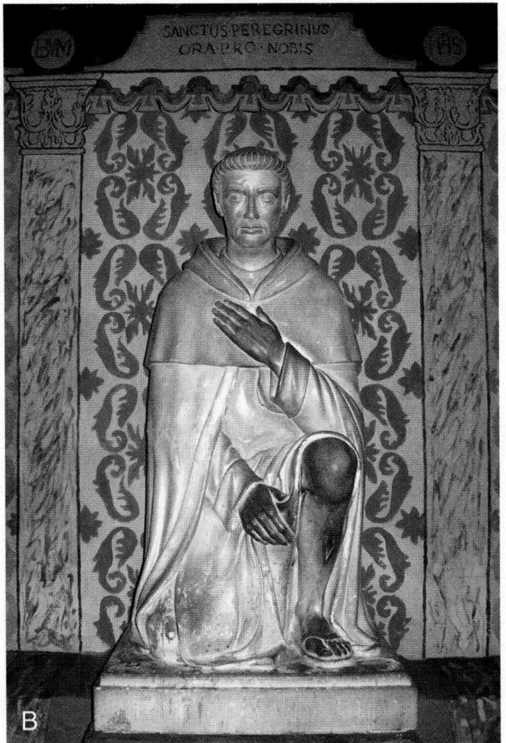

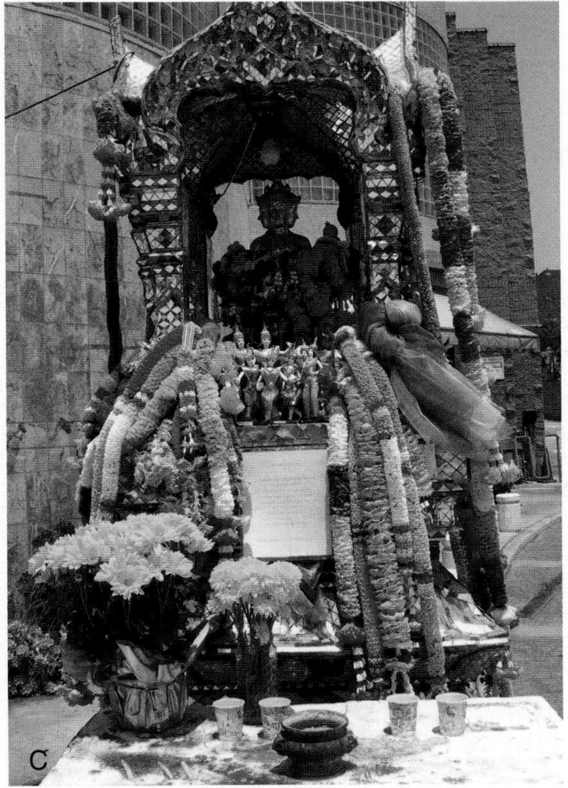

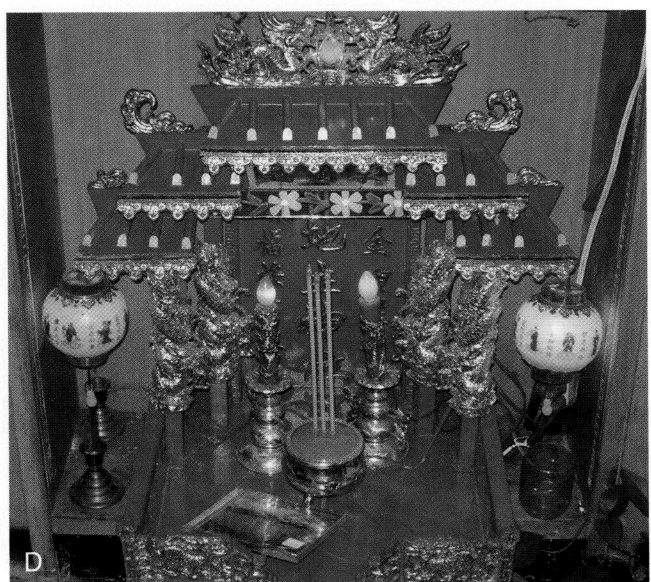

2-3 **A,** The Vietnam Wall.[20] **B,** Saint Peregrine.[20] **C,** Thai Spirit House.[20] **D,** Buddhist Shrine.

HERITAGE ASSESSMENT

The following are the factors indicative of heritage consistency, with examples, that may be explored to determine the depth to which you and the given patient identify with a traditional heritage; that is, the cultural beliefs and practices of the family, the extended family, and an ethnoreligious community[20]:

1. Childhood development occurred in the country of origin or in an immigrant neighborhood in the United States of like ethnic and religious group: *Where were you born? Where did you grow up?*

   Both you and the person were raised in a specific ethnic neighborhood, such as an Italian, Black, Hispanic, or Jewish one, in a given part of a city and were exposed only to the culture, language, foods, and customs of that particular group.
2. Extended family members encouraged participation in traditional religious and cultural activities: *Did your parents encourage you to participate in religious or ethnic activities? What kind of school did you go to? Did you go to a special religious school after regular school hours?*

   Parents and members of the extended family and ethnoreligious community encouraged the person to know

Heritage Assessment

The following set of questions can be used by caregivers to begin to determine a person's ethnic, cultural, or religious heritage and its relationship to his or her personal and health care traditions. The stronger the association of these items to a person's identification, the more traditional is his or her heritage.

1. Where were you born? ______
2. Where were your parents/grandparents born?
   a. Mother: ______
   b. Father: ______
   c. Mother's mother: ______
   d. Mother's father: ______
   e. Father's mother: ______
   f. Father's father: ______
3. How many brothers ______ and sisters ______ do you have?
4. What setting did you grow up in? Urban ______ Rural ______ Suburban ______
   Where? ______
5. What country did your parents/grandparents grow up in?
   a. Mother: ______
   b. Father: ______
   c. Mother's mother: ______
   d. Mother's father: ______
   e. Father's mother: ______
   f. Father's father: ______
6. How old were you when you came to the United States? ______
7. How old were your parents/ grandparents when they came to the United States?
   a. Mother: ______
   b. Father: ______
   c. Mother's mother: ______
   d. Mother's father: ______
   e. Father's mother: ______
   f. Father's father: ______
8. When you were growing up, who lived with you? ______
9. Have you maintained contact with:
   a. Aunts, uncles, cousins? ______ Yes ______ No
   b. Brothers and sisters? ______ Yes ______ No
   c. Parents? ______ Yes ______ No
   d. Your own children? ______ Yes ______ No
10. Does most of your family live near you? ______ Describe: ______
11. Approximately how often did you visit your family members who lived outside your home? ______ Daily ______ Weekly ______ Monthly ______ <Once a year ______ Never
12. Was your original family name changed? ______ Yes ______ No
13. What is your religious preference? ______ Catholic ______ Jewish ______ Protestant–Denomination ______ Other ______ None
14. Is your spouse of the same religion? ______ Yes ______ No
    Describe: ______
15. Is your spouse of the same ethnic background as you? ______ Yes ______ No
    Describe: ______
16. What kind of school did you go to? ______ Public ______ Private ______ Parochial
17. As an adult, do you live in a neighborhood where the neighbors are the same religion and ethnic background as yourself? ______ Yes ______ No
18. Do you belong to a religious institution? ______ Yes ______ No
    Describe: ______
19. Would you describe yourself as an active member? ______ Yes ______ No
20. How often do you attend your religious institution? ______ More than once a week ______ Weekly ______ Monthly ______ Special holidays only ______ Never
21. Do you practice your religion or other spiritual practices in your home? ______ Yes ______ No
    If yes, please specify: ______ Praying ______ Bible reading ______ Diet ______ Celebrating religious holidays ______ Meditating ______ Other: describe ______
22. Do you prepare foods of your ethnic background? ______ Yes ______ No
    Describe: ______
23. Do you participate in ethnic activities? ______ Yes ______ No
    If yes, specify: ______ Singing ______ Holiday celebrations ______ Dancing ______ Costumes ______ Festivals ______ Other
    Describe: ______
24. Are your friends from the same religious background? ______ Yes ______ No
25. Are your friends of the same ethnic background as you? ______ Yes ______ No
26. What is your native language? ______
    Do you speak this language? ______ Prefer ______ Occasionally ______ Rarely
27. Do you read in your native language? ______ Prefer ______ Occasionally ______ Rarely

From Spector, R.E. (2009). *Cultural diversity in health and illness* (7th ed.). Upper Saddle River, NJ: Prentice Hall, pp. 365-367.

2-4

his or her ethnocultural heritage and sent the person to religious (parochial) school, and most social activities were church related.

3. The person engages in frequent visits to the country of origin or returns to the "old neighborhood" in the United States: *Have you visited the nation(s) or neighborhoods where your family originated?*

   The desire to return to the old country or to the old neighborhood is expressed by many people; however, many people, for various reasons, cannot return to the "old country or neighborhood." The people who came here to escape religious persecution or whose families were killed during World War II, during the Holocaust, in the killing fields of Cambodia, or other recent massacres may not want to return to European or other homelands. Other reasons why people may not return to their native countries include political conditions in the homeland or lack of relatives or friends in that land.

4. The person's family home is within the ethnic community of which he or she is a member: *Who are the people living in the neighborhood where you now live?*

   As an adult, the person has elected to live with his or her family in the ethnic neighborhood or community wherein the people are from a similar heritage.

5. The person participates in ethnic cultural events, such as religious festivals or national holidays, sometimes with singing, dancing, and costumes: *Do you participate in ethnic celebrations from your heritage?*

   The person is active in social and cultural groups and participates in festivities of his or her family. One example is the August festival of Saint Anthony that is celebrated by people of Italian descent in the Northeast.

6. The person was raised in an extended family setting: *Who lived in your home? Were they related to you?*

   When the person was growing up, there may have been grandparents living in the same household or aunts and uncles living in the same house or close by. The person's social frame of reference was the family and the extended family.

7. The person maintains regular contact with the extended family: *Do you maintain ties to family?*

   The person maintains close ties, either with visits or telephone contact, with family members of the same generation, surviving members of the older generation, and members of the younger generation. This includes aunts, uncles, and cousins.

8. The person's name has not been Americanized: *Was your family name changed when the family came to the United States? Was the name changed to facilitate assimilation?*

   Many people's surnames were changed, either by immigration officials when they entered the country or by personal choice to make their names more "American" as an attempt to assimilate to the dominant culture more fully.

9. The person was educated in a parochial (nonpublic) school with a religious or ethnic philosophy similar to the family's background: *What school did you go to? Was it public or private?*

   The person's education plays an enormous role in socialization, and the major purpose of education is to socialize a given person into the dominant culture. Children learn English and the customs and norms of American life in the schools. In the parochial or private schools, they not only learn English but also are socialized in the culture and norms of the particular religious or ethnic group that is sponsoring the school.

10. The person engages in social activities primarily with others of the same religious or ethnic background: *Who are your friends, and how often do you spend time with them?*

    For example, the major portion of the person's personal time is spent with family and friends from his or her ethnocultural or religious community.

11. The person has knowledge of the culture and language of origin: *Do you speak or read the language of your parents or grandparents?*

    For example, the person has been socialized in the traditional ways of the family and expresses this as a central theme of life.

12. The person expresses pride in his or her heritage: *Do you identify as an ethnic American or as an American?*

    For example, the person may identify himself or herself as ethnic American and be supportive of ethnic activities to a great extent.

Fig. 2-4, the Heritage Assessment tool, lists all of the questions that may be asked. It is important to ask the questions slowly over time. If the person appears anxious, it is best to postpone asking the questions or to weave the questions into other parts of the health history. The responses can be scored, and an image arises as to whether the person identifies with his or her traditional heritage or whether the person is acculturated and assimilated into the mainstream of modern American culture.

There are four short questions that may be asked in addition to the background information:

1. Do you mostly participate in social activities with members of your family?
2. Do you mostly have friends from a similar cultural background as you?
3. Do you mostly eat the foods of your family's tradition?
4. Do you mostly participate in the religious traditions of your family?

If the person answers two to four of these questions positively, the probability of being more likely to use health practices relevant to their traditional heritage is high.

HEALTH-RELATED BELIEFS AND PRACTICES

Earlier in this chapter, HEALTH was defined as the **balance** of the person, both within one's being (physical, mental, or spiritual) and in the outside world (natural, communal, or metaphysical) as a complex, interrelated phenomenon. Before determining whether cultural practices are helpful, harmful, or neutral, you must first understand the logic of the traditional belief systems underlying the beliefs and practices that are derived from a person's heritage; then be certain that you fully grasp the nature and meaning of the HEALTH practice from the person's cultural perspective.

Wide cultural variation exists in the manner in which certain symptoms and disease conditions are perceived, diagnosed, labeled, and treated. You should not assume that the perceived symptoms or complaints of patients are equivalent to the names of recognized diseases or syndromes familiar to nurses, physicians, and other health care professionals.[23] The same disease that is considered grounds for social ostracism in one culture may be reason for increased status in another. For example, epilepsy is seen as contagious and untreatable among Ugandans, as a cause for family shame among Greeks, as a reflection of a physical imbalance among Mexican Americans, as the entry of a "spirit" into the person's body by the Hmong, and as a sign of having gained favor by enduring a trial by God among the Hutterites.

Bodily symptoms are also perceived and reported in a variety of ways. For example, people of Mediterranean descent tend to report common physical symptoms more often than persons of Northern European or Asian heritage. Among Chinese, no translation exists for the English word "sadness," yet all people experience the feeling of sadness at some time in life. To express emotion, Chinese patients somaticize their symptoms, or convert mental experiences or states into bodily symptoms (e.g., complain of cardiac symptoms because the center of emotion in the Chinese culture is the heart). You may collect in-depth data about the cardiovascular system only to learn subsequently that all diagnostic tests are negative. On further assessment, you may determine that the person has experienced a loss and is grieving (e.g., has experienced the death of a close relative or friend or has been divorced or separated). This is recognized as a culturally acceptable somatic expression of emotional disharmony.

For patients, symptom labeling and diagnosis depend on the degree of difference between the person's behaviors and those the group has defined as normal, beliefs about the causation of illness, level of stigma attached to a particular set of symptoms, prevalence of the pathologic condition, and the meaning of the illness to the person and his or her family.

Throughout history, humankind has attempted to understand the cause of illness and disease. Theories of causation have been formulated on the basis of ethnic identity, religious beliefs, social class, philosophic perspectives, and level of knowledge. You need to determine what the person believes has caused the illness. Many people who maintain traditional beliefs would define HEALTH in terms of balance and ILLNESS a loss of this balance. The understanding tends to include the balance of mind, body, and spirit in the overall definitions of HEALTH and ILLNESS.

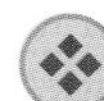 DEVELOPMENTAL COMPETENCE

Illness during childhood may be an especially difficult clinical situation. Children and adults have spiritual needs that vary according to the child's developmental level and the religious climate that exists in the family. Parental perceptions about the illness of the child may be partially influenced by religious beliefs. For example, some parents may believe that a transgression against a religious law is responsible for a congenital anomaly in their offspring. Other parents may delay seeking medical care because they believe that prayer should be tried first. Certain types of treatment (e.g., administration of blood; medications containing caffeine, pork, or other prohibited substances) and selected procedures may be perceived as *cultural taboos*—that is, practices to be avoided (by both children and adults).

Values held by the dominant United States and Canadian culture, such as emphasis on independence, self-reliance, and productivity, influence aging members of society. North Americans define people as old at the chronologic age of 65 years and then limit their work, in contrast to other cultures in which persons are first recognized as being unable to work and then are identified as being "old." The generation born just before or at the end of World War II (1940-1949) comprises the early range of older adults who are eligible for Social Security and Medicare.

In adopting a cultural perspective in working with aging individuals from culturally diverse backgrounds, you should consider that the main task of the person is to achieve a sense of integrity in accepting responsibility for his or her own life and in gaining a sense of accomplishment. Individuals who achieve integrity see aging as a positive experience, make adjustments in their personal space and social relationships, maintain a sense of usefulness, and begin closure and life review.

Older persons may develop their own means of coping with illness through self-care, assistance from family members, and support from social groups. Some cultures have developed attitudes and specific behaviors for older adults that may include humanistic care and identification of family members as care providers. The older adults may have special family responsibilities—for example, providing hospitality to visitors among Amish cultures and communicating to members of younger generations skills and accrued wisdom among Filipinos.

Older immigrants who have made major lifestyle adjustments in their move from their homelands to the United States or from a rural to an urban area (or vice versa) may not be aware of health care alternatives, preventive programs, health care benefits, and screening programs for which they are eligible. The people may also be in various stages of *culture shock;* that is, the state of disorientation or inability to respond to the behavior of a different cultural group because of its sudden strangeness, unfamiliarity, and incompatibility to the newcomer's perceptions and expectations. For example, in order to maintain ties with their native heritage, people may seek to purchase food in stores that specialize in selling products from their homelands.

TRADITIONAL CAUSES OF ILLNESS

Disease causation may be viewed in three major ways: from a biomedical or scientific, a naturalistic or holistic, or a magicoreligious perspective.

Biomedical

The first, called the **biomedical** or **scientific** theory of illness causation, is based on the assumption that all events in life have a cause and effect, that the human body functions more or less mechanically (i.e., the functioning of the human body is analogous to the functioning of an automobile), that all life can be reduced or divided into smaller parts (e.g., the reduction of the human person into body, mind, and spirit), and that all of reality can be observed and measured (e.g., intelligence tests and psychometric measures of behavior). Among the biomedical explanations for disease is the germ theory, which posits that microscopic organisms such as bacteria and viruses are responsible for specific disease conditions. Most educational programs for physicians, nurses, and other health care providers embrace the biomedical or scientific theories that explain the causes of both physical and psychological illnesses.

Naturalistic

The second way in which people explain the cause of illness is from the **naturalistic** or **holistic** perspective, found most frequently among American Indians, Asians, and others who believe that human life is only one aspect of nature and a part of the general order of the cosmos. The people may believe that the forces of nature must be kept in natural balance or harmony.

Some Asians believe in the **yin/yang theory,** in which health is believed to exist when all aspects of the person are in perfect balance. Rooted in the ancient Chinese philosophy of *Tao,* the yin/yang theory states that all organisms and objects in the universe consist of yin and yang energy forces. The seat of the energy forces is within the autonomic nervous system where balance between the opposing forces is maintained during health. Yin energy represents the female and negative forces, such as emptiness, darkness, and cold, whereas yang forces are male and positive, emitting warmth and fullness. Foods are classified as hot and cold in this theory and are transformed into yin and yang energy when metabolized by the body. Yin foods are cold, and yang foods are hot. Cold foods are eaten with a hot illness, and hot foods are eaten with a cold illness. The yin/yang theory is the basis for *Eastern* or *Chinese* medicine and is commonly embraced by many Asian Americans.

The naturalistic perspective posits that the laws of nature create imbalances, chaos, and disease. People embracing the naturalistic view use metaphors such as the healing power of nature, and they call the earth "Mother." From the perspective of the Chinese, for example, illness is not seen as an intruding agent but as a part of life's rhythmic course and as an outward sign of disharmony within.

Many Hispanic, Arab, Black, and Asian groups embrace the **hot/cold theory** of health and illness, an explanatory model with origins in the ancient Greek humoral theory. The four humors of the body—blood, phlegm, black bile, and yellow bile—regulate basic bodily functions and are described in terms of temperature, dryness, and moisture. The treatment of disease consists of adding or subtracting cold, heat, dryness, or wetness to restore the balance of the humors.

Beverages, foods, herbs, medicines, and diseases are classified as hot or cold according to their perceived effects on the body, not on their physical characteristics. Illnesses believed to be caused by cold entering the body include earache, chest cramps, paralysis, gastrointestinal discomfort, rheumatism, and tuberculosis. Among those illnesses believed to be caused by overheating are abscessed teeth, sore throats, rashes, and kidney disorders.

According to the hot/cold theory, the person is whole, not just a particular ailment. Those who embrace the hot/cold theory maintain that health consists of a positive state of total well-being, including physical, psychological, spiritual, and social aspects of the person. Paradoxically, the language used to describe this artificial dissection of the body into parts is itself a reflection of the biomedical/scientific perspective, not a naturalistic or holistic one.

Magicoreligious

The third major way in which people explain the causation of ILLNESS is from a **magicoreligious** perspective. The basic premise is that the world is seen as an arena in which supernatural forces dominate. The fate of the world and those in it depends on the action of supernatural forces for good or evil. Examples of magical causes of illness include belief in voodoo or witchcraft among some African Americans and others from circum-Caribbean countries. *Faith healing* is based on religious beliefs and is most prevalent among certain Christian religions, including Christian Scientists, whereas various healing rituals may be found in many other religions such as Roman Catholicism and Mormonism.

Of course, it is possible to have a combination of worldviews, and many people are likely to offer more than one explanation for the cause of their illness, the means of protecting themselves from such an illness, and the means to recovery. As a profession, nursing largely embraces the scientific/biomedical worldview, but some other aspects are gaining popularity, including techniques for management of chronic pain, such as acupuncture, herbal therapies, hypnosis, therapeutic touch, and biofeedback.

Amulets are objects, such as charms, that may be worn on a string or chain around the neck, wrist, or waist to protect the wearer from the "evil eye" or the "evil spirits" that could

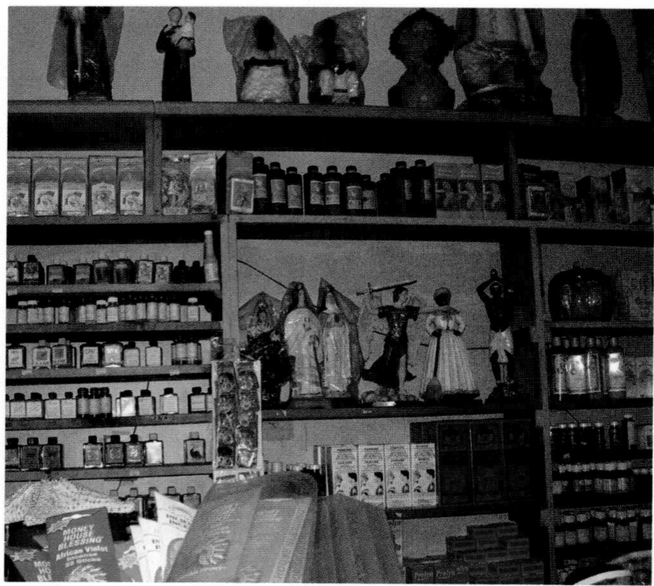

2-5 The interior of a *botanica*.[20]

be transmitted from one person to another or that could have supernatural origins. They may also be hung in the home, car, or workplace. Natural folk medicine uses remedies from the natural environment—herbs, plants, minerals, and animal substances—to treat illnesses. Amulets and remedies have come to the United States from every corner of the world, the East and the West. They may be purchased in pharmacies, markets, and natural food stores. Fig. 2-5 illustrates the interior of a *botanica,* a store in which a person can purchase amulets and remedies used by people from many *Latino* heritages. Others may be objects or substances used externally. Fig. 2-6 presents samples of traditional amulets.

Healing and Culture

When self-treatment is unsuccessful, the person might turn to the lay or folk healing systems, to spiritual or religious healing, or to scientific biomedicine. All cultures have their

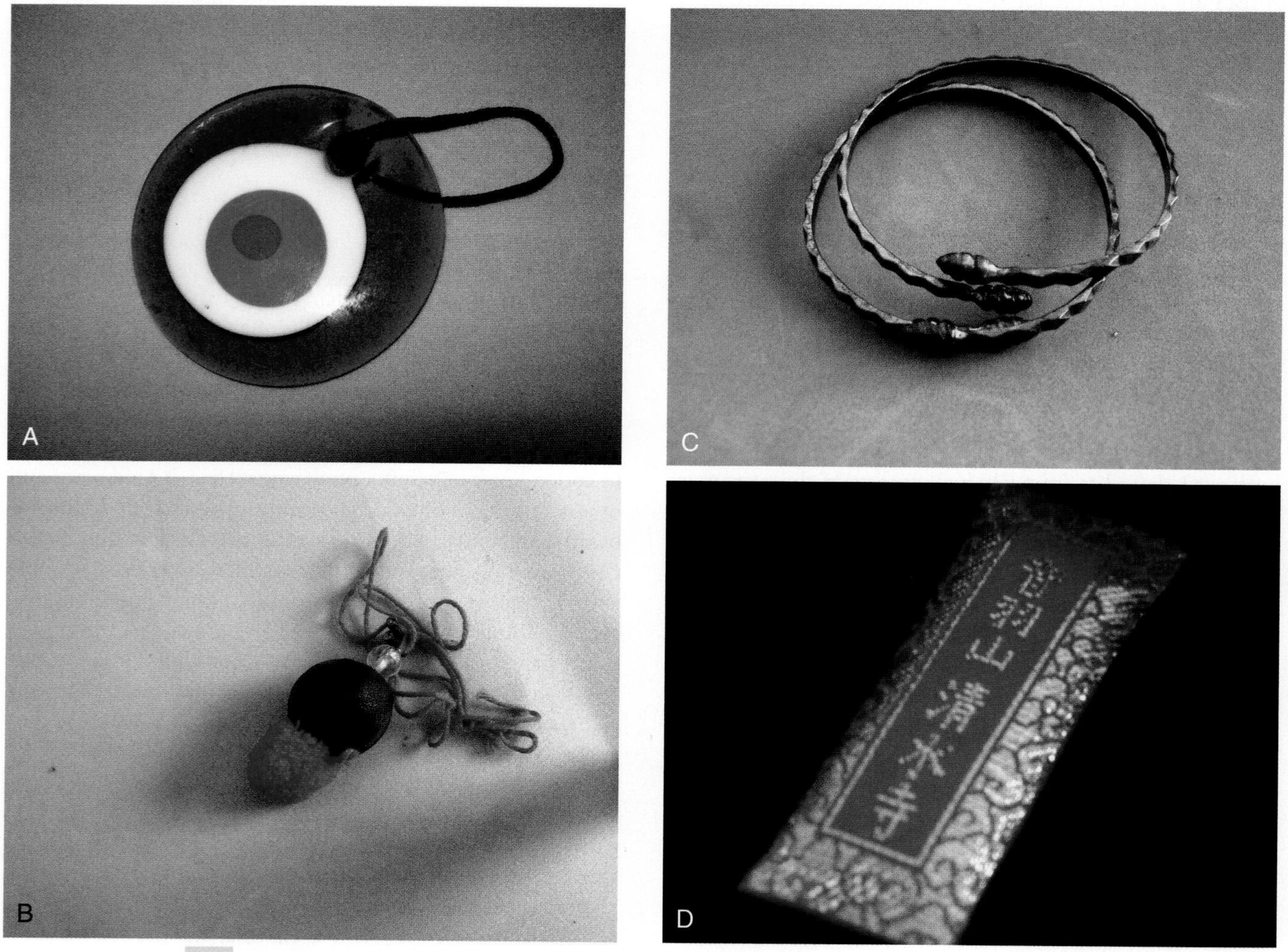

2-6 **A,** The glass blue eye from Turkey, seen here, is an example of an amulet that may be hung in the home.[20] **B,** A seed with a red string may be placed on the crib of a baby of Mexican heritage.[20] **C,** These bangles may be worn for protection by a person of Caribbean heritage.[20] **D,** This small packet is placed on a crib or baby's room of a baby of Japanese heritage.[20]

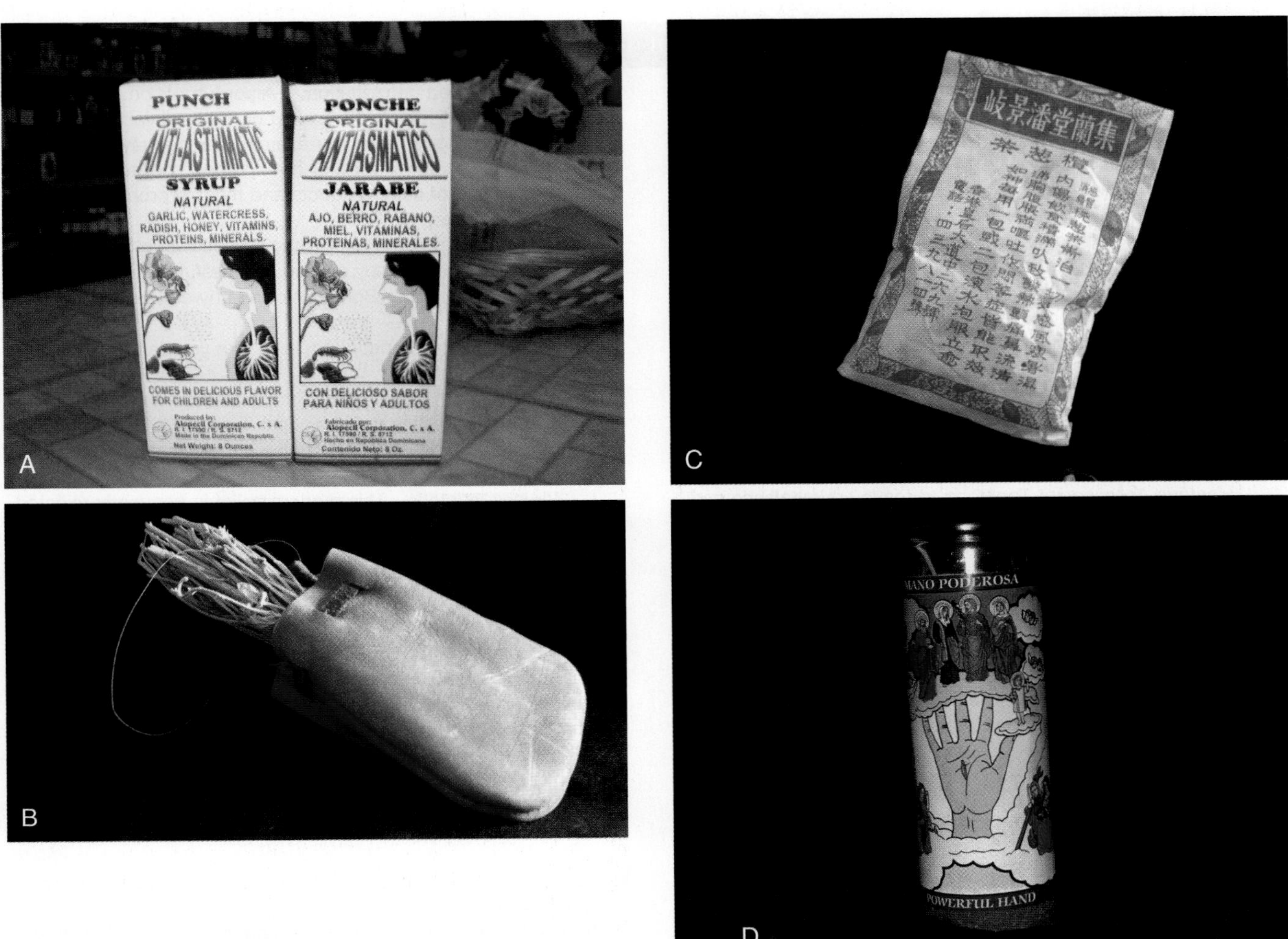

2-7 **A,** This "tonic" sold in a *botanica* is used to treat asthma.[20] **B,** The traditional medicine bag of an American Indian shaman is used to carry necessary medicines.[20] **C,** The leaves in this package may be used by a person of Chinese heritage to treat indigestion.[20] **D,** This candle may be burned for cleansing by a person of Mexican heritage.[20]

own preferred lay or popular healers, recognized symptoms of ill health, acceptable sick role behavior, and treatments. In addition to seeking help from you as a biomedical/scientific health care provider, patients may also seek help from folk or religious healers. Some people, such as those of Hispanic or American Indian origins, may believe that the cure is incomplete unless healing of body, mind, and spirit are all carried out. The division of the person into parts is itself a Western concept. For example, a Hispanic person with a respiratory infection may take the antibiotics prescribed by a physician or nurse practitioner and herbal teas recommended by a *curandero* and may say prayers for healing suggested by a Catholic priest. Many people from different faith traditions practice prayer or visit healing shrines, as discussed earlier in this chapter. There are countless shrines in the United States and the rest of the world where people make pilgrimages for this purpose, including Chimayo in New Mexico, Fatima in Portugal, and Lourdes in France.

The variety of healing beliefs and practices used by the many ethnocultural populations found in this country far exceeds the limitations of this chapter. It is important, however, that you be aware of the existence of traditional practices and recognize that, in addition to folk practices, many other complementary healing practices exist. Although it is dangerous to assume that all indigenous approaches to healing are innocuous, the majority of practices are quite harmless, regardless of whether they are effective cures. Fig. 2-7 presents samples of traditional remedies used for recovery.

Table 2-2 lists questions to ask and sample answers for this phase of assessment.

Folk Healers

People from most traditional heritages tend to use traditional healers from their own background. Although numerous folk healers exist, you may find Hispanics turning to a *curandero(ra), espiritualista* (spiritualist), *yerbo(ba)* (herbalist), *partera* (lay midwife), or *sabedor* (healer who manipulates bones and muscles). African Americans may mention having received assistance from a *hougan* (a voodoo priest

TABLE 2-2 Health Beliefs and Practices Assessment

1. How do you define health?
   When asked this question, people who score high on the Heritage Assessment Tool tend to focus on balance and holistic definitions of HEALTH, whereas people who have been socialized in modern ways within the dominant culture tend to see health as a relationship between mind-body and mainly focus on being able to move and do what they must in terms of work and so forth.

2. How do you rate your health?
   When asked this question, most nurses tend to rate their health as excellent or good, whereas many lay people rate their health as good to poor.

3. How do you describe illness?
   When asked this question, people who score high on the Heritage Assessment Tool tend to focus on imbalance and holistic definitions of ILLNESS, whereas people who have been socialized in modern ways tend to see health as a relationship between mind-body and mainly focus on being able to move and do what they must in terms of work and so forth.

4. What do you believe causes illness?
   a. Environmental change—The belief that going from a hot place to a cold one and vice versa may cause illness.
   b. Evil eye—The evil eye is an ancient belief that still persists. People believe that illness may be caused by a person or spirit looking at them with malice. It can be prevented by wearing amulets and cured with various remedies and practices.
   c. Exposure to drafts—This European belief holds that cold air blowing on the body may make one ill. The prevention is to wear a shawl.
   d. God's punishment—This is a common belief among many traditional people.
   e. Grief and loss—This is both a modern and traditional cause of illness.
   f. Hexes and spells—People may cast a hex or spell on another person. Often the person who is able to do this may be the person who knows the way to remove the spell.
   g. Incorrect food combinations—Among traditional people, Asian and Hispanic, the mixing of foods of various compositions is taboo; for example, foods may be classified as *yin* or *yang* or hot and cold, not temperature. The mixing of dairy products and meat is prohibited in Jewish dietary law.
   h. Jealousy or envy—People may believe that others may cast illness on them if they are too successful or rich.
   i. Not enough work—Boredom or apathy can be a cause of illness.
   j. Overwork—Many people believe that you can become ill by too much work.
   k. Poor eating habits—Among many traditional people, nutrition excesses or imbalances tend to be factors that contribute to illness. This is also a causative agent in modern health care.
   l. Viruses, bacteria—This modern belief is frequently rejected by traditional people.
   m. Witchcraft—This ancient cause of illness still persists where people may believe that the practices of people known as "witches" can harm them.

5. What did your mother do to keep you from getting sick, and what home remedies did your mother use to restore your health?
   Contemporary nursing students may find that their mothers followed modern methods of health care; however, immigrants and traditional people may have a much different response to this question in terms of folk beliefs and practices.

6. How do you keep yourself from getting sick, and what home remedies do you use?
   In all probability, you answer with modern remedies; however, patients from a traditional heritage may tell you of the folk remedies they use. There may be a problem when people are using folk remedies rather than or in addition to modern medicines. It is important that, when this information is gathered, the interactions of the folk remedy and the modern remedy be researched.

or priestess), *spiritualist,* or "*old lady*" (an older woman who has successfully raised a family and who specializes in childcare and folk remedies). American Indians may seek assistance from a *shaman* or *medicine (wo)man.* Asians may mention that they have visited *herbalists, acupuncturists,* or *bone setters.* Among the Amish, the term *braucher* refers to folk healers who use herbs and tonics in the home or community context. *Brauche,* a folk healing art, refers to sympathy curing, which is sometimes called *powwowing* in English.

The treatments used by a traditional healer may be provided in conjunction with massage; foot treatments; acupressure; reflexology; or, less frequently, iridology.[20] Each culture has its own healers, most of whom speak the person's native tongue, make house calls, understand the person's cultural HEALTH beliefs, and cost significantly less than healers practicing in the biomedical/scientific health care system. Table 2-3 lists examples of traditional HEALTH and ILLNESS beliefs and practices, causes of illness, and examples of traditional healers.

In some religions, spiritual healers may be found among the ranks of the ordained and official religious hierarchy and may be known by a variety of names such as *priest, bishop, elder, deacon, rabbi, brother,* and *sister.* In other religions, a separate category of healer may be found—e.g., Christian Science "nurses" (not licensed by states) or practitioners. Spirituality is included in the perceptions of health and illness.

TABLE 2-3 Selected Examples of Traditional HEALTH and ILLNESS Beliefs and Practices

Origin	HEALTH Beliefs	ILLNESS Beliefs	ILLNESS Causation	HEALTH Maintenance	HEALTH Protection	HEALTH Restoration	Traditional Healers
ASIAN HERITAGES							
China India Japan Korea Philippines Southeast Asia Laos Cambodia Vietnam	Balance of *"yin and yang"*	Imbalance of *"yin and yang"*	Upset in the balance of *"yin and yang"* Overexertion Prolonged sitting Lying in bed	Prevent imbalances of *"yin and yang"* and changes in climate	Wear amulets, such as jade Eat correct and compatible foods	Traditional remedies such as ginseng root Acupuncture Moxibustion Cupping	Chinese physicians Herbalists
AFRICAN HERITAGES							
Africa—west coast (as slaves) Ghana Nigeria, etc. Haiti Jamaica West Indian islands	Harmony with nature	Disharmony with nature	Demons Evil spirits Voodoo Hexes	Prevent disharmony; respect cleanliness Religion Avoid sick people	Wear bangles Faith	*Asafoetida,* herbs and roots	Root worker Spiritualists "Old Lady"
EUROPEAN HERITAGES							
England France Germany Poland Russia Others	Physical and emotional well-being; feeling okay	Absence of well-being; feeling bad	Evil eye Evil spirits Hexes	Proper nutrition, exercise, cleanliness, and faith in God	Wear amulets Shawls	Home remedies, such as swamp root and *Olbas*	Homeopathic physicians Brauchers
AMERICAN INDIAN/ALASKA NATIVE HERITAGES							
North American Indians/Alaska Natives 550+ federally or state recognized nations	Living in harmony with nature Balance of the mind, emotions, body, and spirit	Disharmony with nature	Evil spirits Ghosts Displeasing Holy people	Respect nature; avoid evil spirits Masks	Use of amulets and sweet grass	Sand paintings Herbs	Medicine man (shaman)
IBERIAN, CENTRAL AND SOUTH AMERICAN HERITAGES							
Spain and Portugal Brazil Cuba Mexico Puerto Rico Colombia	Reward for good behavior Balance of "hot and cold" humors	Punishment for wrongdoing Imbalance of hot and cold	Evil eye Envy of other people Jealousy	Use proper diet to maintain balance of "hot and cold" Faith	Amulets, such as a *mano negro,* soaps, candles	Prayers Promises to saints Herbs, *Anis* and *Manzanilla*	Folk healers, such as the *santro/a, partera,* or *curandero/a*

TRANSCULTURAL EXPRESSION OF ILLNESS

Transcultural Expression of Pain

To illustrate the manner in which symptom expression may reflect the person's cultural background, let us use an extensively studied symptom—pain. Pain is a universally recognized phenomenon, and it is an important aspect of assessment for people of various ages. Pain is a very private, subjective experience that is greatly influenced by cultural heritage. Expectations, manifestations, and management of pain are all embedded in a cultural context. The definition of pain, like that of health or illness, is culturally determined.

The word *pain* is derived from the Greek word for *penalty,* which helps explain the long association between pain and punishment in Judeo-Christian thought. The meaning of painful stimuli, the way people define their situation, and the impact of personal experience all help determine the experience of pain.

Much cross-cultural research has been conducted on pain. Pain has been found to be a highly personal experience, depending on cultural learning, the meaning of the situation, and other factors unique to the person. Silent suffering has been identified as the most valued response to pain by health care professionals. The majority of nurses have been socialized to believe that in virtually any situation, self-control is better than open displays of strong feelings.

In addition to expecting variations in pain perception and tolerance, you also should expect variations in the expression of pain. It is well known that people turn to their social environment for validation and comparison. A first important comparison group is the family, which transmits cultural norms to its children.

TABLE 2-4 Examples of Culture-Bound Syndromes

Origin	Culture-Bound Syndrome	Presenting Symptoms
ASIAN HERITAGES		
China India Japan Korea Philippines Southeast Asia Laos Cambodia Vietnam	Shenkui (China)	Marked anxiety or panic symptoms with dizziness, backache, general weakness, insomnia, frequent dreams, and complaints of sexual dysfunction (premature ejaculation and impotence). Believed to be caused by excessive semen loss. Feared because it represents a loss of vital essence and is believed to be life threatening.
	Dhat (India)	Semen-loss syndrome. Characterized by severe anxiety and hypochondriac concerns about semen discharge. Whitish discoloration of the urine and feelings of weakness.
AFRICAN HERITAGES		
Africa—west coast (as slaves) Ghana Nigeria, etc. Haiti Jamaica West Indian islands	Low blood	Not enough blood or weakness of the blood, which is often treated with diet.
	High blood	Blood that is too rich in certain nutrients as a result of ingestion of too much red meat or rich foods.
	Thin blood	Occurs in women, children, and old people; susceptible to illness in general.
EUROPEAN HERITAGES		
England France Germany Poland Russia Others	Hysteria (Greece)	Bizarre complaints and behavior because the uterus leaves the pelvis for another part of the body.
	Involutional paraphrenia (Germany)	Paranoid disorder occurring in midlife.
	Rodina (Russia)	Malaise, depression.
AMERICAN INDIAN/ALASKA NATIVE HERITAGES		
North American Indians/Alaska Natives 550+ federally or state recognized nations	Ghost	Tremor, hallucinations, sense of danger.
	Hi-Wa itck	Insomnia, depression, loss of appetite. Associated with unwanted separation from a loved one.
IBERIAN, CENTRAL AND SOUTH AMERICAN HERITAGES		
Spain and Portugal Brazil Cuba Mexico Puerto Rico Colombia	*Empacho*	Food forms into a ball and clings to the stomach or intestines, causing pain and cramping.
	Mal ojo ("evil eye")	Fitful sleep, crying, diarrhea in children caused by a stranger's attention; sudden onset.
	Susto	Anxiety, trembling, phobias from sudden fright.

Culture-Bound Syndromes

Some people may have a condition that is culturally defined, known as a *culture-bound syndrome.* Some of these conditions have no equivalent from a biomedical/scientific perspective, whereas others, such as anorexia nervosa and bulimia, are examples of the cultural aspects of illness among members of a dominant cultural population in North America. Table 2-4 summarizes selected examples from among the more than 150 culture-bound syndromes that have been documented by medical anthropologists, mental health providers, or community spokespeople.

Culture and Treatment

After a symptom is identified, the first effort at treatment is often self-care. In the United States, an estimated 38% of adults use some form of complementary therapy to treat an illness. Furthermore, U.S. adults spent $33.9 billion out-of-pocket on visits to complementary and alternative medicine practitioners and the purchase of related products.[13a] The availability of over-the-counter medications, the relatively high literacy level of Americans, the growing availability of herbal remedies, and the influence of the Internet and mass media in communicating health-related information to the general population have contributed to the high percentage of cases of self-treatment. Home treatments are attractive for their accessibility, especially compared with the inconvenience associated with traveling to a physician, nurse practitioner, or pharmacist, particularly for people from rural or sparsely populated areas. Furthermore, home treatment may mobilize the person's social support network and provide the sick person with a caring environment in which to convalesce. You should be aware, however, that not all home remedies are inexpensive. For example, urban Black populations in the Southeast sometimes use medicinal potions that cost much more than the equivalent treatment with a biomedical intervention.

A wide variety of alternative, complementary, or traditional interventions are gaining the recognition of health care professionals in the biomedical/scientific health care system. Acupuncture, acupressure, therapeutic touch, massage, therapeutic use of music, biofeedback, relaxation techniques, meditation, hypnosis, distraction, imagery, iridology, reflexology, herbal remedies, and others are interventions that people may use either alone or in combination with other treatments. Many pharmacies and grocery stores routinely carry herbal treatments for a wide variety of common illnesses. The efficacy of complementary and alternative interventions for specific health problems has been studied extensively (see National Center for Complementary and Alternative Medicine at www.nccam.nih.gov). The frequency of use of traditional remedies, such as herbs purchased in *botanicas* and Chinese herbal drugs, is unknown at this time. However, personal observations in these settings indicate great popularity within the traditional members of the ethnocultural community. Fig. 2-7 illustrates examples of the remedies.

Culture and Disease Prevalence

For the past generation, the United States and Canada have enjoyed improvement in the health status of the population. Despite this fact, there continues to be disparities in deaths and illnesses experienced by racial and ethnic emerging majority populations, and it is well known that diseases are not distributed equally among all segments of the population. Abnormal biocultural variations may be genetic or acquired. Information about disease prevalence for various racial and ethnic groups is useful because you are able to focus your assessment according to the increased statistical probability that a particular condition may occur. For example, if you are examining an African-American child with gastrointestinal symptoms, you may focus more on the possibility of lactose intolerance or sickle-cell anemia while considering cystic fibrosis, known primarily among white children, a much less likely source of the problem. Poverty also plays a role in the disparities. Thus, in your assessment, you will want to be certain that you have gathered the appropriate data needed to support or to refute your suspicions. Information regarding several health disparities is included in the CULTURE AND GENETICS section of chapters in this text.

STEPS TO CULTURAL COMPETENCY

There are several steps that you must climb on the journey to CULTURAL COMPETENCY. The integration of this knowledge into day-to-day practice will take time because many practitioners in the health care system are hesitant to adopt new ideas. CULTURAL COMPETENCY does not come instantly, certainly not after reading a chapter or several chapters or books on this highly specialized area. It is complex and multifaceted, and many facets change over time. The areas of knowledge include sociology, psychology, theology, cultural anthropology, demography, folklore, and immigration history and policies. One must also have an understanding of poverty and environmental health. CULTURAL COMPETENCY also involves soul searching about your own heritage and HEALTH.

The first step in understanding the HEALTH care needs of others is to understand your own heritage based on cultural values, beliefs, attitudes, and practices that are relevant to HEALTH and ILLNESS (Table 2-5). Sometimes this requires considerable searching and necessitates that you explore your family's heritage and traditional beliefs and practices. Your mother or maternal grandmother is a familial resource whom you may want to interview to determine the meaning of these terms within your family. The reason for suggesting that you interview your maternal side is that, in the past, mothers tended to be the family gatekeepers and the persons who determined whether you were healthy or sick.

You are now learning the modern, scientific meanings of health and illness, and at the same time, you must develop a frame of reference as to the traditional beliefs and practices relevant to these concepts. In addition, many of your patients will come from socioeconomic and religious backgrounds different from your own, so you must confront your own biases, preconceptions, and prejudices about specific racial, ethnic, religious, sexual, or socioeconomic groups.

The second phase is to identify the meaning of HEALTH to the other person, remembering that concepts are derived, in part, from the way in which members of a cultural group define health. Considerable research has been conducted on the various definitions of HEALTH that may be held by various groups. For example, one traditional American Indian belief is that HEALTH reflects living in total harmony with nature; illness is the result of a lack of prevention. Some Jamaicans may define health as having a good appetite, feeling strong and energetic, performing activities of daily living without difficulty, and being sexually active and fertile. For Italian women, health may mean the ability to interact socially and to perform routine tasks such as cooking, cleaning, and caring for self and others. On the other hand, some people of Mexican heritage believe that coughing, sweating, and diarrhea are a normal part of living, not symptoms of ill health—perhaps because of the high frequency of these conditions in the country of origin. Thus individuals may define themselves or others in their group as healthy even though you identify them as having symptoms of disease.

Third, you must understand the health care delivery system, how it works, what it does, the meanings of various procedures, and the costs and consequences to the patients and to you as a nurse. Fourth, you must be knowledge-

TABLE 2-5 Guide for CULTURAL CARE

PREPARING

- Discover and understand your own heritage, cultural values, biases, and traditional HEALTH beliefs and practices.
- Acquire basic knowledge of cultural values and health/HEALTH beliefs and practices for patient groups you serve.

R.E.S.P.E.C.T.

Realize that you MUST know and understand your heritage and that of your patient.
Examine the patient within the context of his or her cultural HEALTH and ILLNESS practices.
Select questions that are not complex, and do not ask questions rapidly.
Pace questions throughout the physical examination.
Encourage the patient to discuss the meanings of health and illness with you.
Check for the patient's understanding and acceptance of recommendations, and build on cultural HEALTH practices when indicated.
Touch the patient within the cultural boundaries of his or her heritage—manners are a vital component of the nurse-patient relationship.

able about the social backgrounds of your patients—the meanings of immigration, racism, socioeconomic status, welfare reform, and aging. Fifth, you must be familiar with the language people speak, the resources available to help with interpretation, and the resources within the community.

The bibliography lists several books and selected websites that can provide you with introductory material related to this content. Remember, everything is connected to CULTURAL COMPETENCY: heritage, culture, ethnicity, religion, socialization, population diversity, immigration, religion, demographic change, globalization, health and illness, modern and traditional beliefs and practices, sociopolitical issues, sanitation, housing, and infrastructure. CULTURAL CARE is the goal to strive for. As stated in the beginning of the chapter, it is a long journey.

BIBLIOGRAPHY

1. Abramson, H. J. (1980). Religion. In S. Thernstrom (Ed.), *Harvard encyclopedia of American ethnic groups.* Cambridge: Harvard University Press.

1a. American Religious Identification Survey 2001. (2001). The City University of New York. Accessed June 9, 2009, from http://www.gc.cuny.edu/faculty/research_studies/aris.pdf.

2. Andrews, M. M., & Boyle, J. S. (2003). *Transcultural concepts in nursing care* (4th ed.). Philadelphia: Lippincott Williams & Wilkins.

3. Bernstein, R. *U. S. Hispanic population surpasses 45 million: now is 15 percent of total.* Public Information Office. Accessed June 9, 2009, from www.census.gov/PressRelease/www/releases/archives/population/011910.html.

4. Estes, G., & Zitzow, D. (1980). *Heritage consistency as a consideration in counseling Native Americans.* Presented at the National Indian Education Association Convention, Dallas: The Association.

5. Fix, M. E., & Passel, J. S. (2001). *U.S. immigration at the beginning of the 21st century:* Testimony before the Subcommittee on Immigration and Claims Hearing on "The U.S. Population and Immigration" Committee on the Judiciary U.S. House of Representatives Accessed August 2, 2001, from: www.urban.org/url.cfm?ID=900417.

6. Flores, G. (2006). Language barriers to health care in the United States. *New England Journal of Medicine, 355,* 229-231.

7. Giger, J. N., & Davidhizar, R. E. (2008). *Transcultural nursing: assessment and intervention* (5th ed.). St. Louis: Mosby.

8. Giger, J., Davidhizar, R., Purnell, L., et al. (2007). American Academy of Nursing Expert Panel Report: Developing cultural competence to eliminate health disparities in ethnic minorities and other vulnerable populations. *Journal of Transcultural Nursing, 18*(2), 95-102.

9. Hoefer, M., Rytina, N., & Baker, B. B. (2008). *Estimates of the unauthorized immigrant population residing in the United States: January, 2008.* Accessed June 8, 2009, from www.dhs.gov/xlibrary/assets/statistics/publications/ois_ill_pe_2008.pdf.

10. Homeland Security. (2008). *Definition of terms, 2008.* Accessed June 5, 2009, from www.dhs.gov/ximgtn/statistics/stdfdef.shtm#11.

11. LaFrombose, T., Coleman, L. K., & Gerton, J. (1993). Psychological impact of biculturalism: Evidence and theory. *Psychological Bulletin, 114,* 395.

12. Levin, J. (2001). *God, faith and health: Exploring the spirituality-healing connection.* New York: John Wiley & Sons.

13. Ludwig-Beymer, P. A. (2002). Transcultural aspects of pain. In M. M. Andrews & J. S. Boyle (Eds.), *Transcultural concepts in nursing care* (4th ed.). Philadelphia: Lippincott Williams & Wilkins.

13a. Nahin, R. L., Barnes, P. M., Stussman, B. J., et al. (2009). Costs of complementary and alternative medicine (CAM) and frequency of visits to CAM practitioners: United States, 2007. *National health statistics reports; no 18.* Hyattsville, MD: National Center for Health Statistics.

14. *National standards for culturally and linguistically appropriate services in health care, final report,* March 2001, Washington, DC, Office of Minority Health, Department of Health and Human Services.

15. Novak, M. (1972). *The rise of the unmeltable ethnics.* New York: Macmillan.

16. Pew Forum on Religion and Public Life. *U. S. Religious Landscape Survey, 2007.* Accessed June 9, 2009, from http://religions.pewforum.org/pdf/report2religious-landscape-study-key-findings.pdf.

17. Randall, M., & Rytina, N. *U.S. legal permanent residents, 2008.* Accessed June 7, 2009, from www.dhs.gov/xlibrary/assets/statistics/publications/lpr_fr_2008.pdf.

18. Skalla, K. A., & McCoy, J. P. (2006). Spiritual assessment of patients with cancer: The mortal authority, vocational, aesthetic, social, and transcendent model. *Oncology Nursing Forum, 33,* 752.

19. Spector, R. E. (2004). *Culture care: Guide to heritage assessment and health traditions* (3rd ed.). Upper Saddle River, NJ: Prentice Hall.

20. Spector, R. E. (2009). *Cultural diversity in health and illness* (7th ed.). Upper Saddle River, NJ: Prentice Hall.

21. U.S. Census Bureau, Public Information Office (301) 763-3030. *U.S. Census. 2008. Population and housing narrative profile: 2005-2007.* Accessed June 8, 2009, from http://factfinder.census.gov/servlet/NPTable?_bm=y&-qr_name=ACS_2007_3YR_G00_NP01&-geo_id=01000US&-ds_name=ACS_2007_3YR_G00_&-_lang=en.

22. *U.S. Census Bureau.* Home page. Accessed June 3, 2009, from www.census.gov/.

23. Wenger, A. F. (1993). Cultural meaning of symptoms. *Holistic Nursing Practice, 7,* 22-35.

24. Wenger, A. F. (1995). Cultural context, health, and health care decision making. *Journal of Transcultural Nursing, 7,* 3-14.

Websites of Interest

www.census.gov/—A complete demographic profile at national, state, and local levels.

www.tcns.org/—The Transcultural Nursing Society.

www.healthpowerforminorities.org/resources/national.cfm—A directory and links to resources for minority health programs.

www.hhs-stat.net/omh/index.htm—Links to programs developed to reduce health disparities.

www.hhs.gov/ocr/hospitalcommunication.html—Information regarding Title VI of the Civil Rights Act.

www.thinkculturalhealth.org/ccnm/—Self-study program in cultural competency.

www.omhrc.gov/—The division in the government that is developing standards and educational programs in cultural competency.

www.census.gov/hhes/www/poverty/poverty.html—Facts and figures regarding economic poverty.

http://nccam.nih.gov/news/camstats/costs/.

www.kaiseredu.org/topics_index.asp—An online health policy resource that includes the following topics: Health and the Law, Health System, HIV/AIDS, Medicare, Minority Health, Uninsured, and Women's Health.

www.cdc.gov/nchs/data/hus/hus08.pdf—This publication, *Health United States: 2008,* is the 32nd report on the health status of the Nation. The report is published annually and is an invaluable resource for health statistics in four major areas—health status and determinants, health care utilization, health care resources, and health care expenditures.

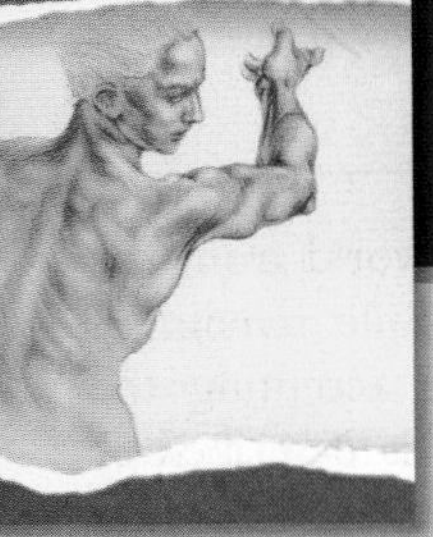

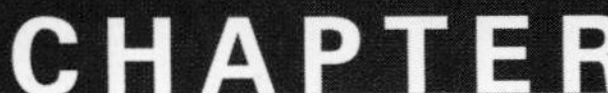

CHAPTER 3

The Interview

evolve WEBSITE

http://evolve.elsevier.com/Jarvis/

- Audio Key Points
- NCLEX Review Questions

The interview is a meeting between you and your patient. The meeting's goal is to record a complete health history. The health history is important in beginning to identify the person's health strengths and problems and as a bridge to the next step in data collection, the physical examination.

The interview is the first and really the most important part of data collection. It collects **subjective data**—what the person says about himself or herself. The interview is the first and the best chance a person has to tell you what *he or she* perceives the health state to be. Once people enter the health care system, they relinquish some control. At the interview, however, the patient is still in charge. The individual knows everything about his or her own health state, and you know nothing. Your skill in interviewing will glean all the necessary information as well as build rapport for a successful working relationship. When you have a successful interview, you:

1. Gather complete and accurate data about the person's health state, including the description and chronology of any symptoms of illness.
2. Establish rapport and trust so the person feels accepted and thus free to share all relevant data.
3. Teach the person about the health state so that the person can participate in identifying problems.
4. Build rapport for a continuing therapeutic relationship; this rapport facilitates future diagnoses, planning, and treatment.
5. Begin teaching for health promotion and disease prevention.

Consider the interview as being similar to forming a **contract** between you and your patient. A contract consists of spoken or unspoken rules for behavior. In this case, the contract concerns what the person needs and expects from health care and what you, the health professional, have to offer. Your mutual goal is optimal health for the patient. The contract's terms include:

- Time and place of the interview and succeeding physical examination
- Introduction of yourself and a brief explanation of your role
- The purpose of the interview
- How long it will take
- Expectation of participation for each person
- Presence of any other people (e.g., patient's family, other health professionals, students)
- Confidentiality and to what extent it may be limited
- Any costs that the patient must pay

Although the patient already may know some of this information through telephone contact with receptionists or the admitting office, the remaining points need to be stated clearly at the outset. Any confusion could produce resentment and anger, rather than the openness and trust you need to facilitate the interview.

THE PROCESS OF COMMUNICATION

The vehicle that carries you and your patient through the interview is communication. Communication is exchanging information so that each person clearly understands the other. If you do not understand each other, if you have not *conveyed meaning,* no communication has occurred.

It is challenging to teach the skill of interviewing because initially most students think little needs to be learned. They assume that if they can talk and hear, they can communicate. But much more than talking and hearing is necessary. Communication is all behavior, conscious and unconscious, verbal and nonverbal. *All behavior has meaning.*

Sending

Likely, you are most aware of *verbal* communication—the words you speak, vocalizations, the tone of voice. *Nonverbal* communication also occurs. This is your body language—posture, gestures, facial expression, eye contact, foot tapping, touch, even where you place your chair. Because nonverbal communication is under less conscious control than verbal communication, nonverbal communication probably is more reflective of your true feelings.

Receiving

Being aware of the messages you send is only part of the process. Your words and gestures must be interpreted in a *specific context* to have meaning. You have a specific context in mind when you send your words. The receiver puts his or her own interpretation on them. The receiver attaches meaning determined by his or her past experiences, culture, and self-concept, as well as current physical and emotional state. Sometimes these contexts do not coincide. Remember how frustrating it may have been to try to communicate something to a friend, only to have your message totally misunderstood? Your message can be sabotaged by the listener's bias. It takes mutual understanding by the sender and receiver to have successful communication.

Even greater risk for misunderstanding exists in the health care setting than in a social setting. The patient's frame of reference is narrowed and focused on illness. The patient usually has a health problem, and this factor emotionally charges your professional relationship. It *intensifies* the communication because the person feels dependent on you to get better.

Communication is a *basic skill* that can be learned and polished when you are a beginning practitioner. It is a tool, as basic to quality health care as the tools of inspection or palpation. To maximize your communicating skill, first you need to be aware of internal and external factors and their influence.

Internal Factors

Internal factors are those particular to the examiner, what you bring into the interview. Cultivate the three inner factors of liking others, empathy, and the ability to listen.

Liking Others. One essential factor for an examiner's "goodness of fit" into a helping profession is a genuine liking of other people. This means a generally optimistic view of people—an assumption of their strengths and a tolerance for their weaknesses. An atmosphere of warmth and caring is necessary. The patient must feel that he or she is accepted unconditionally.

The respect for other people extends to respect for their own control over their health. Your goal is *not* to make your patients dependent on you, but to help them to be increasingly responsible for themselves. You wish to promote their growth. You have the health care resources to offer. Patients must choose how to apply those resources to their own lives.

Empathy. Empathy means viewing the world from the other person's inner frame of reference while remaining yourself. Empathy means recognizing and accepting the other person's feelings without criticism. It is described as "feeling *with* the person rather than feeling *like* the person." It does not mean you become lost in the other person at the expense of your own self. If this occurred, you would cease to be helpful. Rather, it is to *understand with* the person how *he or she* perceives his or her world.

The Ability to Listen. Listening is not a passive role in the communication process; it is active and demanding. Listening requires your complete attention. You cannot be preoccupied with your own needs or the needs of other patients, or you will miss something important with this one. For the time of this interview, no one is more important than this person. This person's needs are your sole concern.

Active listening is the route to understanding. You cannot be thinking of what you are going to say as soon as the person stops for breath. Listen to *what* the person says. The story may not come out in the order you would ask it or will record it later. Let the person talk from his or her own outline; nearly everything that is said will be relevant. Listen to *the way* a person tells the story, such as difficulty with language, impaired memory, the tone of the person's voice, and even to what the person is leaving out (see the Clinical Illustration below.)

CLINICAL ILLUSTRATION

Sandra B., 32 years of age, sought care for headaches she had during the past 3 months, which were unresponsive to aspirin and were interfering with her job. She was interviewed for 30 minutes. Through this time, she never mentioned her husband, although they had been married only 5 months earlier. Finally, the examiner asked, "I haven't heard you mention your husband. Tell me about him." It unfolded that Sandra's husband lost his job a few months after they were married because of alcohol-related work errors. Although Sandra related extreme personal stress and worry, she never thought that her headaches might be related to the stressful situation.

External Factors

Prepare the physical setting. The setting may be in a hospital room, an examination room in an office or clinic, or the person's home (where you have less control). In any location, optimal conditions are important to have a smooth interview.

Ensure Privacy. Aim for geographic privacy—a private room in the hospital, clinic, office, or home. This may involve asking an ambulatory roommate to step out for a while or finding an unoccupied room or an empty lounge. If geographic privacy is not available, "psychological privacy" by curtained partitions may suffice as long as the person feels sure no one can overhear the conversation or interrupt.

Refuse Interruptions. Most people resent interruptions except in cases of an emergency. Inform any support staff of your interview, and ask that they not interrupt you during this time. Discourage other health professionals from interrupting you with *their* need for access to the patient. You need to concentrate and to establish rapport. An interruption can destroy in seconds what you have spent many minutes building up.

Physical Environment

- Set the room temperature at a comfortable level.
- Provide sufficient lighting so that you can see each other clearly. Avoid facing the patient directly toward a strong light where the patient must squint as if on stage.
- Reduce noise. Multiple stimuli are confusing. Turn off the television, radio, and any unnecessary equipment.
- Remove distracting objects or equipment. It is appropriate to leave some professional equipment (oto/ophthalmoscope, blood pressure manometer) in view. However, clutter, stacks of mail, files of other patients, or your lunch should not be seen. The room should advertise the professional nature of the interviewer.
- Place the distance between you and the patient at 4 to 5 feet (twice arm's length). If you place the patient any closer, you may invade his or her private space and you may create anxiety. If you place the patient farther away, you seem distant and aloof. (See the section on Culture and Genetics for more information.)
- Arrange **equal-status seating** (Fig. 3-1). Both you and the patient should be comfortably seated, at eye level. Avoid facing a patient across a desk or table because that feels like a barrier. Placing the chairs at 90 degrees is good because it allows the person either to face you or to look straight ahead from time to time. Most important, avoid standing. Standing does two things: (1) it communicates your haste, and (2) it assumes superiority. Standing makes you loom over the patient as an authority figure. When you are sitting, the person feels some control in the setting.
- Arrange a face-to-face position when interviewing the hospitalized bedridden person. The person should not have to stare at the ceiling, because this causes him or her to lose the visual message of your communication.

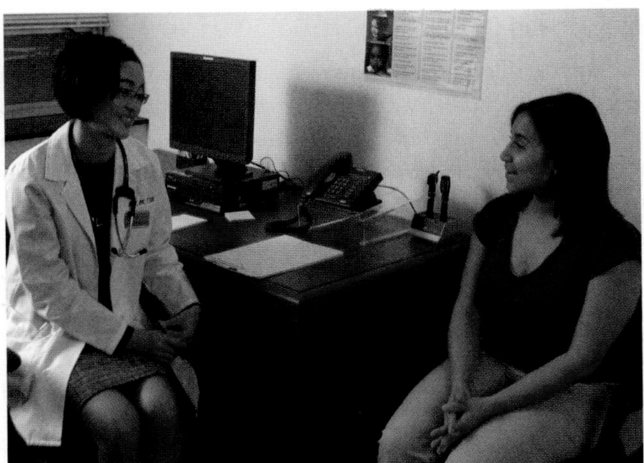

3-1 Equal status seating.

3-2

Dress

- The patient should remain in street clothes except in the case of an emergency.
- Your appearance and clothing should be appropriate to the setting and should meet conventional professional standards: a uniform or lab coat over conservative clothing, a name tag, and neat hair. Avoid extremes.

Note-Taking. Some use of history forms and note-taking may be unavoidable (Fig. 3-2). When you sit down later to record the interview, you cannot rely completely on memory to furnish details of previous hospitalizations or the review of body systems, for example. But be aware that note-taking during the interview has disadvantages:

- It breaks eye contact too often.
- It shifts your attention away from the person, diminishing his or her sense of importance.
- It can interrupt the patient's narrative flow. You may say, "Please slow down; I'm not getting it all." Or, the patient may see you recording furiously, and in an effort to please you, adjust his or her tempo to your writing. Either way, the patient's natural mode of expression is lost.
- It impedes your observation of the patient's nonverbal behavior.
- It is threatening to the patient during the discussion of sensitive issues (e.g., amount of alcohol and drug use, number of sexual partners, or incidence of physical abuse).

So keep note-taking to a minimum, and try to focus your attention on the person. Any recording you do should be secondary to the dialogue and should not interfere with the person's spontaneity. With experience, you will not rely on note-taking as much.

Tape and Video Recording. An audio tape documents a complete record of what was said during the interview. You cannot refer to it as easily as you can to your notes, but the tape is an excellent teaching tool to study objectively your performance as an interviewer. After listening, other students have commented:

"I never realized how much I talked. I really dominated the patient."

"I have to watch my interrupting. I cut her off that time."

"There. That response really worked. She opened up. I want to be that effective more often."

Tapes demonstrate how you can improve your communication. And, as you gain experience, the tapes also document your advancing skills. This process is very rewarding.

A video recording takes the teaching-learning tool one step further because you can study both verbal and nonverbal communication at the same time. Initial anxiety is common among students who feel self-conscious and fear "making a fool" of themselves on camera, but the video can detect richer detail in nonverbal behavior.

"I must have crossed and uncrossed my legs 20 times! I never realized I did that. My fidgeting sure made Mr. J. look distracted."

"It was good that I leaned toward her when she paused that time. I think it helped her continue."

"I talked for five minutes nonstop about how to perform a breast self-examination, without ever letting Mrs. S. ask a question!"

If you use any tape recording, some ethical considerations are necessary. Explain to the person the purpose of the recording (whether for teaching, supervision, research), exactly who will hear it (you, your supervisor), and that it will then be destroyed. Obtain consent before you start. Be thoroughly familiar with the equipment; fumbling with the controls is distracting. Arrange the microphone between you and the patient, and place the rest of the recording equipment out of sight. It is likely that after a few moments, neither of you will be aware of the recording.

Electronic Health Recording (EHR). Direct computer recording of the patient health record has moved into many outpatient offices and hospital rooms in the twenty-first century. This eliminates handwritten clinical data as well as provides access to patient education materials and Internet searches. Although computer entry facilitates data retrieval from numerous locations, this new technology poses problems for the provider-patient relationship. In the worst case scenario, the patient sits idly by while the examiner interacts silently with the computer.[29]

If this technology is used in your setting, do not let the computer screen become a barrier between you and the patient. Begin the interview as you usually would by greeting the person, establishing rapport, and collecting the person's narrative story in a direct face-to-face manner. Only after the narrative is fully explored should you type data into the computer. Ask the person if you may now type some notes into the computer, and position the monitor so the patient can see it. Typing directly into the computer may ease entry of some sections of history such as past health occurrences, family history, and review of systems (see Chapter 4). However, be aware that the patient narrative, emotional issues, and complex health problems can only be addressed by the reciprocal communication techniques and patient-centered interviewing presented in this chapter.

TECHNIQUES OF COMMUNICATION

Introducing the Interview

The patient is here, and you are ready for the interview. If you are nervous about how to begin, remember to keep the beginning short. Probably the patient is nervous, too, and is anxious to start. Address the person using his or her surname, and shake hands if that seems comfortable. Except for a child or adolescent, avoid using the first name in this interview; automatic use of the first name is too familiar for most adults and lessens their dignity.

Introduce yourself, and state your role in the agency (if you are a student, say so). If you are gathering a complete history, give the reason for this interview:

"Mrs. Sanchez, I would like to talk about your illness that caused you to come to the hospital."

"Ms. Taft, I want to ask you some questions about your health so that we can identify what is keeping you healthy and explore any problems."

"Mr. Craig, I want to ask you some questions about your health and your usual daily activities so that we can plan your care here in the hospital."

If the person is in the hospital, more than one health team member may be collecting a history. Patients are apt to feel exasperated because they believe they are repeating the same thing unless you give a reason for this interview.

After this brief introduction, ask an open-ended question (see the following section) and then let the person proceed. You do not need much friendly small talk to build rapport. This is not a social visit; the person has some concern to talk about and wants to get on with it. You will build rapport best by letting him or her discuss the concern early.

The Working Phase

The working phase is the data-gathering phase. Verbal skills for this phase include your questions to the patient and your responses to what the patient has said. Two types of questions exist: open-ended and closed. Each type has a different place and function in the interview.

Open-Ended Questions

The **open-ended** question asks for narrative information. It states the topic to be discussed but only in **general** terms. Use it to begin the interview and to introduce a new section of questions; use it also whenever the person introduces a new topic.

"Tell me how I can help you."

"What brings you to the hospital?"

"Tell me why you have come here today."

"How have you been getting along?"

"You mentioned shortness of breath. Tell me more about that."

"How have you been feeling since your last appointment?"

The open-ended question is unbiased; it leaves the person free to answer in any way. This question encourages the person to respond in paragraphs and to give a spontaneous account in any order chosen. It lets the person express himself or herself fully.

As the person answers, stop and *listen.* What usually happens is that the patient answers with a short phrase or sentence, pauses, and then looks at you expecting some direction of how to go on. What you do next is the key to the interview. If you pose new questions on other topics, you may lose much of the initial story. Instead, respond to the first statement with "Tell me about it" or "Anything else?" or merely look acutely interested. Lean forward slightly toward the patient, and make eye contact. The person then will tell the story.

Closed or Direct Questions

Closed or **direct** questions ask for specific information. They elicit a short, one- or two-word answer, a "yes" or "no," or a forced choice. Whereas the open-ended question allows the patient to have free rein, the direct question limits his or her answer (Table 3-1).

Use the direct questions after the person's opening narrative to fill in any details he or she left out. Also use direct questions when you need many specific facts, such as when asking about past health problems or during the review of systems. You need direct questions to speed up the interview. Asking all open-ended questions would be unwieldy and may take hours. But be careful not to overuse closed questions. Follow these guidelines:

1. Ask only one direct question at a time. Avoid bombarding the person with long lists: "Have you ever had pain, double vision, watering, or redness in the eyes?" Avoid double-barreled questions, such as "Do you exercise and follow a diet for your weight?" The person will not know which question to answer. And if the person answers "yes," you will not know which question the person has answered.
2. Choose language the person understands. You may need to use regional phrases or colloquial expressions. For example, "running off" means running away in standard English, but it means diarrhea to Appalachian mountain people.

TABLE 3-1 Comparison of Open-Ended and Closed Questions

Open-Ended	Direct, Closed
Use for narrative information	Use for specific information
Calls for long paragraph answers	Calls for short one- to two-word answers
Elicits feelings, opinions, ideas	Elicits cold facts
Builds and enhances rapport	Limits rapport and leaves interaction neutral
Tell me all about your headaches.	*Are your headaches on one side or both?*

Responses—Assisting the Narrative

You have asked the first open-ended question, and the patient answers. As the person talks, your role is to encourage free expression but not let the person wander off course. Your responses help the teller amplify the story.

Some people seek health care for short-term or relatively simple needs. Their history is direct and uncomplicated; for these people, two responses (facilitation and silence) may be all you need to get a complete picture. Other people have a complex story, a long history of a chronic condition, or accompanying emotions. Additional responses help you gather data without cutting them off.

There are nine types of verbal responses in all. The first five responses (facilitation, silence, reflection, empathy, clarification) involve your *reactions* to the facts or feelings the person has communicated. Your response focuses on the patient's frame of reference. Your own frame of reference does not enter into the response. In the last four responses (confrontation, interpretation, explanation, summary), you start to express your *own* thoughts and feelings. The frame of reference shifts from the patient's perspective to yours. In the first five responses, the patient leads; in the last four responses, you lead.

Facilitation. These responses encourage the patient to say more, to continue with the story ("mm-hmm, go on, continue, uh-huh"). Also called *general leads,* these responses show the person you are interested and will listen further. Simply maintaining eye contact, shifting forward in your seat with increased attention, nodding "Yes," or using your hand to gesture, "Yes, go on, I'm with you," encourage the person to continue talking.

Silence. Silence is golden after open-ended questions. Your silent attentiveness communicates that the patient has time to think, to organize what he or she wishes to say without interruption from you. This "thinking silence" is the one health professionals interrupt most often. The interruption destroys the person's train of thought. The patient is often interrupted because silence is uncomfortable to beginning examiners. They feel responsible for keeping the dialogue going and feel at fault if it stops. But silence has advantages. One advantage is letting the person collect his or her thoughts. Also, silence gives you a chance to observe the person unobtrusively and to note nonverbal cues. Finally, silence gives you time to plan your next approach.

Reflection. This response echoes the patient's words. Reflection is repeating part of what the person has just said. In this example, it focuses further attention on a specific phrase and helps the person continue in his own way:

Patient: I'm here because of my water. It was cutting off.
Response: It was cutting off?
Patient: Yes, yesterday it took me 30 minutes to pass my water. Finally I got a tiny stream, but then it just closed off.

Reflection also can help express feeling behind a person's words. The feeling is already in the statement. You focus on it and encourage the person to elaborate:

Patient: It's so hard having to stay flat on my back in the hospital with this pregnancy. I have two more little ones at home. I'm so worried they are not getting the care they need.

Response: You feel worried and anxious about your children?

Think of yourself as a mirror reflecting the person's words or feelings. This helps the person elaborate on the problem.

Empathy. A physical symptom, condition, or illness often has accompanying emotions. Many people have trouble expressing these feelings, perhaps because of confusion or embarrassment. In the reflecting example above, the person already had stated her feeling and you echoed it. But in the following example, he has not said it yet. An empathic response recognizes a feeling and puts it into words. It names the feeling and allows the expression of it. When the empathic response is used, the patient feels accepted and can deal with the feeling openly.

Patient (sarcastically): This is just great. I have my own business, I direct 20 employees every day, and now here I am having to call on you for every little thing.

Response: It must be hard—one day having so much control, and now feeling dependent on someone else.

Your response does not cut off further communication as would happen by giving false reassurance ("Oh, you'll be back to work in no time"). Also, it does not deny the feeling and indicate that it is not justified ("Now I don't do *everything* for you. Why, you are feeding yourself."). An empathic response recognizes the feeling, accepts it, and allows the person to express it without embarrassment. It strengthens rapport. The patient feels understood, which by itself is therapeutic because it opens the isolation of illness. Other empathic responses are "This must be very hard for you" or "I understand" or just placing your hand on the person's arm (Fig. 3-3).

Clarification. Use this when the person's word choice is ambiguous or confusing (e.g., "Tell me what you mean by 'tired blood.'"). Clarification also is used to summarize the person's words, simplify the words to make them clearer, and then ask if you are on the right track. You are asking for agreement, and the person can then confirm or deny your understanding.

Response: Now as I understand you, this heaviness in your chest comes when you shovel snow or climb stairs, and it goes away when you stop doing those things. Is that correct?

Patient: Yes, that's pretty much it.

Confrontation. Recall that in these last four responses, (confrontation, interpretation, explanation, summary), the frame of reference shifts from the patient's perspective to yours. These responses now include your own thoughts and feelings. Use the last four responses only when merited by the situation. If you use them too often, you take over at the patient's expense. In the case of confrontation, you have observed a certain action, feeling, or statement and you now focus the person's attention on it. You give your honest feedback about what you see or feel. This may focus on a discrepancy: "You say it doesn't hurt, but when I touch you here, you grimace." Or, it may focus on the person's affect: "You look sad" or "You sound angry." Or, you may confront the person when you notice parts of the story are inconsistent: "Earlier you said you were laying off alcohol and just now you said you had a few drinks after work."

Interpretation. This statement is not based on direct observation as with confrontation, but it is based on your inference or conclusion. It links events, makes associations, or implies cause: "It seems that every time you feel the stomach pain, you have had some kind of stress in your life." Interpretation also ascribes feelings and helps the person understand his or her own feelings in relation to the verbal message.

Patient: I have decided I don't want to take any more treatments. But I can't seem to tell my doctor that. Every time she comes in, I tighten up and can't say anything.

Response: Could it be that you're afraid of her reaction?

You do run a risk of making the wrong inference. If this is the case, the person will correct it. But even if the inference is corrected, interpretation helps prompt further discussion of the topic.

Explanation. With these statements, you inform the person. You share factual and objective information. This may be for orientation to the agency setting: "Your dinner comes at 5:30 PM." Or, it may be to explain cause: "The reason you cannot eat or drink before your blood test is that the food will change the test results."

Summary. This is a final review of what you understand the person has said. It condenses the facts and presents a survey of how you perceive the health problem or need. It is a type of validation in that the person can agree with it or correct it. Both you and the patient should participate. When the summary occurs at the end of the interview, it signals that termination of the interview is imminent.

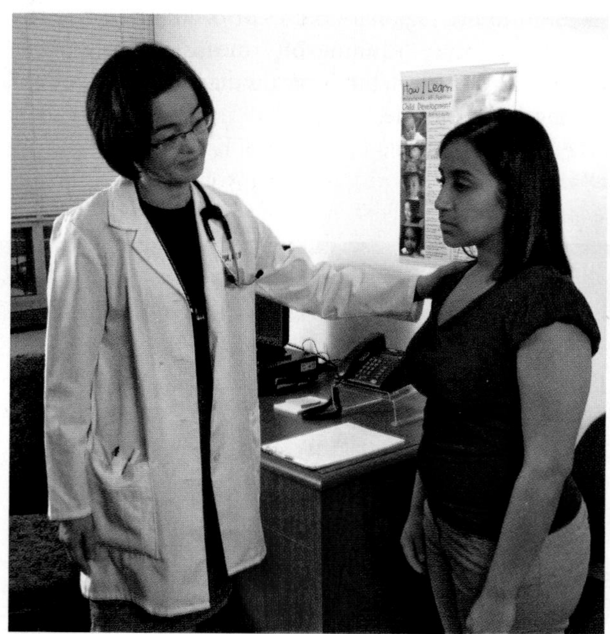

3-3 Showing empathy.

Ten Traps of Interviewing

The verbal skills just discussed are productive and enhance the interview. Now take time to consider nonproductive, defeating verbal messages, or *traps.* It is easy to fall into these traps because you are anxious to help. The danger is that they restrict the patient's response. The following traps are obstacles to obtaining complete data and to establishing rapport.

1. Providing False Assurance or Reassurance. A woman says, "Oh I just know this lump is going to turn out to be cancer." What happens inside you? The automatic response of many clinicians is to say, "Now don't worry; I'm sure you will be all right." This "courage builder" relieves *your* anxiety and gives you the false sense of having provided comfort. But for the woman, it actually closes off communication. It trivializes her anxiety and effectively denies any further talk of it. (Also, it promises something that may not happen—that is, she may *not* be all right.) Consider instead these responses:

"You are really worried about the lump, aren't you?"
"It must be hard to wait for the biopsy results."

These responses acknowledge the feeling and open the door for more communication.

A genuine, valid form of reassurance does exist. You *can* reassure patients that you are listening to them, that you understand them, that you have hope for them, and that you will take good care of them.

Patient: I feel so lost here since they transferred me to the medical center. No one comes to see me. No one here cares what happens to me.
Response: I care what happens to you. I am here today, and I want you to know that I'll be here all week.

This type of reassurance makes a commitment to the patient, and it can have a powerful impact.

2. Giving Unwanted Advice. Know when to give advice and when to avoid giving it. Often, people seek health care because they do want your professional advice and information on the management of a health problem: "My child has chickenpox; how should I take care of him?" This is a straightforward request for information that you have that the parent needs. You respond by giving a health prescription, a therapeutic plan based on your knowledge and experience.

In other situations, advice is different; it is based on a hunch or feeling. It is your personal opinion. Consider the woman who has just left a meeting with her consultant physician: "Dr. Kline just told me my only chance of getting pregnant is to have an operation. I just don't know. What would you do?" Does the woman really want your advice? If you answer, "If I were you, I'd … ," then you would be making a mistake. You are not her. If you give your answer, you have shifted the accountability for decision making from her to you. She has not worked out her own solution. She has learned nothing about herself.

Does the woman really want to know what you would do? Probably not. Instead, a better response is reflection:

Response: Have an operation?
Woman: Yes, and I'm terrified of being put to sleep. What if I don't wake up?

Now you know her *real* concern and can help her deal with it. She will have grown in the process and may be better equipped to make her next decision.

When asked for advice, other preferred responses are:

"What are the pros and cons of ________ [this choice] for you?"
"What concerns do you have?"
"What is holding you back?"

Although it is quicker just to give advice, take the time to involve the patient in a problem-solving process. When a patient participates, he or she is more likely to learn and to change behavior.

3. Using Authority. "Your doctor/nurse knows best" is a response that promotes dependency and inferiority. The communication pathway looks something like this:

Interviewer: ↘
Patient: ↗

with your talk coming "down" and little from the patient going back "up." A better approach is to avoid using authority. Although you and the patient cannot have equality of professional skill and experience, you do have equally worthy roles in the health process, with each respecting the other.

4. Using Avoidance Language. People use euphemisms such as "passed on" to avoid reality or to hide their feelings. They think if they just say the word "death," it might really happen. So to protect themselves, they evade the issue. Although it seems this will make comfortable potentially fearful topics, it does not. Not talking about the fear does not make it go away; it just suppresses the fear and makes it even more frightening. Using direct language is the best way to deal with frightening topics.

5. Engaging in Distancing. Distancing is the use of impersonal speech to put space between a threat and the self: "My friend has a problem; she is afraid she.…" or "There is a lump in the left breast." By using "the" instead of "my," the woman can deny any association with her diseased breast and protect herself from it. Health professionals use distancing, too, to soften reality. This does not work because it communicates to the other person that you also are afraid of the procedure. The use of blunt specific terms actually is preferable to defuse anxiety.

6. Using Professional Jargon. What is called a *myocardial infarction* in the health profession is called a *heart attack* by most laypeople. Use of jargon sounds exclusionary and paternalistic. You need to adjust your vocabulary to the person, but avoid sounding condescending.

If a patient uses medical jargon, do not assume he or she always knows the correct meaning. For example, some people think "hypertensive" means that they are very tense. As a result, they take their medication only when feeling stressed and not when they feel relaxed. This misinformation must be corrected. They need to understand that hypertension is a chronic condition that needs consistent medication to avoid side effects. On the other hand, you do not need to feel that it is a moral imperative to correct all misstatements (e.g., when a patient says "prostrate" for prostate gland).

7. Using Leading or Biased Questions. Asking a man, "You don't smoke, do you?" implies that one answer is "better" than another. If the person wants to please you, either he is forced to answer in a way corresponding to your values or he feels guilty when he must admit the other answer. He risks your disapproval. And if he feels dependent on you for care, the last thing he wants to do is alienate you.

8. Talking Too Much. Some examiners positively associate helpfulness with verbal productivity. If the air has been thick with their oratory and advice, these examiners leave thinking they have met the patient's needs. Just the opposite is true. Anxious to please the examiner, the patient lets the professional talk at the expense of his or her need to express himself or herself. A good rule for every interviewer is to *listen more than you talk.*

9. Interrupting. Often, when you think you know what the person will say, you interrupt and cut the person off. This does not show that you are clever. Rather, it signals that you are impatient or bored with the interview.

A related trap is preoccupation with yourself by thinking of your next remark while the person is talking. The communication pathway looks like this:

Patient: ⟶ Interviewer: ⟶

As the patient speaks, you are thinking about what to say next. Thus you cannot fully understand what the person says. You are so preoccupied with your own role as the interviewer that you are not really listening. Aim for a second of silence between the person's statement and your next response. Ideally, your communication pathway should look like this:

⟷ ⟷

with two people talking, and two people listening.

10. Using "Why" Questions. A young child asks, "Why does the moon look like the end of my fingernail?" The motive behind this question is an innocent search for information. This is quite different from that of an adult's "why" question, such as "*Why* were you so late for your appointment?" The adult's use of "why" questions usually implies blame and condemnation; it puts the person on the defensive.

Consider your use of "why" questions in the health care setting. "Why did you take so much medication?" Or, let's say you ask a man who has just come to the emergency department, "Why did you wait so long before coming to the hospital?" The only possible answer to a "why" question is "because ..." and the man may not know the answer. He may not have worked it out. You sound whining, accusatory, and judgmental. And the man now must produce an excuse to rationalize his own behavior. To avoid this trap, say, "I see you started to have chest pains early in the day. What was happening between the time the pains started and the time you came to the emergency department?"

Nonverbal Skills

Learn to listen with your eyes as well as with your ears. Nonverbal modes of communication include physical appearance, posture, gestures, facial expression, eye contact, voice, and touch. Nonverbal messages are very important in establishing rapport and in conveying information, especially about feelings. Nonverbal messages provide clues to understanding feelings. When nonverbal and verbal messages are congruent, the verbal is reinforced. When they are incongruent, the nonverbal message tends to be the true one, because it is under less conscious control.

Physical Appearance. In his classic work *The Stress of Life,* Hans Selye[23] reports his interest in the body's total response to stress began as a student. Unbiased as yet by medical knowledge, he noted that some patients just "looked sick," even though they did not exhibit the specific characteristic signs that would lead to a precise medical diagnosis. Such people simply felt and looked ill or feverish. The same view can work for you. Inattention to dressing or grooming suggests the person is too sick to maintain self-care or has an emotional dysfunction such as depression. Choice of clothing also sends a message, projecting such varied images as role (student, worker, or professional) or attitude (casual, suggestive, or rebellious).

Your own appearance sends a message to the patient. Professional dress varies among agencies and settings. Depending on the setting, the use of a professional uniform may create a positive stereotype (comfort, expertise, or ease of identification) or a negative stereotype (distance, authority, or formality). Whatever your personal choice in clothing or grooming, the aim should be to convey a competent, professional image.

Posture. Note the patient's position. An open position with extension of large muscle groups shows relaxation, physical comfort, and a willingness to share information. A closed position with arms and legs crossed looks defensive and anxious. Note any change in posture. If a person in a relaxed position suddenly tenses, it suggests discomfort with the new topic.

Your own calm, relaxed posture creates a feeling of warmth and trust and conveys an interest in the person. Standing and hastily filling out a history form with periodic peeks at your watch communicates that you are busy with many more important things than interviewing this person. Even when your time is limited, appear calm and unhurried. Sit down, even if it is only for a few minutes, and look as if nothing else mattered except this person.

Gestures. Gestures send messages. For example, nodding or an open turning out of the hand shows acceptance, attention, or agreement. A wringing of the hands often indicates anxiety. Pointing a finger occurs with anger and vehemence. Also, hand gestures can reinforce a person's description of pain. When a crushing substernal chest pain is described, the person often holds the hand twisted into a fist in front of the sternum. Or, pain that is bright and sharply localized may be shown by pointing one finger to the exact spot: "It hurts right here."

Facial Expression. The face reflects a wide variety of relevant emotions and conditions. The expression may look alert, relaxed, and interested, or it may look anxious, angry, and suspicious. Physical conditions such as pain or shortness of breath also show in the expression.

Your own expression should reflect a professional who is attentive, sincere, and interested in the patient. Any expression of boredom, distraction, disgust, criticism, or disbelief is picked up by the other person, and rapport will dissolve.

Eye Contact. Lack of eye contact suggests that the person is shy, withdrawn, confused, bored, intimidated, apathetic, or depressed. This applies to examiners, too. You should aim to maintain eye contact, but do not "stare down" the person. Do not have a fixed, penetrating look but, rather, an easy gaze toward the person's eyes, with occasional glances away. One exception to this is when you are interviewing someone from a culture that avoids direct eye contact (see the section on Culture and Genetics).

Voice. Besides the spoken words, meaning comes through the tone of voice, the intensity and rate of speech, the pitch, and any pauses. These are just as important as words in conveying meaning. For example, the tone of a person's voice may show sarcasm, disbelief, sympathy, or hostility. An anxious person often speaks in a loud, fast voice. A whining voice is similar; it has a high-pitched, wavering quality and long, drawn-out syllables. A soft voice may indicate shyness or fear. A hearing-impaired person may use a loud voice.

Even the use of pauses conveys meaning. When your question is easy and straightforward, a patient's long, unexpected pause indicates the person is taking time to think of an answer. This raises some doubt as to the honesty of the answer. Unusually frequent and long pauses, when combined with speech that is slow and monotonous and a weak, breathy voice, indicate depression.

Touch. The meaning of physical touch is influenced by the person's age, gender, cultural background, past experience, and current setting. The meaning of touch is easily misinterpreted. In most Western cultures, physical touch is reserved for expressions of love and affection or for rigidly defined acts of greeting (see the section on Culture and Genetics). Do not use touch during the interview unless you know the person well and are sure how it will be interpreted. When appropriate, touch communicates effectively, such as a touch of the hand or arm to signal empathy.

In sum, an examiner's nonverbal messages that are productive and enhancing to the relationship are those that show attentiveness and unconditional acceptance. Defeating, nonproductive nonverbal behaviors are those of inattentiveness, authority, and superiority (Table 3-2).

TABLE 3-2 Nonverbal Behaviors of the Interviewer

Positive	Negative
Appropriate professional appearance	Appearance objectionable to patient
Equal-status seating	Standing
Close proximity to patient	Sitting behind desk, far away, turned away
Relaxed, open posture	Tense posture
Leaning slightly toward person	Slouched back
Occasional facilitating gestures	Critical or distracting gestures: pointing finger, clenched fist, finger-tapping, foot-swinging, looking at watch
Facial animation, interest	Bland expression, yawning, tight mouth
Appropriate smiling	Frowning, lip biting
Appropriate eye contact	Shifty, avoiding eye contact, focusing on notes
Moderate tone of voice	Strident, high-pitched tone
Moderate rate of speech	Rate too slow or too fast
Appropriate touch	Too frequent or inappropriate touch

Closing the Interview

The session should end gracefully. An abrupt or awkward closing can destroy rapport and leave the person with a negative impression of the whole interview. To ease into the closing, ask the person:

"Is there anything else you would like to mention?"
"Are there any questions you would like to ask?"
"Are there any other areas I should have asked about?"
"We have covered a number of concerns today. What would you most like to accomplish?"

This gives the person the final opportunity for self-expression. Then, to indicate that closing is imminent, say something like "Our interview is just about over." No new topic should be introduced now. This is a good time to give your **summary** or a recapitulation of what you have learned during the interview. The summary is a final statement of what you and the patient agree the health state to be. It should include positive health aspects, any health problems that have been identified, any plans for action, and an explanation of the following physical examination. As you part from patients, thank them for the time spent and for their cooperation.

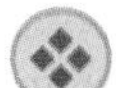

DEVELOPMENTAL COMPETENCE

Interviewing the Parent

When your patient is a child, you must build rapport with two people—the child and the accompanying parent. Greet both by name, but with a younger child (1 to 6 years old), focus more on the parent. By ignoring the child temporarily, you allow the child to size you up from a safe distance. The child can observe your interaction with the parent, see that the parent accepts and likes you, and relax (Fig. 3-4).

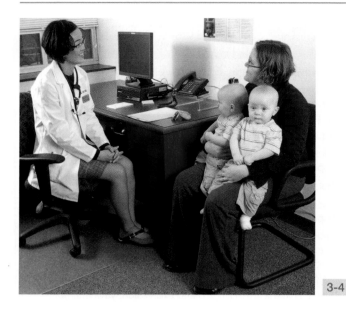
3-4

Begin by interviewing the parent and child together. If any sensitive topics arise (e.g., the parents' troubled relationship or the child's problems at school or with peers), explore them later when the parent is alone. Provide toys to occupy the child as you and the parent talk. This frees the parent to concentrate on the history. Also, it indicates the child's level of attention span or independent play. Through the interview, be alert to ways the parent and child interact.

For younger children, the parent will provide all or most of the history. Thus you are collecting the child's health data from the parent's frame of reference. Usually, this viewpoint is reliable because most parents have the child's well-being as a priority and see cooperation with you as a way to enhance this well-being. But the possibilities exist for parental bias. Bias can occur when parents are asked to describe the child's achievements or when their own parenting ability seems called into question. For example, if you say "His fever was 103 and you did not bring him in?" you are implying a lack of parenting skill. This puts the parent on the defensive and increases anxiety. Instead, use open-ended questions that increase description and defuse threat, such as "What happened when the fever went up?"

A parent with more than one child has more than one set of data to remember. Be patient as the parent sorts through his or her memory to pull out facts of developmental milestones or past history. A comprehensive history may be lacking if the child is accompanied by a family friend or daycare provider instead of the parent.

In collecting developmental data, avoid being judgmental about the age of achievement of certain milestones. Parents are understandably proud of their child's achievements and are sensitive to inferences that these milestones may occur late.

Refer to the child by name—not as "the baby." Refer to the parent by name—not the demeaning "Mother" or "Dad." Also, be clear when identifying the parents. The mother's present husband may not necessarily be the child's father. Instead of asking about "your husband's" health, ask "Is Joan's father in good health?"

Although most of your communication is with the parent, do not ignore the child completely. You need to make contact to ease into the physical examination later. Begin by asking about the toys the child is playing with or about a special doll or teddy bear brought from home: "Does your doll have a name?" or "What can your truck do?" Stoop down to meet the child at his or her eye level. Adult size can be overwhelming to young children and can emphasize their smallness.

Nonverbal communication is even more important to children than it is to adults. Children are quick to pick up feelings, anxiety, or comfort from nonverbal cues. Keep your physical appearance neat and clean, and avoid formal uniforms that distance you. Keep your gestures slow, deliberate, and close to your body. Children are frightened by quick or grandiose gestures. Do not try to maintain constant eye contact; this feels threatening to a small child. Use a quiet, measured voice, and choose simple words in your speech. Considering the child's level of language development is valuable in planning your communication.

The Infant

Nonverbal communication is the primary method of communicating with infants. Most infants look calm and relaxed when all their needs are met, and they cry when they are frightened, hungry, tired, or uncomfortable. They respond best to firm, gentle handling and a quiet, calm voice. Your voice is comforting, even though they do not understand the words. Older infants have anxiety toward strangers. They are more cooperative when the parent is kept in view.

The Preschooler

A 2- to 6-year-old is egocentric. He or she sees the world mostly from his or her own point of view. Everything revolves around him or her. It may not work to cite the example of another child's behavior to get the child to cooperate. It has no meaning. Only the child's own experience is relevant.

Language progresses from a vocabulary of about two words at 1 year to a spurt of about 200 words by 2 years. Then the 2-year-old combines words into simple two-word phrases—"all gone," "me up," "baby crying." This is **telegraphic speech,** which is usually a combination of a noun and a verb and includes only words that have concrete meaning. Interest in language is high during the second year, and a 2-year-old seems to understand all that is said to him or her. A 3-year-old uses more complex sentences with more parts of speech. Between 3 and 4 years of age, the child uses three- to four-word **telegraphic** sentences containing only essential words. By 5 to 6 years, the sentences are six to eight words long and grammar is well developed.

Preschoolers' communication is direct, concrete, literal, and set in the present. Avoid expressions such as "climbing the walls," because they are easily misinterpreted by young children. Use short, simple sentences with a concrete explanation. Take time to give a short, simple explanation for any unfamiliar equipment that will be used on the child. Preschoolers can have *animistic* thinking about unfamiliar objects. They may imagine that unfamiliar inanimate objects can come alive and have human characteristics (e.g., that a blood pressure cuff can wake up and bite or pinch).

The School-Age Child

A child 7 to 12 years old can tolerate and understand others' viewpoints. This child is more objective and realistic. He or she wants to know functional aspects—how things work and why things are done.

The school-age child can read. By using printed symbols (words) for objects and events, the child can process a significant amount of information. At this age, thinking is more stable and logical. The school-age child can **decenter** and consider all sides of a situation to form a conclusion. The school-age child is able to reason, but this reasoning capacity still is limited because he or she cannot yet deal with abstract ideas.

Children of this age-group have the verbal ability to add important data to the history. Interview the parent and child together, but when a presenting symptom or sign exists, ask the child about it first and then gather data from the parent. For the well child seeking a checkup, pose questions about school, friends, or activities directly to the child.

The Adolescent

Adolescence begins with puberty. Puberty is a time of dramatic physiologic change. It includes the growth spurt—rapid growth in height, weight, and muscular development; development of primary and secondary sex characteristics; and maturation of the reproductive organs. A changing body affects a person's self-concept.

Adolescents want to be adults, but they do not have the cognitive ability yet to achieve their goal. They are between two stages. Sometimes they are capable of mature actions, and other times they fall back on childhood response patterns, especially in times of stress. You cannot treat adolescents as children, yet you cannot overcompensate and assume that their communication style, learning ability, and motivation are consistently at an adult level.

Adolescents value their peers. They crave acceptance and sameness with their peers. Adolescents think no adult can understand them. Because of this, some act with aloof contempt, answering only in monosyllables. Others make eye contact and tell you what they think you want to hear, but inside they are thinking "You'll never know the full story about me."

This knowledge about adolescents is apt to paralyze you in communicating with them. However, successful communication is possible and rewarding. The guidelines are simple.

The first consideration is your attitude, which must be one of respect. Respect is the most important thing you can communicate to the adolescent. The adolescent needs to feel validated as a human being, accepted, and worthy.

Second, your communication must be totally honest. The adolescent's intuition is highly tuned and can detect phoniness or when information is withheld. Always give them the truth. Play it straight or you will lose them. They will cooperate if they understand your rationale.

Stay in character. Avoid using language that is absurd for your age or professional role. It is helpful to understand some of the jargon used by adolescents, but you cannot use those words yourself simply to try to bond with the adolescent. Do not try to be his or her peer. You are not, and the adolescent will not accept you as such.

Use icebreakers. Focus first on the adolescent, not on the problem. Although an adult just wants to get on with it and talk about the health concern immediately, the adolescent responds best when the focus is on him or her as a person. Show an interest in the adolescent. Ask open, friendly questions about school, activities, hobbies, friends. "*How are things at school?*" "*Are you in any sports? Any activities?*" "*Do you have any pets at home?*" Refrain from asking questions about parents and family for now—these topics can be emotionally charged during adolescence.

Do not assume adolescents know *anything* about a health interview or a physical examination. Explain every step, and give the rationale. They need direction. They will cooperate when they know the reason for the questions or actions. Encourage their questions. Adolescents are afraid they will sound "dumb" if they ask a question to which they assume everybody else knows the answer.

Keep your questions short and simple. "Why are you here?" sounds brazen to you, but it is effective with the adolescent. Be prepared for the adolescent who does *not* know why he or she is there. Some adolescents are pushed into coming to the examination by a parent.

The communication responses described for the adult need to be reconsidered when talking with the adolescent. Silent periods usually are best avoided. Giving adolescents a little time to collect their thoughts is acceptable, but a silence for other reasons is threatening. Also, avoid reflection. If you use reflection, the adolescent is likely to answer, "What?" They just do not have the cognitive skills to respond to that indirect mode of questioning. Also, adolescents are more sensitive to nonverbal communication than are adults. Be aware of your expressions and gestures. They are also more sensitive to any comment they take to mean criticism from you and will withdraw.

Later in the interview, after you have developed rapport with the adolescent, you can address the topics that are emotionally charged, including smoking, alcohol and drug use, sexual behaviors, suicidal thoughts, and depression. Adolescents undertake risky behaviors that may yield serious consequences. Many of these behaviors are carried forward to adulthood.

Adolescents will assume that health professionals have similar values and standards of behavior as most of the other authority figures in their lives, and they may be reluctant to share this information. You can assure them that your questions are not intended to be curious or intrusive, but cover topics that are important for most teens and on which you have relevant health information to share.

If confidential material is uncovered during the interview, consider what can remain confidential and what you feel you must share for the well-being of the adolescent. State laws vary about confidentiality with minors, and in some states, parents are not notified about, for example, birth control prescriptions or treatment for sexually transmitted infections (STIs). However, if the adolescent talks about an abusive home situation or risk of imminent physical harm, state that you must share this information with other health professionals for his or her own protection. Ask the adolescent, "*Do you have a problem with that?*" and then talk it through. Tell the adolescent, "*You will have to trust that I will handle this information professionally and in your best interest.*"

Finally, take every opportunity for positive reinforcement. Praise every action regarding healthy lifestyle choices: "*That's great that you don't smoke. You get lots of gold stars in my book for staying off the cigarettes. It will save you lots of money that you can use on other things, makes you smell good, and your skin won't be so wrinkled when you get older.*"

For those lifestyle choices that are risky, this is a premium opportunity for discussion and early intervention. "*Have you ever tried to quit smoking?*" "*I am concerned about your extra weight for someone so young. What kind of exercise you do like?*" "*What do you like to drink when you are at a party with your friends?*" "*Did you use a condom the last time you had sex?*" Providing information alone is not enough. Listen to their stories in an open, nonjudgmental way. Give them a small, achievable goal, and encourage another visit in a few weeks for follow-up on the behaviors of concern.

The Older Adult

The aging adult has the developmental task of finding the meaning of life and the purpose of his or her own existence, and adjusting to the inevitability of death. Some people have developed comfortable and satisfying answers and greet you with a calm demeanor and self-assurance. Be alert for the occasional person who sounds hopeless and despairing about life at present and in the future. Symptoms of illness and worries over finances are even more frightening when they mean physical limitation or threaten independence.

Always address the person by the last name (e.g., "Hello, Mr. Choi;" "Good morning, Mrs. Smith"). Some older adults resent being called by their first name by younger persons and almost all cringe at the ignominious "Grandma" or "Pop." Above all, avoid "elderspeak,"[30] which consists of (1) diminutives (honey, sweetie, dearie); (2) inappropriate plural pronouns ("*Are we ready for our interview?*"); (3) tag questions ("*You would rather sit in this nice soft chair, wouldn't you?*"); and (4) shortened sentences, slow speech rate, and simple vocabulary that sounds like baby talk.

The interview usually takes longer with older adults because they have a longer story to tell. You may need to break up the interview into more than one visit, collecting the most important historical data first. Or certain portions of the data, such as past history or the review of systems, can be provided on a form that is filled out at home, as long as the person's vision and handwriting are adequate. Take time to review these parts with the person during the interview.

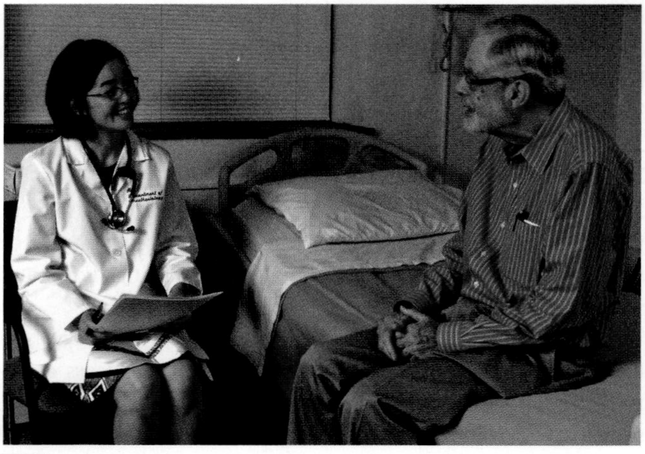

3-5

It is important to adjust the pace of the interview to the aging person (Fig. 3-5). The older person has a great amount of background material to sort through, and this takes some time. Also, some aging persons need a greater amount of response time to interpret the question and process their answer. Avoid trying to hurry them along. This approach only affirms their stereotype of younger persons in general and health care providers in particular—that is, people who are interested merely in numbers of patients and filling out forms. Any urge from you to get on with it will surely make them retreat. You will lose valuable data, and their needs will not be met.

Consider physical limitations when planning the interview. An aging person may fatigue earlier and may require that the interview be broken up into shorter segments. For the person with impaired hearing, face directly so that your mouth and face are fully visible. Do not shout; it does not help and actually distorts speech.

Touch is a nonverbal skill that is very important to older persons. Their other senses may be diminished, and touch grounds you in reality. Also, a hand on the arm or shoulder is an empathic message that communicates you empathize with the person and want to understand his or her problem (see the Culture and Genetics section for exceptions).

INTERVIEWING PEOPLE WITH SPECIAL NEEDS

Hearing-Impaired People

As the population ages, you will encounter more people who are deaf or hard of hearing. They see themselves as a linguistic minority, not as disabled.[8] Many feel marginalized by professionals and that their intelligence is questioned. How should you provide high-quality care to these individuals? Although many will tell you in advance that they have a hearing deficit, others must be recognized by clues, such as staring at your mouth and face, not attending unless looking at you, or speaking in a voice unusually loud or with guttural or garbled sounds. The deaf person may be familiar with some equipment in the hospital or office setting or may have had previous experience with health care settings. But without full communication, the hearing-impaired person is sure to feel isolated and anxious. Ask his or her preferred way to communicate—by signing, lip reading, or writing, "*How can I best communicate with you*?"

A complete health history requires a sign language interpreter. Because most health care professionals are not proficient in signing, try to find an interpreter through a social service agency or the person's own social network. You may use family members, but be aware that they sometimes edit for the person. Use the same guidelines as for the bilingual interpreter (see p. 46).

If the person prefers lip reading, be sure to face him or her squarely and have good lighting on your face. Examiners with a beard, mustache, or foreign accents are less effective. Do not exaggerate your lip movements because this distorts your words. Similarly, shouting distorts the reception of a hearing aid the person may wear. Speak slowly, and supplement your voice with appropriate hand gestures or pantomime. Nonverbal cues are important adjuncts because the lip reader understands at best only 50% of your speech when relying solely on vision. Be sure the person understands your questions. Many hearing-impaired people nod "yes" just to be friendly and cooperative but really do not understand.

Written communication is efficient in sections such as past health history or review of systems. For the present history of illness, writing is very time consuming and laborious. The syntax of the person's written words will read like English if the hearing impairment occurred after speech patterns developed. If the deafness occurred before speech patterns developed, the grammar and written syntax follow that of sign language, which is different from that of English.

Acutely Ill People

An emergency demands your prompt action. You must combine interviewing with physical examination skills to determine lifesaving actions. Although life-support measures may be paramount, still try to interview the person as much as possible. Subjective data are crucial to determine the cause and course of the emergency. Abbreviate your questioning. Identify the main area of distress, and inquire about that. Family or friends often can provide important data.

A hospitalized person with a critical or severe illness is usually too weak, too short of breath, or in too much pain to talk. First attend to the comfort of the person. Then establish a priority; find out immediately what parts of the history are the most relevant. Explore the first concern the person mentions. Begin to use closed, direct questions earlier. Finally, watch that your statements are very clear. When a person is very sick, even the simplest sentence can be misconstrued. The person will react according to preconceived ideas about what a serious illness means, so anything you say should be direct and precise.

People Under the Influence of Street Drugs or Alcohol

It is common for persons under the influence of alcohol or other mood-altering drugs to be admitted to a hospital; all of these drugs affect the central nervous system, increasing the risk for overdose, accidents, and injuries. Also, chronic use creates complex medical problems that require increasing care.

Many substance abusers are poly-drug abusers. You may be faced with a wide range of patient behaviors due to current influence. Alcohol, benzodiazepines, and the opioids (heroin, meperidine, morphine, oxycodone, Vicodin) are central nervous system depressants. Stimulants of the central nervous system (cocaine, amphetamine) can cause an intense high, agitation, and paranoid behavior. Hallucinogens cause bizarre, inappropriate, sometimes even violent behavior accompanied by superhuman strength and insensitivity to pain.

When interviewing a person currently under the influence of alcohol or illicit drugs, ask simple and direct questions. Take care to make your manner and questions nonthreatening. Avoid confrontation at this point. Furthermore, avoid any display of scolding or disgust, because this person may become belligerent.

The top priority is to find out the time of the person's last drink or drug and how much he or she drank at this episode, as well as the name and amount of other drugs taken. This information will help assess any withdrawal patterns. For your own protection, be aware of hospital security or other personnel who could be called on for assistance.

Once he or she has been detoxified and is sober, the hospitalized substance abuser should be assessed for the extent of the problem and the meaning of the problem for the person and family. Initially you will encounter denial and increased defensiveness; special interview techniques are needed (see Chapter 6).

Personal Questions

Occasionally, people will ask you questions about *your* personal life or opinions, such as "Are you married?" "Do you have children?" or "Do you smoke?" You do not need to answer every question. You may supply brief information when you feel it is appropriate, but be sensitive to the possibility that there may be a motive behind the personal questions such as loneliness or anxiety. Try directing your response back to the person's frame of reference. You might say something like "No, I don't have children; I wonder if your question is related to how I can help you care for little Jamie?"

Sexually Aggressive People

On some occasions, personal questions extend to flirtatious compliments, seductive innuendo, or advances. Some people experience serious or chronic illness as a threat to their self-esteem and sexual adequacy. This creates anxiety that makes them act out in sexually aggressive ways.

Your response must make it clear that you are a health professional who can best care for the person by maintaining a professional relationship. At the same time, you should communicate that you accept the person and you understand the person's need to be self-assertive but that you cannot tolerate sexual advances. This may be difficult, considering that the person's words or gestures may have left you shocked, embarrassed, or angry. Your feelings are normal. You need to set appropriate verbal boundaries by saying, "I am uncomfortable when you talk to me that way; please don't." A further response that would open communication is "I wonder if the way you're feeling now relates to your illness or to being in the hospital?"

Crying

A beginning examiner usually feels horrified when the patient starts crying. But crying actually is a big relief to a person. Health problems come with powerful emotions. Worries about illness, death, or loss take a great amount of energy to keep bottled up inside. When you say something that "makes the person cry," do not think you have hurt the person. You have just hit on a topic that is important. Do not go on to a new topic. Just let the person cry and express his or her feelings fully. You can offer a tissue and wait until the crying subsides to talk. The person will regain control soon.

Sometimes your patient looks as if he or she is on the verge of tears but is trying hard to suppress them. Again, instead of moving on to something new, acknowledge the expression by saying, "You look sad." Do not worry that you will open an uncontrollable floodgate. The person may cry but will be relieved, and you will have gained insight to a serious concern (see the Clinical Illustration below).

CLINICAL ILLUSTRATION

Alice P., a 49-year-old, white, divorced female with chronic alcoholism and skin yellow with jaundice has entered treatment for substance abuse. Today, she needs a pelvic examination and Pap smear.

Alice: I haven't had a pelvic exam in 5 years. I had a hysterectomy 18 years ago. They said I had "preinvasive" cancer cells. (At this, Alice's lips fold in, her eyes squeeze shut, and she puts hand to mouth and breathes in audibly in jerks.)

Response: Alice, you look sad. (Puts hand on upper arm.)

Alice: (Crying freely now.) What if you find more cancer now? They can't operate on me with my liver so big. I'd never survive the anesthesia. And my father died of cancer. He had cirrhosis too, and they opened him up and he was full of cancer. He never woke up from surgery, and he died 2 weeks later.

Response: I understand how worried you are. I think you have done the right thing to come in for treatment. That took courage. As for today, let's take one step at a time. Today we need to do the pelvic exam and Pap smear. There is no reason today to assume you need an operation. I'll do your exam today, and I'll be here all week. We'll work together to help you get through this.

Alice: (Breathing deeply, sitting up straight, arms down and open at sides, making eye contact.) All right. I'm better now. Let's go ahead.

Anger

Occasionally you will try to interview a person who is already angry. Try not to personalize this anger; usually it does not relate to you. The person is showing aggression as a response to his or her own feelings of anxiety or helplessness. Do ask about the anger and hear the person out. Deal with the angry feelings before you ask anything else. An angry person cannot be an effective participant in a health interview.

Maybe because of an unrelated incident, *you* are angry when you come into the interview. When you are angry, say so and tell the patient that you are angry at something or someone else. Otherwise the patient, unusually vulnerable and dependent on you, thinks you are angry at him or her.

Threat of Violence

The health care setting is not immune to violent behavior. An individual may act with such angry gestures that you feel a threat to your personal safety. Other red-flag behaviors of a potentially disruptive person include fist clenching, pacing back and forth, a vacant stare, confusion, statements out of touch with reality, statements that do not make sense, a history of recent drug use (alcohol, hallucinogen, methamphetamine, cocaine), or perhaps even a recent history of intense bereavement (loss of spouse, loss of job). Trust your instincts. If you sense any suspicious or threatening behavior, act immediately to defuse the situation. Leave the examining room door open, and position yourself between the person and the door. Many departments have a prearranged sign or signal so that a co-worker can call 911 and the security department to send help to the setting. Do not raise your own voice or try to argue with the threatening person. Act quite calm, and talk to the person in a soft voice. Act interested in what the person is saying, and behave in an unhurried way. Your most important goal is safety; avoid taking any risks.

Anxiety

Finally, take it for granted that nearly all sick people have some anxiety. This is a normal response to being sick. It makes some people aggressive and others dependent. Remember that the person is not reacting as typically as when he or she is healthy.

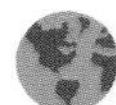

CULTURE AND GENETICS

CROSS-CULTURAL COMMUNICATION

When two people come from different cultural backgrounds, the probability of miscommunication increases. Verbal and nonverbal communications are influenced by the cultural background of both the health care professional and the patient. *Cross-cultural communication* refers to the process occurring between a health care professional and a patient, each with different cultural backgrounds, in which both attempt to understand the other's point of view (Fig. 3-6).

As was discussed in Chapter 2, people who have limited English proficiency (LEP) should have an interpreter who is

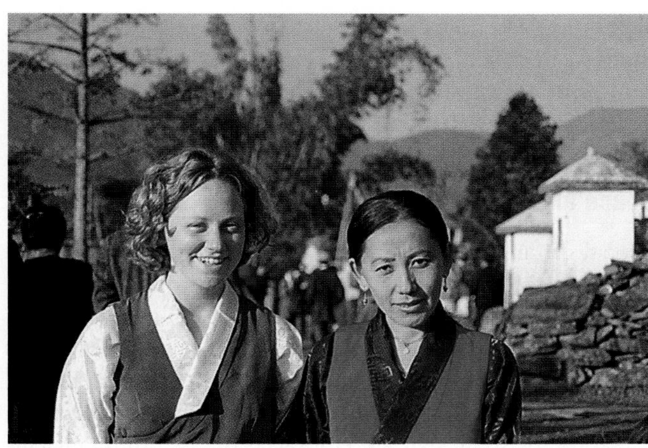

3-6

not a family member or friend. Carefully document that the patient and family fully understand what is happening to them; what their diagnosis and the implications of this diagnosis are; what procedures, diagnostic and therapeutic, are going to be done, how the procedures will be done, and what they mean; how medications are to be taken and when; and the prognosis derived from the given problem(s).

Cultural Perspectives on Professional Interactions

Your professional interaction depends on the patient's cultural perception of health care providers and the degree of formality/informality that is considered appropriate. For example, some Southeast Asians expect those in authority, such as health care providers, to be authoritarian, directive, and detached. In seeking health care, some Asian Americans may expect the health care provider to intuitively know what is wrong with them, and you may actually lose some credibility by asking a fairly standard interview question such as, "What brings you here?" The Asian person may be thinking, "Don't you know why I'm here? You're supposed to be the one with all the answers."

The emphasis on social harmony among Asians and American Indians may prevent the full expression of concerns or feelings during the interview. Such reserved behavior suggests that the person agrees with or understands your explanation. Nodding or smiling by Asians may only reflect their cultural value for interpersonal harmony, not agreement with you. It may also be done to "save face," for when the patient is expected to understand something and does not understand, it is a "loss of face" to admit this. You may distinguish between socially compliant patient responses and genuine concurrence by validating your assumptions. Invite the person to respond frankly to your suggestions, or give the person "permission" to disagree.

In contrast, Appalachians traditionally have close family interaction patterns, which often lead them to expect close personal relationships with health care providers. The Appalachian may evaluate your effectiveness by your interpersonal skills rather than professional competencies. Appalachians may dislike the impersonal, bureaucratic orientation of most health care institutions. People of Latin-American or Mediterranean origin often expect an even higher degree of intimacy and may attempt to involve you in their family system by expecting you to participate in personal activities and social functions. Some individuals might expect personal favors that extend beyond the scope of your professional practice and feel it is their privilege to contact you at home during any time of the day or night for care.

Etiquette

Etiquette refers to the conventional code of good manners that governs behavior and varies cross-culturally. Consider the cultural perceptions of some people from American Indian, Hispanic, Middle Eastern, and African cultures who expect personal or social conversation before they feel comfortable entering into the more intimate aspects of the health history and physical examination. For these people, there is a high value placed on developing interpersonal relationships and getting to know about a person's family, personal concerns, and interests before they allow you to interact therapeutically. Recognizing that time constraints affect the social interchange expected, you should strive to incorporate the person's cultural needs with the health history data categories. For example, using a conversational tone of voice, you might begin the health history by inquiring about the patient's family members and their health.

You should be prepared for the converse; that is, individuals from some cultures may want to interview *you*. They may ask questions about your family, marital status, salary, home address, telephone number, and so forth. Remember that you are not obligated to answer questions that you deem too personal and always have a right to protect your personal safety. For example, you are **never** to provide your home address, e-mail, or telephone number. Rather, you should provide the patient with the hospital, clinic, or agency's business number. If you want the patient to be able to contact you while you are at home, you should ask a secretary or other third party at the health care facility to call your home number. Consider in advance which categories of questions you are willing to discuss and which ones you will politely avoid. If you refuse to answer certain questions about yourself, remember that the person may perceive your behavior as aloof and uncaring. Thus the *manner* in which you reply to personal inquiries should be carefully worded, sensitive to the cultural needs of the patient, and congruent with your own cultural beliefs.

When meeting a patient for the first time, it is best to be formal, respectful, and polite. Unless a physical disability or handicap prevents, you should be standing when you first greet the person and those accompanying him or her. To establish a mutually respectful relationship, introduce yourself and indicate how you prefer to be called—that is, by first name, last name, and/or title. Elicit the same information from the patient because this enables you to address the person in a manner that is culturally appropriate and could actually spare you considerable embarrassment. Everyone likes to be called by his or her correct name.

Among Chinese, Vietnamese, and many other Asian groups, the family or surname is written and spoken first, followed by the first or given name. This is the opposite of most European-American cultures. Because politeness and formality frequently are valued by those from Asian cultures, you should address the person using the correct title followed by the family or surname. Be aware that some Asians, particularly those who are members of Christian religions, also may have English names. Most Asian women do not use their husband's last name after marriage. Be mindful of this when examining children in the presence of both parents. In most Asian cultures, the child is given the father's last name. Depending on the degree of acculturation, some Asian Americans switch the order of their names in order to be consistent with the European-American custom.

In traditional Chinese, Japanese, and other Asian cultures, when people are introduced, they show each other respect by bowing. The more profound the bow is, the deeper the respect. For example, it would be appropriate to bow very low to an older adult whose wisdom is highly regarded and to bow less profoundly to an adolescent or a young adult. With Westernization, handshakes are now customary throughout most parts of Asia and among Asian Americans, but shaking someone's hand too firmly or vigorously is considered rude or intrusive.

Because of the importance of family for people from Central and South America, two surnames are used, representing their father's and mother's last names. The paternal name is first, then the maternal name. For example, if the patient's name is Juan Diaz Hernandez, his father's last name is Diaz and his mother's last name is Hernandez. With immigration to the United States or Canada, some people with Spanish surnames drop their mother's name for the sake of brevity.

Although there are dozens of Arab cultures and subcultures, customs pertaining to names are similar. Both males and females are given a first name as infants. The father's first name is used as the middle name and the last name is the family name. Some may prefer to be addressed as father *(abu)* or mother *(um)* of their oldest son (e.g., abu Walid or father of Walid). Because formality is emphasized in most Arab cultures, you should call patients Mr., Mrs., Ms., Miss, or Dr. followed by their last name unless invited to use more familiar first names or the *abu/um* form of the name. In most Arab cultures, etiquette requires either a gentle kiss on the cheeks or a handshake on arrival and departure for people of the same gender. When an Arab man is introduced to a woman, he will prefer to not be touched by her; that is, no handshaking. This is respectful of the traditional beliefs about modesty in male-female relationships. Women may back off from strange men and not touch at all. When a handshake is not exchanged, the Muslim woman usually faces the man while bowing her head slightly and crossing her arms across her chest.

With more than 510 federal and/or state-recognized American Indian tribes, there is wide variation in the customs pertaining to names, titles, and etiquette. The majority tend to follow the European-American cultural norms. In the Navajo culture, a health care provider may call an older adult "grandfather" or "grandmother" as a sign of respect after getting to know him or her but should be more formal during the initial introduction. Some American Indians and Alaska natives have anglicized traditional names into surnames such as Running Deer, Flying Eagle, or Swift Bear, often reflecting the clan to which the person belongs. You should extend a gentle, nonaggressive handshake when introduced to an American Indian patient.

Space and Distance

Spatial distance is significant throughout the interview and physical examination, with culturally appropriate distance zones varying widely. Some cultural groups value close physical proximity and may perceive a health care provider who is distancing as being aloof and unfriendly. Summarized in Table 3-3 are the four distance zones identified for the functional use of space that are embraced by the dominant cultural group, including that of most health care professionals.

Cultural Considerations on Gender

Violating cultural norms related to appropriate male-female relationships may jeopardize a professional relationship. Among some Arab Americans, an adult male is never alone with a female (except his wife) and is generally accompanied by one or more other males when interacting with females. This behavior is culturally very significant; a lone male could be accused of sexual impropriety. Ask the person about culturally relevant aspects of male-female relationships at the beginning of the interview. When gender differences are important to the patient, try strategies such as offering to have a third person present. If a family member or friend has accompanied the patient, inquire whether the patient would like that person to be in the examination room during the history and/or physical examination. It is not unusual for a female to refuse to be examined by a male and vice-versa. Modesty is another issue. It is imperative to ensure that the patient is carefully draped at all times, that curtains are closed,

TABLE 3-3 Functional Use of Space

Zone	Remarks
Intimate zone (0 to 1½ ft)	Visual distortion occurs Best for assessing breath and other body odors
Personal distance (1½ to 4 ft)	Perceived as an extension of the self similar to a bubble Voice is moderate Body odors inapparent No visual distortion Much of the physical assessment occurs at this distance
Social distance (4 to 12 ft)	Used for impersonal business transactions Perceptual information much less detailed Much of the interview occurs at this distance
Public distance (12+ ft)	Interaction with others impersonal Speaker's voice must be projected Subtle facial expressions imperceptible

From Hall, E. (1963). Proxemics: The study of man's spatial relations. In Galdston, I. (Ed.), *Man's image in medicine and anthropology,* New York: International University Press, pp. 109-120.

and, when possible, doors should also be closed. Do not enter a room without knocking first and announcing yourself.

Cultural Considerations on Sexual Orientation

Lesbian, gay, and bisexual individuals are always aware of heterosexist biases and the communication of these biases during the interview and physical examination. *Heterosexism* refers to the institutionalized belief that heterosexuality is the only natural choice and assumes it is the norm. For example, most health histories include a question concerning marital status. Although many same-sex couples are in committed, long-term, monogamous relationships, seldom is there a category on the standard form that acknowledges this type of relationship. Although technically and legally the person may be single, this trivializes the relationship with his or her significant other. It also may have health-related implications if the person is diagnosed, for example, with a communicable disease, which may range in severity from a minor sore throat to a life-threatening condition such as HIV/AIDS. In extreme cases, lesbians have been subjected to unnecessary diagnostic procedures when the heterosexual assumption was made.

OVERCOMING COMMUNICATION BARRIERS

Health care providers tend to have stereotypical expectations of the patient's behavior during the interview and physical examination: undemanding compliance, an attitude of respect for the health care provider, and cooperation with requested behavior throughout the examination. Although patients may ask a few questions for the purpose of clarification, slight deference to recognized authority figures (i.e., health care providers) is expected. Individuals from culturally diverse backgrounds, however, may have significantly different perceptions about the appropriate role of the individual and his or her family when seeking health care.

During illness, culturally acceptable sick-role behavior may range from aggressive, demanding behavior to silent passivity. Complaining, demanding behavior during illness is often rewarded with attention among American Jewish and Italian groups, whereas Asians and American Indians are likely to be quiet and compliant during illness. During the interview, Asians may provide the answers they think are expected, behavior consistent with the dominant cultural value for harmonious relationships with others. Appalachian people may reject an interviewer whom they perceive as prying or nosey as a result of a cultural ethic of neutrality that mandates minding one's own business and avoiding assertive or argumentative behavior.

Working With (and Without) an Interpreter

Nearly 52 million people in the United States speak a language other than English at home.[26] Many also can read and write other languages. One of the greatest challenges in cross-cultural communication occurs when you and the patient speak different languages (Fig. 3-7). After assessing the language skills of non–English-speaking people, you may find yourself in one of two situations: trying to communicate effectively through an interpreter or trying to communicate effectively when there is no interpreter.

Interviewing the non–English-speaking person requires a bilingual interpreter for full communication. Even the person from another culture or country who has a basic command of English (those for whom English is a second language) may need an interpreter when faced with the anxiety-provoking situation of entering a hospital, describing a strange symptom, or discussing sensitive topics such as those related to reproductive or urologic concerns.

It is tempting to ask an "ad hoc" interpreter—a relative, friend, or even another patient—to interpret because this person is readily available and probably would like to help. This is disadvantageous because it violates confidentiality for the patient, who may not want personal information shared with another. Furthermore, the friend or relative, although fluent in ordinary language usage, is likely to be unfamiliar with medical terminology, hospital or clinic procedures, and medical ethics. Having a relative interpret adds stress to an already stressful situation and may disrupt family relationships. In some cultures, talk about death or cancer is taboo and a family interpreter may edit out this language.[7]

Whenever possible, work with a bilingual team member or a trained medical interpreter. This person knows interpreting techniques, has a health care background, and understands patients' rights. The trained interpreter also is knowledgeable about cultural beliefs and health practices. This "cultural broker" can help you bridge the cultural gap and can advise you concerning the cultural appropriateness of your recommendations.

Many patients with limited English proficiency do not have access to interpreters. It is your responsibility to ensure that the provisions of Title VI as discussed in Chapter 2 are met. It is well known that few clinicians are receiving the necessary preparation to practice with interpreters; only 23% of teaching hospitals in the United States provide this training.[4] As a first preference, language services should include the availability of a bilingual staff that can communicate directly with patients in their preferred language and dialect. Also, become familiar with telephone translation services

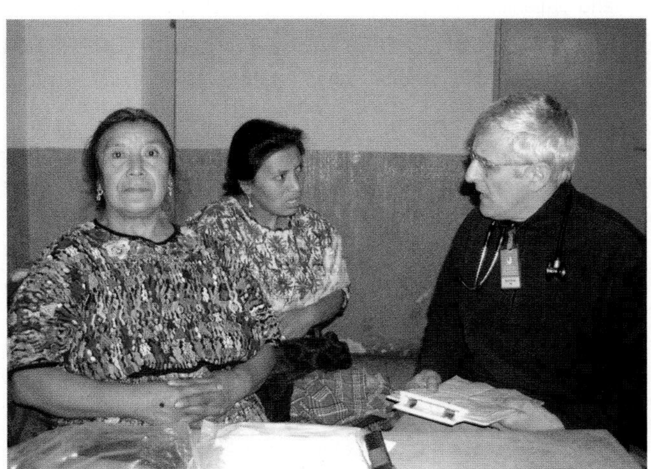

3-7

such as the AT&T Language Line (www.languageline.com) that are available 24 hours a day.

Although interpreters are trained to remain neutral, they can influence both the content of information exchanged and the nature of the interaction. Many trained medical interpreters are members of the linguistic community they serve. Although this is largely beneficial, it has limitations. For example, interpreters often know patients and details of their circumstances before the interview begins. Although acceptance of a code of ethics governing confidentiality and conflicts of interest is part of the training interpreters receive, discord may arise when they relate information that the patient has not volunteered to the examiner.

Note that being bilingual does not always mean the interpreter is culturally aware. The Hispanic culture, for example, is so diverse that a Spanish-speaking interpreter from one country, class, race, and gender does not necessarily understand the cultural background of a Spanish-speaking person from another country and different circumstances. Even trained interpreters, who are often from urban areas and represent a higher socioeconomic class than the patients for whom they interpret, may be unaware of or embarrassed by rural attitudes and practices.

Although you will be in charge of the focus and flow of the interview, view yourself and the interpreters as a team. Ask the interpreter to meet the patient beforehand to establish rapport and to determine the patient's age, occupation, educational level, and attitude toward health care. This enables the interpreter to communicate on the patient's level. Place the interpreter next to the patient, and make eye contact mostly with the patient. Do not address your questions to the interpreter; that is, do not say, "*Ask him if he has pain,*" but, rather, ask the patient directly, "*Do you have pain?*"

Allow more time for this interview. With the third person repeating everything, it can take considerably longer than interviewing English-speaking people. You need to focus on priority data.

There are two styles of interpreting—line-by-line and summarizing. Translating line-by-line takes more time, but it ensures accuracy. Use this style for most of the interview. Both you and the patient should speak only a sentence or two, and then allow the interpreter some time. Use simple language yourself, not medical jargon that the interpreter must simplify before it can be translated. Summary translation progresses faster and is useful for teaching relatively simple health techniques with which the interpreter is already familiar. Be alert

TABLE 3-4 Use of an Interpreter

CHOOSING AN INTERPRETER

- Before locating an interpreter, identify the language the person speaks at home. Be aware that it may differ from the language spoken publicly (e.g., French is sometimes spoken by well-educated and upper-class members of certain Asian, African, or Middle Eastern cultures, but it is not the language spoken in the home).
- Whenever possible, use a *trained* interpreter, preferably one who knows medical terminology.
- Avoid interpreters from a rival tribe, state, region, or nation (e.g., a Palestinian who knows Hebrew may not be the best interpreter for a Jewish person).
- Be aware of gender differences between interpreter and patient. In general, the same gender is preferred.
- Be aware of age differences between interpreter and patient. In general, an older, more mature interpreter is preferred to a younger, less experienced one.
- Be aware of socioeconomic differences between interpreter and patient.

STRATEGIES FOR EFFECTIVE USE OF AN INTERPRETER

- Plan what you want to say ahead of time. Meet privately with the interpreter before the interview. Avoid confusing the interpreter by backing up, hesitating, or inserting a proviso.
- Ask the interpreter to provide a line-by-line verbatim account of the conversation. Ask for a detailed interpretation when provided with brief summaries of longer exchanges between interpreter and patient.
- Be patient. When using an interpreter, interviews often take two to three times longer.
- Longer-than-expected explanatory exchanges are often required to convey the meaning of words such as *stress, depression, allergy, preventive medicine, and physical therapy* because there may not be comparable terms in the language the patient understands.
- When discussing diagnostic tests such as mammograms, magnetic resonance imaging (MRI), computed tomography (CT) scans, or those involving body fluids such as blood, urine, stool, spinal fluid, or saliva, be sure to clarify the nature of the test to the interpreter. Indicate the purpose of the test, exactly what will happen to the patient, approximately how long the test will take, whether the procedure is invasive or noninvasive, and what part(s) of the body will be tested.
- Be aware that the interpreter may modify or edit some aspects of the conversation, especially if he or she thinks you might not understand the cultural context of the patient's response (e.g., traditional or folk beliefs and practices related to healing).
- Avoid ambiguous statements and questions. Refrain from using conditional or indefinite phrasing such as "if," "would," and "could," especially for target languages, such as Khmer (Cambodia), that lack nuances of conditionality or distinctions of time other than simple past and present. Conditional statements may be mistaken for actual agreement or approval of a course of action.
- Avoid abstract expressions, idioms, similes, metaphors, and medical jargon.
- To ensure confidentiality and privacy, avoid using as interpreters children or strangers who may be visiting other patients.
- Be aware that an interpreter who is a nonrelative may seek compensation for services rendered. Be sure to negotiate fees ahead of time.

RECOMMENDATIONS FOR INSTITUTIONS

- Maintain a current, computerized list of interpreters who may be contacted as needed.
- Network with area hospitals, colleges, universities, and other organizations that may serve as resources.
- Utilize over-the-telephone interpretation services provided by telephone companies. For example, since 1989, AT&T has operated the Language Line Services, which provides interpretation in more than 140 languages. Services are available around-the-clock every day of the year. Call (800) 628-8486 or visit www.languageline.com for further information on services and charges.

TABLE 3-5 What to Do When No Language Interpreter is Available

1. Be polite and formal.
2. Pronounce name correctly. Use proper titles of respect, such as "Mr.," "Mrs.," "Ms.," "Dr." Greet the person using the last or complete name.
   Gesture to yourself and say your name.
   Offer a handshake or nod. Smile.
3. Proceed in an unhurried manner. Pay attention to any effort by the patient or family to communicate.
4. Speak in a low, moderate voice. Avoid talking loudly. Remember that there is a tendency to raise the volume and pitch of your voice when the listener appears not to understand. The listener may perceive that you are shouting and/or angry.
5. Use any words you might know in the person's language. This indicates that you are aware of and respect his or her culture.
6. Use simple words, such as "pain" instead of "discomfort." Avoid medical jargon, idioms, and slang. Avoid using contractions (e.g., don't, can't, won't). Use nouns repeatedly instead of pronouns.
   Example:
   Do not say: "He has been taking his medicine, hasn't he?"
   Do say: "Does Juan take medicine?"
7. Pantomime words and simple actions while you verbalize them.
8. Give instructions in the proper sequence.
   Example:
   Do not say: "Before you rinse the bottle, sterilize it."
   Do say: "First wash the bottle. Second, rinse the bottle."
9. Discuss one topic at a time. Avoid using conjunctions.
   Example:
   Do not say: "Are you cold and in pain?"
   Do say: "Are you cold (while pantomiming)? Are you in pain?"
10. Validate if person understands by having him or her repeat instructions, demonstrate the procedure, or act out the meaning.
11. Write out several short sentences in English and determine the person's ability to read them.
12. Try a third language. Many Indochinese speak French. Europeans often know two or more languages. Try Latin words or phrases.
13. Ask who among the person's family and friends could serve as an interpreter.
14. Obtain phrase books from a library or bookstore, make or purchase flash cards, contact hospitals for a list of interpreters, and use both a formal and an informal network to locate a suitable interpreter.

for nonverbal cues as the patient talks. These cues can give valuable data. A good interpreter also notes nonverbal messages and passes them on to you. Summarized in Table 3-4 are suggestions for the selection and use of an interpreter.

Although use of an interpreter is the ideal, you may find yourself in a situation with a non–English-speaking patient when no interpreter is available. Table 3-5 summarizes some suggestions for overcoming language barriers when no interpreter is present. Communicating with these patients may require that you combine verbal and nonverbal communication.

Nonverbal Cross-Cultural Communication

There are five types of nonverbal behaviors that convey information about the person: (1) *vocal cues,* such as pitch, tone, and quality of voice, including moaning, crying, and groaning; (2) *action cues,* such as posture, facial expression, and gestures; (3) *object cues,* such as clothes, jewelry, and hair styles; (4) *use of personal and territorial space* in interpersonal transactions and care of belongings; and (5) *touch,* which involves the use of personal space and action.[12]

Unless you make an effort to understand the patient's nonverbal behavior, you may overlook important information such as facial expressions, silence, eye contact, touch, and other body language. Communication patterns vary widely transculturally, even for such conventional social behaviors as smiling and handshaking. Among many Hispanic people, for example, smiling and handshaking are considered an integral part of sincere interactions and essential to establishing trust, whereas a Russian person might perceive the same behavior as insolent and frivolous.

Wide cultural variation exists when interpreting **silence.** Some individuals find silence extremely uncomfortable and make every effort to fill conversational lags with words. Conversely, many American Indians consider silence essential to understanding and respecting the other person. A pause following your question signifies that what has been asked is important enough to be given thoughtful consideration. In traditional Chinese and Japanese cultures, silence may mean that the speaker wishes the listener to consider the content of what has been said before continuing. The English and Arabs may use silence out of respect for another's privacy, whereas the French, Spanish, and Russians may interpret it as a sign of agreement. Asian cultures often use silence to demonstrate respect for older adults.

Eye contact is perhaps among the most culturally variable nonverbal behaviors. People from European cultures are taught to maintain eye contact when speaking with others. Asian, American Indian, Indochinese, Arab, and Appalachian people may consider direct eye contact impolite or aggressive, and they may avert their eyes when talking with you. American Indians often stare at the floor during conversations, a culturally appropriate behavior indicating that the listener is paying close attention to the speaker. Among Hispanics, respect dictates appropriate deferential behavior in the form of downcast eyes toward others on the basis of age, gender, social position, economic status, and position of authority. Older adults expect respect from younger individuals, adults from children, men from women, teachers from students, and employers from employees.

In some cultures—including Arab, Latino, and Black groups—*modesty for both women and men* is interrelated with eye contact. For Muslim-Arab women, modesty is achieved in part by avoiding eye contact with males (except for one's husband in private settings) and keeping the eyes downcast when encountering members of the opposite gender in public situations. Hasidic Jewish males also have culturally based norms concerning eye contact with females. You may observe the male avoiding direct eye contact and turning his head in the opposite direction when walking past or speaking to a woman.

Touch

Without doubt, touching the patient is a necessary component of a comprehensive assessment. While recognizing the benefits reported by many in establishing rapport with patients through touch, physical contact with patients conveys various meanings cross-culturally. In many cultures, such as Arab and Latino societies, male health care providers may be prohibited from touching or examining either all or certain parts of the female body. In many cultures, adolescent girls may prefer female health care providers or refuse to be examined by a male. The patient's significant others also may exert pressure on nurses by enforcing these culturally meaningful norms in the health care setting.

Touching children also may have associated meaning transculturally. For example, many of the world's people believe in *mal ojo,* which literally translated means "evil of the eye." In this culture-bound syndrome, a child's illness may be attributed to excessive admiration by another person. *Mal ojo* is especially prevalent in Latino cultures. Many Asians believe that one's strength resides in the head and that touching the head is a sign of disrespect. The clinical significance of this is that you need to be aware that patting the child on the head or examining the fontanel of a Southeast Asian infant, for example, should be avoided or done only with parental permission.

BIBLIOGRAPHY

1. Aboul-Enein, F. H., & Ahmed, F. (2006). How language barriers impact patient care: A commentary. *Journal of Cultural Diversity, 13*(3), 169.
2. Arnold, E., & Boggs, K. (2007). *Interpersonal relationships: Professional communication skills for nurses* (5th ed.). Philadelphia: Saunders.
3. Berry, J. A. (2006). Pilot study: Nurse practitioner communication and the use of recommended clinical preventive services. *Journal of the American Academy of Nurse Practitioners, 18,* 277-283.
4. Flores, G. (2006). Language barriers to health care in the United States. *New England Journal of Medicine, 355*(3), 229-231.
5. Gerrish, K., Chau, R., Sobowale, A., et al. (2004). Bridging the language barrier: the use of interpreters in primary care nursing. *Health and Social Care in the Community, 12*(5), 407-413.
6. Goldenring, J. M., & Rosen, D. S. (2004). Getting into adolescent heads: An essential update. *Contemporary Pediatrics, 21*(1), 64-74.
7. Ho, A. (2008). Using family members as interpreters in the clinical setting. *Journal of Clinical Ethics, 19*(3), 223-233.
8. Iezzoni, L. I., O'Day, B. L., Killeen, M., et al. (2004). Communicating about health care: observations from persons who are deaf or hard of hearing. *Annals of Internal Medicine, 140*(5), 356-362.
9. Jacobs, E. A., Sadowski, L. S., & Rathouz, R. J. (2007). The impact of an enhanced interpreter service intervention on hospital costs and patient satisfaction. *Journal of General Internal Medicine, 22*(Suppl 2), 306-311, 2007.
10. Jolly, K., Weiss, J. A., & Liehr, P. (2007). Understanding adolescent voice as a guide for nursing practice and research. *Issues in Comprehensive Pediatric Nursing, 30*(1-2), 3-13.
11. Lange, N., Tigges, B. B. (2005). Influence positive change with motivational interviewing. *Nurse Practitioner, 30*(3), 44-53.
12. Lapierre, E. D., & Padgett, J. (1991). How can we become more aware of culturally specific body language and use this awareness therapeutically? *Journal of Psychosocial Nursing & Mental Health Services, 29*(11), 38-41.
13. Levensky, E. R., Forcehimes, A., O'Donohue, W. T., et al. (2007). Motivational interviewing. *American Journal of Nursing, 107*(10), 50-59.
14. Nordby, H. (2006). Nurse-patient communication: Language mastery and concept possession, *Nursing Inquiry, 13*(1), 64-72.
15. Oliva, N. L. (2008). When language intervenes: Improving care for patients with limited English proficiency. *American Journal of Nursing, 108*(3), 73-75.
16. Pullen, R. L. (2007). Tips for communicating with a patient from another culture. *Nursing, 37*(10), 48-49.
17. Purtilo, R., & Haddad, A. (2007). *Health professional and patient interaction* (7th ed.). Philadelphia: Saunders.
18. Rhodes, K. V., Frankel, R. M., Levinthal, N., et al. (2007). "You're not a victim of domestic violence, are you?": provider-patient communication about domestic violence. *Annals of Internal Medicine, 147*(9), 620-627.
19. Roche, M., Diers, D., Duffield, C., et al. (2010). Violence toward nurses, the work environment and patient outcomes, *Journal of Nursing Scholarship, 42*(1), 13-22.
20. Rosenzweig, M., Hravnak, M., Magdic, K., et al. (2008). Patient communication simulation laboratory for students in an acute care nurse practitioner program. *American Journal of Critical Care, 17*(4), 364-371.
21. Rudy, S. F. (2007). Working effectively with live language interpreters. *ORL Head and Neck Nursing, 25*(4), 17-21.
22. Schwartzberg, J. G., Cowett, A., Van Geest, J., et al. (2007). Communication techniques for patients with low health literacy: A survey of physicians, nurses, and pharmacists. *American Journal of Health Behavior, 31*(Suppl 1), S96-S104.
23. Selye, H. (1956). *The stress of life.* New York: McGraw-Hill.
24. Sheldon, L. K., Barrett, R., & Ellington, L. (2006). Difficult communication in nursing. *Journal of Nursing Scholarship, 38*(2), 141-147.
25. Taylor, J. L. (2010). Workplace violence. *American Journal of Nursing, 110*(3), 11.
26. U.S. Bureau of the Census. *2005 American community survey.* Accessed November 27, 2006, from www.factfinder.census.gov.
27. U.S. Department of Health and Human Services. *The Health Insurance Portability and Accountability Act of 1996 (HIPAA) Privacy Rule.* Website: www.hhs.gov/ocr/privacy/index.html.
28. U.S. Preventive Services Task Force (USPSTF). *Screening for family and intimate partner violence.* Agency for Healthcare Research and Quality. Website: www.ahrq.gov/clinic/3rduspstf/famviolence/famviolrs.htm.
29. Ventres, W., Kooienga, S., Vuckovic, N., et al. (2006). Physicians, patients, and the electronic health record: An ethnographic analysis. *Annals of Family Medicine, 4*(2), 124-131.
30. Williams, K., Kemper, S., & Vockevic, N. (2005). Enhancing communication with older adults: Overcoming elderspeak. *Journal of Psychosocial Nursing, 43*(5), 12-16.
31. Wu, H. W., Nishimi, R. Y., Paige-Lopez, C. M., et al. *Improving patient safety through informed consent for patients with limited health literacy: an implementation report.* Washington, DC: National Quality Forum 2005. Website: www.qualityforum.org/publications/reports/informed_consent.asp.

Websites of Interest

Health History and Assessment Skills

Diversity Rx website: www.diversityrx.org
Deaf Library website: www.deaflibrary.org
HSTAT: National Library of Medicine website: www.ncbi.nlm.nih.gov/books/bv.fcgi?rid=hstat
I Love Languages website: www.ilovelanguages.com/index.php
Interactive Patient website: http://healthweb.org

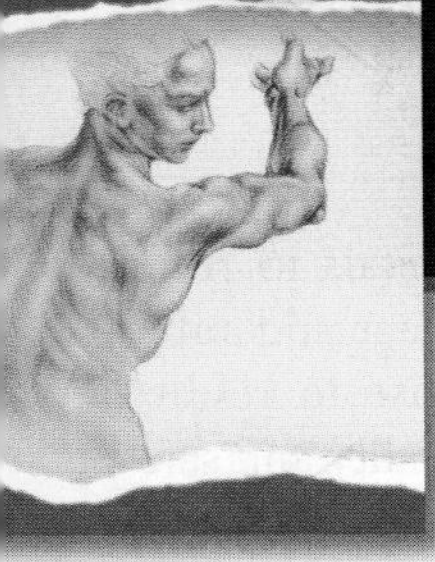

CHAPTER

4

The Complete Health History

evolve WEBSITE

http://evolve.elsevier.com/Jarvis/

- Audio Key Points
- Comprehensive Older Person's Evaluation
- NCLEX Review Questions

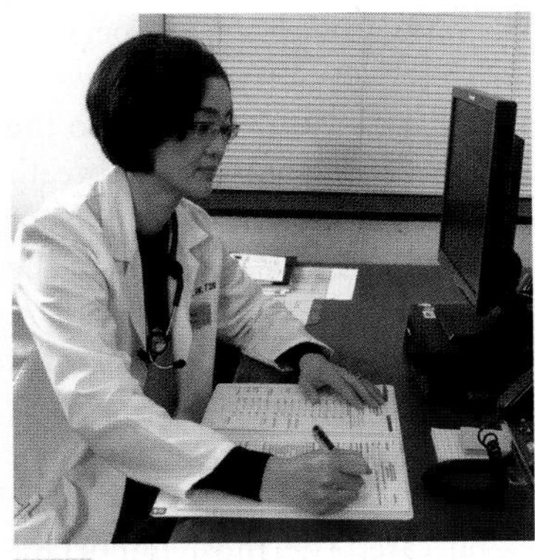

4-1

The purpose of the health history is to collect **subjective data**—what the person says about himself or herself. This is different from **objective data**—what you observe through measurement, inspection, palpation, percussion, and auscultation. The history is combined with the objective data from the physical examination and laboratory studies to form the database. The database is used to make a judgment or a diagnosis about the health status of the individual (Fig. 4-1).

The following health history provides a complete picture of the person's past and present health. It describes the individual as a whole and how the person interacts with the environment. It records health strengths and coping skills. The history should recognize and affirm what the person is *doing right:* what he or she is doing to help stay well. For the well person, the history is used to assess his or her lifestyle, including such factors as exercise, healthy diet, substance use, risk reduction, and health promotion behaviors.

For the ill person, the health history includes a detailed and chronologic record of the health problem. For all, the health history is a screening tool for abnormal symptoms, health problems, and concerns, and it records ways of responding to the health problems.

In many settings, the patient fills out a printed history form or checklist. This allows the person ample time to recall and consider such items as dates of health landmarks and relevant family history. The interview is then used to validate the written data and to collect more data on lifestyle management and current health problems.

Although history forms vary, most contain information in the sequence of categories listed to the left. This health history format presents a generic database for all practitioners. Those in primary care settings may use all of it, whereas those in a hospital may focus primarily on the history of present illness and the functional, or patterns of living, data.

Health History Sequence

1. Biographic data
2. Reason for seeking care
3. Present health or history of present illness
4. Past history
5. Family history
6. Review of systems
7. Functional assessment or activities of daily living (ADLs)

THE HEALTH HISTORY—THE ADULT

Record the date and time of day of the interview.

Biographic Data

Biographic data include name, address and phone number, age and birth date, birthplace, gender, marital status, race, ethnic origin, and occupation (usual and present; an illness or disability may have prompted change in occupation). Note that 2010 standards from The Joint Commission (formerly known as *JCAHO*) require hospitals to record language and communication needs. Therefore the person's primary language and authorized representative, if any, should be recorded here. This is in response to research showing differences in language and culture may have an impact on the quality and safety of care.[12]

Source of History

Sample Statements:
Patient herself, who seems reliable.
Patient's son, John Ramirez, who seems reliable.
Mrs. R. Fuentes, interpreter for Theresa Castillo, who does not speak English.

1. Record who furnishes the information—usually the person himself or herself, although the source may be a relative, friend, or caseworker.
2. Judge how reliable the informant seems and how willing he or she is to communicate. What is reliable? A reliable person always gives the same answers, even when questions are rephrased or are repeated later in the interview.
3. Note any special circumstances, such as the use of an interpreter.

See sample recordings at left.

Reason for Seeking Care*

Sample Statements:
"Chest pain" for 2 hours.
"Sore throat for 3 days now and just getting worse."
"Earache and fussy all night."
"Need yearly physical for work."
"Want to start jogging and need checkup."

This is a brief, spontaneous statement in the person's own words that describes the reason for the visit. Think of it as the "title" for the story to follow. It states one (possibly two) symptoms or signs and their duration. A **symptom** is a subjective sensation that the person feels from the disorder. A **sign** is an objective abnormality that you as the examiner could detect on physical examination or in laboratory reports. Try to record whatever the person says is the reason for seeking care, enclose it in quotation marks to indicate the person's exact words, and record a time frame. See examples at left.

The reason for seeking care is not a diagnostic statement. Avoid translating it into the terms of a medical diagnosis. For example, Mr. J. Schmidt enters with shortness of breath and you ponder writing "emphysema." Even if he is known to have emphysema from previous visits, it is not the chronic emphysema that prompted *this visit* but, rather, the "increasing shortness of breath" for 4 hours.

Some people try to self-diagnose based on similar signs and symptoms in their relatives or friends or based on conditions they know they have. Rather than record a woman's statement that she has "strep throat," ask her what symptoms she has that make her think this is present and record those symptoms.

Occasionally a person may list *many* reasons for seeking care. The most important reason to the person may not necessarily be the one stated first. Try to focus on which is the most pressing concern by asking the person which one prompted him or her to seek help *now*.

Present Health or History of Present Illness

For the well person, this is a short statement about the general state of health: *"I feel healthy right now." "I am healthy and active."*

For the ill person, this section is a chronologic record of the reason for seeking care, from the time the symptom first started until now. Isolate each reason for care identified by the person and say, for example, "Please tell me all about your headache, from the time it started until the time you came to the hospital." If the concern started months or years ago, record what occurred during that time and find out why the person is seeking care *now*.

As the person talks, do not jump to conclusions and bias the story by adding your opinion. Collect *all* the data first. Although you want the person to respond in a narrative format without interruption from you, your final summary of any symptom the person has should include these *eight critical characteristics:*

1. **Location.** Be specific; ask the person to point to the location. If the problem is pain, note the precise site. "Head pain" is vague, whereas descriptions such as "pain behind

*In the past, this statement was called the "Chief Complaint" (CC). Avoid this title because it labels the person a "complainer" and, more important, does not include wellness needs.

the eyes," "jaw pain," and "occipital pain" are more precise and are diagnostically significant. Is the pain localized to this site or radiating? Is the pain superficial or deep?

2. **Character** or **Quality.** This calls for specific descriptive terms such as burning, sharp, dull, aching, gnawing, throbbing, shooting, viselike. Use similes: Does blood in the stool look like sticky tar? Does blood in vomitus look like coffee grounds?
3. **Quantity** or **Severity.** Attempt to quantify the sign or symptom such as "profuse menstrual flow soaking five pads per hour." Quantify the symptom of pain using the scale shown on the right. With pain, avoid adjectives and ask how it affects daily activities. Then record if the person says, "I was so sick I was doubled up and couldn't move," or "I was able to go to work, but then I came home and went to bed."
4. **Timing** (Onset, Duration, Frequency). When did the symptom first appear? Give the specific date and time, or state specifically how long ago the symptom started prior to arrival (PTA). "The pain started yesterday" will not mean much when you return to read the record in the future. The report must include questions such as How long did the symptom last (duration)? Was it steady (constant), or did it come and go during that time (intermittent)? Did it resolve completely and reappear days or weeks later (cycle of remission and exacerbation)?
5. **Setting.** Where was the person or what was the person doing when the symptom started? What brings it on? For example, "Did you notice the chest pain after shoveling snow, or did the pain start by itself?"
6. **Aggravating** or **Relieving Factors.** What makes the pain worse? Is it aggravated by weather, activity, food, medication, standing bent over, fatigue, time of day, season, and so on? What relieves it (e.g., rest, medication, or ice pack)? What is the effect of any treatment? Ask, "What have you tried?" or "What seems to help?"
7. **Associated Factors.** Is this primary symptom associated with any others (e.g., urinary frequency and burning associated with fever and chills)? Review the body system related to this symptom now rather than wait for the Review of Systems section later. Many clinicians review the person's medication regimen now (including alcohol and tobacco use) because the presenting symptom may be a side effect or toxic effect of a chemical.
8. **Patient's Perception.** Find out the meaning of the symptom by asking how it affects daily activities. "How has this affected you?" "Is there anything you cannot do now that you could do before?" Also ask directly, "What do you think it means?" This is crucial because it alerts you to potential anxiety if the person thinks the symptom may be ominous.

Pain Scale

Quantify the symptom of pain by asking: *"On a 10-point scale, with 10 being the most pain you can possibly imagine and 1 being mild pain you barely notice, tell me how your pain feels right now."* (See Chapter 10 for a full description.)

You may find it helpful to organize this same question sequence into the mnemonic **PQRSTU** to help remember all the points. Note that you still need to address the patient's perception of the problem.

P: Provocative or Palliative. What brings it on? What were you doing when you first noticed it? What makes it better? Worse?
Q: Quality or Quantity. How does it look, feel, sound? How intense/severe is it?
R: Region or Radiation. Where is it? Does it spread anywhere?
S: Severity Scale. How bad is it (on a scale of 1 to 10)? Is it getting better, worse, staying the same?
T: Timing. Onset—Exactly when did it first occur? Duration—How long did it last? Frequency—How often does it occur?
U: Understand Patient's Perception of the problem. What do you think it means?

Past Health

Past health events are important because they may have residual effects on the current health state. Also, the previous experience with illness may give clues as to how the person responds to illness and to the significance of illness for him or her.

Childhood Illnesses. Measles, mumps, rubella, chickenpox, pertussis, and strep throat. Avoid recording "usual childhood illnesses," because an illness common in the person's childhood (e.g., measles) may be unusual today. Ask about serious illnesses that may have sequelae for the person in later years (e.g., rheumatic fever, scarlet fever, poliomyelitis).

Accidents or Injuries. Auto accidents, fractures, penetrating wounds, head injuries (especially if associated with unconsciousness), and burns.

Serious or Chronic Illnesses. Asthma, depression, diabetes, hypertension, heart disease, HIV infection, hepatitis, sickle-cell anemia, cancer, and seizure disorder.

Hospitalizations. Cause, name of hospital, how the condition was treated, how long the person was hospitalized, and name of the physician.

Operations. Type of surgery, date, name of the surgeon, name of hospital, and how the person recovered.

Recorded as:
Grav 3
Term 2
Preterm 1
Ab 0
Living 3

Obstetric History. Number of pregnancies (gravidity), number of deliveries in which the fetus reached full term (term), number of preterm pregnancies (preterm), number of incomplete pregnancies (abortions), and number of children living (living). For each complete pregnancy, note the course of pregnancy; labor and delivery; gender, weight, and condition of each infant; and postpartum course. For any incomplete pregnancies, record the duration and whether the pregnancy resulted in spontaneous (S) or induced (I) abortion.

Immunizations. Measles-mumps-rubella, polio, diphtheria-pertussis-tetanus, varicella, hepatitis A and B, meningococcal disease, human papilloma virus, *Haemophilus influenzae* type b, pneumococcal vaccine, influenza.[3] Note the date of the last tetanus immunization and last tuberculosis skin test. The 2010 guidelines for adult immunizations published by the Centers for Disease Control and Prevention (CDC) contain several changes. First, the CDC recommends either the quadrivalent or the newer bivalent human papillomavirus (HPV) vaccine for young adult women ages 19 to 26 years.[1a] In addition, the HPV vaccine is now recommended for young men ages 9 to 26 years to reduce HPV-associated genital warts. For the measles, mumps, rubella (MMR) vaccine, the CDC clairifies that most adults born after 1957 do not need a second vaccination if they can document receiving at least one dose. However, health care workers, college students, international travelers, and adults exposed to measles in an outbreak setting still need to have a second MMR vaccination.

Last Examination Date. Physical, dental, vision, hearing, electrocardiogram, chest x-ray, mammogram, Pap test, stool occult blood, serum cholesterol.

Allergies. Note both the allergen (medication, food, or contact agent, such as fabric or environmental agent) and the reaction (rash, itching, runny nose, watery eyes, difficulty breathing). With a drug, this symptom should not be a side effect but a true allergic reaction.

Current Medications. Note all prescription and over-the-counter medications. Ask specifically about vitamins, birth control pills, aspirin, and antacids, because many people do not consider these to be medications. For each medication, note the name, dose, and schedule, and ask, "How often do you take it each day?" "What is it for?" and "How long have you been taking it?"

Inquire about substances (alcohol, tobacco, street drugs) here or later in social history (see p. 58). Finally, note any home or herbal remedies.

Family History

Family History Tools in Electronic and Print Format
U.S. Surgeon General (My Family Health Portrait): www.hhs.gov/familyhistory/
Utah Health Family Tree: www.health.utah.gov/genomics
American Medical Association: www.ama-assn.org/ama/pub/category/2380.html

In the age of genomics, an accurate family history will highlight those diseases and conditions for which a particular patient may be at increased risk. A person who sees he or she may be vulnerable for a certain condition may seek early screening and periodic surveillance and may be influenced to adopt a healthy lifestyle when possible to mitigate that risk.

The most fruitful way to compile a complete family history is to send home a detailed questionnaire before the health care/hospital encounter because the information takes time to compile and often comes from multiple family members. Then you can use the health visit to complete the pedigree. A **pedigree** or **genogram** is a graphic family tree that uses symbols to depict the gender, relationship, and age of immediate blood relatives in at least three generations, such as parents, grandparents, siblings (Fig. 4-2). The health of close family members, such as spouse and children, is equally important to highlight the patient's prolonged contact with any communicable disease or environmental

Drawing Your Family Tree

- Make a list of all of your family members.
- Use this sample family tree as a guide to draw your own family tree.
- Write your name at the top of your paper and the date you drew your family tree.
- In place of the words *father, mother* etc., write the names of your family members.
- When possible, draw your brothers and sisters and your parents' brothers and sisters starting from oldest to the youngest, going from left to right across the paper.
- If dates of birth or ages are not known, then estimate or guess ("50s," "late 60s").

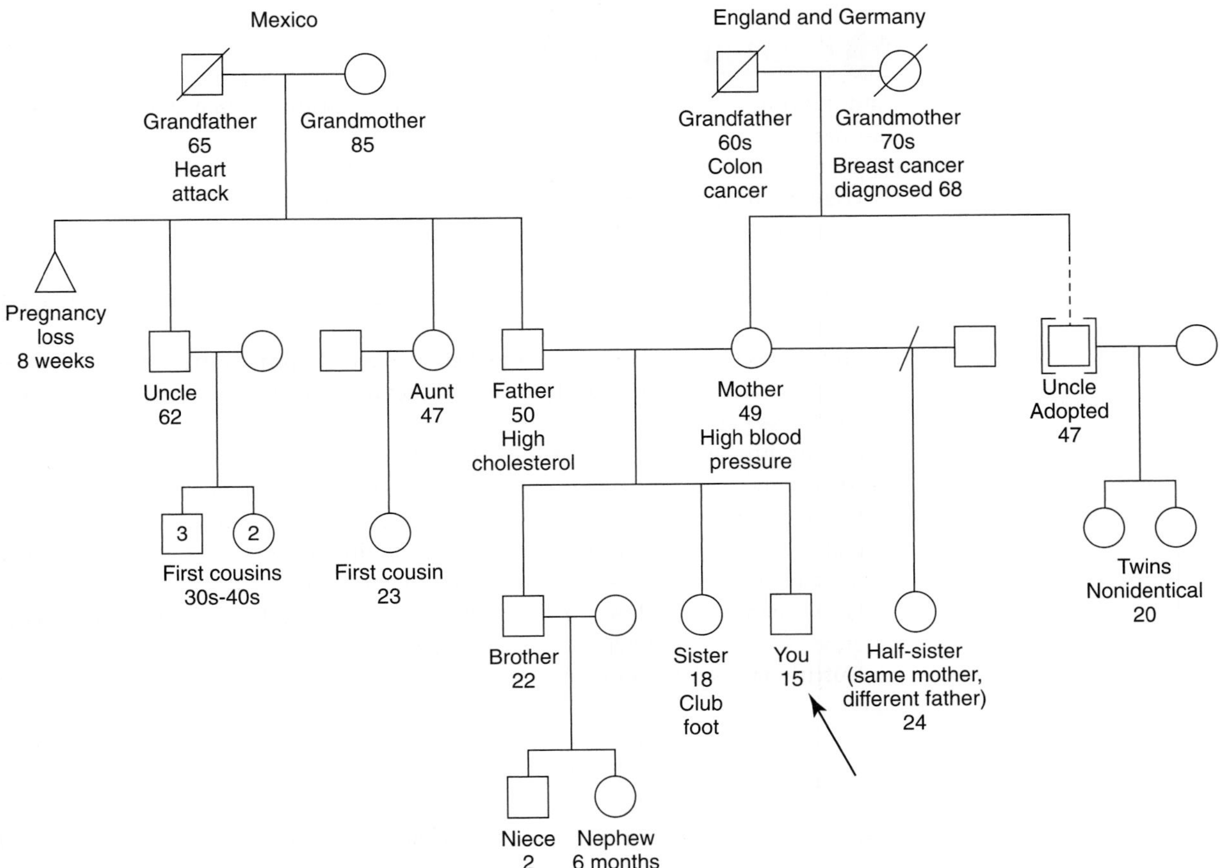

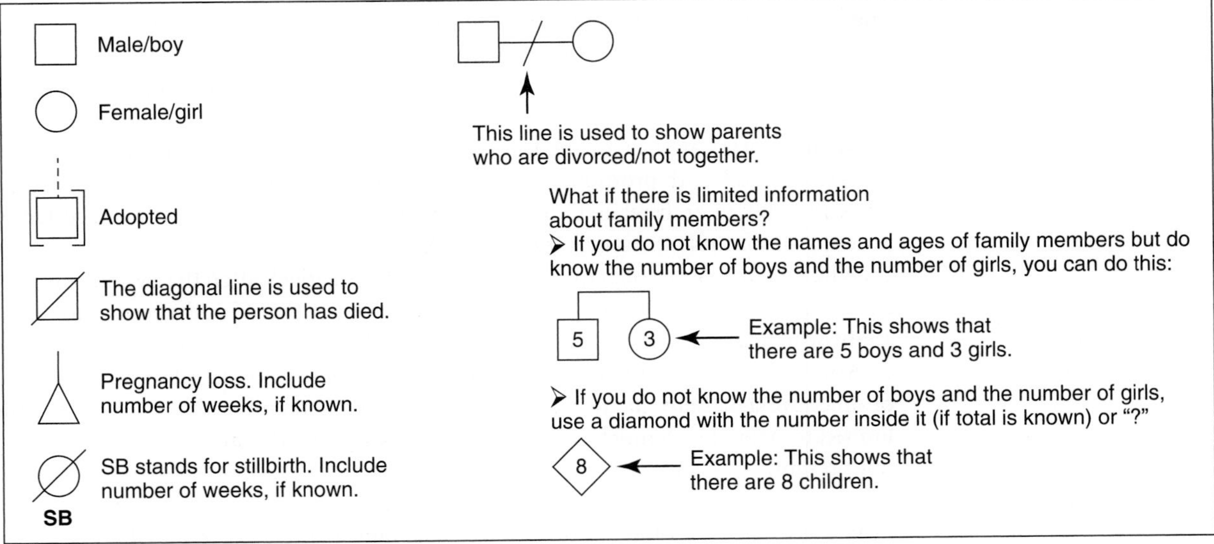

4-2 Genogram or family tree.

hazard such as tobacco smoke or to flag the effect of a family member's illness on this person.

Record the medical condition of each relative as well as other significant health data, such as age and cause of death, twinning, tobacco use, and heavy alcohol use. When reviewing the family history data, ask specifically for coronary heart disease, high blood pressure, stroke, diabetes, obesity, blood disorders, breast/ovarian cancer, colon cancer, sickle-cell anemia, arthritis, allergies, alcohol or drug addiction, mental illness, suicide, seizure disorder, kidney disease, and tuberculosis.

CULTURE AND GENETICS

Add several questions to the complete health history when the person is a new immigrant:

- Biographical data—when did the persons enter the United States and from what country; if they are refugees, what were the conditions under which they came here, whether they had been harassed or tortured.
    - The older adult may have come to this country after World War II and may be a Holocaust survivor—questions regarding family and past history may evoke painful memories and must be asked carefully.
- Spiritual resources/religion—assess whether certain procedures cannot be done, such as administering blood to a Jehovah's Witness or drawing large amounts of blood from a Chinese patient.
- Past health—what immunizations were given in their homeland; for example, was the person given *Bacillus Calmette-Guérin* (BCG). This vaccine is used in many countries to prevent tuberculosis; it is not administered in the United States. If the person has had BCG, he or she will have a positive tuberculin test and further diagnostic procedures must be done, including a sputum test and chest x-ray.
- Health perception—how does the person describe health and illness and what does he or she see as the problem he or she is now experiencing?
- Nutritional—what foods and food combinations are taboo?

Review of Systems

The purposes of this section are (1) to evaluate the past and present health state of each body system, (2) to double-check in case any significant data were omitted in the Present Illness section, and (3) to evaluate health promotion practices. The order of the examination of body systems is roughly head-to-toe. The items within each system are not inclusive, and only the most common symptoms are listed. If the Present Illness section covered one body system, you do not need to repeat all the data here. For example, if the reason for seeking care is earache, the Present Illness section describes most of the symptoms listed for the auditory system. Just ask now what was not asked in the Present Illness section.

Medical terms are listed here, but they need to be translated for the patient. (Note that symptoms and health promotion activities are merely listed here. These terms are repeated and expanded in each related physical examination chapter, along with suggested ways to pose questions and a rationale for each question.)

When recording information, avoid writing "negative" after the system heading. You need to record the *presence* or *absence* of all symptoms; otherwise, the reader does not know about which factors you asked.

A common mistake made by beginning practitioners is to record some physical finding or objective data here, such as "skin warm and dry." Remember that the history should be limited to patient statements, or subjective data—factors that the person *says* were or were not present.

General Overall Health State. Present weight (gain or loss, over what period of time, by diet or other factors), fatigue, weakness or malaise, fever, chills, sweats or night sweats.

Skin. History of skin disease (eczema, psoriasis, hives), pigment or color change, change in mole, excessive dryness or moisture, pruritus, excessive bruising, rash or lesion.

Hair. Recent loss, change in texture. Nails: change in shape, color, or brittleness.
Health Promotion. Amount of sun exposure; method of self-care for skin and hair.

Head. Any unusually frequent or severe headache, any head injury, dizziness (syncope) or vertigo.

Eyes. Difficulty with vision (decreased acuity, blurring, blind spots), eye pain, diplopia (double vision), redness or swelling, watering or discharge, glaucoma or cataracts.
Health Promotion. Wears glasses or contacts; last vision check or glaucoma test; and how coping with loss of vision if any.

Ears. Earaches, infections, discharge and its characteristics, tinnitus or vertigo.
Health Promotion. Hearing loss, hearing aid use, how loss affects the daily life, any exposure to environmental noise, and method of cleaning ears.

Nose and Sinuses. Discharge and its characteristics, any unusually frequent or severe colds, sinus pain, nasal obstruction, nosebleeds, allergies or hay fever, or change in sense of smell.

Mouth and Throat. Mouth pain, frequent sore throat, bleeding gums, toothache, lesion in mouth or tongue, dysphagia, hoarseness or voice change, tonsillectomy, altered taste.
Health Promotion. Pattern of daily dental care, use of dentures, bridge, and last dental checkup.

Neck. Pain, limitation of motion, lumps or swelling, enlarged or tender nodes, goiter.

Breast. Pain, lump, nipple discharge, rash, history of breast disease, any surgery on the breasts.
Health Promotion. Performs breast self-examination, including its frequency and method used, last mammogram.

Axilla. Tenderness, lump or swelling, rash.

Respiratory System. History of lung diseases (asthma, emphysema, bronchitis, pneumonia, tuberculosis), chest pain with breathing, wheezing or noisy breathing, shortness of breath, how much activity produces shortness of breath, cough, sputum (color, amount), hemoptysis, toxin or pollution exposure.
Health Promotion. Last chest x-ray study, TB skin test.

Cardiovascular. Precordial or retrosternal pain, palpitation, cyanosis, dyspnea on exertion (specify amount of exertion [e.g., walking one flight of stairs, walking from chair to bath, or just talking]), orthopnea, paroxysmal nocturnal dyspnea, nocturia, edema, history of heart murmur, hypertension, coronary artery disease, anemia.
Health Promotion. Date of last ECG or other heart tests, cholesterol screening.

Peripheral Vascular. Coldness, numbness and tingling, swelling of legs (time of day, activity), discoloration in hands or feet (bluish red, pallor, mottling, associated with position, especially around feet and ankles), varicose veins or complications, intermittent claudication, thrombophlebitis, ulcers.
Health Promotion. Does the work involve long-term sitting or standing? Avoid crossing legs at the knees. Wear support hose.

Gastrointestinal. Appetite, food intolerance, dysphagia, heartburn, indigestion, pain (associated with eating), other abdominal pain, pyrosis (esophageal and stomach burning sensation with sour eructation), nausea and vomiting (character), vomiting blood, history of abdominal disease (ulcer, liver or gallbladder, jaundice, appendicitis, colitis), flatulence, frequency of bowel movement, any recent change, stool characteristics, constipation or diarrhea, black stools, rectal bleeding, rectal conditions (hemorrhoids, fistula).

Health Promotion. Use of antacids or laxatives. (Alternatively, diet history and substance habits can be placed here.)

Urinary System. Frequency, urgency, nocturia (the number of times the person awakens at night to urinate, recent change), dysuria, polyuria or oliguria, hesitancy or straining, narrowed stream, urine color (cloudy or presence of hematuria), incontinence, history of urinary disease (kidney disease, kidney stones, urinary tract infections, prostate), pain in flank, groin, suprapubic region, or low back.

Health Promotion. Measures to avoid or treat urinary tract infections, use of Kegel exercises after childbirth.

Male Genital System. Penis or testicular pain, sores or lesions, penile discharge, lumps, hernia.

Health Promotion. Perform testicular self-examination? How frequently?

Female Genital System. Menstrual history (age at menarche, last menstrual period, cycle and duration, any amenorrhea or menorrhagia, premenstrual pain or dysmenorrhea, intermenstrual spotting), vaginal itching, discharge and its characteristics, age at menopause, menopausal signs or symptoms, postmenopausal bleeding.

Health Promotion. Last gynecologic checkup and last Papanicolaou (Pap) test.

Sexual Health. Begin with: "I usually ask all patients about their sexual health." Then ask: Are you presently in a relationship involving intercourse? Are the aspects of sex satisfactory to the patient and partner? Routine use of condoms? Any dyspareunia (for female), any changes in erection or ejaculation (for male), and use of contraceptive? Is the contraceptive method satisfactory? Aware of contact with a partner who has any sexually transmitted infection (gonorrhea, herpes, chlamydia, venereal warts, HIV/AIDS, or syphilis)?

Musculoskeletal System. History of arthritis or gout. In the joints: pain, stiffness, swelling (location, migratory nature), deformity, limitation of motion, noise with joint motion? In the muscles: any pain, cramps, weakness, gait problems or problems with coordinated activities? In the back: any pain (location and radiation to extremities), stiffness, limitation of motion, or history of back pain or disk disease?

Health Promotion. How much walking per day? What is the effect of limited range of motion on daily activities, such as on grooming, feeding, toileting, dressing? Are any mobility aids used?

Neurologic System. History of seizure disorder, stroke, fainting, blackouts. In motor function: weakness, tic or tremor, paralysis, or coordination problems. In sensory function: numbness and tingling (paresthesia). In cognitive function: memory disorder (recent or distant, disorientation). In mental status: any nervousness, mood change, depression, or any history of mental health dysfunction or hallucinations.

Health Promotion. Alternatively, data about interpersonal relationships; coping patterns placed here.

Hematologic System. Bleeding tendency of skin or mucous membranes, excessive bruising, lymph node swelling, exposure to toxic agents or radiation, blood transfusion and reactions.

Endocrine System. History of diabetes or diabetic symptoms (polyuria, polydipsia, polyphagia), history of thyroid disease, intolerance to heat and cold, change in skin pigmentation or texture, excessive sweating, relationship between appetite and weight, abnormal hair distribution, nervousness, tremors, and need for hormone therapy.

Functional Assessment (Including Activities of Daily Living)

Functional assessment measures a person's self-care ability in the areas of general physical health or absence of illness; ADLs, such as bathing, dressing, toileting, eating, walking; instrumental activities of daily living (IADLs), or those needed for independent living, such as housekeeping, shopping, cooking, doing laundry, using the telephone, managing finances; nutrition; social relationships and resources; self-concept and coping; and home environment.

Functional assessment may mean organizing the entire assessment around functional "pattern areas."[6] Instruments that emphasize functional categories may help in leading to a nursing diagnosis.

Functional assessment may also mean that the health history may be supplemented by a standardized instrument on functional assessment. These instruments objectively measure a person's present functional status and monitor any changes over time (see Chapter 30 for more information).

Whether or not you use any of these formalized instruments, functional assessment questions such as those listed in the following section should be included in the standard health history. These questions provide data on the lifestyle and type of living environment to which the person is accustomed. Because some of the data may be judged private by the individual, the questions are best asked at this later point in the interview after you have had time to establish rapport.

Self-Esteem, Self-Concept. Education (last grade completed, other significant training), financial status (income adequate for lifestyle and/or health concerns), value-belief system (religious practices and perception of personal strengths).

Activity/Exercise. A daily profile reflecting usual daily activities: ask "Tell me how you spend a typical day." Note ability to perform ADLs: independent or needs assistance with feeding, bathing, hygiene, dressing, toileting, bed-to-chair transfer, walking, standing, or climbing stairs. Any use of wheelchair, prostheses, or mobility aids?

Record leisure activities enjoyed and the exercise pattern (type, amount per day or week, method of warm-up session, method of monitoring the body's response to exercise).

Sleep/Rest. Sleep patterns, daytime naps, any sleep aids used.

Nutrition/Elimination. Record the diet by a recall of all food and beverages taken over the past 24 hours (see Chapter 11 for suggested method of inquiry). "Is that menu typical of most days?" Describe eating habits and current appetite. Ask "Who buys food and prepares food?" "Are your finances adequate for food?" "Who is present at mealtimes?" Indicate any food allergy or intolerance. Record daily intake of caffeine (coffee, tea, cola drinks).

Ask about usual pattern of bowel elimination and urinating including problems with mobility or transfer in toileting, continence, use of laxatives.

Interpersonal Relationships/Resources. Social roles: "How would you describe your role in the family?" "How would you say you get along with family, friends, and co-workers?" Ask about support systems composed of family and significant others: "To whom could you go for support with a problem at work, with your health, or a personal problem?" Include contact with spouse, siblings, parents, children, friends, organizations, workplace: "Is time spent alone pleasurable and relaxing, or isolating?"

Spiritual Resources. Many people believe in a relationship between spirituality and health, and they may wish to have spiritual matters addressed in the traditional health care setting. Use the faith, influence, community, and address (FICA) questions to incorporate the person's spiritual values into the health history.[10a] *Faith:* "Does religious faith or spirituality play an important part in your life? Do you consider yourself to be a religious or spiritual person?" *Influence:* "How does your religious faith or spirituality influence the way you think about your health or the way you care for yourself?" *Community:* "Are you a part of any religious or spiritual community or congregation?" *Address:* "Would you like me to address any religious or spiritual issues or concerns with you?"

Coping and Stress Management. Kinds of stresses in life, especially in the past year, any change in lifestyle or any current stress, methods tried to relieve stress, and whether these have been helpful.

Personal Habits. Tobacco, alcohol, street drugs: "Do you smoke cigarettes (pipe, use chewing tobacco)?" "At what age did you start?" "How many packs do you smoke per day?" "How many years have you smoked?" Record the number of packs smoked per day (PPD) and duration (e.g., 1 PPD × 5 years). Then ask, "Have you ever tried to quit?" and "How did it go?" to introduce plans about smoking cessation.

Alcohol. Health care professionals often fail to question about alcohol unless problems are obvious. However, alcohol interacts adversely with all medications; is a factor in many social problems such as assaults, rapes, high-risk sexual behavior, and child abuse; contributes to half of all fatal traffic accidents; and accounts for 5% of all deaths in the United States. The latter figure is actually an underestimate because alcohol-related conditions are underreported on death certificates.

Be alert, then, to early signs of hazardous alcohol use. Ask whether the person drinks alcohol. If yes, ask specific questions about the amount and frequency of alcohol use: "When was your last drink of alcohol?" "How much did you drink that time?" "Out of the past 30 days, about how many days would you say that you drank alcohol?" Has anyone ever said you had a drinking problem?"

You may wish to use a screening questionnaire to identify excessive or uncontrolled drinking, such as the Cut down, Annoyed, Guilty, and Eye-opener (**CAGE**) test.[4]

- Have you ever thought you should **C**ut down your drinking?
- Have you ever been **A**nnoyed by criticism of your drinking?
- Have you ever felt **G**uilty about your drinking?
- Do you drink in the morning? (i.e., an **E**ye opener?)

If the person answers "yes" to two or more CAGE questions, you should suspect alcohol abuse and continue with a more complete substance abuse assessment (see Chapter 6, p. 93). If the person answers "no" to drinking alcohol, ask the reason for this decision (psychosocial, legal, health). Any history of alcohol treatment? Involvement in recovery activities? History of family member with problem drinking?

Illicit or Street Drugs. Ask specifically about marijuana, cocaine, crack cocaine, amphetamines, heroin, pain killers like OxyContin or Vicodin, and barbiturates. Indicate frequency of use and how usage has affected work or family.

Environment/Hazards. Housing and neighborhood (living alone, knowledge of neighbors), safety of area, adequate heat and utilities, access to transportation, and involvement in community services. Note environmental health, including hazards in workplace, hazards at home, use of seatbelts, geographic or occupational exposures, and travel or residence in other countries, including time spent abroad during military service.

Intimate Partner Violence. Begin with open-ended questions: "How are things at home?" and "Do you feel safe?" These are valuable initial screening questions, because some people may not recognize that they are in abusive situations or may be reluctant to admit it due to guilt, fear, shame, or denial. If the person responds to feeling unsafe, follow up with closed-ended questions: "Have you ever been emotionally or physically abused by your partner or someone important to you?" "Within the past year, have you been hit, slapped, kicked, pushed, or shoved or otherwise physically hurt by your partner or ex-partner?" "If yes, by whom?" "Number of times?" "Does your partner ever force you into having sex?" "Are you afraid of your partner or ex-partner?" See Chapter 7 for more information.

Occupational Health. Ask the person to describe his or her job. Ever worked with any health hazard, such as asbestos, inhalants, chemicals, repetitive motion? Wear any protective equipment? Any work programs in place that monitor exposure? Aware of any health problems now that may be related to work exposure?

Note the timing of the reason for seeking care and whether it may be related to change in work or home activities, job titles, or exposure history. Take a careful smoking history, which may contribute to occupational hazards. Finally, ask the person what he or she likes or dislikes about the job.

Perception of Health

Ask the person questions such as: "How do you define health?" "How do you view your situation now?" "What are your concerns?" "What do you think will happen in the future?" "What are your health goals?" "What do you expect from us as nurses, physicians, (or other health care providers)?"

DEVELOPMENTAL COMPETENCE

Children

The health history is adapted to include information specific for the age and developmental stage of the child (e.g., the mother's health during pregnancy, labor and delivery, and the perinatal period) (Fig. 4-3). Note that the developmental history and nutritional data are listed as separate sections because of their importance for current health.

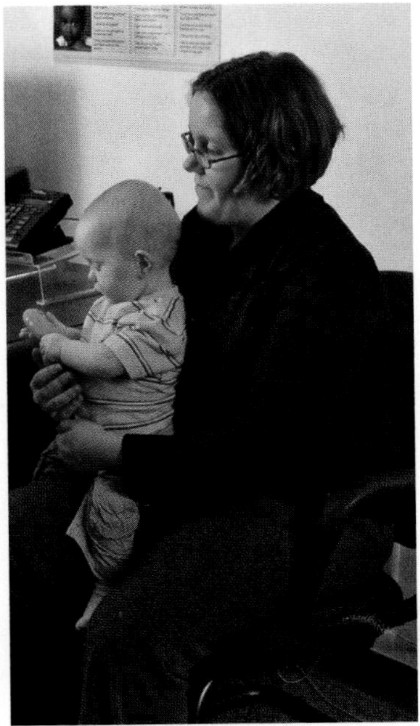

4-3

Biographic Data

Include the child's name, nickname, address and phone number, parents' names and work numbers, child's age and birth date, birthplace, gender, race, ethnic origin, and information on other children and family members at home.

Source of History

1. Person providing information and relation to child
2. Your impression of reliability of information
3. Any special circumstances (e.g., the use of an interpreter)

Reason for Seeking Care

Record the parent's spontaneous statement. Because of the frequency of well-child visits for routine health care, there will be more reasons such as "time for the child's checkup" or "she needs the next baby shot." Reasons for health problems may be initiated by the child, the parent, or a third party such as the classroom teacher or social worker.

Sometimes the reason stated may not be the real reason for the visit. A parent may have a "hidden agenda," such as the mother who brought her 4-year-old child in because "she looked pale." Further questioning revealed that the mother had heard recently from a former college friend whose own 4-year-old child had just been diagnosed with leukemia.

Present Health or History of Present Illness

If the parent or child seeks routine health care, include a statement about the usual health of the child and any common health problems or major health concerns.

Describe any presenting symptom or sign, using the same format as for the adult. Some additional considerations include:

- Severity of pain: "How do you know the child is in pain" (e.g., pulling at ears alerts parent to ear pain)? Note effect of pain on usual behavior (e.g., does it stop child from playing?).
- Associated factors, such as relation to activity, eating, and body position.
- The parent's intuitive sense of a problem. As the constant caregiver, this intuitive sense is often very accurate. Even if proved otherwise, this factor gives you an idea of the parent's area of concern.
- Parent's coping ability and reaction of other family members to child's symptoms or illness.

Past Health

Prenatal Status. Start with an open-ended question: "Tell me about your pregnancy." Then ask: How was this pregnancy spaced? Was it planned? What was the mother's attitude toward the pregnancy? What was the father's attitude? Was there medical supervision for the mother? At what month was the supervision started? What was the mother's health during pregnancy? Were there any complications (bleeding, excessive nausea and vomiting, unusual weight gain, high blood pressure, swelling of hands and feet, falls, infections—rubella or sexually transmitted infections)? During what month were diet and medications prescribed and/or taken during pregnancy (dose and duration)? Record the mother's use of alcohol, street drugs, or cigarettes and any x-ray studies taken during pregnancy.

Labor and Delivery. Parity of the mother, duration of the pregnancy, name of the hospital, course and duration of labor, use of anesthesia, type of delivery (vertex, breech, cesarean section), birth weight, Apgar scores, onset of breathing, any cyanosis, need for resuscitation, and use of special equipment or procedures.

Postnatal Status. Any problems in the nursery, length of hospital stay, neonatal jaundice, whether the baby was discharged with the mother, whether the baby was breastfed or bottle-fed, weight gain, any feeding problems, "blue spells," colic, diarrhea, patterns of crying and sleeping, the mother's health postpartum, and the mother's reaction to the baby.

Childhood Illnesses. Age and any complications of measles, mumps, rubella, chickenpox, whooping cough, strep throat, and frequent ear infections; also, any recent exposure to illness.

Serious Accidents or Injuries. Age of occurrence, extent of injury, how the child was treated, and complications of auto accidents, falls, head injuries, fractures, burns, and poisonings.

Serious or Chronic Illnesses. Age of onset, how the child was treated, and complications of meningitis or encephalitis; seizure disorders; asthma, pneumonia, and other chronic lung conditions; rheumatic fever; scarlet fever; diabetes; kidney problems; sickle-cell anemia; high blood pressure; and allergies.

Operations or Hospitalizations. Reason for care, age at admission, name of surgeon or primary care providers, name of hospital, duration of stay, how child reacted to hospitalization, and any complications. (If child reacted poorly, he or she may be afraid now and will need special preparation for the examination that is to follow.)

Immunizations. Age when administered, date administered, and any reactions following immunizations. Appendix A on the *Evolve* website lists suggested immunization schedules. Because of outbreaks of measles across the United States, the American Academy of Pediatrics recommends two doses of the measles-mumps-rubella vaccine, one at 12 to 15 months and one at age 4 to 6 years.[1]

Allergies. Any drugs, foods, contact agents, and environmental agents to which the child is allergic, and reaction to allergen. Note allergic reactions particularly common in childhood, such as allergic rhinitis, insect hypersensitivity, eczema, and urticaria.

Medications. Any prescription and over-the-counter medications (or vitamins) the child takes, including the dose, daily schedule, why the medication is given, and any problems.

Developmental History

Growth. Height and weight at birth and at 1, 2, 5, and 10 years, any periods of rapid gain or loss, and process of dentition (age of tooth eruption and pattern of loss).

Milestones. Age when child first held head erect, rolled over, sat alone, walked alone, cut his or her first tooth, said his or her first words with meaning, spoke in sentences, was toilet trained, tied shoes, dressed without help. Does the parent believe this development has been normal? How does this child's development compare with siblings or peers?

Current Development (Children 1 Month Through Preschool). Gross motor skills (rolls over, sits alone, walks alone, skips, climbs), fine motor skills (inspects hands, brings hands to mouth, pincer grasp, stacks blocks, feeds self, uses crayon to draw, uses scissors), language skills (vocalizes, first words with meaning, sentences, persistence of baby talk, speech problems), and personal-social skills (smiles, tracks movement with eyes to midline, past midline, attends to sound by turning head, recognizes own name). If the child is undergoing toilet training, indicate the method used, age of bladder/bowel control, parents' attitude toward toilet training, and terms used for toileting.

School-Age Child. Gross motor skills (runs, jumps, climbs, rides bicycle, general coordination), fine motor skills (ties shoelace, uses scissors, writes name and numbers, draws pictures), and language skills (vocabulary, verbal ability, able to tell time, reading level).

Nutritional History

The amount of nutritional information needed depends on the child's age; the younger the child, the more detailed and specific the data should be. For the infant, record whether breastfeeding or bottle-feeding is used. If the child is breastfed, record nursing frequency and duration, any supplements (vitamin, iron, fluoride, bottles), family support for nursing, and age and method of weaning. If the child is bottle-fed, record type of formula used, frequency and amount, any problems with feeding (spitting up, colic, diarrhea), supplements used, and any bottle propping. Record introduction of solid foods (age when the child began eating solids, which foods, whether foods are home or commercially made, amount given, child's reaction to new food, parent's reaction to feeding).

For preschool- and school-age children and adolescents, record the child's appetite, 24-hour diet recall (meals, snacks, amounts), vitamins taken, how much junk food is eaten, who eats with the child, food likes and dislikes, and parent's perception of child's nutrition.

A week-long diary of food intake may be more accurate than a spot 24-hour recall. Also, consider cultural practices in assessing child's diet.

Family History

As with the adult, diagram a family tree for the child, including siblings, parents, and grandparents (see p. 53). Ask specifically for the family history of heart disease, high blood pressure, diabetes, blood disorders, cancer, sickle-cell anemia, arthritis, allergies, obesity, cystic fibrosis, alcoholism, mental illness, seizure disorder, kidney disease, mental retardation, learning disabilities, birth defects, and sudden infant death. (When interviewing the mother, ask about the "child's father," not "your husband," in case of the separation of the child's biologic parents.)

Review of Systems

General. Significant gain or loss of weight, failure to gain weight appropriate for age, frequent colds, ear infections, illnesses, energy level, fatigue, overactivity, and behavior change (irritability, increased crying, nervousness).

Skin. Birthmarks, skin disease, pigment or color change, mottling, change in mole, pruritus, rash, lesion, acne, easy bruising or petechiae, easy bleeding, and changes in hair or nails.

Head. Headache, head injury, dizziness.

Eyes. Strabismus, diplopia, pain, redness, discharge, cataracts, vision changes, reading problems. Is the child able to see the board at school? Does the child sit too close to the television?

Health Promotion. Use of eyeglasses, date of last vision screening.

Ears. Earaches, frequency of ear infections, myringotomy tubes in ears, discharge (characteristics), cerumen, ringing or crackling, and whether parent perceives any hearing problems.

Health Promotion. How does the child clean his or her ears?

Nose and Sinuses. Discharge and its characteristics, frequency of colds, nasal stuffiness, nosebleeds, and allergies.

Mouth and Throat. History of cleft lip or palate, frequency of sore throats, toothache, caries, sores in mouth or tongue, tonsils present, mouth breathing, difficulty chewing, difficulty swallowing, and hoarseness or voice change.

Health Promotion. Child's pattern of brushing teeth and last dental checkup.

Neck. Swollen or tender glands, limitation of movement, or stiffness.

Breast. For preadolescent and adolescent girls, when did they notice that their breasts were changing? What is the girl's self-perception of development? For older adolescents, does the girl perform breast self-examination? (See Chapter 17 for suggested phrasing of questions.)

Respiratory System. Croup or asthma, wheezing or noisy breathing, shortness of breath, chronic cough.

Cardiovascular System. Congenital heart problems, history of murmur, and cyanosis (what prompts this condition). Is there any limitation of activity, or can the child keep up with peers? Is there any dyspnea on exertion, palpitations, high blood pressure, or coldness in the extremities?

Gastrointestinal System. Abdominal pain, nausea and vomiting, history of ulcer, frequency of bowel movements, stool color and characteristics, diarrhea, constipation or stool-holding, rectal bleeding, anal itching, history of pinworms, and use of laxatives.

Urinary System. Painful urination, polyuria/oliguria, narrowed stream, urine color (cloudy, dark), history of urinary tract infection, whether toilet trained, when toilet training was planned, any problems, bedwetting (when the child started, frequency, associated with stress, how child feels about it).

Male Genital System. Penis or testicular pain, whether told if testes are descended, any sores or lesions, discharge, hernia or hydrocele, or swelling in scrotum during crying. For the preadolescent and adolescent boy, has he noticed any change in the penis and scrotum? Is the boy familiar with normal growth patterns, nocturnal emissions, and sex education? Screen for sexual abuse. (See Chapter 24 for suggested phrasing of questions.)

Female Genital System. Has the girl noted any genital itching, rash, vaginal discharge? For the preadolescent and adolescent girl, when did menstruation start? Was she prepared? Screen for sexual abuse. (See Chapter 26 for suggested phrasing of questions.)

Sexual Health. What is the child's attitude toward the opposite sex? Who provides sex education? How does the family deal with sex education, masturbation, dating patterns? Is the adolescent in a relationship involving intercourse? Does he or she have information on birth control and sexually transmitted infections? (See Chapters 24 and 26 for suggested phrasing of questions.)

Musculoskeletal System. In bones and joints: arthritis, joint pain, stiffness, swelling, limitation of movement, gait strength and coordination. In muscles: pain, cramps, and weakness. In the back: pain, posture, spinal curvature, and any treatment.

Neurologic System. Numbness and tingling. (Behavior and cognitive issues are covered in the sections on development and interpersonal relationships.)

Hematologic Systems. Excessive bruising, lymph node swelling, and exposure to toxic agents or radiation.

Endocrine System. History of diabetes or thyroid disease; excessive hunger, thirst, or urinating; abnormal hair distribution; and precocious or delayed puberty.

Functional Assessment (Including Activities of Daily Living)

Interpersonal Relationships. Within the family constellation, record the child's position in family; whether the child is adopted; who lives with the child; who is the primary caregiver; who is the caregiver if both parents work outside of the home; any support from relatives, neighbors, or friends; and the ethnic or cultural milieu.

Indicate family cohesion. Does the family enjoy activities as a unit? Has there been a recent family change or crisis (death, divorce, move)? Record information on child's self-image and level of independence. Does the child use a security blanket or toy? Is there any repetitive behavior (bed-rocking, head-banging), pica, thumb-sucking, or nail-biting? Note method of discipline used. Indicate type used at home. How effective is it? Who disciplines the child? Is there any occurrence of negativism, temper tantrums, withdrawal, or aggressive behavior?

Provide information on the child's friends: whether the child makes friends easily. How does the child get along with friends? Does he or she play with same-age or older or younger children?

Activity and Rest. Record the child's play activities. Indicate amount of active and quiet play, outdoor play, time watching television, and special hobbies or activities. Record sleep and rest. Indicate pattern and number of hours at night and during the day and the child's routine at bedtime. Is the child a sound sleeper, or is he or she wakeful? Does the child have nightmares, night terrors, or somnambulation? How does the parent respond? Does the child have naps during the day?

Record school attendance. Any experience with daycare or nursery school? In what grade is the child in school? Has the child ever skipped a grade or been held back? Does the child seem to like school? What is his or her school performance? Are the parent and child satisfied with the performance? Were days missed in school? Provide a reason for the absence. (These questions give an important index to the child's functioning outside the home.)

Economic Status. Ask about the mother's occupation and father's occupation. Indicate the number of hours each parent is away from home. Do parents perceive their income as adequate? What is the effect of illness on financial status?

Home Environment. Where does family live (house, apartment)? Is the size of the home adequate? Is there access to an outdoor play area? Does the child share a room, have his or her own bed, and have toys appropriate for his or her age?

Environmental Hazards. Inquire about home safety (precautions for poisons, medications, household products, presence of gates for stairways, and safe yard equipment). Inquire about the home structure (adequate heating, ventilation, bathroom facilities), neighborhood (residential or industrial, age of neighbors, safe play areas, playmates available, distance to school, amount of traffic, is area remote or congested and overcrowded, is crime a problem, presence of air or water pollution), and automobile (child safety seat, seatbelts).

Coping/Stress Management. Is the child able to adapt to new situations? Record recent stressful experiences (death, divorce, move, loss of special friend). How does the child cope with stress? Any recent change in behavior or mood? Has counseling ever been sought?

Habits. Has the child ever tried cigarette smoking? How much did he or she smoke? Has the child ever tried alcohol? How much alcohol did he or she drink weekly or daily? Has the child ever tried other drugs (marijuana, cocaine, amphetamines, barbiturates)?

Health Promotion. Who is the primary health care provider? When was the child's last checkup? Who is the dental care provider, and when was the last dental checkup? Provide date and result of screening for vision, hearing, urinalysis, phenylketonuria, hematocrit, tuberculosis skin test, sickle-cell trait, blood lead, and other tests specific for high-risk populations.

The Adolescent

This section presents a psychosocial review of symptoms intended to maximize communication with youth. The **HEEADSSS** method of interviewing focuses on assessment of the **H**ome environment, **E**ducation and employment, **E**ating, peer-related **A**ctivities **D**rugs, **S**exuality, **S**uicide/depression, and **S**afety from injury and violence (Fig. 4-4). The tool minimizes adolescent stress because it moves from expected and less-threatening questions to those that are more personal. The tool presents the questions in three colors: green are considered essential to explore with every adolescent; blue are important for you to ask if time permits; red questions delve in more deeply if the situation demands it.[5] Interview the youth alone, while the parent can wait outside and fill out past health questionnaires.

The HEEADSSS Psychosocial Interview for Adolescents

Home
Who lives with you? Where do you live? Do you have your own room?
What are relationships like at home?
To whom are you closest at home?
To whom can you talk at home?
Is there anyone new at home? Has someone left recently?
Have you moved recently?
Have you ever had to live away from home? (Why?)
Have you ever run away? (Why?)
Is there any physical violence at home?

Education and Employment
What are your favorite subjects at school? Your least favorite subjects?
How are your grades? Any recent changes? Any dramatic changes in the past?
Have you changed schools in the past few years?
What are your future education/employment plans/goals?
Are you working? Where? How much?
Tell me about your friends at school.
Is your school a safe place? (Why?)
Have you ever had to repeat a class? Have you ever had to repeat a grade?
Have you ever been suspended? Expelled? Have you ever considered dropping out?
How well do you get along with the people at school? Work?
Have your responsibilities at work increased?
Do you feel connected to your school? Do you feel as if you belong?
Are there adults at school you feel you could talk to about something important? (Who?)

Eating
What do you like and not like about your body?
Have there been any recent changes in your weight?
Have you dieted in the past year? How? How often?
Have you done anything else to try to manage your weight?
How much exercise do you get in an average day? Week?
What do you think would be a healthy diet? How does that compare with your current eating patterns?
Do you worry about your weight? How often?
Do you eat in front of the TV? Computer?
Does it ever seem as though your eating is out of control?
Have you ever made yourself throw up on purpose to control your weight?
Have you ever taken diet pills?
What would it be like if you gained (lost) 10 pounds?

Activities
What do you and your *friends* do for fun? (with whom, where, and when?)
What do you and your *family* do for fun? (with whom, where, and when?)
Do you participate in any sports or other activities?
Do you regularly attend a church group, club, or other organized activity?
Do you have any hobbies?
Do you read for fun? (What?)
How much TV do you watch in a week? How about video games?
What music do you like to listen to?

Drugs
Do any of your friends use tobacco? Alcohol? Other drugs?
Does anyone in your family use tobacco? Alcohol? Other drugs?
Do you use tobacco? Alcohol? Other drugs?
Is there any history of alcohol or drug problems in your family?
Do you ever drink or use drugs when you're alone?
(Assess frequency, intensity, patterns of use or abuse, and how youth obtains or pays for drugs, alcohol, or tobacco.)

Sexuality
Have you ever been in a romantic relationship?
Tell me about the people that you've dated. *OR* Tell me about your sex life.
Have any of your relationships ever been sexual relationships?
Are your sexual activities enjoyable?
What does the term "safer sex" mean to you?
Are you interested in boys? Girls? Both?
Have you ever been forced or pressured into doing something sexual that you didn't want to do?
Have you ever been touched sexually in a way that you didn't want?
Have you ever been raped, on a date or any other time?
How many sexual partners have you had altogether?
Have you ever been pregnant or worried that you may be pregnant? (females)
Have you ever gotten someone pregnant or worried that that might have happened? (males)
What are you using for birth control? Are you satisfied with your method?
Do you use condoms every time you have intercourse?
Does anything ever get in the way of always using a condom?
Have you ever had a sexually transmitted infection (STI) or worried that you had an STI?

Suicide and Depression
Do you feel sad or down more than usual? Do you find yourself crying more than usual?
Are you "bored" all the time?
Are you having trouble getting to sleep?
Have you thought a lot about hurting yourself or someone else?
Does it seem that you've lost interest in things that you used to really enjoy?
Do you find yourself spending less and less time with friends?
Would you rather just be by yourself most of the time?
Have you ever tried to kill yourself?
Have you ever had to hurt yourself (by cutting yourself, for example) to calm down or feel better?
Have you started using alcohol or drugs to help you relax, calm down, or feel better?

Safety (Savagery)
Have you ever been seriously injured? (How?) How about anyone else you know?
Do you always wear a seatbelt in the car?
Have you ever ridden with a driver who was drunk or high? When? How often?
Do you use safety equipment for sports and/or other physical activities (e.g., helmets for biking or skateboarding)?
Is there any violence in your home? Does the violence ever get physical?
Is there a lot of violence at your school? In your neighborhood? Among your friends?
Have you ever been physically or sexually abused? Have you ever been raped, on a date or at any other time? (If not asked previously)
Have you ever been in a car or motorcycle accident? (What happened?)
Have you ever been picked on or bullied? Is that still a problem?
Have you gotten into physical fights in school or your neighborhood? Are you still getting into fights?
Have you ever felt that you had to carry a knife, gun, or other weapon to protect yourself? Do you still feel that way?

Green = essential questions
Blue = as time permits
Red = optional or when situation requires

4-4

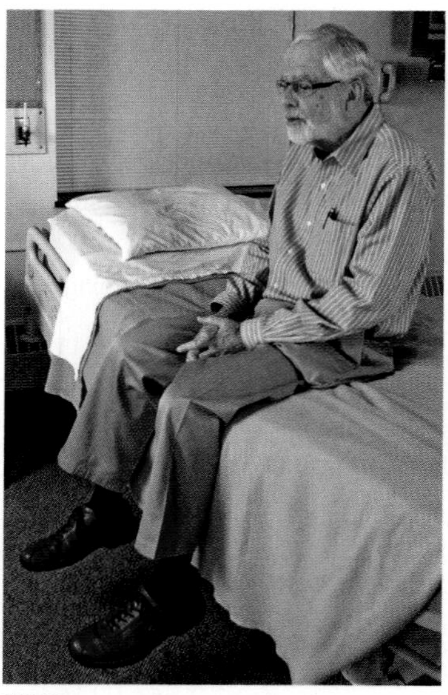

4-5

The Older Adult

This health history includes the same format as that described for the younger adult, as well as some additional questions. These questions address ways in which the ADLs may have been affected by normal aging processes or by the effects of chronic illness or disability. There is no specific age at which to ask these additional questions. Use them when it seems appropriate (Fig. 4-5).

It is important for you to recognize positive health measures: what the person has been doing to help himself or herself stay well and to live to an older age. Older people have spent a lifetime with a traditional health care system that searches only for pathology and what is wrong with their health. It may be a pleasant surprise to have a health professional affirm the things that they are "doing right" and to note health strengths.

As you study the following, keep in mind the format for the "younger" older adult. Only additional questions or a varying focus is addressed here.

Reason for Seeking Care

It may take time to figure out the reason that the older person has come in for an examination. An aging person may shrug off a symptom as evidence of growing old and may be unsure whether it is "worth mentioning." Also, some older people have a conservative philosophy toward their health status: "If it isn't broken, don't fix it." These people come for care only when something is disturbingly wrong.

An older person may have many chronic problems, such as diabetes, hypertension, or constipation. It is challenging to filter out what brought the person in this time. The final statement should be the *person's* reason for seeking care, not your assumption of what the problem is.

Past Health

General Health. Health state in the past 5 years.

Accidents or Injuries, Serious or Chronic Illnesses, Hospitalizations, Operations. These areas may produce lengthy responses, and the person probably will not relate them in chronologic order. Let the person talk freely; you can reorder the events later when you do the write-up. The amount of data included here can indicate the amount of stress the person has faced during his or her lifetime. This section of the history can be filled out at home or before the interview if the person's vision and writing ability are adequate. Then you can concentrate remaining time of the interview on reviewing pertinent data and on the present health of the person.

Last Examination. Most recent mammography, colonoscopy, and tonometry.

Obstetric Status. It is *not* necessary to collect a detailed account of each pregnancy and delivery if the woman has passed menopause and has no gynecologic symptoms. Merely record the number of pregnancies and the health of each newborn.

Current Medications. For each medication, record the name, purpose, and daily schedule. Does the person have a system to remember to take the medicine? Does medicine seem to work? Are there any side effects? If so, does the person feel like skipping medicine because of them? Also, consider the following issues:

- Some older persons take a large number of drugs, prescribed by different physicians.
- The person may not know the drug name or purpose. When this occurs, ask the person to bring in the drug to be identified.
- Is cost a problem? When the person is unable to afford a drug, he or she may decrease the dosage, take one pill instead of two, or not refill the empty bottle immediately.
- Is traveling to the pharmacy to refill a prescription a problem?
- Is the person taking any over-the-counter medications? Some people use a local pharmacist for self-treatment.
- Has the person ever shared medications with neighbors or friends? Some establish "lay referral" networks by comparing symptoms and thus medications.

Family History

This is not as useful in predicting which familial diseases the person may contract, because most of those will have occurred at an earlier age. But these data are useful to assess which diseases or causes of death of relatives the person has experienced. Also, it describes the person's existing social network.

Review of Systems

Remember that these are *additional* items to ask the older adult. Refer to the history for the younger adult for the basic list.

Eyes. Use of bifocal glasses, any trouble adjusting to far vision (problems with stairs).

Ears. Increased sensitivity to background noise and whether conversation sounds garbled or distorted.

Mouth. Use of dentures, when the person wears them (always, all day, only at meals, only at social occasions, or never), method of cleaning, any difficulty wearing the dentures (loose, pain, makes whistling or clicking noise), cracks at corners of the mouth.

Respiratory System. Shortness of breath and level of activity that produces it. Shortness of breath often is an early sign of cardiac dysfunction, but many older people dismiss it as "a cold" or getting "winded" because of old age.

Cardiovascular System. If chest pain occurs, the person may not feel it as intensely as a younger person may. Instead, the older adult may feel dyspnea on exertion.

Peripheral Vascular System. Wears constrictive clothing or garters or rolls stockings at knees. Any color change at feet or ankles.

Urinary System. Urinary retention, incomplete emptying, straining to urinate, change in force of stream. If a weakened stream occurs, men may note the need to stand closer to the toilet. Women may note incontinence when coughing, laughing, or sneezing.

Sexual Health. Ask about any changes in sexual relationship the person has experienced. Note for men it is normal for an erection to develop slowly. (See Chapter 24.) Note for women any vaginal dryness or pain with intercourse. Note for all whether aspects of sex are satisfactory and whether adequate privacy exists for a sexual relationship.

Musculoskeletal System. Gait change (balance, weakness, difficulty with steps, fear of falling), use of any assistive device (cane, walker). Any joint stiffness? During what part of the day does the stiffness occur? Does pain or stiffness occur with activity or rest?

Neurologic System. Any problem with memory (recent or remote) or disorientation (time of day, in what settings)?

Functional Assessment (Including Activities of Daily Living)

Functional assessment measures how a person manages day-to-day activities. For older people, the meaning of health becomes those activities that they can or cannot do. The *impact* of a disease on their daily activities and overall quality of life (called the *disease burden*) is more important to older people than the actual disease diagnosis or pathology. Thus the functional assessment—because it emphasizes function—is very important in assessing older people.

Many functional assessment instruments are available that objectively measure a person's present functional status and monitor any changes over time. Most instruments measure the performance of specific tasks such as the ADLs and IADLs. The Comprehensive Older Person's Evaluation (on the *Evolve* website) is particularly useful because it contains the basic ADL/IADL functional assessment as well as physical, social, psychological, demographic, financial, and legal issues.

Whether or not a standardized instrument is used, the following functional assessment questions are important additions to the older adult's health history.

Self-Concept, Self-Esteem. When the aging person was an adolescent, educational opportunities were not as available as they are today nor were they equally available for women. The aging person may be sensitive about having achieved only the level of elementary school education or less.

Occupation. Past positions, volunteer activities, and community activities. Many people continue to work past the age of 65; they grew up with a strong work ethic and are proud to continue. If the person is retired, how has he or she adjusted to the change in role? It may mean loss of social role or social status, loss of personal relationships formed at work, and reduced income.

Activity and Exercise. How does the person spend a typical day in work, hobbies, and leisure activities? Is there any day this routine changes (e.g., Sunday visits from family)? Note that the person suffering from chronic illness or disability may have a self-care deficit, musculoskeletal changes such as arthritis, and mental confusion.

List significant leisure activities, hobbies, sports, and community activities. Is there a community senior citizen center available for nutrition, social network, and screening of health status?

What are the type, amount, and frequency of the exercise? Is a warm-up included? How does the body respond?

Sleep and Rest. Usual sleep pattern: feel rested during the day? Is energy sufficient to carry out daily activities? Need naps? Is there a problem with night wakenings (nocturia, shortness of breath, light sleep, insomnia [difficulty falling asleep, awakening during night, early morning wakening])? If no routine, do you tend to nap all afternoon? Does insomnia worsen with lack of a daily schedule?

Nutrition/Elimination. Record a 24-hour recall. Is this typical of most days? (Nutrition may vary greatly. Ask the person to keep a weekly log to bring in.) What are the meal patterns? Are there three full meals or five or six smaller meals per day? How many convenience foods and soft foods are used? Who prepares meals? Eat alone? Who shops for food? How are groceries transported home? Is the income adequate for groceries? Is there a problem preparing meals (adequate vision, motor deficit, adequate energy)? Are the appliances and water and utilities adequate for meal preparation? Is there any difficulty chewing or swallowing? What are the food preferences (aging persons often eat high amounts of carbohydrates because these foods are cheaper, easier to make, and easier to chew)?

Interpersonal Relationships/Resources. Who else is at home with you? Live alone? Is this satisfactory? Have a pet? How close is family or friends? How often do you see family or friends? If infrequent, do you experience this as a loss?

Do you live with family, such as a spouse, children, or a sibling? Is this a satisfactory arrangement? What is the role in family for preparation of meals, housework, and other activities? Are there any conflicts?

On whom do you depend for emotional support? For help with problems? Who meets affection needs?

Coping and Stress Management. Has there been a recent change in lifestyle, such as loss of occupation, spouse, friends, move from home, illness of self or family member, or has income been decreased? How dealing with stress? If a loved one has died, how responding to the loss? "How do you feel about being 'alone' and having to take on unfamiliar responsibilities now?"

Environmental/Hazards. Home safety: one floor or are there stairs, state of repair, is money adequate to maintain home, exits for fire, heating and utilities adequate, how long in the present home? Transportation: own automobile, last driver's test, consider self a safe driver, income adequate for maintenance, public transportation access, receive drives from community resources, friends? Neighborhood: secure in personal safety at day or night; danger of loss of possessions; amount of noise and pollution; access to family and friends, grocery store, drug store, laundry, church, temple, mosque, health care facilities?

BIBLIOGRAPHY

1. American Academy of Pediatrics. *Recommended childhood and adolescent immunization schedule United States, 2006*. Accessed January 2010, from www.cispimmunize.org.

1a. Advisory Committee on Immunization Practices. (2010). Recommended adult immunization schedule: United States, 2010. *Annals of Internal Medicine, 152*(1), 36-39.

2. Bennett, R. L., Steinhaus, K. A., Uhrich, S. B., et al. (1995). Recommendations for standardized human pedigree nomenclature. Pedigree Standardization Task Force of the National Society of Genetic Counselors. *American Journal of Human Genetics, 56*(3), 745-752.

3. Carlson, L. H. (2007). Immunization update: Neonates to adolescents. *Nurse Practitioner, 32*(3), 49-56.

4. Ewing, J. A. (1984). Detecting alcoholism: The CAGE questionnaire. *Journal of the American Medical Association, 252*, 1905-1907.

5. Goldenring, J. M., & Rosen, D. S. (2004). Getting into adolescent heads: An essential update. *Contemporary Pediatrics, 21*(1), 64-75.

6. Gordon, M. (2002). *Manual of nursing diagnosis.* (10th ed.) St Louis: Mosby.

7. Hanson, C., Novilla, M. L. B., Barnes, M. D., et al. (2007). Using family health history for chronic disease prevention in the age of genomics: translation to health education practice. *American Journal of Health Education, 38*(4), 219-229.

8. Hinton, R. B. (2008). The family history: Reemergence of an established tool. *Critical Care Nursing Clinics of North America, 20*(2), 149-158.

9. Johnson, A. (2009). What's your food allergy familiarity? *Nurse Practitioner, 34*(4), 29-35.

10. McNeill, J. A., Cook, J., Mahon, M., et al. (2008). Family history: Value-added information in assessing cardiac health. *American Association of Occupational Health Nurses Journal, 56*(7), 297-306.

10a. Post, S. G., Puchalski, C. M., Larson, D. B., et al. (2000). Physician and patient spirituality: Professional boundaries, competency, and ethics. *Annals of Internal Medicine, 132*, 578-583.

11. Reece, S. M. (2006). The 3rd National Family History Initiative: Thanksgiving 2006. *Nurse Practitioner, 31*(11), 57-59, 2006.

12. The Joint Commission (formerly JCAHO). *Hospitals, language, and culture: A snapshot of the nation.* Accessed August 2010 from www.jointcommission.org/PatientSafety/HLC/.

13. Zurakowski, T. (2009). The practicalities and pitfalls of polypharmacy. *Nurse Practitioner, 34*(4), 36-41.

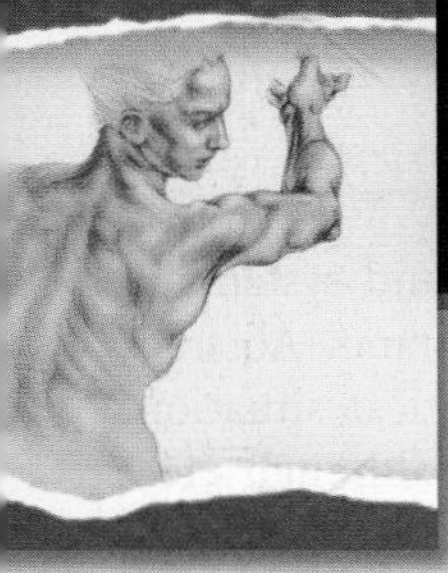

CHAPTER 5

Mental Status Assessment

evolve WEBSITE

http://evolve.elsevier.com/Jarvis/

- Animations
- Audio Key Points
- Bedside Assessment Summary Checklist
- Case Study
  Mood Assessment
- Health Promotion Guide
  Depression
- NCLEX Review Questions
- Physical Examination Summary Checklist
- Quick Assessment for Common Conditions
  Alzheimer Disease
  Depression

OUTLINE

Structure and Function, 71

Defining Mental Status
Components of the Mental Status Examination

Objective Data, 73

Appearance
Behavior
Cognitive Functions
Thought Processes and Perceptions
Supplemental Mental Status Examination
Summary Checklist: Mental Status Assessment

Documentation and Critical Thinking, 82

Abnormal Findings, 83

Abnormal Findings for Advanced Practice, 86

STRUCTURE AND FUNCTION

DEFINING MENTAL STATUS

Mental status is a person's emotional (feeling) and cognitive (knowing) function. Optimal functioning aims toward simultaneous life satisfaction in work, in caring relationships, and within the self. Mental health is relative and ongoing. Everyone has "good" days and "bad" days. Usually, mental status strikes a balance, allowing the person to function socially and occupationally.

The stress surrounding a traumatic life event (death of a loved one, serious illness) tips the balance, causing transient dysfunction. This is an expected response to a trauma. Mental status assessment during a traumatic life event can identify remaining strengths and can help the individual mobilize resources and use coping skills.

A **mental disorder** is apparent when a person's response is much greater than the expected reaction to a traumatic life event. A mental disorder is defined as a significant behavioral or psychological *pattern* that is associated with distress (a painful symptom) or disability (impaired functioning) and has a significant risk of pain, disability, or death or a loss of freedom.[2] Mental disorders include **organic disorders** (due to brain disease of *known* specific organic cause [e.g., delirium, dementia, alcohol and drug intoxication and withdrawal]) and **psychiatric mental illness** (in which an organic etiology has not yet been established [e.g., anxiety disorder or schizophrenia]). Mental status assessment documents a dysfunction and determines how that dysfunction affects self-care in everyday life.

Mental status cannot be scrutinized directly like the characteristics of skin or heart sounds. Its functioning is *inferred* through assessment of an individual's behaviors:

Consciousness: Being aware of one's own existence, feelings, and thoughts and aware of the environment. This is the most elementary of mental status functions.

Language: Using the voice to communicate one's thoughts and feelings. This is a basic tool of humans, and its loss has a heavy social impact on the individual.

Mood and affect: Both of these elements deal with the prevailing feelings; **affect** is a temporary expression of feelings or state of mind, and **mood** is more durable, a prolonged display of feelings that color the whole emotional life.

Orientation: The awareness of the objective world in relation to the self.

Attention: The power of concentration, the ability to focus on one specific thing without being distracted by many environmental stimuli.

Memory: The ability to lay down and store experiences and perceptions for later recall. *Recent* memory evokes day-to-day events; *remote* memory brings up years' worth of experiences.

Abstract reasoning: Pondering a deeper meaning beyond the concrete and literal.

Thought process: The *way* a person thinks, the logical train of thought.

Thought content: *What* the person thinks—specific ideas, beliefs, the use of words.

Perceptions: An awareness of objects through the five senses.

DEVELOPMENTAL COMPETENCE

Infants and Children

Emotional and cognitive functioning mature progressively from simple reflex behavior into complex logical and abstract thought. It is difficult to separate and trace the development of just one aspect of mental status. All aspects are interdependent. For example, consciousness is rudimentary at birth because the cerebral cortex is not yet developed; the infant cannot distinguish the self from the mother's body. Consciousness gradually develops along with language so that by 18 to 24 months, the child learns that he or she is separate from objects in the environment and has words to express this. We also can trace language development: from the differentiated crying at 4 weeks, the cooing at 6 weeks, through one-word sentences at 1 year to multi-word sentences at 2 years. Yet the concept of language as a social tool of communication occurs around 4 to 5 years of age, coincident with the child's readiness to play cooperatively with other children.

Attention gradually increases in span through preschool years so that by school age, most children are able to sit and concentrate on their work for a period of time. Some children are late in developing concentration. School readiness coincides with the development of the thought process; around age 7 years, thinking becomes more logical and systematic and the child is able to reason and understand. Abstract thinking, the ability to consider a hypothetical situation, usually develops between ages 12 and 15 years, although a few adolescents never achieve it.

The Aging Adult

The aging process leaves the parameters of mental status mostly intact. There is no decrease in general knowledge and little or no loss in vocabulary. Response time is slower than in youth; it takes a bit longer for the brain to process information and react to it. Thus performance on timed intelligence tests may be lower for the aging person—not because intelligence has declined, but because it takes longer to respond to the questions. The slower response time affects new learning; if a new presentation is rapidly paced, the older person does not have time to respond to it.[4]

Recent memory, which requires some processing (e.g., medication instructions, 24-hour diet recall, names of new acquaintances), is somewhat decreased with aging. Remote memory is not affected.

Age-related changes in sensory perception can affect mental status. For example, vision loss (as detailed in Chapter 14) may result in apathy, social isolation, and depression. Hearing changes are common in older adults (see the discussion of presbycusis in Chapter 15). Age-related hearing loss involves high-frequency sounds. Consonants are high-frequency sounds, so older people who have difficulty hearing them have problems with normal conversation. This problem produces frustration, suspicion, and social isolation and makes the person look confused.

The era of older adulthood contains more potential for loss than do earlier eras, such as loss of loved ones, loss of job status and prestige, loss of income, and loss of an energetic and resilient body. Also, living with chronic diseases (heart failure, cancer, diabetes, osteoporosis) includes the fear of loss of life itself. The grief and despair surrounding these losses can affect mental status. These losses can result in disorientation, disability, or depression.

COMPONENTS OF THE MENTAL STATUS EXAMINATION

The full mental status examination is a systematic check of emotional and cognitive functioning. The steps described here, however, rarely need to be taken in their entirety. Usually, you can assess mental status through the context of the health history interview. During that time, keep in mind the four main headings of mental status assessment:

Appearance, **Behavior**, **Cognition**,
and **Thought processes**, or
A, B, C, T

Integrating the mental status examination into the health history interview is sufficient for most people. You will collect ample data to be able to assess mental health strengths and coping skills and to screen for any dysfunction.

It is necessary to perform a full mental status examination when you discover any abnormality in affect or behavior, and in the following situations:

- Patients whose initial brief screening suggests an anxiety disorder or depression.
- Family members concerned about a person's behavioral changes, such as memory loss, inappropriate social interaction.
- Brain lesions (trauma, tumor, brain attack [also known as *cerebrovascular accident* or *stroke*]). A mental status assessment documents any emotional or cognitive change associated with the lesion. Not recognizing these changes hinders care planning and creates problems with social readjustment.
- Aphasia (the impairment of language ability secondary to brain damage). A mental status examination assesses language dysfunction as well as any emotional problems associated with it, such as depression or agitation.
- Symptoms of psychiatric mental illness, especially with acute onset.

In every mental status examination, note these factors from the health history that could affect your interpretation of the findings:

- Any known illnesses or health problems, such as alcoholism or chronic renal disease.
- Current medications whose side effects may cause confusion or depression.
- The usual educational and behavioral level—note that factor as the normal baseline, and do not expect performance on the mental status examination to exceed it.
- Responses to personal history questions, indicating current stress, social interaction patterns, sleep habits, drug and alcohol use.

In the following examination, the sequence of steps forms a *hierarchy* in which the most basic functions (consciousness, language) are assessed first. The first steps must be accurately assessed to ensure validity for the steps to follow. That is, if consciousness is clouded, then the person cannot be expected to have full attention and to cooperate with new learning. Or, if language is impaired, subsequent assessment of new learning or abstract reasoning (anything that requires language functioning) can give erroneous conclusions.

OBJECTIVE DATA

EQUIPMENT NEEDED

(Occasionally)
Pencil, paper, reading material

Normal Range of Findings	Abnormal Findings
APPEARANCE	
Posture. *Posture* is erect, and *position* is relaxed.	Sitting on edge of chair or curled in bed, tense muscles, frowning, darting watchful eyes, restless pacing occur with anxiety and with hyperthyroidism. Sitting slumped in chair, slow walk, dragging feet occur with depression and some organic brain diseases.
Body Movements. *Body movements* are voluntary, deliberate, coordinated, and smooth and even.	Restless, fidgety movements or hyperkinetic appearance occurs with anxiety. Apathy and psychomotor slowing occur with depression and dementia. Abnormal posturing and bizarre gestures occur with schizophrenia. Facial grimaces.
Dress. *Dress* is appropriate for setting, season, age, gender, and social group. Clothing fits and is put on appropriately.	Inappropriate dress can occur with organic brain syndrome. Eccentric dress combination and bizarre makeup occur with schizophrenia or manic syndrome.

Normal Range of Findings	Abnormal Findings
Grooming and Hygiene. The person is clean and well groomed; hair is neat and clean; women have moderate or no makeup; men are shaved, or beard or mustache is well groomed. Nails are clean (although some jobs leave nails chronically dirty). Note: A disheveled appearance in a previously well-groomed person is significant. Use care in interpreting clothing that is disheveled, bizarre, or in poor repair, piercings, and tattoos, because these sometimes reflect the person's economic status or a deliberate fashion trend (especially among adolescents).	Unilateral neglect (total inattention to one side of body) occurs following some cerebrovascular accidents. Inappropriate dress, poor hygiene, and lack of concern with appearance occur with depression and severe Alzheimer disease. Meticulously dressed and groomed appearance and fastidious manner may occur with obsessive-compulsive disorders.

BEHAVIOR

Normal Range of Findings	Abnormal Findings
Level of Consciousness. The person is awake, alert, aware of stimuli from the environment and within the self, and responds appropriately and reasonably soon to stimuli.	Loses track of conversation, falls asleep. Lethargic (drowsy), obtunded (confused) (see Table 5-3, Levels of Consciousness, p. 83).
Facial Expression. The look is appropriate to the situation and changes appropriately with the topic. There is comfortable eye contact unless precluded by cultural norm (e.g., American Indian).	Flat, masklike expression occurs with parkinsonism and with depression.
Speech. Judge the quality of speech by noting that the person makes laryngeal sounds effortlessly and shares conversation appropriately.	Dysphonia is abnormal volume, pitch (see Table 5-4, Speech Disorders, p. 84). Monopolizes interview. Silent, secretive, or uncommunicative.
The pace of the conversation is moderate, and stream of talking is fluent.	Slow, monotonous speech with parkinsonism, depression. Rapid-fire, pressured, and loud talking occurs with manic syndrome.
Articulation (ability to form words) is clear and understandable.	Dysarthria is distorted speech (see Table 5-4). Misuses words; omits letters, syllables, or words; transposes words; occurs with aphasia. Circumlocution, or repetitious abnormal patterns: neologism, echolalia (see Table 5-6, p. 86).
Word choice is effortless and appropriate to educational level. The person completes sentences, occasionally pausing to think.	Unduly long word-finding or failure in word search occurs with aphasia.
Mood and Affect. Judge this by body language and facial expression and by asking directly, "How do you feel today," or "How do you usually feel?" The mood should be appropriate to the person's place and condition and change appropriately with topics. The person is willing to cooperate with you.	See Table 5-5, Abnormalities of Mood and Affect. Wide mood swings occur with manic syndrome. Bizarre mood is apparent in schizophrenia.

COGNITIVE FUNCTIONS

Orientation. You can discern orientation through the course of the interview by asking about the person's address, phone number, health history. Or ask for it directly, using tact, "Some people have trouble keeping up with the dates while in the hospital. Do you know today's date?" Assess:

Normal Range of Findings	Abnormal Findings
Time: Day of week, date, year, season *Place: Where person lives, present location, type of building, name of city and state* *Person: Own name, age, who examiner is, type of worker* Many hospitalized people normally have trouble with the exact date but are fully oriented on the remaining items.	Disorientation occurs with delirium and dementia. Orientation is usually lost in this order—first to time, then to place, and rarely to person.
Attention Span. Check the person's ability to concentrate by noting whether he or she completes a thought without wandering. Note any distractibility or difficulty attending to you. Or give a series of directions to follow and note the correct sequence of behaviors, such as "Please take this glass of water with your left hand, drink from it, shift it to your right hand, and set it on the table." Note that attention span commonly is impaired in people who are anxious, fatigued, or drug intoxicated.	Digression from initial thought. Irrelevant replies to questions. Easily distracted; "stimulus bound" (i.e., any new stimulus quickly draws attention). Confusion, negativism.
Recent Memory. Assess recent memory in the context of the interview by the 24-hour diet recall or by asking the time the person arrived at the agency. Ask questions you can corroborate. This screens for the occasional person who confabulates or makes up answers to fill in the gaps of memory loss.	Recent memory deficit occurs with delirium, dementia, amnestic syndrome, or Korsakoff's syndrome in chronic alcoholism.
Remote Memory. In the context of the interview, ask the person verifiable past events; for example, ask to describe past health, the first job, birthday and anniversary dates, and historical events that are relevant for that person.	Remote memory is lost when cortical storage area for that memory is damaged (e.g., Alzheimer dementia or any disease that damages the cerebral cortex).
New Learning—The Four Unrelated Words Test. This tests the person's ability to lay down new memories. It is a highly sensitive and valid memory test. It requires more effort than does the recall of personal or historic events. It also avoids the danger of unverifiable material. To the person, say, "I am going to say four words. I want you to remember them. In a few minutes I will ask you to recall them." To be sure the person has understood, have the words repeated. Pick four words with semantic and phonetic diversity: 1. brown / 1. fun 2. honesty / 2. carrot 3. tulip / 3. ankle 4. eyedropper / 4. loyalty	
After 5 minutes, ask for the recall of the four words. To test the duration of memory, ask for a recall at 10 minutes and at 30 minutes. The normal response for persons younger than 60 years is an accurate three- or four-word recall after a 5-, 10-, and 30-minute delay.[33]	People with Alzheimer dementia score a zero- or one-word recall. Impaired new learning ability also occurs with anxiety (due to inattention and distractibility) and depression (due to lack of effort mobilized to remember).
Additional Testing for Persons with Aphasia	
Word Comprehension. Point to articles in the room, parts of the body, articles from pockets, and ask the person to name them.	Aphasia is the loss of the ability to speak or write coherently or to understand speech or writing, due to a brain attack (see Table 5-4, Speech Disorders).
Reading. Ask the person to read available print. Be aware that reading is related to educational level. Use caution that you are not just testing literacy.	
Writing. Ask the person to make up and write a sentence. Note coherence, spelling, and parts of speech (the sentence should have a subject and a verb).	Reading and writing are important in planning health teaching and rehabilitation.

Objective Data

Normal Range of Findings	Abnormal Findings

Higher Intellectual Function

These tests measure problem-solving and reasoning abilities. Results are closely related to the person's general intelligence and must be assessed considering educational and cultural background. Tests of higher intellectual functioning have been used to discriminate between organic brain disease and psychiatric disorders; errors on the tests indicate organic dysfunction.

Although they have been widely used, there is little evidence that most of these tests are valid in detecting organic brain disease. Furthermore, most of these tests have little relevance for daily clinical care. Thus many time-honored, standard tests of higher intellectual function are not discussed here, such as fund of general knowledge, digit span repetition, calculation, proverb interpretation and similarities to test abstract reasoning, or hypothetical situations to test judgment.

Judgment

A person exercises judgment when he or she can compare and evaluate the alternatives in a situation and reach an appropriate course of action. Rather than testing the person's response to a hypothetical situation (e.g., "What would you do if you found a stamped, addressed envelope lying on the sidewalk?"), you should be more interested in the person's judgment about daily or long-term life goals, the likelihood of acting in response to delusions or hallucinations, and the capacity for violent or suicidal behavior.

To assess judgment in the context of the interview, note what the person says about job plans, social or family obligations, and plans for the future. Job and future plans should be realistic, considering the person's health situation. Also, ask the person to describe the rationale for personal health care and how he or she decided about whether or not to comply with prescribed health regimens. The person's actions and decisions should be realistic.

Impaired judgment (unrealistic or impulsive decisions, wish fulfillment) occurs with mental retardation, emotional dysfunction, schizophrenia, and organic brain disease.

THOUGHT PROCESSES AND PERCEPTIONS

Thought Processes. Ask yourself, "Does this person make sense? Can I follow what the person is saying?" The *way* a person thinks should be logical, goal directed, coherent, and relevant. The person should complete a thought.

Illogical, unrealistic thought processes. Digression from initial thought. Ideas run together. Evidence of blocking (person stops in middle of thought) (see Table 5-6, Abnormalities of Thought Process).

Thought Content. *What* the person says should be consistent and logical.

Obsessions, compulsions (see Table 5-7, Abnormalities of Thought Content).

Perceptions. The person should be consistently aware of reality. The perceptions should be congruent with yours. Ask the following questions:

- How do people treat you?
- Do other people talk about you?
- Do you feel like you are being watched, followed, or controlled?
- Is your imagination very active?
- Have you heard your name when alone?

Illusions, hallucinations (see Table 5-8, Abnormalities of Perception). Auditory and visual hallucinations occur with psychiatric and organic brain disease and with psychedelic drugs. Tactile hallucinations occur with alcohol withdrawal.

Normal Range of Findings | **Abnormal Findings**

GAD-7

Over the last 2 weeks, how often have you been bothered by the following problems?	Not at all	Several days	More than half the days	Nearly every day
1. Feeling nervous, anxious or on edge	0	1	2	3
2. Not being able to stop or control worrying	0	1	2	3
3. Worrying too much about different things	0	1	2	3
4. Trouble relaxing	0	1	2	3
5. Being so restless that it is hard to sit still	0	1	2	3
6. Becoming easily annoyed or irritable	0	1	2	3
7. Feeling afraid as if something awful might happen	0	1	2	3

Total score ___ = Add columns ___ + ___ + ___

If you checked off any problems, how difficult have these problems made it for you to do your work, take care of things at home, or get along with other people?

Not difficult at all	Somewhat difficult	Very difficult	Extremely difficult
☐	☐	☐	☐

5-1 Screen for anxiety symptoms.

Screen for Anxiety Disorders. Anxiety and depression are the two most common mental health problems seen in people seeking general medical care. Anxiety disorders are common, disabling, and often untreated. However, you can screen for core anxiety symptoms by asking the first two questions from the 7-item GAD scale listed in Fig. 5-1.[22] Scores on this GAD subscale range from 0 to 6; a score of 0 suggests no anxiety disorder is present.

If these first 2 items yield positive results, Kroenke et al.[22] suggest following with the other 5 items. The full scale identifies probable presentations of GAD and also is a severity measure in that increasing scores are associated with increasing impairment and disability.[31]

The four most common anxiety disorders: generalized anxiety disorder (GAD), panic disorder, social anxiety disorder, posttraumatic stress disorder (PTSD) (see Table 5-12, Anxiety Disorders).

A score of 10 on the GAD-7 identifies GAD; scores of 5, 10, and 15 represent mild, moderate, and severe levels of anxiety.

Screen for Depression. There are many formal screening tools available. However, a shorter method, simply asking two simple questions about depressed mood and anhedonia (little interest or pleasure in doing things) will detect a majority of depressed patients.[35] Thus you can ask: "Over the past 2 weeks, have you felt down, depressed, or hopeless? And "Over the past 2 weeks, have you felt little interest or pleasure in doing things?"

Finding positive answers to these questions then requires further diagnostic interviews that use criteria such as the DSM-IV-TR to assess specific depressive disorders (see Table 5-11, Mood Disorders, p. 89).

Screen for Suicidal Thoughts. When the person expresses feelings of sadness, hopelessness, despair, or grief, it is important to assess any possible risk of physical harm to himself or herself. Begin with more general questions. If you hear affirmative answers, continue with more specific questions:

Suicide is a preventable health problem; it is the 11th leading cause of death in the United States and the third leading cause of death in young people ages 10 to 24 years.[28]

Normal Range of Findings	Abnormal Findings

- Have you ever felt so blue you thought of hurting yourself?
- Do you feel like hurting yourself now?
- Do you have a plan to hurt yourself?
- How would you do it?
- What would happen if you were dead?
- How would other people react if you were dead?

It is very difficult to question people about possible suicidal wishes, especially for beginning examiners. Examiners fear invading privacy and may have their own normal denial of death and suicide. However, the risk is far greater if you skip these questions when you have the slightest clue that they are appropriate. You may be the only health professional to pick up clues of suicide risk. You are responsible for encouraging the person to talk about suicidal thoughts.

Depression is painful and debilitating, and sometimes a depressed person really wishes to kill himself or herself. However, the majority of suicidal people are ambivalent, and for them, you can buy time so they can be helped to find an alternate route to the stressful situation. Promptly share any concerns you have about a person's suicide ideation with a mental health professional.

A precise suicide plan to take place in the next 24 to 48 hours using a lethal method constitutes high risk. Important clues and warning signs of suicide:

- Prior suicide attempts
- Depression, hopelessness
- Firearms in the home
- Family history of suicide
- Incarceration
- Family violence including physical or sexual abuse
- Self-mutilation
- Anorexia
- Verbal suicide messages (defeat, failure, worthlessness, loss, giving up, desire to kill self)
- Death themes in art, jokes, writing, behaviors
- Saying goodbye (giving away prized possessions)

Additional content on mental disorders is listed in Table 5-9, Schizophrenia; Table 5-10, Delirium, Dementia, and Amnestic Disorders; Table 5-11, Mood Disorders; and Table 5-12, Anxiety Disorders.

Objective Data

SUPPLEMENTAL MENTAL STATUS EXAMINATION

The Mini-Mental State is a simplified scored form of the cognitive functions of the mental status examination (memory, orientation to time and place, naming, reading, copying or visuospatial orientation, writing, and the ability to follow a three-stage command)[10,13] (Table 5-1).

The Mini-Mental State Examination (MMSE) quick and easy, includes a standard set of only 11 questions, and requires only 5 to 10 minutes to administer. It is useful for both initial and serial measurement, so you can demonstrate

Table 5-1 Sample Items from the Mini-Mental State Examination (MMSE)

ORIENTATION TO TIME
"What is the date?"

REGISTRATION
"Listen carefully, I am going to say three words. You say them back after I stop.
Ready? Here they are ...
HOUSE (pause), CAR (pause), LAKE (pause). Now repeat those words back to me."
(Repeat up to five times, but score only the first trial.)

NAMING
"What is this?" (Point to a pencil or pen.)

READING
"Please read this and do what it says." (Show examinee the words on the stimulus forms.)
CLOSE YOUR EYES

Normal Range of Findings	Abnormal Findings

worsening or improvement of cognition over time and with treatment. It concentrates only on cognitive functioning, not on mood or thought processes. It is a valid detector of organic disease; thus it is a good screening tool to detect dementia and delirium and to differentiate these from psychiatric mental illness.

The maximum score on the test is 30; people with normal mental status average 27. Scores between 24 and 30 indicate no cognitive impairment.

Scores that occur with dementia and delirium are classified as follows: 18-23 = mild cognitive impairment; 0-7 = severe cognitive impairment.

DEVELOPMENTAL COMPETENCE

Infants and Children

The mental status assessment of infants and children covers behavioral, cognitive, and psychosocial development and examines how the child is coping with his or her environment. Essentially, you will follow the same A-B-C-T guidelines as for the adult, with special consideration for developmental milestones. Your best examination "technique" arises from thorough knowledge of developmental milestones. Abnormalities are often problems of *omission;* the child does not achieve a milestone you would expect.

The parent's health history, especially the sections on the developmental history and personal history, yields most of the mental status data.

In addition, the **Denver II screening** test gives you a chance to interact directly with the young child to assess mental status. The Denver II is designed to detect developmental delays in infants and preschoolers within four functions: gross motor, language, fine motor–adaptive, and personal-social skills. For mental status assessment, the Denver II helps identify young children who may be slow in development in behavioral, language, cognitive, and psychosocial areas. The test has 125 items arranged in chronologic order and displayed in groupings corresponding to recommended ages for health maintenance visits.

Denver II scoring avoids diagnostic labeling (e.g., mental retardation, language disorder). Instead, the child's performance is scored either "normal," "abnormal," or "questionable."

For school-age children, ages 7 to 11, who have grown beyond the age when developmental milestones are very useful, the "Behavioral Checklist" (Table 5-2) is an additional tool that can be given to the parent along with the history. It covers five major areas: mood, play, school, friends, and family relations. It is easy to administer and lasts about 5 minutes.

TABLE 5-2 Behavioral Checklist

1. Prefers to play alone
2. Gets hurt in major accidents
3. Does he/she ever play with fire?
4. Has difficulties with teachers
5. Gets poor grades in school
6. Is absent from school
7. Becomes angry easily
8. Daydreams
9. Feels unhappy
10. Acts younger than other children his/her age
11. Does not listen to parents
12. Does not tell the truth
13. Unsure of himself/herself
14. Has trouble sleeping
15. Seems afraid of someone or something
16. Is nervous and jumpy
17. Has a nervous habit
18. Does not show feelings
19. Fights with other children
20. Is understanding of other people's feelings
21. Refuses to share
22. Shows jealousy
23. Takes things that are not his/hers
24. Blames others for his/her troubles
25. Prefers to play with children not his/her age
26. Gets along well with grownups
27. Teases others

Scoring is a point system: 0—never; 1—sometimes; 2—often. Scoring is reversed for items 20 and 26. Scores between 15 and 22 indicate closer following; scores above 22 warrant psychiatric evaluation.

From Jellinek, M., Evans, N., & Knight, R. (1979). Use of a behavior checklist on a pediatric inpatient unit. *Journal of Pediatrics,* 94,156-158.

Normal Range of Findings	Abnormal Findings

For the adolescent, follow the same A-B-C-T guidelines as described for the adult.

The Aging Adult

It is important to conduct even a brief examination of all older people admitted to the hospital. Confusion is common in aging people and is easily misdiagnosed. Up to 25% of older adults are hospitalized with acute delirium, and up to 56% develop acute delirium during their hospitalization.[21a] In comparison, about 10% of adults older than 65 years and 50% of adults older than 90 years have chronic dementia.[1]

Delirium is an acute confusional change or loss of consciousness and perceptual disturbance, may accompany acute illness (e.g., pneumonia, alcohol/drug intoxication), and is usually resolved when the underlying cause is treated.

In contrast, **dementia** is a gradual progressive process, causing decreased cognitive function, even though the person is fully conscious and awake, and is not reversible. Alzheimer disease accounts for about two thirds of cases of dementia in older adults (see Table 5-10). Dementia is not part of normal aging.

Check sensory status before assessing any aspect of mental status. Vision and hearing changes due to aging may alter alertness and leave the person looking confused. When older people cannot hear your questions, they may test worse than they actually are. Older people with psychiatric mental illness test significantly better when wearing hearing aids.

Follow the same A-B-C-T guidelines as described for the younger adult with these *additional* considerations:

Objective Data

Behavior

Level of Consciousness. In a hospital or extended care setting, the Glasgow Coma Scale (see Chapter 23) is a quantitative tool that is useful in testing consciousness in aging persons in whom confusion is common. It gives a numerical value to the person's response in eye-opening, best verbal response, and best motor response. This system avoids ambiguity when numerous examiners care for the same person.

Cognitive Functions

Orientation. Many aging persons experience social isolation, loss of structure without a job, a change in residence, or some short-term memory loss. These factors affect orientation, and this person may not provide the precise date or complete name of agency. You may consider aging persons oriented if they know *generally* where they are and the present period. That is, consider them oriented to time if the year and month are correctly stated. Orientation to place is accepted with the correct identification of the type of setting (e.g., the hospital) and the name of the town.

New Learning. In people of normal cognitive function, an age-related decline occurs in performance in the Four Unrelated Words Test described on p. 75. Persons in the eighth decade average two of four words recalled over 5

Normal Range of Findings	Abnormal Findings
minutes. They will improve their performance at 10 and 30 minutes after being reminded by verbal cues (e.g., "one word was a color; a common flower in Holland is ____________________").	People with Alzheimer dementia do not improve their performance on subsequent trials.

Supplemental Mental Status Examination

The Mini-Cog. Because the Mini-Mental State Examination described earlier is available only by copyright, the Mini-Cog is a newly developed, reliable, quick, and easily available instrument to screen for cognitive impairment in otherwise healthy older adults (Fig. 5-2).[5,7] It can be used with various language, culture, and literacy levels and takes only 3 to 5 minutes to administer.

The Mini-Cog consists of a 3-item recall test and a clock-drawing test. Begin by asking the older adult to listen carefully to, remember, and then repeat three words that you will say. Make sure the person can hear you and that no distracting noises are present. Keep the words short and unrelated: *"Listen carefully, I am going to say three words. You say them back after I stop. Ready? Cup (pause), train (pause), blue. Now repeat those words to me. Good."* Next, give the adult a blank sheet of paper, saying, *"Now I want you to draw the face of a clock and write the numbers on the clock face. That is fine. Next, I want you to draw the hands of the clock so it shows the time of 11:10." "Remember the three words I told you earlier? Now I want you to repeat them."*

The Mini-Cog tests the person's executive function, including the ability to plan, manage time, organize activities, and manage working memory.[11] A person with no cognitive impairment or dementia can recall all three words and can draw a complete, round, closed clock circle, with all face numbers present and in correct position and sequence, and with the hour and minute hands indicating the time you requested.

Abnormal Findings: Recalling 1 or 2 words indicates possible dementia; recalling none of the words indicates dementia. Drawing an abnormal clock (numbers misplaced, crowded, or out of sequence; short hour hand or long minute hand in wrong spot) indicates cognitive impairment.

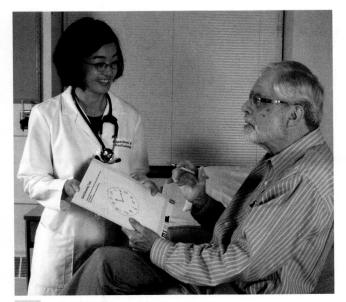

5-2 Clock drawing for the Mini-Cog.

DOCUMENTATION AND CRITICAL THINKING

Sample Charting

Appearance: Person's posture is erect, with no involuntary body movements. Dress and grooming are appropriate for season and setting.

Behavior: Person is alert, with appropriate facial expression and with fluent, understandable speech. Affect and verbal responses are appropriate.

Cognitive functions: Oriented to time, person, place. Able to attend cooperatively with examiner. Recent and remote memory intact. Can recall four unrelated words at 5-, 10-, and 30-minute testing intervals. Future plans include returning to home and to local university once individual therapy is established and medication is adjusted.

Thought processes: Perceptions and thought processes are logical and coherent. No suicide ideation.

Score on Mini-Mental State Examination is 28.

Focused Assessment: Clinical Case Study

Lola P. is a 79-year-old married, white woman, with a recent hospitalization for evaluation of increasing memory loss, confusion, and socially inappropriate behavior. Her family reports that Mrs. P.'s hygiene and grooming have decreased; she eats very little and has lost weight, does not sleep through the night, has angry emotional outbursts that are unlike her former demeanor, and does not recognize her younger grandchildren. Her husband reports that she has drifted away from the stove while cooking, allowing food to burn on the stovetop. He has found her wandering through the house in the middle of the night, unsure of where she was. She used to "talk on the phone for hours" but now he has to push her into conversations. During this hospitalization, Mrs. P. has undergone a series of medical tests, including a negative lumbar puncture test, normal electroencephalogram (EEG), and a benign head computed tomography (CT) scan. Her physician now suggests a diagnosis of Alzheimer dementia.

Appearance: Sitting quietly, somewhat slumped, picking on loose threads on her dress. Hooded, zippered sweatshirt top worn over dress. Hair is gathered in loose ponytail with stray wisps. No makeup.

Behavior: Awake and gazing at hands and lap. Expression is flat and vacant. Will make eye contact when called by name, although gaze quickly shifts back to lap. Speech is a bit slow but articulate; some trouble with word choice.

Cognitive functions: Oriented to person and place. Can state the season but not the day of the week or the year. Is not able to repeat the correct sequence of complex directions involving lifting and shifting glass of water to the other hand. Scores a one-word recall on the Four Unrelated Words Test. Cannot tell examiner how she would plan a grocery shopping trip.

Thought processes: Experiences blocking in train of thought. Thought content is logical. Acts cranky and suspicious with family members. No suicide ideation.

Mini-Mental State Examination score is 17 and shows poor recall ability and marked difficulty with serial 7s.

ASSESSMENT

Chronic confusion
Impaired social interaction
Impaired memory
Wandering

ABNORMAL FINDINGS

TABLE 5-3 Levels of Consciousness

These terms are commonly used in clinical practice. They spread over a continuum from full alertness to deep coma. The terms are qualitative and therefore are not always reliable. (A *quantitative* tool that serves the same purpose and eliminates ambiguity is the Glasgow Coma Scale in Chapter 23.) These terms are widely accepted, however, and are useful as long as all co-workers agree on definitions and are consistent in their application. To increase clarity when using these terms, record also:

1. The level of stimulus used, ranging progressively from
   a. Name called in normal tone of voice
   b. Name called in loud voice
   c. Light touch on person's arm
   d. Vigorous shake of shoulder
   e. Pain applied
2. The person's response
   a. Amount and quality of movement
   b. Presence and coherence of speech
   c. Opening of eyes and making eye contact
3. What the person does on cessation of your stimulus

(1) Alert
Awake or readily aroused, oriented, fully aware of external and internal stimuli and responds appropriately, conducts meaningful interpersonal interactions.

(2) Lethargic (or Somnolent)
Not fully alert, drifts off to sleep when not stimulated, can be aroused to name when called in normal voice but looks drowsy, responds appropriately to questions or commands but thinking seems slow and fuzzy, inattentive, loses train of thought, spontaneous movements are decreased.

(3) Obtunded
(Transitional state between lethargy and stupor; some sources omit this level.)
Sleeps most of time, difficult to arouse—needs loud shout or vigorous shake, acts confused when is aroused, converses in monosyllables, speech may be mumbled and incoherent, requires constant stimulation for even marginal cooperation.

(4) Stupor or Semi-Coma
Spontaneously unconscious, responds only to persistent and vigorous shake or pain; has appropriate motor response (i.e., withdraws hand to avoid pain); otherwise can only groan, mumble, or move restlessly; reflex activity persists.

(5) Coma
Completely unconscious, no response to pain or to any external or internal stimuli (e.g., when suctioned, does not try to push the catheter away), light coma has some reflex activity but no purposeful movement, deep coma has no motor response.

Acute Confusional State (Delirium)
Clouding of consciousness (dulled cognition, impaired alertness); inattentive; incoherent conversation; impaired recent memory and confabulatory for recent events; often agitated and having visual hallucinations; disoriented, with confusion worse at night when environmental stimuli are decreased.

Adapted from Strub, R.L., Black, F.W. (2000). *Mental status examination in neurology* (4th ed.). Philadelphia: Davis, with permission.

TABLE 5-4 Speech Disorders

Condition	Disorder of	Description
Dysphonia	Voice	Difficulty or discomfort in talking, with abnormal pitch or volume, due to laryngeal disease. Voice sounds hoarse or whispered, but articulation and language are intact.
Dysarthria	Articulation	Distorted speech sounds; speech may sound unintelligible; basic language (word choice, grammar, comprehension) intact.
Aphasia	Language comprehension and production secondary to brain damage	True language disturbance, defect in word choice and grammar or defect in comprehension; defect is in *higher* integrative language processing.

Types of Aphasia

An earlier dichotomy classified aphasias as *expressive* (difficulty producing language) or *receptive* (difficulty understanding language). Because all people with aphasia have some difficulty with expression, beginning examiners tend to classify them all as expressive. The following system is more descriptive.

Condition	Description
Global aphasia	The most common and severe form. Spontaneous speech is absent or reduced to a few stereotyped words or sounds. Comprehension is absent or reduced to only the person's own name and a few select words. Repetition, reading, and writing are severely impaired. Prognosis for language recovery is poor. Caused by a large lesion that damages most of combined anterior and posterior language areas.
Broca's aphasia	Expressive aphasia. The person can understand language but cannot express himself or herself using language. This is characterized by nonfluent, dysarthric, and effortful speech. The speech is mostly nouns and verbs (high-content words) with few grammatic fillers, termed "agrammatic" or "telegraphic" speech. Repetition and reading aloud are severely impaired. Auditory and reading comprehensions are surprisingly intact. Lesion is in anterior language area called the *motor speech cortex* or *Broca's area.*
Wernicke's aphasia	Receptive aphasia. The linguistic opposite of Broca's aphasia. The person can hear sounds and words but cannot relate them to previous experiences. Speech is fluent, effortless, and well articulated but has many paraphasias (word substitutions that are malformed or wrong) and neologisms (made-up words) and often lacks substantive words. Speech can be totally incomprehensible. Often there is a great urge to speak. Repetition, reading, and writing also are impaired. Lesion is in posterior language area called the *association auditory cortex* or *Wernicke's area.*

(For a discussion of other types of aphasia (e.g., conduction, anomic, transcortical), please consult a neurology text.)

Abnormal Findings

TABLE 5-5 Abnormalities of Mood and Affect

Type of Mood or Affect	Definition	Clinical Example
Flat affect (blunted affect)	Lack of emotional response; no expression of feelings; voice monotonous and face immobile	Topic varies, expression does not
Depression	Sad, gloomy, dejected; symptoms may occur with rainy weather, after a holiday, or with an illness; if the situation is temporary, symptoms fade quickly	"I've got the blues."
Depersonalization (lack of ego boundaries)	Loss of identity, feels estranged, perplexed about own identity and meaning of existence	"I don't feel real." "I feel like I'm not really here."
Elation	Joy and optimism, overconfidence, increased motor activity, not necessarily pathologic	"I'm feeling very happy."
Euphoria	Excessive well-being, unusually cheerful or elated, which is inappropriate considering physical and mental condition, implies a pathologic mood	"I am high." "I feel like I'm flying." "I feel on top of the world."
Anxiety	Worried, uneasy, apprehensive from the anticipation of a danger whose source is unknown	"I feel nervous and high strung." "I worry all the time." "I can't seem to make up my mind."
Fear	Worried, uneasy, apprehensive; external danger is known and identified	Fear of flying in airplanes
Irritability	Annoyed, easily provoked, impatient	Person internalizes a feeling of tension, and a seemingly mild stimulus "sets him (or her) off"
Rage	Furious, loss of control	Person has expressed violent behavior toward self or others
Ambivalence	The existence of opposing emotions toward an idea, object, person	A person feels love and hate toward another at the same time
Lability	Rapid shift of emotions	Person expresses euphoric, tearful, angry feelings in rapid succession
Inappropriate affect	Affect clearly discordant with the content of the person's speech	Laughs while discussing admission for liver biopsy

ABNORMAL FINDINGS
FOR ADVANCED PRACTICE

TABLE 5-6 Abnormalities of Thought Process

Type of Process	Definition	Clinical Example
Blocking	Sudden interruption in train of thought, unable to complete sentence, seems related to strong emotion	"Forgot what I was going to say."
Confabulation	Fabricates events to fill in memory gaps	Gives detailed description of his long walk around the hospital although you know Mr. J. remained in his room all afternoon.
Neologism	Coining a new word; invented word has no real meaning except for the person; may condense several words	"I'll have to turn on my thinkilator."
Circumlocution	Round-about expression, substituting a phrase when cannot think of name of object	Says "the thing you open the door with" instead of "key."
Circumstantiality	Talks with excessive and unnecessary detail, delays reaching point; sentences have a meaningful connection but are irrelevant (this occurs normally in some people)	"When was my surgery? Well I was 28, I was living with my aunt, she's the one with psoriasis, she had it bad that year because of the heat, the heat was worse then than it was the summer of '92, …"
Loosening associations	Shifting from one topic to an unrelated topic; person seems unaware that topics are unconnected	"My boss is angry with me and it wasn't even my fault. *(pause)* I saw that movie too, Lassie. I felt really bad about it. But she kept trying to land the airplane and she never knew what was going on."
Flight of ideas	Abrupt change, rapid skipping from topic to topic, practically continuous flow of accelerated speech; topics usually have recognizable associations or are plays on words	"Take this pill? The pill is blue. I feel blue. *(sings)* She wore blue velvet."
Word salad	Incoherent mixture of words, phrases, and sentences; illogical, disconnected, includes neologisms	"Beauty, red-based five, pigeon, the street corner, sort of."
Perseveration	Persistent repeating of verbal or motor response, even with varied stimuli	"I'm going to lock the door, lock the door. I walk every day and I lock the door. I usually take the dog and I lock the door."
Echolalia	Imitation, repeats others' words or phrases, often with a mumbling, mocking, or mechanical tone	Nurse: "I want you to take your pill." Patient *(mocking)*: "Take your pill. Take your pill."
Clanging	Word choice based on sound, not meaning, includes nonsense rhymes and puns	"My feet are cold. Cold, bold, told. The bell tolled for me."

TABLE 5-7 Abnormalities of Thought Content

Type of Content	Definition	Clinical Example
Phobia	Strong, persistent, irrational fear of an object or situation; feels driven to avoid it	Cats, dogs, heights, enclosed spaces
Hypochondriasis	Morbid worrying about his or her own health, feels sick with no actual basis for that assumption	Preoccupied with the fear of having cancer; any symptom or physical sign means cancer
Obsession	Unwanted, persistent thoughts or impulses; logic will not purge them from consciousness; experienced as intrusive and senseless	Violence (parent having repeated impulse to kill a loved child); contamination (becoming infected by shaking hands)
Compulsion	Unwanted repetitive, purposeful act; driven to do it; behavior thought to neutralize or prevent discomfort or some dreaded event	Handwashing, counting, checking and rechecking, touching
Delusions	Firm, fixed, false beliefs; irrational; person clings to delusion despite objective evidence to contrary	Grandiose—person believes he or she is God; famous, historical, or sports figure; or other well-known person Persecution—"They are out to get me."

TABLE 5-8 Abnormalities of Perception

Type of Perception	Definition	Clinical Example
Hallucination	Sensory perceptions for which there are no external stimuli; may strike any sense: visual, auditory, tactile, olfactory, gustatory	Visual: seeing an image (ghost) of a person who is not there; auditory: hearing voices or music
Illusion	*Mis*perception of an actual existing stimulus, by any sense	Folds of bed sheets appear to be animated

TABLE 5-9 Schizophrenia*

A. Characteristic Symptoms

Two (or more) of the following, each present for a significant part of a 1-month period:

1. Delusions (i.e., involving a phenomenon that the person's culture would regard as totally implausible, such as thought broadcasting, being controlled by a dead person)
2. Hallucinations (auditory are more common) (e.g., voices speaking directly to the person or commenting on his or her ongoing behavior)
3. Disorganized speech (e.g., frequent derailment or incoherence)
4. Grossly disorganized or catatonic behavior
5. Negative symptoms (i.e., affective flattening, alogia [inability to speak], or avolition)

B. Social/Occupational Dysfunction

One or more major areas of functioning such as work, interpersonal relations, or self-care are markedly below the level achieved prior to onset of the disturbance

C. Duration

Continuous signs persist for at least 6 months, including at least 1 month of symptoms from criterion A (i.e., active phase) and may include periods of prodromal or residual symptoms

Adapted from the American Psychiatric Association. (2000). *Diagnostic and statistical manual of mental disorders* (4th ed.). Washington, DC: The Association. Reprinted with permission from the American Psychiatric Association.

*These diagnostic categories are meant to be illustrative, not inclusive. Please see the original source or a psychiatry textbook for further categories and schizophrenia subtypes, such as paranoid type, catatonic type, disorganized type.

TABLE 5-10 Delirium, Dementia, and Amnestic Disorders*

Delirium

A. **Disturbance of consciousness** (i.e., reduced clarity of awareness of the environment) with reduced ability to focus, sustain, or shift attention.

B. A **change in cognition** (e.g., memory deficit, disorientation, language disturbance) or the development of a perceptual disturbance.

C. The disturbance **develops over a short period of time** (usually hours to days) and tends to fluctuate during the course of the day.

Delirium may be due to a **general medical condition:** systemic infections, metabolic disorders (e.g., hypoxia, hypercarbia, hypoglycemia), fluid or electrolyte imbalances, liver or kidney disease, thiamine deficiency, postoperative states, hypertensive encephalopathy, or following seizures or head trauma.

Delirium also may be **substance-induced** (i.e., due to a drug of abuse, a medication, or toxin exposure).

Dementia

A. The development of multiple cognitive deficits manifested by both:
   1. **Memory impairment** (impaired ability to learn new information or to recall previously learned information), and
   2. One (or more) of the following cognitive disturbances:
      a. Aphasia (language disturbance)
      b. Apraxia (impaired ability to carry out motor activities despite intact motor function)
      c. Agnosia (failure to recognize or identify objects despite intact sensory function)
      d. Disturbance in executive functioning (i.e., planning, organizing, sequencing, abstracting)

B. The cognitive deficits must be sufficiently severe to cause **impairment in occupational or social functioning** and must represent a decline from a previously higher level of functioning.

Dementias have a common symptom presentation but are differentiated based on etiology, which include senile dementia of the Alzheimer's type or SDAT (course is characterized by gradual onset and continuing cognitive decline); dementia due to cerebrovascular disease (characterized by focal neurologic signs and symptoms [e.g., exaggeration of deep tendon reflexes, extensor plantar response, gait abnormalities, weakness of an extremity]); human immunodeficiency virus disease; head trauma; Parkinson disease; and others.

Amnestic Disorder

A. The development of **memory impairment** (inability to learn new information or to recall previously learned information) in the absence of other significant cognitive impairments.

B. The memory disturbance causes significant **impairment in social or occupational functioning** and represents a significant decline from a previous level of functioning.

This may be due to pathology (closed head trauma, penetrating missile wounds, surgical intervention, hypoxia, infarction of the posterior cerebral artery, herpes simplex encephalitis), or it may be substance induced (e.g., alcohol-induced amnestic disorder due to thiamine deficiency associated with prolonged, heavy ingestion of alcohol).

Adapted from the American Psychiatric Association. (2000). *Diagnostic and statistical manual of mental disorders* (4th ed.). Washington, DC: The Association. Reprinted with permission from the American Psychiatric Association.

*The terms *organic mental disorder* and *organic brain syndrome* are no longer used for these disorders. These diagnostic categories are meant to be illustrative, not inclusive. Please refer to the original source for additional details and for further categories.

TABLE 5-11 Mood Disorders*

Major Depressive Episode
Characteristics

A. Five (or more) of the following symptoms present during the same 2-week period and represent a change from previous functioning; at least one of the symptoms is either (1) depressed mood, or (2) loss of interest or pleasure. Note: Do not include symptoms that are clearly caused by a general medical condition or delusions or hallucinations.
   1. **Depressed mood** most of the day nearly every day, as indicated by either subjective report (e.g., feels sad or empty) or by observation by others (e.g., appears tearful)
      Note: In children and adolescents, can be irritable mood.
   2. Markedly **diminished interest or pleasure** in all, or almost all, activities most of the day nearly every day
   3. Significant **weight loss** when not dieting, weight gain (e.g., a change of >5% body weight in a month), or decrease or increase in appetite nearly every day
      Note: In children, consider failure to make expected weight gains.
   4. **Insomnia** or hypersomnia nearly every day
   5. **Psychomotor agitation** or retardation nearly every day
   6. **Fatigue** or loss of energy nearly every day
   7. Feelings of **worthlessness** or excessive or inappropriate guilt nearly every day
   8. **Diminished ability to think** or concentrate or indecisiveness nearly every day
   9. Recurrent **thoughts of death** (not just fear of dying), recurrent suicidal ideation without a specific plan, or a suicide attempt or a specific plan for committing suicide

B. The symptoms cause clinically significant distress or impairment in social, occupational, or other important areas of functioning.

C. The symptoms are not due to the direct physiologic effects of a substance (e.g., drug of abuse, a medication) or a general medical condition (e.g., hypothyroidism) and are not better accounted for by bereavement, as with loss of a loved one (unless persist for longer than 2 months or are characterized by functional impairment, morbid preoccupation with worthlessness, suicidal ideation, psychotic symptoms, or psychomotor retardation).

Manic Episode
Characteristics

A. A distinct period of abnormally and **persistently elevated, expansive, or irritable mood,** lasting at least 1 week (or any duration if hospitalization is necessary).

B. During this period of mood disturbance, three (or more) of the following symptoms have persisted (four if the mood is only irritable):
   1. Inflated self-esteem or grandiosity
   2. Decreased need for sleep (e.g., feels rested after only 3 hours of sleep)
   3. More talkative than usual or pressure to keep talking
   4. Flight of ideas or subjective experience that thoughts are racing
   5. Distractibility (i.e., attention too easily drawn to unimportant or irrelevant external stimuli)
   6. Increase in goal-directed activity (either socially, at work or school, or sexually) or psychomotor agitation
   7. Excessive involvement in pleasurable activities that have a high potential for painful consequences (e.g., engaging in unrestrained buying sprees, sexual indiscretions, or foolish business investments)

C. The mood disturbance is sufficiently severe to cause marked impairment in occupational functioning or in usual social activities or relationships with others or to necessitate hospitalization to prevent harm to self or others, or there are psychotic features.

D. The symptoms are not due to the direct physiologic effects of a substance (e.g., a drug of abuse, a medication) or a general medical condition (e.g., hyperthyroidism).

Major depressive disorder is characterized by one or more major depressive episodes (i.e., at least 2 weeks of depressed mood or loss of interest accompanied by at least four additional symptoms of depression); **dysthymic disorder** is characterized by at least 2 years of depressed mood for more days than not, accompanied by additional depressive symptoms; **bipolar disorder** is characterized by one or more manic episodes usually accompanied by major depressive episodes.

Adapted from the American Psychiatric Association. (2000). *Diagnostic and statistical manual of mental disorders* (4th ed.). Washington, DC: The Association. Reprinted with permission from the American Psychiatric Association.

*These diagnostic categories are meant to be illustrative, not inclusive. Please see the original source or a psychiatry textbook for further categories, such as personality disorders or somatoform disorders.

TABLE 5-12 Anxiety Disorders*

Panic Attack

A discrete period of **intense fear or discomfort,** in which four (or more) of the following symptoms developed abruptly and reached a peak within 10 minutes:

1. Palpitations, pounding heart, or accelerated heart rate
2. Sweating
3. Trembling or shaking
4. Sensations of shortness of breath or smothering
5. Feeling of choking
6. Chest pain or discomfort
7. Nausea or abdominal distress
8. Feeling dizzy, unsteady, light-headed, or faint
9. Derealization (feelings of unreality) or depersonalization (being detached from oneself)
10. Fear of losing control or going crazy
11. Fear of dying
12. Paresthesias (numbness or tingling sensations)
13. Chills or hot flashes

Agoraphobia

A. Anxiety about being in places or situations from which escape might be difficult (or embarrassing) or in which help may not be available in the event of having a panic attack or panic-like symptoms—agoraphobic fears typically involve being outside the home alone; being in a crowd or standing in a line; being on a bridge; and traveling in a bus, train, or automobile.

B. The situations are avoided (e.g., travel is restricted), are endured with marked distress or with anxiety about having a panic attack or panic-like symptoms, or require the presence of a companion.

Panic Disorder

A. Both 1 and 2 occur:
   1. Recurrent unexpected panic attacks (see above)
   2. At least one of the attacks has been followed by 1 month (or more) of one (or more) of the following:
      a. Persistent concern about having additional attacks
      b. Worry about the implications of the attack or its consequences (e.g., losing control, having a heart attack, "going crazy")
      c. A significant change in behavior related to the attacks

B. Agoraphobia may be present or absent.

Specific Phobia

A. Marked and persistent fear that is excessive or unreasonable, cued by a specific object or situation (e.g., flying, heights, animals, receiving an injection, seeing blood).

B. Exposure to the phobic stimulus almost invariably provokes an immediate anxiety response, which may be a panic attack.

Note: In children, the anxiety may be expressed by crying, tantrums, freezing, or clinging.

C. The person recognizes that the fear is excessive or unreasonable.

D. The phobic situation is avoided or is endured with intense anxiety or distress.

E. This interferes significantly with the person's normal routine, occupational (or academic) functioning, or social activities or relationships.

Social Phobia

A. A marked and persistent fear of one or more social or performance situations in which the person is exposed to unfamiliar people or to possible scrutiny by others; the individual fears that he or she will act in a way (or show anxiety symptoms) that will be humiliating or embarrassing.

B.–E.: The same as in specific phobia.

Obsessive-Compulsive Disorder

A. Person has either **obsessions:**
   1. Recurrent and persistent thoughts, impulses, or images that are experienced as intrusive and inappropriate and that cause marked anxiety or distress
   2. The thoughts, impulses, or images are not simply excessive worries about real-life problems
   3. The person attempts to ignore or suppress such thoughts, impulses, or images or to neutralize them with some other thought or action
   4. The person recognizes that the obsessional thoughts are a product of his or her own mind (not imposed from without)

TABLE 5-12 Anxiety Disorders*—cont'd

Or **compulsions:**

1. Repetitive behaviors (e.g., handwashing, ordering, checking) or mental acts (e.g., praying, counting, repeating words silently) that the person feels driven to perform in response to an obsession or according to rules that must be applied rigidly
2. The behaviors or mental acts are aimed at preventing or reducing distress or at preventing some dreaded event or situation

B. At some point, the person has recognized that the obsessions or compulsions are excessive or unreasonable.
C. The obsessions or compulsions cause marked distress; are time consuming; or significantly interfere with the person's normal routine, occupational (or academic) functioning, or usual social activities or relationships.

Posttraumatic Stress Disorder

A. The person has been exposed to a traumatic event in which:
   1. The person experienced, witnessed, or was confronted with the actual or threatened death or serious injury of self or others
   2. The person's response involved intense fear, helplessness, or horror
B. The traumatic event is persistently reexperienced by:
   1. Recurrent and intrusive distressing recollections of the event, including images, thoughts, or perceptions
   2. Recurrent distressing dreams of the event
   3. Acting or feeling as if the traumatic event were recurring
C. Persistent avoidance of stimuli associated with the trauma and numbing of general responsiveness (e.g., feeling of detachment or estrangement from others, unable to have loving feelings, sense of a foreshortened future).
D. Persistent symptoms of increased arousal:
   1. Difficulty falling or staying asleep
   2. Irritability or outbursts of anger
   3. Difficulty concentrating
   4. Hypervigilance
   5. Exaggerated startle response

Generalized Anxiety Disorder

A. Excessive anxiety and worry occurring more days than not for at least 6 months about a number of events or activities (e.g., work or school performance).
B. The person finds it difficult to control the worry.
C. The anxiety and worry are associated with three (or more) of the following:
   1. Restlessness or feeling keyed up or on edge
   2. Being easily fatigued
   3. Difficulty concentrating or mind going blank
   4. Irritability
   5. Muscle tension
   6. Sleep disturbance

Adapted from the American Psychiatric Association. (2000). *Diagnostic and statistical manual of mental disorders* (4th ed.). Washington, DC: The Association. Reprinted with permission from the American Psychiatric Association.
*These diagnostic categories are meant to be illustrative, not inclusive. Please see the original source or a psychiatry textbook for further details and categories of anxiety disorders.

Abnormal Findings

BIBLIOGRAPHY

1. Adelman, A. M., & Daly, M. P. (2005). Initial evaluation of the patient with suspected dementia. *American Family Physician, 71*(9), 1745-1750.

1a. Alverzo, J. P. (2006). A review of the literature on orientation as an indicator of level of consciousness. *Journal of Nursing Scholarship, 38*(2), 159-164.

2. American Psychiatric Association. (2000). *Diagnostic and statistical manual of mental disorders* (4th ed.). Text Revision, Washington, DC: The Association.

3. Beatty, G. E. (2006). Shedding light on Alzheimer's. *Nurse Practitioner, 31*(9), 32-45.

4. Birren, J. E., & Schaie, K. W. (Eds.). (2006). *Handbook of the psychology of aging* (6th ed.). San Diego: Academic Press.

5. Borson, S., Scanlan, J. M., Watanabe, J., et al. (2006). Improving identification of cognitive impairment in primary care. *International Journal of Geriatric Psychiatry, 21*(4), 349-355.

6. Bradway, C., & Hirschman, K. B. (2008). Working with families of hospitalized older adults with dementia. *American Journal of Nursing, 108*(10), 52-61.

7. Brodaty, H., Low, L. F., Gibson, L., et al. (2006). What is the best dementia screening instrument for general practitioners to use? *American Journal of Geriatric Psychiatry, 14*(5), 391-400.

8. Centers for Disease Control and Prevention: *Suicide facts at a glance.* Website: www.cdc.gov/ncipc/dvp/suicide/SuicideDataSheet.pdf.

9. De Nisco, S., Tiago, C., & Kravitz, C. (2005). Evaluation and treatment of pediatric ADHD. *Nurse Practitioner, 30*(8), 14-25.

10. Depaulo, J. R. Jr., & Folstein, M. F. (1978). Psychiatric disturbances in neurological patients: Detection, recognition and hospital course. *Annals of Neurology, 4*(3), 225-228.

11. Doerflinger, D. M. C. (2007). The Mini-Cog. *American Journal of Nursing, 107*(12), 62-72.

12. Fick, D. M., & Mion, L. C. (2008). Delirium superimposed on dementia. *American Journal of Nursing, 108*(1), 52-61.
12a. Fisher, D., & Valente, S. (2009). Evaluating and managing insomnia. *Nurse Practitioner, 34*(8), 21-26.
13. Folstein, M. F., Folstein, S. E., & McHugh, P. R. (1975). "Mini-Mental State": A practical method for grading the cognitive state of patients for the clinician. *Journal of Psychiatric Research, 12*:189-198.
14. Forrest, J., Willis, L., Holm, K., et al. (2007). Recognizing quiet delirium. *American Journal of Nursing, 107*(4), 35-39.
15. Fricchione, G. (2004). Generalized anxiety disorder. *New England Journal of Medicine, 351*(7), 675-676.
16. Garand, L., Mitchell, A. M., Dietrick, A., et al. (2006). Suicide in older adults: Nursing assessment of suicide risk. *Issues in Mental Health Nursing, 29*(4), 355-370.
17. Gary, F. A. (2005). Stigma: barrier to mental health care among ethnic minorities. *Issues in Mental Health Nursing, 26*(10), 979-999.
18. Gill, J. M., & Saligan, L. N. (2008). Don't let SAD get you down this season. *Nurse Practitioner, 33*(12), 22-26.
18a. Gill, J., Saligan, L. N., Henderson, W. A., et al. (2009). PTSD—Know the warning signs. *Nurse Practitioner, 34*(7), 30-37.
19. Greenberg, S. A. (2007). The geriatric depression scale: Short form. *American Journal of Nursing, 107*(10), 60-70.
20. Guess, K. F. (2006). Posttraumatic stress disorder. *Nurse Practitioner, 31*(3), 26-35.
21. Holcomb, S. S. (2006). Identification and treatment of depression. *Nurse Practitioner, 31*(12), 42-44.
21a. Inouye, S. K. (2006). Delirium in older persons. *New England Journal of Medicine, 354*(11), 1157-1165.
22. Kroenke, K., Spitzer, R. L., Williams, J. B., et al. (2007). Anxiety disorders in primary care: Prevalence, impairment, comorbidity, and detection. *Annals of Internal Medicine, 146*(5), 317-325.
23. Lemiengre, J., Nelis, T., Jooston, E., et al. (2006). Detection of delirium by bedside nurses using the confusion assessment method. *Journal of the American Geriatrics Society, 54*(4), 685-689.
24. Lumby, B. (2007). Guide schizophrenia patients to better physical health. *Nurse Practitioner, 32*(7), 30-38.
25. Maslow, K., & Mezey, M. (2008). Recognition of dementia in hospitalized older adults. *American Journal of Nursing, 108*(1), 40-50.
26. McCravy, S., Johnson, A., Wetsel, M. A., et al. (2010). Speak the language of autism. *Nurse Practitioner, 35*(4), 26-33.
27. Mynatt, S., & Cunningham, P. (2007). Unraveling anxiety and depression. *Nurse Practitioner, 32*(8), 28-37.
28. National Institute of Mental Health. *Suicide in the U.S.: statistics and prevention.* Website: www.nimh.nih.gov/health/publications/suicide-in-the-us-statistics-and-prevention.shtml.
29. Rabins, P. V. (2004). Research update: Mild cognitive impairment (MCI)—definition, diagnosis, and treatment possibilities. *Advanced Studies in Medicine, 4*(6), 290-296.
30. Roux, S. L., & Overcash, J. (2008). Scratching the surface: Addressing self-harm in adolescents, *Nurse Practitioner, 33*(6), 30-36.
31. Spitzer, R. L., Kroenke, K., Williams, J. B. W., et al. (2006). A brief measure for assessing generalized anxiety disorder. *Archives of Internal Medicine, 166*(10), 1092-1097.
32. Stanton, K. (2007). Communicating with ED patients who have chronic mental illness. *American Journal of Nursing, 107*(2), 61-65.
33. Strub, R. L., & Black, F. W. (2000). *Mental status examination in neurology* (4th ed.). Philadelphia: Davis.
34. Thayer, K. M., & Bruce, M. L. (2006). Recognition and management of major depression. *Nurse Pract, 31*(5), 12-25.
35. U.S. Preventive Services Task Force. *Screening for depression in adults: recommendations and rationale*, Agency for Healthcare Research and Quality. Website: www.ahrq.gov/clinic/3rduspstf/depression/depressrr.htm.
36. U.S. Preventive Services Task Force. *Screening for suicide risk in adults: recommendations and rationale*, Agency for Healthcare Research and Quality. Website: www.ahrq.gov/clinic/3rduspstf/suicide/suiciderr.htm.
36a. Valente, S. (2008). Suicide risk in elderly patients. *Nurse Practitioner, 33*(8), 34-40.
37. Waszynski, C. M. (2007). Detecting delirium. *American Journal of Nursing, 107*(12), 50-60.
38. Weber, K. (2008). Asperger's syndrome: From hiding to thriving. *Nurse Practitioner, 33*(7), 14-22.

Summary Checklist: Mental Status Assessment

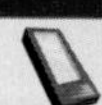 For a PDA-downloadable version, go to http://evolve.elsevier.com/Jarvis/.

1. Appearance
- Posture
- Body movements
- Dress
- Grooming and hygiene

2. Behavior
- Level of consciousness
- Facial expression
- Speech (quality, pace, articulation, word choice)
- Mood and affect

3. Cognitive functions
- Orientation
- Attention span
- Recent and remote memory
- New learning—the Four Unrelated Words Test
- Judgment

4. Thought processes
- Thought processes
- Thought content
- Perceptions
- Screen for suicidal thoughts (when indicated)

5. Perform the Mini-Mental State Examination

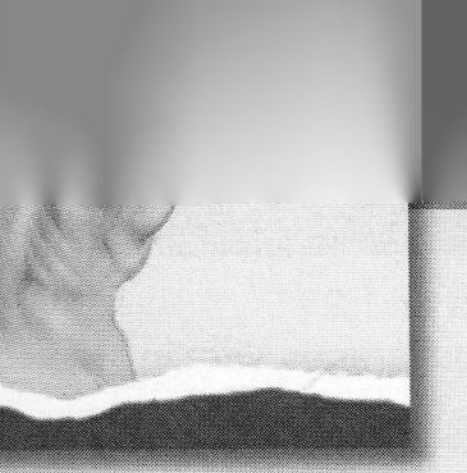

6

Substance Use Assessment

evolve WEBSITE

http://evolve.elsevier.com/Jarvis/

- Animations
- Audio Key Points
- NCLEX Review Questions

OUTLINE

Subjective Data, 96

Health History Questions

Objective Data, 99

Abnormal Findings, 100

ALCOHOL USE AND ABUSE

In 2008, slightly more than half (51.6%) of Americans ages 12 and older reported being current alcohol drinkers.[32] More than one fifth (23.3%) of persons ages 12 and older were binge drinkers (≥5 drinks/occasion) and 6.9% reported heavy drinking (binge drinking on at least 5 days in the past 30 days). Thus alcohol is the most used and abused psychoactive drug. People like to drink! Given the rates of alcohol use, it is not surprising that many patients in the hospital and in primary care offices find themselves with alcohol-related disorders.

Morbidity and mortality data reflect the adverse consequences of excessive alcohol use. Alcohol is involved in 40% of the 41,000 annual deaths due to traffic crashes.[23] The number of emergency department (ED) visits attributable to alcohol from the period 1992 to 2000 was about 68.6 million,[19] with an increasing trend of 18% during that time. In the general population, alcohol consumption of at least 4 standard drinks per day (each containing 12 g alcohol, see Table 6-1) is associated with increased rates of death from cirrhosis and alcoholism; cancers of the mouth, esophagus, pharynx, and liver combined; and injuries and other external causes in men.[30] In women, alcohol consumption increases the risk for breast cancer in a dose-response relation, starting at an alcohol intake of 24 g (about 2 drinks) a day.[15] The link between chronic alcohol use and alcohol liver disease is well known. Cirrhosis accounted for 27,000 deaths in the United States in 2004, or the 12th leading cause of death.[6] There are multiple alcohol effects on the heart. Chronic heavy use increases the risk for alcoholic cardiomyopathy, with an increase in left ventricular mass, dilation of ventricles, and wall thinning.[31] Hypertension is a common detrimental effect, with a causal association between consumption of 30 to 60 g alcohol per day (3 to 5 standard drinks) and blood pressure (BP) elevation in men and women.[13] Finally, alcohol and illicit drugs are arrhythmogenic and are associated with the rapid heart rate of atrial fibrillation.[14]

Because of alcohol-related morbidity, many patients you encounter in primary care settings and in the hospital will have a significant drinking history. Persons visiting primary care providers have a significantly higher rate of past or present alcohol abuse (23%) than those in the general population (9%).[17,21a] Surveys of hospital ICU admissions show a range of 12% to 21% prevalence of alcohol dependence among their patients.[18,24] Excessive alcohol use increases risk for ICU admissions due to trauma, hypothermia, and pancreatitis. Once in the hospital, heavy alcohol use can lead to respiratory failure from acute alcohol intoxication and alcohol withdrawal syndrome. Alcohol dependence increases risk for sepsis, septic shock, and hospital mortality among ICU patients.[24]

DEFINING ILLICIT DRUG USE

In 2008, about 8% of Americans ages 12 years and older reported current (past month) illicit drug use.[33] Illicit drugs include marijuana/hashish, cocaine (including crack), heroin, hallucinogens, inhalants, and prescription-type drugs used nonmedically. Marijuana was the most commonly used illicit drug, with 6.1% of persons ages 12 years and older reporting

TABLE 6-1 What is a Standard Drink?

A standard drink in the United States is any drink that contains about 14 grams of pure alcohol (about 0.6 fluid ounces or 1.2 tablespoons). Below are U.S. standard drink equivalents. These are approximate, since different brands and types of beverages vary in their actual alcohol content.

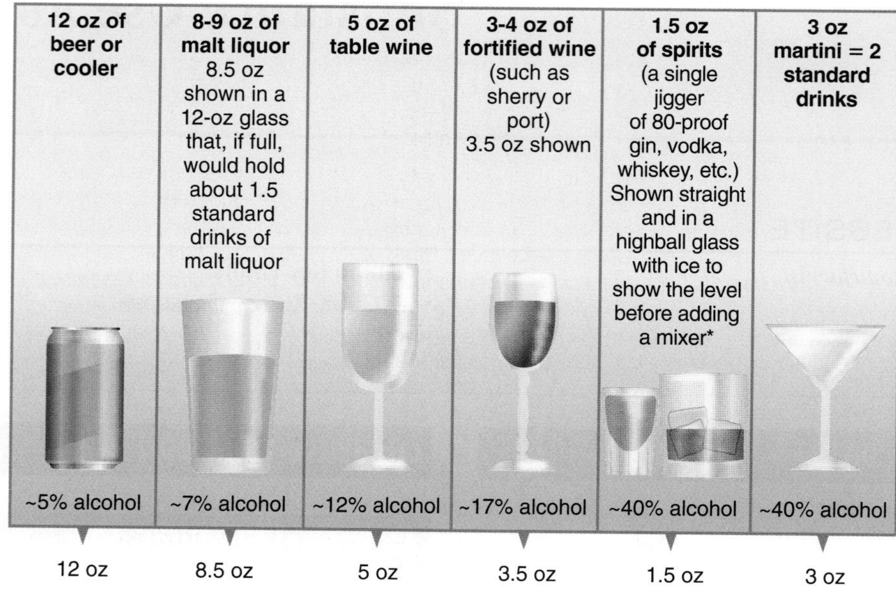

Many people do not know what counts as a standard drink and so they do not realize how many standard drinks are in the containers in which these drinks are often sold. Some examples:

For **beer,** the approximate number of standard drinks in:
- 12 oz. = 1
- 16 oz. = 1.3
- 22 oz. = 2
- 40 oz. = 3.3

For **malt liquor,** the approximate number of standard drinks in:
- 12 oz. = 1.5
- 16 oz. = 2
- 22 oz. = 2.5
- 40 oz. = 4.5

For **table wine,** the approximate number of standard drinks in:
- A standard 750-mL (25-oz.) bottle = 5

For **80-proof spirits,** or "hard liquor," the approximate number of standard drinks in:
- A mixed drink = 1 to 3 or more*
- A pint (16 oz.) = 11
- A fifth (25 oz.) = 17
- 1.75 L (59 oz.) = 39

Adapted from National Institute on Alcohol Abuse and Alcoholism (NIAAA). (Reprinted 2007). Helping patients who drink too much: a clinician's guide. Available at http://pubs.niaaa.nih.gov/publications/Practitioner/CliniciansGuide2005/clinicians_guide.htm.

*__Note:__ It can be difficult to estimate the number of standard drinks in a single mixed drink made with hard liquor. Depending on factors such as the type of spirits and the recipe, a mixed drink can contain from one to three or more standard drinks.

past-month use. Among youth ages 12 to 17 years, between 2002 and 2008, the rates of use of illicit drugs in general declined significantly (from 11.6% to 9.3%). Still, that represents 1 out of 10 adolescents as illicit drug users. This warrants our attention and intervention. Any amount of illicit drug use has serious legal consequences, as well as consequences for health, relationships, and future jobs, school, and career.

The abuse of prescription drugs is the fastest growing drug problem in the United States. Between 2004 and 2008, visits to hospital EDs for the nonmedical use of narcotic pain relievers more than doubled, rising 111%.[7] The three most frequently abused prescription opioid pain relievers were products using oxycodone, hydrocodone, and methadone. The misuse of prescription drugs has a huge impact not only on health and safety but also on burdens to the ED system.

TABLE 6-2 Categories and Definitions for Patterns of Alcohol Use

Category	Organization	Definition
Moderate drinking	NIAAA	Men, ≤2 drinks/day; women, ≤1 drink/day; >65 years, ≤1 drink/day
At-risk drinking	NIAAA	Men, >14 drinks/wk or >4 drinks/occasion; women, >7 drinks/wk or >3 drinks/occasion
Hazardous drinking	WHO	At risk for adverse consequences from alcohol
Harmful drinking	WHO	Alcohol is causing physical or psychological harm
Alcohol abuse	APA	≥1 of the following events in a year: recurrent use resulting in failure to fulfill major role obligations; recurrent use in hazardous situations; recurrent alcohol-related legal problems (e.g., DUI); continued use despite social or interpersonal problems caused or exacerbated by alcohol
Alcohol dependence	APA	≥3 of the following events in a year: tolerance (increased amounts to achieve effect; diminished effect from same amount); withdrawal; a great deal of time spent obtaining alcohol, using it, or recovering from its effect; important activities given up or reduced because of alcohol; drinking more or longer than intended; persistent desire or unsuccessful efforts to cut down or control alcohol use; use continued despite knowledge of having a psychological problem caused or exacerbated by alcohol

APA, American Psychiatric Association; *DUI,* driving under the influence; *NIAAA,* National Institute on Alcohol Abuse and Alcoholism; *WHO,* World Health Organization.

DIAGNOSING SUBSTANCE ABUSE

The rate of Americans classified with substance abuse or dependence is 9.2 % of the population ages 12 years and older; of these persons, 68% were dependent on or abused alcohol but not illicit drugs and 14% used both alcohol and illicit drugs. There is a continuum of alcohol drinking ranging from special occasion use, through moderate drinking, to harmful drinking (Table 6-2). Alcohol dependence or alcoholism is a chronic progressive disease that is not curable but is highly treatable. Accurate diagnosis is needed in order to provide advice, brief intervention, appropriate treatment, and follow-up. The gold standard of diagnosis is well defined by the American Psychiatric Association (APA) in their *Diagnostic and Statistical Manual of Mental Disorders,* 4th edition *(DSM-IV-TR).* Tables 6-3 and 6-4 give the criteria for these diagnoses. Unfortunately, alcohol problems are underdiagnosed both

TABLE 6-3 Criteria for Substance Abuse

A maladaptive pattern of substance use with ≥1 of the following events in a year:

1. Recurrent substance use resulting in a failure to fulfill major role obligations at work, school, or home (e.g., repeated absences or poor work performance related to substance use; substance-related absences, suspensions, or expulsions from school; neglect of children or household)
2. Recurrent substance use in situations in which it is physically hazardous (e.g., driving an automobile or operating a machine when impaired by substance use)
3. Recurrent substance-related legal problems (e.g., arrests for substance-related disorderly conduct)
4. Continued substance use despite having persistent or recurrent social or interpersonal problems caused or exacerbated by the effects of the substance (e.g., arguments with spouse about consequences of intoxication, physical fights)

Adapted from American Psychiatric Association. (2000). *Diagnostic and statistical manual of mental disorders, DSM-IV-TR* (4th ed., pp. 182-183). Washington, DC: Author.

TABLE 6-4 Criteria for Substance Dependence

A maladaptive pattern of substance use with ≥3 of the following events in a year:

1. Tolerance
   a. A need for markedly increased amounts of the substance to achieve intoxication or desired effect, or
   b. Markedly diminished effect with continued use of the same amount of the substance
2. Withdrawal
   a. The characteristic withdrawal syndrome for the substance, or
   b. The same (or a closely related) substance is taken to relieve or avoid withdrawal symptoms
3. The substance is often taken in larger amounts or over a longer period than was intended.
4. There is a persistent desire or unsuccessful efforts to cut down or control substance use.
5. A great deal of time is spent in activities necessary to obtain the substance (e.g., visiting multiple doctors or driving long distances), use the substance (e.g., chain-smoking), or recover from its effects.
6. Important social, occupational, or recreational activities are given up or reduced because of substance use.
7. The substance use is continued despite knowledge of having a persistent or recurrent physical or psychological problem that is likely to have been caused or exacerbated by the substance (e.g., current cocaine use despite recognition of cocaine-induced depression or continued drinking despite recognition that an ulcer was made worse by alcohol consumption).

Adapted from American Psychiatric Association. (2000). *Diagnostic and statistical manual of mental disorders, DSM-IV-TR* (4th ed., p. 181). Washington, DC: Author.

in primary care settings and in hospitals. Excessive alcohol use often is unrecognized until patients develop serious complications.

DEVELOPMENTAL COMPETENCE

The Pregnant Woman

Among pregnant women ages 15 to 44 years, about 10.6% report current alcohol use, with 4.5% reporting binge drinking and 0.8% reporting heavy drinking.[32] These rates are much lower than their age-matched counterparts who are not pregnant (54%, 24.2%, and 5.5%, respectively). However, no amount of alcohol has been determined safe for pregnant women. The potential adverse consequences of alcohol use to the fetus are well known. Thus all women contemplating pregnancy and who are pregnant should be screened for alcohol use, and abstinence should be recommended.

The Aging Adult

The prevalence of current alcohol use decreases with increasing age, from 67.4% among those ages 26 to 29 years; down to 50.3% in those ages 60 to 64 years; and to 39.7% in adults ages 65 years and older.[32] However, older adults have numerous characteristics that can increase the risk for alcohol use. Liver metabolism and kidney function are decreased, which increases the bioavailability of alcohol in the blood for longer time periods. Aging people lose muscle mass; less tissue for the alcohol to be distributed to means an increased alcohol concentration in the blood. Older adults may be on multiple medications, which can interact adversely with alcohol (e.g., benzodiazepines, antidepressants, antihypertensives, aspirin, to name just a few). Drinking alcohol increases risk for falls, depression, and gastrointestinal problems. Finally, older adults may avoid detection of their alcohol problems; they may avoid alcohol-related consequences such as a DUI just because they no longer drive, or they may avoid job problems just because they no longer work.

SUBJECTIVE DATA

If the patient currently is intoxicated or going through substance withdrawal, collecting any history data is difficult and unreliable. However, when sober, most people are willing and able to give reliable data, provided that the setting is private, confidential, and nonconfrontational.

Examiner Asks	Rationale
1. Ask about alcohol use: "Do you sometimes drink beer, wine, or other alcoholic beverages?" If the answer is "Yes," ask the screening question about heavy drinking days: "How many times in the past year have you had 5 or more drinks a day *(for men)* or 4 or more drinks a day?"*(for women)*	One or more heavy drinking days means this person is an "at-risk" drinker.
To complete a picture of the person's drinking pattern, ask: "On average, how many days a week do you have an alcoholic drink?" and "On a typical drinking day, how many drinks do you have?" Recommend the person stay at **moderate** drinking patterns: for men, ≤2 drinks/day; for women, ≤1 drink/day; for older than 65 years, ≤1 drink/day.[22] Recommend even lower limits or abstinence for patients who take medications that interact with alcohol, have a health condition exacerbated by alcohol, or are pregnant (advise abstinence here).	For men, ≥14 drinks/week or ≥4 drinks/occasion = **at risk** drinking. For women, ≥7 drinks/week or ≥3 drinks/occasion = **at-risk** drinking.[22]
2. Use brief screening instruments to help identify problem drinking and those persons who need a more thorough assessment. Ask the patient to respond to the AUDIT questionnaire (Table 6-5). A quantitative form has the advantage of letting you document a number for a response so it is not open to individual interpretation. The AUDIT will help detect less severe alcohol problems (hazardous and harmful drinking) as well as alcohol abuse and dependence disorders. It is helpful with ED and trauma patients because it is sensitive to current as opposed to past alcohol problems. It is useful in primary care settings, with adolescent and older adults. It is relatively free of gender and cultural bias.	Hazardous drinking—pattern is high risk for future damage to physical or mental health. Harmful drinking—alcohol use already results in problems.

Examiner Asks	Rationale

TABLE 6-5 The Alcohol Use Disorders Identification Test—AUDIT*

Questions	0	1	2	3	4
1. How often do you have a drink containing alcohol?	Never	Monthly or less	2 to 4 times a month	2 to 3 times a week	4 or more times a week
2. How many drinks containing alcohol do you have on a typical day when you are drinking?	1 or 2	3 or 4	5 or 6	7 to 9	10 or more
3. How often do you have 5 or more drinks on one occasion?	Never	Less than monthly	Monthly	Weekly	Daily or almost daily
4. How often during the last year have you found that you were not able to stop drinking once you had started?	Never	Less than monthly	Monthly	Weekly	Daily or almost daily
5. How often during the last year have you failed to do what was normally expected of you because of drinking?	Never	Less than monthly	Monthly	Weekly	Daily or almost daily
6. How often during the last year have you needed a first drink in the morning to get yourself going after a heavy drinking session?	Never	Less than monthly	Monthly	Weekly	Daily or almost daily
7. How often during the last year have you had a feeling of guilt or remorse after drinking?	Never	Less than monthly	Monthly	Weekly	Daily or almost daily
8. How often during the last year have you been unable to remember what happened the night before because of your drinking?	Never	Less than monthly	Monthly	Weekly	Daily or almost daily
9. Have you or someone else been injured because of your drinking?	No		Yes, but not in the last year		Yes, during the last year
10. Has a relative, friend, doctor, or other health care worker been concerned about your drinking or suggested you cut down?	No		Yes, but not in the last year		Yes, during the last year
					Total

***Note:** This questionnaire (the AUDIT) is reprinted with permission from the World Health Organization. To reflect standard drink sizes in the United States, the number of drinks in question 3 was changed from 6 to 5. A free AUDIT manual with guidelines for use in primary care settings is available online at www.who.org.

Note that the AUDIT covers three domains: alcohol consumption (questions 1-3); drinking behavior or dependence (questions 4-6); and adverse consequences from alcohol (questions 7-10). Record the score at the end of each line and total; the maximum total is 40.

A cutpoint of ≥8 points for men or ≥4 points for women, adolescents, and those older than 60 years indicates hazardous alcohol consumption.

The AUDIT-C is a shorter form that is helpful for acute and critical care units. The AUDIT-C is a valid screening test for heavy drinking and/or active alcohol abuse.[5] It uses the three alcohol consumption questions (numbers 1-3), including question number 3 that is itself a brief screening test for heavy drinking. This helps you discriminate heavy, at-risk drinking from low-risk drinking in a very short time (less than 2 minutes). The possible score is 0 to 12; a low-risk response is ≤2 points.

A cutpoint of ≥3 is a measure of heavy or at-risk drinking. Also, a "Yes" to drinking 6 or more drinks on one occasion *ever* in the past year warrants further assessment.

Examiner Asks	Rationale

The CAGE questionnaire (**C**utdown, **A**nnoyed, **G**uilty, **E**ye-opener) as described in Chapter 4 works well in busy primary care settings because it takes less than 1 minute to complete and the four straightforward yes/no questions are easy for clinicians to remember. The CAGE tests for lifetime alcohol abuse and/or dependence but does not distinguish past problem drinking from active present drinking.[5] It may not detect low but risky levels of drinking and is less effective with women and minority groups.[29]

Answering "Yes" to ≥2 CAGE questions signals possible alcohol abuse and a need for further assessment.

3. Assess for alcohol use disorders using the standard clinical diagnostic criteria. Determine whether there is a maladaptive pattern of alcohol use causing clinically significant impairment or distress.[2,22] Ask whether, in the past 12 months, "Has your drinking repeatedly caused or contributed to:

- **Risk** for bodily harm (drinking and driving, operating machinery, swimming)
- **Relationship** trouble (family or friends)
- **Role failure** (interference with home, work, or school obligations)
- **Run-ins** with the law (arrests or other legal problems)?"

If "Yes" to one or more points, it means that the patient meets criteria for Alcohol Abuse diagnosis. Warrants advice and brief intervention for assistance.

Ask whether, in the past 12 months, "Have you:

- **Not been able to stick to drinking limits** (repeatedly gone over them)
- **Not been able to cut down or stop** (repeated failed attempts)
- **Shown tolerance** (needed to drink a lot more to get the same effect)
- **Shown signs of withdrawal** (tremors, sweating, nausea, or insomnia when trying to quit or cut down)
- **Kept drinking despite problems** (recurrent physical or psychological problems)
- **Spent a lot of time drinking** (or anticipating or recovering from drinking)
- **Spent less time on other matters** (activities than had been important or pleasurable)?"

If "Yes" to three or more → patient meets criteria for Alcohol Dependence diagnosis.

If "No" → patient still at risk for developing alcohol-related problems. Warrants advice and brief intervention for assistance.

Ask about use of illicit substances: "Do you sometimes take illicit drugs or street drugs, such as marijuana, cocaine, hallucinogens, narcotics?" If "Yes," "When was the last time you used drugs? How much did you take that time?"

Screening Women for Alcohol Problems

The TWEAK questions[25a] are a combination of items of two other questionnaires that help identify at-risk drinking in women, especially pregnant women. Instead of the guilt question from the CAGE questionnaire, the TWEAK includes a question that measures tolerance:

- **Tolerance:** How many drinks can you hold? Or how many drinks does it take to make you feel high?
- **Worry:** Have close friends or relatives worried or complained about your drinking in the past year?
- **Eye-opener:** Do you sometimes take a drink in the morning when you first get up?
- **Amnesia:** Has a friend or family member ever told you about things you said or did that you could not remember?
- **Kut down:** Do you sometimes feel the need to cut down on your drinking?

Taking ≥3 drinks to feel high = tolerance.

Score 2 points each for Tolerance and Worry, 1 point each for the rest. A low-risk response is ≤1 point.

≥2 points = a drinking problem.

Screening Aging Adults

Use the SMAST-G questionnaire for older adults who report social or regular drinking of any amount of alcohol.[20] Older adults have specific emotional responses and physical reactions to alcohol and the 10 questions with yes/no responses address these factors. A low-risk response is zero or 1 point (Table 6-6).

Scoring ≥2 points indicates an alcohol problem and a need for more in-depth assessment.

Examiner Asks	Rationale

TABLE 6-6 Short Michigan Alcoholism Screening Test—Geriatric Version (SMAST-G)

	Yes (1)	No (0)
1. When talking with others, do you ever underestimate how much you drink?		
2. After a few drinks, have you sometimes not eaten or been able to skip a meal because you didn't feel hungry?		
3. Does having a few drinks help decrease your shakiness or tremors?		
4. Does alcohol sometimes make it hard for you to remember parts of the day or night?		
5. Do you usually take a drink to relax or calm your nerves?		
6. Do you drink to take your mind off your problems?		
7. Have you ever increased your drinking after experiencing a loss in your life?		
8. Has a doctor or nurse ever said they were worried or concerned about your drinking?		
9. Have you ever made rules to manage your drinking?		
10. When you feel lonely, does having a drink help?		
TOTAL SMAST-G-SCORE (0-10)	______	
SCORING: 2 OR MORE **"YES"** RESPONSES IS INDICATIVE OF AN ALCOHOL PROBLEM.		

4. Advise and Assist (Brief intervention). Although it is beyond the scope of this text to present treatment plans, the consequences of substance abuse are so debilitating and destructive to patients and their families that a short statement of assistance and concern is given here. If your assessment has determined the patient to have at-risk drinking or illicit substance use, state your conclusion and recommendation clearly[22]:

"You are drinking more than is medically safe." Relate to the person's concerns and medical findings, if present. "I strongly recommend that you cut down (or quit), and I'm willing to help."

Or, if you determine the person to have an alcohol use disorder, state your conclusion and recommendation clearly:

"I believe that you have an alcohol use disorder. I strongly recommend that you quit drinking, and I'm willing to help." Relate to the person's concerns and medical findings if present.

OBJECTIVE DATA

Normal Range of Findings

Clinical laboratory findings give objective evidence of problem drinking. These are less sensitive and specific than self-report questionnaires, but they are useful data to corroborate the subjective data. The serum protein *gamma glutamyl transferase (GGT)* is the most commonly used biochemical marker of alcohol drinking. Occasional alcohol drinking will not raise this measure, but chronic heavy drinking will. Be aware that nonalcoholic liver disease also can increase GGT levels in the absence of alcohol.

Serum aspartate aminotransferase (AST) is an enzyme found in high concentrations in the heart and liver.

From the complete blood count, the mean corpuscular volume (MCV) is an index of red blood cell (RBC) size. MCV is not sensitive enough to use as the only biomarker, but it can detect earlier drinking after a long period of abstinence.[21]

Abnormal Findings

Chronic alcohol drinking of ≥4 drinks/day for 4 to 8 weeks significantly raises GGT. It takes 4 to 5 weeks of abstinence for GGT levels to return to normal range.[21]

Months of chronic drinking increases AST.

Heavy alcohol drinking for 4 to 8 weeks increases MCV.

Objective Data

Normal Range of Findings	Abnormal Findings
Breath alcohol analysis detects any amount of alcohol in the end of exhaled air following a deep inhalation until all ingested alcohol is metabolized. This measure can be correlated with blood alcohol concentration (BAC) and is the basis for legal interpretation of drinking. Normal values indicating no alcohol are 0.00. Clinical appearance and behavioral signs of commonly abused substances are presented in Table 6-7. Note that clinical signs are described both for the intoxicated person and for the person in withdrawal.	A BAC ≥0.08% = legal intoxication in most states (3 standard drinks), with loss of balance and loss of motor coordination.

PROMOTING A HEALTHY LIFESTYLE

Prescription AD/HD Medication Abuse

Prescription attention-deficit/hyperactivity disorder (AD/HD) medications are among the most commonly abused prescription medications. In a recent study, Setlik et al. (2009) documented an 86% increase in the number of prescriptions written for AD/HD medications in 10- to 19- year-olds, as well as a 76% rise in poison center calls for adolescent abuse of AD/HD medication. They also noted the significant increase in prescription AD/HD medication abuse far exceeded other substance abuse in teens, suggesting a rising problem with teen and young adult AD/HD medication abuse.

Prescription AD/HD medication abuse occurs when an individual takes a medication that was prescribed for someone else OR takes their own prescription in a manner or dosage other than what was prescribed. These medications are known to health care providers by their chemical names, *dextroamphetamine* and *methylphenidate*, or by their brand names, *Dexedrine* or *Adderall* and *Ritalin* or *Concerta*. Among teens and young adults, these medications are also referred to by their street names, which include *Skippy*, *Vitamin R*, *Cramming Drug*, *R-Ball*, *The Smart Drug*, *Bennies*, *Black Beauties*, *Roses*, *Speed*, or *Uppers*. Methylphenidate and amphetamines are stimulant medications that are often prescribed to treat individuals with AD/HD. The therapeutic action of these stimulant medications is a slow and steady increase in dopamine—a neurotransmitter associated with attention. The prescription doses are typically started at low levels and increased gradually until a therapeutic effect is achieved for the individual that mimics levels in the brain unaffected by AD/HD and allows individuals with AD/HD to focus. When these medications are taken in doses and/or routes other than those prescribed, such as crushing the pill and snorting or injecting it, dopamine levels increase in a rapid, highly amplified manner, disrupting normal neurotransmission and often creating a state of euphoria. When prescription AD/HD medications are taken orally either in higher doses or by individuals without AD/HD, students report they can stay awake and maintain abnormally high levels of concentration for long nights of studying. However, continued abuse or an overdose of stimulants can cause anxiety, panic, tremors, irregular heartbeat, dangerously high body temperatures, and even heart attack. Further, teens and young adults who stop taking stimulants may suffer from fatigue and depression, which may set the stage for further medication use, abuse, and addiction.

The primary mission of the National Institutes of Health (NIH) National Institute on Drug Abuse (NIDA) is to lead the nation in bringing the power of science to bear on drug abuse and addiction. The NIDA *InfoFacts: Stimulant ADHD Medications: Methylphenidate and Amphetamines* provides an overview of current science on these prescriptions, including their use and abuse. It is available at www.nida.nih.gov/infofacts/ADHD.html.

The NIDA also has a site for teens about prescription medication abuse and the science behind addiction. It includes information aimed at teens, parents, and teachers, as well as an ongoing blog. It is available at http://teens.drugabuse.gov/facts/facts_rx1.php.

Resources

Setlik, J., Bond, R. B., & Ho, M. (2009). Adolescent prescription ADHD medication abuse is rising along with prescriptions for these medications. *Pediatrics*, *124*(3), 875-880.

ABNORMAL FINDINGS

TABLE 6-7 Clinical Signs of Substance Use Disorders

"Substances" refer to those agents taken nonmedically to alter mood or behavior.

Intoxication: ingestion of substance produces maladaptive behavior changes due to effects on the central nervous system

Abuse: daily use needed to function, inability to stop, impaired social and occupational functioning, recurrent use when it is physically hazardous, substance-related legal problems

Dependence: physiologic dependence on substance

Tolerance: requires increased amount of substance to produce same effect

Withdrawal: cessation of substance produces a syndrome of physiologic symptoms

TABLE 6-7 Clinical Signs of Substance Use Disorders—cont'd		
Substance	Intoxication	Withdrawal
Alcohol	**Appearance.** Unsteady gait, incoordination, nystagmus, flushed face **Behavior.** Sedation, relief of anxiety, dulled concentration, impaired judgment, expansive, uninhibited behavior, talkativeness, slurred speech, impaired memory, irritability, depression, emotional lability	**Uncomplicated.** (Shortly after cessation of drinking, peaks at 2nd day, improves by 4th to 5th day.) Coarse tremor of hands, tongue, eyelids; anorexia; nausea and vomiting; malaise; autonomic hyperactivity (tachycardia, sweating, elevated blood pressure); headache; insomnia; anxiety; depression or irritability; transient hallucinations or illusions **Withdrawal delirium, "delirium tremens."** (Much less common than uncomplicated, occurs within 1 week of cessation.) Coarse, irregular tremor; marked autonomic hyperactivity (tachycardia, sweating); vivid hallucinations; delusions; agitated behavior; fever
Sedatives, hypnotics (benzodiazepines)	Similar to alcohol **Appearance.** Unsteady gait, incoordination **Behavior.** Talkativeness, slurred speech, inattention, impaired memory, irritability, emotional lability, sexual aggressiveness, impaired judgment, impaired social or occupational functioning	Anxiety or irritability; nausea or vomiting; malaise; autonomic hyperactivity (tachycardia, sweating); orthostatic hypotension; coarse tremor of hands, tongue, and eyelids; marked insomnia; grand mal seizures
Nicotine	**Appearance.** Alert, increased systolic blood pressure, increased heart rate, vasoconstriction **Behavior.** Nausea, vomiting, indigestion (first use); loss of appetite, head rush, dizziness, jittery feeling, mild stimulant	Vasodilation, headaches, anger, irritability, frustration, anxiety, nervousness, awakening at night, difficulty concentrating, depression, hunger, impatience or restlessness, desire to smoke
Cannabis (marijuana)	**Appearance.** Reddened eyes; tachycardia; dry mouth; increased appetite, especially for "junk" food; loss of coordination and balance **Behavior.** Euphoria, pleasant state of relaxation and tranquility, slowed time perception, increased perceptions, impaired judgment, social withdrawal, anxiety, suspiciousness or paranoid ideation	No withdrawal with occasional use. Chronic heavy use may → mild withdrawal: irritability, sleep disturbances, weight loss, loss of appetite, sweating
Cocaine (including crack)	**Appearance.** Pupillary dilation, tachycardia or bradycardia, elevated or lowered blood pressure, sweating, chills, nausea, vomiting, weight loss **Behavior.** Euphoria, talkativeness, hypervigilance, pacing, psychomotor agitation, impaired social or occupational functioning, fighting, grandiosity, visual or tactile hallucinations	Dysphoric mood (anxiety, depression, irritability), fatigue, insomnia or hypersomnia, psychomotor agitation
Amphetamines	Similar to cocaine **Appearance.** Pupillary dilation, tachycardia or bradycardia, elevated or lowered blood pressure, sweating or chills, nausea and vomiting, weight loss **Behavior.** Elation, talkativeness, hypervigilance, psychomotor agitation, fighting, grandiosity, impaired judgment, impaired social and occupational functioning	Dysphoric mood (anxiety, depression, irritability), fatigue, insomnia or hypersomnia, psychomotor agitation
Opiates (morphine, heroin, meperidine)	**Appearance.** Pinpoint pupils; decreased blood pressure, pulse, respirations, and temperature **Behavior.** Lethargy; somnolence; slurred speech; initial euphoria followed by apathy, dysphoria, and psychomotor retardation; inattention; impaired memory; impaired judgment; impaired social or occupational functioning	Dilated pupils, lacrimation, runny nose, tachycardia, fever, elevated blood pressure, piloerection, sweating, diarrhea, yawning, insomnia, restlessness, irritability, depression, nausea, vomiting, malaise, tremor, muscle and joint pains; symptoms are remarkably similar to clinical picture of influenza

BIBLIOGRAPHY

1. Allen, N. E., Beral, V., Casabonne, D., et al. (2009). Moderate alcohol intake and cancer incidence in women. *Journal of the National Cancer Institute, 101*(5), 296-305.
2. American Psychiatric Association (APA). (1994). *Diagnostic and statistical manual of mental disorders, DSM-IV-TR* (4th ed.). Washington, DC: Author.
3. Becker, K. L., & Walton-Moss, B. (2001). Detecting and addressing alcohol abuse in women. *Nurse Practitioner, 26*(10), 13-25.
4. Bohn, M. J., Babor, T. F., & Kranzler, H. R. (1995). The alcohol use disorders identification test (AUDIT). *Journal of Studies on Alcohol, 56*(4), 423-432.
5. Bush, K., Kivlahan, D. R., McDonell, M. B., et al. (1998). The AUDIT alcohol consumption questions. *Archives of Internal Medicine, 158*, 1789-1795.
6. Centers for Disease Control and Prevention. (2007). Deaths: final data for 2004. *National Vital Statistics Reports, 55*(19). Retrieved July 2010 from www.cdc.gov/nchs/data/nvsr.
7. Centers for Disease Control and Prevention. (2010). Emergency department visits involving nonmedical use of selected prescription drugs. *MMWR Morbidity and Mortality Weekly Report, 59*(23). Retrieved July 2010 from www.cdc.gov/mmwr/pdf/wk/mm5923.
8. Compton, W. M., Thomas, Y. F., Stinson, F. S., et al. (2007). Prevalence, correlates, disability, and comorbidity of DSM-IV drug abuse and dependence in the United States. *Archives of General Psychiatry, 64*(5), 566-576.
9. Ewing, J. A. (1984). Detecting alcoholism: the CAGE questionnaire. *Journal of the American Medical Association, 252*(14), 1905-1907.
10. Fiellin, D. A., Reid, M. C., & O'Connor, P. G. (2000). Screening for alcohol problems in primary care: a systematic review. *Archives of Internal Medicine, 160*(13), 1977-1989.
11. Harwood, G. A. (2005). Alcohol abuse: screening in primary care. *Nurse Practitioner, 30*(2), 56-61.
12. Keegan, J., Parva, M., Finnegan, M., et al. (2010). Addiction in pregnancy. *Journal of Addictive Diseases, 29*(2), 175-191.
13. Keil, U., Liese, A., Filipiak, B., et al. (1998). *Alcohol, blood pressure and hypertension*. Chichester, UK: Wiley, Novartis Foundation Symposium.
14. Krishnamoorthy, S., Lip, G. Y. H., & Lane, D. A. (2009). Alcohol and illicit drug use as precipitants of atrial fibrillation in young adults. *American Journal of Medicine, 122*, 851-856.
15. Longnecker, M. P., Berlin, J. A., Orza, M. J., et al. (1988). A meta-analysis of alcohol consumption in relation to risk of breast cancer. *Journal of the American Medical Association, 260*(5), 652-656.
16. Lucey, M. R., Mathurin, P., & Morgan, T. R. (2009). Alcoholic hepatitis. *New England Journal of Medicine, 360*(26), 2758-2769.
17. Manwell, L. B., Fleming, M. F., Johnson, K., et al. (1998). Tobacco, alcohol, and drug use in a primary care sample. *Journal of Addictive Diseases, 17*(1), 67-81.
18. Marik, P., & Mohedin, B. (1996). Alcohol-related admissions to an inner city hospital intensive care unit. *Alcohol and Alcoholism, 31*(4), 393-396.
19. McDonald, A. J., Wang, N., & Camargo, C. A. (2004). U.S. emergency department visits for alcohol-related diseases and injuries between 1992 and 2000. *Archives of Internal Medicine, 164*, 531-537.
20. Naegle, M. A. (2008). Screening for alcohol use and misuse in older adults. *American Journal of Nursing, 108*(11), 50-59.
21. National Institute on Alcohol Abuse and Alcoholism. (2002). *Alcohol alert #56—screening for alcohol problems: an update*. Retrieved July 2010 from http://pubs.niaaa.nih.gov/publications/aa56.htm.

21a. National Institute on Alcohol Abuse and Alcoholism. (January 2003). Helping patients with alcohol problems: a health practitioner's guide. NIH Pub. No. 03-3769. Rockville, MD: Author.

22. National Institute on Alcohol Abuse and Alcoholism. (2005). (Reprinted 2007). *Helping patients who drink too much: a clinician's guide*. Retrieved July 2010 from http://pubs.niaaa.nih.gov/publications/Practitioner/CliniciansGuide2005/Clinicians_guide.htm.
23. National Institutes of Health. (2006). *Alcohol-related traffic deaths*. Retrieved July 2010 from www.nih.gov/about/researchresultforthepublic.
24. O'Brien, J. M., Lu, B., Ali, N. A., et al. (2007). Alcohol dependence is independently associated with sepsis, septic shock, and hospital mortality among adult intensive care unit patients. *Critical Care Medicine, 35*(2), 345-450.
25. Rehm, J., Gmel, G., Sempos, C. T., et al. (2002). Alcohol-related morbidity and mortality. *Alcohol Research & Health, 27*(1), 39-51.

25a. Russell, M., Materier, S. S., & Sokol, R. J. (1994). Screening for pregnancy risk drinking. *Alcoholism: Clinical and Experimental Research, 18*(5), 1156-1161.

26. Saitz, R. (2005). Unhealthy alcohol use. *New England Journal of Medicine, 352*(6), 596-607.
27. Saitz, R., Horton, N. J., Sullivan, L. M., et al. (2003). Addressing alcohol problems in primary care. *Annals of Internal Medicine, 138*(5), 372-382.
28. Sommers, M. S., Wray, J., Savage, C., et al. (2003). Assessing acute and critically ill patients for problem drinking. *Dimensions of Critical Care Nursing, 22*(2), 76-88.
29. Steinbauer, J. R., Cantor, S. B., Holzer, C. E., et al. (1998). Ethnic and sex bias in primary care screening tests for alcohol use disorders. *Annals of Internal Medicine, 129*(5), 353-362.
30. Thun, M. J., Peto, R., Lopez, A. D., et al. (1997). Alcohol consumption and mortality among middle-aged and elderly U.S. adults. *New England Journal of Medicine, 337*(24), 1705-1714.
31. Urbano-Marquez, A., Estruch, R., Fernandez-Sola, J., et al. (1995). The greater risk of alcoholic cardiomyopathy and myopathy in women compared with men. *Journal of the American Medical Association, 274*(2), 149-154.
32. U.S. Department of Health and Human Services, Substance Abuse and Mental Health Services Administration. (2009). *Results from the 2008 national survey on drug use and health*. Rockville, MD: USDHHS Pub. No. SMA 09-4434. Retrieved July 2010 from www.oas.samhsa.gov/nsduh/2k8nsduh/2k8Results.pdf .
33. Volicer, B. J., Quattrochi, N., Candelieri, R., et al. (2006). Depression and alcohol abuse in asthmatic college students. *Nurse Practitioner, 31*(2), 49-54.

7

Domestic Violence Assessment

evolve WEBSITE

http://evolve.elsevier.com/Jarvis/

- Audio Key Points
- Case Study
  Bruising
  Confusion and Paranoia
- NCLEX Review Questions

OUTLINE

Intimate Partner Violence Defined, 103
Child Abuse and Neglect Defined, 103
Elder Abuse and Neglect Defined, 104
Health Effects of Violence, 104
Assessing for Intimate Partner Violence, 105
Assessing for Elder and Vulnerable Person Abuse and Neglect, 107
History, 108
Screening for Child Abuse and Neglect, 108
Physical Examination, 108
Documentation, 110
Assessing for Risk of Homicide, 112
When She Says "No" to the AAS but There Are Other IPV Health Indicators, 113

Intimate partner violence, child abuse, and **elder abuse** are important health problems that health care professionals must recognize and assess. The Joint Commission (formerly known as *JCAHO*) requires that all health care settings have policies and procedures to assess, document, and make referrals for all kinds of family violence, including child abuse. All of the major nursing and medical organizations such as the American Nurses Association (ANA) and the American Medical Association (AMA) have policy statements recognizing the need for health care professionals to assess family violence.

INTIMATE PARTNER VIOLENCE DEFINED

The Centers for Disease Control and Prevention (CDC) definition for intimate partner violence (IPV) will be used throughout this chapter. The definition identifies two types of IPV[46]:

- Physical and/or sexual violence (use of physical force) or threat of such violence
- Psychological/emotional abuse and/or coercive tactics when there has been prior physical and/or sexual violence between persons who are spouses or nonmarital partners (dating, boyfriend/girlfriend) or former spouses or nonmarital partners

CHILD ABUSE AND NEGLECT DEFINED

Child abuse and neglect are defined at both the federal and state levels. The Child Abuse and Prevention Treatment Act (CAPTA) dictates the minimum standards that must be incorporated into the state statutes. Most of the state statutes incorporate the following definitions:

- **Neglect** is failure to provide for a child's basic needs (physical, educational, medical, and emotional).
- **Physical abuse** is physical injury due to punching, beating, kicking, biting, burning, shaking, or otherwise harming a child. Even if the parent or caregiver did not intend to harm the child, such acts are considered abuse when done purposefully.
- **Sexual abuse** includes fondling a child's genitals, incest, penetration, rape, sodomy, indecent exposure, and commercial exploitation through prostitution or the production of pornographic materials.
- **Emotional abuse** is any pattern of behavior that harms a child's emotional development or sense of self-worth. It

includes frequent belittling, rejection, threats, and withholding of love and support.

ELDER ABUSE AND NEGLECT DEFINED

Almost every state has some form of mandatory reporting of abused older adults and other vulnerable patients (the developmentally disabled and the mentally ill). You need to be familiar with specific state reporting requirements in your state of practice. Those who work in communities that border two states will need to be informed about mandatory reporting statutes in both states. In some communities, the reporting mechanism is established county by county, while some states have a statewide hotline. As mandatory reporters of abuse, you need only have suspicion that elder abuse and/or neglect may have occurred in order to generate a call to the authorities. Many nurses, physicians, and social workers are erroneously under the assumption that they must have proof of abuse before calling the hotline. Although exact definitions of elder abuse and neglect vary from state to state, the AMA has developed a generic list of definitions that are clinically useful (Table 7-1).[5] The National Research Council defines elder abuse as[8]:

1. Intentional actions that cause harm or create a serious risk of harm (whether or not harm is intended) to a vulnerable elder by a caregiver or person who stands in a trust relationship to the elder

   or
2. Failure by a caregiver to satisfy the elder's basic needs or to protect the elder from harm

HEALTH EFFECTS OF VIOLENCE

Although estimates vary, approximately 1 million women in the United States report being physically and/or sexually assaulted by an intimate partner annually.[56] Lifetime estimates of intimate violence vary from 5% to 51%,[56] with the most usual range between 25% and 35%. Women are significantly more likely to be physically or sexually assaulted by a current or former intimate partner than by an acquaintance, family member, friend, or stranger.[45,56] As high as these figures are, it is commonly accepted that they (particularly crime data) represent *under*estimates of the true incidence and prevalence of IPV.

In 2007, 794,000 children in the Unites States were determined by Child Protective Services to have been maltreated. Of these children, approximately 59% were neglected, 11% were physically abused, 8% were sexually abused, 8% were emotionally or psychologically abused, and fewer than 1% were medically neglected.[57] Although a number of children are injured by non-related caregivers, approximately 80% of children are injured by a parent or parents. Approximately 1760 children were confirmed to have died from maltreatment. Young children account for most of these deaths. Over 75% of the deaths due to child maltreatment were in children younger than 4 years. In deaths due to child maltreatment, nearly 70% were caused by one or both parents.[57]

Aside from minor differences, the reporting laws across the United States are essentially the same. As in cases of elder abuse, only a reasonable suspicion that a child has been maltreated is needed in order to make a report to the appropriate authorities. Waiting until a conclusive diagnosis of abuse is made can put children at risk of further abuse and injury.

A persuasive body of knowledge accumulated in the past decade has established that violent experiences have significant effects on women's health. The most obvious health care problem for abused women is injury. Cutaneous injuries can be caused by blunt, squeezing, and/or sharp mechanisms of injury.[52] Blunt-force injury is the most common form of intimate partner violence, with being struck by a hand (closed fist or slap) the most common mechanism of blunt-force trauma.[51] When blunt injuries cause the skin to tear, the wound is best described as a *laceration*.[50-52] When a sharp instrument (knife, razor, scalpel, glass) slices through the tissue, the wound is best described as a *cut* or *incision*.[50-52] Strangulation (often referred to by patient as "being choked") can be caused by the manual compression of the neck by any body part (usually hands) or by tightening a cordlike object around the neck (ligature compression).[50,52,55] Many of the mechanisms of injury just mentioned have particular patterns that can be recognized.[6,50-52]

In many controlled investigations of women in a variety of health care settings, abused women also have been found to have significantly more chronic health problems, including significantly more neurologic, gastrointestinal, and gynecologic symptoms and chronic pain.[9,12,39] Abused women have also been shown to visit health care professionals more often than women not battered and to incur more health care costs. In terms of mental health, abused women also have significantly more depression, suicidality, and post-traumatic stress disorder (PTSD) symptoms, as well as problems with substance abuse.[59] The forced sex that accompanies physical abuse in 40% to 45% of the cases contributes to a host of

TABLE 7-1 AMA Definitions for Elder Abuse and Neglect

Physical abuse	Violent acts that result or could result in injury, pain, impairment, and/or disease
Physical neglect	Failure of the family member and/or caregiver to provide basic goods and/or services such as food, shelter, health care, and medications
Psychological abuse	Behaviors that result in mental anguish
Psychological neglect	Failing to provide basic social stimulation
Financial abuse	Intentional misuse of the elderly person's financial/material resources without the informed consent of the person
Financial neglect	Failure to use the assets of the elderly person to provide services needed by the elderly person

Adapted from Arvanis, S. C., Adelman, R. D., Breckman, R., et al. (1993). Diagnostic and treatment guidelines on elder abuse and neglect. *Archives of Family Medicine*, *2*(4), 371-388.

reproductive health problems including chronic pelvic pain, unintended pregnancy, STIs (including HIV), and urinary tract infections.[10] Abuse during pregnancy is also a significant health problem, with serious consequences for both the pregnant mother (e.g., depression, substance abuse) and infant (low birth weight, increased risk of child abuse).[23,35]

Although more than half of battered women say they have been injured, only 25% to 30% of abused women say they have actually sought health care for one of the injuries.[47] Even so, the majority of abused women (80%) say they have been in the health care setting for some reason, either for regular checkups or for one of the long-term health problems described previously. Because many abused women are not yet ready to seek help from a shelter or from the criminal justice system, the health care system can be an extremely important early point of contact. By uncovering abuse in its early stages, it is hoped that the pattern of violence can be stopped and long-term health problems avoided or minimized.

The health effects of elder abuse are not nearly as well studied. Complications from intentional injury can range from minor pain and discomfort to life-threatening injuries.[18] Bleeding from intentional trauma can cause significant changes in circulatory homeostasis, leading to marked fluctuations in blood pressure and pulse, shock, and then death. Localized infections can progress to generalized sepsis and then death in aging patients who are immunocompromised. The actual assault or the stress leading up to or following an assault can contribute to cardiac complications. All of the sexually transmitted infections and sexually related complications that are sequelae of abuse for the younger women are present in the older sexually assaulted women. In addition, postmenopausal women have more friable vaginal mucosal tissue secondary to de-estrogenation.[42]

Abuse of older adults often is coupled with neglect. Neglect can manifest itself with symptoms of dehydration and malnutrition. Neglect can be intentional or unintentional. Many family members or caregivers working with an aging person consciously, and with malice, withhold food, water, medication, and appropriate necessities, while often stealing the financial assets of the older, dependent person. This type of neglect is often, by definition, criminal in nature.

Other family members or caregivers working with an older person struggle with their own severe physical and cognitive health challenges. Their intentions are good; however, the older patient may experience profound unintentional neglect. Although unintentional neglect is usually not viewed as a crime, it is still reportable to adult protective service agencies. Self-neglect raises often unanswerable questions about one's right to live autonomously versus society's obligation to care for a person who is not able to care for herself or himself. Suspected self-neglect is also a mandatory reportable activity to adult protective services.

There are many possible long-term physical and psychological effects of child maltreatment. The immediate consequences can include a spectrum of physical injuries such as bruises, fractures, and lacerations and can involve more severe injury such as inflicted traumatic brain injury (shaken baby syndrome). More severe forms of maltreatment can lead to death or long-term disability such as mental retardation, blindness, and physical disability.

Child maltreatment can have deleterious effects on a child's quality of life and overall poor health, which can last into adulthood.[4,16] Ongoing child maltreatment can lead to changes in brain structure and chemistry, which may lead to long-term physical, psychological, emotional, social, and cognitive dysfunction.[24] Childhood physical abuse is reported to be the most consistent predictor of youth violence.[30] Children who are abused are 11 times more likely to be arrested for violent crime as a juvenile and 2.7 times more likely to be arrested for violent crime as an adult.[19] Approximately one third of abused children will abuse their own children.[43] Two out of three people in drug treatment programs report abuse as children.[29]

Examples of risk factors that may contribute to child maltreatment[14]:

- Disabilities or mental retardation in children that may increase caregiver burden
- Social isolation of families
- Parents' lack of understanding of children's needs and child development
- Parents' history of domestic abuse
- Poverty and other socioeconomic disadvantages, such as unemployment
- Family disorganization, dissolution, and violence, including intimate partner violence
- Lack of family cohesion
- Substance abuse in family
- Young, single, nonbiological parents
- Poor parent-child relationships and negative interactions
- Parental thoughts and emotions supporting maltreatment behaviors
- Parental stress and distress, including depression or other mental health conditions
- Community violence

Although there are identified risk factors for child maltreatment, a study on missed cases of abusive head trauma conducted by Jenny et al.[26] found several factors significant for missed injuries. They found that missed cases of abusive head injury occurred more often in white children than children of minority races, in children with both parents living with the child, in younger children, and in children with less severe presenting symptoms.

ASSESSING FOR INTIMATE PARTNER VIOLENCE

Routine, universal assessments for intimate partner violence means asking every woman at every health care encounter if she has been abused by a husband, boyfriend, or other intimate partner or ex-partner. The majority of both abused and nonabused women say that they are in favor of routine assessments and that they believe it would assist women in getting help for the problem.[3,22] Routine, universal assessment for IPV has been called for by most nursing professional organizations (e.g., ANA; American College of Nurse Midwives

[ACNM]; Association of Women's Health and Obstetrics and Neonatal Nursing [AWHONN]; Emergency Nurses Association [ENA]; International Association of Forensic Nurses [IAFN]; Nursing Network on Violence Against Women, International [NNVAWI]).[33]

How to Assess

The Abuse Assessment Screen (AAS) has been used in many different health care settings, has been translated into at least seven languages, and has strong support for reliability and validity.[53] It has never been copyrighted, with the intention that nurses be able to revise and reformat its content to be adaptable to their own health care setting (Fig. 7-1).

Many health care professionals precede the questions with an introduction such as: "Because domestic violence is so common in our society, we are asking all women the following questions." or "Because domestic violence has such serious health care consequences, we are asking all of our female patients the questions that follow." This both alerts the woman that questions about domestic violence are coming and makes sure that the woman knows she is not being singled out for these questions.

The Family Violence Prevention Fund[20] has developed a protocol for the recommended frequency of screening (Fig. 7-2).

Assessment

If a woman answers "yes" to any of the AAS questions, you need to ask questions designed to assess how recent and how serious the abuse was. Asking the woman to "tell me about this abuse in your relationship" is a good way to start. Even if the woman says "yes" only to the first question and calls the abuse "only emotional" or "not that bad" or says "we just fight a lot" at first, more abuse may be revealed as you gently assess the situation. This type of assessment is often like "peeling layers of an onion," with more violence being uncovered as the assessment continues. This is not "denial" on the woman's part but, rather, the normal minimization that often accompanies trauma from violence.

It is appropriate for you to show that you are concerned and even distressed about the degree of violence. One message that needs to be conveyed during the assessment is that the abuse is not the woman's fault; this can be said several times. Another important message is that you are concerned and that help is possible. Still another is that several health problems can occur because of domestic violence and that is why it is necessary to conduct a thorough assessment. In fact, in a recent survey of 265 abused women who accepted a referral to a social worker, 59% said it was because the medical provider expressed concern that their presenting health problem was related to IPV.[32]

Abuse Assessment Screen
NRCVA (1988)

Violence is very common in today's world, and it can overlap into our homes. Because violence affects so many people, I now routinely ask all my patients (clients) a few questions about violence in their lives.

All couples argue now and again, even the best of couples.

1. When you and your partner argue, are you ever afraid of him (her)?
2. When you and your partner verbally argue, do you think he (she) tries to emotionally hurt/abuse you?
3. Does your partner try to control you? Where you go? Who you see? How much money you can have?
4. Has your partner (or anyone) ever slapped you, pushed you, hit you, kicked you, or otherwise physically hurt you?
5. Since you have been pregnant (when you were pregnant), has your partner ever bit you, slapped you, pushed you, hit you, kicked you, or otherwise physically hurt you?
6. Has your partner ever forced you into sex when you did not want to participate?

With any yes, say, "Thank you for sharing. Can you tell me more about the last time?"

The Nursing Research Consortium on Violence and Abuse (NRCVA) (1988) encourages the reproduction, modification, and/or use of the Abuse Assessment Screen in routine screening for domestic violence.

7-1 Abuse Assessment Screen (AAS).

Protocol for Screening Summary: Women Over 14 Years of Age

Setting
Frequency of IPV screening

Primary Care
Every first visit for a new chief complaint, every new patient encounter, every new intimate relationship, and all periodic examinations

Emergency Department and Urgent Care
All women, all visits

OB/GYN
Each prenatal and postpartum visit, each new intimate relationship, all routine gynecologic visits (periodic and symptom based), all family planning visits, and all visits in STI and abortion clinics

Mental Health
Every initial assessment, each new intimate relationship, and annually if ongoing or periodic treatment

Inpatient
Part of all admissions and discharge

Source: Family Violence Prevention Fund, 1999. (www.fvpf.org)

7-2 Protocol for screening summary—women over 14 years of age.

ASSESSING FOR ELDER AND VULNERABLE PERSON ABUSE AND NEGLECT

Routine assessment for possible elder abuse and neglect can be more complicated than assessments for IPV. Older adults can present for health care cognitively and physically intact or with multiple health, physical, and cognitive challenges. Assessing for intimate partner violence in older adults is very similar to screening for IPV among younger women if the patient is cognitively intact.[27] The AAS can be a useful screen for assessing domestic violence among older women. You may modify the introductory statement as follows: "Because domestic violence has such serious health care consequences, we are asking women of all ages the following questions."

Whereas some aging women have been in abusive relationships for decades, others are experiencing for the first time physical and sexual violence from normally nonabusive partners who themselves are afflicted with behavior-altering neurologic illness (Alzheimer disease, organic brain syndromes). An older battered woman in a long-term abusive relationship may be trying to outlive her abuser, whereas the newly abused older woman may be reluctant to disclose because of embarrassment, shame, and fears that her partner will be institutionalized.

Older adults are vulnerable to abuse from other family members and caregivers. The AMA nine-question clinically effective screen can be used with older persons who are cognitively intact (Table 7-2). Chapter 3 gives further direction for assessment.

Assessment of physical abuse and/or neglect in the cognitively challenged person is much more complicated. Physical findings that are inconsistent with the history provided by the patient, family member, or caregiver are significant red flags of possible abuse and neglect. Almost all states have some form of mandatory reporting of suspected abuse of patients ages 65 years and older. To report abuse, you need not have proof of abuse or neglect, only reasonable cause to suspect that elder abuse or neglect may have occurred.

TABLE 7-2 AMA Elder Abuse Screening Questions

1. Has anyone ever touched you inappropriately without your consent?
2. Has anyone ever made you do things you didn't want to do?
3. Has anyone taken things that were yours without first asking?
4. Has anyone ever physically hurt you?
5. Has anyone ever scolded or threatened you?
6. Have you ever signed any documents you did not understand?
7. Are you afraid of anybody at home or who enters your home?
8. Are you alone a lot?
9. Has anyone ever failed to help you take care of yourself when you needed help?

Adapted from Arvanis, S. C., Adelman, R. D., Breckman, R., et al. (1993). Diagnostic and treatment guidelines on elder abuse and neglect. *Archives of Family Medicine*, 2(4), 371-388.

HISTORY

It is important also to assess and document prior abuse, including prior IPV, childhood physical and sexual abuse, and prior rapes of all kinds (stranger, date, intimate partner). Cumulative trauma has been associated with more severe mental and physical health problems.[59] Also important to determine is the history of traumatic injuries, because these may have an impact on the current health condition. For instance, a woman may have experienced prior episodes of head trauma and strangulation, both of which may be related to chronic but subtle neurologic symptoms and problems. Another extremely important area of history and examination in cases of IPV or elder abuse is a mental status examination, both for potential head trauma and neurologic symptoms and also for mental health problems. All survivors of violence should be given a mental status examination, with particular attention to the most frequent mental health problems associated with violence: depression, suicidality, PTSD, substance abuse, and anxiety. Chapter 5 gives direction for conducting this part of the history.

SCREENING FOR CHILD ABUSE AND NEGLECT

The American Academy of Pediatrics[1] recommends screening for IPV as an active means to prevent child maltreatment. There is a significant co-occurrence between child abuse and IPV, and it is suggested that when exposed to both, children may have more significant long-term health effects.[25] Child abuse is reported in 33% to 77% of homes where there is ongoing abuse of an adult.[1] Positive responses should prompt you to involve additional members of the health care team (e.g., physician, social worker).

An important part of evaluating any child for suspected abuse is to determine the child's age and developmental level. Could the child have suffered the injury that is being reported based on his or her developmental level? For example, the history that a 3-week-old child rolled off a bed causing injury is not yet developmentally plausible. Because you may not be able to directly observe the child's motor and cognitive milestones during the history taking, it is important to ask the caregivers directly. Is your child crawling, pulling to stand, or walking? What other developmental issues are currently being faced at home: for example, tantrums, potty training?

If the child is verbal, a history should be obtained away from the caregivers through open-ended questions or spontaneous statements. It is important to remember that children may have suffered significant trauma yet respond only minimally to open-ended questions.[36] Keeping the questions short and using age-appropriate language and familiar words can help enrich the history taking. Children older than 11 years can generally be expected to provide a history at the level of most adults.[36]

The medical history is also an important part of your evaluation. Has the child had previous hospitalizations or injuries, or does he or she suffer from any chronic medical conditions? Does the child take any medication that may cause easy bruising? Does the child have a history of repeated visits to the hospital? Was there a delay in seeking care for anything other than a minor injury? Is there a history of substance abuse in the family or any financial or social stressors in the home? What are the typical methods of discipline used in the home?

PHYSICAL EXAMINATION

Important components of the physical examination of the known survivor of IPV and/or elder abuse include a complete head-to-toe visual examination, especially if the patient is receiving health services secondary to reported abuse. When the examination reveals physical findings, knowledge of basic medical forensic terminology is essential in all documentation. Table 7-3 lists the most common forensic terms with definitions. Note that the most commonly misused terms are *ecchymosis* and *laceration*. Ecchymoses are not directly related to blunt-force trauma that results in bruising, and not all open wounds should be called *lacerations* (only those related to splitting of tissue from blunt-force impact and/or tearing of tissue should be).

Keep in mind the following guidelines when documenting the physical examination[50-52]:

- *Bruise* can be used interchangeably with *contusion*.
- *Laceration* is related to *avulsion*.
- *Ecchymosis* is related to *(senile) purpura*.
- *Petechia* is related to *purpura*.
- *Rug burn* is more accurately described as a *friction abrasion*.
- *Incision* can be used interchangeably with *cut*.
- *Cut* can be used interchangeably with *sharp injury*.
- *Stab wounds* are penetrating, deep, sharp injuries.
- *Hematoma* is a collection of blood that is often but not always caused by blunt-force trauma.

Many practitioners try to date bruises based on the color; however, there is no scientific evidence to support the accurate dating of injuries based on color of the contusion.[28,37] Therefore trying to accurately date injuries solely by examination is forensically futile. However, some guidelines can assist in determining if the approximate age of the bruise is consistent with the history being provided by the patient and/or caregiver.

A new bruise is usually red and will often develop a purple or purple-blue appearance 12 to 36 hours after blunt-force trauma. The color of bruises (and ecchymoses) generally progresses from purple-blue to bluish green to greenish brown to brownish yellow before fading away. This process will be the same on all people; however, depending on the color of a person's skin, the process may be more or less visible and more or less able to be photographed. In general, newer bruises will be mostly reddish purple, whereas bruises that are beginning to age will be more greenish brown or brownish yellow.[37]

Multiple factors can contribute to older adults bruising more readily or more severely than younger people. Medications and abnormal blood values related to medication side effects and underlying hematologic disorders can affect ease

TABLE 7-3 Forensic Terminology

Abrasion A wound caused by rubbing the skin or mucous membrane.
Avulsion The tearing away of a structure or part.
Bruise Superficial discoloration due to hemorrhage into the tissues from ruptured blood vessels beneath the skin surface, without the skin itself being broken; also called a *contusion.*
Contusion A bruise; injury to tissues without breakage of skin; blood from broken blood vessels accumulates, producing pain, swelling, tenderness.
Cut See "Incision."
Ecchymosis A hemorrhagic spot or blotch, larger than petechia, in the skin or mucous membrane, forming a nonelevated, rounded or regular, blue or purplish patch.
Hematoma A localized collection of extravasated blood, usually clotted in an organ, space, or tissue.
Hemorrhage The escape of blood from a ruptured vessel, which can be external, internal, and/or into the skin or other organ.
Incision A cut or wound made by a sharp instrument; the act of cutting.
Laceration The act of tearing or splitting; a wound produced by the tearing and/or splitting of body tissue, usually from blunt impact over a bony surface.
Lesion A broad term referring to any pathologic or traumatic discontinuity of tissue or loss of function of a part.
Patterned injury An injury caused by an object that leaves a distinct pattern on the skin and/or organ (e.g., being whipped with an extension cord) or an injury caused by a unique mechanism of injury (e.g., immersion burns to the hands [glove burns] or feet [sock burns]).
Pattern of injuries Injuries, usually bruises and fractures, in various stages of healing.
Petechiae Minute, pinpoint, nonraised, perfectly round, purplish red spots caused by intradermal or submucous hemorrhage, which later turn blue or yellow.
Puncture The act of piercing or penetrating with a pointed object or instrument.
Stab wound A penetrating, sharp, cutting injury that is deeper than it is wide.
Traumatic alopecia Loss of hair from pulling and yanking or by other traumatic means.
Wound A general term referring to a bodily injury caused by physical means.

Adapted from Miller, B. F., Keane, C. B., O'Toole, M. (2005). *Miller-Keane encyclopedia & dictionary of medicine, nursing, and allied health* (7th ed.). Philadelphia: Saunders; Sheridan, D. J. (2001). Treating survivors of intimate partner abuse: forensic identification and documentation. In Olshaker, J. S., Jackson, M. L., Smock, W. S., editors: *Forensic emergency medicine,* Philadelphia: Saunders; *Taber's cyclopedic medical dictionary*. (1997). Philadelphia: Davis.

of bruising or the formation of ecchymosis. Common medications that increase risk for bruising or bleeding complications include but are not limited to the following: aspirin, ibuprofen, any of the nonsteroidal anti-inflammatory drugs, warfarin, heparin, valproic acid, prednisone, and clopidogrel. Vitamin nutritional supplements also may contribute to hematologic complications, especially if the person is already taking a blood-thinning or platelet-altering medication. Bilberry, garlic, ginger, and ginkgo are among the more common supplements linked to increased risk of bruising and/or bleeding complications.[17]

Any health evaluation for known or suspected elder abuse and neglect should include baseline laboratory tests, including, at a minimum, a complete blood count (CBC) with platelet level, basic blood chemistries (including blood urea nitrogen [BUN], creatinine, protein, and albumin), serum liver function tests, a coagulation panel, and a urinalysis.[21]

Physical Examination of Children

The forensic terminology used in documentation of IPV/elder abuse applies similarly to children. A visual inspection of the child from head to toe is important in any physical examination. Significant injuries can be hidden under clothing, diapers, socks, and long hair. The American Academy of Pediatrics[2] defines significant trauma as any injury beyond temporary redness of the skin. Bruising in children is one of the most common physical findings in child abuse. Unfortunately, it can also be easily overlooked and may be a missed opportunity for intervention and prevention of further injury. Pierce et al.[41] found that bruising was a missed warning sign in up to 44% of fatal and near-fatal cases of physical child abuse. Accidental bruising in healthy, active children is common, yet the presence of bruises in babies has significance in evaluating a child for abuse. Children who are not yet walking with support—"cruising"—typically should not have bruises.[54] Bruising in infants who are not yet cruising, usually infants younger than 9 months, should alert you to possible abusive mechanisms to the injury or an underlying medical illness.

Once children begin to walk, bruising, particularly on the bony prominences, is common.[54] Reece and Ludwig[44] found that in children who were walking, 40% to 50% had bruises over the bony prominences of the front of their bodies. Sugar, Taylor, and Feldman[54] found that bruising in "atypical" places such as the buttocks, hands, feet, and abdomen was exceedingly rare and should arouse concern. This is further supported by Pierce et al.,[41] who found that in children younger than 4 years, bruising on the torso, ears, and neck as well as any bruising on a pre-cruising infant was significantly correlated with abuse, in absence of a compelling history. Similarly, Mosqueda et al.[34] studied older adults who had accidental bruises and found that nearly 90% of their bruises were on their extremities and no accidental bruises were found on the neck, ears, genitalia, buttocks, or soles of the feet. Furthermore, any bruise that takes the shape of an object should be considered highly specific for abuse. Bruising found in non-mobile children should raise the concern for further injury, including fractures and intracranial injury.

Health care providers are often asked to estimate the ages of bruises, particularly as it relates to an inflicted injury. This should be avoided, because published evidence does not support the ability to date a bruise by color alone, either by visual assessment or photography.[31]

In addition to bruising, lacerations, abrasions, bite marks, and burns are commonly seen in abused children. These findings, taken into context of the child's developmental

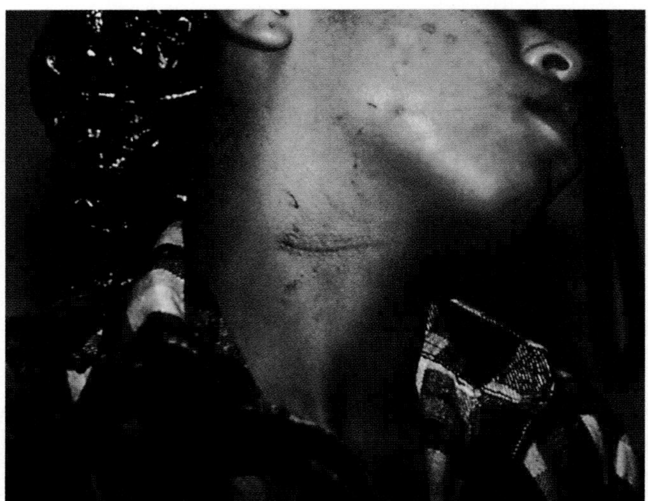

7-3 Patterned fingernail-like scratch abrasions to the left lateral neck from a manual strangulation mechanism of injury.

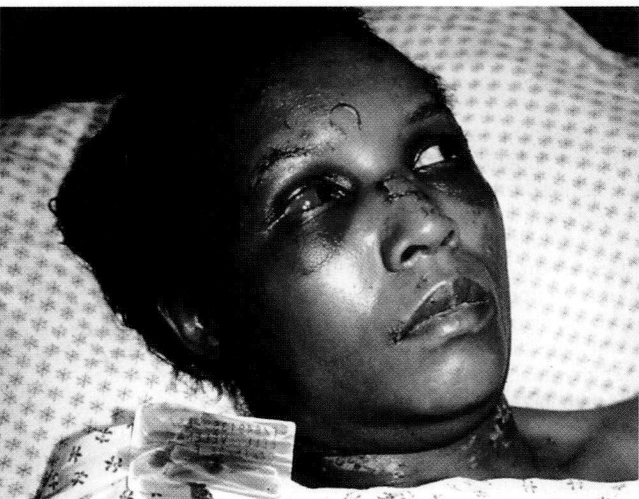

7-4 Patterned punchlike abrasion to the mid-forehead from an assailant wearing a ring with a stone; sutured laceration to the left eyebrow; sutured partial-avulsion injury to the nose, punchlike contusion to the left eye involving the sclera, and manual strangulation–related abrasion to the neck.

level, history and mechanism of injury, location of injury, and social history, can help guide in determining if an injury is concerning for abuse.

DOCUMENTATION

Documentation of intimate partner violence and elder abuse must include detailed, nonbiased progress notes, the use of injury maps, and photographic documentation in the health record. Examples of photographic documentation of patients of one of the authors are included in this chapter (Figs. 7-3 through 7-9*).

Written documentation of histories of IPV and elder abuse need to be verbatim but within reason. It is clinically unrealistic to document verbatim every statement made by an abused patient. However, it is critical to document exceptionally poignant statements made by the victim that identify the reported perpetrator and severe threats of harm made by the reported perpetrator. Other aspects of the abuse history, including reports of past abusive incidents, can be paraphrased with the use of partial direct quotations.

When quoting or paraphrasing the history, you should not sanitize the words reportedly heard by the victim. Verbatim documentation of the reported perpetrator's threats interlaced with curses and expletives can be extremely useful in future court proceedings. Also, be careful to use the exact terms an abused patient may use to describe sexual organs or sexually assaultive behaviors.

Photographic documentation in the medical record can be invaluable. Prior written consent to take photographs should be obtained from all cognitively intact, competent adults. Most health facilities have standardized consent to photograph forms. If a patient is unconscious or cognitively impaired, the taking of photographs without consent is generally viewed as ethically sound because it is a noninvasive, painless intervention that has high potential to help a suspected abuse victim. There are advantages and disadvantages to the different photographic systems (35-mm versus

*Many of these photos were first published in Sheridan, 2001.[49] Reprinted here with the author's permission.

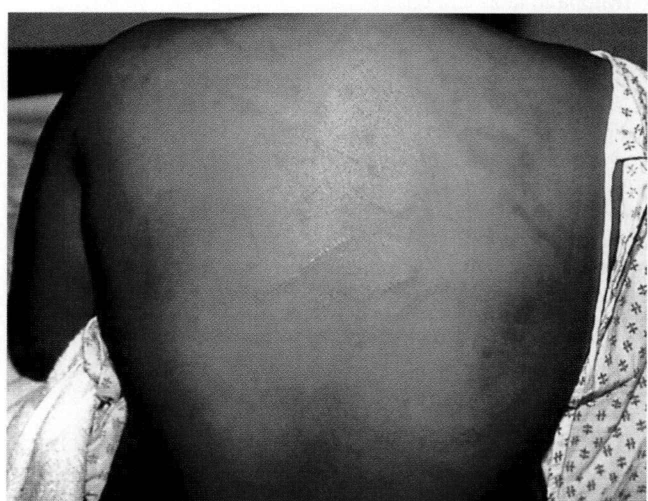

7-5 Newer patterned looped, cordlike contusions to the right upper posterior shoulder and left lower posterior shoulder; patterned looped, cordlike scar to the right mid-lateral back; scabbed, cordlike abrasions to the mid-back; patterned kick/stomplike heel contusion to the left mid-back; and patterned foot/kick/stomplike heel and sole bruise imprint to the upper left posterior shoulder.

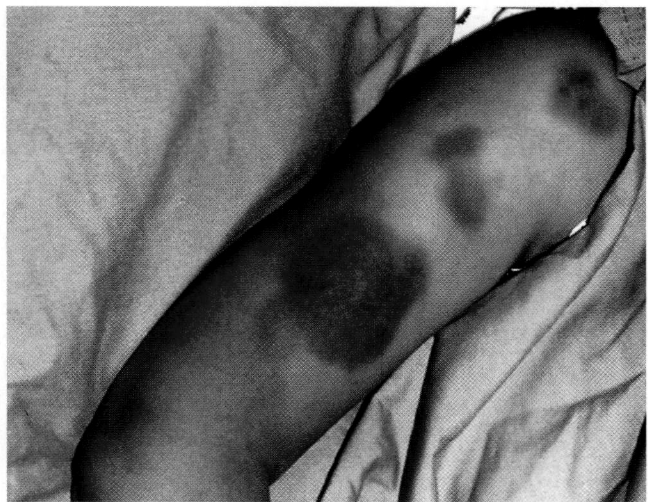

7-6 Multiple patterned punchlike contusions to the right upper arm.

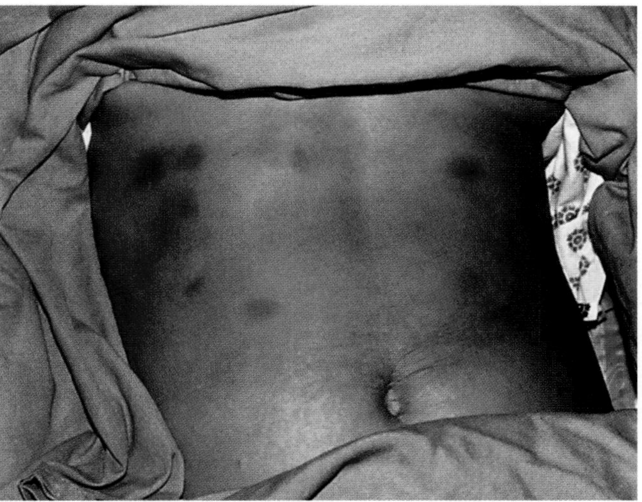

7-7 Multiple patterned "hidden" punchlike contusions to the upper abdomen and lower anterior chest.

digital) commonly in use.[7,50] In general, any in-focus picture of injury is better than no picture, regardless of what system is used.

When documenting the history and physical findings of child abuse and neglect, use the words the child has given to describe how his or her injury occurred. Remember that the possibility arises that the abuser may be accompanying the child. If the child is nonverbal, use statements from caregivers. It is important to know your employer/institutional protocol for obtaining a history in cases of suspected child maltreatment. Some protocols may delay a full interview until it can be done by a forensically trained interviewer.

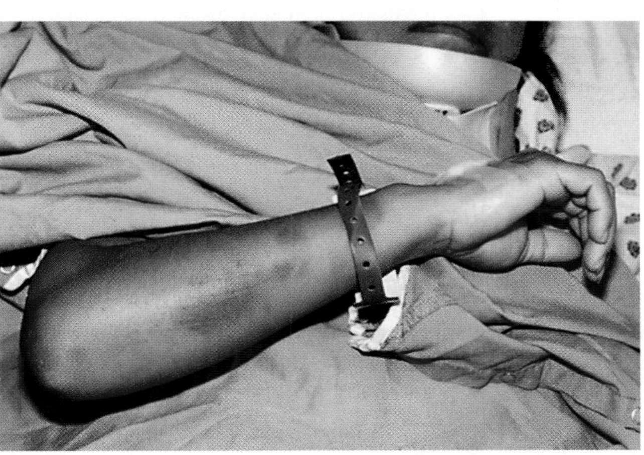

7-8 Patterned defensive posture–like bruises to the right forearm.

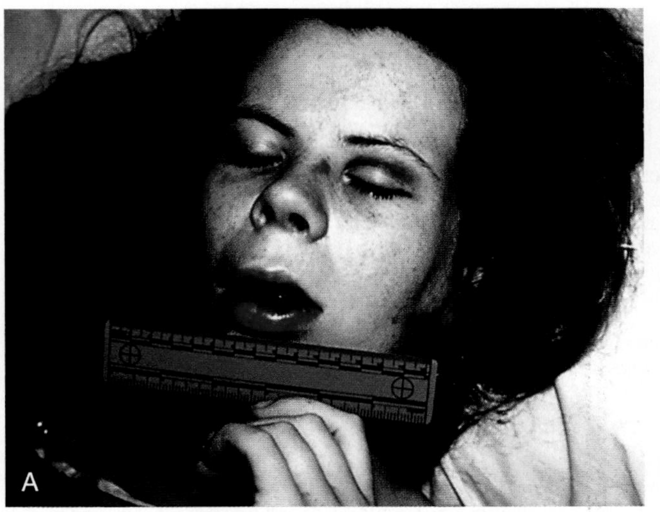

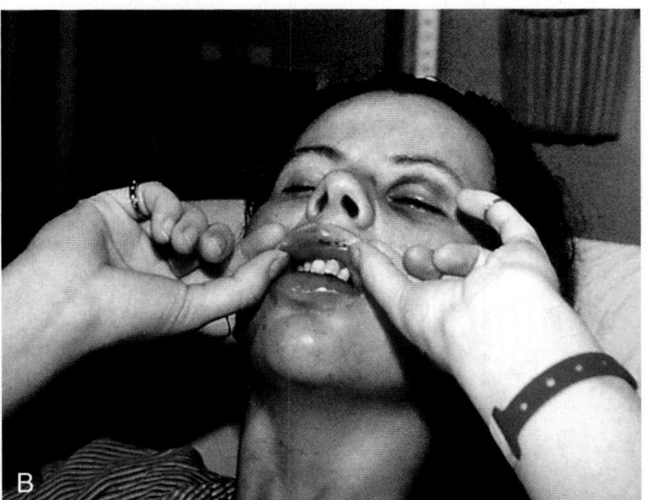

7-9 Series of two photographs to illustrate how photographs can be used to demonstrate mechanisms of injuries. **A,** Victim has obvious facial trauma to her left eyelid, left lateral nose, and mouth. The left lateral nose contusion was caused by the nosepiece of her glasses being forcefully pushed into her skin from a punch injury to the left eye. The patient's glasses absorbed much of the punch force and were broken (not pictured). A second punch produced the mouth trauma. **B,** The force of the mouth punch caused the upper teeth to leave patterned contusions, abrasions, and minor lacerations to the oral mucosa of the upper lip.

ASSESSING FOR RISK OF HOMICIDE

Women in this country are more often killed by a husband, boyfriend, or ex-husband than by anyone else, and about three fourths of these women had been abused by the man who subsequently killed them.[13] In a multicity study of intimate partner homicide of women, 42% of the women killed had been seen somewhere in the health care system (the ED in the majority of cases but also in primary care, prenatal care, and other settings) for something in the year before she was killed.[48] These encounters were missed opportunities for health care professionals to identify IPV and intervene to decrease the danger. The same study found reliability and validity support for the Danger Assessment (DA), a 19-item yes/no instrument that has been used extensively by nurses in the health care system as well as advocates in other settings with battered women[13] (Fig. 7-10). The instrument starts with a calendar so that women can more accurately see for themselves how frequent and severe the violence has become over the past year. This is also an excellent assessment of frequency and severity for the health care provider. Although there are no predetermined cutoff scores on the DA, the more "yes" answers there are, the more serious the danger of the woman's situation. In the previously described

DANGER ASSESSMENT
Jacquelyn C. Campbell, Ph.D., R.N.

Several risk factors have been associated with homicides (murders) of both batterers and battered women in research conducted after the murders have taken place. We cannot predict what will happen in your case, but we would like you to be aware of the danger of homicide in situations of severe battering and for you to see how many of the risk factors apply to your situation.

Using the calendar, please mark the approximate dates during the past year when you were beaten by your husband or partner. Write on that date how bad the incident was according to the following scale:

1. Slapping, pushing; no injuries and/or lasting pain
2. Punching, kicking; bruises, cuts, and/or continuing pain
3. "Beating up"; severe contusions, burns, broken bones
4. Threat to use weapon; head injury, internal injury, permanent injury
5. Use of weapon; wounds from weapon

(If **any** of the descriptions for the higher number apply, use the higher number.)

Mark **Yes** or **No** for each of the following. ("He" refers to your husband, partner, ex-husband, ex-partner, or whoever is currently physically hurting you.)

____ 1. Has the physical violence increased in severity or frequency over the past year?
____ 2. Has he ever used a weapon against you or threatened you with a weapon?
____ 3. Does he ever try to choke you?
____ 4. Does he own a gun?
____ 5. Has he ever forced you to have sex when you did not wish to do so?
____ 6. Does he use drugs? By drugs, I mean "uppers" or amphetamines, speed, angel dust, cocaine, "crack", street drugs or mixtures.
____ 7. Does he threaten to kill you and/or do you believe he is capable of killing you?
____ 8. Is he drunk every day or almost every day? (In terms of quantity of alcohol.)
____ 9. Does he control most or all of your daily activities? For instance: does he tell you who you can be friends with, when you can see your family, how much money you can use, or when you can take the car? (If he tries, but you do not let him, check here: ____)
____ 10. Have you ever been beaten by him while you were pregnant? (If you have never been pregnant by him, check here: ____)
____ 11. Is he violently and constantly jealous of you? (For instance, does he say "If I can't have you, no one can"?)
____ 12. Have you ever threatened or tried to commit suicide?
____ 13. Has he ever threatened or tried to commit suicide?
____ 14. Does he threaten to harm your children?
____ 15. Do you have a child that is not his?
____ 16. Is he unemployed?
____ 17. Have you left him during the past year? (If you have *never* lived with him, check here: ____)
____ 18. Do you currently have another (different) intimate partner?
____ 19. Does he follow or spy on you, leave threatening notes, destroy your property, or call you when you don't want him to?

____ Total "Yes" Answers

Thank you. Please talk to your nurse, advocate, or counselor about what the Danger Assessment means in terms of your situation.

7-10 Danger Assessment.

multicity study, abused women who were the victims of a homicide had an average score of 7.1 on the original 15-item DA. The DA is copyrighted, so users need to use it intact and are asked to communicate with the author if they are planning to use it in research. It can also be downloaded from www.son.jhmi.edu.

WHEN SHE SAYS "NO" TO THE AAS BUT THERE ARE OTHER IPV HEALTH INDICATORS

In addition to the AAS, providers need to be alert for the conditions particularly associated with IPV, including gynecologic problems (especially STIs, pelvic pain, and complaints of sexual dysfunction), chronic irritable bowel syndrome, back pain, depression, and the presenting symptoms of PTSD (especially problems sleeping and "panic" attacks or problems with "nerves"). When these problems occur, and especially when they persist, a thorough and repeated assessment for domestic violence is needed. In this case, an instrument such as the Women's Experience with Battering (WEB)[15] scale might be used in addition to the AAS, or gentle indirect queries may be used (e.g., "I am concerned about your health conditions. Is there any chance that stress at home is contributing to these problems?").

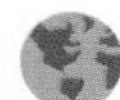

CULTURE AND GENETICS

Domestic violence is a phenomenon that occurs cross-culturally.[58] It may be more difficult to determine in many cultural groups. For example, the battering may be hidden, covered by clothing and heavy facial makeup, by many Chinese women. Indicators that domestic violence may be a problem include higher reported rates of alcoholism, suicide, and homicide in American Indian and other communities.

Domestic violence has a profound effect on the person, family, and community, and the roots or outcomes are seen in the following examples[38]:

- The reporting of serious psychological distress among persons 18 years of age and older was 3.0% for the general population, 3.0% for whites, 7.1% for American Indians, and 3.0% for African Americans.
- The heavy use of alcohol by persons 12 years of age and older for the white population was 7.5%, African Americans 4.4%, and American Indians 8.7% of the population.
- Death rates from suicide among the general male population was 10.9 per 100,000 residents, but 16.4 per 100,000 male American Indians and 9.8 per 100,000 African Americans.
- Death rates for homicide among the general male population was 9.4 per 100,000 residents, but 11.6 per 100,000 male American Indians and 36.4 per 100,000 African Americans.

BIBLIOGRAPHY

1. American Academy of Pediatrics. (1998). The role of the pediatrician in recognizing and intervening on behalf of abused women. *Pediatrics, 101*(6), 1091-1092.
2. American Academy of Pediatrics. (2002). When inflicted skin injuries constitute child abuse. *Pediatrics, 110*, 644-645.
3. Anglin, D. (2009). Diagnosis through disclosure and pattern recognition. In C. Mitchell & D. Anglin (Eds.), *Intimate partner violence: A health-based perspective*. New York: Oxford University Press.
4. Arnow, B. A. (2004). Relationships between childhood maltreatment, adult health and psychiatric outcomes and medical utilization. *The Journal of Clinical Psychiatry, 65*(Suppl. 12), 10-15.
5. Arvanis, S. C., Adelman, R. D., Breckman, R., et al. (1993). Diagnostic and treatment guidelines on elder abuse and neglect. *Archives of Family Medicine, 2*(4), 371-388.
6. Besant-Matthews, P. E. (2006). Blunt and sharp injuries. In V. Lynch & J. B. Duval (Eds.), *Forensic nursing*. St. Louis: Mosby.
7. Besant-Matthews, P. E., & Smock, W. S. (2001). Forensic photography in the emergency department. In J. S. Olshaker, M. C. Jackson, & W. S. Smock (Eds.), *Forensic emergency medicine* (pp. 257-282). Philadelphia: Lippincott Williams & Wilkins.
8. Bonnie, R. J., & Wallace, R. B. (Eds.). (2003). *Elder mistreatment: Abuse, neglect, and exploitation in an aging America*. Washington, DC: National Academies Press.
9. Campbell, J., Jones, A. S., Dienemann, J., et al. (2002). Intimate partner violence and physical health consequences. *Archives of Internal Medicine, 162*, 1157-1163.
10. Campbell, J., & Soeken, K. (1999). Forced sex and intimate partner violence: Effects on women's health. *Violence Against Women, 5*, 1017-1035.
11. Campbell, J., & Soeken, K. L. (1999). Women's responses to battering: a test of the model. *Research in Nursing & Health, 22*, 49-58.
12. Campbell, J. C. (2002). Health consequences of intimate partner violence. *Lancet, 359*(9314), 1331-1336.
13. Campbell, J. C., et al. (2001). Risk assessment for intimate partner homicide. In G. F. Pinard & L. Pagani (Eds.), *Clinical assessment of dangerousness: Empirical contributions*. New York: Cambridge University Press.
14. Child Welfare Information Gateway. (2007). *Common risk and protective factors*. Retrieved September 8, 2007, from www.childwelfare.gov/preventing/overview/commonfactors.cfm.
15. Coker, A., Smith, P. H., McKeown, R. E., et al. (2000). Frequency and correlates of intimate partner violence by type: physical, sexual, and psychological battering. *American Journal of Public Health, 90*(4), 553-559.
16. Corso, P. S., Edwards, V. J., Fang, X., et al. (2008). Health related quality of life among adults who experienced maltreatment during childhood. *American Journal of Public Health, 98*(6), 1094-1100.
17. Doyle, R. M., Harold, C., & Johnson, P. (Eds.). (2001). *Nursing herbal medicine handbook*. Springhouse, PA: Springhouse.
18. Dyer, C. B., Connolly, M. T., & McFeeley, P. (2003). The clinical and medical forensics of elder abuse and neglect. In R. J. Bonnie & R. B. Wallace (Eds.), *Elder mistreatment: Abuse, neglect and exploitation in an aging America*. Washington, DC: National Academies Press.
19. English, D. J., Widom, C. S., & Brandford, C. (2004). Another look at the effects of child abuse. *National Institute of Justice Journal, 251*, 23-24.

20. Family Violence Prevention Fund. (1999). *Preventing domestic violence: Clinical guidelines on routine screening*. San Francisco: Author (www.fvpf.org).
21. Geroff, A. J., & Olshaker, J. S. (2001). Elder abuse. In J. S. Olshaker, M. C. Jackson, & W. S. Smock (Eds.), *Forensic emergency medicine*. Philadelphia: Lippincott Williams & Wilkins.
22. Glass, N. E., Dearwater, S., & Campbell, J. C. (2001). Intimate partner violence screening and intervention: Data from eleven Pennsylvania and California community hospital emergency departments. *Journal of Emergency Nursing, 27*(2), 141-149.
23. Goodman, P. E. (2009). Intimate partner violence and pregnancy. In C. Mitchell & D. Anglin (Eds.), *Intimate partner violence: A health-based perspective*. New York: Oxford University Press.
24. Hagele, D. M. (2005). The impact of maltreatment on the developing child. *North Carolina Medical Journal, 66*(5), 356-359.
25. Herrenkohl, T. I., Sousa, C, Tajima, E. A., et al. (2008). Intersection of child abuse and children's exposure to domestic violence. *Trauma, Violence & Abuse, 9*(2), 84-99.
26. Jenny, C., Hymel, K. P., Ritzen, A., et al. (1999). Analysis of missed cases of abusive head trauma. *JAMA: The Journal of the American Medical Association, 281*, 621-626.
27. Koin, D. (2009). Intimate partner violence among the elderly and people with disabilities. In C. Mitchell & D. Anglin (Eds.), *Intimate partner violence: A health-based perspective*. New York: Oxford University Press.
28. Langlois, N. E.I., & Greshman, G. A. (2001). The aging of bruises: A review and study of the colour changes with time. *Forensic Science International, 50*, 227-238.
29. Leshner, A. I. (2007). NIDA probes the elusive link between child abuse and later drug use. *NIDA Notes* (serial online). Retrieved September 8, 2007, from www.nida.nih.gov/NIDA_Notes/NNVol13N2/DirrepVol13N2.html.
30. Maas, C., Herrenkohl, T. I., & Sousa, C. (2008). Review of research on child maltreatment and violence in youth. *Trauma, Violence & Abuse, 9*(1), 56-67.
31. Maguire, S., Mann, M. K., Sibert, J., et al. (2005). Can you age bruises accurately in children? A systematic review. *Archives of Disease in Childhood, 90*(2), 187-189.
32. McCaw, B., Bauer, H. M., Berman, W. H., et al. (2002). Women referred for on-site domestic violence services in a managed care organization. *Women & Health, 35*(2/3), 23-40.
33. Mitchell, C., & James, L. (2009). Evolving health policy on intimate partner violence. In C. Mitchell & D. Anglin (Eds.), *Intimate partner violence: A health-based perspective*. New York: Oxford University Press.
34. Mosqueda, L., Burnight, K., & Liao, S. (2005). The life cycle of bruises in older adults. *Journal of the American Geriatrics Society, 53*(8), 1339-1343.
35. Murphy, C. C., Schei, B., Myhr, T. L., et al. (2001). Abuse: a risk factor for low birth weight? A systematic review and meta-analysis. *Canadian Medical Association Journal, 164*(11), 1567-1572.
36. Myers, J. E., Berliner, L. A., Briere, J., et al. (2002). *The APSAC handbook on child maltreatment*. Thousand Oaks, CA: Sage Publications.
37. Nash, K. R., & Sheridan, D. J. (2009). Can one accurately date a bruise: State of the science, *Journal of Forensic Nursing, 5*, 31-37.
38. National Center for Health Statistics. (2006). *Health, United States, 2005, with chartbook on trends in the health of Americans* (USDHHS Publication No. 2005-1232). Hyattsville, MD: Author.
39. Nicolaidis, C., & Liebschutz, J. (2009). Chronic physical symptoms in survivors of intimate partner violence. In C. Mitchell & D. Anglin (Eds.), *Intimate partner violence: A health-based perspective*. New York: Oxford University Press.
40. O'Toole, M. T. (2005). *Miller-Keane encyclopedia and dictionary of medicine, nursing, and allied health* (7th ed.). Philadelphia: Saunders.
41. Pierce, M. C., Kaczor, K., Aldridge, S., et al. (2010). Bruising characteristics discriminating physical child abuse from accidental trauma. *Pediatrics, 125*(1), 67-74.
42. Poulos, C., & Sheridan, D. J. (2008). Genital injuries in postmenopausal women after sexual assault. *Journal of Elder Abuse & Neglect, 20*(4), 323-335.
43. Prevent Child Abuse New York. (2003). *The costs of child abuse and the urgent need for prevention*. Retrieved April 8, 2010, from http://preventchildabuseny.org/pdf/cancost.pdf.
44. Reece, R. M., & Ludwig, S. (2001). *Child abuse: medical diagnosis and management* (2nd ed.). Philadelphia: Lippincott Williams & Wilkins.
45. Rennison, C. M. (2003). *Intimate partner violence 1993-2001 (NCJ-197838)*. Washington, DC: Bureau of Justice Statistics.
46. Saltzman, L. E., Fanslow, J. L., McMahon, P. M., et al. (1999). *Intimate partner violence surveillance: uniform definitions and recommended data elements (Version 1.0)*. Atlanta: National Center for Injury Prevention and Control, Centers for Disease Control and Prevention.
47. Saltzman, L. E., & Houry, D. (2009). Prevalence of nonfatal and fatal intimate partner violence in the Unites States. In C. Mitchell & D. Anglin (Eds.), *Intimate partner violence: A health-based perspective*. New York: Oxford University Press.
48. Sharps, P., Koziol-McLain, J., Campbell, J., et al. (2001). Health care providers' missed opportunities for preventing femicide. *Preventive Medicine, 33*, 373-380.
49. Sheridan, D. J. (2001). Treating survivors of intimate partner abuse: forensic identification and documentation. In J. S. Olshaker, M. C. Jackson, & W. S. Smock (Eds.), *Forensic emergency medicine*. Philadelphia: Lippincott Williams & Wilkins.
50. Sheridan, D. J. (2007). Treating survivors of intimate partner abuse: forensic identification and documentation. In J. S. Olshaker, M. C. Jackson, & W. S. Smock (Eds.). (2007). *Forensic emergency medicine* (2nd ed.). Philadelphia: Lippincott Williams & Wilkins.
51. Sheridan, D. J., & Nash, K. R. (2007). Acute injury patterns of intimate partner violence. *Trauma, Violence & Abuse, 8*(3), 281-289.
52. Sheridan, D. J., Nash, K. R., Poulos, C. A., et al. (2009). Soft tissue and cutaneous injury patterns. In C. Mitchell & D. Anglin (Eds.), *Intimate partner violence: a health-based perspective*, New York: Oxford University Press.
53. Soeken, K., McFarlane, J., Parker, B., et al. (1998). The abuse assessment screen: a clinical instrument to measure frequency, severity, and perpetrator of abuse against women. In J. C. Campbell (Ed.), *Empowering survivors of abuse: Health care for battered women and their children*. Newbury Park, CA: Sage.
54. Sugar, N. F., Taylor, J. A., & Feldman, K. W. (1999). Bruises in infants and toddlers: Those who don't cruise rarely bruise. *Archives of Pediatrics & Adolescent Medicine, 153*(4), 399-403.
55. Taliaferro, E., Hawley, D., McClane, G., et al. (2009). Strangulation in intimate partner violence. In C. Mitchell & D. Anglin (Eds.). *Intimate partner violence: a health-based perspective*. New York: Oxford University Press.
56. Tjaden, P., & Thoennes, N. (2000). *Full report of the prevalence, incidence, and consequences of violence against women (NCJ-183781)*. Washington, DC: National Institute of Justice.
57. U.S. Department of Health and Human Services, Administration on Children, Youth and Families. (2009). *Child maltreatment 2007*. Washington, DC: U.S. Government Printing Office. Retrieved January 26, 2010, from www.acf.hhs.gov/programs/cb/stats_research/index.htm#can.
58. Warrier, S. (2009). Culture and cultural competency in addressing intimate partner violence. In C. Mitchell & D. Anglin (Eds.). (2009). *Intimate partner violence: A health-based perspective*. New York: Oxford University Press.
59. Warsaw, C., Brashler, P., & Gil, J. (2009). Mental health consequence of intimate partner violence. In C. Mitchell & D. Anglin (Eds.). (2009). *Intimate partner violence: A health-based perspective*. New York: Oxford University Press.

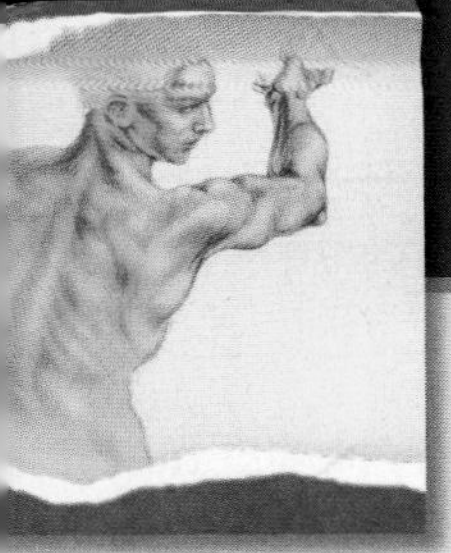

CHAPTER 8

Assessment Techniques and the Clinical Setting

evolve WEBSITE

http://evolve.elsevier.com/Jarvis/

- Audio Key Points
- NCLEX Review Questions

OUTLINE

Cultivating Your Senses, 115
Setting, 118
Equipment, 119
A Safer Environment, 120
The Clinical Setting, 121

The physical examination requires you to develop technical skills and a knowledge base. The technical skills are the tools to gather data. You will relate those data to your knowledge base and to your previous experience. A sturdy knowledge base enables you to look *for,* rather than merely look *at.* Consider a statement by the eighteenth century German poet Goethe: "We see only what we know." To recognize a significant finding, you need to know what to look for.

CULTIVATING YOUR SENSES

You will use your senses—sight, smell, touch, and hearing—to gather data during the physical examination. You always have perceived the world through your senses, but now they will be focused in a new way. The skills requisite for the physical examination are **inspection, palpation, percussion,** and **auscultation.** The skills are performed one at a time and in this order.

Inspection

Inspection is concentrated watching. It is close, careful scrutiny, first of the individual as a whole and then of each body system. Inspection begins the moment you first meet the person and develop a "general survey." (Specific data to consider for the general survey are presented in the following chapter.) Then as you proceed through the examination, start the assessment of each body system with inspection.

Inspection always comes first. Initially you may feel embarrassed "staring" at the person without also "doing something." But do not be too eager to touch the person. A focused inspection takes time and yields a surprising amount of data. Train yourself not to rush through inspection by holding your hands behind your back.

Learn to use each person as his or her own control, and compare the right and left sides of the body. The two sides are nearly symmetric. Inspection requires good lighting, adequate exposure, and occasional use of certain instruments (otoscope, ophthalmoscope, penlight, nasal and vaginal specula) to enlarge your view.

Palpation

Palpation follows and often confirms points you noted during inspection. Palpation applies your sense of touch to assess these factors: texture, temperature, moisture, organ location and size, as well as any swelling, vibration or pulsation, rigidity or spasticity, crepitation, presence of lumps or masses, and presence of tenderness or pain. Different parts of the hands are best suited for assessing different factors:

- Fingertips—best for fine tactile discrimination, as of skin texture, swelling, pulsation, and determining presence of lumps
- A grasping action of the fingers and thumb—to detect the position, shape, and consistency of an organ or mass

- The dorsa (backs) of hands and fingers—best for determining temperature because the skin here is thinner than on the palms
- Base of fingers (metacarpophalangeal joints) or ulnar surface of the hand—best for vibration

Your palpation technique should be slow and systematic. A person stiffens when touched suddenly, making it difficult for you to feel very much. Use a calm, gentle approach. Warm your hands by kneading them together or holding them under warm water. Identify any tender areas, and palpate them last.

Start with light palpation to detect surface characteristics and to accustom the person to being touched. Then perform deeper palpation, perhaps by helping the person use relaxation techniques such as imagery or deep breathing. Your sense of touch becomes blunted with heavy or continuous pressure. When deep palpation is needed (as for abdominal contents), intermittent pressure is better than one long, continuous palpation. Avoid any situation in which deep palpation could cause internal injury or pain.

Bimanual palpation requires the use of both of your hands to envelop or capture certain body parts or organs—such as the kidneys, uterus, or adnexa—for more precise delimitation (see Chapters 21 and 26).

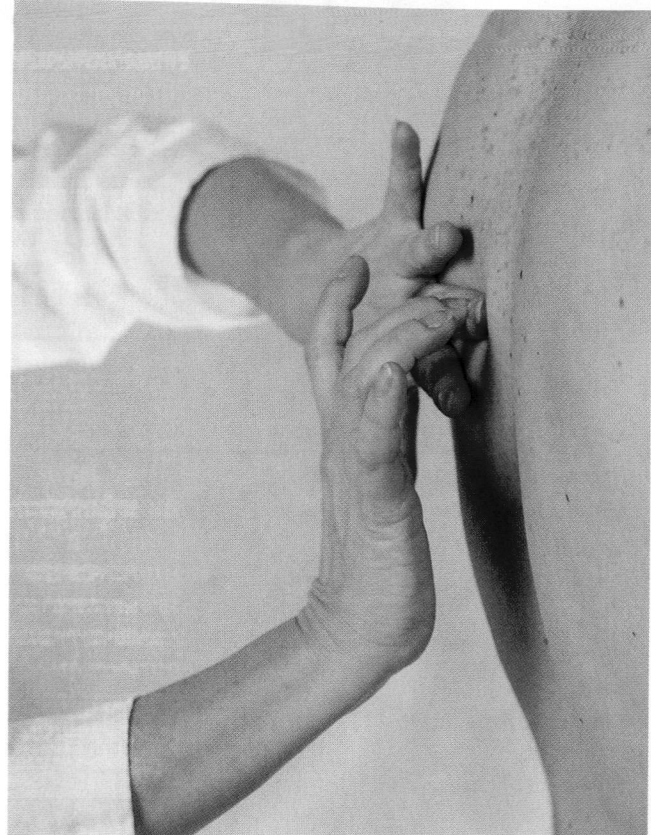

8-1

Percussion

Percussion is tapping the person's skin with short, sharp strokes to assess underlying structures. The strokes yield a palpable vibration and a characteristic sound that depicts the location, size, and density of the underlying organ. Why learn percussion when an x-ray study is so much more accurate? It's because your percussing hands are always available, are easily portable, and give instant feedback. Percussion has the following uses:

- Mapping out the *location* and *size* of an organ by exploring where the percussion note changes between the borders of an organ and its neighbors.
- Signaling the *density* (air, fluid, or solid) of a structure by a characteristic note.
- Detecting an abnormal mass if it is fairly superficial; the percussion vibrations penetrate about 5 cm deep—a deeper mass would give no change in percussion.
- Eliciting a deep tendon reflex using the percussion hammer.

The Stationary Hand

Hyperextend the middle finger (sometimes called the *pleximeter*) and place its distal portion, the phalanx and distal interphalangeal joint, *firmly* against the person's skin. Avoid the person's ribs and scapulae. Percussing over a bone yields no data because it always sounds "dull." Lift the rest of the stationary hand up off the person's skin (Fig. 8-1). Otherwise the resting hand will dampen off the produced vibrations, just as a drummer uses the hand to halt a drum roll.

The Striking Hand

Use the middle finger of your dominant hand as the *striking finger* (sometimes called the *plexor*) (Fig. 8-2). Hold your forearm close to the skin surface, with your upper arm and shoulder steady. Scan your muscles to make sure they are steady but not rigid. The action is all in the wrist, and it *must* be relaxed. Spread your fingers, swish your wrist, and bounce your middle finger off the stationary one. Aim for just behind the nail bed or at the distal interphalangeal joint; the goal is to hit the portion of the finger that is pushing the hardest into the skin surface. Flex the striking finger so that its tip, not the finger pad, makes contact. It hits directly at right angles to the stationary finger.

Percuss two times in this location using even, staccato blows. Lift the striking finger off quickly; a resting finger dampens vibrations. Then move to a new body location and repeat, keeping your technique even. The force of the blow determines the loudness of the note. You do not need a very loud sound; use just enough force to achieve a clear note. The thickness of the person's body wall will be a factor. You will need a stronger percussion stroke for persons with obese or very muscular body walls.

Percussion can be an awkward technique for beginning examiners. You may feel surprised and embarrassed if your striking finger misses your stationary hand completely. You may wince if the fingernail of your striking finger is too long and painfully gouges your stationary finger. As with all new skills, refinement follows practice. After a few weeks, your

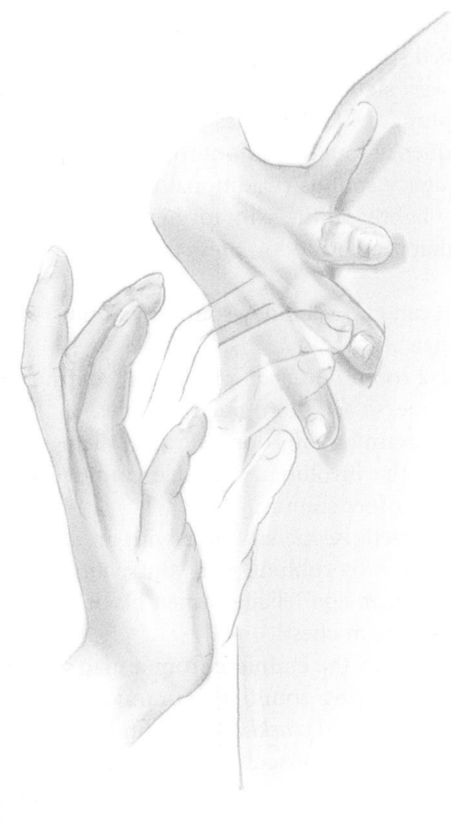

8-2

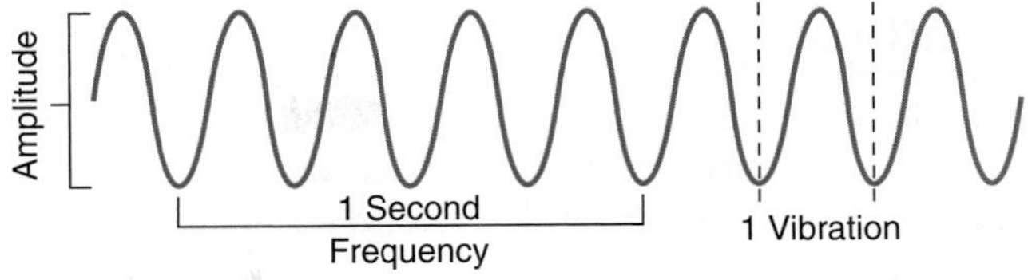

8-3 Sound wave.

hand placement becomes precise and feels natural and your ears learn to perceive the subtle difference in percussion notes.

Production of Sound

All sound results from vibration of some structure (Fig. 8-3). Percussing over a body structure causes vibrations that produce characteristic waves and are heard as "notes" (Table 8-1), which are differentiated by the following components:

1. **Amplitude** (or intensity), a loud or soft sound. Loudness depends on the force of the blow and the structure's ability to vibrate.
2. **Pitch** (or frequency), the number of vibrations per second. More rapid vibrations produce a high-pitched tone; slower vibrations yield a low-pitched tone.
3. **Quality** (timbre), a subjective difference due to a sound's distinctive overtones. Variations within a sound wave produce overtones. Overtones allow you to distinguish a C on a piano from a C on a violin.
4. **Duration,** the length of time the note lingers.

A basic principle is that a structure with relatively more air (e.g., the lungs) produces a louder, deeper, and longer sound because it vibrates freely, whereas a denser, more solid structure (e.g., the liver) gives a softer, higher, shorter sound because it does not vibrate as easily. Although Table 8-1 describes five "normal" percussion notes, variations occur in clinical practice. The "note" you hear depends on the nature of the underlying structure, as well as the thickness of the body wall and your correct technique. Do not learn these various notes just from written description. Practice on a willing partner.

TABLE 8-1 Characteristics of Percussion Notes

	Amplitude	Pitch	Quality	Duration	Sample Location
Resonant	Medium-loud	Low	Clear, hollow	Moderate	Over normal lung tissue
Hyperresonant	Louder	Lower	Booming	Longer	Normal over child's lung Abnormal in the adult, over lungs with increased amount of air, as in emphysema
Tympany	Loud	High	Musical and drumlike (like the kettle drum)	Sustained longest	Over air-filled viscus (e.g., the stomach, the intestine)
Dull	Soft	High	Muffled thud	Short	Relatively dense organ, as liver or spleen
Flat	Very soft	High	A dead stop of sound, absolute dullness	Very short	When no air is present, over thigh muscles, bone, or over tumor

Auscultation

Auscultation is listening to sounds produced by the body, such as the heart and blood vessels and the lungs and abdomen. Likely you already have heard certain body sounds with your ear alone—for example, the harsh gurgling of very congested breathing. However, most body sounds are very soft and must be channeled through a **stethoscope** for you to evaluate them. The stethoscope does not magnify sound but does block out extraneous room sounds. Of all the equipment you will use, the stethoscope quickly becomes a very personal instrument. Take time to learn its features and to fit one individually to yourself.

The fit and quality of the stethoscope are important. You cannot assess what you cannot hear through a poor instrument. The slope of the earpiece should point forward toward your nose. This matches the natural slope of your ear canal and efficiently blocks out environmental sound. If necessary, twist the earpieces to parallel the slope of your ear canals. The earpieces should fit snugly, but if they hurt, they are inserted too far. Adjust the tension and experiment with different rubber or plastic earplugs to achieve the most comfort. The tubing should be of thick material, with an internal diameter of 4 mm (⅛ in), and about 36 to 46 cm (14 to 18 in) long. Longer tubing may distort the sound.

Choose a stethoscope with two endpieces—a diaphragm and a bell (Fig. 8-4). You will use the **diaphragm** most often because its flat edge is best for high-pitched sounds—breath, bowel, and normal heart sounds. Hold the diaphragm firmly against the person's skin—firm enough to leave a slight ring afterward. The **bell** endpiece has a deep, hollow, cuplike shape. It is best for soft, low-pitched sounds such as extra heart sounds or murmurs. Hold it lightly against the person's skin—just enough that it forms a perfect seal. Any harder causes the person's skin to act as a diaphragm, obliterating the low-pitched sounds.

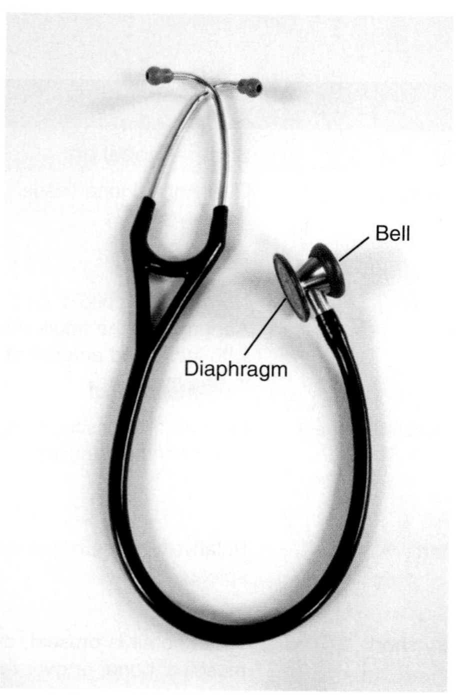

8-4 Stethoscope diaphragm *(left)* and bell *(right)*.

Some newer stethoscopes have one endpiece with a "tunable diaphragm." This enables you to listen to both low- and high-frequency sounds without rotation of the endpiece. For low-frequency sounds (traditional bell mode), hold the endpiece very lightly on the skin; for high-frequency sounds (traditional diaphragm mode), press the endpiece firmly on the skin.

Before you can evaluate body sounds, you must eliminate any confusing artifacts:

- Any extra room noise can produce a "roaring" in your stethoscope, so the room must be quiet.
- Keep the examination room warm. If the person starts shivering, the involuntary muscle contractions could drown out other sounds.
- Clean the stethoscope endpiece with an alcohol wipe. Then warm it by rubbing it in your palm. This avoids the "chandelier sign" elicited when placing a cold endpiece on a warm chest!
- The friction on the endpiece from a man's hairy chest causes a crackling sound that mimics an abnormal breath sound called *crackles.* To minimize this problem, wet the hair before auscultating the area.
- **Never listen through a gown.** Listening through clothing creates artifactual sound and muffles any diagnostically valuable sound from the heart or lungs. So, reach under a gown to listen, but take care that no clothing rubs on the stethoscope.
- Finally, avoid your own "artifact," such as breathing on the tubing, or the "thump" from bumping the tubing together.

Auscultation is a skill that beginning examiners are eager to learn, but one that is difficult to master. First you must learn the wide range of normal sounds. Once you can recognize normal sounds, you can distinguish the abnormal sounds and "extra" sounds. Be aware that in some body locations, you may hear more than one sound; this can be confusing. You will need to listen selectively, to only one thing at a time. As you listen, ask yourself: What am I *actually hearing?* … What *should* I be hearing at this spot?

SETTING

The examination room should be warm and comfortable, quiet, private, and well lit. When possible, stop any distracting noises—such as humming machinery, radio or television, or people talking—that could make it difficult to hear body sounds. Your time with the individual should be secure from interruptions from other health care personnel.

Lighting with natural daylight is best, although it is often not available; artificial light from two sources will suffice and will prevent shadows. A wall-mounted or gooseneck stand lamp is needed for high-intensity lighting. This provides *tangential* lighting (directed at an angle), which will highlight pulsations and body contours better than perpendicular lighting.

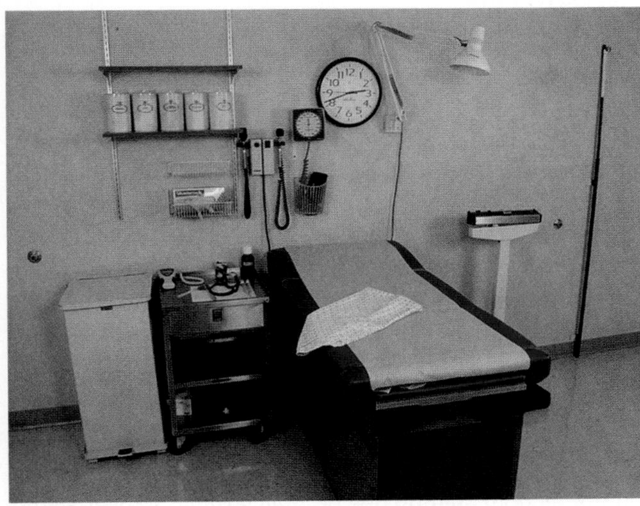

8-5

Position the examination table so that both sides of the person are easily accessible (Fig. 8-5). The table should be at a height at which you can stand without stooping and should be equipped to raise the person's head up to 45 degrees. A roll-up stool is used for the sections of the examination for which you must be sitting. A bedside stand or table is needed to lay out all your equipment.

EQUIPMENT

During the examination, you do not want to be searching for equipment or to have to leave the room to find an item. Have all your equipment at easy reach and laid out in an organized fashion (Fig. 8-6). The following items are usually needed for a screening physical examination:

- Platform scale with height attachment
- Sphygmomanometer
- Stethoscope with bell and diaphragm endpieces
- Thermometer
- Pulse oximeter (in hospital setting)
- Paper and pencil or pen
- Flashlight or penlight
- Otoscope/ophthalmoscope
- Tuning fork

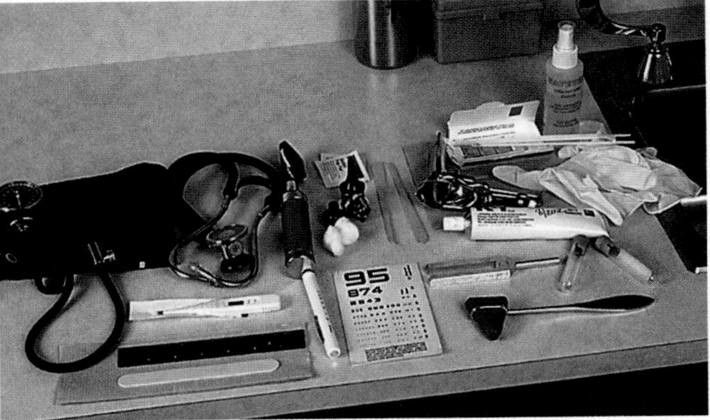

8-6

- Nasal speculum (if a short, broad speculum is not included with the otoscope)
- Tongue depressor
- Pocket vision screener
- Skin-marking pen
- Flexible tape measure and ruler marked in centimeters
- Reflex hammer
- Sharp object (split tongue blade)
- Cotton balls
- Bivalve vaginal speculum
- Clean gloves
- Materials for cytologic study
- Lubricant
- Fecal occult blood test materials

Most of the equipment is described as it comes into use throughout the text. However, consider these introductory comments on the otoscope and ophthalmoscope.

The **otoscope** funnels light into the ear canal and onto the tympanic membrane. The base serves both as the power source by holding a battery and as the handle. To attach the head, press it down onto the male adaptor end of the base and turn clockwise until you feel a stop. To turn the light on, press the red button rheostat down and clockwise. (Always turn it off after use to increase the life of the bulb and battery.) Five specula, each a different size, are available to attach to the head (Fig. 8-7). (The short, broad speculum is for viewing the nares.) Choose the largest one that will fit comfortably into the person's ear canal. See Chapter 15 for technique on use of the otoscope.

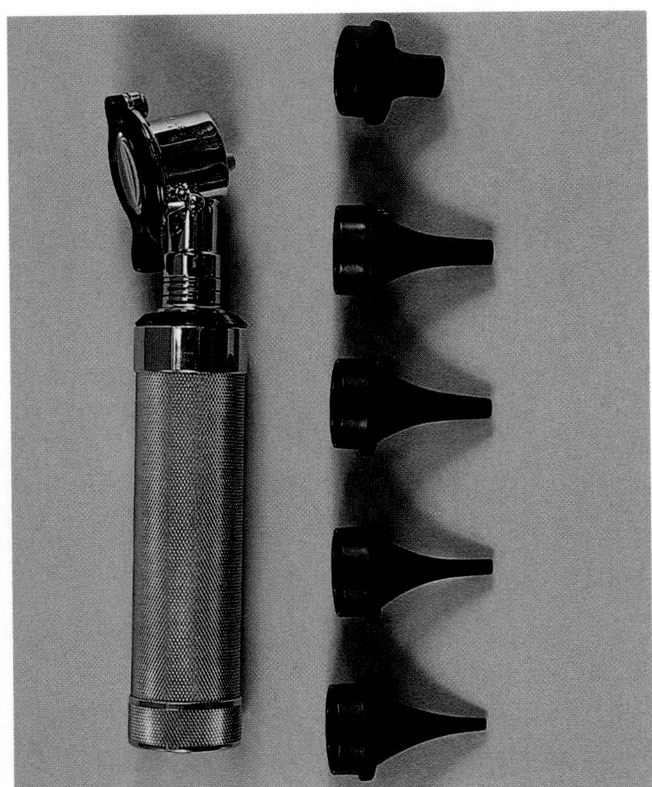

8-7 Otoscope.

The **ophthalmoscope** illuminates the internal eye structures. Its system of lenses and mirrors enables you to look through the pupil at the fundus (background) of the eye, much like looking through a keyhole at a room beyond. The ophthalmoscope head attaches to the base male adaptor just as the otoscope head does (Fig. 8-8). The head has five different parts:

1. Viewing aperture, with five different apertures
2. Aperture selector dial on the front
3. Mirror window on the front
4. Lens selector dial
5. Lens indicator

Select the aperture to be used (Fig. 8-9).

Rotating the lens selector dial brings the object into focus. The lens indicator shows a number, or *diopter,* that indicates the value of the lens in position. The black numbers indicate a positive lens, from 0 to +40. The red numbers indicate a negative lens, from 0 to −20. The ophthalmoscope can compensate for myopia (nearsightedness) or hyperopia (farsightedness) but will not correct for astigmatism. See Chapter 14 for details on how to hold the instrument and what to inspect.

The following equipment occasionally will be used, depending on the individual's needs: goniometer to measure joint range of motion, Doppler sonometer to augment pulse or blood pressure measurement, fetoscope for auscultating fetal heart tones, and pelvimeter to measure pelvic width.

For a child, you also will need appropriate pediatric-size endpieces for stethoscope and otoscope specula, materials for developmental assessment, age-appropriate toys, and a nipple or pacifier for an infant.

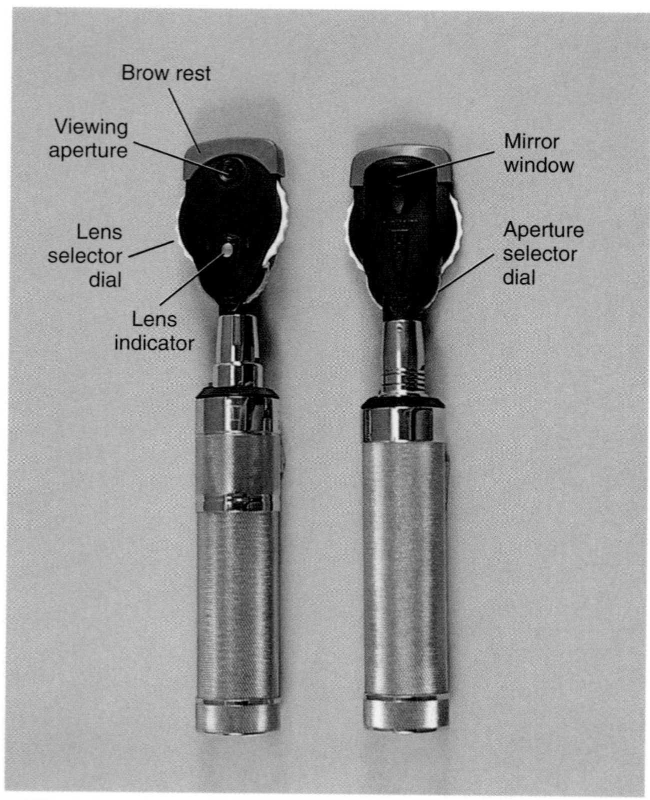

8-8 Ophthalmoscope.

- Large (full spot) for dilated pupils
- Small for undilated pupils
- Red-free filter — a green beam, used to examine the optic disc for hemorrhage (which looks black) and melanin deposits (which look gray)
- Grid — to determine fixation pattern and to assess size and location of lesions on the fundus
- Slit — to examine the anterior portion of the eye and to assess elevation or depression of lesions on the fundus

8-9 Otoscope apertures.

A Clean Field

Do not let your stethoscope become a *staph*-oscope! Stethoscopes and other equipment that are frequently used on many patients are a common vehicle for transmission of infection. Clean your stethoscope endpiece with an alcohol wipe before and after every patient contact. The best routine is to combine stethoscope rubbing with every hand hygiene.

Designate a "clean" versus a "used" area for handling of your equipment. In a hospital setting, you may use the bedside stand for your clean surface and the overbed table for the used equipment surface. Or in a clinic setting, use two separate areas of the pull-up table. Distinguish the clean area by one or two disposable paper towels. On the towels, place all the new or newly alcohol-swabbed equipment that you will use on this patient (e.g., your stethoscope endpieces, the reflex hammer, ruler). As you proceed through the examination, pick up each piece of equipment from the clean area, and after use on the patient, relegate it to the used area, or (as in the case of tongue blades, gloves) throw it directly in the trash.

A SAFER ENVIRONMENT

In addition to monitoring the cleanliness of your equipment, take all steps to avoid any possible transmission of infection between patients or between patient and examiner (Table 8-2). A **nosocomial** infection (an infection acquired during hospitalization) is a hazard because hospitals have sites that are reservoirs for virulent microorganisms. Some of these microorganisms are resistant to antibiotics, such as methicillin-resistant *Staphylococcus aureus* (MRSA), vancomycin-resistant *Enterococcus* (VRE), or multidrug-resistant tuberculosis, or are microorganisms for which there is currently no known cure, such as human immunodeficiency virus (HIV).

The single most important step to decrease risk of microorganism transmission is to wash your hands promptly and thoroughly: (1) before and after every physical patient encounter; (2) after contact with blood, body fluids, secretions, and excretions; (3) after contact with any equipment contaminated with body fluids; and (4) after removing gloves (see Table 8-2). Using alcohol-based hand rubs takes less time than soap-and-water handwashing; it also kills more organisms more quickly and is less damaging to the skin

TABLE 8-2 Standard Precautions for Use with All Patients

STANDARD PRECAUTIONS are based on the principle that all blood, body fluids, secretions, excretions except sweat, nonintact skin, and mucous membranes may contain transmissible infectious agents. Precautions apply to all patients, regardless of suspected or confirmed infection status, and in any setting in which health care is delivered. Components are:

- **Hand hygiene.** (1) Avoid unnecessary touching of surfaces in close proximity to the patient. (2) When hands are visibly dirty, contaminated with proteinaceous material, or visibly soiled with blood or body fluids, wash hands with soap and water. (3) If not visibly soiled, decontaminate hands with an alcohol-based hand rub. Perform hand hygiene: (a) before having direct contact with patients; (b) after contact with blood, body fluids or excretions, mucous membranes, nonintact skin, or wound dressings; (c) after contact with a patient's intact skin (e.g., taking a pulse or BP or lifting a patient); (d) after contact with medical equipment in the immediate vicinity of the patient; (e) after removing gloves.
- **Use of gloves, gown, mask, eye protection, or face shield.** (1) Wear gloves when you anticipate contact with blood or other potentially infectious materials, mucous membranes, nonintact skin, or potentially contaminated intact skin (e.g., patient incontinent of stool or urine) could occur. (2) Wear a gown to protect skin and clothing when you anticipate contact with blood, body fluids, secretions, or excretions. (3) Use mouth, nose, and eye protection to protect the mucous membranes during procedures that are likely to generate splashes or sprays of blood, body fluids, secretions, and excretions.
- **Safe injection practices.** (1) Use aseptic technique to avoid contamination of sterile injection equipment. (2) Needles, cannulae, and syringes are sterile, single-use items; do not reuse for another patient.
- **Respiratory hygiene/Cough etiquette** is targeted at patients and accompanying persons with undiagnosed transmissible respiratory infections. Elements include: (1) education of staff, patients, and visitors; (2) posted signs in language(s) appropriate to the population; (3) source control measures (e.g., covering the mouth/nose with a tissue when coughing and prompt disposal of used tissues, using surgical masks on the coughing person); (4) hand hygiene after contact with respiratory secretions; and (5) spatial separation of >3 feet of persons with respiratory infections in common waiting areas.

Adapted from Centers for Disease Control and Prevention. (2007). *Standard precautions—Excerpt from the guidelines for isolation precautions: preventing transmissions of infectious agents in healthcare settings 2007*, Centers for Disease Control and Prevention. Available at www.cdc.gov/ncidod/dhqp/gl_isolation_standard.html.

because of emollients added to the product. Alcohol is highly effective against both gram-positive and gram-negative bacteria, *Mycobacterium tuberculosis,* and most viruses, including hepatitis B and C viruses, HIV, and enteroviruses.[5] Use the mechanical action of soap-and-water handwashing when hands are visibly soiled and when patients are infected with spore-forming organisms (e.g., *Clostridium difficile* or *Bacillus anthracis*).

Wear gloves when the potential exists for contact with any body fluids (e.g., blood, mucous membranes, body fluids, drainage, open skin lesions). Wearing gloves is *not* a protective substitute for washing hands, however, because gloves may have undetectable holes or may become torn during use or hands may become contaminated as gloves are removed. Wear a gown, mask, and protective eyewear when the potential exists for any blood or body fluid spattering (e.g., suctioning, arterial puncture).

THE CLINICAL SETTING

General Approach

Consider your emotional state and that of the person being examined. The patient is usually anxious due to the anticipation of being examined by a stranger and the unknown outcome of the examination. If anxiety can be reduced, the person will feel more comfortable and the data gathered will more closely describe the person's natural state. Anxiety can be reduced by an examiner who is confident and self-assured, as well as considerate and unhurried.

Usually, a beginning examiner feels anything *but* self-assured! Most worry about their technical skill, about missing something significant, or about forgetting a step. Many are embarrassed themselves about encountering a partially dressed individual. All these fears are natural and common. The best way to minimize them is with much tutored practice on a healthy willing subject, usually a fellow student. You have to feel comfortable with your motor skills before you can absorb what you are actually seeing or hearing in a "real" patient. This comes with practice under the guidance of an experienced tutor, in an atmosphere in which it is acceptable to make mistakes and to ask questions. Your subject should "act like a patient" so that you can deal with the "real" situation while still in a safe setting. After you feel comfortable with the laboratory setting, accompany your tutor as he or she examines an actual patient so that you can observe an experienced examiner.

Hands On

With this preparation, it is possible to interact with your own patient in a confident manner. Begin by measuring the person's height, weight, blood pressure, temperature, pulse, and respirations (see Chapter 9). If needed, measure visual acuity at this time using the Snellen eye chart. All of these are familiar, relatively nonthreatening actions; they will gradually accustom the person to the examination. Then ask the person to change into an examining gown, leaving his or her underpants on. This will feel more comfortable, and the underpants can easily be removed just before the genital

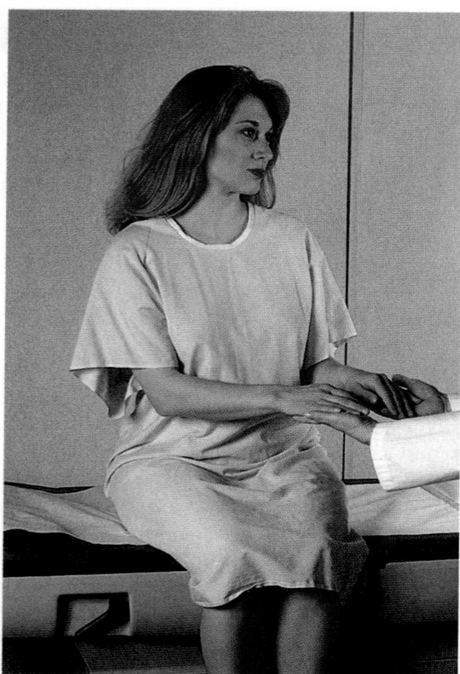

8-10

examination. Unless your assistance is needed, leave the room as the person undresses.

As you reenter the room, clean your hands in the person's presence. This indicates you are protective of this person and are starting fresh for him or her. Explain each step in the examination and how the person can cooperate. Encourage the person to ask questions. Keep your own movements slow, methodical, and deliberate.

Begin by touching the person's hands, checking skin color, nail beds, and metacarpophalangeal joints (Fig. 8-10; see Chapters 12 and 22). Again, this is a less threatening way to ease a person into being touched. Most people are used to having relative strangers touch their hands.

As you proceed through the examination, avoid distractions and concentrate on one step at a time. The sequence of the steps may differ depending on the age of the person and your own preference. However, you should establish a system that works for you and stick to it to avoid omissions. Organize the steps so the person does not change positions too often. Although proper exposure is necessary, use additional drapes to maintain the person's privacy and to prevent chilling.

Do not hesitate to write out the examination sequence and refer to it as you proceed. The patient will accept this as quite natural if you explain you are making brief notations to ensure accuracy. Many agencies use a printed form. You will find that you will glance at the form less and less as you gain experience. Even with a form, you sometimes may forget a step in the examination. When you realize this, perform the maneuver in the next logical place in the sequence. (See Chapter 27 for the sequence of steps in the complete physical examination.)

As you proceed through the examination, occasionally offer some brief teaching about the person's body. For example, you might say, "Everyone has two sounds for each heartbeat, something like this—lub-dup. Your own beats sound normal." Do not do this with every single step, or you will be hard pressed to make a comment when you do come across an abnormality. But some sharing of information builds rapport and increases the person's confidence in you as an examiner. It also gives the person a little more control in a situation in which it is easy to feel completely helpless.

At some point, you will want to linger in one location to concentrate on some complicated findings. To avoid anxiety, tell the person, "I always listen to heart sounds on a number of places on the chest. Just because I am listening a long time does not necessarily mean anything is wrong with you." And it follows that sometimes you *will* discover a finding that may be abnormal and you want another examiner to double-check. You need to give the person some information, yet you should not alarm the person unnecessarily. Say something like, "I do not have a complete assessment of your heart sounds. I want Ms. Wright to listen to you too."

At the end of the examination, summarize your findings and share the necessary information with the person. Thank the person for the time spent. In a hospital setting, apprise the person of what is scheduled next. Before you leave a hospitalized person, lower the bed to avoid risk for falls; make the person comfortable and safe; and return the bedside table, television, or any equipment to the way it was originally, with the call button available.

DEVELOPMENTAL COMPETENCE

Children are different from adults. Their difference in size is obvious. Their bodies grow in a predictable pattern that is assessed during the physical examination. However, their behavior is also different. Behavior grows and develops through predictable stages, just as the body does.

With all children, the goal is to increase their comfort in the setting. This approach reveals their natural state as much as possible and will give them a more positive memory of health care providers. Remember that a "routine" examination is anything but routine to the child. You can increase their comfort by attending to the following developmental principles and approaches. The *order* of the developmental stages is more meaningful than the exact chronological age. Each child is an individual and will not fit exactly into one category. For example, if your efforts to "play games" with the preschooler are rebuffed, modify your approach to the security measures used with the toddler.

The Infant

Erikson defines the major task of infancy as establishing trust. An infant is completely dependent on the parent for his or her basic needs. If these needs are met promptly and consistently, the infant feels secure and learns to trust others.

Position

- The parent always should be present to understand normal growth and development and for the child's feeling of security.

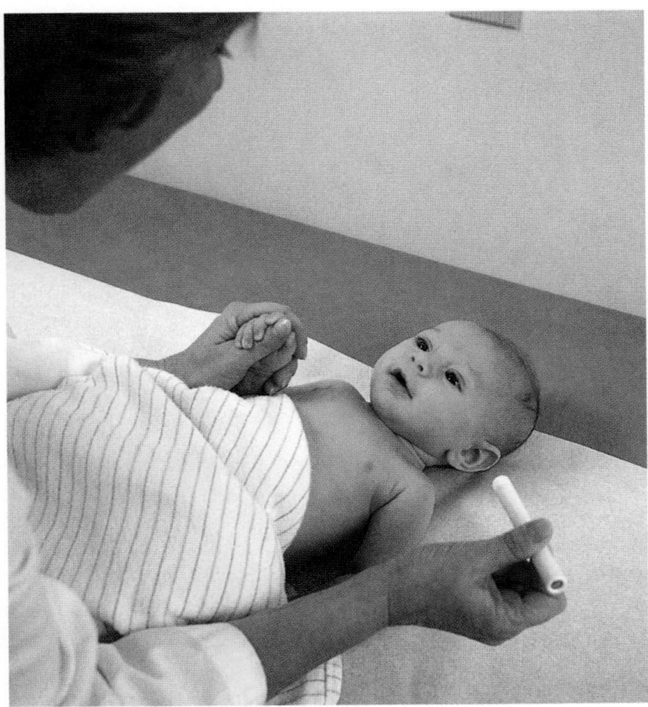

8-11

- Place the neonate or young infant flat on a padded examination table (Fig. 8-11). The infant also may be held against the parent's chest for some steps.
- Once the baby can sit without support (around 6 months), as much of the examination as possible should be performed while the infant is in the parent's lap.
- By 9 to 12 months, the infant is acutely aware of the surroundings. Anything outside the infant's range of vision is "lost," so the parent must be in full view.

Preparation

- Timing should be 1 to 2 hours after feeding, when the baby is not too drowsy or too hungry.
- Maintain a warm environment. A neonate may require an overhead radiant heater.
- An infant will not object to being nude. Have the parent remove outer clothing, but leave a diaper on a boy.
- An infant does not mind being touched, but make sure your hands and stethoscope endpiece are warm.
- Use a soft, crooning voice during the examination; the baby responds more to the feeling in the tone of the voice than to what is actually said.
- An infant likes eye contact; lock eyes from time to time.
- Smile; a baby prefers a smiling face to a frowning one. (Often beginning examiners are so absorbed in their technique that they look serious or stern.) Take time to play.
- Keep movements smooth and deliberate, not jerky.
- Use a pacifier for crying or during invasive steps.
- Offer brightly colored toys for a distraction when the infant is fussy.
- Let an older baby touch the stethoscope or tongue blade.

Sequence

- Seize the opportunity with a sleeping baby to listen to heart, lung, and abdominal sounds first.
- Perform least distressing steps first. (See the sequence in Chapter 27.) Save the invasive steps of examination of the eye, ear, nose, and throat until last.
- If you elicit the Moro or "startle" reflex, do it at the end of the examination because it may cause the baby to cry.

The Toddler

This is Erikson's stage of developing autonomy. However, the need to explore the world and be independent is in conflict with the basic dependency on the parent. This often results in frustration and negativism. The toddler may be difficult to examine; do not take this personally. Because he or she is acutely aware of the new environment, the toddler may be frightened and cling to the parent. Also, the toddler has fear of invasive procedures and dislikes being restrained (Fig. 8-12).

Position

- The toddler should be sitting up on the parent's lap for all of the examination. When the toddler must be supine (as in the abdominal examination), move chairs to sit knee-to-knee with parent. Have the toddler lie in the parent's lap with the toddler's legs in your lap.
- Enlist the aid of a cooperative parent to help position the toddler during invasive procedures, such as using the otoscope or taking a rectal temperature.

Preparation

- Children 1 or 2 years of age can understand symbols, so a security object, such as a special blanket or teddy bear, is helpful.
- Begin by greeting the child and the accompanying parent by name, but with a child 1 to 6 years old, focus more on the parent. By essentially "ignoring" the child at first, you allow the child to adjust gradually and to size you up from a safe distance. Then turn your attention gradually to the

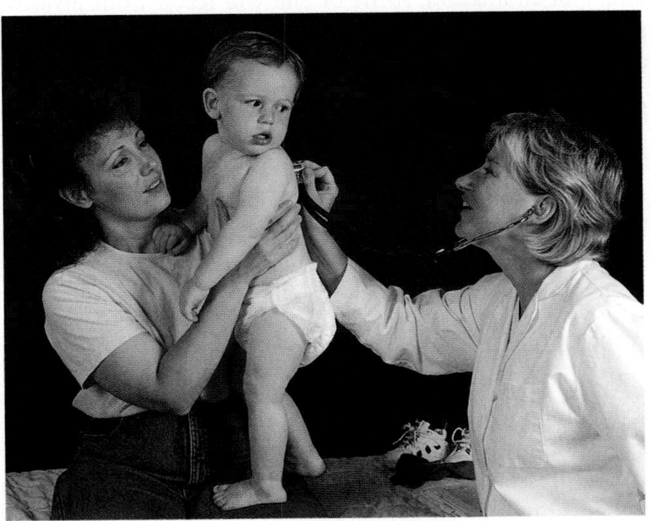

8-12

child, at first to a toy or object the child is holding, or perhaps to compliment a dress, the hair, or what a big girl or boy the child is. If the child is ready, you will note these signals: eye contact with you, smiling, talking with you, or accepting a toy or a piece of equipment.

- A 2-year-old child does not like to take off his or her clothes; have the parent undress the child one part at a time.
- Children 1 or 2 years of age like to say "No." Do not offer a choice when there really is none. Avoid saying, "May I listen to your heart now?" When the 1- or 2-year-old child says "No" and you go ahead and do it anyway, you lose trust. Instead, use clear, firm instructions, in a tone that expects cooperation, "Now it is time for you to lie down so I can check your tummy."
- Also, 1- or 2-year-old children like to make choices. When possible, enhance autonomy by offering the *limited option:* "Shall I listen to your heart next, or your tummy?"
- Demonstrate the procedures on the parent (see Fig. 15-11).
- Praise the child when he or she is cooperative.

Sequence

- Collect some objective data during the history, which is a less stressful time. While you are focusing on the parent, note the child's gross motor and fine motor skills and gait.
- Begin with "games," such as the Denver II test or cranial nerve testing.
- Start with nonthreatening areas. Save distressing procedures—such as examination of the head, ear, nose, or throat—for last.

The Preschool Child

The child at this stage displays developing initiative. The preschooler takes on tasks independently and plans the task and sees it through. A child of this age is often cooperative, helpful, and easy to involve. However, children of this age have fantasies and may see illness as punishment for being "bad." The concept of body image is limited. The child fears any body injury or mutilation, so he or she will recoil from invasive procedures (e.g., tongue blade, rectal temperature, injection, and venipuncture).

Position

- With a 3-year-old child, the parent should be present and may hold the child on his or her lap (Fig. 8-13).
- A 4- or 5-year-old child usually feels comfortable on the Big Girl or Big Boy (examining) table, with the parent present.

Preparation

- A preschooler can talk. Verbal communication becomes helpful now, but remember that the child's understanding is still limited. Use short, simple explanations.
- The preschooler is usually willing to undress. Leave underpants on until the genital examination.

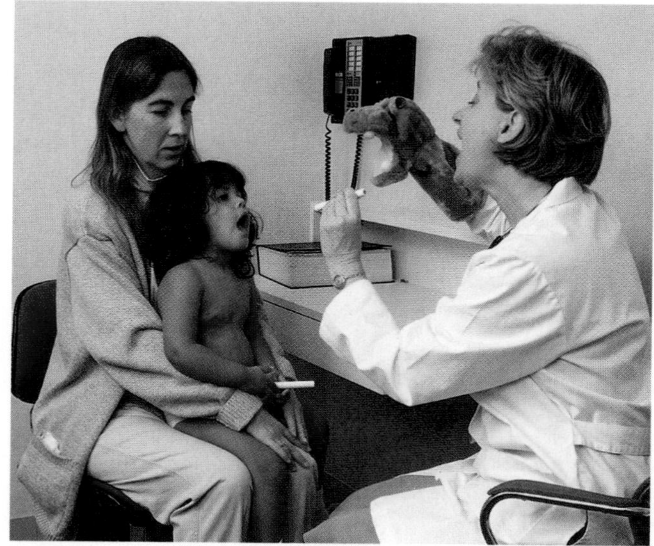

8-13

- Talk to the child and explain the steps in the examination exactly.
- Do not allow a choice when there is none.
- As with the toddler, enhance the autonomy of the preschooler by offering choice when possible.
- Allow the child to play with equipment to reduce fears (Fig. 8-14).
- A preschooler likes to help; have the child hold the stethoscope for you.
- Use games. Have the child "blow out" the light on the penlight as you listen to the breath sounds. Or, pretend to listen to the heart sounds of the child's teddy bear first. One technique that is absorbing to a preschooler is to trace his or her shape on the examining table paper. You can comment on how big the child is, then fill in the outline with a heart or stomach and listen to the paper doll first.

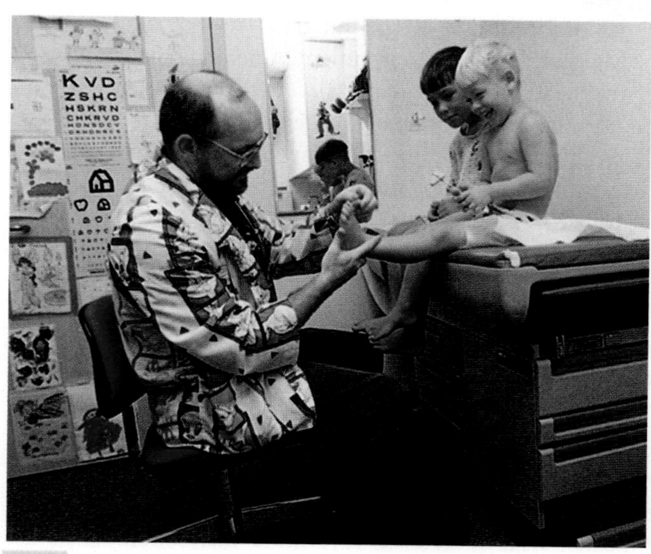

8-14

After the examination, the child can take the paper doll home as a souvenir.
- Use a slow, patient, deliberate approach. Do not rush.
- During the examination, give the preschooler needed feedback and reassurance: "Your tummy feels just fine."
- Compliment the child on his or her cooperation.

Sequence

- Examine the thorax, abdomen, extremities, and genitalia first. Although the preschooler is usually cooperative, continue to assess head, eye, ear, nose, and throat last.

The School-Age Child

During the school-age period, the major task of the child is developing industry. The child is developing basic competency in school and in social networks and desires the approval of parents and teachers. When successful, the child has a feeling of accomplishment. During the examination, the child is cooperative and is interested in learning about the body. Language is more sophisticated now, but do not overestimate and treat the school-age child as a small adult. The child's level of understanding does not match that of his or her speech.

Position

- The school-age child should be sitting or lying on the examination table (Fig. 8-15).
- A 5-year-old child has a sense of modesty. To maintain privacy, let the older child (an 11- or 12-year-old child) decide whether parents or siblings should be present.

Preparation

- Break the ice with small talk about family, school, friends, music, or sports.

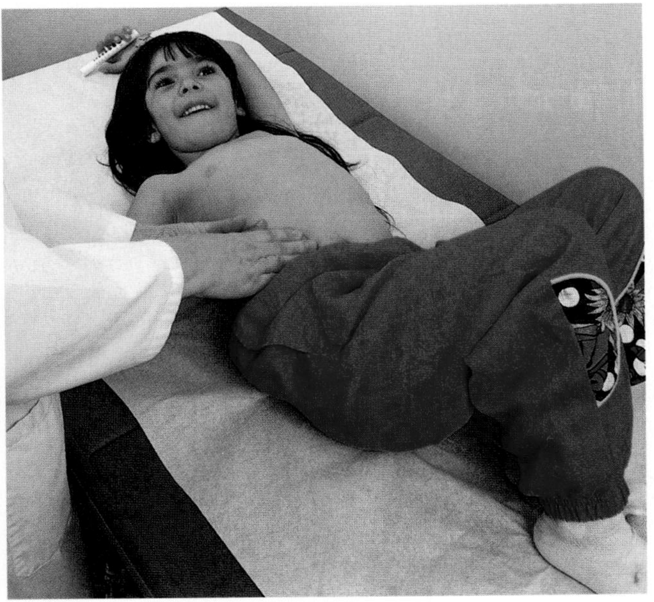

8-15

- The child should undress himself or herself, leave underpants on, and use a gown and drape.
- Demonstrate equipment—a school-age child is curious to know how equipment works.
- Comment on the body and how it works. An 8- or 9-year-old child has some understanding of the body and is interested to learn more. It is rewarding to see the child's eyes light up when he or she hears the heart sounds.

Sequence

- As with the adult, progress from head to toes.

The Adolescent

The major task of adolescence is developing a self-identity. This takes shape from various sets of values and different social roles (son or daughter, sibling, and student). In the end, each person needs to feel satisfied and comfortable with who he or she is. In the process, the adolescent is increasingly self-conscious and introspective. Peer group values and acceptance are important.

Position

- The adolescent should be sitting on the examination table.
- Examine the adolescent alone, without parent or sibling present.

Preparation

- The body is changing rapidly. During the examination, the adolescent needs feedback that his or her own body is healthy and developing normally.
- The adolescent has keen awareness of body image, often comparing himself or herself to peers. Apprise the adolescent of the wide variation among teenagers on the rate of growth and development (see Sexual Maturity Rating [SMR], Chapters 17, 24, and 26).
- Communicate with some care. Do not treat the teenager like a child, but do not overestimate and treat him or her like an adult either.
- Because the person is idealistic at this age, the adolescent is ripe for health teaching. Positive attitudes developed now may last through adult life. Focus your teaching on ways the adolescent can promote wellness.

Sequence

- As with the adult, a head-to-toe approach is appropriate. Examine genitalia last, and do it quickly.

The Aging Adult

During later years, the tasks are developing the meaning of life and one's own existence and adjusting to changes in physical strength and health.

Position

- The older adult should be sitting on the examination table; a frail older adult may need to be supine.

- Arrange the sequence to allow as few position changes as possible.
- Allow rest periods when needed.

Preparation

- Adjust examination pace to meet the possible slowed pace of the aging person. It is better to break the complete examination into a few visits than to rush through the examination and turn off the person.
- Use physical touch (unless there is a cultural contraindication). This is especially important with the aging person because other senses, such as vision and hearing, may be diminished.
- Do not mistake diminished vision or hearing for confusion. Confusion of sudden onset may signify a disease state. It is noted by short-term memory loss, diminished thought process, diminished attention span, and labile emotions (see Mental Status Assessment in Chapter 5).
- Be aware that aging years contain more of life's stress. Loss is inevitable, including changes in physical appearance of the face and body, declining energy level, loss of job through retirement, loss of financial security, loss of longtime home, and death of friends or spouse. How the person adapts to these losses significantly affects health assessment.

Sequence

- Use the head-to-toe approach as in the younger adult.

The Ill Person

For the person in some distress, alter the position during the examination. For example, a person with shortness of breath or ear pain may want to sit up, whereas a person with faintness or overwhelming fatigue may want to be supine. Initially it may be necessary just to examine the body areas appropriate to the problem, collecting a **mini-database.** You may return to finish a complete assessment after the initial distress is resolved.

BIBLIOGRAPHY

1. Amella, E. J. (2004). Presentation of illness in older adults. *The American Journal of Nursing, 104*(10), 40-52.
2. Anderson, F. (2007). Finding HIPPA in your soup: decoding the privacy rule. *The American Journal of Nursing, 107*(2), 66-72.
3. Bates, B. (July/August 2005). Study: bacteria bloom on hospital stethoscopes. *The Journal for Nurse Practitioners, 1*(1), 44-46.
4. Berk, L. E. (2007). *Development through the lifespan* (4th ed.). Boston: Allyn & Bacon.
5. Boyce, J. M., & Pittet, D. (2002). Guideline for hand hygiene in health-care settings. *MMWR Recommendation and Reports, 51*(RR16), 1-44. Retrieved June 4, 2009, from www.cdc.gov/mmwr/preview/mmwrhtml/rr5116a1.htm.
6. Centers for Disease Control and Prevention (CDC). (2007). *Standard precautions—Excerpt from the guidelines for isolation precautions: preventing transmission of infectious agents in health-care settings 2007.* Retrieved June 4, 2009, from http://cdc.gov/ncidod/dhqp/gl_isolation_standard.html.
7. Centers for Disease Control and Prevention (CDC). (2007). *Information about MRSA for healthcare personnel.* Retrieved June 4, 2009, from www.cdc.gov/ncidod/dhqp/ar_mrsa_healthcareFS.html.
8. Haas, J. P., & Larson, E. L. (2008). Compliance with hand hygiene. *The American Journal of Nursing, 108*(8), 40-45.
9. Hockenberry, M., & Wilson, D. (2006). *Wong's nursing care of infants and children* (8th ed.). St. Louis: Mosby.
10. Romero, D. V., Treston, J., & O'Sullivan, A. L. (2006). Hand-to-hand preventing MRSA. *The Nurse Practitioner, 31*(3), 16-25.
11. Romig, L. E. (2001). PREP for peds: size-up & approach tips for pediatric calls. *JEMS: A Journal of Emergency Medical Services, 26*(5), 24-33.
12. Schneiderman, H. (2009). Auscult the skin, not the sweater. *Consultant, 49*(3), 167.

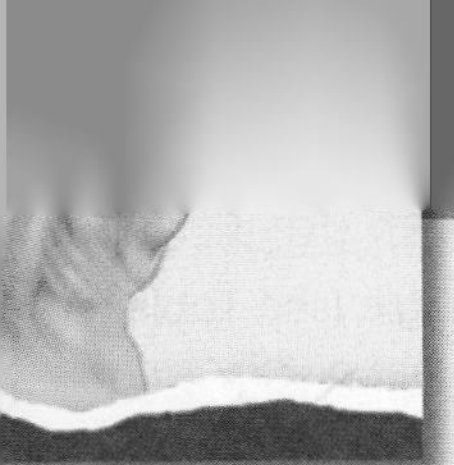

9

General Survey, Measurement, Vital Signs

evolve WEBSITE

http://evolve.elsevier.com/Jarvis/

- Animations
- Audio Key Points
- Case Study
  Dizziness
  Vital Signs
- NCLEX Review Questions
- Quick Assessment for Common Conditions
  Alzheimer Disease
  Iron Deficiency Anemia
  Sepsis
- Video—Assessment
  Approach
  General Appearance
  Measurements
  Vital Signs

OUTLINE

Objective Data, 127

The General Survey
Measurement
Vital Signs
Additional Techniques
Promoting Health and Self-Care

Documentation and Critical Thinking, 153

Abnormal Findings, 154

OBJECTIVE DATA

The general survey is a study of the whole person, covering the general health state and any obvious physical characteristics. It is an introduction for the physical examination that will follow; it should give an overall impression, a "gestalt," of the person (see Sample Charting on p. 153). Objective parameters are used to form the general survey, but these apply to the whole person, not just to one body system.

Launch a general survey at the moment you first encounter the person. What leaves an immediate impression? Does the person stand promptly as his or her name is called and walk easily to meet you? Or does the person look sick, rising slowly or with effort, with shoulders slumped and eyes without luster or downcast? Is the hospitalized patient conversing with visitors, involved in reading or television, or lying perfectly still? Even as you introduce yourself and shake hands, you collect data. Does the person fully extend the arm, shake your hand firmly, make eye contact, or smile? Are the palms dry or wet and clammy? As you proceed through the health history, the measurements, and the vital signs, note the following points that will add up to the general survey. Consider these four areas: **physical appearance, body structure, mobility,** and **behavior.**

Normal Range of Findings	Abnormal Findings
THE GENERAL SURVEY	
Physical Appearance	
Age—The person appears his or her stated age.	Appears older than stated age, as with chronic illness, chronic alcoholism.
Sex—Sexual development is appropriate for gender and age.	Delayed or precocious puberty.

Normal Range of Findings	Abnormal Findings
Level of consciousness—The person is alert and oriented, attends to your questions and responds appropriately.	Confused, drowsy, lethargic (see Table 5-3, Levels of Consciousness, p. 83).
Skin color—Color tone is even, pigmentation varying with genetic background, skin is intact with no obvious lesions.	Pallor, cyanosis, jaundice, erythema, any lesions (see Chapter 12).
Facial features—Facial features are symmetric with movement.	Immobile, masklike, asymmetric, drooping (see Table 13-5, Abnormal Facies with Chronic Illnesses, pp. 275-277).
No signs of acute distress are present.	Cardiac or respiratory signs— diaphoresis, clutching the chest, shortness of breath, wheezing. Pain, indicated by facial grimace, holding body part.
Body Structure	
Stature—The height appears within normal range for age, genetic heritage (see Measurement, p. 130).	Excessively short or tall (see Table 9-5, Abnormalities in Body Height and Proportion, p. 154).
Nutrition—The weight appears within normal range for height and body build; body fat distribution is even.	Cachectic, emaciated. Simple obesity, with even fat distribution. Centripetal (truncal) obesity—fat concentrated in face, neck, trunk, with thin extremities, as in Cushing syndrome (hyperadrenalism) (see Table 9-5).
Symmetry—Body parts look equal bilaterally and are in relative proportion to each other.	Unilateral atrophy or hypertrophy. Asymmetric location of a body part.
Posture—The person stands comfortably erect as appropriate for age. Note the normal "plumb line" through anterior ear, shoulder, hip, patella, ankle. Exceptions are the standing toddler who has a normally protuberant abdomen ("toddler lordosis") and the aging person who may be stooped with kyphosis.	Rigid spine and neck; moves as one unit (e.g., arthritis). Stiff and tense, ready to spring from chair, fidgety movements. Shoulders slumped; looks deflated (e.g., depression).
Position—The person sits comfortably in a chair or on the bed or examination table, arms relaxed at sides, head turned to examiner.	Tripod—leaning forward with arms braced on chair arms; occurs with chronic pulmonary disease. Sitting straight up and resists lying down (e.g., congestive heart failure). Curled up in fetal position (e.g., acute abdominal pain).
Body build, contour—Proportions are: 1. Arm span (fingertip to fingertip) equals height. 2. Body length from crown to pubis roughly equal to length from pubis to sole. Obvious physical deformities—note any congenital or acquired defects.	Elongated arm span, arm span greater than height (e.g., Marfan's syndrome hypogonadism) (see Table 9-5). Missing extremities or digits; webbed digits; shortened limb.

Normal Range of Findings	Abnormal Findings
Mobility	
Gait—Normally, the base is as wide as the shoulder width; foot placement is accurate; the walk is smooth, even, and well-balanced; and associated movements, such as symmetric arm swing, are present.	Exceptionally wide base. Staggered, stumbling. Shuffling, dragging, nonfunctional leg. Limping with injury. Propulsion—difficulty stopping (see Table 23-6, Abnormal Gaits, pp. 672-673).
Range of motion—Note full mobility for each joint and that movement is deliberate, accurate, smooth, and coordinated. (See Chapter 22 for information on more detailed testing of joint range of motion.) No involuntary movement.	Limited joint range of motion. Paralysis—absent movement. Movement jerky, uncoordinated. Tics, tremors, seizures (see Table 23-5, Abnormalities in Muscle Movement, pp. 670-671).
Behavior	
Facial expression—The person maintains eye contact (unless a cultural taboo exists), expressions are appropriate to the situation (e.g., thoughtful, serious, or smiling). (Note expressions both while the face is at rest and while the person is talking.)	Flat, depressed, angry, sad, anxious. However, note that anxiety is common in ill people. Also, some people smile when they are anxious.
Mood and affect—The person is comfortable and cooperative with the examiner and interacts pleasantly.	Hostile, distrustful, suspicious, crying.
Speech—Articulation (the ability to form words) is clear and understandable.	Dysarthria and dysphagia (see Table 5-4, Speech Disorders, p. 84). Speech defect, monotone, garbled speech.
The stream of talking is fluent, with an even pace. The person conveys ideas clearly. Word choice is appropriate to culture and education. The person communicates in prevailing language easily by himself or herself or with an interpreter.	Extremes of few words or of constant talking.
Dress—Clothing is appropriate to the climate, looks clean and fits the body, and is appropriate to the person's culture and age-group; for example, normally, Amish women wear clothing from the nineteenth century, Indian women may wear saris. Culturally determined dress should not be labeled as bizarre by Western standards or by adult expectations.	Clothing too large and held up by belt suggests weight loss, as does the addition of new holes in belt. Clothing too tight may indicate obesity or ascites. Consistent wear of certain clothing may provide clues: long sleeves may conceal needle marks of drug abuse or thin arms of anorexia; Velcro fasteners instead of buttons may indicate chronic motor dysfunction.
Personal hygiene—The person appears clean and groomed appropriately for his or her age, occupation, and socioeconomic group. (Note that a wide variation of dress and hygiene is "normal." Many cultures do not include use of deodorant or women shaving legs.) Hair is groomed, brushed. Women's makeup is appropriate for age and culture.	In a previously carefully groomed woman, unkempt hair and absent makeup may indicate malaise or illness.

Normal Range of Findings	Abnormal Findings

MEASUREMENT

Weight

Use a standardized *balance* or electronic standing scale (Fig. 9-1). Instruct the person to remove his or her shoes and heavy outer clothing before standing on the scale. When a sequence of repeated weights is necessary, aim for approximately the same time of day and the same type of clothing worn each time. Record the weight in kilograms and in pounds.

An unexplained weight loss may be a sign of a short-term illness (e.g., fever, infection, disease of the mouth or throat) or a chronic illness (e.g., endocrine disease, malignancy, depression, anorexia nervosa, bulimia).

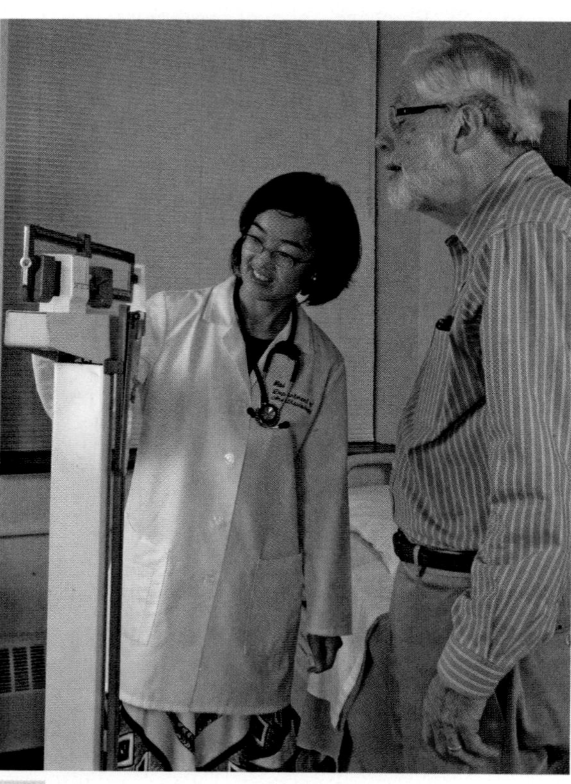

9-1

Height

Use a wall-mounted device or the measuring pole on the balance scale. Align the extended headpiece with the top of the head. The person should be shoeless, standing straight with gentle traction under the jaw, and looking straight ahead. Feet, shoulders, and buttocks should be in contact with the hard surface.

Body Mass Index

Body mass index (BMI) is a practical marker of optimal healthy weight for height and an indicator of obesity or malnutrition. Evidence supports using BMI in obesity risk assessment because it provides a more accurate measure of total body fat compared with the measure of body weight alone.[26]

Weight gain usually is due to excess caloric intake; occasionally it is due to endocrine disorders, drug therapy (e.g., corticosteroids), or depression. BMI classifications for adults[26]:

- Underweight <18.5 kg/m^2
- Normal weight 18.5-24.9 kg/m^2
- Overweight 25-29.9 kg/m^2
- Obesity (Class 1) 30-34.9 kg/m^2
- Obesity (Class 2) 35-39.9 kg/m^2
- Extreme obesity (Class 3) ≥40

Normal Range of Findings

A healthy BMI is a level of 19 or greater to less than 25. Show the person how his or her own weight matches up to the national guidelines for optimal BMI (Table 9-1). Compare the person's current weight with that from the previous health visit. A recent weight loss may be explained by successful dieting. A weight gain usually reflects overabundant caloric intake, unhealthy eating habits, and sedentary lifestyle. Note that BMI overestimates body fat in persons who are very muscular, and it underestimates body fat in older adults who have lost muscle mass.

Abnormal Findings

TABLE 9-1 Body Mass Index Table

	Normal						Overweight					Obese									
BMI	19	20	21	22	23	24	25	26	27	28	29	30	31	32	33	34	35	36	37	38	39
Height (inches)	Body Weight (pounds)																				
58	91	96	100	105	110	115	119	124	129	134	138	143	148	153	158	162	167	172	177	181	186
59	94	99	104	109	114	119	124	128	133	138	143	148	153	158	163	168	173	178	183	188	193
60	97	102	107	112	118	123	128	133	138	143	148	153	158	163	168	174	179	184	189	194	199
61	100	106	111	116	122	127	132	137	143	148	153	158	164	169	174	180	185	190	195	201	206
62	104	109	115	120	126	131	136	142	147	153	158	164	169	175	180	186	191	196	202	207	213
63	107	113	118	124	130	135	141	146	152	158	163	169	175	180	186	191	197	203	208	214	220
64	110	116	122	128	134	140	145	151	157	163	169	174	180	186	192	197	204	209	215	221	227
65	114	120	126	132	138	144	150	156	162	168	174	180	186	192	198	204	210	216	222	228	234
66	118	124	130	136	142	148	155	161	167	173	179	186	192	198	204	210	216	223	229	235	241
67	121	127	134	140	146	153	159	166	172	178	185	191	198	204	211	217	223	230	236	242	249
68	125	131	138	144	151	158	164	171	177	184	190	197	203	210	216	223	230	236	243	249	256
69	128	135	142	149	155	162	169	176	182	189	196	203	209	216	223	230	236	243	250	257	263
70	132	139	146	153	160	167	174	181	188	195	202	209	216	222	229	236	243	250	257	264	271
71	136	143	150	157	165	172	179	186	193	200	208	215	222	229	236	243	250	257	265	272	279
72	140	147	154	162	169	177	184	191	199	206	213	221	228	235	242	250	258	265	272	279	287
73	144	151	159	166	174	182	189	197	204	212	219	227	235	242	250	257	265	272	280	288	295
74	148	155	163	171	179	186	194	202	210	218	225	233	241	249	256	264	272	280	287	295	303
75	152	160	168	176	184	192	200	208	216	224	232	240	248	256	264	272	279	287	295	303	311
76	156	164	172	180	189	197	205	213	221	230	238	246	254	263	271	279	287	295	304	312	320

	Extreme Obesity														
BMI	40	41	42	43	44	45	46	47	48	49	50	51	52	53	54
Height (inches)	Body Weight (pounds)														
58	191	196	201	205	210	215	220	224	229	234	239	244	248	253	258
59	198	203	208	212	217	222	227	232	237	242	247	252	257	262	267
60	204	209	215	220	225	230	235	240	245	250	255	261	266	271	276
61	211	217	222	227	232	238	243	248	254	259	264	269	275	280	285
62	218	224	229	235	240	246	251	256	262	267	273	278	284	289	295
63	225	231	237	242	248	254	259	265	270	278	282	287	293	299	304
64	232	238	244	250	256	262	267	273	279	285	291	296	302	308	314
65	240	246	252	258	264	270	276	282	288	294	300	306	312	318	324
66	247	253	260	266	272	278	284	291	297	303	309	315	322	328	334
67	255	261	268	274	280	287	293	299	306	312	319	325	331	338	344
68	262	269	276	282	289	295	302	308	315	322	328	335	341	348	354
69	270	277	284	291	297	304	311	318	324	331	338	345	351	358	365
70	278	285	292	299	306	313	320	327	334	341	348	355	362	369	376
71	286	293	301	308	315	322	329	338	343	351	358	365	372	379	386
72	294	302	309	316	324	331	338	346	353	361	368	375	383	390	397
73	302	310	318	325	333	340	348	355	363	371	378	386	393	401	408
74	311	319	326	334	342	350	358	365	373	381	389	396	404	412	420
75	319	327	335	343	351	359	367	375	383	391	399	407	415	423	431
76	328	336	344	353	361	369	377	385	394	402	410	418	426	435	443

Adapted from *Clinical Guidelines on the Identification, Evaluation, and Treatment of Overweight and Obesity in Adults: The Evidence Report.* Accessed June 9, 2009, from www.nhlbi.nih.gov/guidelines/obesity/bmi_tbl.pdf.

Normal Range of Findings	Abnormal Findings

You also may calculate BMI by using the "BMI Calculator" at the NIH website: www.nhlbisupport.com/bmi/bmicalc.htm.

Or, you can calculate with the following formulae:

$$\text{BMI} = \frac{\text{Weight (in pounds)}}{\text{Height (in inches)}^2} \times 703$$

Or

$$\text{BMI} = \frac{\text{Weight (in kilograms)}}{\text{Height (in meters)}^2}$$

Waist Circumference

Excess abdominal fat is an important independent risk factor for disease, over and above that of BMI.[26] With the person standing, locate the hip bone and the top of its right iliac crest. Place a measuring tape around the waist, parallel to the floor, at the level of the iliac crest. The tape should be snug but not pinch in the skin. Note the measurement at the end of a normal expiration (Fig. 9-2).

A weight circumference (WC) ≥35 inches in women and ≥40 inches in men increases the risk for type 2 diabetes, dyslipidemia, hypertension, and cardiovascular disease (CVD) in persons with a BMI between 25 and 35 kg/m^2.

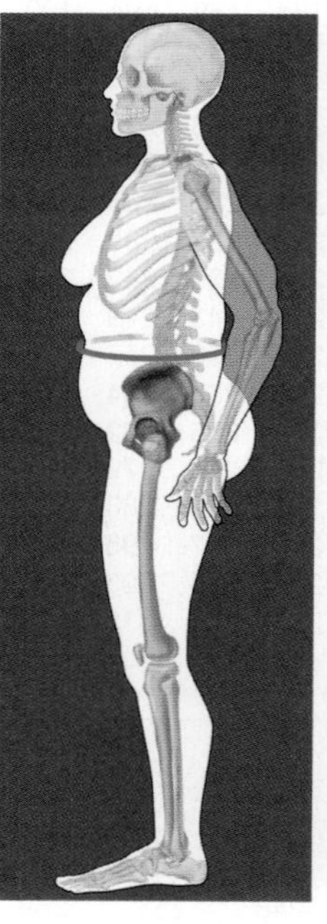

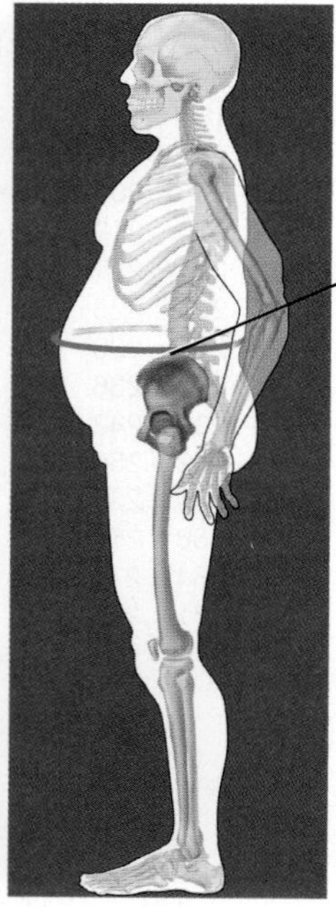

9-2 Measuring tape position for abdominal circumference

VITAL SIGNS

Temperature

Cellular metabolism requires a stable core, or "deep body," temperature of a mean of 37.2° C (99° F). The body maintains a steady temperature through a thermostat, or feedback mechanism, regulated in the hypothalamus of the brain. The thermostat balances heat production (from metabolism, exercise, food digestion, external factors) with heat loss (through radiation, evaporation of sweat, convection, conduction).

The various routes of temperature measurement reflect the body's core temperature. The normal oral temperature in a resting person is 37° C (98.6° F), with a range of 35.8° to 37.3° C (96.4° to 99.1° F). The rectal temperature measures 0.4° to 0.5° C (0.7° to 1° F) higher.

The thermostatic function of the hypothalamus may become scrambled during illness or central nervous system disorders.

Normal Range of Findings

The normal temperature is influenced by:

- A diurnal cycle of 1° to 1.5° F, with the trough occurring in the early morning hours and the peak occurring in late afternoon to early evening.
- The menstruation cycle in women. Progesterone secretion, occurring with ovulation at midcycle, causes a 0.5° to 1.0° F rise in temperature that continues until menses.
- Exercise. Moderate to hard exercise increases body temperature.
- Age. Wider normal variations occur in the infant and young child due to less effective heat control mechanisms. In older adults, temperature is usually lower than in other age-groups, with a mean of 36.2° C (97.2° F).

The **oral** temperature is accurate and convenient. The oral sublingual site has a rich blood supply from the carotid arteries that quickly responds to changes in inner core temperature.

Due to environmental concerns of mercury pollution from medical waste incinerators, mercury-containing oral thermometers and sphygmomanometers have been replaced with electronic equipment. Shake a mercury-free glass thermometer down to 35.5° C (96° F) and place it at the base of the tongue in either of the posterior sublingual pockets—*not* in front of the tongue. Instruct the person to keep his or her lips closed. Leave in place 3 to 4 minutes if the person is afebrile, and up to 8 minutes if febrile. (Take other vital signs during this time.) Wait 15 minutes if the person has just taken hot or iced liquids and 2 minutes if he or she has just smoked.

The **electronic thermometer** has the advantages of swift and accurate measurement (usually in 20 to 30 seconds) as well as safe, unbreakable, disposable probe covers. The instrument must be fully charged and correctly calibrated. Most children enjoy watching their temperature numbers advance on the box.

Take a **rectal** temperature only when the other routes are not practical—for example, for comatose or confused persons, for persons in shock, or for those who cannot close the mouth because of breathing or oxygen tubes, wired mandible, or other facial dysfunction or if no tympanic membrane thermometer equipment is available. Wear gloves and insert a lubricated rectal probe cover on an electronic thermometer only 2 to 3 cm (1 in) into the adult rectum, directed toward the umbilicus. (For a glass thermometer, leave in place for 2½ minutes.) Disadvantages to the rectal route are patient discomfort and the time-consuming and disruptive nature of the activity.

The **tympanic membrane thermometer (TMT)** senses infrared emissions of the tympanic membrane (eardrum). The tympanic membrane shares the same vascular supply that perfuses the hypothalamus (the internal carotid artery); thus it is an accurate measurement of core temperature.

The tympanic membrane thermometer is a noninvasive, nontraumatic device that is extremely quick and efficient. The probe tip has the shape of an otoscope, the instrument used to inspect the ear. Gently place the covered probe tip in the person's ear canal and aim the infrared beam at the tympanic membrane (see Fig. 9-16 on p. 147). Do not occlude the canal. Activate the device, and read the temperature in 2 to 3 seconds.

There is minimal chance of cross-contamination with the tympanic thermometer because the ear canal is lined with skin and not mucous membrane. This thermometer is used with unconscious patients or with those in emergency departments, recovery areas, labor and delivery units). Current evidence is conflicting; some studies do not support use of tympanic thermometry in critically ill patients.[9,11,20] These groups primarily studied normothermic patients; we need more research under conditions common in acute care settings. A newer noninvasive measurement uses infrared emissions from the *temporal* artery. This device yields measures that agree closely with core temperature,[20] but accuracy can be affected by diaphoresis in patients.

Abnormal Findings

Hyperthermia, or fever, is caused by pyrogens secreted by toxic bacteria during infections or from tissue breakdown such as that following myocardial infarction, trauma, surgery, or malignancy. Neurologic disorders (e.g., a cerebral vascular accident, cerebral edema, brain trauma, tumor, or surgery) also can reset the brain's thermostat at a higher level, resulting in heat production and conservation.

Hypothermia is usually due to accidental, prolonged exposure to cold. It also may be purposefully induced to lower the body's oxygen requirements during heart or peripheral vascular surgery, neurosurgery, amputation, or gastrointestinal hemorrhage.

Normal Range of Findings | **Abnormal Findings**

Report the temperature in degrees Celsius unless your agency uses the Fahrenheit scale. Familiarize yourself with both scales. Note that it is far easier to learn to *think* in the centigrade scale than to take the time for paper-and-pencil conversions. Begin by memorizing these convenient equivalents:

104.0° F = 40.0° C; 98.6° F = 37.0° C; 95.0° F = 35.0° C

Pulse

With every beat, the heart pumps an amount of blood—the **stroke volume**—into the aorta. This is about 70 mL in the adult. The force flares the arterial walls and generates a pressure wave, which is felt in the periphery as the **pulse.** Palpating the peripheral pulse gives the rate and rhythm of the heartbeat, as well as local data on the condition of the artery.

Using the pads of your first three fingers, palpate the radial pulse at the flexor aspect of the wrist laterally along the radius bone (Fig. 9-3). If the rhythm is regular, count the number of beats in 30 seconds and multiply by 2. Although the 15-second interval is frequently practiced, any one-beat error in counting results in a recorded error of four beats per minute. The 30-second interval is the most accurate and efficient when heart rates are normal or rapid and when rhythms are regular. However, if the rhythm is irregular, count for a full minute. As you begin the counting interval, start your count with "zero" for the first pulse felt. The second pulse felt is "one," and so on. Assess the pulse, including (1) rate, (2) rhythm, and (3) force.

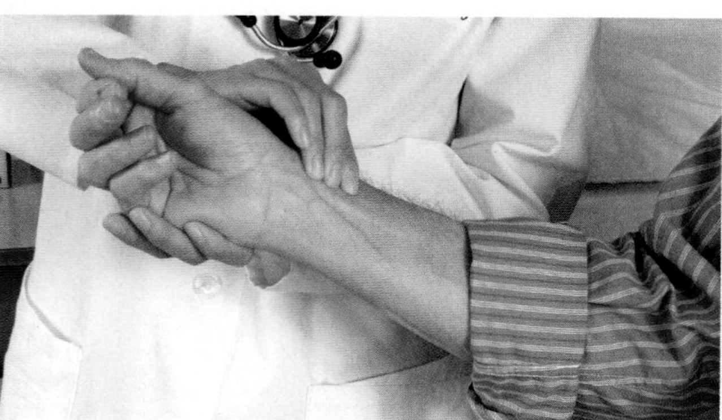

9-3

Rate

In the adult at physical and mental rest, clinical evidence shows the normal resting heart range at 50 to 90 beats per minute (bpm).[34] This differs from the conventional rate limits—60 to 100 bpm—that were established by consensus in the 1950s and never formally examined.

The rate normally varies with age, being more rapid in infancy and childhood and more moderate during adult and older years. The rate also varies with gender; after puberty, females have a slightly faster rate than males.

In the adult, a resting heart rate less than 50 bpm is **bradycardia.** Heart rates in the 50s/min occur normally in the well-trained athlete whose heart muscle develops along with the skeletal muscles. The stronger, more efficient heart muscle pushes out a larger stroke volume with each beat, thus requiring fewer beats per minute to maintain a stable cardiac output.

For descriptions of abnormal rates and rhythms, see Table 20-1, Variations in Pulse Contour, p. 519).

A more rapid resting heart rate, over 90 bpm, is **tachycardia.** Rapid rates occur normally with anxiety or with increased exercise to match the body's demand for increased metabolism.

Tachycardia occurs with fever, sepsis, and following myocardial infarction.

Objective Data

Normal Range of Findings	Abnormal Findings

Rhythm

The rhythm of the pulse normally has an even tempo. However, one irregularity that is commonly found in children and young adults is **sinus arrhythmia.** Here the heart rate varies with the respiratory cycle, speeding up at the peak of inspiration and slowing to normal with expiration. Inspiration momentarily causes a decreased stroke volume from the left side of the heart; to compensate, the heart rate increases. (See Chapter 19 for a full discussion on sinus arrhythmia.) If any other irregularities are felt, auscultate heart sounds for a more complete assessment (see Chapter 19).

Force

The force of the pulse shows the strength of the heart's stroke volume. A "weak, thready" pulse reflects a decreased stroke volume (e.g., as occurs with hemorrhagic shock). A "full, bounding" pulse denotes an increased stroke volume (e.g., as with anxiety, exercise, and some abnormal conditions). The pulse force is recorded using a three-point scale:

3+—Full, bounding
2+—Normal
1+—Weak, thready
0—Absent

Some agencies use a four-point scale; make sure your system is consistent with that used by the rest of your staff. Either scale is somewhat subjective. Experience will increase your clinical judgment.

Respirations

Normally, a person's breathing is relaxed, regular, automatic, and silent. Because most people are unaware of their breathing, do not mention that you will be counting the respirations, because sudden awareness may alter the normal pattern. Instead, maintain your position of counting the radial pulse and unobtrusively count the respirations. Count for 30 seconds or for a full minute if you suspect an abnormality. Avoid the 15-second interval. The result can vary by a factor of +4 or −4, which is significant with such a small number.

Note that respiratory rates presented in Table 9-2 normally are more rapid in infants and children. Also, a fairly constant ratio of pulse rate to respiratory rate exists, which is about 4:1. Normally, both pulse and respiratory rates rise as a response to exercise or anxiety. More detailed assessment on respiratory status is presented in Chapter 18.

TABLE 9-2 Normal Respiratory Rates

Age	Breaths per Minute
Neonate	30-40
1 yr	20-40
2 yr	25-32
8-10 yr	20-26
12-14 yr	18-22
16 yr	12-20
Adult	10-20

Normal Range of Findings	Abnormal Findings

Blood Pressure

Blood pressure (BP) is the force of the blood pushing against the side of its container, the vessel wall. The strength of the push changes with the event in the cardiac cycle. The **systolic** pressure is the maximum pressure felt on the artery during left ventricular contraction, or systole. The **diastolic** pressure is the elastic recoil, or resting, pressure that the blood exerts constantly between each contraction. The **pulse pressure** is the difference between the systolic and diastolic pressures and reflects the stroke volume (Fig. 9-4).

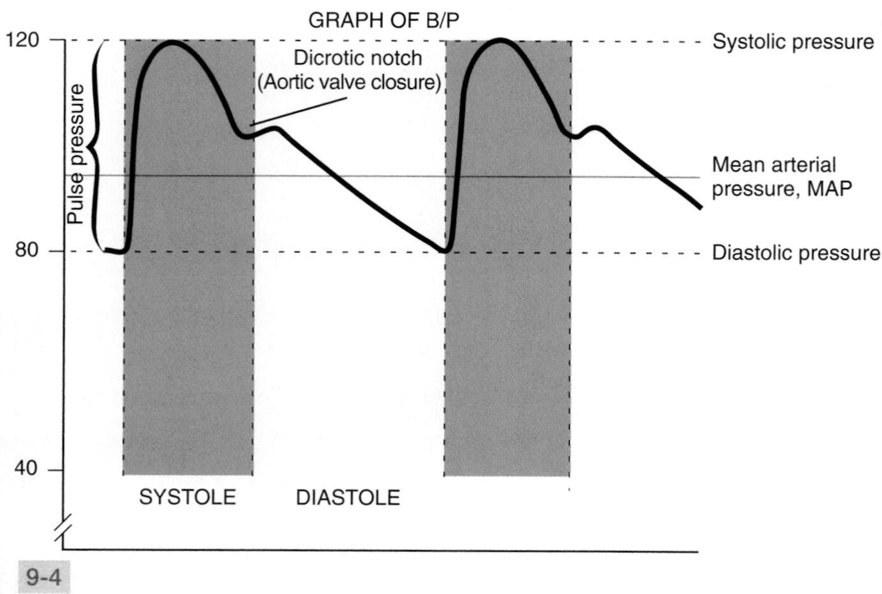

9-4

The **mean arterial pressure (MAP)** is the pressure forcing blood into the tissues, averaged over the cardiac cycle. This is not an arithmetic average of systolic and diastolic pressures because diastole lasts longer. Rather, it is a value closer to diastolic pressure plus one-third the pulse pressure.

The average BP in the young adult varies with many factors, such as:

- **Age.** Normally, a gradual rise occurs through childhood and into the adult years.
- **Gender.** Before puberty, no difference exists between males and females. After puberty, females usually show a lower BP reading than do male counterparts. After menopause, BP in females is higher than in male counterparts.
- **Race.** In the United States, an African American adult's BP is often higher than that of a white person of the same age. The incidence of hypertension is twice as high in African Americans as in whites. The reasons for this difference are not understood fully, but we do know genetic profile and environmental factors are involved.
- **Diurnal rhythm.** A daily cycle of a peak and a trough occurs: the BP climbs to a high in late afternoon or early evening and then declines to an early morning low.
- **Weight.** BP is higher in obese persons than in persons of normal weight of the same age (including adolescents).
- **Exercise.** Increasing activity yields a proportionate increase in BP. Within 5 minutes of terminating the exercise, the BP normally returns to baseline.

Normal Range of Findings	Abnormal Findings

- **Emotions.** The BP momentarily rises with fear, anger, and pain as a result of stimulation of the sympathetic nervous system.
- **Stress.** The BP is elevated in persons feeling continual tension because of lifestyle, occupational stress, or life problems.

The level of **BP** is determined by five factors:

1. **Cardiac output.** If the heart pumps more blood into the container (i.e., the blood vessels), the pressure on the container walls increases (Fig. 9-5).

FACTORS CONTROLLING BLOOD PRESSURE

FACTOR	CONDITION	RESULT
Cardiac output	↑ with heavy exercise to meet body demand for increased metabolism	↑BP
	↓ with pump failure (weak pumping action after myocardial infarction, or in shock)	↓BP
Vascular resistance	↑ resistance (vasoconstriction)	↑BP
	↓ resistance (vasodilation)	↓BP
Volume	↓ volume (hemorrhage)	↓BP
	↑ volume (increased sodium and water retention, intravenous fluid overload)	↑BP
Viscosity	↑ viscosity (increased hematocrit in polycythemia)	↑BP
Elasticity of arterial walls	↑ rigidity, hardening as in arteriosclerosis (heart pumping against greater resistance)	↑BP

9-5

2. **Peripheral vascular resistance.** Peripheral vascular resistance is the opposition to blood flow through the arteries. When the container becomes smaller (e.g., with constricted vessels), the pressure needed to push the contents becomes greater.
3. **Volume of circulating blood.** Volume of circulating blood refers to how tightly the blood is packed into the arteries. Increasing the contents in the container increases the pressure.
4. **Viscosity.** The "thickness" of blood is determined by its formed elements, the blood cells. When the contents are thicker, the pressure increases.
5. **Elasticity of vessel walls.** When the container walls are stiff and rigid, the pressure needed to push the contents increases.

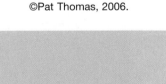

Blood pressure is measured with a stethoscope and an aneroid *sphygmomanometer.* The aneroid gauge is subject to drift; it must be recalibrated at least once each year, and it must rest at zero.

The cuff consists of an inflatable rubber bladder inside a cloth cover. The width of the rubber bladder should equal 40% of the circumference of the person's arm. The length of the bladder should equal 80% of this circumference.

Normal Range of Findings

Available cuffs include six sizes that fit newborn infants to the extra-large adult, as well as tapered cuffs for the cone-shaped obese arm and thigh cuffs. Match the appropriate-size cuff to the person's arm size and shape and not to the person's age (Fig. 9-6).

Thigh cuff or large arm cuff

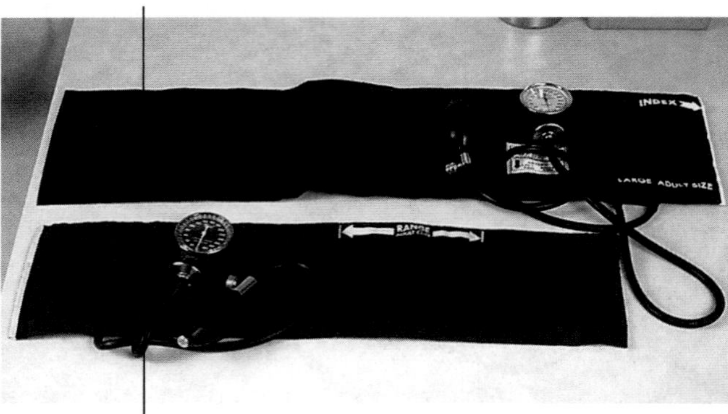

Standard adult arm cuff

9-6

Arm Pressure

A comfortable, relaxed person yields a valid blood pressure. Many people are anxious at the beginning of an examination; allow at least a 5-minute rest before measuring the BP. Then take two or more BP measurements separated by 2 minutes.

For each person, verify BP in both arms once, either on admission or for the first complete physical examination. It is not necessary to continue to check both arms for screening or monitoring. Occasionally a 5– to 10–mm Hg difference may occur in BP in the two arms (if values are different, use the higher value) and is due to artifact or to subtle differences in technique.

The person may be sitting or lying, with the bare arm supported at heart level. (If used, place the mercury manometer so that it is vertical and at your eye level.) When sitting, the patient's feet should be flat on the floor because BP has a false high measurement when legs are crossed versus uncrossed.[17]

Palpate the brachial artery, which is located just above the antecubital fossa, medial to the biceps tendon. With the cuff deflated, center it about 2.5 cm (1 in) above the brachial artery and wrap it evenly.

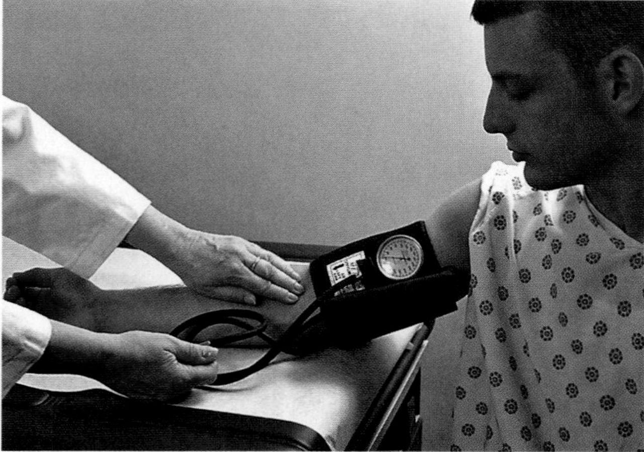

9-7

Now palpate the brachial or the radial artery (Fig. 9-7). Inflate the cuff until the artery pulsation is obliterated and then 20 to 30 mm Hg beyond. This will avoid missing an **auscultatory gap,** which is a period when Korotkoff sounds disappear during auscultation (Table 9-3).

Abnormal Findings

The cuff size is important; using a cuff that is too narrow yields a falsely high BP because it takes extra pressure to compress the artery.

A reproducible difference in the two arms of more than 10 to 15 mm Hg may indicate arterial obstruction on the side with the lower reading.

An auscultatory gap occurs in about 5% of people, most often in hypertension caused by a noncompliant arterial system.

Normal Range of Findings | Abnormal Findings

TABLE 9-3 Korotkoff Sounds

Phase	Quality	Description	Rationale
Cuff correctly inflated	No sound		Cuff inflation compresses brachial artery. Cuff pressure exceeds heart's systolic pressure, occluding brachial artery blood flow.
I	Tapping	Soft, clear tapping, increasing in intensity	The **systolic** pressure. As the cuff pressure lowers to reach intraluminal systolic pressure, the artery opens and blood first spurts into the brachial artery. Blood is at very high velocity because of small opening of artery and large pressure difference across opening. This creates turbulent flow, which is audible.
Auscultatory gap	No sound	Silence for 30-40 mm Hg during deflation, an abnormal finding	Sounds temporarily disappear during end of phase I and then reappear in phase II. Common with hypertension. If undetected, results in falsely low systolic or falsely high diastolic reading.
II	Swooshing	Softer murmur follows tapping	Turbulent blood flow through still partially occluded artery.
III	Knocking	Crisp, high-pitched sounds	Longer duration of blood flow through artery. Artery closes just briefly during late diastole.
IV	Abrupt muffling	Sound mutes to a low-pitched, cushioned murmur; blowing quality	Artery no longer closes in any part of cardiac cycle. Change in quality, not intensity.
V	Silence		Decreased velocity of blood flow. Streamlined blood flow is silent. The last audible sound (marking the disappearance of sounds) is **diastolic** pressure. The fifth Korotkoff sound is now used to define diastolic pressure in all age-groups.[4]

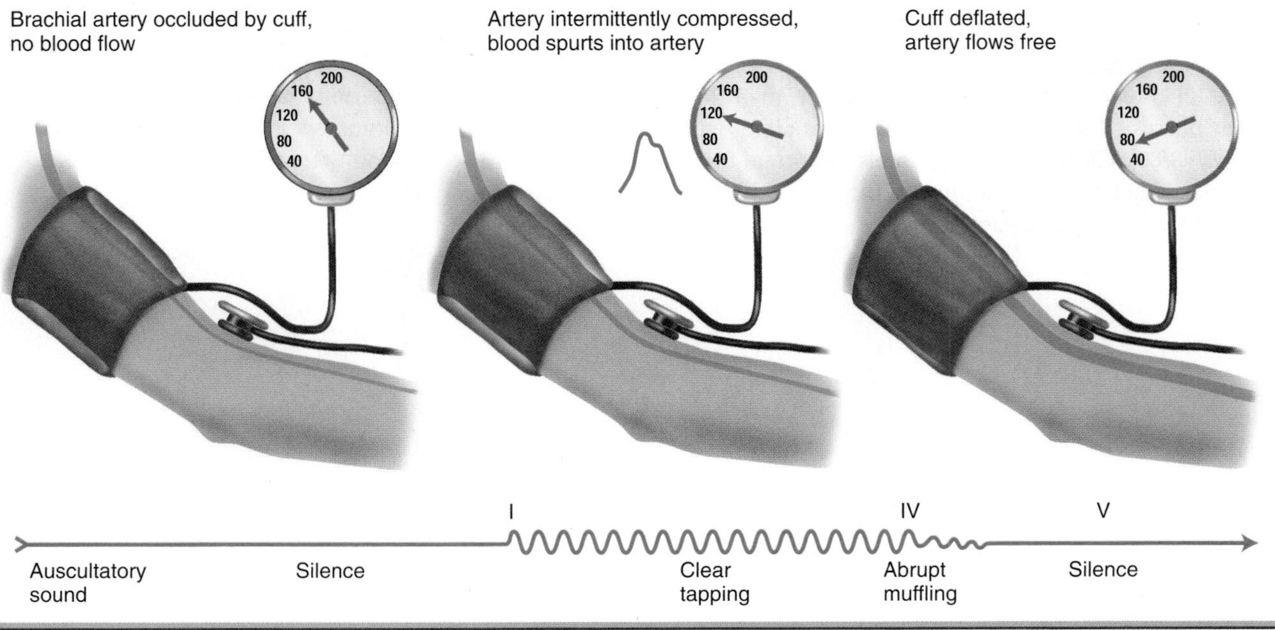

Objective Data

Normal Range of Findings

Deflate the cuff quickly and completely; then wait 15 to 30 seconds before reinflating so that the blood trapped in the veins can dissipate. Place the bell of the stethoscope over the site of the brachial artery, making a light but airtight seal (Fig. 9-8). The diaphragm endpiece is usually adequate, but the bell is designed to pick up low-pitched sounds such as the sounds of a blood pressure reading. So if you have a bell, use it.

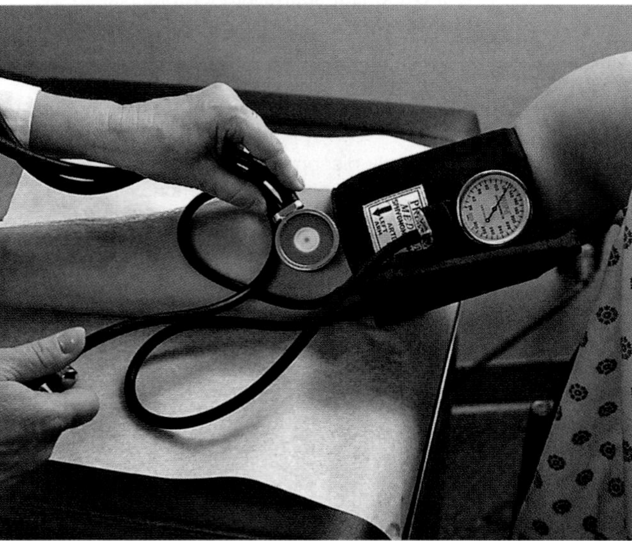

9-8

Rapidly inflate the cuff to the maximal inflation level you determined. Then deflate the cuff slowly and evenly, about 2 mm Hg per heartbeat. Note the points at which you hear the first appearance of sound, the muffling of sound, and the final disappearance of sound. These are phases I, IV, and V of **Korotkoff sounds,** which are the components of a BP reading first described by a Russian surgeon in 1905 (see Table 9-3).

For all age-groups, the fifth Korotkoff phase is now used to define diastolic pressure.[4] However, when a variance greater than 10 to 12 mm Hg exists between phases IV and V, record *both* phases along with the systolic reading (e.g., 142/98/80). Clear communication is important because the results significantly affect diagnosis and planning of care. See Table 9-4 for a list of common errors in blood pressure measurement.

Abnormal Findings

Hypotension, abnormally low BP; **hypertension,** abnormally high BP (see parameters in Table 9-6, Abnormalities in Blood Pressure, on p. 156).

Objective Data

Normal Range of Findings | **Abnormal Findings**

TABLE 9-4 Common Errors in Blood Pressure Measurement

Common Error	Result	Rationale
Taking blood pressure reading when person is anxious or angry or has just been active.	Falsely high	Sympathetic nervous system stimulation
Faulty arm position:		
Above level of heart	Falsely low	Eliminates effect of hydrostatic pressure
Below level of heart	Falsely high	Additional force of gravity added to brachial artery pressure
Person supports own arm	Falsely high diastolic	Sustained isometric muscular contraction
Faulty leg position (e.g., person's legs are crossed)	Falsely high systolic and diastolic	Translocation of blood volume from dependent legs to thoracic area
Examiner's eyes are not level with meniscus of mercury column:		
Looking up at meniscus	Falsely high	Parallax
Looking down on meniscus	Falsely low	
Inaccurate cuff size (this is the most common error):		
Cuff too narrow for extremity	Falsely high	Needs excessive pressure to occlude brachial artery
Cuff wrap is too loose or uneven, or bladder balloons out of wrap	Falsely high	Needs excessive pressure to occlude brachial artery
Failure to palpate radial artery while inflating:		
Inflating not high enough	Falsely low systolic	Miss initial systolic tapping or may tune in during *auscultatory gap* (tapping sounds disappear for 10 to 40 mm Hg and then return; common with hypertension)
Inflating cuff too high	Pain	
Pushing stethoscope too hard on brachial artery	Falsely low diastolic	Excessive pressure distorts artery and the sounds continue
Deflating cuff:		
Too quickly	Falsely low systolic or falsely high diastolic	Insufficient time to hear tapping
Too slowly	Falsely high diastolic	Venous congestion in forearm makes sounds less audible
Halting during descent and reinflating cuff to recheck systolic	Falsely high diastolic	Venous congestion in forearm
Failure to wait 1-2 min before repeating entire reading	Falsely high diastolic	Venous congestion in forearm
Any observer error:		
Examiner's "subconscious bias"; a preconceived idea of what blood pressure reading *should* be due to person's age, race, gender, weight, history, or condition	Error anywhere	
Examiner's haste	Error anywhere	
Faulty technique		
Examiner's digit preference, "hears" more results that end in zero than would occur by chance alone (e.g., 130/80)		
Diminished hearing acuity		
Defective or inaccurately calibrated equipment		

Orthostatic (or Postural) Vital Signs

Take serial measurements of pulse and blood pressure when (1) you suspect volume depletion; (2) when the person is known to have hypertension or is taking antihypertensive medications; or (3) when the person reports fainting or syncope. Have the person rest supine for 2 or 3 minutes, take baseline readings of pulse and BP, and then repeat the measurements with the person sitting and

Normal Range of Findings	Abnormal Findings
then standing. For the person who is too weak or dizzy to stand, assess supine and then sitting with legs dangling. When the position is changed from supine to standing, normally a slight decrease (less than 10 mm Hg) in systolic pressure may occur.	**Orthostatic hypotension,** a drop in systolic pressure of more than 20 mm Hg or orthostatic pulse increases of 20 bpm or more occurs with a quick change to a standing position. These changes are due to abrupt peripheral vasodilation without a compensatory increase in cardiac output. Orthostatic changes also occur with prolonged bedrest, older age, hypovolemia, and some drugs.

Record the BP by using even numbers. Also record the person's position, the arm used, and the cuff size if different from the standard adult cuff. Record the pulse rate and rhythm, noting whether the pulse is regular.

Thigh Pressure

When BP measured at the arm is excessively high, particularly in adolescents and young adults, compare it with the thigh pressure to check for **coarctation** of the aorta (a congenital form of narrowing). Normally, the *thigh pressure is higher* than that in the arm. If possible, turn the person to the prone position on the abdomen. (If the person must remain in the supine position, bend the knee slightly.) Wrap a large cuff, 18 to 20 cm, around the lower third of the thigh, centered over the popliteal artery on the back of the knee. Auscultate the popliteal artery for the reading (Fig. 9-9). Normally, the systolic value is 10 to 40 mm Hg higher in the thigh than in the arm, and the diastolic pressure is the same.

With **coarctation of the aorta,** arm pressures are high. Thigh pressure is *lower* because the blood supply to the thigh is below the constriction.

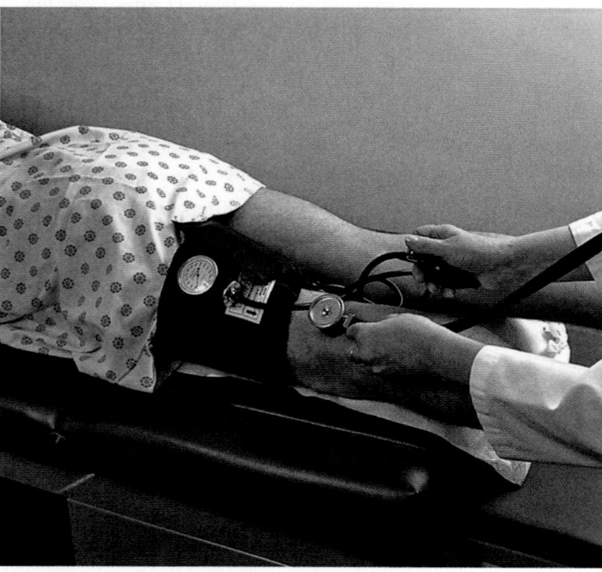

9-9

DEVELOPMENTAL COMPETENCE

Infants and Children

General Survey

Physical appearance, body structure, mobility—Note the same basic elements as with the adult, with consideration to age and development.
Behavior—Note the response to stimuli and level of alertness appropriate for age.

Normal Range of Findings	Abnormal Findings
Parental bonding—Note the child's interactions with parents, that parent and child show a mutual response and are warm and affectionate, appropriate to the child's condition. The parent provides appropriate physical care of child and promotes new learning.	Some signs of child abuse are that the child avoids eye contact; the child exhibits no separation anxiety when you would expect it for age; the parent is disgusted by child's odor, sounds, drooling, or stools. Deprivation of physical or emotional care (see Chapter 7).

Measurement

Weight. Weigh an infant on a platform-type balance scale (Fig. 9-10). To check calibration, set the weight at zero and observe the beam balance. Guard the baby so that he or she does not fall. Weigh to the nearest 10 g (½ oz) for infants and 100 g (¼ lb) for toddlers.

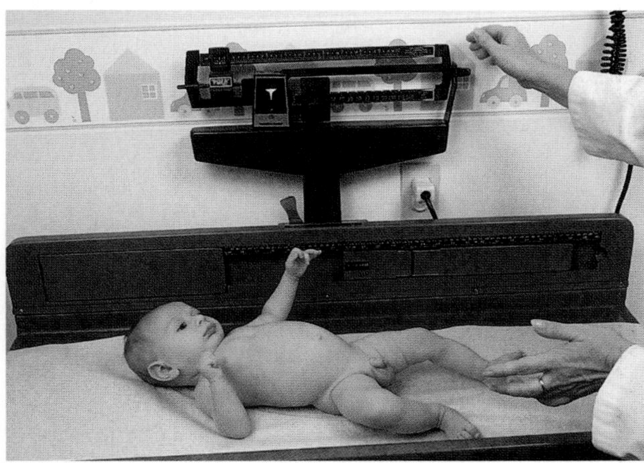

9-10

By age 2 or 3 years, use the upright scale. Leave underpants on the child. Some young children are fearful of the rickety standing platform and may prefer sitting on the infant scale. Use the upright scale with preschoolers and school-age children, maintaining modesty with light clothing (Fig. 9-11).

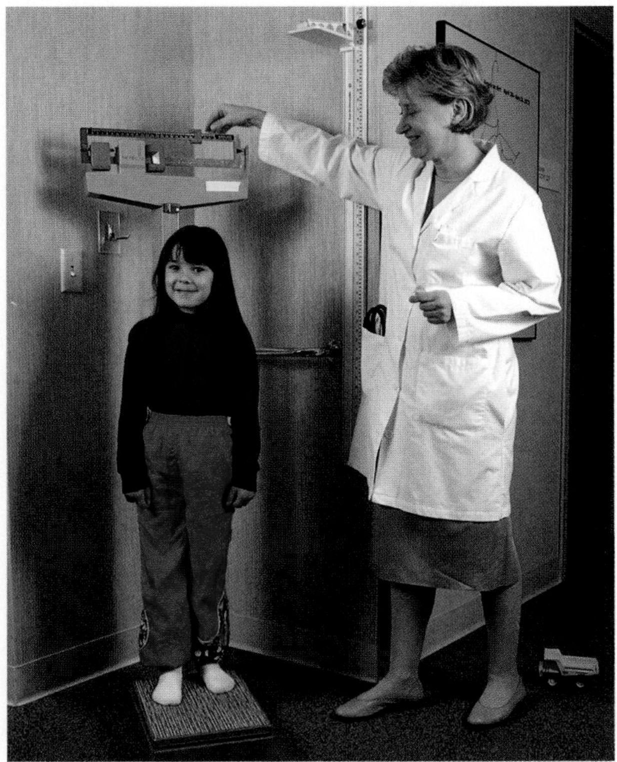

9-11

Normal Range of Findings	Abnormal Findings

Length. Until age 2 years, measure the infant's body length supine by using a horizontal measuring board (Fig. 9-12). One person holds the top of the head against the head plate. Because the infant normally has flexed legs, extend them momentarily by gently stretching the spine and legs with the feet touching the perpendicular foot plate. You may need to repeat the measure to ensure accuracy.

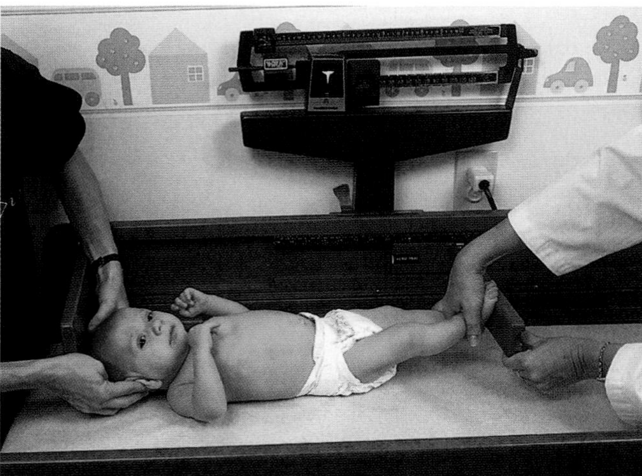

9-12

For age 2 or 3 years, measure the child's height by standing the child against a stadiometer (flat ruler) mounted on the wall (Fig. 9-13). Encourage the child to stand straight and tall and to look straight ahead without tilting the head. The shoulders, buttocks, and heels should touch the wall. Hold a level on the child's head at a right angle to the wall. Mark just under the level, noting the measure to the nearest 1 mm (⅛ in).

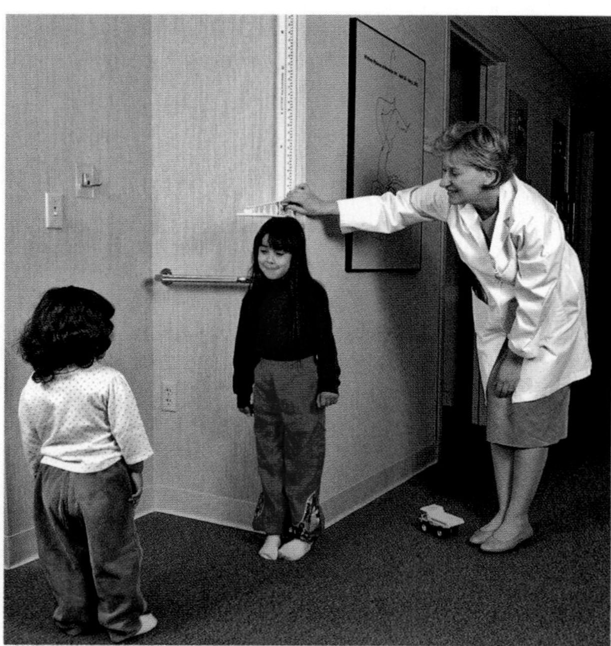

9-13

Normal Range of Findings	Abnormal Findings

Physical growth is perhaps the best index of a child's general health. The child's height and weight are recorded at every health care visit to determine normal growth patterns. The results are plotted on growth charts based on data from the Centers for Disease Control and Prevention (CDC).[3] You can view these charts in Appendix D on the *Evolve* website or at www.cdc.gov/growthcharts. In addition to the weight, height, and head circumference charts, body mass index–for-age charts are available for boys and girls ages 2 to 20 years.

Healthy childhood growth is continuous but uneven, with rapid growth spurts occurring during infancy and adolescence. Results are more reliable when comparing numerous growth measures over a long time. These charts also compare the individual child's measurements against the general population. Normal limits range from the 5th to the 95th percentile on the standardized charts.

Further explore any growth measure that:

- Falls below the 5th or above the 95th percentile with no genetic explanation
- Shows a wide percentile difference between height and weight—for example, a 10th percentile height with a 95th percentile weight
- Shows that growth has suddenly stopped when it had been steady
- Fails to show normal growth spurts during infancy and adolescence

Use your judgment and consider the genetic background of the small-for-age child. Explore the growth patterns of the parents and siblings. The differences in size and growth among the major racial/ethnic groups in the United States appear to be small and inconsistent.[3] You can use the revised 2000 CDC growth charts on all infants and children in the United States, regardless of race or ethnicity. The CDC notes the most important evidence for growth potential appears to be economic, nutritional, and environmental.[3]

Head Circumference. Measure the infant's head circumference at birth and at each well-child visit up to age 2 years and then yearly up to 6 years (Fig. 9-14). Use a retractable plastic tape rather than a paper tape measure. Circle the tape around the head aligned with the eyebrows at the prominent frontal and occipital bones; the widest span is correct. Plot the measurement on standardized growth charts. Compare the infant's head size with that expected for age. A series of measurements is more valuable than a single figure to show the *pattern* of head growth.

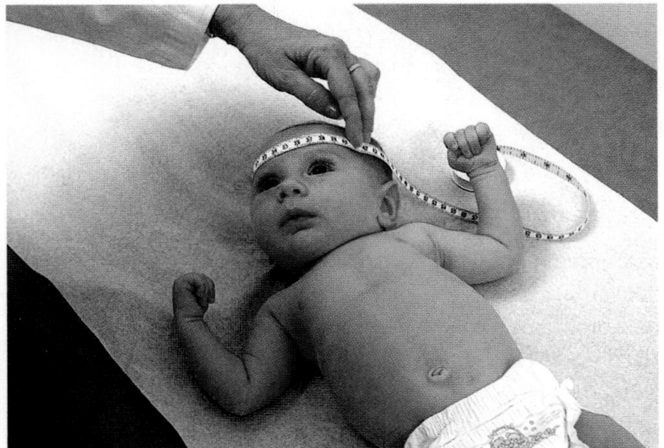

9-14

The newborn's head measures about 32 to 38 cm (average around 34 cm) and is about 2 cm larger than the chest circumference. The chest grows at a faster rate than the cranium; at some time between 6 months and 2 years, both measurements are about the same, and after age 2 years, the chest circumference is greater than the head circumference.

Enlarged head circumference occurs with increased intracranial pressure (see Chapter 13).

Normal Range of Findings | **Abnormal Findings**

Measurement of the chest circumference is valuable in a comparison with the head circumference, but not necessarily by itself. Encircle the tape around the chest at the nipple line. It should be snug, but not so tight that it leaves a mark (Fig. 9-15).

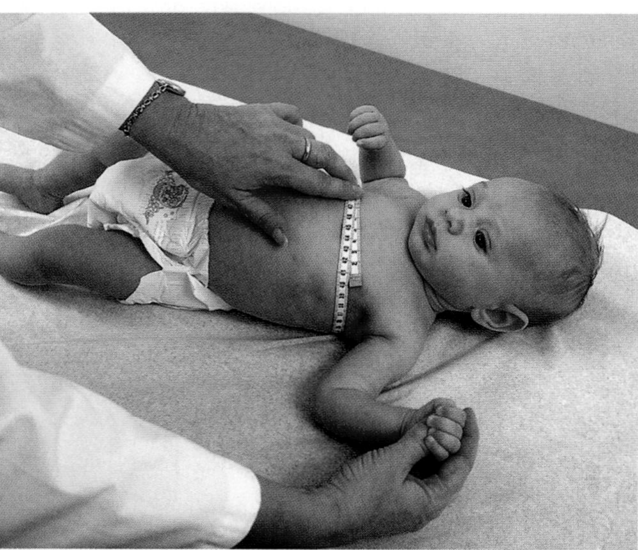

9-15

Vital Signs

Measure vital signs with the same purpose and frequency as you would in an adult. With an *infant,* reverse the order of vital sign measurement to respiration, pulse, and temperature. Taking a rectal temperature may cause the infant to cry, which will increase the respiratory and pulse rate, thus masking the normal resting values. A *preschooler's* normal fear of body mutilation is increased with any invasive procedure. Whenever possible, avoid the rectal route and take a tympanic temperature. Promote the cooperation of the *school-age child* by explaining the procedure completely and encouraging the child to handle the equipment. Your approach to measuring vital signs with the *adolescent* is much the same as with the adult.

Temperature

Tympanic. Tympanic membrane temperature (TMT) measurement is useful with toddlers who squirm at the restraint needed for the rectal route, and it is useful with preschoolers who are not yet able to cooperate for an oral temperature yet fear the disrobing and invasion of a rectal temperature. The TMT measurement is so rapid that it is over before the child realizes it (Fig. 9-16).

Normal Range of Findings	Abnormal Findings

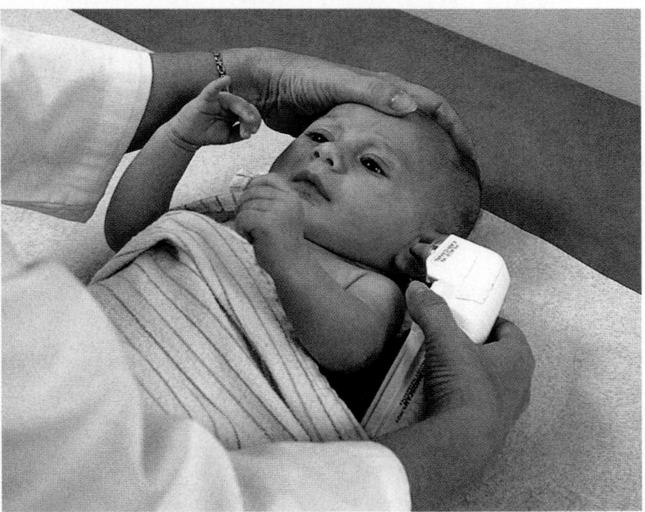

9-16

The data on TMT use with newborn infants and young children are conflicting. In a study of infants ages 3 to 36 months in outpatient settings, Jean-Mary[16] found the TMT useful for noninvasive screening, but if the history or physical examination suggests a possible febrile illness, the rectal value should be used for clinical accuracy. However, Nimah et al.[27] studied critically ill hospitalized children younger than 7 years and concluded that TMT measurements more accurately reflect core temperatures during febrile and nonfebrile states.

Axillary. The axillary route is safer and more accessible than the rectal route; however, its accuracy and reliability have been questioned.[6] When cold receptors are stimulated, brown fat tissue in the area releases heat through chemical energy, which artificially raises skin temperature. When the axillary route is used, place the tip well into the axilla and hold the child's arm close to the body.

Oral. Use the oral route when the child is old enough to keep his or her mouth closed. This is usually at age 5 or 6 years, although some 4-year-old children can cooperate. When available, use an electronic thermometer because it is unbreakable and it registers quickly.

Rectal. Use this route with infants or with other age-groups when other routes are not feasible, such as with the child who is unable to cooperate, agitated, unconscious, critically ill, or prone to seizure. An infant may be supine or side-lying, with the examiner's hand flexing the knees up onto the abdomen. (When supine, cover the boy's penis with a diaper.) An infant also may lie prone across the adult's lap. Separate the buttocks with one hand, and insert the lubricated electronic rectal probe *no farther than* 2.5 cm (1 in). Any deeper insertion risks rectal perforation because the colon curves posteriorly at 3 cm (1¼ in). (In a glass thermometer, a temperature will register by 3 minutes.)

Normally, rectal temperatures measure higher in infants and young children than in adults, with an average of 37.8° C (100° F) at 18 months. Also, the temperature normally may be elevated in the late afternoon, after vigorous playing, or after eating.

Up to ages 6 to 8 years, children have higher fevers with illness than adults do. Even with minor infections, fevers may elevate to 39.5° to 40.5° C (103° to 105° F).

Pulse

Palpate or auscultate an apical rate with infants and toddlers. (See Chapter 19 for location of apex and technique.) In children older than 2 years, use the radial site. Count the pulse for a full minute to take into account normal irregularities, such as sinus dysrhythmia. The heart rate normally fluctuates more with infants and children than with adults in response to exercise, emotion, and illness.

Normal Range of Findings | Abnormal Findings

Respirations

Watch the infant's abdomen for movement, because the infant's respirations are normally more diaphragmatic than thoracic (Fig. 9-17). The sleeping respiratory rate is the most accurate. Count a full minute because the pattern varies significantly from rapid breaths to short periods of apnea. Note the normal rate in Table 9-2.

Tachypnea, or rapid respiratory rate, is >60/min for newborns to 2 months, and >50/min for 2 to 12 months. This occurs with fever and may indicate infection. Tachypnea and labored respirations may indicate pneumonia.

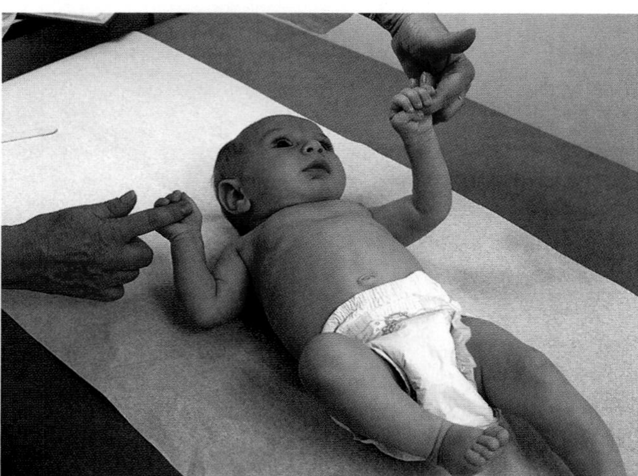

9-17

Blood Pressure

In children ages 3 years and older and in younger children at risk, measure a routine BP at least annually. For accurate measurement in children, make some adjustment in the choice of equipment and technique. The most common error is to use the incorrect size cuff. The cuff width must cover two thirds of the upper arm, and the cuff bladder must completely encircle it.

Use a pediatric-size endpiece on the stethoscope to locate the sounds. If possible, allow a crying infant to become quiet for 5 to 10 minutes before measuring the BP; crying may elevate the systolic pressure by 30 to 50 mm Hg. Use the disappearance of sound (phase V Korotkoff) for the diastolic reading in children as well as adults. Note the revised guidelines for BP standards based on gender, age, and height[25] (Appendixes E-1 and E-2 on the *Evolve* website). These standards give a more precise classification of BP according to body size and avoid misclassifying children who are very tall or very short.

Developing evidence shows primary hypertension is detectable in children and occurs commonly.[25] BP between the 90th and 95th percentiles is prehypertension. In adolescents, BP ≥120/80 mm Hg is prehypertension, even if this is <90th percentile. BP >95th percentile may be hypertension. It should be remeasured on two more occasions. But if BP is >99th percentile, make a prompt referral for evaluation and therapy.

Children younger than 3 years have such small arm vessels that it is difficult to hear Korotkoff sounds with a stethoscope. Instead, use an electronic BP device that uses *oscillometry,* such as Dinamap, and gives a digital readout for systolic, diastolic, and MAP and pulse. Or use a *Doppler* ultrasound device to amplify the sounds. This instrument is easy to use and can be used by one examiner. (Note the technique for using the Doppler device on p. 151.)

The Aging Adult

General Survey

Physical appearance—By the eighth and ninth decades, body contour is sharper, with more angular facial features, and body proportions are redistributed. (See measuring weight and height, p. 130.)

Normal Range of Findings	Abnormal Findings

Posture—A general flexion occurs by the eight or ninth decade.

Gait—Older adults often use a wider base to compensate for diminished balance, arms may be held out to help balance, and steps may be shorter or uneven.

Measurement

Weight. The aging person appears sharper in contour with more prominent bony landmarks than the younger adult. Body weight decreases during the 80s and 90s. This factor is more evident in males, perhaps because of greater muscle shrinkage. The distribution of fat also changes during the 80s and 90s. Even with good nutrition, subcutaneous fat is lost from the face and periphery (especially the forearms), whereas additional fat is deposited on the abdomen and hips (Fig. 9-18).

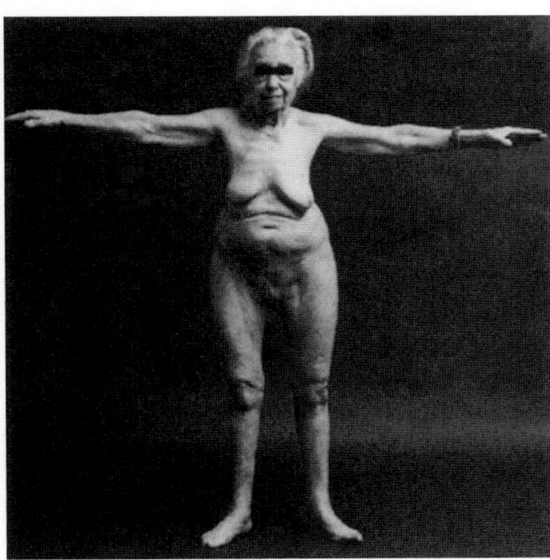

9-18

This change in fat distribution and loss in muscle mass can affect the BMI interpretation in older adults. For any given BMI, an older adult has more fat tissue than lean tissue when compared with a younger adult. As an aging person becomes shorter (see below), the BMI reflecting the shorter height may overestimate the body fat content. However, these factors do not affect the validity of BMI classification in order to monitor the person's weight status.[26]

Height. By their 80s and 90s, many people are shorter than they were in their 70s. This results from shortening in the spinal column from thinning of the vertebral disks and shortening of the individual vertebrae and from the postural changes of kyphosis and slight flexion in the knees and hips. Because long bones do not shorten with age, the overall body proportion looks different—a shorter trunk with relatively long extremities (see Fig. 9-18).

Vital Signs

Temperature. Changes in the body's temperature regulatory mechanism leave the aging person less likely to have fever but at a greater risk for hypothermia. Thus the temperature is a less reliable index of the older person's true health state. Sweat gland activity is also diminished.

Pulse. The normal range of heart rate is 50 to 90 bpm, but the rhythm may be slightly irregular. The radial artery may feel stiff, rigid, and tortuous in an older person, although this condition does not necessarily imply vascular disease in the heart or brain. The increasingly rigid arterial wall needs a faster upstroke of blood, so the pulse is actually easier to palpate.

Normal Range of Findings	Abnormal Findings

Respirations. Aging causes a decrease in vital capacity and a decreased inspiratory reserve volume. You may note a shallower inspiratory phase and an increased respiratory rate.

Blood Pressure. The aorta and major arteries tend to harden with age. As the heart pumps against a stiffer aorta, the systolic pressure increases, leading to a widened pulse pressure. With many older people, both the systolic and diastolic pressures increase, making it difficult to distinguish normal aging values from abnormal hypertension.

ADDITIONAL TECHNIQUES

Measurement of Oxygen Saturation

The **pulse oximeter** is a noninvasive method to assess arterial oxygen saturation (SpO_2). A sensor attached to the person's finger or earlobe has a diode that emits light and a detector that measures the relative amount of light absorbed by oxyhemoglobin (Hbo_2) and unoxygenated (reduced) hemoglobin (Hb). The pulse oximeter compares the ratio of light emitted with light absorbed and converts this ratio into the percentage of oxygen saturation. Because it only measures light absorption of pulsatile flow, the result is arterial oxygen saturation. A healthy person with no lung disease and no anemia normally has an SpO_2 of 97% to 100% saturation.

Select the appropriate pulse oximeter probe. The finger probe is spring loaded and feels like a clothespin attached to the finger but does not hurt (Fig. 9-19). At lower oxygen saturations, the earlobe probe is more accurate and is less affected by peripheral vasoconstriction.

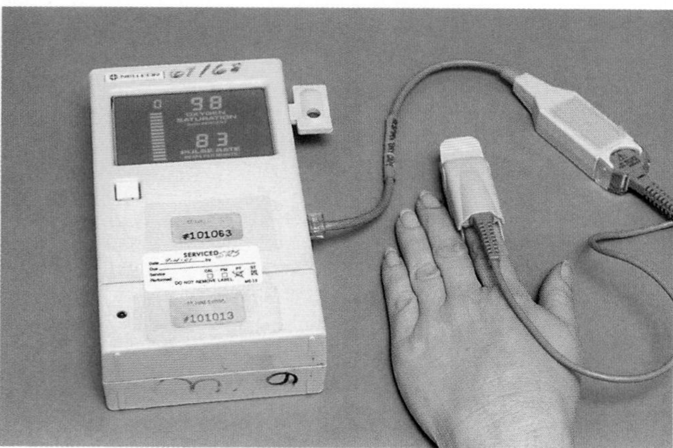

9-19

Electronic Vital Signs Monitor

An automated vital signs monitor is in frequent use in hospital and clinic settings, especially when frequent BP measurement is needed. The artery pulsations create vibrations that are detected by an electronic sensor. The blood pressure mode is noninvasive and fast and has automatic measurement intervals and a bright numeric display. As with manual BP equipment, accuracy depends on correct cuff selection and placement.

The electronic BP monitor cannot sense vibrations of low BP; do not use it with a patient who has a systolic BP of <90 mm Hg nor with conditions of an irregular heart rate, shivering, tremors, or seizures. If the numeric display does not fit with the patient's clinical picture, always validate the measurement with a manual sphygmomanometer and your own stethoscope. Some electronic BP devices also have probes for thermometry and pulse oximetry (Fig. 9-20).

Normal Range of Findings	Abnormal Findings

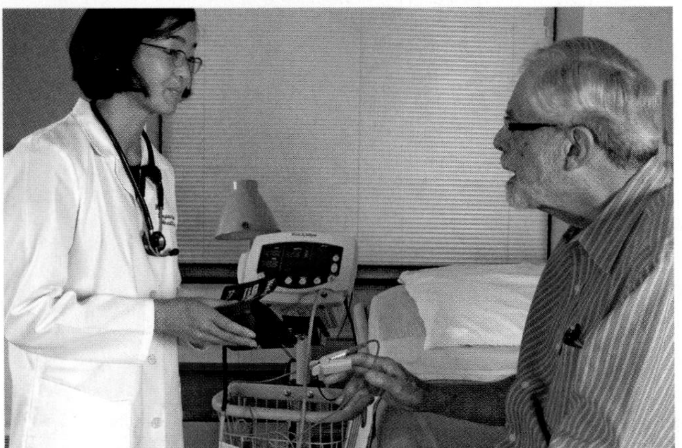

9-20

The Doppler Technique

In many situations, pulse and BP measurement are enhanced by using an electronic device, the *Doppler ultrasonic flowmeter.* The Doppler technique works by a principle discovered in the nineteenth century by an Austrian physicist, Johannes Doppler. Sound varies in pitch in relation to the distance between the sound source and the listener; the pitch is higher when the distance is small, and the pitch lowers as the distance increases. Think of a railroad train speeding toward you; its train whistle sounds higher the closer it gets, and the pitch of the whistle lowers as the train fades away.

In this case, the sound source is the blood pumping through the artery in a rhythmic manner. A handheld transducer picks up changes in sound frequency as the blood flows and ebbs, and it amplifies them. The listener hears a whooshing pulsatile beat.

The Doppler technique is used to locate the peripheral pulse sites (see Chapter 20 for further discussion of this technique). For BP measurement, the Doppler technique will augment Korotkoff sounds (Fig. 9-21). Through this technique, you can evaluate sounds that are hard to hear with a stethoscope, such as those in critically ill individuals with a low BP, in infants with small arms, and in obese persons in whom the sounds are muffled by layers of fat. Also, proper cuff placement is difficult on the obese person's cone-shaped upper arm. In this situation, you can place the cuff on the more even forearm and hold the Doppler probe over the radial artery. For either location, use the following procedure:

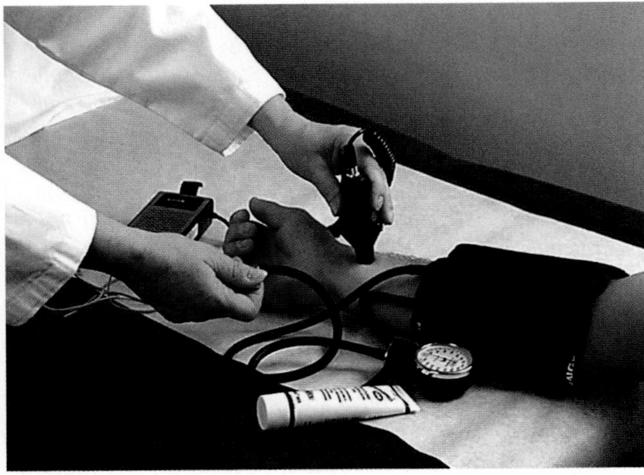

9-21

Normal Range of Findings	Abnormal Findings

- Apply coupling gel to the transducer probe.
- Turn Doppler flowmeter on.
- Touch the probe to the skin, holding the probe perpendicular to the artery.
- A pulsatile whooshing sound indicates location of the artery. You may need to rotate the probe, but maintain contact with the skin. Do not push the probe too hard or you will wipe out the pulse.
- Inflate the cuff until the sounds disappear; then proceed another 20 to 30 mm Hg beyond that point.
- Slowly deflate the cuff, noting the point at which the first whooshing sounds appear. This is the systolic pressure.
- It is difficult to hear the muffling of sounds or a reliable disappearance of sounds indicating the diastolic pressure (phases IV and V of Korotkoff sounds). However, the systolic pressure alone gives valuable data on the level of tissue perfusion and on blood flow through patent vessels.

PROMOTING HEALTH AND SELF-CARE

As you measure height and weight and collect vital signs, it is a good time to begin a teaching plan to help the individual keep these physical signs within normal limits. The 2003 Joint National Committee on Detection, Evaluation, and Treatment of High Blood Pressure considers the following **lifestyle modifications** to be the foundation of hypertension control. Even if your patient is normotensive and has body weight in normal limits, the following lifestyle modifications will help keep blood pressure under control:[4]

- Lose weight if you are more than 10% above ideal weight.
- Limit alcohol intake to no more than 1 oz of ethanol (i.e., 24 oz [720 mL] of beer, 10 oz [300 mL] of wine, or 2 oz [60 mL] of 100-proof whiskey) per day for men, or 0.5 oz (15 mL) of ethanol per day for women and lighter-weight people.
- Get regular aerobic exercise (e.g., a 30- to 45-minute brisk walk) most days of the week.
- Cut sodium intake from the average 150 mmol/L (150 mEq/L) to less than 100 mmol/L (100 mEq/L) per day (less than 2.3 g of sodium or 6 g of sodium chloride).
- Include the recommended daily allowances of potassium, calcium, and magnesium in your diet.
- Stop smoking.
- Reduce dietary saturated fat and cholesterol.

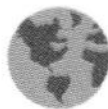

CULTURE AND GENETICS

General Appearance

Genetic differences are found in the body proportions of individuals. In general, white males are 1.27 cm (0.5 in) taller than Black males, whereas white women and Black women are, on the average, the same height. Sitting-to-standing height ratios reveal that Blacks of both genders have longer legs and shorter trunks than whites.[13] Because proportionately most of the weight is in the trunk, white men appear more obese than Black men. Asians are markedly shorter, weigh less, and have smaller body frames.

However, genes are not destiny. In the twentieth century, people grew taller in developed countries than they did in developing countries, largely because of environmental influences.[1] This is most apparent among children of immigrants[1]:

Japanese-born men living in Japan are shorter than those living in Hawaii, and shorter still than those living in California, and Hawaiian-born children of Japanese immigrants were significantly taller than their parents. Similarly, Guatemala Mayan refugee children born in the United States were significantly taller than their peers born in Guatemala or in Mexico en route to the United States. In total, Mayan children growing up in the United States are on average 5.5 cm taller than their cohort remaining in Guatemala. In general, subsequent generations of children of immigrants tend to increase in stature until they attain the height of the host population.

Bone length, as revealed by stature, shows definite genetic differences, with Blacks having longer legs and arms than whites. Asians and American Indians have, on the average, proportionately longer trunks and shorter limbs than whites. Blacks tend to be wide shouldered and narrow hipped, whereas Asians tend to be wide hipped and narrow shouldered. Shoulder width is largely produced by the clavicle.

Because the clavicle is a long bone, taller people have wide shoulders, whereas shorter people have narrower shoulders.

Obesity. Data from the most recent National Health and Nutrition Examination Survey (NHANES) show that 32.2% of U.S. adults are obese.[28] Obesity rates by racial groups include 30% non-Hispanic white adults; 45% non-Hispanic Blacks; and 37% Mexican Americans. When studied by gender, among adult men, no differences in weight are found between racial/ethnic groups. However, Mexican American and non-Hispanic Black women are significantly more likely to be obese than non-Hispanic white women. Trends in children over the past 30 years show that Black children have had larger increases in BMI, weight, and height than white children, with increases for Mexican American children in between.[28] What causes the increase in obesity? Probably an interaction of biologic and social factors, but notably a U.S. environment with few opportunities for physical activity and an overabundance of high-calorie food.[28]

DOCUMENTATION AND CRITICAL THINKING

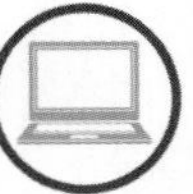

Sample Charting

A.J. is a 47-year-old Black female high school principal, who appears healthy and of her stated age. She is alert, oriented, cooperative, with no signs of pain or difficulty breathing. Ht 163 cm (5′4″), Wt 57 kg (126 lb), TPR 37° C - 76 - 14, BP 146/84 right arm, sitting.

Focused Assessment: Clinical Case Study*

Mrs. Grazia Sanchez is a 76-year-old Hispanic female retired secretary, in previous good health, who is brought to the emergency department by her 83-year-old husband. They have both been ill during the night with nausea, vomiting, abdominal pain, and diarrhea, which they attribute to eating "bad food" at a buffet-style restaurant the night before. Mr. Sanchez's condition has improved during the next day, but Mrs. Sanchez is worse, with severe vomiting, diarrhea, weakness, dizziness, and abdominal pain.

SUBJECTIVE

Extreme fatigue. Weakness and dizziness occur whenever patient tries to sit or stand up: "Feels like I'm going to black out." Severe nausea and vomiting, thirsty but cannot keep anything down; even sips of water result in "dry heaves." Abdominal pain is moderate aching, intermittent. Diarrhea is watery brown stool, profuse during the night, somewhat diminished now.

OBJECTIVE

Vital signs: Temp 99° F; BP (supine) 102/64 mm Hg; pulse (supine) 70, regular rhythm; respirations 18.

Helped to seated, leg-dangling position; vitals: BP 74/52 mm Hg; pulse 138, regular rhythm; respirations 20. Skin pale and moist (diaphoretic).

Reports light-headed and dizzy in seated position. Returned to supine.

Respiratory: Breath sounds clear in all fields, no adventitious sounds.

Cardiovascular: Regular rate (70 bpm) and rhythm when supine, S_1 and S_2 are not accentuated or diminished, no extra sounds. All pulses present, 2+ and equal bilaterally. Carotids 2+ with no carotid bruit.

Abdomen: Bowel sounds hyperactive, skin pale and moist, abdomen soft and mildly tender to palpation. No enlargement of liver or spleen.

Neuro: Level of consciousness alert and oriented; pupils equal, round, react to light and accommodation. Sensory status normal. Mild weakness in arms and legs. Gait and standing leg strength not tested due to inability to stand. Deep tendon reflexes 2+ and equal bilaterally. Babinski reflex → down-going toes.

ASSESSMENT

Orthostatic hypotension, orthostatic pulse increase, and syncopal symptoms, R/T hypovolemia
Diarrhea, possibly R/T ingestion of contaminated food
Risk for hyperthermia, R/T dehydration and aging
Deficient fluid volume

*Please note that space does not allow a detailed plan for each clinical case study in this text. Please consult the appropriate text for current treatment plan.

TABLE 9-5 Abnormalities in Body Height and Proportion

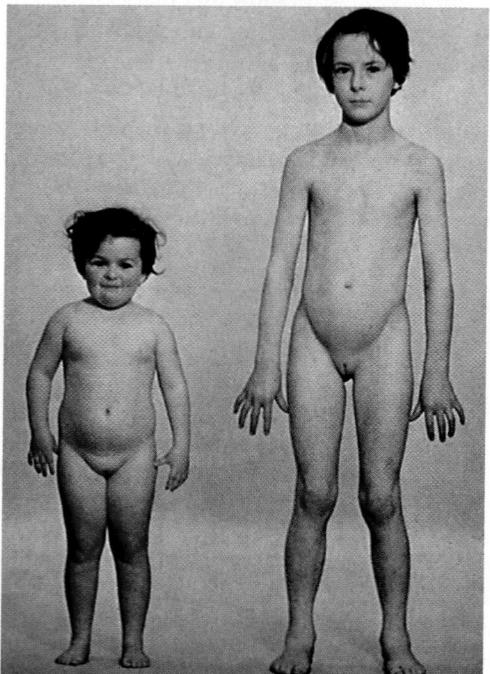

Hypopituitary Dwarfism

Deficiency in growth hormone in childhood results in retardation of growth below the 3rd percentile, delayed puberty, hypothyroidism, and adrenal insufficiency. The 9-year-old girl at left appears much younger than her chronological age, with infantile facial features and chubbiness. The age-matched girl at right shows increased height, more mature facies, and loss of infantile fat.

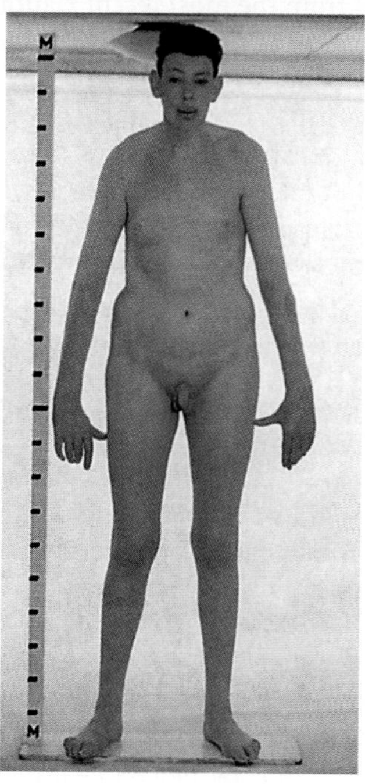

Gigantism

Excessive secretion of growth hormone by the anterior pituitary resulting in overgrowth of entire body. When this occurs during childhood, before closure of bone epiphyses in puberty, it causes increased height (here 2.09 m, or 6 ft 9 in) and weight and delayed sexual development.

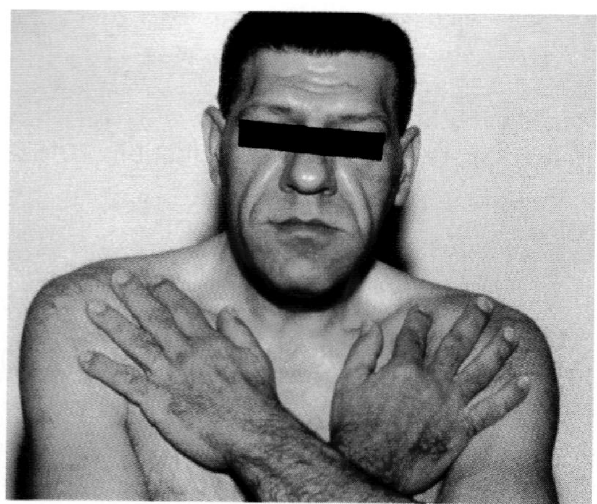

Acromegaly (Hyperpituitarism)

Excessive secretion of growth hormone in adulthood, after normal completion of body growth, causes overgrowth of bone in the face, head, hands, and feet but no change in height. Internal organs also enlarge (e.g., cardiomegaly), and metabolic disorders (e.g., diabetes mellitus) may be present.

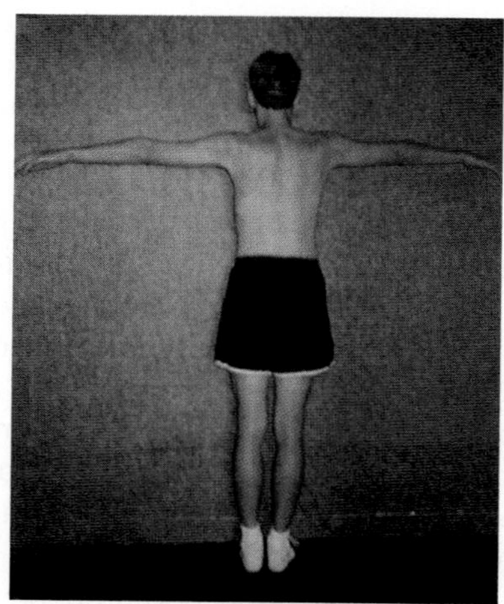

Marfan's Syndrome

Abraham Lincoln, Paganini, and Rachmaninoff are thought to have had this inherited connective tissue disorder, characterized by tall, thin stature (greater than 95th percentile), arachnodactyly (long, thin fingers), hyperextensible joints, arm span greater than height, pubis-to-sole measurement exceeding crown-to-pubis measurement, sternal deformity, high-arched narrow palate, and pes planus. Early morbidity and mortality occur as a result of cardiovascular complications such as mitral regurgitation and aortic dissection.

TABLE 9-5 Abnormalities in Body Height and Proportion—cont'd

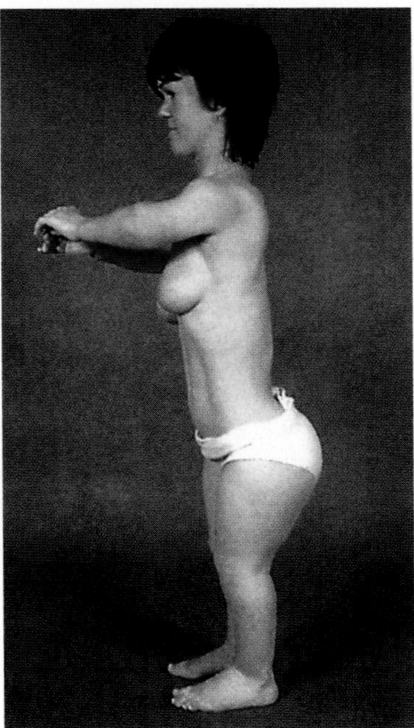

Achondroplastic Dwarfism

A genetic disorder in converting cartilage to bone results in normal trunk size, short arms and legs, and short stature. It is characterized by a relatively large head with frontal bossing and midplace hypoplasia and, often, thoracic kyphosis, prominent lumbar lordosis, and abdominal protrusion. The mean adult height in men is about 131.5 cm (51.8 in) and in women about 125 cm (49.2 in).

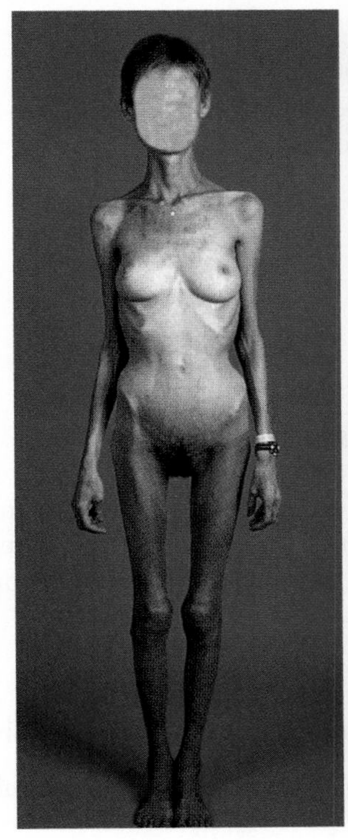

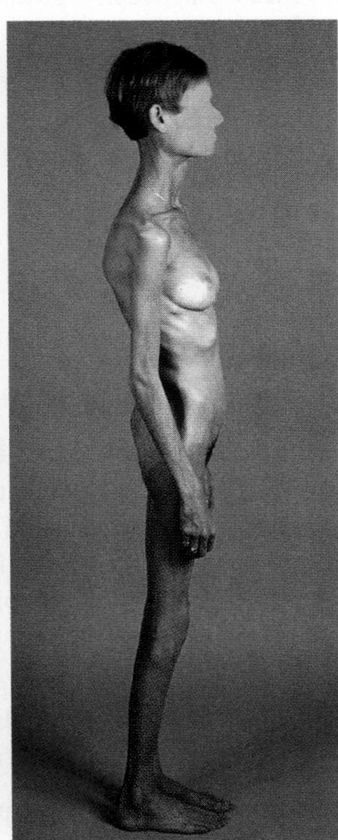

Anorexia Nervosa

A serious psychological disorder characterized by severe and life-threatening weight loss and amenorrhea in an otherwise healthy adolescent or young woman. Behavior is characterized by fanatic concern about weight, aversion to food, distorted body image (perceives self as fat despite skeletal appearance), starvation diets, frenetic exercise patterns, and striving for perfection.

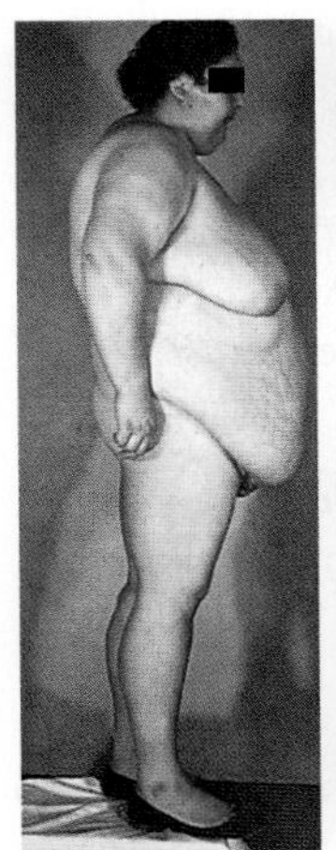

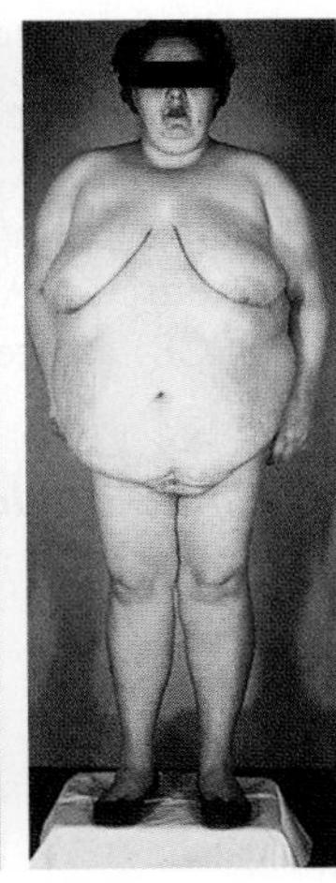

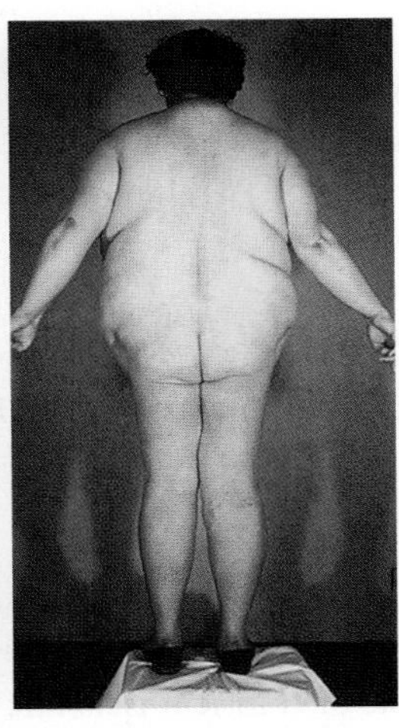

◀ Endogenous Obesity—Cushing Syndrome

Either administration of adrenocorticotropin (ACTH) or excessive production of ACTH by the pituitary will stimulate the adrenal cortex to secrete excess cortisol. This causes Cushing syndrome, characterized by weight gain and edema with central trunk and cervical obesity (buffalo hump) and round, plethoric face (moon face). Excessive catabolism causes muscle wasting; weakness; thin arms and legs; reduced height; and thin, fragile skin with purple abdominal striae, bruising, and acne. Note the obesity here is markedly different from *exogenous obesity* due to excessive caloric intake, in which body fat is evenly distributed and muscle strength is intact.

TABLE 9-6 Abnormalities in Blood Pressure

Hypotension

In normotensive adults: <95/60 mm Hg
In hypertensive adults: <the person's average reading, but >95/60 mm Hg
In children: <expected value for age

Occurs With	Rationale
Acute myocardial infarction	Decreased cardiac output
Shock	Decreased cardiac output
Hemorrhage	Decrease in total blood volume
Vasodilation	Decrease in peripheral vascular resistance
Addison's disease (hypofunction of adrenal glands)	

Associated Symptoms and Signs
In conditions of decreased cardiac output, a low BP is accompanied by an increased pulse, dizziness, diaphoresis, confusion, and blurred vision. The skin feels cool and clammy because the superficial blood vessels constrict to shunt blood to the vital organs. An individual having an acute myocardial infarction (MI) may also complain of crushing substernal chest pain, high epigastric pain, and shoulder or jaw pain.

Hypertension

Essential or Primary Hypertension
This occurs from no known cause but is responsible for about 95% of cases of hypertension in adults.

Classification and Follow-Up of Blood Pressure for Adults Ages 18 and Older*

BP Classification	SBP (mm Hg)*	DBP (mm Hg)*	Lifestyle Modification	Initial Drug Therapy	
				Without Compelling Indication	With Compelling Indication
Normal	<120	and <80	Encourage		
Prehypertension	120-139	or 80-89	Yes	No antihypertensive drug indicated.	Drug(s) for the compelling indications.‡
Stage 1 hypertension	140-159	or 90-99	Yes	Thiazide-type diuretics for most. May consider ACEI, ARB, BB, CCB, or combination.	Drug(s) for the compelling indications.‡ Other antihypertensive drugs (diuretics, ACEI, ARB, BB, CCB) as needed.
Stage 2 hypertension	≥160	or ≥100	Yes	Two-drug combination for most† usually thiazide-type diuretic and ACEI, or ARB or BB or CCB.	Drug(s) for the compelling indications.‡ Other antihypertensive drugs (diuretics, ACEI, ARB, BB, CCB) as needed.

Cardiovascular Risk Stratification in Patients With Hypertension

Major Risk Factors
Smoking
Dyslipidemia
Diabetes mellitus
Age >60 yr
Gender (men and postmenopausal women)
Family history of cardiovascular disease: women <65 yr or men <55 yr

Target Organ Damage/Clinical Cardiovascular Disease
Heart diseases
Left ventricular atrophy
Angina or prior myocardial infarction
Prior coronary revascularization
Heart failure
Stroke or transient ischemic attack
Nephropathy
Peripheral arterial disease
Retinopathy

TABLE 9-6 Abnormalities in Blood Pressure—cont'd

Lifestyle Modifications for Hypertension Prevention and Management

- Lose weight if overweight
- Limit alcohol intake to no more than 1 oz (30 mL) of ethanol (e.g., 24 oz [720 mL] of beer, 10 oz [300 mL] of wine, or 2 oz [60 mL] of 100-proof whiskey) per day or 0.5 oz (15 mL) of ethanol per day for women and lighter-weight people.
- Increase aerobic physical activity (30-45 min most days of the week).
- Reduce sodium intake to no more than 100 mmol/d (2.4 g of sodium or 6 g of sodium chloride).
- Maintain adequate intake of dietary potassium (approximately 90 mmol/day).
- Maintain adequate intake of dietary calcium and magnesium for general health.
- Stop smoking and reduce intake of dietary saturated fat and cholesterol for overall cardiovascular health.

Data on classification of hypertension in adults adapted from Chobanian, A. V., Bakris, G. L., Black, H. R., et al: National Heart, Lung, and Blood Institute Joint National Committee on Prevention, Detection, Evaluation, and Treatment of High Blood Pressure; National High Blood Pressure Education Program Coordinating Committee. (2003). The Seventh Report of the Joint National Committee on Prevention, Detection, Evaluation, and Treatment of High Blood Pressure: The JNC 7 report. *The Journal of the American Medical Association*, 289(19):2560-2572; www.nhlbi.nih.gov/guidelines/hypertension.

ACEI, Angiotensin-converting enzyme inhibitor; *ARB,* angiotensin receptor blocker; *BB,* beta-blocker; *CCB,* calcium channel blocker; *DBP,* diastolic blood pressure; *SBP,* systolic blood pressure.

*Treatment determined by highest BP category.

†Initial combined therapy should be used cautiously in those at risk for orthostatic hypotension.

‡Treat patients with chronic kidney disease or diabetes to BP goal of <130/80 mm Hg.

Abnormal Findings

BIBLIOGRAPHY

1. Beard, A. S., & Blaser, M. J. (2002). The ecology of height: the effect of microbial transmission on human height. *Perspectives in Biology and Medicine, 45*(4), 475-498.
2. Canzanello, V. J., Jensen, P. L., & Schwartz, G. L. (2001). Are aneroid sphygmomanometers accurate in hospital and clinic settings? *Archives of Internal Medicine, 161*(5), 729-731.
3. Centers for Disease Control and Prevention. (2000). *Growth charts.* National Center for Health Statistics in collaboration with the National Center for Chronic Disease Prevention and Health Promotion. Retrieved June 17, 2009, from www.cdc.gov/growth_charts.
4. Chobanian, A. V., Bakris, G. L., Black, H. R., et al. National Heart, Lung, and Blood Institute Joint National Committee on Prevention, Detection, Evaluation, and Treatment of High Blood Pressure; National High Blood Pressure Education Program Coordinating Committee (2003). The Seventh Report of the Joint National Committee on Prevention, Detection, Evaluation and Treatment of High Blood Pressure: The JNC 7 Report. *JAMA, 289*(19), 2560-2572.
5. Craig, J. V., Lancaster, G. A., Taylor, S. (2002). Infrared ear thermometry compared with rectal thermometry in children: a systematic review. *Lancet, 360*(9333), 603-609.
6. Cusson, R. M., Madonia, J. A., & Taekmen, J. B. (1997). The effect of environment on body site temperatures in full-term neonates. *Nursing Research, 46*(4), 202-207.
7. DeMeulenaere, S. (2007). Pulse oximetry: uses and limitations, *The Journal for Nurse Practitioners, 3*(5), 312-317.
8. Falkenstern, S. K., & Bauer, L. A. (2009). Helping kids grow. *The Nurse Practitioner, 34*(3), 31-41.
9. Fountain, C., Goins, L., Hartman, M., et al. (2008). Evaluating the accuracy of four temperature instruments on an adult inpatient oncology unit. *Clinical Journal of Oncology Nursing, 12*(6), 983-987.
10. Freedman, D. S., Khan, L. K., Serdula, M. K., et al. (2006). Racial and ethnic differences in secular trends for childhood BMI, weight, and height. *Obesity, 14*(2), 301-307.
11. Frommelt, T., Ott, C., & Hays, V. (2008). Accuracy of different devices to measure temperature. *Medsurg Nursing, 17*(3), 171-176.
12. Gidding, S. S. (2008). Measuring children's blood pressure matters. *Circulation, 117*, 3163-3164.
13. Gilsanz, V., Skaggs, D. L., Kovanlikaya, A., et al. (1998). Differential effect of race on the axial and appendicular skeletons of children. *The Journal of Clinical Endocrinology and Metabolism, 83*(5), 1420-1427.
14. Hwu, Y., Coates, V. E., & Lin, F. (2000). A study of the effectiveness of different measuring times and counting methods of human radial pulse rates. *Journal of Clinical Nursing, 9*(1), 146-152.
15. Jarosz, P. A., & Bellar, A. (2008). Age-appropriate obesity treatment. *The Nurse Practitioner, 33*(5), 24-32.
16. Jean-Mary, M. B., DiCanzio, J., Shaw, J., et al. (2002). Limited accuracy and reliability of infrared axillary and aural thermometers in a pediatric outpatient population. *The Journal of Pediatrics, 141*(5), 671-676.
17. Keele-Smith, R., & Price-Daniel, C. (2001). Effects of crossing legs on blood pressure measurement. *Clinical Nursing Research, 10*(2), 202-213.
18. Kiekkas, P., & Brokalaki, H. (2008). Physical antipyresis in critically ill adults. *The American Journal of Nursing, 108*(7), 40-50.
19. Kimbro, R. T., Brooks-Gunn, J., & McLanahan, S. (2007). Racial and ethnic differentials in overweight and obesity among 3-year-old children. *American Journal of Public Health, 97*(2), 298-305.
20. Lawson, L., Bridges, E. J., Ballou, I., et al. (2007). Accuracy and precision of noninvasive temperature measurement in adult intensive care patients. *American Journal of Critical Care, 16*(5), 485-496.
21. Lewis, C. E., McTigue, K. M., Burke, L. E., et al. (2009). Mortality, health outcomes, and body mass index in the overweight range. *Circulation, 119*(25), 3263.
22. Lipman, T. H., McGinley, A., & Hughes, J. (2006). Evaluation of the accuracy of height assessment of premenopausal and menopausal women. *Journal of Obstetric, Gynecologic, and Neonatal Nursing, 35*, 516-522.
23. Mitsnefes, M. M. (2006). Hypertension in children and adolescents. *Pediatric Clinics of North America, 53*(3), 493-512.
24. Moore, J. (2005). Hypertension: catching the silent killer. *The Nurse Practitioner, 30*(10), 16-35.

25. National High Blood Pressure Education Program (NHBPEP). (2004). Working Group on High Blood Pressure in Children and Adolescents. The Fourth Report on the Diagnosis, Evaluation, and Treatment of High Blood Pressure in Children and Adolescents. *Pediatrics, 114*(2), 555-576.
26. National Institutes of Health (NIH). (2000). *The practical guide to identification, evaluation, and treatment of overweight and obesity in adults.* Retrieved June 10, 2009, from www.nhlbi.nih.gov/guidelines/obesity/ob_home_htm.
27. Nimah, M. M., Bshesh, K., Callahann, J. D., et al. (2006). Infrared tympanic thermometry in comparison with other temperature measurement techniques in febrile children. *Pediatric Critical Care Medicine, 7*(1), 48-55.
28. Ogden, C. L., Ogden, C. L., Curtin, L. R., et al. (2006). Prevalence of overweight and obesity in the United States, 1999-2004. *JAMA: The Journal of the American Medical Association, 295*(13), 1549-1555.
29. Pesola, G. R., Pesola, H. R., Nelson, M. J., et al. (2001). The normal difference in bilateral indirect blood pressure recordings in normotensive individuals. *The American Journal of Emergency Medicine, 19*(1), 43-45.
30. Pickering, T. G., Hall, J. E., Appel, L. J., et al. (2005). Blood pressure measurement in humans. *Hypertension, 45,* 142-161.
31. Quatrara, B., Coffman, J., Jenkins, T., et al. (2007). The effect of respiratory rate and ingestion of hot and cold beverages on the accuracy of oral temperatures measured by electronic thermometers. *Medsurg Nursing, 16*(2), 105-108.
32. Schell, K. A. (2006). Evidence-based practice: noninvasive blood pressure measurement in children. *Pediatric Nursing, 32*(3), 263-267.
33. Schell, K., Lyons, D., Bradley, E., et al. (2006). Clinical comparison of autonomic, noninvasive measurements of blood pressure in the forearm and upper arm with the patient supine or with the head of the bed raised 45 degrees: a follow-up study. *American Journal of Critical Care, 15*(2), 196-205.
34. Spodick, D. H. (1996). Normal sinus heart rate: appropriate rate thresholds for sinus tachycardia and bradycardia. *Southern Medical Journal, 89*(7), 666-667.
35. Todd, B. (2006). *Clostridium difficile:* familiar pathogen, changing epidemiology. *The American Journal of Nursing, 106*(5), 33-36.

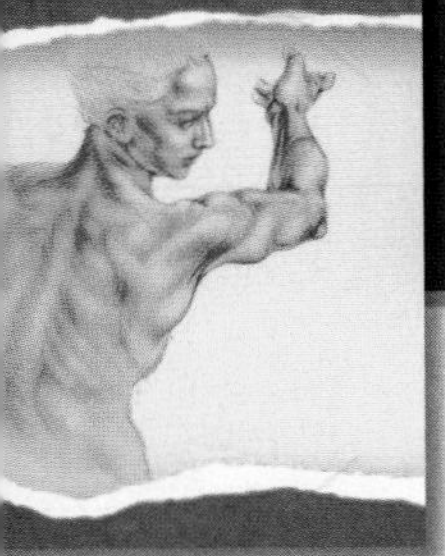

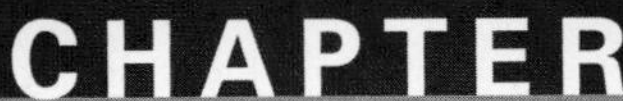

CHAPTER 10

Pain Assessment: The Fifth Vital Sign

evolve WEBSITE

http://evolve.elsevier.com/Jarvis/

- Audio Key Points
- Case Study
  Pain of Unknown Origin
- NCLEX Review Questions
- Quick Assessment for Common Conditions
  Sepsis
  Sickle Cell Anemia

OUTLINE

Structure and Function, 159

Neuropathic Processing of Pain
Neuroanatomic Pathway
Nociceptive Pain
Neuropathic Pain
Sources of Pain
Types of Pain (by Duration)

Subjective Data, 164

Initial Pain Assessment
Pain Assessment Tools
Infants and Children

Objective Data, 168

Preparation
Joints
Muscles and Skin
Abdomen
Nonverbal Behaviors of Pain

Documentation and Critical Thinking, 171

Abnormal Findings, 172

STRUCTURE AND FUNCTION

NEUROANATOMIC PROCESSING OF PAIN

Currently, we understand pain to develop by two main processes: **nociceptive** and/or **neuropathic** processing. It is important to understand how these two types of pain develop because patients will present with distinguishing sensations and respond differently to analgesics. When we are better able to assess the type(s) of pain, clinicians can more accurately select effective pharmacologic and nonpharmacologic strategies to interrupt the pain processing along multiple points within the pain messaging system and ultimately provide improved pain relief.[38]

NEUROANATOMIC PATHWAY

Pain is a highly complex and subjective experience that originates from the central nervous system (CNS) or peripheral nervous system (PNS), or both. Specialized nerve endings called **nociceptors** are designed to detect painful sensations from the periphery and transmit them to the CNS. Nociceptors are located within the skin, connective tissue, muscle, and the thoracic, abdominal, and pelvic viscera. These nociceptors can be stimulated directly by trauma or injury or secondarily by chemical mediators that are released from the site of tissue damage.

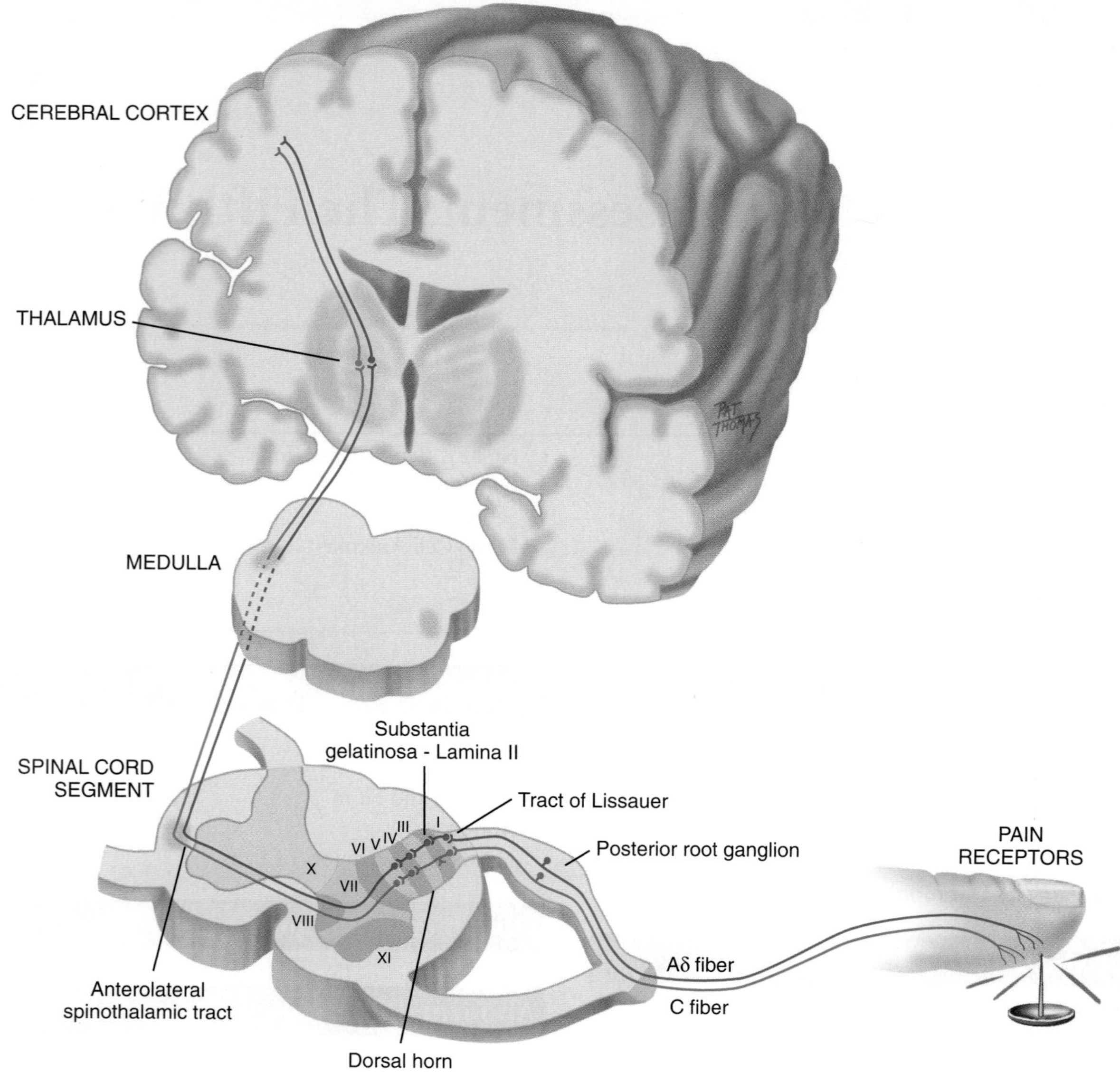

10-1

Nociceptors carry the pain signal to the central nervous system by two primary sensory (or afferent) fibers: **Aδ and C fibers** (Fig. 10-1). Aδ fibers are myelinated and larger in diameter, so they transmit the pain signal rapidly to the CNS. The sensation is very localized, short-term, and sharp in nature because of the Aδ fiber stimulation. In contrast, C fibers are unmyelinated and smaller and they transmit the signal more slowly. The "secondary" sensations are diffuse and aching, and they last longer after the initial injury.

Peripheral sensory Aδ and C fibers enter the spinal cord by posterior nerve roots within the dorsal horn by the tract of Lissauer. The fibers synapse with **interneurons** located within a specified area of the cord called the **substantia gelatinosa.** A cross section shows that the gray matter of the spinal cord is divided into a series of consecutively numbered laminae (layers of nerve cells) (see Fig. 10-1). The substantia gelatinosa is lamina II, which receives sensory input from various areas of the body. The pain signals then cross over to the other side of the spinal cord and ascend to the brain by the **anterolateral spinothalamic tract.** Pain researchers are demonstrating that when pain is poorly controlled over an extended period, cells within the dorsal horn become altered in size and function and this damage ultimately turns future pain signals into more exaggerated or hypersensitive processing.[6,8]

NOCICEPTIVE PAIN

Nociceptive pain develops when nerve fibers in the periphery and in the central nervous system are *functioning and intact.* Nociceptive pain starts outside of the nervous system from actual or potential tissue damage. Nociception can be divided into four phases: (1) transduction, (2) transmission, (3) perception, and (4) modulation (Fig. 10-2).

Initially, the first phase of **transduction** occurs when a noxious stimulus in the form of traumatic or chemical injury, burn, incision, or tumor takes place in the periphery. The periphery includes the skin, as well as somatic and visceral structures. These injured tissues then release a variety of chemicals, including substance P, histamine, prostaglandins, serotonin, and bradykinin. These chemicals are neurotransmitters that propagate a pain message, or action potential, along sensory afferent nerve fibers to the spinal cord. These nerve fibers terminate in the dorsal horn of the spinal cord. Because the initial afferent fibers stop in the dorsal horn, a second set of neurotransmitters carries the pain impulse across the synaptic cleft to the dorsal horn neurons. These neurotransmitters include substance P, glutamate, and adenosine triphosphate (ATP).

In the second phase, known as **transmission,** the pain impulse moves from the level of the spinal cord to the brain. Within the spinal cord, at the site of the synaptic cleft, are opioid receptors that can block this pain signaling with our own endogenous opioids or with exogenous opioids if they are administered. However, if not stopped, the pain impulse moves to the brain via various ascending fibers within the spinothalamic tract to the thalamus. Once the pain impulse moves through the thalamus, the message is dispersed to higher cortical areas via mechanisms that are not clearly understood at this time.

The third phase, **perception,** indicates the conscious awareness of a painful sensation. Cortical structures such as the limbic system account for the emotional response to pain, and somatosensory areas can characterize the sensation. Only when the noxious stimuli are interpreted in these higher cortical structures can this sensation be identified as "pain."

Last, the pain message is inhibited through the phase of **modulation**. Fortunately, our bodies have a built-in system that will eventually slow down and stop the processing of a painful stimulus. If not, we would continue to experience pain from childhood injuries and beyond. Descending pathways from the brainstem to the spinal cord produce a third set of neurotransmitters that slow down or impede the pain impulse, producing an analgesic effect. These neurotransmitters include serotonin, norepinephrine, neurotensin, γ-aminobutyric acid (GABA), and our own endogenous opioids—β-endorphins, enkephalins, and dynorphins.

This type of nociceptive processing is protective.[10] It is a warning signal that injury is about to or has taken place. We quickly learn to move our hand away from a burning flame. Other examples of nociceptive pain include a skinned knee, kidney stones, menstrual cramps, muscle strain, venipuncture, or arthritic joint pain. Nociceptive pain is typically predictable and time limited based on the extent of the injury.

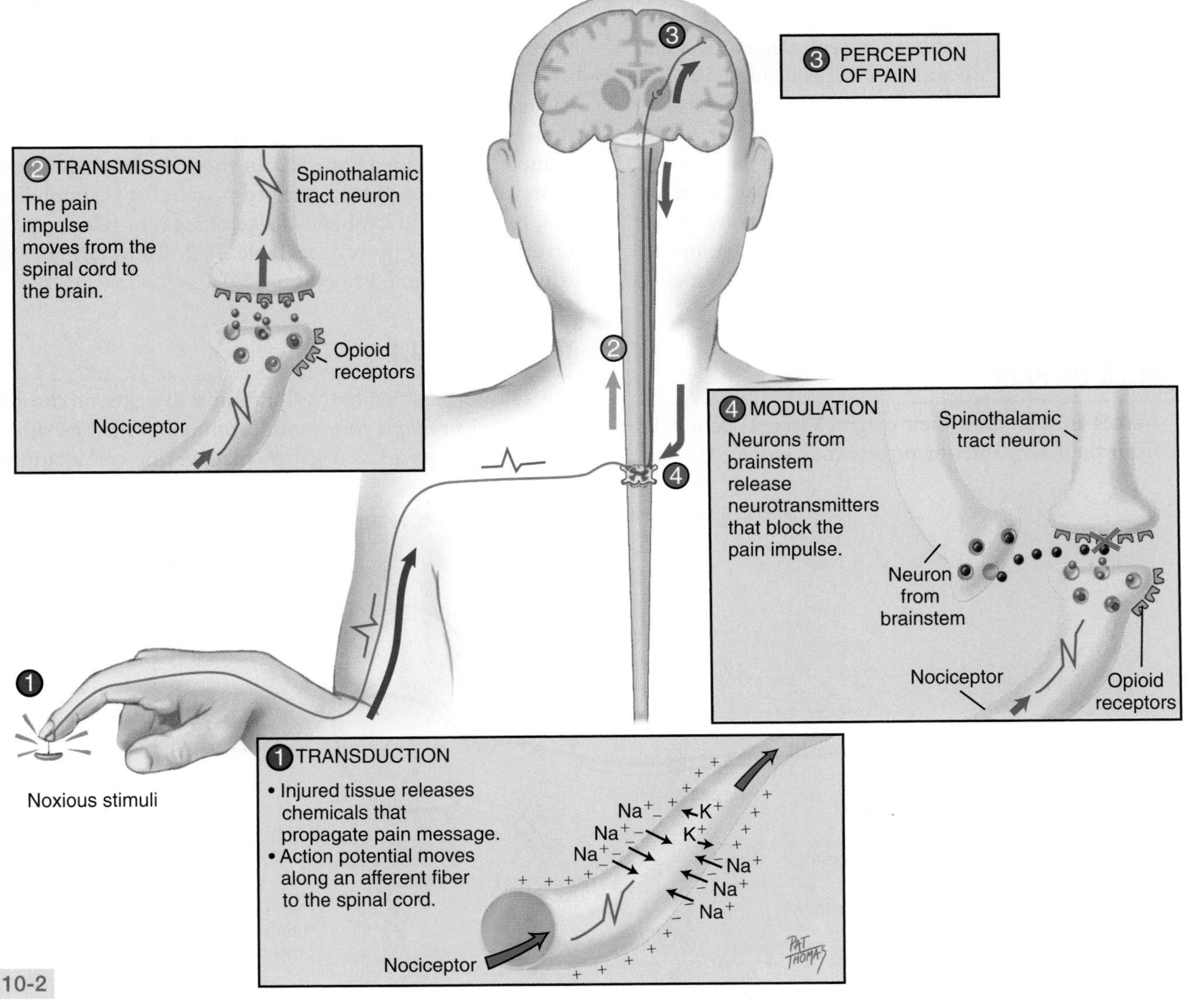

10-2

NEUROPATHIC PAIN

Neuropathic pain is pain that does not adhere to the typical and rather predictable phases in nociceptive pain. Neuropathic pain implies an abnormal processing of the pain message from an injury to the nerve fibers. It is this type of pain that is most difficult to assess and treat. Pain is often perceived long after the site of injury heals and can start 2 to 3 years after an initial injury.

We are learning that the nociceptive pattern can change into a neuropathic pattern over time when pain has been poorly controlled. Because of the constant irritation and inflammation caused by a pain stimulus, the form of the nerve cells alters, making them more sensitive to any stimulus. The constant irritation also decreases the number of opioid receptors.

Conditions that may cause neuropathy include diabetes mellitus, herpes zoster (shingles), HIV/AIDS, sciatica, trigeminal neuralgia, phantom limb pain, and chemotherapy. Further examples include CNS lesions such as stroke, multiple sclerosis, and tumor. Pain is sustained on a neurochemical level that cannot be identified by x-ray, computerized axial tomography (CAT) scan, or magnetic resonance imaging (MRI); electromyography and nerve-conduction studies are needed.[6,39]

The abnormal processing of the neuropathic pain impulse can be continued by the peripheral or central nervous system. Exact mechanisms are unclear to date. A proposed mechanism is that injury to peripheral neurons can result in spontaneous and repetitive firing of nerve fibers, almost seizurelike in activity (Fig. 10-3). Neuropathic pain may be sustained centrally in a phenomenon known as neuronal "wind-up." Within the dorsal horn of the spinal cord, neurons are thought to be transformed into a hyperexcitable state and a minimal stimulus can ultimately spiral into a much larger painful effect.

SOURCES OF PAIN

Pain sources are based on their origin. **Visceral** pain originates from the larger interior organs (i.e., kidney, stomach, intestine, gallbladder, pancreas). The pain can stem from direct injury to the organ or from stretching of the organ from tumor, ischemia, distention, or severe contraction. Examples of visceral pain include ureteral colic, acute appendicitis, ulcer pain, and cholecystitis. The pain impulse is transmitted by ascending nerve fibers along with nerve fibers of the autonomic nervous system. That is why visceral pain often presents along with autonomic responses such as vomiting, nausea, pallor, and diaphoresis.

Deep somatic pain comes from sources such as the blood vessels, joints, tendons, muscles, and bone. Injury may result from pressure, trauma, or ischemia. **Cutaneous pain** is derived from skin surface and subcutaneous tissues. The injury is superficial, with a sharp, burning sensation.

In past literature, you may have come across the term *psychogenic pain*. This term was attributed to pain with no known physical cause and assumed to have a psychiatric or emotional cause. It often was used as a derogatory label. *Psychogenic* is an obsolete term and is not accepted by the International Association for the Study of Pain. Linking pain to a mental disorder negates the person's pain report. A clinician's lack of awareness and understanding of neuropathic pain may contribute to this mislabeling.

Pain that is felt at a particular site but originates from another location is known as **referred pain.** Both sites are innervated by the same spinal nerve, and it is difficult for the brain to differentiate the point of origin. Referred pain may originate from visceral or somatic structures. Various structures maintain their same embryonic innervation. For example, an inflamed appendix in the right lower quadrant of the abdomen may have referred pain in the periumbilical area. It is useful to have knowledge of areas of referred pain for diagnostic purposes (see Table 21-2, Common Sites of Referred Abdominal Pain, on p. 559).

TYPES OF PAIN

Pain can be classified by its duration into acute or chronic categories (*chronic* is now more commonly called *persistent* because it carries a less negative, malingering connotation).

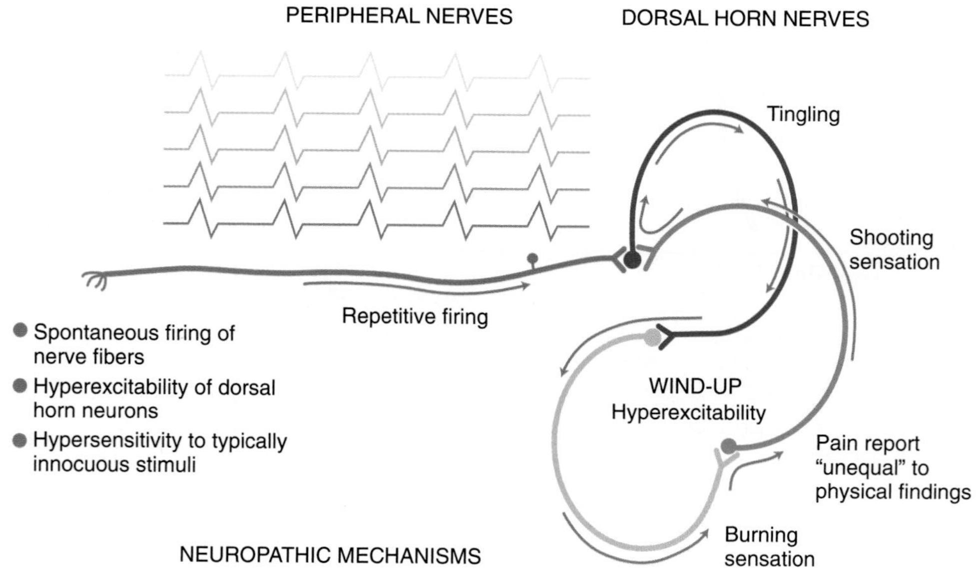

10-3 NEUROPATHIC MECHANISMS

The duration provides information on possible underlying mechanisms and treatment decisions.

Acute pain is short-term and self-limiting, often follows a predictable trajectory, and dissipates after an injury heals. Examples of acute pain include surgery, trauma, and kidney stones. Acute pain serves a self-protective purpose; acute pain warns the individual of actual or potential tissue damage. *Incident pain* is an acute type that happens predictably when certain movements take place. Examples include pain in the lower back upon standing or shoulder pain when arms are raised.

In contrast, **persisten**t (or **chronic**) **pain** is diagnosed when the pain continues for 6 months or longer. It can last 5, 15, or 20 years and beyond. Persistent pain can be further divided into *malignant* (cancer-related) and *nonmalignant.* Malignant pain often parallels the pathology created by the tumor cells. The pain is induced by tissue necrosis or stretching of an organ by the growing tumor. The pain fluctuates within the course of the disease. Chronic nonmalignant pain is often associated with musculoskeletal conditions, such as arthritis, low back pain, or fibromyalgia.

Chronic pain does not stop when the injury heals. It persists after the predicted trajectory. Chronic pain outlasts its protective purpose, and the level of pain intensity does not correspond with the physical findings. Unfortunately, many patients with chronic pain are not believed and often are labeled as malingers, attention seekers, drug seekers, and so forth. Chronic pain originates from abnormal processing of pain fibers from peripheral or central sites. Because the pain is transmitted on a cellular level, our current technology cannot reliably detect this process. Therefore the most important and reliable indicator for pain is the patient's self-report.

Finally, *breakthrough pain* is pain that starts again or escalates before the next scheduled analgesic dose. Pain breaks through when it is expected to be controlled by pain medications.[21,26]

DEVELOPMENTAL COMPETENCE

Infants

Infants have the same capacity for pain as adults. By 20 weeks' gestation, ascending fibers, neurotransmitters, and the cerebral cortex are developed and functioning to the extent that the fetus is capable of feeling pain.[29,30] However, inhibitory neurotransmitters are in insufficient supply until birth at full term. Therefore the preterm infant is rendered more sensitive to painful stimuli.

Preverbal infants are at high risk for undertreatment of pain because of persistent myths and beliefs that infants do not remember pain. In fact, new research indicates that repetitive and poorly controlled pain in infants (e.g., daily heel sticks, venipunctures) can result in lifelong adverse consequences such as neurodevelopmental problems, poor weight gain, learning disabilities, psychiatric disorders, and alcoholism.[28]

The Aging Adult

No evidence exists to suggest that older individuals perceive pain to a lesser degree or that sensitivity is diminished. Although pain is a common experience among individuals 65 years of age and older, it is *not* a normal process of aging. Pain indicates pathology or injury. Pain should never be considered something to tolerate or accept in one's later years.

Unfortunately, many clinicians and older adults wrongfully assume that pain should be expected in aging, which leads to less aggressive treatment. Older adults have additional fears about becoming dependent, undergoing invasive procedures, taking pain medications, and having a financial burden. The most common pain-producing conditions for aging adults include pathologies such as arthritis, osteoarthritis, osteoporosis, peripheral vascular disease, cancer, peripheral neuropathies, angina, and chronic constipation.

People with dementia do feel pain. The somatosensory cortex is generally unaffected by dementia of the Alzheimer type. Sensory discrimination is preserved in cognitively intact and impaired adults.[1] Because the limbic system is affected by Alzheimer disease, current research focuses on how the person interprets and reports these pain messages.[24] See further discussion on pain assessment with dementia on p. 170.

Gender Differences

Gender differences are influenced by societal expectations, hormones, and genetic makeup. Traditionally, men have been raised to be more stoic about pain and more affective or emotional displays of pain are accepted for women. Hormonal changes are found to have strong influences on pain sensitivity for women. Women are two to three times more likely to experience migraines during childbearing years, are more sensitive to pain during the premenstrual period, and are six times more likely to have fibromyalgia.[18] With recent findings from the Human Genome Project, genetic differences between both genders may account for the differences in pain perception.[19] A pain gene exists, which helps explain why some people feel more/less pain even with the same stimulus. Efforts are being made to tailor pharmacologic agents to improve pain treatment based on genetic sequencing.

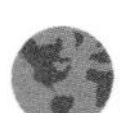

CULTURE AND GENETICS

Please review the cultural variations in Chapter 2. As clinicians, adopt the habit of asking each patient how he or she typically behaves when in pain.

Most of the research conducted on racial differences and pain has focused on the disparity in management of pain for various racial groups—comparing pain treatment for individuals of color (e.g., Blacks, Hispanics) with the standard treatment for all individuals with similar injuries or diseases. Various studies describe how Black and Hispanic patients are often prescribed and administered less analgesic therapy than whites, although the majority of these differences is quite small.[16]

SUBJECTIVE DATA

Pain is defined as an "unpleasant sensory and emotional experience associated with actual or potential tissue damage or described in terms of such damage. Pain is always subjective."[2]

The subjective report is the most reliable indicator of pain. Because pain occurs on a neurochemical level, the diagnosis of pain cannot be made exclusively on physical examination findings, although these findings can lend support.

Examiner Asks	Rationale
INITIAL PAIN ASSESSMENT	
1. **Do you have pain?** Discomfort or soreness? Ouch?	Some people will report pain only when it is severe. Try a variety of words.
2. **Where is your pain?** Tell me about *all* of the places that have pain.	Pain may be localized or occurring in *multiple* sites.
3. **When did your pain start?**	Identifies onset and duration. Chronic pain persists after injury heals; it is pain that occurs for 6 months or longer.
4. **What does your pain feel like?** • Burning, stabbing, aching • Throbbing, firelike, squeezing • Cramping, sharp, itching, tingling • Shooting, crushing, sharp, dull	Identifies quality of pain and helps differentiate between nociceptive and neuropathic pain mechanisms. Neuropathic pain is described as burning, shooting, and tingling. Nociceptive pain originating from visceral sites is described as aching if localized and cramping if poorly localized; from somatic sites, it is described as throbbing/aching.
5. **How much pain do you have now?**	Identifies intensity (refer to various intensity scales).
6. **What makes your pain better or worse?** (Include behavioral, pharmacologic, and nonpharmacologic interventions.)	Identifies alleviating and aggravating factors. Evaluates effectiveness of current treatment.
7. **How does pain limit your function or activities?** What does pain prevent you from doing?	Identifies degree of impairment and quality of life.
8. **How do you usually react when you are in pain?** How would others know you are in pain?	Nonverbal behaviors are extremely variable, especially for chronic pain syndromes. Will aid in detection and assessment.
9. **What does this pain mean to you?** Why do you think you are having pain?	Can identify myths, misconceptions, beliefs, such as "I'm getting old"; "It's a punishment from God."

PAIN ASSESSMENT TOOLS

Pain is multidimensional in scope, encompassing physical, affective, and functional domains. Various tools have been developed to capture unidimensional aspects (i.e., intensity) or multidimensional components. Select the pain assessment tool based on its purpose, time involved in administration, and the patient's ability to comprehend and complete the tool. First, teach patients how to use each tool, with practice sessions to strengthen the validity and reliability of the response. Enlarge the print when appropriate for individuals with impaired vision. The printed language should be translated to the native language of the patient. Ask the patient to rate and evaluate all of the pain sites. Some forms allow for only one number, so be sure to add to your documentation. Finally, use the pain tool consistently before and after treatment to see if the treatment has been effective.

Standardized **overall pain assessment tools** are more useful for chronic pain conditions or particularly problematic acute pain problems. A few examples include the Initial Pain Assessment, the Brief Pain Inventory, and the McGill Pain Questionnaire.

In the **Initial Pain Assessment,**[31] the clinician asks the patient to answer eight questions concerning location, duration, quality, intensity, and aggravating/relieving factors. Further, the clinician adds questions about the manner of expressing pain and the effects of pain that impair one's quality of life (Fig. 10-4).

Initial Pain Assessment Tool

Date________
Patient's Name________ Age________ Room________
Diagnosis________ Physician________
Nurse________

1. LOCATION: Patient or nurse mark drawing.

Right Left Right Left Left Right Left Right
R L L R
Left Right
Right Left Left Right

2. INTENSITY: Patient rates the pain. Scale used________
   Present:________
   Worst pain gets:________
   Best pain gets:________
   Acceptable level of pain:________
3. QUALITY: (Use patient's own words, e.g., prick, ache, burn, throb, pull, sharp.)________
4. ONSET, DURATION, VARIATION, RHYTHMS:________
5. MANNER OF EXPRESSING PAIN:________
6. WHAT RELIEVES THE PAIN?________
7. WHAT CAUSES OR INCREASES THE PAIN?________
8. EFFECTS OF PAIN: (Note decreased function, decreased quality of life.)
   Accompanying symptoms (e.g., nausea)________
   Sleep________
   Appetite________
   Physical activity________
   Relationship with others (e.g., irritability)________
   Emotions (e.g., anger, suicidal, crying)________
   Concentration________
   Other________
9. OTHER COMMENTS:________
10. PLAN:________

10-4

The Brief Pain Inventory[15] asks the patient to rate the pain within the past 24 hours using graduated scales (0-10) with respect to its impact on areas such as mood, walking ability, and sleep (Fig. 10-5). **The short-form McGill Pain Questionnaire**[33] (not illustrated) asks the patient to rank a list of descriptors in terms of their intensity and to give an overall intensity rating to his or her pain.

Pain rating scales are unidimensional and are intended to reflect pain intensity. They come in various forms. Pain rating scales can indicate a baseline intensity, track changes, and give some degree of evaluation to a treatment modality. **Numeric rating scales** ask the patient to choose a number that rates the level of pain for each painful site, with 0 being no pain and the highest anchor 10 indicating the worst pain ever

Brief Pain Inventory

Date:____/____/____ Time: ____________

Name:_______________________________________

Last First Middle initial

1. Throughout our lives, most of us have had pain from time to time (such as minor headaches, sprains, and toothaches). Have you had pain other than these everyday kinds of pain today?
   1. Yes 2. No

2. On the diagram, shade in the areas where you feel pain. Put an X on the area that hurts the most.

   Right Left Left Right

3. Please rate your pain by circling the one number that best describes your pain at its **worst** in the past 24 hours.

0	1	2	3	4	5	6	7	8	9	10
No pain										Pain as bad as you can imagine

4. Please rate your pain by circling the one number that best describes your pain at its **least** in the past 24 hours.

0	1	2	3	4	5	6	7	8	9	10
No pain										Pain as bad as you can imagine

5. Please rate your pain by circling the one number that best describes your pain on the **average**.

0	1	2	3	4	5	6	7	8	9	10
No pain										Pain as bad as you can imagine

6. Please rate your pain by circling the one number that tells how much pain you have **right now**.

0	1	2	3	4	5	6	7	8	9	10
No pain										Pain as bad as you can imagine

7. What treatments or medications are you receiving for your pain?

   ____

   ____

8. In the past 24 hours, how much **relief** have pain treatments or medications provided? Please circle the one percentage that most shows how much relief you have received.

0%	10	20	30	40	50	60	70	80	90	100%
No relief										Complete relief

9. Circle the one number that describes how, during the past 24 hours, pain has **interfered** with your:

A: General activity

0	1	2	3	4	5	6	7	8	9	10
Does not interfere										Completely interferes

B: Mood

0	1	2	3	4	5	6	7	8	9	10
Does not interfere										Completely interferes

C: Walking ability

0	1	2	3	4	5	6	7	8	9	10
Does not interfere										Completely interferes

D: Normal work (includes both work outside the home and housework)

0	1	2	3	4	5	6	7	8	9	10
Does not interfere										Completely interferes

E: Relations with other people

0	1	2	3	4	5	6	7	8	9	10
Does not interfere										Completely interferes

F: Sleep

0	1	2	3	4	5	6	7	8	9	10
Does not interfere										Completely interferes

G: Enjoyment of life

0	1	2	3	4	5	6	7	8	9	10
Does not interfere										Completely interferes

10-5

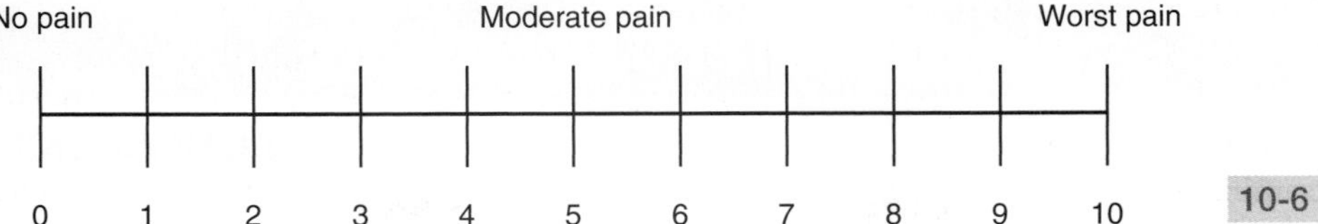

10-6

experienced. It can be administered verbally or visually along a vertical or horizontal line (Fig. 10-6).

In general, older adults find the numeric rating scale abstract and have difficulty responding, especially with a fluctuating chronic pain experience. An alternative is the simple **descriptor scale** that lists words that describe different levels of pain intensity, such as *no pain, mild pain, moderate pain,* and *severe pain*. Older adults will often respond to scales in which words are selected. Again, it is essential to teach the person how to use the scale to enhance accuracy.

INFANTS AND CHILDREN

Because infants are preverbal and incapable of self-report, pain assessment depends on behavioral and physiologic cues. Refer to the Objective Data section. It is important to underscore the understanding that infants do feel pain.

Children 2 years of age can report pain and point to its location. They cannot rate pain intensity at this developmental level. It is helpful to ask the parent or caregiver what words the child uses to report pain (e.g., boo–boo, owie). Be aware that some children will try to be "grown up and brave" and often deny having pain in the presence of a stranger or if they are fearful of receiving a "shot."

Rating scales can be introduced at 4 to 5 years of age. The Faces Pain Scale–Revised (FPS-R) has six drawings of faces that show pain intensity, from "no pain" on the left (score of 0) to "very much pain" on the right (score of 10) (Fig. 10-7). Numbers are not shown to children, but the number scoring makes this tool compatible with the widely used 0-to-10 metric for numeric pain scales.[23] This revised drawing has more realistic facial expressions with a furrowed brow and horizontal mouth stretch to rate pain. It avoids smiles or tears, so that children will not confuse pain intensity with happiness or sadness.

Similarly, the Oucher Scale[7] has six photographs of young boys' faces with different expressions of pain, ranked on a 0-to-5 scale of increasing intensity. The child is asked to point at the face that best matches his or her hurt/pain. You may use Oucher Scale variations for girls and diverse ethnic groups.

Subjective Data

Faces Pain Scale — Revised (FPS-R)

In the following instructions, say "hurt" or "pain," whichever seems right for a particular child.

"These faces show how much something can hurt. This face [point to left-most face] **shows no pain. The faces show more and more pain** [point to each from left to right] **up to this one** [point to right-most face] **— it shows very much pain. Point to the face that shows how much you hurt** [right now]."

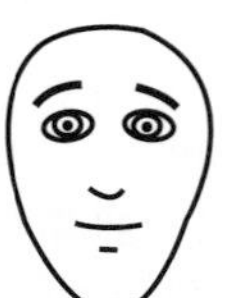 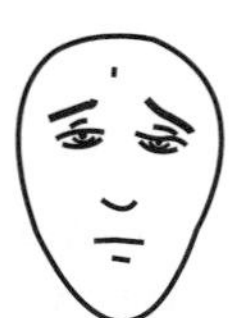 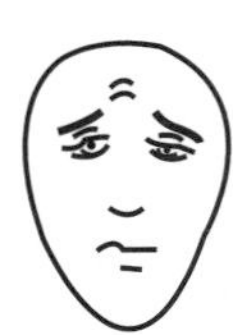 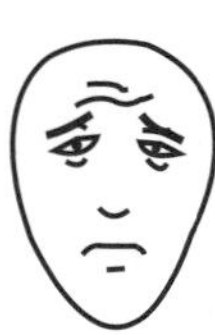 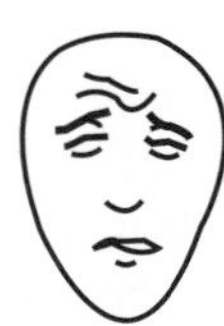 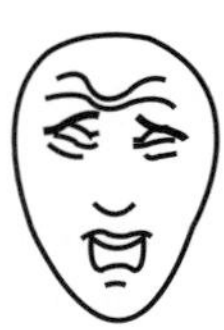

Score the chosen face 0, 2, 4, 6, 8, or 10, counting left to right, so '0' = 'no pain' and '10' = 'very much pain.' Do not use words like 'happy' and 'sad'. This scale is intended to measure how children feel inside, not how their face looks.

Sources. Hicks CL, von Baeyer CL, Spafford P, van Korlaar I, Goodenough B. The Faces Pain Scale— Revised: Toward a common metric in pediatric pain measurement. *Pain* 2001; 93: 173-183. Bieri D, Reeve R, Champion GD, Addicoat L, Ziegler J. The Faces Pain Scale for the self-assessment of the severity of pain experienced by children: Development, initial validation and preliminary investigation for ratio scale properties. *Pain* 1990; 41: 139-150.

10-7

OBJECTIVE DATA

PREPARATION

The physical examination process can help you understand the nature of the pain. Consider whether this is an acute or a chronic condition. Recall that physical findings may not always support the patient's pain complaints, particularly for chronic pain syndromes. Pain should not be discounted when objective physical evidence is not found. Based on the patient's pain report, make every effort to reduce or eliminate the pain with appropriate analgesic and nonpharmacologic intervention. According to the American Pain Society[2]:

> *In cases in which the cause of acute pain is uncertain, establishing a diagnosis is a priority, but symptomatic treatment of pain should be given while the investigation is proceeding. With occasional exceptions (e.g., the* initial *examination of the patient with an acute condition of the abdomen), it is rarely justified to defer analgesia until a diagnosis is made. In fact, a comfortable patient is better able to cooperate with diagnostic procedures. (p. 3)*

EQUIPMENT NEEDED

Tape measure to measure circumference of swollen joints or extremities
Tongue blade

Normal Range of Findings	Abnormal Findings
THE JOINTS	
Note the size and contour of the joint. Measure the circumference of the involved joint for comparison with baseline. Check active or passive range of motion (see discussion of complete technique beginning on p. 578 in Chapter 22). Joint motion normally causes no tenderness, pain, or crepitation.	Swelling, inflammation, injury, deformity, diminished range of motion, increased pain on palpation. Crepitation is an audible and palpable crunching that accompanies movement.
THE MUSCLES AND SKIN	
Inspect the skin and tissues for color, swelling, and any masses or deformity.	Bruising, lesions, open wounds, tissue damage, atrophy, bulging, change in hair distribution.
To assess for changes in sensation, ask the person to close his or her eyes. Test the person's ability to perceive sensation by breaking a tongue blade in two lengthwise. Lightly press the sharp and blunted ends on the skin in a random fashion and ask to identify it as sharp or dull (see Fig. 23-23). This test will help you identify location and extent of altered sensation.	Absent pain sensation (analgesia); increased pain sensation (hyperalgesia); or if a severe pain sensation is evoked with a stimulus that does not normally induce pain (e.g., the blunt end of the tongue blade; cotton ball; clothing) (allodynia).
THE ABDOMEN	
Observe for contour and symmetry. Palpate for muscle guarding and organ size (see discussion of complete technique beginning on p. 545 in Chapter 21). Note any areas of referred pain (see Table 21-2).	Swelling, bulging, herniation, inflammation, organ enlargement.

Table 10-1 lists physiologic changes resulting from poorly controlled pain.

NONVERBAL BEHAVIORS OF PAIN

When the individual cannot verbally communicate the pain, you can (to a limited extent) identify pain using behavioral cues. Recall that individuals react to painful stimuli with a wide variety of behaviors. Behaviors are influenced by a wide variety of factors, including the nature of the pain (acute vs. chronic), age, and cultural and gender expectations.

Acute Pain Behaviors

Because acute pain involves autonomic responses and has a protective purpose, individuals experiencing moderate to intense levels of pain *may* exhibit the following behaviors: guarding, grimacing, vocalizations such as moaning, agitation, restlessness, stillness, diaphoresis, or change in vital signs. This list of behaviors is not exhaustive because they should not be used exclusively to deny or confirm the presence of pain. For example, in a postoperative patient, pulse and blood pressure can be altered by fluid volume, medications, and blood loss.

TABLE 10-1 Physiologic Changes from Poorly Controlled Pain

Pain is not a benign symptom. Poorly controlled acute pain and chronic pain have a negative impact on physiologic systems.

Physiologic System	Acute Pain Responses
Cardiac	Tachycardia Elevated blood pressure Increased myocardial oxygen demand Increased cardiac output
Pulmonary	Hypoventilation Hypoxia Decreased cough Atelectasis
Gastrointestinal	Nausea Vomiting Ileus
Renal	Oliguria Urinary retention
Musculoskeletal	Spasm Joint stiffness
Endocrine	Increased adrenergic activity
Central nervous system	Fear Anxiety Fatigue
Immune	Impaired cellular immunity Impaired wound healing
Poorly controlled chronic pain	Depression Isolation Limited mobility and function Confusion Family distress Diminished quality of life

Persistent (Chronic) Pain Behaviors

Persons with persistent pain often live with the experience for months and years. One cannot function physiologically and go on with life in a repetitive state of behaviors such as grimacing, diaphoresis, and guarding. The person adapts over time, and clinicians cannot look for or anticipate the same acute pain behaviors to exist in order to confirm a pain diagnosis.

Chronic pain behaviors have even more variability than acute pain behaviors. Persons with chronic pain typically try to give little indication that they are in pain and therefore are at higher risk for underdetection (Fig. 10-8). Behaviors that have been associated with chronic pain include bracing, rubbing, diminished activity, sighing, and change in appetite. Whenever possible, it is best to ask the person how he or she acts or behaves when in pain. Chronic pain behaviors, such as being with other people, movement, exercise, prayer, sleeping, or inactivity, underscore the more subtle, less anticipated ways in which persons behave when they are experiencing chronic pain. Sleeping is one way persons behave in response to chronic pain in order to self-distract. Unfortunately, clinical staff may inadvertently interpret this behavior as "comfort" and do not follow up with an appropriate pharmacologic intervention.

DEVELOPMENTAL COMPETENCE

Infants

Most pain research on infants has focused on acute procedural pain. We have a limited understanding of how to assess chronic pain in the infant. At this time, no one assessment tool adequately identifies pain in the infant. Using a multidimensional approach for the whole infant is encouraged. Changes in facial activity and body movements may help assess pain. Much effort and time is spent on decoding facial expressions (e.g., taut tongue, bulging brow, closing of eye fissures), which may be difficult for the general practitioner to carry out in a busy clinical setting.

One tool that has been developed for postoperative pain in preterm and term neonates is the CRIES score developed by Krechel and Bildner.[27] It measures physiologic and behavioral indicators on a 3-point scale (Fig. 10-9).

Because the sympathetic nervous system is engaged particularly in acute episodes of pain, physiologic changes take place that may indicate the presence of pain. These include sweating, increases in blood pressure and heart rate, vomiting, nausea, and changes in oxygen saturation. However, like the adult, these physiologic changes cannot be used exclusively to confirm or deny pain because of other factors such as stress, medications, and fluid changes.

Note that these measures target acute pain. No biological markers have been identified for long-term chronic pain in infants or children. Therefore evaluate the whole individual. Look for changes in temperament, expression, and activity. If a procedure or disease process is known to induce pain in adults (e.g., circumcision, surgery, sickle cell disease, cancer), it *will* induce pain in the infant or child.

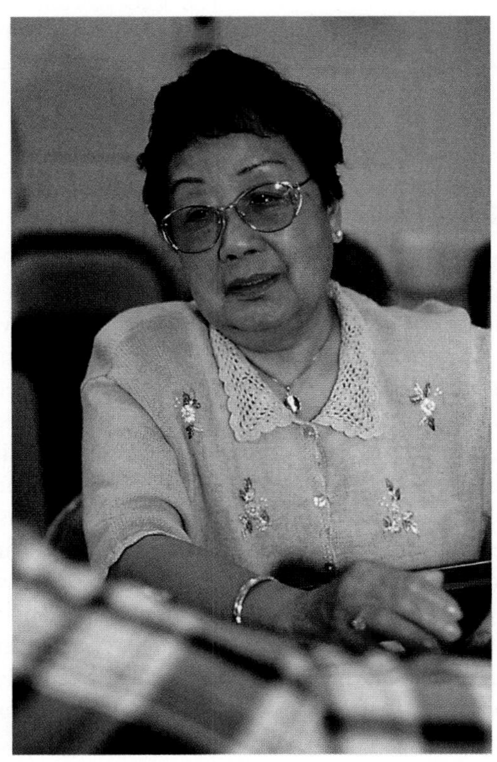

10-8

CRIES Neonatal Postoperative Pain Measurement Score

	0	1	2
Crying	No	High pitched	Inconsolable
Requires O_2 for sat $>95\%$	No	$<30\%$	$>30\%$
Increased vital signs	HR and BP $=$ or $<$ preop	HR or BP $\uparrow$ $<20\%$ of preop	HR or BP $\uparrow$ $>20\%$ of preop
Expression	None	Grimace	Grimace/grunt
Sleepless	No	Wakes at frequent intervals	Constantly awake

CODING TIPS FOR USING CRIES

Crying	The characteristic cry of pain is *high pitched.* If no cry or cry that is not high pitched, score 0. If cry is high pitched but baby is easily consoled, score 1. If cry is high pitched and baby is inconsolable, score 2.
Requires O_2 for sat $>95\%$	Look for *changes* in oxygenation. Babies experiencing pain manifest decreases in oxygenation as measured by Tco_2 or oxygen saturation. If no oxygen is required, score 0. If $<30\%$ O_2 is required, score 1. If $>30\%$ O_2 is required, score 2. (Consider other causes of changes in oxygenation, such as atelectasis, pneumothorax, over-sedation)
Increased vital signs	NOTE: Take blood presssure last as this may wake child, causing difficulty with other assessments. Use baseline preoperative parameters from a nonstressed period. Multiply baseline HR $\times$ 0.2 and then add this to baseline HR to determine the HR, which is 20% over baseline. Do likewise for BP. Use mean BP. If HR and BP are both unchanged or less than baseline, score 0. If HR or BP is increased but increase is $<20\%$ of baseline, score 1. If either one is increased $>20\%$ over baseline, score 2.
Expression	The facial expression most often associated with pain is a grimace. This may be characterized by brow lowering, eyes squeezed shut, deepening of the nasolabial furrow, open lips and mouth. If no grimace is present, score 0. If grimace alone is present, score 1. If grimace and noncry vocalization grunt are present, score 2.
Sleepless	This parameter is scored based on the infant's state during the hour preceding this recorded score. If the child has been continuously asleep, score 0. If he or she has awakened at frequent intervals, score 1. If he or she has been awake constantly, score 2.

10-9

The Aging Adult

Although pain should not be considered a "normal" part of aging, it is prevalent. When the older adult reports a history of conditions such as osteoarthritis, peripheral vascular disease, cancer, osteoporosis, angina, or chronic constipation, be alert and anticipate a pain problem. Older adults will often deny having pain for fear of dependency, further testing or invasive procedures, cost, and fear of taking pain killers or becoming a drug addict. During the interview, you must establish an empathic and caring rapport to gain trust.

When you look for behavioral cues, look at changes in functional status. Observe for changes in dressing, walking, toileting, or involvement in activities. A slowness and rigidity may develop, and fatigue may occur. Look for a sudden onset of acute confusion, which may indicate poorly controlled pain. However, you will need to rule out other competing explanations such as infection or adverse reaction from medications.

People with dementia become less able to identify and describe pain over time although pain is still present and destructive. The way people with dementia communicate pain is through their behavior. Agitation, pacing, and repetitive yelling may indicate pain and not a worsening of the dementia. People who are comfortable do not yell, cry, moan, hit, or kick. So when these behaviors occur, consider pain as a primary explanation.

When asked if they are having pain, people with dementia may say "No" when in fact they are very uncomfortable. Words have lost their meaning. Use the PAINAD scale (Fig. 10-10), which evaluates five common behaviors of breathing, vocalization, facial expression, body language, and consolability. Specific behaviors in these categories are quantified from 0 to 2, with a total score ranging from 0 to 10. This is consistent with the commonly used 0-to-10 metric on other pain tool scores. For the PAINAD, a score of 4 or more indicates a need for pain management.

Pain Assessment In Advanced Dementia (PAINAD) Scale

	0	1	2	Score
Breathing Independent of Vocalization	Normal	Occasional labored breathing, short period of hyperventilation	Noisy labored breathing, long period of hyperventilation, Cheyne-Stokes respirations	
Negative Vocalization	None	Occasional moan or groan, low level of speech with a negative or disapproving quality	Repeated troubled calling out, loud moaning or groaning, crying	
Facial Expression	Smiling or inexpressive	Sad, frightened, frown	Facial grimacing	
Body Language	Relaxed	Tense, distressed pacing, fidgeting	Rigid, fists clenched, knees pulled up, pulling or pushing away, striking out	
Consolability	No need to console	Distracted or reassured by voice or touch	Unable to console, distract or reassure	
			TOTAL	

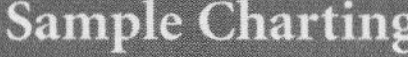
10-10

A score of 4 or greater should be reported to the RN for pain intervention

DOCUMENTATION AND CRITICAL THINKING

Sample Charting

SUBJECTIVE

Starting within the past 2 weeks, states having severe epigastric pain within a half-hour of eating greasy, fatty foods. Pain is stabbing and squeezing in nature with radiation to right shoulder blade. Rates pain as a 10 on a 0-to-10 scale. Nausea accompanies pain. Takes antacids with minimal relief. Pain diminishes after bringing knees to chest and "not moving" for a 1-hour period.

OBJECTIVE

Patient diaphoretic, grimacing, and having difficulty concentrating. Breathless during history. Arms guarding upper abdominal area. Abdomen distended. Severe tenderness noted upon light left upper quadrant and epigastric palpation. Bowel sounds hyperactive in all four quadrants.

ASSESSMENT

Acute episodic pain

Focused Assessment: Clinical Case Study 1

R.M. is a 20-year-old African-American male diagnosed with sickle cell crisis. Admitted to the emergency department.

SUBJECTIVE

Within the past 48 hours, R.M. reports increasing pain in upper and lower extremity joints and swelling of right knee. States having "stomach flu" 1 week before with periods of vomiting and diarrhea. Pain is aching and constant in nature. Rates pain as +10 on a 0-to-10 scale. Reports difficulty walking and climbing stairs. Taking ibuprofen, two tablets every 4 hours, and using ice packs with no relief.

OBJECTIVE

Requiring assistance to sit on exam table. Unable to bear weight on right leg. Affect flat, clenches jaw during position changes. Tenderness localized in elbow, wrist, finger, and knee joints. Diminished range of motion in wrists and knees (right knee 36 cm, left knee 30 cm diameter). Right knee warm and boggy to touch.

ASSESSMENT

Acute pain

Focused Assessment: Clinical Case Study 2

A.G. is an 85-year-old Irish-American female with a 20-year history of osteoarthritis.

SUBJECTIVE

A.G. reports increased pain and stiffness in her neck, arms, and lower back for the past month. Denies radiation of pain. Denies tingling or numbness in upper or lower extremities.

Having difficulty getting in and out of bathtub and dressing herself. Describes pain as aching, with good and bad days. Becomes frustrated when asked to rate her pain intensity. Replies, "I don't know what number to give; it hurts a lot, on and off." Takes acetaminophen, extra strength, two tablets, when the pain "really gets the best of me," with some degree of relief. Does not take part in "field trips" offered by assisted living facility because she "hurts too much."

OBJECTIVE

Localized tenderness noted upon palpation to C3 and C4; unable to flex neck to chest. Crepitus noted in both shoulder joints. No swelling noted. Muscle strength 1+ and equal for upper extremities. Lumbar area tender to moderate palpation. Rubs lower back frequently; limited flexion at the waist. Gait slow and unsteady. Facial expression stoic.

ASSESSMENT

Chronic pain

ABNORMAL FINDINGS

TABLE 10-2 Summary of Pain Types

Types of Pain	Etiology	Pain Descriptors	Associated Disorders	Treatment Options
Nociceptive (somatic or visceral)	Activity of nociceptors in cutaneous and deep musculoskeletal tissue in response to tissue-damaging stimuli Inflammation	**Somatic:** Dull Aching Well-localized Nocturnal **Visceral:** Deep squeezing pressure Local tenderness and referred Poorly localized	**Somatic:** Postoperative pain Bone metastases Arthritis Sports injury Mechanical back pain **Visceral:** Liver metastases Pancreatic cancer	Treat the underlying cause Nonsteroidal anti-inflammatory drug (NSAID) Opioid Muscle relaxant Corticosteroid Bisphosphonate
Neuropathic	Primary lesion (neuroma) or dysfunction in nervous system causing ectopic charges within the nervous system	Constant dull ache Burning Stabbing Vice-like Electric shock–like Numbness Tingling Allodynia Hyperalgesia Hyperpathia	Distal polyneuropathy (diabetes, HIV) Central poststroke pain Herpes zoster Trigeminal neuralgia Neuropathic back pain Complex regional pain syndrome	Tricyclic antidepressant (TCA) Anticonvulsant Antidepressant Antineuroleptic Local anesthetic Bisphosphonate Corticosteroid Opioid Interventional techniques
Cancer pain	Infiltration of lesion Nerve injury from periphery, or central nervous system	Dependent on underlying pathology	Bone metastases neuropathy	Symptom control—any of the above

Data from Miller-Saultz, D. (2008). Identifying chronic pain: Awareness important. *Nurse Practitioner* 33(9):7.

TABLE 10-3 Reflective Sympathetic Dystrophy

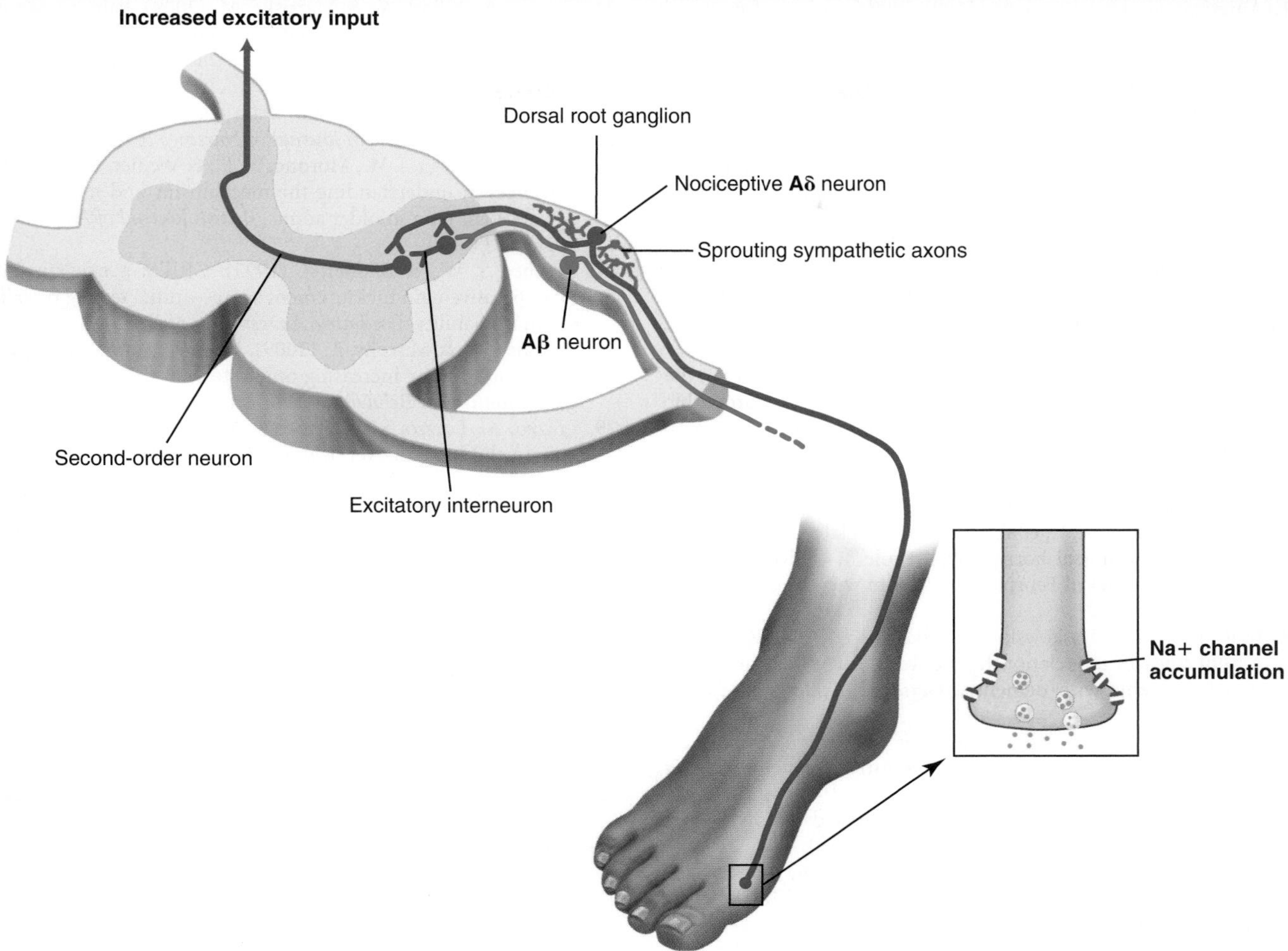

REFLEXIVE SYMPATHETIC DYSTROPHY (RSD) OR COMPLEX REGIONAL PAIN SYNDROME (CRPS)

RSD/CRPS is a chronic progressive nerve condition, characterized by burning pain, swelling, stiffness, and discoloration of the affected extremity. It affects both men and women, usually around 40 to 60 years old, and occurs weeks to months after a nerve injury (e.g., carpal tunnel syndrome, broken leg, cerebral lesions). Pathophysiology involves a complex interaction of sensory, motor, and autonomic nerves, as well as the immune system. The nerve injury may modify the usual pain pathway, causing a neuropathic "wind-up" or "short-circuit" mechanism.

A key feature is that a typically innocuous stimulus (e.g., a light brush of a cotton ball or clothing) can create a severe, intense painful response. Other subjective data include burning pain often disproportionate to the degree of injury and joint pain during movement. Objective data include swelling, disappearance of skin wrinkles, cool skin temperature, discoloration, brittle nails, and, finally, atrophic changes (pale, dry, shiny skin and muscle atrophy). Treatment is beyond the scope of this text but initially includes oral medication to decrease symptoms and physical therapy to regain limb function.

BIBLIOGRAPHY

1. American Geriatrics Society. (2009). Pharmacological management of persistent pain in older persons. *Journal of the American Geriatrics Society, 57*(8), 1331-1346.
2. American Pain Society (APS). (1992). *Principles of analgesic use in the treatment of acute and cancer pain* (3rd ed.). Glenview, IL: Author.
3. Anand, K. J. S. (1993). The applied physiology of pain. In K. J. S. Anand & R. J. McGrath (Eds.), *Pain in neonates*. Amsterdam: Elsevier.
4. Anand, K. J. S. (2000). Effects of perinatal pain and stress. *Progress in Brain Research, 122*, 117-119.
5. Anderson, K. O., Green, C. R., & Payne, R. (2009). Racial and ethnic disparities in pain: causes and consequences of unequal care. *The Journal of Pain, 10*(12), 1187-1204.
6. Balasubramanyan, S., & Smith, P. (2007). Cellular changes in the superficial dorsal horn in nerve-injury models of neuropathic pain. *Journal of Neuropathic Pain & Symptom Palliation, 2*(2), 9-42.
7. Beyer, J. E. (1983). *The Oucher: a user's manual and technical report*. Evanston, IL: Judson.
8. Bird, G., Han, J., Fu, Y., et al. (2006). Pain-related synaptic plasticity in spinal dorsal horn neurons: role of CGRP. *Molecular Pain, 2*, 31. Retrieved February 2010 from www.molecularpain.com/content/2/1/31.
9. Buffum, M. D., Miaskowski, C., Sands, L., & Brod, M. (2001). A pilot study of the relationship between discomfort and agitation in patients with dementia. *Geriatric Nursing, 22*(2), 80-85.
10. Cervero, F. (2009). Pain: friend or foe? A neurobiologic perspective—the 2008 Bonica award lecture. *Regional Anesthesia and Pain Medicine, 34*(6), 569-574.
11. Chen, Y., & Kelly, J. (2007). Reflex sympathetic dystrophy: a case of total body pain. *The Nurse Practitioner, 32*(9), 8-10.
12. Cruccu, G., & Truini, A. (2009). Tools for assessing neuropathic pain. *PLoS Medicine, 6*(4), e1000045. doi:10.1371/journal/pmed.1000045.
13. D'Arcy, Y. (2005). Field guide to pain. Part 1. Screening for pain in primary care. *The Nurse Practitioner, 30*(9), 46-48.
14. D'Arcy, Y. (2008). Pain in the older adult. *The Nurse Practitioner, 33*(3), 18-24.
15. Daut, R. L., & Cleeland, C. S. (1982). The prevalence and severity of pain in cancer. *Cancer, 50*, 1913-1918.
16. Ezenwa, M. O., Ameringer, S., Ward, S. E., et al. (2006). Racial and ethnic disparities in pain management in the United States. *Journal of Nursing Scholarship, 38*(3), 225-233.
17. Fillingim, R. B. (2000). *Sex, gender and pain*. Seattle: IASP Press.
18. Fillingim, R. B., Wallace, M. R., Herbstaman, D. M., et al. (2008). Genetic contributions to pain: a review of findings in humans. *Oral Diseases, 14*(8), 673-682.
19. Fillingim, R. B., King, C. D., Ribeiro-Dasilva, M. C., et al. (2009). Sex, gender, and pain: a review of recent clinical and experimental findings. *The Journal of Pain, 10*(5), 447-485.
20. Flaherty, E. (2008). Using pain-rating scales with older adults. *The American Journal of Nursing, 108*(6), 40-48.
21. Helms, J. E., & Barone, C. P. (2008). Physiology and treatment of pain. *Critical Care Nurse, 28*(6), 38-50.
22. Herr, K., Coyne, P. J., Tonya, K., et al. (2006). Pain assessment in the nonverbal patient: position statement with clinical practice recommendations. *Pain Management Nursing, 7*(2), 44-52.
23. Hicks, C. L., von Baeyer, C. L., Spafford, P., et al. (2001). The Faces pain scale—revised: toward a common metric in pediatric pain measurement. *Pain, 93*, 173-183.
24. Horgas, A., Elliott, A., & Marsiske, M. (2009). Pain assessment in persons with dementia: relationship between self-report and behavioral observation. *Journal of the American Geriatrics Society, 57*(1), 126-132.
25. Horgas, A., & Miller, L. (2008). Pain assessment in people with dementia. *The American Journal of Nursing, 108*(7), 62-71.
26. Karp, J. F., Shega, J. W., Morone, N. E., & Weiner, D. K. (2008). Advances in understanding the mechanisms and management of persistent pain in older adults. *British Journal of Anaesthesia, 101*(1), 111-120.
27. Krechel, S. W., & Bildner, J. (1995). CRIES: a new neonatal postoperative pain measurement score—initial testing of validity and reliability. *Paediatric Anaesthesia, 5*(1), 53-61.
28. LaPrairie, J., & Murphy, A. (2009). Neonatal injury alters adult pain sensitivity by increasing opioid tone in the periaqueductal gray. *Frontiers in Behavioral Neuroscience, 3*, 31.
29. Loizzo, A., Loizzo, S., & Capasso, A. (2009). Neurobiology of pain in children: an overview. *The Open Biochemistry Journal, 3*, 18-25.
30. Lowery, C. L., Hardman, M. P., Manning, N., et al. (2007). Neurodevelopmental changes of fetal pain. *Seminars in Perinatology, 31*, 275-282.
31. McCaffery, M., & Pasero, C. (1999). *Pain: clinical manual* (2nd ed.). St. Louis: Mosby.
32. McCarberg, B., & D'Arcy, Y. (2007). Target pain with topical peripheral analgesics. *The Nurse Practitioner, 32*(7), 44-49.
33. Melzack, R. (1987). The short-form McGill Pain Questionnaire. *Pain, 30*, 191-197.
34. Mendell, J. R., & Sahenk, Z. (2003). Painful sensory neuropathy. *The New England Journal of Medicine, 348*(13), 1243-1255.
35. Miller-Saultz, D. (2008). Identifying chronic pain: awareness important. *The Nurse Practitioner, 33*(9), 6-9.
36. Mogil, J. S. (2002). Pain genetics: pre- and post-genomic findings. *International Association for the Study of Pain Technical Corner Newsletter, 2*, 3-6.
37. Polomano, R. C., & Farrar, J. T. (2006). Pain and neuropathy in cancer survivors. *The American Journal of Nursing, 106*(3), 39-47.
38. Rosenblum, A., Marsch, L., Herman, J., & Portenoy, R. (2008). Opioids and the treatment of chronic pain: controversies, current status, and future directions. *Experimental and Clinical Psychopharmacology, 16*(5), 405-416.
39. Schestatsky, P., & Nascimento, O. J. (2009). What do general neurologists need to know about neuropathic pain? *Arquivos de Neuro-psiquiatria, 67*(3-A), 741-749.
40. Solano, J. P., Gomes, B., & Higginson, I. J. (2006). A comparison of symptom prevalence in far advanced cancer, AIDS, heart disease, chronic obstructive pulmonary disease and renal disease. *Journal of Pain and Symptom Management, 31*(1), 58-69.
41. Spagrud, L. J., Piira, T., & von Baeyer, C. L. (2003). Children's self-report of pain intensity. *The American Journal of Nursing, 103*(12), 62-64.
42. Turk, D. C., & Melzack, R. (Eds.). (1992). *Handbook of pain assessment*. New York: Guilford Press.
43. Vreeling, F. W., Houx, P. J., Jolles, J., & Verhey, F. R. (1995). Primitive reflexes in Alzheimer's disease and vascular dementia. *Journal of Geriatric Psychiatry and Neurology, 8*(2), 111-117.

Website of Interest

International Association for the Study of Pain (IASP): www.IASP.org

11

Nutritional Assessment

evolve WEBSITE

http://evolve.elsevier.com/Jarvis/

- Animations
- Audio Key Points
- Bedside Assessment Summary Checklist
- Case Study
  Irregular Pulse
  Stomach Pains
- Health Promotion Guide
  Type 2 Diabetes Mellitus
- NCLEX Review Questions
- Physical Examination Summary Checklist

OUTLINE

Structure and Function, 175

Defining Nutritional Status
Dietary Practices of Selected Cultural Groups
Purposes and Components of Nutritional Assessment

Subjective Data, 182

Health History Questions

Objective Data, 186

Clinical Signs
Anthropometric Measures
Laboratory Studies
Serial Assessment

Documentation and Critical Thinking, 195

Abnormal Findings, 196

Abnormal Findings for Advanced Practice, 200

STRUCTURE AND FUNCTION

DEFINING NUTRITIONAL STATUS

Nutritional status refers to the degree of balance between nutrient intake and nutrient requirements. This balance is affected by many factors, including physiologic, psychosocial, developmental, cultural, and economic.

Optimal nutritional status is achieved when sufficient nutrients are consumed to support day-to-day body needs and any increased metabolic demands due to growth, pregnancy, or illness. Persons having optimal nutritional status are more active, have fewer physical illnesses, and live longer than persons who are malnourished.

Undernutrition occurs when nutritional reserves are depleted and/or when nutrient intake is inadequate to meet day-to-day needs or added metabolic demands. Vulnerable groups—infants, children, pregnant women, recent immigrants, persons with low incomes, hospitalized people, and aging adults—are at risk for impaired growth and development, lowered resistance to infection and disease, delayed wound healing, longer hospital stays, and higher health care costs.

Overnutrition is caused by the consumption of nutrients—especially calories, sodium, and fat—in excess of body needs. A major nutritional problem today, overnutrition can lead to obesity and is a risk factor for heart disease, type 2 diabetes, hypertension, stroke, gallbladder disease, sleep apnea, certain cancers, and osteoarthritis.[24]

An estimated 17% of children and adolescents (ages 2 to 19 years) are overweight, and 66% of adults in the United States are either overweight or obese.[7,27] For children, overweight is a body mass index (BMI) equal to or greater than the 95th percentile based on age- and gender-specific BMI charts. For adults, overweight is a BMI of 25 or greater and obesity is a BMI of 30 or greater.[7] Although obesity rates in both children and adults seem to be leveling off after several years of increases, these data are alarming. Being overweight during childhood and adolescence is associated with increased risk for becoming overweight during adulthood.[24]

 DEVELOPMENTAL COMPETENCE

Infants and Children

The time from birth to 4 months of age is the most rapid period of growth in the life cycle. Although infants lose weight during the first few days of life, they usually regain birth weight by the 7th to 10th day after birth. Thereafter, infants double their birth weight by 4 months and triple it by 1 year of age. The number of pounds gained during the second year approximates the birth weight.

Breastfeeding is recommended for full-term infants for the 1st year of life because breast milk is ideally formulated to promote normal infant growth and development and natural immunity. Other advantages of breastfeeding are (1) fewer food allergies and intolerances, (2) reduced likelihood of overfeeding, (3) less cost than commercial infant formulas, and (4) increased mother-infant interaction time. Because cow's milk may cause gastrointestinal and kidney problems and is a poor source of iron and vitamins C and E, it is not recommended for infants until 1 year of age. Although relatively few contraindications to breastfeeding exist, women who are human immunodeficiency virus (HIV) positive should not breastfeed because HIV can be transmitted through breast milk.

Infants increase their length by 50% during the first year of life and double it by 4 years of age. Brain size also increases very rapidly during infancy and childhood. By age 2 years, the brain has reached 50% of its adult size; by age 4, 75%; and by age 8, 100%. For this reason, infants and children younger than 2 years should not drink skim or low-fat milk or be placed on low-fat diets—fat (calories and essential fatty acids) is required for proper growth and central nervous system development.

Adolescence

After a period of slow growth in late childhood, adolescence is characterized by a rapid physical growth and endocrine and hormonal changes. Caloric and protein requirements increase to meet this demand, and because of bone growth and increasing muscle mass (and, in girls, the onset of menarche), calcium and iron requirements also increase. Typically, these increased requirements cannot be met by three meals per day; therefore nutritious snacks play an important role in achieving adequate nutrient intake. The following are some factors to consider when working with adolescents to select healthier food choices: skipped meals, excessive fast food and sweetened beverage consumption, limited fruit and vegetable intake, peer pressure, alternative dietary patterns, eating disorders, hectic schedules, and possible experimentation with drugs and alcohol.

In general, boys grow taller and have less body fat than girls. The percent of body fat increases in females to about 25% and decreases in males (replaced by muscle mass) to about 12%. Typically, girls double their body weight between the ages of 8 and 14 years; boys double their body weight between the ages of 10 and 17 years.

Pregnancy and Lactation

To support the synthesis of maternal and fetal tissues, sufficient calories, protein, vitamins, and minerals must be consumed. In particular, iron, folate, and zinc are essential for fetal growth, and vitamin and mineral supplements are often required. The National Academy of Sciences (NAS) recommends a weight gain of 25 to 35 lb for women of normal weight, 28 to 40 lb for underweight women, 15 to 25 lb for overweight women, and 11 to 20 lb for obese women, a new weight gain category. See Appendix F on the *Evolve* website for increased requirements of pregnancy and lactation. Appendix G on the *Evolve* website gives recommended weight gain guidelines based on body mass index and illustrates curves of desirable weight gain during pregnancy, as recommended by the Subcommittee on Nutritional Status and Weight Gain During Pregnancy.[23]

Adulthood

During adulthood, growth and nutrient needs stabilize. Most adults are in relatively good health. However, lifestyle factors such as cigarette smoking, stress, lack of exercise, excessive alcohol intake, and diets high in saturated fat, cholesterol, salt, and sugar and low in fiber can be factors in the development of hypertension, obesity, atherosclerosis, cancer, osteoporosis, and diabetes mellitus. The adult years, therefore, are an important time for education, to preserve health and to prevent or delay the onset of chronic disease.

The Aging Adult

Older adults have increased risk for undernutrition or overnutrition. Poor physical or mental health, social isolation, alcoholism, limited functional ability, poverty, and polypharmacy are the major risk factors for malnutrition in older adults.[30]

Normal physiologic changes in aging adults that directly affect nutritional status include poor dentition, decreased visual acuity, decreased saliva production, slowed gastrointestinal motility, decreased gastrointestinal absorption, and diminished olfactory and taste sensitivity. Important nutritional features of the older years are a decrease in energy requirements due to loss of lean body mass (the most metabolically active tissue) and an increase in fat mass. Because protein and vitamin and mineral needs remain the same or increase (e.g., vitamin D and calcium), nutrient-dense food choices (e.g., milk, eggs, cheese, and peanut butter) are important to offset lower energy/calorie needs.

Socioeconomic conditions frequently affect the nutritional status of the aging adult. The decline of extended families and increased mobility of families reduce available support systems. Facilities for meal preparation and eating, transportation to grocery stores, physical limitations, income, and social isolation are frequent problems that interfere with acquiring a balanced diet. Medications must also be considered, because aging adults frequently take multiple medications that have a potential for interaction with nutrients and with one another.

CULTURE AND GENETICS

Because foods and eating customs are culturally distinct, each person has a unique cultural heritage that may affect nutritional status. Immigrants commonly maintain traditional eating customs long after the language and manner of dress of an adopted country become routine (especially for holidays and observance of religious customs). Occupation, class, religion, gender, and health awareness also have a great bearing on eating customs. Within the past decade, hundreds of thousands of individuals from Mexico, the Caribbean, Central and South America, Asia, Africa, and the Middle East have immigrated to the United States. Their food habits not only change to accommodate their new cultures but also influence their adoptive country. The popularity of tortillas, salsa, plantains, tofu, pita bread, hummus, and curry is just one example of these influences on American eating habits (Fig. 11-1).

Newly arriving immigrants may be at nutritional risk for a variety of reasons. They frequently come from countries with limited food supplies caused by poverty, poor sanitation, war, or political strife. General undernutrition, hypertension, diarrhea, lactose intolerance, osteomalacia (soft bones), scurvy, and dental caries are among the more common nutrition-related problems of new immigrants from developing countries.

When immigrants arrive in the United States, other factors contribute to their nutritional problems:

- They are in a new country with a completely new language, culture, and society.
- They are faced with unfamiliar foods, food storage, food preparation, and food-buying habits.
- Many familiar foods are difficult or impossible to obtain.
- Low income may also limit their access to familiar foods.

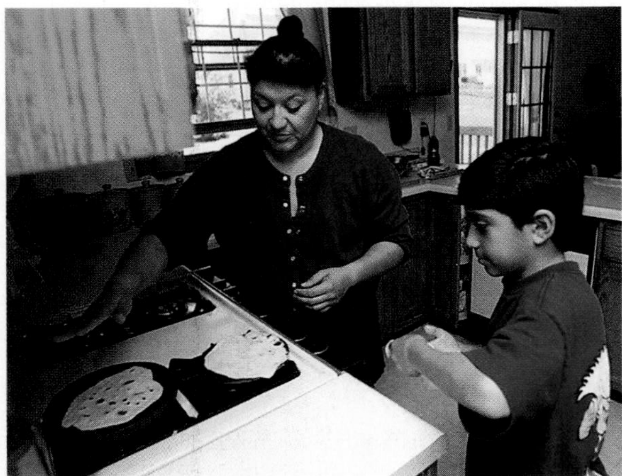

11-1

When traditional food habits are disrupted by a new culture, borderline deficiencies or adverse nutritional consequences may result. As an example, Hispanic immigrants to the United States have increased risk of becoming overweight and obese as they adapt to a diet in the United States that is higher in saturated fats and calories.[2]

Cultural heritage also plays a role in nutrient needs. For example, studies have shown that Black women have lower hemoglobin levels than white women independent of iron intake and that their risk for osteoporosis is significantly less despite lower overall calcium intake. Or, cultural values may conflict with optimum nutrition (e.g., many cultures worldwide consider obesity an indication of beauty, affluence, and well-being).

Because eating patterns and customs are changing rapidly in all countries, what are considered customs today may not be considered traditional in a few years. The best way to learn about the eating patterns of a people is to talk with them, eat with them, and ask about their dietary customs. It is important to keep in mind that recent immigrant groups, such as Southeast Asians, are often shorter and weigh less than their Western counterparts, so American standard tables of weight for age, height for age, and weight for height may not work to evaluate growth and development of immigrant children. At present, no reliable standards to evaluate every immigrant group exist.

The cultural factors to consider are the cultural definition of food, frequency and number of meals eaten away from home, form and content of ceremonial meals, amount and types of foods eaten, and regularity of food consumption. The 24-hour dietary recalls or 3-day food records used traditionally for assessment may be inadequate when dealing with people from culturally diverse backgrounds. Standard dietary handbooks may not provide culture-specific diet information because nutritional content and exchange tables are generally based on Western diets. Another source of error may be cultural patterns of eating. For example, many low-income ethnic groups eat sparingly or moderately during the week (i.e., simple rice or bean dishes), whereas weekend meals are markedly more elaborate (i.e., meats, fruits, vegetables, and sweets are added).

Although you may assume that the term "food" is a universal concept, you should have the person clarify what is meant by the term. For example, Latino groups do not consider chili peppers—an important source of vitamins A and C—to be food and thus fail to list them as vegetables on daily food records. Among Vietnamese refugees, the dietary intake of calcium may appear inadequate, particularly with the low consumption of dairy products. But daily soups prepared by soaking bones in acidified broth or pickled or sweet-and-sour meats such as pork ribs (vinegar leaches calcium from the bones and makes it available to the body) are commonly consumed, thus providing adequate quantities of calcium to meet daily requirements. Tofu is also a good source of calcium if calcium salts are used to precipitate the curd. For Mexican Americans, tortillas prepared from corn treated with lime water significantly increase dietary calcium. In Middle Eastern countries, yogurt and feta cheese are the major dietary sources of calcium since milk is not commonly consumed by adults. The reason for this is lactose intolerance, a condition found in many African Americans, American Indians, and Asian Americans.

Food itself is only one part of eating. In some cultures, social contacts during meals are restricted to members of the immediate or extended family. For example, in some Middle Eastern cultures, men and women eat meals separately or women may be permitted to eat with their husbands but not with other males. Among some Hispanic groups, the male breadwinner is served first, then women and children. Etiquette during meals, the use of hands, type of eating utensils (e.g., chopsticks, special flatware), and protocols governing the order in which foods are consumed during a meal all vary cross-culturally.

Dietary Practices of Selected Cultural Groups

It is necessary to avoid **cultural stereotyping,** the tendency to view individuals of common cultural backgrounds similarly and according to a preconceived notion of how they "ought" to behave. For example, despite widely held stereotypes, we know that some Chinese do not like rice, some Italians dislike spaghetti, some Irish dislike corned beef and cabbage, and so forth. Aggregate dietary preferences among people from certain cultural groups, however, can be described (e.g., characteristic ethnic dishes, methods of food preparation). Refer to nutrition texts on the topic for detailed information about culture-specific diets and the nutritional value of ethnic foods.

Cultural food preferences are often interrelated with religious dietary beliefs and practices. Many religions use foods as symbols in celebrations and rituals. Knowing the person's religious practices related to food enables you to suggest improvements or modifications that do not conflict with dietary laws. Table 11-1 summarizes dietary practices for selected religious groups.

Other issues are fasting and other religious observations that may limit a person's food or liquid intake during specified times (e.g., many Catholics fast and abstain from meat on Ash Wednesday and the Fridays of Lent; Muslims fast from dawn to sunset during the month of Ramadan in the Islamic calendar and eat only twice a day—before dawn and after sunset; Jews observe a 24-hour fast on Yom Kippur).

Kosher is the term that refers to the dietary laws of observant Jews; not mixing milk and meat products at the same meal and not eating pork and pork products are examples of the many practices within the system. *Halal* is the term that refers to the Islamic dietary laws (here, too, the prohibition of pork is one of many dietary practices).

TABLE 11-1 Religious Dietary Practices

Religious Group	Food Restrictions
Buddhism	All meat
Catholicism	Meat by some denominations on Ash Wednesday, Good Friday, and other holy days Alcoholic beverages by some denominations
Hinduism	Beef, pork, and some fowl Alcohol Garlic and onions by some Red-colored foods (e.g., tomatoes) by some
Islam	All pork and pork products Meat not slaughtered according to ritual Alcoholic beverages and alcohol products (e.g., vanilla extract), coffee, and tea Food and beverages before sunset during Ramadan
Mormon	Alcoholic beverages Caffeinated beverages (e.g., coffee, tea, sodas) and medicines containing caffeine, stimulants, or alcohol (e.g., Anacin, NoDoz, Nyquil) Food and beverages on first Sunday of each month
Orthodox Judaism	All pork and pork products Meat not slaughtered according to ritual All shellfish (e.g., crab, lobster, shrimp, oysters) Dairy products and meat at the same meal Leavened bread and cake during Passover Food and beverages on Yom Kippur
Seventh-Day Adventist	All pork and pork products Shellfish Meat, dairy products, and eggs by some Alcoholic beverages, coffee, and tea Highly seasoned foods

PURPOSES AND COMPONENTS OF NUTRITIONAL ASSESSMENT

Nutritional assessment techniques are noninvasive, inexpensive, and easy to perform. The purposes of nutritional assessment are to (1) identify individuals who are malnourished or are at risk for developing malnutrition, (2) provide data for designing a nutrition plan of care that will prevent or minimize the development of malnutrition, and (3) establish baseline data for evaluating the efficacy of nutritional care.

Nutrition screening, the first step in assessing nutritional status, is required for all patients in all health care settings within 24 hours of admission.[21] Based on easily obtained data, nutrition screening is a quick and easy way to identify individuals at nutrition risk, such as those with weight loss,

TABLE 11-2 Malnutrition Screening Tool (MST)

Have you lost weight recently without trying?	
No	0
Unsure	2
If yes, how much weight (in kilograms) have you lost?	
1-5	1
6-10	2
11-15	3
>15	4
Unsure	2
Have you been eating poorly because of a decreased appetite?	
No	0
Yes	1
Total	

Score of 2 or more = patient at risk for malnutrition.

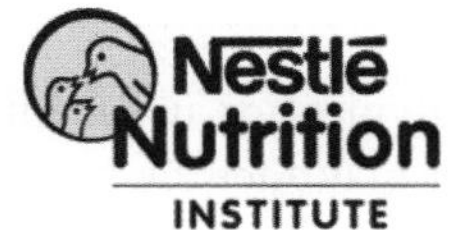

Mini Nutritional Assessment
MNA®

Last name: First name: Sex: Date:

Age: Weight, kg: Height, cm: I.D. number:

Complete the screen by filling in the boxes with the appropriate numbers. Total the numbers for the final screening score.

Screening

A Has food intake declined over the past 3 months due to loss of appetite, digestive problems, chewing or swallowing difficulties?

0 = severe decrease in food intake
1 = moderate decrease in food intake
2 = no decrease in food intake ☐

B Weight loss during the last 3 months

0 = weight loss greater than 3 kg (6.6 lbs)
1 = does not know
2 = weight loss between 1 and 3 kg (2.2 and 6.6 lbs)
3 = no weight loss ☐

C Mobility

0 = bed or chair bound
1 = able to get out of bed / chair but does not go out
2 = goes out ☐

D Has suffered psychological stress or acute disease in the past 3 months?

0 = yes 2 = no ☐

E Neuropsychological problems

0 = severe dementia or depression
1 = mild dementia
2 = no psychological problems ☐

F1 Body Mass Index (BMI) (weight in kg) / (height in m^2)

0 = BMI less than 19
1 = BMI 19 to less than 21
2 = BMI 21 to less than 23
3 = BMI 23 or greater ☐

IF BMI IS NOT AVAILABLE, REPLACE QUESTION F1 WITH QUESTION F2.
DO NOT ANSWER QUESTION F2 IF QUESTION F1 IS ALREADY COMPLETED.

F2 Calf circumference (CC) in cm

0 = CC less than 31
3 = CC 31 or greater ☐

Screening score
(max. 14 points) ☐☐

12-14 points: Normal nutritional status
8-11 points: At risk of malnutrition
0-7 points: Malnourished

For a more in-depth assessment, complete the full MNA® which is available at www.mna-elderly.com

Ref. Vellas B, Villars H, Abellan G, et al. *Overview of the MNA® - Its History and Challenges.* J Nutr Health Aging 2006;10:456-465.

Rubenstein LZ, Harker JO, Salva A, Guigoz Y, Vellas B. *Screening for Undernutrition in Geriatric Practice: Developing the Short-Form Mini Nutritional Assessment (MNA-SF).* J. Geront 2001;56A: M366-377.

Guigoz Y. The Mini-Nutritional Assessment (MNA®) Review of the Literature - What does it tell us? J Nutr Health Aging 2006; 10:466-487.

For more information: www.mna-elderly.com

11-2

inadequate food intake, or recent illness. Parameters used for nutrition screening typically include weight and weight history, conditions associated with increased nutritional risk, diet information, and routine laboratory data. A variety of valid tools are available for screening different populations. For example, the Malnutrition Screening Tool[12] (Table 11-2) was validated for use in adult acute care patients and the Mini Nutritional Assessment (MNA®) (Fig. 11-2) was designed and validated for use in older adults in long-term care and community settings.[36]

Individuals identified at nutritional risk during screening should undergo a **comprehensive nutritional assessment,** which includes dietary history and clinical information, physical examination for clinical signs, anthropometric measures, and laboratory tests. The skills needed to collect the clinical and dietary history and to perform the physical examination are described in the Subjective Data and Objective Data sections that follow. Table 11-3 is an example of a Subjective Global Assessment form for compiling comprehensive nutritional assessment data.

Various methods for collecting current dietary intake information are available—24-hour recall, food frequency questionnaire, and food diary. During hospitalization, documentation of nutritional intake is achieved through calorie counts of nutrients consumed and/or infused.

The easiest and most popular method for obtaining information about dietary intake is the **24-hour recall.** The individual or family member completes a questionnaire or is interviewed and asked to recall everything eaten within the last 24 hours. An advantage of the 24-hour recall is that it can elicit specific information about dietary intake over a specific period of time. However, there are several significant sources of error: (1) the individual or family member may not be able to recall the type or amount of food eaten; (2) intake within the last 24 hours may be atypical of usual intake; (3) the individual or family member may alter the truth for a variety of reasons; and (4) snack items and use of gravies, sauces, and condiments may be underreported.

To counter some of the difficulties inherent in the 24-hour recall method, you can use a **food frequency questionnaire.** With this tool, information is collected on how many times per day, week, or month the individual eats particular foods, providing an estimate of usual intake. Drawbacks to the use of the food frequency questionnaire are (1) it does not always quantify amount of intake and (2) like the 24-hour recall, it relies on the individual's or family member's memory for how often a food was eaten.

Food diaries or records ask the individual or family member to write down everything consumed for a certain period of time. Three days—two weekdays and one weekend day—are customarily used. A food diary is most complete and accurate if you teach the individual to record information immediately after eating. Potential problems with the food diary include (1) noncompliance, (2) inaccurate recording, (3) atypical intake on the recording days, and (4) conscious alteration of diet during the recording period.

Direct observation of the feeding and eating process can detect problems not readily identified through standard

TABLE 11-3 Features of Subjective Global Assessment (SGA)

(Select appropriate category with a checkmark, or enter numerical value where indicated by "#".)

A. HISTORY

1. Weight change
   Overall loss in past 6 mos: amount = # ________ kg; % loss = # ________
   Change in past 2 wks: ____ increase, ____ no change, ____ decrease
2. Dietary intake change (relative to normal)
   ____ No change
   ____ Change ____ duration = # ________ weeks
   ____ Type: ____ suboptimal solid diet ____ full liquid diet ____ hypocaloric liquids ____ starvation
3. Gastrointestinal symptoms (that persisted for >2 wks)
   ____ None ____ Nausea ____ Vomiting
   ____ Diarrhea ____ Anorexia
4. Functional capacity
   ____ No dysfunction (e.g., full capacity)
   ____ Dysfunction ____ duration = # ________ wks
   ____ Type: ____ working suboptimally ____ ambulatory ____ bedridden
5. Disease and its relation to nutritional requirements
   Primary diagnosis (specify)
   Metabolic demand (stress): ____ no stress ____ low stress ____ moderate stress ____ high stress

B. PHYSICAL

(for each trait, specify 0 = normal, 1+ = mild, 2+ = moderate, 3+ = severe)
____ loss of subcutaneous fat (triceps, chest)
____ muscle wasting (quadriceps, deltoids)
____ ankle edema
____ sacral edema
____ ascites

C. SGA RATING

(select one)
____ A = Well nourished
____ B = Moderately malnourished (or suspected of being malnourished)
____ C = Severely malnourished

nutrition interviews. For example, observing the typical feeding techniques used by a parent or caregiver and the interaction between the individual and caregiver can help when assessing failure to thrive in children or unintentional weight loss in older adults.

MyPyramid, Dietary Guidelines, and the Daily Reference Intakes (DRIs) are three guides commonly used to determine an adequate diet. MyPyramid and Dietary Guidelines were released in 2005 (Fig. 11-3 and Table 11-4). Please access the website at www.mypyramid.gov for additional information

TABLE 11-4 Summary of 2010 Dietary Guidelines

1. Control total calorie intake to manage body weight.
2. Increase physical activity and reduce time spent in sedentary behaviors.
3. Consume less than 2300 mg/day of sodium.
4. Consume less than 10% of calories from saturated fatty acids; replace with monounsaturated and polyunsaturated fatty acids.
5. Consume less than 300 mg/day of cholesterol.
6. Consume at least half of all grains as whole grains.
7. Increase vegetable and fruit intake.
8. Reduce calories from solid fats and added sugars.
9. Increase intake of fat-free or low-fat milk/milk products.
10. Choose foods with potassium, fiber, calcium, and vitamin D, including vegetables, fruits, whole grains, and milk/milk products.
11. Choose a variety of protein foods, including seafood, lean meat, poultry, eggs, beans, peas, soy products, and unsalted nuts and seeds.
12. If alcohol is consumed, do so in moderation.

From U.S. Department of Agriculture and U.S. Department of Health and Human Services. (2011). *Dietary guidelines for Americans, 2010*. Washington, DC: USDA and USDHHS. www.dietaryguidelines.gov.

A

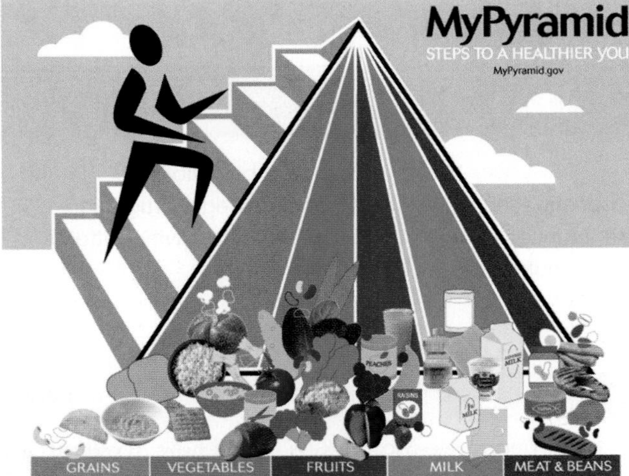

GRAINS Make half your grains whole	VEGETABLES Vary your veggies	FRUITS Focus on fruits	MILK Get your calcium-rich foods	MEAT & BEANS Go lean with protein
Eat at least 3 oz. of whole-grain cereals, breads, crackers, rice, or pasta every day 1 oz. is about 1 slice of bread, about 1 cup of breakfast cereal, or ½ cup of cooked rice, cereal, or pasta	Eat more dark-green veggies like broccoli, spinach, and other dark leafy greens Eat more orange vegetables like carrots and sweet potatoes Eat more dry beans and peas like pinto beans, kidney beans, and lentils	Eat a variety of fruit Choose fresh, frozen, canned, or dried fruit Go easy on fruit juices	Go low-fat or fat-free when you choose milk, yogurt, and other milk products If you don't or can't consume milk, choose lactose-free products or other calcium sources such as fortified foods and beverages	Choose low-fat or lean meats and poultry Bake it, broil it, or grill it Vary your protein routine – choose more fish, beans, peas, nuts, and seeds
For a 2,000-calorie diet, you need the amounts below from each food group. To find the amounts that are right for you, go to MyPyramid.gov.				
Eat 6 oz. every day	Eat 2½ cups every day	Eat 2 cups every day	Get 3 cups every day; for kids aged 2 to 8, it's 2	Eat 5½ oz. every day

Find your balance between food and physical activity

- Be sure to stay within your daily calorie needs.
- Be physically active for at least 30 minutes most days of the week.
- About 60 minutes a day of physical activity may be needed to prevent weight gain.
- For sustaining weight loss, at least 60 to 90 minutes a day of physical activity may be required.
- Children and teenagers should be physically active for 60 minutes every day, or most days.

Know the limits on fats, sugars, and salt (sodium)

- Make most of your fat sources from fish, nuts, and vegetable oils.
- Limit solid fats like butter, stick margarine, shortening, and lard, as well as foods that contain these.
- Check the Nutrition Facts label to keep saturated fats, *trans* fats, and sodium low.
- Choose food and beverages low in added sugars. Added sugars contribute calories with few, if any, nutrients.

B

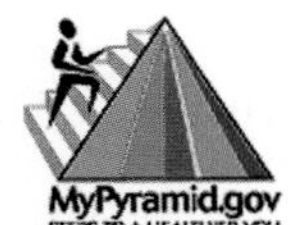

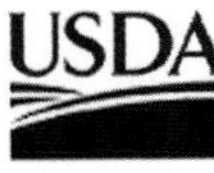

11-3, A & B

MyPyramid has been replaced by MyPlate (www.choosemyplate.gov).

plus interactive features that allow you and your patients to create individualized nutrition and health plans. It can be easily adapted to people with various cultural backgrounds, lifestyles, and health problems. For example, the recommended calorie intake for an active 2-year-old is 1400 kcal/day versus 1000 kcal/day for a sedentary 2-year-old. A more detailed report of the 2005 Dietary Guidelines can be accessed at www.health.gov/dietaryguidelines. The DRIs are recommended amounts of nutrients to prevent deficiencies and reduce the risk for chronic diseases. In addition to recommending adequate intakes, they also specify upper limits of nutrients to avoid toxicity. With increased use of dietary supplements, the risk for nutrient toxicities is on the rise. Examples of specific DRIs can be found at http://fnic.nal.usda.gov/nal_display/index.php?info_center=4&tax_level=1&tax_subject= 256.

SUBJECTIVE DATA

1. Eating patterns
2. Usual weight
3. Changes in appetite, taste, smell, chewing, swallowing
4. Recent surgery, trauma, burns, infection
5. Chronic illnesses
6. Vomiting, diarrhea, constipation
7. Food allergies or intolerances
8. Medications and/or nutritional supplements
9. Self-care behaviors
10. Alcohol or illegal drug use
11. Exercise and activity patterns
12. Family history

Examiner Asks	Rationale
1. Eating patterns. • Number of meals/snacks per day? • Kind and amount of food eaten? • Fad, special, or alternative diets? • Where is food eaten? • Food preferences and dislikes? • Religious or cultural restrictions? • Able to feed self?	Most individuals know about or are interested in the foods they consume. If misconceptions are present, begin gradual instruction to modify ethnic/religious beliefs or feeding difficulties that may affect intake of certain foods. Many alternative diets are not supported by scientific safety or efficacy data.
2. Usual weight. What is your usual weight? • 20% below or above desirable weight? • Recent weight change? How much lost or gained? Over what time period? • Reason for loss or gain?	Persons with a recent weight loss or who are obese are at risk. Underweight individuals are vulnerable because their fuel reserves may be depleted. Excess weight is associated with hypertension, diabetes, heart disease, and even cancer. Protein and calorie needs are often overlooked in acutely ill obese persons.
3. Changes in appetite, taste, smell, chewing, swallowing. • Type of change? • When did change occur?	These alterations interfere with adequate nutrient intake.
4. Recent surgery, trauma, burns, infection. • When? Type? How treated? • Conditions that increase nutrient loss (e.g., draining wounds, effusions, blood loss, dialysis)?	These conditions have caloric and nutrient needs that are two or three times greater than normal.
5. Chronic illnesses. • Type? When diagnosed? How treated? • Dietary modifications? • Recent cancer chemotherapy or radiation therapy?	Chronic illnesses that affect nutrient use (e.g., diabetes mellitus, pancreatitis, or malabsorption) or cancer treatment carries twice the risk for nutritional deficits.
6. Nausea, vomiting, diarrhea, constipation. • Any problems? Due to? How long?	Gastrointestinal (GI) symptoms interfere with nutrient intake or absorption.

Examiner Asks	Rationale
7. Food allergies or intolerances. • Any problematic foods? Type of reaction? How long?	Food allergies, especially peanut allergies, are on the rise and are a major health concern. Intolerances may result in nutrient deficiencies, such as diarrhea after milk ingestion.
8. Medications and/or nutritional supplements. • Prescription medications? • Nonprescription? • Use over a 24-hour period?	Analgesics, antacids, anticonvulsants, antibiotics, diuretics, laxatives, antineoplastic drugs, steroids, and oral contraceptives are drugs that interact with nutrients, impairing their digestion, absorption, metabolism, or utilization.
• Type of vitamin/mineral supplement? Amount? Duration of use?	Vitamin/mineral supplements have harmful side effects if taken in large amounts.
• Herbal and botanical products? Functional foods or foods enhanced with nutrients? Specific type/brand and where obtained? How often used? Who recommended? How does it help you? Any problems?	Use of herbal/botanical supplements is often not reported, so ask and discuss proper use and potential adverse effects. Refer to www.nccam.nih.gov.
9. Self-care behaviors. • Meal preparation facilities? • Transportation for travel to market? • Adequate income for food purchase? • Who prepares meals and does shopping? • Environment during mealtimes?	Socioeconomic factors may interfere with ingestion of adequate amounts of food or usual diet.
10. Alcohol or illegal drug use. • When was last drink of alcohol? • Amount taken that episode? • Amount alcohol each day? Each week? • Duration of use? • (Repeat questions for each drug used.)	These agents are substituted for nutritious foods and increase requirements for some nutrients. Also, pregnant women who smoke, drink alcohol, or use illegal drugs give birth to infants with low birth weights, failure to thrive, and other serious complications.
11. Exercise and activity patterns. • Amount? • Type?	Caloric and nutrient needs increase with competitive sports and manual labor. Inactive or sedentary lifestyles often lead to excess weight gain.
12. Family history. Heart disease, osteoporosis, cancer, gout, GI disorders, obesity, or diabetes? • Effect of each on eating patterns? • Effect on activity patterns?	Long-term nutritional deficiencies or excesses may first show as disease, such as these common examples. Early identification permits dietary and activity modifications at a time when the body can recover more fully.

Additional History for Infants and Children

Dietary histories of infants and children are obtained from the parents, guardian, babysitter, or daycare center. Usually, the person responsible for food preparation provides a fairly accurate dietary history. Having the caregivers keep a thorough daily food diary and occasionally requesting 24-hour recalls during clinic visits are the commonly employed techniques.

Subjective Data

Examiner Asks	Rationale
1. Gestational nutrition. • Maternal history of alcohol or illegal drug use? • Any diet-related complications during gestation? • Infant's birth weight? • Any evidence of delayed physical or mental growth?	Low birth weight (<2500 g) is a major factor in infant morbidity and mortality. Poor gestational nutrition, low maternal weight gain, and maternal alcohol and drug use—all factors in low birth weight—can lead to birth defects and delayed growth and development.
2. Infant breastfed or bottle fed. • Type, frequency, amount, and duration of feeding? • Any difficulties encountered? • Timing and method of weaning?	Well-nourished infants have appropriate physical and social growth and development. Inexperienced mothers may have problems with feeding or have questions about whether the infant is receiving adequate food.
3. Child's willingness to eat what you prepare. • Any special likes or dislikes? • How much will child eat? • How do you control non-nutritious snack foods? • How do you avoid food aspiration?	The preschool period has increasing growth. Lifelong food habits form. Use of small portions, finger foods, simple meals, and nutritious snacks improve dietary intake. Avoid foods likely to be aspirated (e.g., hot dogs, nuts, grapes, round candies, popcorn).
4. Overweight and obesity risk factors. • Overweight or obese parent? • Low-income family? • Maternal smoking during pregnancy? • Large-for-gestational-age birth weight? • Rapid weight gain from birth to 5 months?	Risk factors for overweight and obesity may be present during gestation, at birth, or during infancy, progressing to obesity in childhood, adolescence, and adulthood.[31]
Additional History for the Adolescent	
1. Your present weight. • What would you like to weigh? • How do you feel about your present weight? • On any special diet to lose weight? • On other diets to lose weight? If so, were they successful? • Constantly think about "feeling fat?" Constantly exercising? • Intentionally vomit or use laxatives or diuretics after eating?	Obesity, particularly in girls, may precipitate fad dieting and malnutrition. Adolescents' increased body awareness and self-consciousness may cause eating disorders (anorexia nervosa or bulimia) when the real or perceived body image does not compare favorably to an ideal image in advertisements or pictures of fashion models.
2. Use of anabolic steroids or other agents to increase muscle size and physical performance. • When? • How much? • Any problems?	Once confined to male professional athletes, the use of performance-enhancing agents now extends to junior high, high school, and college. Adverse effects include personality disorders (aggressiveness) and liver and other organ damage.
• Use of caffeinated, energy-boosting drinks? When? Type? Duration?	Energy-boosting drinks like Red Bull and Sprint contain large amounts of caffeine, stimulants, and/or herbal products. Side effects include dehydration, high blood pressure and heart rate, and sleep problems.

Examiner Asks	Rationale
3. Overweight and obesity risk factors. • Are large amounts of food eaten in a short period of time or for hours on end? • Which meals do you skip? How often? What snacks, fast foods, and sweetened beverages do you like? How often do you eat them?	Binge eating is now the most common eating disorder across all age-groups. Skipping meals and consuming fast foods and sweetened beverages are associated with increased weight gain from adolescence to adulthood.[26,35]
4. Age first started menstruating. • What is your menstrual flow like?	Malnutrition delays menarche. Likewise, amenorrhea or scant menstrual flow occurs with nutritional deficiency.

Additional History for the Pregnant Woman

Examiner Asks	Rationale
1. Number of pregnancies. • How many times have you been pregnant? • When? • Any problems encountered during previous pregnancies? • Problems this pregnancy? • Do you take prenatal vitamins or supplements?	A multiparous mother with pregnancies less than 1 year apart has risk for depleted nutritional reserves. Note previous complications of pregnancy (excessive vomiting, anemia, or gestational diabetes). Slower GI motility and pressure from the fetus may cause constipation, hemorrhoids, and indigestion. A history of a low-birth-weight infant suggests past nutritional problems. Giving birth to an infant weighing 4.5 kg (10 lbs) or more may signal *latent* diabetes in the mother.
2. Food preferences when pregnant. • What foods do you avoid? • Crave any particular foods?	The expectant mother is vulnerable to familial, cultural, and traditional influences for food choices. Cravings for or aversions to particular foods are common; evaluate their contribution to, or interference with, dietary intake.
• How much fish do you eat?	Large amounts of fish consumption may be associated with maternal, fetal, and newborn mercury toxicity.

Additional History for the Aging Adult

Examiner Asks	Rationale
1. Any diet differences from when you were in your 40s and 50s? • Why? • What factors affect the way you eat?	Note any physiologic or psychological changes of aging or socioeconomic changes that affect nutritional status.
2. Review the Mini Nutritional Assessment (MNA®) tool (see Fig. 11-2).	The MNA® screens for nutrition risk in older adults. It has 6 questions, which indicate risk factors for inadequate nutritional status. Persons at risk for malnutrition (MNA® score 8-11 points) or malnourishment (MNA® score 0-7 points) need a more comprehensive assessment using the full MNA®, available at www.mna.elderly.com.

OBJECTIVE DATA

CLINICAL SIGNS

The general appearance—obese, cachectic (fat and muscle wasting), or edematous—can provide clues to overall nutritional status. More specific clinical signs of nutritional deficiencies can be detected through a physical examination. Because clinical signs are late manifestations of malnutrition, only in areas of rapid turnover of epithelial tissue—skin, hair, mouth, lips, and eyes—are the deficiencies readily detectable. These signs may also be non-nutritional in origin. Therefore laboratory testing is required to make an accurate diagnosis, reviewed later in this chapter. Clinical signs of various nutritional deficiencies are summarized in Table 11-5 and are depicted in the section on abnormalities at the end of this chapter (see Tables 11-6 to 11-8).

EQUIPMENT NEEDED

Lange or Harpenden skinfold calipers
Ross insertion tape or other measurement tape
Anthropometer
Pen or pencil
Nutritional assessment data form

TABLE 11-5 Clinical Signs of Malnutrition

Area of Examination	Normal Appearance	Signs Associated With Malnutrition	Nutrient Deficiency
Skin	Smooth, no signs of rashes, bruises, flaking	Dry, flaking, scaly	Vitamin A, vitamin B–complex, linoleic acid
		Petechiae/ecchymoses	Vitamins C and K
		Follicular hyperkeratosis (dry, bumpy skin)	Vitamin A, linoleic acid
		Cracks in skin, lesions on the hands, legs, face, or neck	Niacin, tryptophan
		Pellagrous dermatosis (hyperpigmentation of skin exposed to sunlight)	Niacin
		Nasolabial seborrhea	Riboflavin, vitamin B_6
		Acneiform forehead rash	Vitamin B_6
		Eczema	Linoleic acid
		Xanthomas (excessive deposits of cholesterol)	Excessive serum levels of LDLs or VLDLs
Hair	Shiny, firm, does not fall out easily, healthy scalp	Dull, dry, sparse	Protein, zinc, linoleic acid
		Color changes	Copper or protein
		Corkscrew hair	Copper
Eyes	Corneas are clear, shiny; membranes are pink and moist; no sores at corners of eyelids	Foamy plaques (Bitot's spots)	Vitamin A
		Dryness (xerophthalmia)	Vitamin A
		Softening (keratomalacia)	Vitamin A
		Pale conjunctivae	Iron, vitamins B_6, B_{12}
		Red conjunctivae	Riboflavin
		Blepharitis	Vitamin B-complex, biotin
Lips	Smooth, not chapped or swollen	Cheilosis (vertical cracks in lips)	Riboflavin, niacin
		Angular stomatitis (red cracks at sides of mouth)	Riboflavin, niacin, iron, vitamin B_6
Tongue	Red in appearance; not swollen or smooth, no lesions	Glossitis (beefy red)	Vitamin B–complex
		Pale	Iron
		Papillary atrophy	Niacin
		Papillary hypertrophy	Multiple nutrients
		Magenta/purplish colored	Riboflavin
Gums	Reddish-pink, firm, no swelling or bleeding	Bleeding	Vitamin C
Nails	Smooth, pink	Brittle, ridged, or spoon shaped (koilonychia)	Iron
		Splinter hemorrhages	Vitamin C
Musculoskeletal	Erect posture, no malformations, good muscle tone, can walk or run without pain	Pain in calves, thighs	Thiamine
		Osteomalacia	Vitamin D, calcium
		Rickets	Vitamin D, calcium
		Joint pain	Vitamin C
		Muscle wasting	Protein, carbohydrate, fat
Neurologic	Normal reflexes, appropriate affect	Peripheral neuropathy	Thiamine, vitamin B_6
		Hyporeflexia	Thiamine
		Disorientation or irritability	Vitamin B_{12}

Normal Range of Findings

ANTHROPOMETRIC MEASURES

These measures evaluate growth, development, and body composition. The most commonly used anthropometric measures are height, weight, triceps skinfold thickness, elbow breadth, and arm and head circumferences. Measurement of height, weight, body mass index, and waist circumference is described in Chapter 9.

Derived Weight Measures

Three derived weight measures are used to depict changes in body weight.

Body weight as a percentage of ideal body weight is calculated using the following formula:

$$\text{Percent ideal body weight} = \frac{\text{Current weight}}{\text{Ideal weight}} \times 100$$

Ideal weight is based on the Metropolitan Life Insurance Tables, 1983. These tables remain the recommended standard.

The **percent usual body weight** is calculated as follows:

$$\text{Percent usual body weight} = \frac{\text{Current weight}}{\text{Usual weight}} \times 100$$

Recent weight change is calculated using the following formula:

$$\frac{\text{Usual weight} - \text{Current weight}}{\text{Usual weight}} \times 100$$

Body Mass Index

Body mass index is a practical marker of optimal weight for height and an indicator of obesity or undernutrition (see p. 131 in Chapter 9). It is calculated by:

$$\text{Body mass index} = \frac{\text{Weight (kilograms)}}{\text{Height (meters)}^2}$$

$$\text{Or} \quad \frac{\text{Weight (pounds)}}{\text{Height (inches)}^2} \times 703$$

Waist-to-Hip Ratio

The waist-to-hip ratio assesses body fat distribution as an indicator of health risk. Obese persons with a greater proportion of fat in the upper body, especially in the abdomen, have android obesity; obese persons with most of their fat in the hips and thighs have gynoid obesity. The equation is:

$$\text{Waist-to-hip ratio} = \frac{\text{Waist circumference}}{\text{Hip circumference}}$$

where waist circumference is measured in inches at the smallest circumference below the rib cage and above the umbilicus, and hip circumference is measured in inches at the largest circumference of the buttocks. In addition, **waist circumference (WC)** alone can be used to predict greater health risk.

Abnormal Findings

A current weight of 80% to 90% of ideal weight suggests mild malnutrition; 70% to 80%, moderate malnutrition; and <70%, severe malnutrition.

A current weight of 85% to 95% of usual body weight indicates mild malnutrition; 75% to 84%, moderate malnutrition; and <75%, severe malnutrition.

An unintentional loss of >5% of body weight over 1 month, >7.5% of body weight over 3 months, or >10% of body weight over 6 months is clinically significant.

BMI interpretation for adults[24]):

<18.5	Underweight
18.5-24.9	Normal weight
25.0-29.9	Overweight
30.0-39.9	Obesity
≥40	Extreme obesity

BMI interpretation for children ages 2-20 years[7]:

<5th percentile	Underweight
5th-85th percentile	Healthy weight
85th-95th percentile	Overweight
≥95th percentile	Obese

A waist-to-hip ratio of 1.0 or greater in men or 0.8 or greater in women is indicative of android (upper body) obesity and increasing risk for obesity-related diseases and early mortality.

A WC >35 inches in women and >40 inches in men increases risk for heart disease, type 2 diabetes mellitus, and metabolic syndrome.

Normal Range of Findings | **Abnormal Findings**

Skinfold Thickness

Skinfold thickness measurements estimate the body fat stores or the extent of obesity or undernutrition. Although other sites can be used (biceps, subcapsular, or suprailiac skinfolds), the triceps skinfold (TSF) is most easily accessible, and standards and techniques are most developed for this site. To measure TSF thickness:

1. Have the ambulatory person stand with arms hanging freely at the sides and back to the examiner. (Non-ambulatory persons should lie on one side. The uppermost arm should be fully extended, with the palm of the hand resting on the thigh.)
2. Using the thumb and forefinger of your left hand, gently grasp a fold of skin and fat on the back of the person's left upper arm, midway between the acromion process of the scapula and the olecranon process (the tip of the elbow). Gently pull the skinfold away from the underlying muscle (Fig. 11-4).

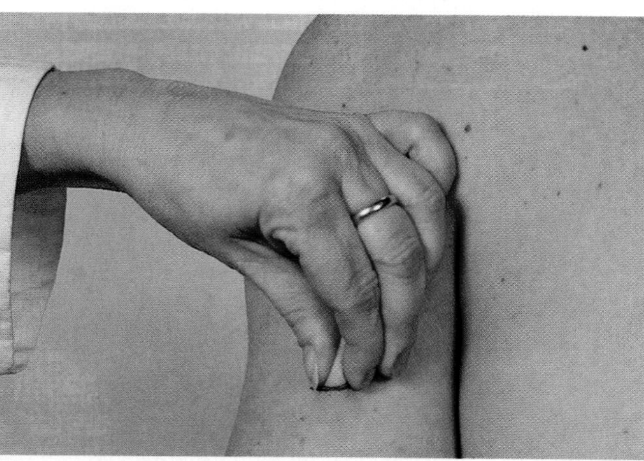

11-4

3. While grasping the skinfold, pick up the calipers with your right hand and depress the spring-loaded lever. Apply caliper jaws horizontally to the fat fold. Release the lever of the calipers while holding the skinfold. Wait 3 seconds, and then take a reading. Repeat three times, and average the three skinfold measurements (Fig. 11-5).

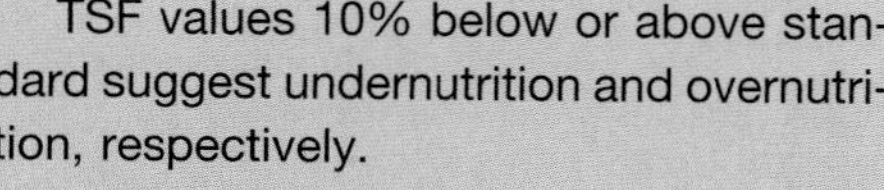

TSF values 10% below or above standard suggest undernutrition and overnutrition, respectively.

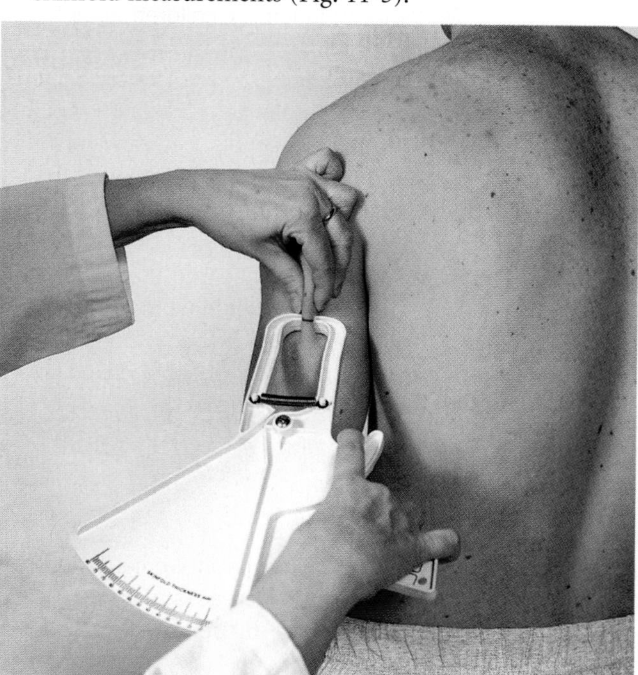

11-5

Normal Range of Findings

4. Record measurements to the nearest 5 mm (0.5 cm) on the nutritional assessment data form. Compare the person's measurements with standards by age, gender, and body frame size (see Appendixes H and J on the *Evolve* website).

Abnormal Findings

Nonreproducible readings may be due to instrument malfunctions, use of plastic calipers (which are less accurate), or examiner error. Edema may produce falsely high readings.

Mid–Upper Arm Circumference

Mid–upper arm circumference (MAC) estimates skeletal muscle mass and fat stores.

1. Have the person stand or sit with arm hanging fully extended and relaxed by the side of the body.
2. Loop the insertion tape or measuring tape around the arm at the midpoint of the upper arm (midway between the acromion and olecranon processes).
3. Position the tape horizontally at the midpoint, and then tighten it firmly around the arm but not so tightly as to cause skin contour indentation or pinching (Fig. 11-6).

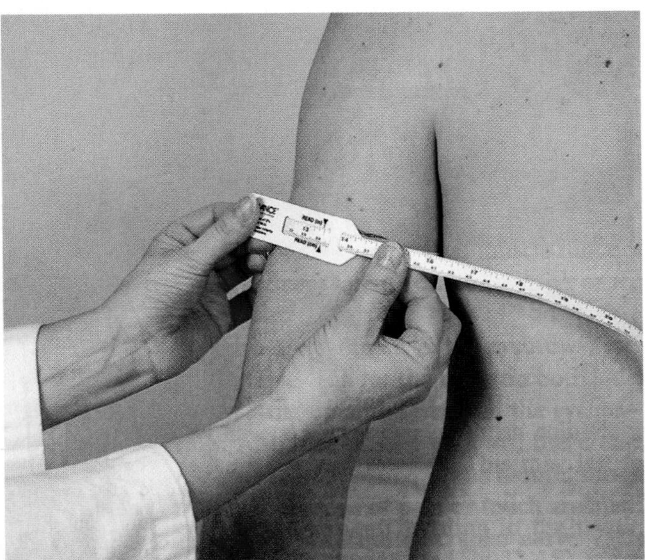

11-6

4. Note and record the measurement (in centimeters) on the appropriate form. Compare with norms (Appendix I on the *Evolve* website).

For example, a normal MAC for a 20-year-old female ranges from 23 to 34.5 cm; for a 20-year-old male, the normal range is 27.2 to 37.2 cm. Remember that accurate MAC and TSF measurements are difficult to obtain and interpret in older adults because of sagging skin, changes in fat distribution, and declining muscle mass.

Measurements below the 10th percentile or above the 95th percentile warrant further medical and nutritional evaluation. Very high or very low readings may be due to examiner error.

Derived Anthropometric Measures

Although the MAC is of little value in and of itself, when combined with the TSF measurement, it is possible to indirectly determine the arm muscle **circumference** and arm muscle **area.**

Normal Range of Findings

Mid–upper arm muscle circumference (MAMC) estimates skeletal muscle reserves or the amount of lean body mass and is derived from the TSF and MAC measures using the following formula:

$$\text{MAMC} = \text{MAC} - (\pi \times \text{TSF})$$

where

$$\pi = 3.14$$
$$\text{MAC} = \text{Mid–upper arm circumference (in cm)}$$
$$\text{TSF} = \text{Triceps skinfold (in mm)}$$
$$\text{MAMC} = \text{Mid–upper arm muscle circumference (in cm)}$$

Record calculation on data forms. Compare with norms (Appendixes I and J on the *Evolve* website).

Mid-arm muscle area (MAMA) is a good indicator of lean body mass and thus skeletal protein reserves. These reserves are important in growing children and are especially valuable in evaluating persons who may be malnourished because of chronic illness, multiple surgeries, or inadequate dietary intake.

The equation for calculating MAMA is

$$\text{MAMA} = \frac{(\text{MAC} - \text{MAMC})^2}{4\pi}$$

where

$$\text{MAMA} = \text{mid-arm muscle area (in cm}^2)$$
$$\text{MAC} = \text{mid–upper arm circumference (in cm)}$$
$$\text{MAMC} = \text{mid–upper arm muscle circumference (in cm)}$$
$$4\pi = 4 \times 3.14 = 12.56$$

Record calculation on data forms. Compare with norms (Appendix I on the *Evolve* website).

Two newer techniques to measure body composition are **bioelectrical impedance analysis (BIA)** and **dual-energy x-ray absorptiometry (DEXA).** Both BIA and DEXA measure fat and lean body mass; in addition, DEXA measures bone mineral density.

Arm Span or Total Arm Length

Measurement of arm span is useful for those situations in which height is difficult to measure, such as in children with cerebral palsy or scoliosis or in aging persons with spinal curvature. Arm span, which is nearly equivalent to height, is sometimes used clinically instead of height. Measure the distance from the sternal notch to the longest finger on the dominant hand, then multiply the number by 2.[8]

Frame Size

Frame size is calculated to determine range of ideal body weight. Most weight standards, such as the Metropolitan Life Insurance Tables of ideal weight for height, contain classifications of weight by frame size. Elbow breadth, a measure of skeletal breadth, is the most accurate method to determine frame size.[16]

1. Instruct the person to extend the right arm forward, perpendicular to the body. Bend the elbow to a 90-degree angle, with the palm of the hand turned laterally (Fig. 11-7).

Abnormal Findings

MAMC is dependent on accurate measurement of the MAC and TSF. In general, a MAMC that is 90% of standard is suggestive of mild malnutrition, 60% to 90% suggests moderate malnutrition, and less than 60% is indicative of severe malnutrition.

MAMA is considered to be a more sensitive measure of long-standing malnutrition than MAMC. A MAMA of 90% of standard reflects mild malnutrition; 60% to 90% moderate malnutrition; and less than 60% severe malnutrition.

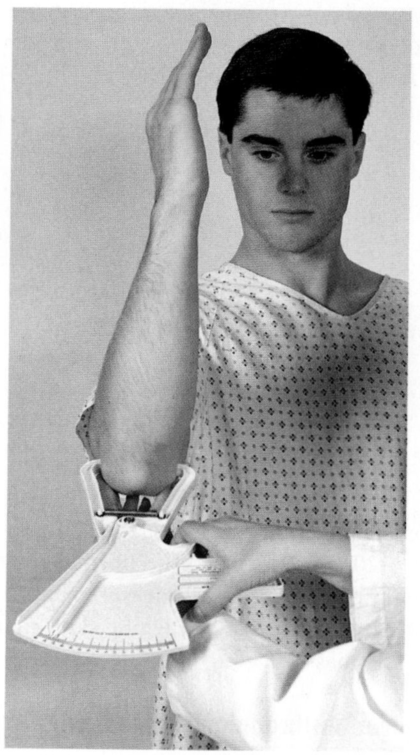

11-7

Normal Range of Findings	Abnormal Findings

2. Facing the person, place the calipers on the condyles of the humerus (a broad-blade anthropometer may be needed if the calipers do not extend to the breadth of the elbow).
3. Read the distance between the condyles; record measurement (in centimeters) on the appropriate form. Using the norms (Appendix J on the *Evolve* website), assess whether the person has small, medium, or large frame size.

DEVELOPMENTAL COMPETENCE

Infants, Children, and Adolescents

Weight. During infancy, childhood, and adolescence, height, weight, and head circumference should be measured at regular intervals, because longitudinal growth is one of the best indices of nutritional status over time. See Chapter 9 for techniques.

Skinfold Thickness and Body Mass Index. Determination of skinfold thickness and/or body mass index may be useful in evaluating childhood and teenage overnutrition.

An estimated 17% of children and adolescents in the United States are obese.

The Pregnant Woman

Weight. Measure weight monthly up to 30 weeks' gestation, then every 2 weeks until the last month of pregnancy, when weight should be measured weekly. Appendix G on the *Evolve* website illustrates approximate weight gain considered normal for each week of pregnancy.

Consider the expectant mother at nutritional risk if her weight is 10% or more below ideal or 20% or more above the norm for her height and age-group.

The Aging Adult

Height. With age, height declines in both men and women very slowly from the early 30s, leading to an average 2.9-cm loss in men and 4.9-cm loss in women.[18,29] Height measures may not be accurate in individuals confined to a bed or wheelchair or those older than 60 years (because of osteoporotic changes). Therefore arm span, which is correlated with height, may be a better measure.

Other Measurements. MAC and TSF measures are difficult to obtain in older adults (because of sagging skin, changes in fat distribution, and declining muscle mass). (See Frisancho[14] for data on weight and TSF thickness by height in U.S. men and women ages 55 to 74 years.) BMI and waist-to-hip ratio are better indicators of obesity in this age-group.

LABORATORY STUDIES

Routine laboratory tests are objective and can detect preclinical nutritional deficiencies. Use caution, however, when interpreting test results that may be outside normal ranges, because they do not always reflect a nutritional problem and because standards for aging adults have not yet been firmly established. The following are some routinely performed laboratory indicators of nutritional status.

Glucose. Plasma glucose level, or the amount of glucose in the serum, is usually a fasting test. Normal fasting plasma glucose levels are: **young children (0-2 yr)**, 60-110 mg/dL; **children (2-18 yr)**, 60-100 mg/dL; and **adults**, <100 mg/dL. Glycosylated hemoglobin, also known as Hb_{A1c}, reflects average blood glucose levels for the prior 2 to 3 months and is useful in managing diabetes mellitus. Normal Hb_{A1c} results range from 5% to 7%.

The term *prediabetes* is used for higher fasting plasma glucose levels (110-125 mg/dL). Hyperglycemia may be due to diabetes mellitus, severe stress such as surgery or trauma, hyperthyroidism, or medications. Hypoglycemia may be caused by hypothyroidism, inadequate food intake, too much insulin, or medications.

Normal Range of Findings

Hemoglobin. The hemoglobin (Hb) determination is used to detect iron deficiency anemia. Normal values are as follows: **infants,** 1 to 3 days—14.5 to 22.5 g/dL, 2 months—9.0 to 14.0 g/dL; **children,** 6 to 12 years—11.5 to 15.5 g/dL; **adults,** males—14 to 18 g/dL, females—12 to 16 g/dL.

Hematocrit. Hematocrit (HCT), a measure of cell volume, also indicates iron status. Normal values are as follows: **infants,** 1 to 3 days—44% to 72%, 2 months—28% to 42%; **children,** 6 to 12 years—35% to 45%; **adults,** males—37% to 49%, females—36% to 46%.

Cholesterol. Total cholesterol evaluates fat metabolism and the risk for cardiovascular disease. Normal cholesterol concentrations vary with age and gender and range from 120 to 200 mg/dL.

Low-density lipoprotein cholesterol (LDL-C), or "bad" cholesterol, is the major carrier of cholesterol in the blood and is closely associated with increased risk for atherosclerosis and coronary heart disease. Desirable LDL-C values are: **children and adolescents**, <110 mg/dL; **adults**, <130 mg/dL. High-density lipoprotein cholesterol (HDL-C), or "good" cholesterol, is inversely related to coronary heart disease risk. Normal values are: **men,** 35-65 mg/dL; **women,** 35-80 mg/dL.

Triglycerides. Serum triglycerides (TGs) or blood fats are used to screen for hyperlipidemia and the risk for coronary artery disease. Triglyceride values are age related. Some controversy exists over the most appropriate normal ranges, but the following fasting levels are fairly widely accepted: **ages 0 to 19,** 10 to 100 mg/dL; **ages 20 to 65,** <150 mg/dL.

Serum Proteins. Serum albumin is a common measurement of visceral protein status. Because of its relatively long half-life (17 to 20 days) and large body pool (4.0 to 5.0 g/kg), albumin is a better indicator of long-term protein status rather than acute protein malnutrition seen during serious illness.

Normal serum albumin concentration in infants and children older than 6 months and adults ranges from 3.5 to 5.5 g/dL.

Levels of **serum transferrin,** an iron-transport protein, can be measured directly or by an indirect measurement of total iron-binding capacity. Serum transferrin, with a half-life of 8 to 10 days, may be a more sensitive indicator of visceral protein status than albumin.

The most widely used formula for computing serum transferrin is

$$\text{Serum transferrin} = (0.8 \times \text{Total iron-binding capacity}) - 43$$

The normal values for serum transferrin are 170 to 250 mg/dL.

Prealbumin, or thyroxine-binding prealbumin, serves as a transport protein for thyroxine (T_4) and retinol-binding protein. With a shorter half-life (48 hours) than either albumin or transferrin, prealbumin is sensitive to acute changes in protein status and sudden demands on protein synthesis. Normal prealbumin levels range from 15 to 25 mg/dL.

C-reactive protein (CRP), a plasma protein marker of inflammatory status produced by the liver, is used to monitor metabolic stress (e.g., trauma, surgery, burns) and to determine when to begin nutritional support in critically ill patients. CRP is generally not detectable in the blood of healthy individuals. High-sensitivity CRP (hs-CRP) is used to assess risk for myocardial infarction. Normal values are <0.1 mg/dL.

Abnormal Findings

Increased Hb levels suggest hemoconcentration due to polycythemia vera or dehydration.

Decreased Hb levels may indicate anemia, recent hemorrhage, or hemodilution caused by fluid retention.

A low value indicates insufficient Hb formation; thus Hct and Hb values should be interpreted together.

Coronary artery disease risk steadily increases as serum cholesterol rises. Serum cholesterol levels of 200 to 239 mg/dL (borderline high) are associated with moderate risk and 240 mg/dL or more (high) with high risk for coronary artery disease, heart attack, stroke, and peripheral vascular disease.

Serum TG levels are also associated with coronary artery disease and are categorized as *borderline* high, 150-199 mg/dL, or *high,* 200-499 mg/dL.

Low serum albumin levels occur with protein-calorie malnutrition, altered hydration status, and decreased liver function.

A serum albumin level of 2.8 to 3.5 g/dL represents moderate visceral protein depletion, and <2.8 g/dL denotes severe depletion.[8a]

Levels of 150 to 170 mg/dL suggest mild protein deficiency; 100 to 150 mg/dL, moderate deficiency; and levels less than 100 mg/dL, severe deficiency.[22] Because many clinical conditions can alter serum albumin and transferrin levels, consider the person's history in conjunction with these values for accurate interpretation.

Prealbumin levels are elevated in renal disease and reduced by surgery, trauma, burns, and infection. Prealbumin levels of 10 to 15 mg/dL indicate mild depletion; 5 to 10 mg/dL, moderate depletion; and less than 5 mg/dL, severe depletion.

Detectable levels of CRP are associated with increased risk for atherosclerosis and may be seen in other inflammatory conditions, such as infections, rheumatoid arthritis, or tuberculosis. The use of oral contraceptives and the last 4 to 5 months of pregnancy may also produce detectable CRP levels.

Normal Range of Findings	Abnormal Findings

 DEVELOPMENTAL COMPETENCE

In infancy and childhood, laboratory tests are performed only when undernutrition is suspected or the child has acute or chronic illnesses that affect nutritional status. However, iron and lead levels should be assessed at 9 to 12 months.

During adolescence, unless overt disease is suspected, laboratory evaluation of Hb and Hct levels and urinalysis for glucose and protein levels are adequate.

In pregnancy, Hb and Hct values can be used to detect deficiencies of protein, folacin, vitamin B_{12}, and iron. Urine is frequently tested for glucose and protein (albumin), which can signal diabetes, preeclampsia, and renal disease.

In older adulthood, all serum and urine data must be interpreted with an understanding of declining renal efficiency and a tendency for aging adults to be overhydrated or underhydrated.

SERIAL ASSESSMENT

To monitor nutritional status in malnourished individuals or in individuals at risk for malnutrition, serial measurements are made at routine intervals. At a minimum, weight and dietary intake should be evaluated weekly. Because the other nutritional assessment parameters change more slowly, data on these indicators may be collected biweekly or monthly.

Based on the findings of the nutritional assessment, the type of malnutrition can be diagnosed. The four major types of malnutrition are obesity, marasmus, kwashiorkor, and marasmus-kwashiorkor mix (see Table 11-6, Classification of Malnutrition, p. 196). Each type of malnutrition has characteristic clinical and laboratory findings and a distinct cause.

Health Promotion

The keys to a healthy diet are as follows:

- Eat a variety of foods from all the basic food groups to ensure nutrient adequacy.
- Consume the recommended amounts of fruits/vegetables, whole grains, and fat-free or low-fat milk products or equivalents.
- Limit intake of foods high in saturated or trans fats, added sugars, starch, cholesterol, salt, and alcohol.
- Match calorie intake with calories expended.
- Be physically active for at least 30 minutes almost every day of the week.
- Follow food safety guidelines for handling, preparing, and storing foods.

Approaches to weight loss for overweight and obesity must be tailored to the individual, be culturally sensitive, and consider the patient's readiness to lose weight and health care and self-care beliefs. Weight loss programs that provide less than 1000 to 1200 calories may not provide adequate nutrients. Regardless of macronutrient composition, any diet that reduces calorie intake or contains 1400 to 1500 calories per day results in weight loss. In other words, it is not eating too much of any particular nutrient such as carbohydrate or fat that makes us gain weight but, rather, the overall number of calories ingested. The **cardinal features** of a successful long-term weight loss plan are (1) getting regular (i.e., 4-5 times/week for 30 minutes) physical exercise; (2) eating a low-calorie (≈1400-1500 kcal/day), low-fat (20%-25% of total calories) diet; and (3) monitoring daily food intake (e.g., food diary, portion size) and weight.

PROMOTING A HEALTHY LIFESTYLE

The Obesity Epidemic

The CDC has identified obesity as a major health risk for obesity-related diseases and a health problem of epidemic proportions. Obesity-related diseases include coronary heart disease; type 2 diabetes; endometrial, breast, and colon cancers; hypertension; stroke; dyslipidemia; liver and gallbladder disease; sleep apnea and respiratory problems; osteoarthritis; and gynecologic problems, including abnormal menses and infertility. On its homepage, the CDC invites health care providers and the public to view a state-by-state breakdown of obesity statistics, trends, and economic impact on the U.S. health system, as well as an interactive map illustrating the growth of obesity in the United States since 1985 to its current epidemic proportions (www.cdc.gov).

For adults, the terms *overweight* and *obese* are determined using weight and height to calculate an individual's body mass index (BMI). For children, BMI calculations must also include age. BMI calculators for children and teens, as well as adults, are available at the CDC website: www.cdc.gov/healthyweight/assessing/index.html. Individuals gain weight when they consume more calories than their body needs. Although this imbalance usually occurs by eating a diet high in fat and calories and/or living a sedentary lifestyle, it can also be caused by physiologic factors, including genetic and endocrine problems. For these reasons, health care providers will need to consider more than just calorie counting and exercise when assessing individuals who are overweight or obese. However, healthy eating and increased activity continue to address the most common causes of obesity. Emphasis on healthy eating and increased activity has even come from the White House, with First Lady Michelle Obama's "Let's Move" initiative that creates online groups for children to track their activity alongside other children and adults across the country. You can visit the "Let's Move" website at www.letsmove.gov/.

Resources

Lean Works! (Leading Employees to Activity and Nutrition) is a web-based resource that offers interactive tool and evidence-based resources for workplace obesity prevention and control programs. Website: www.cdc.gov/leanworks/.

Obesity in America. Website: www.obesityinamerica.org.

The Weight-Control Information Network provides the general public, health professionals, the media, and Congress with up-to-date, science-based information on weight control, obesity, physical activity, and related nutritional issues. Website: http://win.niddk.nih.gov/.

We Can! (Ways to Enhance Children's Activity and Nutrition) is a national movement to help children ages 8 to 13 years stay at a healthy weight by providing parents and caregivers with tools, activities, and resources that focus on eating right, getting active, and reducing TV and computer screen time. Website: www.nhlbi.nih.gov/health/public/heart/obesity/wecan/index.htm.

DOCUMENTATION AND CRITICAL THINKING

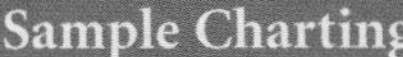

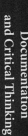

Sample Charting

SUBJECTIVE

No history of diseases or surgery that would alter intake/requirements; no recent weight changes; no appetite changes. Socioeconomic history is noncontributory. Does not smoke; drink alcohol; or use illegal, prescription, or over-the-counter drugs. No food allergies. Sedentary lifestyle; plays golf once per week.

OBJECTIVE

Dietary intake is adequate to meet protein and energy needs. No clinical signs of nutrient deficiencies. Height, weight, and screening laboratory tests within normal ranges.

Focused Assessment: Clinical Case Study 1

Molly is a 14-year-old high school freshman who has been overweight most of her life.

SUBJECTIVE

Molly presents to the school clinic with a weight gain of 10 pounds since starting high school 6 months ago. Daily calorie intake averages 2500 to 3000 calories/day. Skips breakfast and eats lunch at a fast food restaurant across the street from the high school—usually a cheeseburger, fries, and soft drink. Lives in a low-income neighborhood where the nearest grocery store with fresh fruits and vegetables is a bus ride away, and there are few safe places to exercise.

OBJECTIVE

Inspection: General appearance is overweight for age and height.
Anthropometric: Height is 157.4 cm (62 in). Current weight is 63.6 kg (140 lb); BMI is 25.6 (91st percentile—at risk for overweight).
Laboratory: Not available, but fasting plasma glucose should be checked for prediabetes.

ASSESSMENT

Imbalanced nutrition: more than body requirements R/T high fat and calorie intake, undesirable eating patterns, lack of exercise, environmental influences, knowledge deficit.
Overweight with high risk for becoming an obese adult and for developing obesity-related complications, such as type 2 diabetes mellitus, sleep apnea, arthritis, asthma, poor self-esteem and quality of life, and metabolic syndrome.

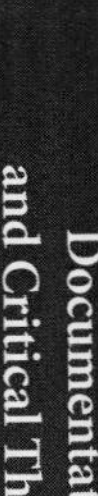

Focused Assessment: Clinical Case Study 2

E.F. is an 87-year-old widow who lives alone in her own home. She has enjoyed good health all of her life.

SUBJECTIVE

During the past year, she has experienced declining memory and no longer cooks or drives. Relies on children to take her grocery shopping and prepare occasional meals. Income adequate. Describes her appetite as excellent. Spends her days watching television and reading. Experiences occasional constipation. Eats a well-balanced diet and enjoys high-carbohydrate foods such as cookies, candy, and doughnuts because they are easy to chew. Caloric intake is 1800 kcal/day.

OBJECTIVE

Inspection: No clinical signs of nutrient deficiencies.
Anthropometric: Height is 160 cm (63 in). Current weight is 56.8 kg (125 lb); usual weight is 56.8 kg (125 lb), and ideal weight is 56.4 kg (124 lb).
Laboratory: Hemoglobin, hematocrit, and albumin values within normal limits.

ASSESSMENT

Normal nutriture
Constipation related to inactivity and diet high in refined carbohydrates

ABNORMAL FINDINGS

TABLE 11-6 Classification of Malnutrition

Type/Etiology	Clinical Features	Anthropometric Measures	Laboratory Findings
Obesity due to caloric excess refers to weight more than 20% above ideal body weight or body mass index (BMI) of 30.0-39.9. The causes are complex and multifaceted; genetic, social, cultural, pathologic, psychological, and physiologic factors are implicated. Regardless of cause, the underlying problem is usually an imbalance of caloric intake and caloric expenditure. In most cases, a small caloric surplus over a long period results in the extra pounds. Although visceral protein levels are normal in the obese individual, anthropometric measures are above normal.	Obese appearance	Weight >120% standard for height BMI >30 Triceps skinfold (TSF) >10% standard Waist-to-hip ratio >1.0 (men) or >0.8 (women) BMI ≥40 is morbid or extreme obesity (see Table 9-1, p. 131)	Serum cholesterol 200 mg/dL Serum triglycerides >250 mg/dL
Marasmus (protein-calorie malnutrition) is due to inadequate intake of protein and calories or prolonged starvation. Anorexia, bowel obstruction, cancer cachexia, and chronic illness are among the clinical conditions leading to marasmus. Marasmus is characterized by decreased anthropometric measures—weight loss and subcutaneous fat and muscle wasting. Visceral protein levels may remain within normal ranges.	Starved appearance 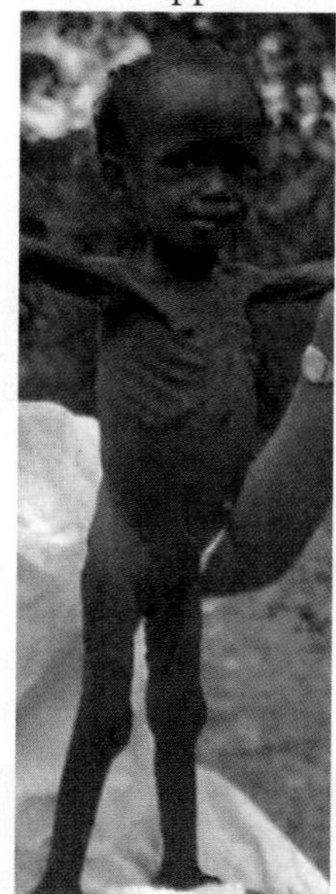	Weight ≤80% standard for height TSF <90% standard Mid–upper arm muscle circumference (MAMC) ≤90% standard	

TABLE 11-6 Classification of Malnutrition—cont'd

Type/Etiology	Clinical Features	Anthropometric Measures	Laboratory Findings
Kwashiorkor (protein malnutrition) is due to diets high in calories but contain little or no protein, e.g., low-protein liquid diets, fad diets, and long-term use of dextrose-containing IV fluids. Individuals with kwashiorkor, in contrast to those with marasmus, have decreased visceral protein levels but adequate anthropometric measures. They may therefore appear well nourished or even obese.	Well-nourished appearance Edematous	Weight ≥100% standard for height TSF ≥100% standard	Serum albumin <3.5 g/dL Serum transferrin <150 mg/dL
Marasmus/kwashiorkor mix is due to prolonged inadequate intake of protein and calories, such as severe starvation and severe catabolic states. This mix combines elements of both marasmus and kwashiorkor. Nutritional assessment findings include muscle, fat, and visceral protein wasting. Individuals have usually undergone acute catabolic stress, such as major surgery, trauma, or burns in combination with prolonged starvation or have AIDS wasting. Without nutritional support, this type of malnutrition is associated with the highest risk for morbidity and mortality.	Emaciated appearance	Weight ≤70% standard TSF ≤80% standard MAMC ≤60% standard	Serum albumin <2.8 g/dL Serum transferrin <100 mg/dL

TABLE 11-7 Abnormalities Due to Nutritional Deficiencies

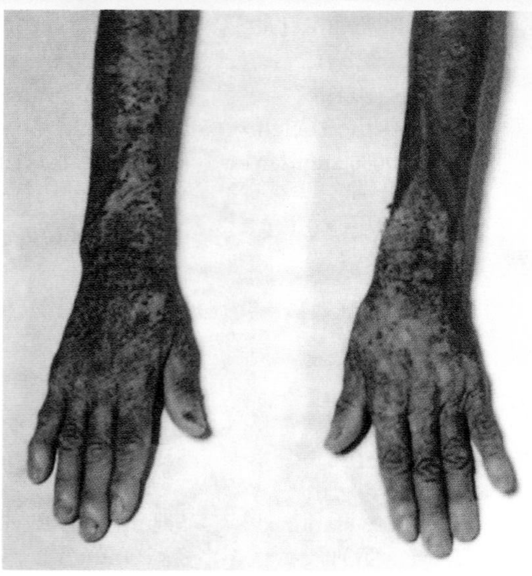

Pellagra

Pigmented keratotic scaling lesions resulting from a deficiency of niacin. These lesions are especially prominent in areas exposed to the sun, such as hands, forearms, neck, and legs.

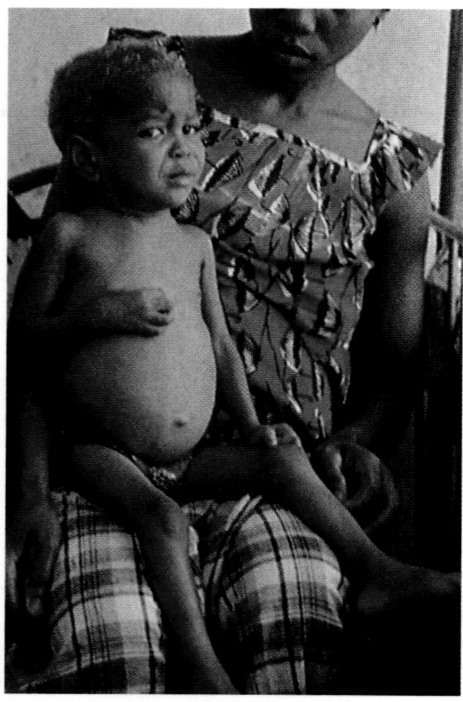

Kwashiorkor

Occurs in children and adults whose diets contain mostly carbohydrate and little or no protein and are under stress (growth, parasitic or viral infections, major surgery, trauma, or burns). Accompanying signs include generalized edema, scaling areas of decreased pigmentation, and decreased hair pigmentation.

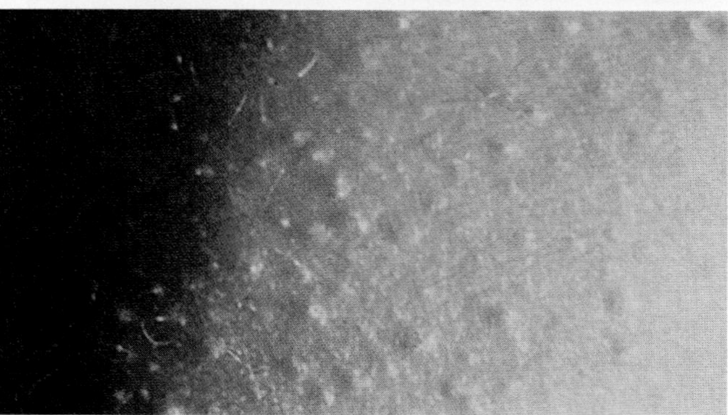

Follicular Hyperkeratosis

Dry, bumpy skin associated with vitamin A and/or linoleic acid (essential fatty acid) deficiency. Linoleic acid deficiency may also result in eczematous skin, especially in infants.

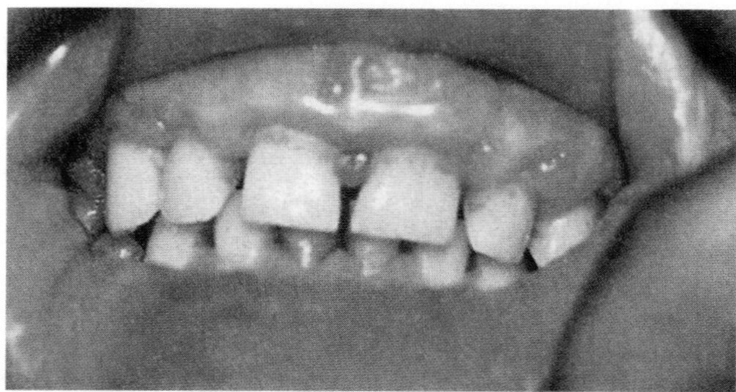

Scorbutic Gums

Deficiency of vitamin C. Gums are swollen, ulcerated, and bleeding due to vitamin C–induced defects in oral epithelial basement membrane and periodontal collagen fiber synthesis.

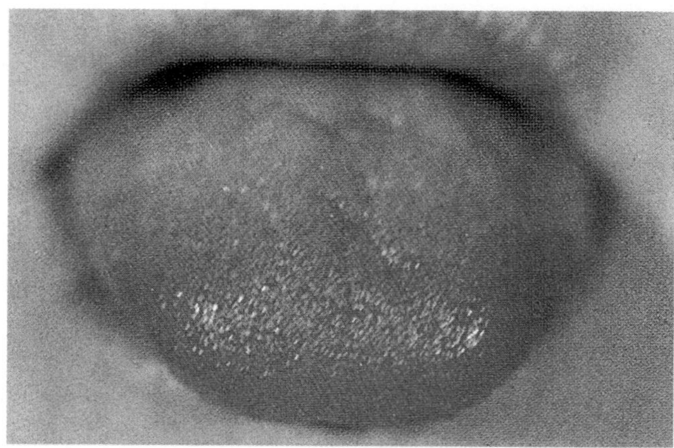

Magenta Tongue

A sign of riboflavin deficiency. In contrast, a pale tongue is probably attributable to iron deficiency; a beefy red–colored tongue is caused by vitamin B–complex deficiency.

TABLE 11-7 Abnormalities Due to Nutritional Deficiencies—cont'd

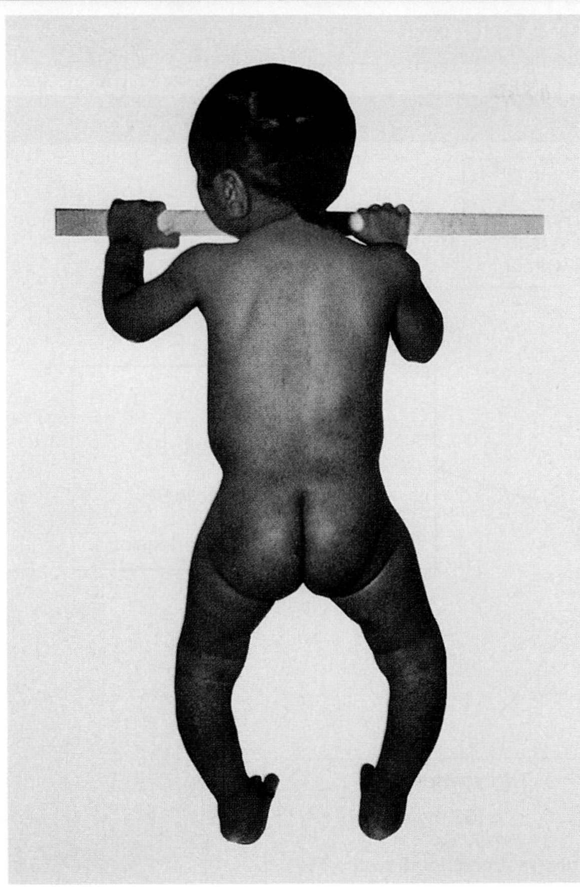

Rickets

Sign of vitamin D and calcium deficiencies in children (disorders of cartilage cell growth, enlargement of epiphyseal growth plates) and adults (osteomalacia).

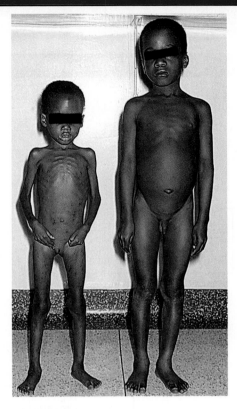

HIV Infection Discordant Twins

An HIV-infected 4½ -year-old girl with her uninfected twin brother. The girl has been sickly since shortly after birth and suffers from HIV-associated malnutrition.

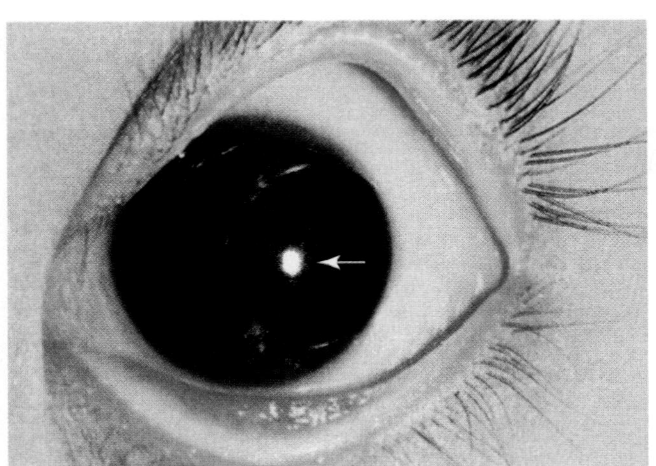

◀ Bitot's Spots

Foamy plaques of the cornea that are a sign of vitamin A deficiency. Severe depletion may result in conjunctival xerosis (drying) and progress to corneal ulceration and, finally, destruction of the eye (keratomalacia).

ABNORMAL FINDINGS FOR ADVANCED PRACTICE

TABLE 11-8 Metabolic Syndrome (MetS)

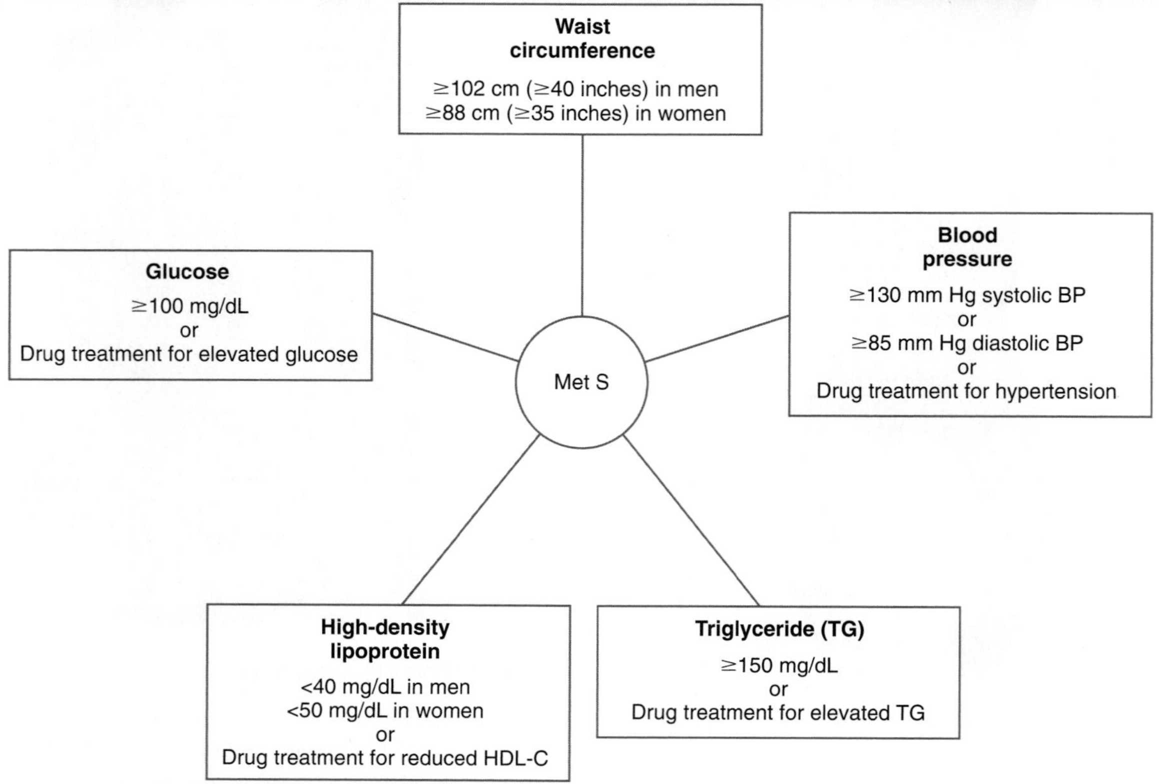

MetS is associated with increased risk for cardiovascular disease, type 2 diabetes mellitus, and mortality, and its prevalence is estimated to be 28% among adolescents and 22% among adults.[13a,37]

Table 11-9 Potential Nutritional Consequences of Bariatric Surgery*† and Related Dietary Changes

Potential Nutritional Consequences	Related Dietary Changes
Malabsorption of protein and calories due to decreased absorptive surface and availability of digestive enzymes	Eating small, nutrient-dense meals
Malabsorption of vitamins and minerals due to achlorhydria or loss of site of absorption	Taking vitamin and mineral supplements
Weight re-gain	Avoiding excessive intake of calorically dense liquids/foods
Obstruction of bypassed sections or pouch	Avoiding chunks of food that could cause blockage

*Vertical and adjustable gastric banding, Roux-en-Y gastric bypass.
†Persons who are 100% or more above ideal body weight or have a BMI ≥40 are categorized as morbidly or extremely obese and are possible candidates for bariatric or weight-loss surgery, as are persons with BMIs ≥35 and comorbid conditions.

BIBLIOGRAPHY

1. Adult Treatment Panel III (ATP III). (2001). Executive summary of the third report of the National Cholesterol Education Program (NCEP) Expert Panel on Detection, Evaluation, and Treatment of High Blood Cholesterol in Adults. *JAMA: The Journal of the American Medical Association, 285*, 2486-2497.
2. Akresh, I. R. (2008). Overweight and obesity among foreign-born and U.S.-born Hispanics. *Biodemography and Social Biology, 54*(2), 183-199.
3. A Scientific Statement from American Heart Association Nutrition Committee of the Council of Nutrition, Physical Activity and Metabolism, Council on Cardiovascular Disease in the Young, Council on Arteriosclerosis, Thrombosis and Vascular Biology, Council on Cardiovascular Nursing, Council on Epidemiology and Prevention, and Council for High Blood Pressure Research. (2009). Implementing American Heart Association pediatric and adult nutrition guidelines. *Circulation, 119*, 1161-1175.
4. Blackburn, G. L., Bistrian, B. R., & Maini, B. S., et al. (1977). Nutritional and metabolic assessment of the hospitalized patient. *JPEN. Journal of Parenteral and Enteral Nutrition, 1*(1), 11-22.
5. Bleyer, A. J., Hire, D., Russell, G. B., et al. (2009). Ethnic variation in the correlation between random serum glucose concentration and glycated haemoglobin. *Diabetic Medicine, 26*(2), 128-133.
6. Centers for Disease Control and Prevention. (2000). *Growth charts.* National Center for Health Statistics in collaboration with the National Center for Chronic Disease Prevention and Health Promotion. Retrieved July 5, 2006, from www.cdc.gov/growth_charts.
7. Centers for Disease Control and Prevention. *Overweight and obesity*. Retrieved July 11, 2009, from www.cdc.gov/obesity/data/index.html.
8. Charney, P., & Malone, A. M. (2009). *ADA pocket guide to nutrition assessment* (2nd ed.). Chicago: American Dietetic Association.

8a. Chernecky, C. C., & Berger, B. J. (2008). *Laboratory tests and diagnostic procedures* (5th ed.). St. Louis: Saunders.

9. Deo, R. C., Reich, D., Tandon, A., et al. (2009). Genetic differences between the determinants of lipid profile phenotypes in African and European Americans: the Jackson Heart Study. *PLoS Genetics, 5*(1), e1000342.
10. Detsky, A. S., McLaughlin, J. R., Baker, J. P., et al. (1987). What is subjective global assessment of nutritional status? *JPEN. Journal of Parenteral and Enteral Nutrition, 11*(1), 8-14.
11. DiMaria-Ghalili, R. A., & Amella, E. (2005). Nutrition in older adults: intervention and assessment can help curb the growing threat of malnutrition. *The American Journal of Nursing, 105*(3), 40-49.
12. Ferguson, M., Capra, S., Bauer, J., & Banks, M. (1999). Development of a valid and reliable malnutrition screening tool for adult acute care hospital patients. *Nutrition, 15*, 458-464.
13. Fischbach, F. T., & Dunning, M. D. (2009). *Manual of laboratory and diagnostic tests* (8th ed.). Philadelphia: Lippincott Williams & Wilkins.

13a. Ford, E. S., Giles, W. H., & Dietz, W. H. (2002). Prevalence of the metabolic syndrome among U.S. adults: findings from the National Health and Nutrition Examination Survey. *JAMA: The Journal of the American Medical Association, 287*, 356-359.

14. Frisancho, A. R. (1984). New standards of weight and body composition by frame size and height for assessment of nutritional status of adults and the elderly. *The American Journal of Clinical Nutrition, 40*, 808-819.
15. Frisancho, A. R. (1990). *Anthropometric standards for the assessment of growth and nutritional status.* Ann Arbor, MI: University of Michigan Press.
16. Frisancho, A. R., & Flegel, P. N. (1983). Elbow breadth as a measure of frame size for U.S. males and females. *The American Journal of Clinical Nutrition, 31*, 311-314.
17. Furman, E. F. (2006). Undernutrition in older adults across the continuum of care: nutritional assessment, barriers, and interventions. *Journal of Gerontological Nursing, 32*(1), 22-27.
18. Gabriella, S. E., & Sinclair, A. J. (1997). Diagnosing undernutrition in elderly people. *Reviews in Clinical Gerontology, 7*, 367-371.
19. Grundy, S. M., Cleeman, J. I., Daniels, S. R., et al. (2005). Diagnosis and management of the metabolic syndrome: an American Heart Association/National Heart, Lung, and Blood Institute scientific statement—Executive Summary. *Circulation, 112*, e285-e290.
20. Jackson, R. T. (1990). Separate hemoglobin standards for blacks and whites: a critical review of the case for separate and unequal hemoglobin standards. *Medical Hypotheses, 32*, 181-189.
21. The Joint Commission. (2009). *Comprehensive accreditation manual for hospitals.* Chicago: Author.
22. Lee, R. D., & Nieman, D. C. (2009). *Nutritional assessment* (5th ed.). New York: McGraw-Hill.
23. National Academy of Sciences, Committee to Reexamine IOM Pregnancy Weight Guidelines, Institute of Medicine, National Research Council, Rasmussen, K. M., & Yaktine, A. L. (Eds.), (2009). *Weight gain during pregnancy: reexamining the guidelines.* Washington, DC: National Academies Press.
24. National Heart, Lung, and Blood Institute, National Institutes of Health, Department of Health and Human Services. Overweight and obesity. Retrieved July 11, 2009, from www.nhlbi.nih.gov/health/dci/Diseases/obe_whatare.html.
25. National Institutes of Health. (2009). *The practical guide: identification, evaluation, and treatment of overweight and obesity in adults (monograph).* Washington, DC: NHLBI Obesity Education Initiative.
26. Niemeier, H. M., Raynor, H. A., Lloyd-Richardson, E. E., et al. (2006). Fast food consumption and breakfast skipping: predictors of weight gain from adolescence to adulthood in a nationally representative sample. *The Journal of Adolescent Health, 29*, 842-849.
27. Ogden, C. L., Carroll, M. D., & Flegal, K. M. (2008). High body mass index for age among U.S. children and adolescents, 2003-2006. *JAMA: The Journal of the American Medical Association, 229*(20), 2401-2405.
28. Pesce-Hammond, K., & Wessel, J. (2005). Nutrition assessment and decision making. In R. Merritt (Ed.), *The A.S.P.E.N. nutrition support practice manual* (2nd ed., pp. 3-26). Silver Spring, MD: The American Society for Parenteral and Enteral Nutrition.
29. Reuben, D. B., Greendale, G. A., & Harrison, G. G. (1995). Nutrition screening in older persons. *Journal of the American Geriatrics Society, 43*(4), 415-425.
30. Silver, H. J. (2009). Oral strategies to supplement older adults' dietary intakes: comparing the evidence. *Nutrition Reviews, 67*(1), 21-31.
31. Trapp, L. W., Ryan, A. A., Ariza, A. J., et al. (2009). Primary care identification of infants at high risk for overweight and obesity. *Clinical Pediatrics, 48*(3), 313-316.
32. U.S. Department of Agriculture, Center for Nutrition Policy and Promotion. (April 2005). *MyPyramid.* Retrieved April 12, 2006, from www.mypyramid.gov.
33. U.S. Department of Agriculture and Department of Health and Human Services. (January 2005). *Dietary guidelines for Americans 2005.* Retrieved April, 12, 2006, from www.health.gov/dietaryguidelines.
34. U.S. Department of Agriculture, Food and Nutrition Information Center. Retrieved July 23, 2009, from http://fnic.nal.usda.gov/nal_display/index.php?info_center=4&tax_level=1&tax_subject= 256.
35. Vartanian, L. R., Schwartz, M. B., & Brownell, K. D. (2007). Effects of soft drink consumption on nutrition and health: a systematic review and meta-analysis. *American Journal of Public Health, 97*, 667-675.

36. Vellas, B., Vellars, H., Abellan, G., et al. (2006). Overview of the MNA®: its history and challenges. *The Journal of Nutrition, Health & Aging, 10*(6), 456-465.
37. Weiss, R., Dziura, J., Burgert, T. S., et al. (2004). Obesity and the metabolic syndrome in children and adolescents. *The New England Journal of Medicine, 350*(23), 2362-2374.

Nutrition-Related Websites

American Cancer Society: www.cancer.org
American Diabetes Association: www.diabetes.org
American Dietetic Association: www.eatright.org
American Heart Association: www.americanheart.org
Centers for Disease Control and Prevention: www.cdc.gov/nccdphp/dnpa/nutrition/index/htm
FDA Food Safety: www.foodsafety.gov
International Food Information Council: www.ific.org/food
Mayo Clinic Food and Nutrition Center: http://mayohealth.org
National Center for Complementary and Alternative Medicine: www.nccam.nih.gov
National Eating Disorders Organization: www.edap.org
National Institutes of Health-Guidelines for Obesity: www.nhlbi.nih.gov/guidelines/obesity/ob_gdlns.htm
USDA Food and Nutrition Information Center: www.nal.usda.gov/fnic/topics_a-z.shtml

Summary Checklist: Nutritional Assessment

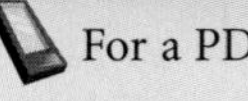
For a PDA-downloadable version, go to http://evolve.elsevier.com/Jarvis/.

1. Obtain a **health history** relevant to nutritional status.
2. Elicit **dietary history**, if indicated.
3. **Inspect** skin, hair, eyes, oral cavity, nails, and musculoskeletal and neurologic systems for clinical signs and symptoms suggestive of nutritional deficiencies.
4. **Measure** height, weight, and other anthropometric parameters, as indicated.
5. Review relevant **laboratory tests.**
6. Offer **health promotion** teaching.

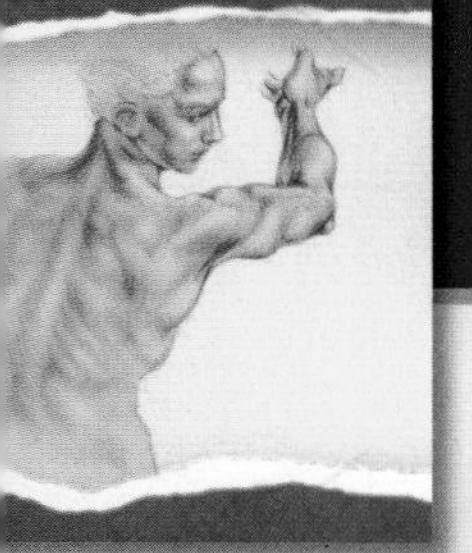

CHAPTER 12

Skin, Hair, and Nails

evolve WEBSITE

http://evolve.elsevier.com/Jarvis/

- Animations
- Audio Key Points
- Bedside Assessment Summary Checklist
- Case Study
  Skin Irritation
  Skin Lesions
- Health Promotion Guide
  Skin Cancer
- Quick Assessment for Common Conditions
  Cellulitis
- NCLEX Review Questions
- Physical Examination Summary Checklist

OUTLINE

Structure and Function, 203

Skin
Epidermal Appendages
Function of the Skin

Subjective Data, 207

Health History Questions

Objective Data, 211

Preparation
Skin
Hair
Nails
Promoting Health and Self-Care

Documentation and Critical Thinking, 227

Abnormal Findings, 229

Abnormal Findings for Advanced Practice, 238

STRUCTURE AND FUNCTION

Think of the skin as the body's largest organ system—it covers 20 square feet of surface area in the average adult. The skin is the sentry that guards the body from environmental stresses (e.g., trauma, pathogens, dirt) and adapts it to other environmental influences (e.g., heat, cold).

SKIN

The skin has two layers—the outer, highly differentiated *epidermis* and the inner, supportive *dermis* (Fig. 12-1). Beneath these layers is a third layer, the *subcutaneous* layer of adipose tissue.

Epidermis

The **epidermis** is thin but tough. Its cells are bound tightly together into sheets that form a rugged protective barrier. It is stratified into several zones. The inner **basal cell layer** forms new skin cells. Their major ingredient is the tough, fibrous protein *keratin.* The melanocytes interspersed along this layer produce the pigment *melanin,* which gives brown tones to the skin and hair. All people have the same number of melanocytes; however, the amount of melanin they produce varies with genetic, hormonal, and environmental influences.

From the basal layer the new cells migrate up and flatten into the outer **horny cell layer.** This consists of dead keratinized cells that are interwoven and closely packed. The cells are constantly being shed, or desquamated, and are replaced with new cells from below. The epidermis is completely replaced every 4 weeks. In fact, each person sheds about 1 pound of skin each year.

The epidermis is uniformly thin except on the surfaces that are exposed to friction, such as the palms and the soles.

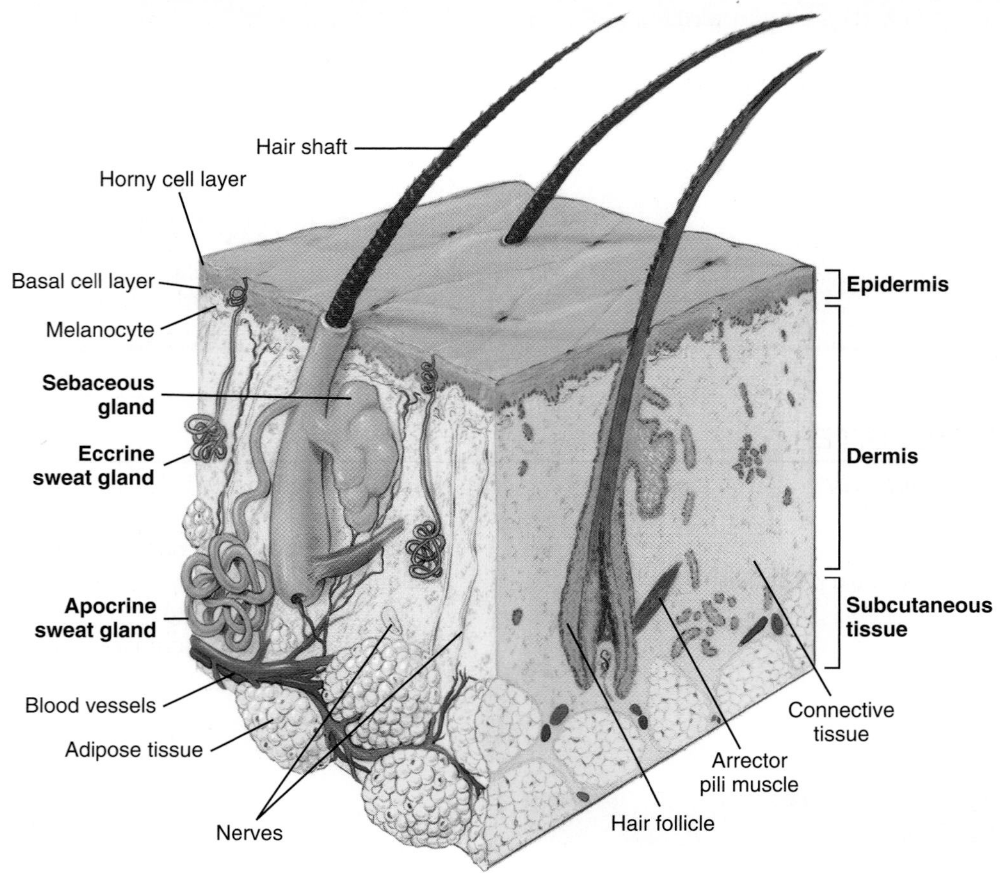

12-1

On these surfaces, skin is thicker because of work and weight bearing. The epidermis is avascular; it is nourished by blood vessels in the dermis below.

Skin color is derived from three sources: (1) mainly from the brown pigment *melanin,* (2) also from the yellow-orange tones of the pigment *carotene,* and (3) from the red-purple tones in the underlying vascular bed. All people have skin of varying shades of brown, yellow, and red; the relative proportion of these shades affects the prevailing color. Skin color is further modified by the thickness of the skin and by the presence of edema.

Dermis

The **dermis** is the inner supportive layer consisting mostly of connective tissue, or *collagen.* This is the tough, fibrous protein that enables the skin to resist tearing. The dermis also has resilient elastic tissue that allows the skin to stretch with body movements. The nerves, sensory receptors, blood vessels, and lymphatics lie in the dermis. Also, appendages from the epidermis—such as the hair follicles, sebaceous glands, and sweat glands—are embedded in the dermis.

Subcutaneous Layer

The *subcutaneous layer* is adipose tissue, which is made up of lobules of fat cells. The subcutaneous tissue stores fat for energy, provides insulation for temperature control, and aids in protection by its soft cushioning effect. Also, the loose subcutaneous layer gives skin its increased mobility over structures underneath.

EPIDERMAL APPENDAGES

These structures are formed by a tubular invagination of the epidermis down into the underlying dermis.

Hair

Hair is *vestigial* for humans; it no longer is needed for protection from cold or trauma. However, hair is highly significant in most cultures for its cosmetic and psychological meaning (see Culture and Genetics, p. 206).

Hairs are threads of keratin. The hair *shaft* is the visible projecting part, and the *root* is below the surface embedded in the follicle. At the root the *bulb matrix* is the expanded area where new cells are produced at a high rate. Hair growth is cyclical, with active and resting phases. Each follicle functions independently so that while some hairs are resting, others are growing. Around the hair follicle are the muscular *arrector pili,* which contract and elevate the hair so that it resembles "goose flesh" when the skin is exposed to cold or in emotional states.

People have two types of hair. Fine, faint **vellus hair** covers most of the body (except the palms and soles, the dorsa of the distal parts of the fingers, the umbilicus, the glans penis, and inside the labia). The other type is **terminal hair,** the darker, thicker hair that grows on the scalp and eyebrows and, after puberty, on the axillae, the pubic area, and the face and chest in the male.

Sebaceous Glands

These glands produce a protective lipid substance, *sebum,* which is secreted through the hair follicles. Sebum oils and lubricates the skin and hair and forms an emulsion with water that retards water loss from the skin. (Dry skin results from loss of water, not directly from loss of oil.) Sebaceous glands are everywhere except on the palms and soles. They are most abundant in the scalp, forehead, face, and chin.

Sweat Glands

There are two types of sweat glands. The **eccrine** glands are coiled tubules that open directly onto the skin surface and produce a dilute saline solution called *sweat.* The evaporation of sweat reduces body temperature. Eccrine glands are widely distributed through the body and are mature in the 2-month-old infant.

The **apocrine** glands produce a thick, milky secretion and open into the hair follicles. They are located mainly in the axillae, anogenital area, nipples, and navel and are vestigial in humans. They become active during puberty, and secretion occurs with emotional and sexual stimulation. Bacterial flora residing on the skin surface react with apocrine sweat to produce a characteristic musky body odor. The functioning of apocrine glands decreases in the aging adult.

Nails

The nails are hard plates of keratin on the dorsal edges of the fingers and toes (Fig. 12-2). The nail plate is clear, with fine longitudinal ridges that become prominent in aging. Nails take their pink color from the underlying nail bed of highly vascular epithelial cells. The lunula is the white, opaque, semilunar area at the proximal end of the nail. It lies over the nail matrix where new keratinized cells are formed. The nail folds overlap the posterior and lateral borders. The cuticle works like a gasket to cover and protect the nail matrix.

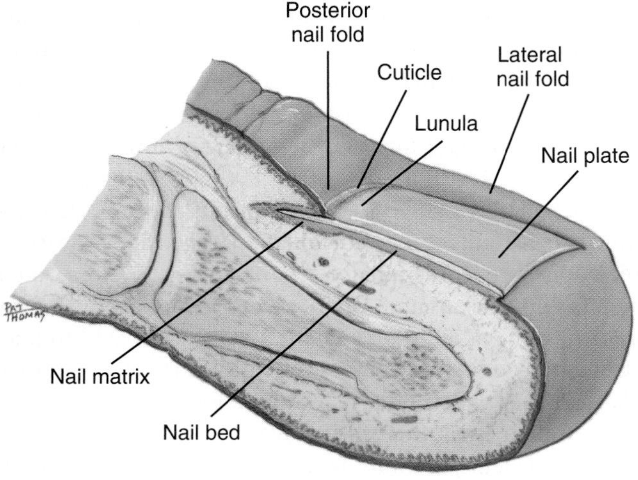

12-2

FUNCTION OF THE SKIN

The skin is a waterproof, almost indestructible, covering that has protective and adaptive properties:

- **Protection.** Skin minimizes injury from physical, chemical, thermal, and light-wave sources.
- **Prevents penetration.** Skin is a barrier that stops invasion of microorganisms and loss of water and electrolytes from within the body.
- **Perception.** Skin is a vast sensory surface holding the neurosensory end-organs for touch, pain, temperature, and pressure.
- **Temperature regulation.** Skin allows heat dissipation through sweat glands and heat storage through subcutaneous insulation.
- **Identification.** People identify one another by unique combinations of facial characteristics, hair, skin color, and even fingerprints. Self-image is often enhanced or deterred by the way society's standards of beauty measure up to each person's perceived characteristics.
- **Communication.** Emotions are expressed in the sign language of the face and in the body posture. Vascular mechanisms such as blushing or blanching also signal emotional states.
- **Wound repair.** Skin allows cell replacement of surface wounds.
- **Absorption and excretion.** Skin allows limited excretion of some metabolic wastes, byproducts of cellular decomposition such as minerals, sugars, amino acids, cholesterol, uric acid, and urea.
- **Production of vitamin D.** The skin is the surface on which ultraviolet light converts cholesterol into vitamin D.

DEVELOPMENTAL COMPETENCE

Infants and Children

The hair follicles develop in the fetus at 3 months' gestation; by midgestation, most of the skin is covered with **lanugo,** the fine downy hair of the newborn infant. In the first few months after birth, this is replaced by fine vellus hair. Terminal hair on the scalp, if present at birth, tends to be soft and to suffer a patchy loss, especially at the temples and occiput. Also present at birth is **vernix caseosa,** the thick, cheesy substance made up of sebum and shed epithelial cells.

The newborn's skin is similar in structure to the adult's, but many of its functions are not fully developed. The newborn's skin is thin, smooth, and elastic and is relatively more permeable than that of the adult, so the infant is at greater risk for fluid loss. Sebum, which holds water in the skin, is present for the first few weeks of life, producing milia (see p. 222) and cradle cap in some babies. Then sebaceous glands decrease in size and production and do not resume functioning until puberty. Temperature regulation is ineffective. Eccrine sweat glands do not secrete in response to heat until the first few months of life and then only minimally throughout childhood. The skin cannot protect much against cold because it cannot contract and shiver and because the subcutaneous layer is inefficient. Also, the pigment system is inefficient at birth.

As the child grows, the epidermis thickens, toughens, and darkens and the skin becomes better lubricated. Hair growth accelerates. At puberty, secretion from apocrine sweat glands increases in response to heat and emotional stimuli, producing body odor. Sebaceous glands become more active—the skin looks oily, and acne develops. Subcutaneous fat deposits increase, especially in females.

Secondary sex characteristics that appear during adolescence are evident in the integument (i.e., skin). In the female, the diameter of the areola enlarges and darkens and breast tissue develops. Coarse pubic hair develops in males and females, then axillary hair, and then coarse facial hair in males.

The Pregnant Woman

The change in hormone levels results in increased pigment in the areolae and nipples, vulva, and sometimes in the midline of the abdomen (**linea nigra**) or in the face (**chloasma**). Hyperestrogenemia probably also causes the common vascular spiders and palmar erythema. Connective tissue develops increased fragility, resulting in **striae gravidarum** (stretch marks), which may develop in the skin of the abdomen, breasts, or thighs. Metabolism is increased in pregnancy; as a way to dissipate heat, the peripheral vasculature dilates and the sweat and sebaceous glands increase secretion. Fat deposits are laid down, particularly in the buttocks and hips, as maternal reserves for the nursing baby.

The Aging Adult

The skin is a mirror that reflects aging changes that proceed in *all* our organ systems; it just happens to be the one organ we can view directly. The aging process carries a slow atrophy of skin structures. The aging skin loses its elasticity; it folds and sags. By the 70s to 80s, it looks parchment thin, lax, dry, and wrinkled.

The epidermis's outer layer thins and flattens. This allows chemicals easier access into the body. Wrinkling occurs because the underlying dermis thins and flattens. A loss of elastin, collagen, and subcutaneous fat occurs as well as a reduction in muscle tone. The loss of collagen increases the risk for shearing, tearing injuries.

Sweat glands and sebaceous glands decrease in number and function, leaving dry skin. Decreased response of the sweat glands to thermoregulatory demand also puts the aging person at greater risk for heat stroke. The vascularity of the skin diminishes while the vascular fragility increases; a minor trauma may produce dark red discolored areas, or **senile purpura.**

Sun exposure and cigarette smoking further accentuate aging changes in the skin. Coarse wrinkling, decreased elasticity, atrophy, speckled and uneven coloring, more pigment changes, and a yellowed, leathery texture occur. Chronic sun damage is even more prominent in pale or light-skinned persons.

An accumulation of factors place the aging person at risk for skin disease and breakdown: the thinning of the skin, the decrease in vascularity and nutrients, the loss of protective cushioning of the subcutaneous layer, a lifetime of environmental trauma to skin, the social changes of aging (e.g., less nutrition, limited financial resources), the increasingly sedentary lifestyle, and the chance of immobility. When skin breakdown does occur, subsequent cell replacement is slower and wound healing is delayed.

In the aging hair matrix, the number of functioning melanocytes decreases, so the hair looks gray or white and feels thin and fine. A person's genetic script determines the onset of graying and the number of gray hairs. Hair distribution changes. Males may have a symmetric W-shaped balding in the frontal areas. Some testosterone is present in both males and females; as it decreases with age, axillary and pubic hair decrease. As the female's estrogen also decreases, testosterone is unopposed and the female may have some bristly facial hairs. Nails grow more slowly. Their surface is lusterless and is characterized by longitudinal ridges resulting from local trauma at the nail matrix.

Because the aging changes in the skin and hair can be viewed directly, they carry a profound psychological impact. For many people, self-esteem is linked to a youthful appearance. This view is compounded by media advertising in Western society. Although sagging and wrinkling skin and graying and thinning hair are normal processes of aging, they prompt a loss of self-esteem for many adults.

CULTURE AND GENETICS

Awareness of normal biocultural differences and the ability to recognize the unique clinical manifestations of disease are especially important for darkly pigmented people. As described earlier, melanin is responsible for the various colors and tones of skin observed among people. Melanin protects the skin against harmful ultraviolet rays, a genetic advantage accounting for the lower incidence of skin cancer among darkly pigmented Blacks and American Indians. The incidence of melanoma is 20 times higher among whites than among Blacks and 4 times higher among whites than among Hispanics.[25]

The apocrine and eccrine sweat glands are important for fluid balance and for thermoregulation. When apocrine gland secretions are contaminated by normal skin flora, odor results. Most Asians and American Indians have a mild body odor or none at all, whereas whites and Blacks tend to have strong body odor. The amount of chloride excreted by sweat glands varies widely, and Blacks have lower salt concentrations in their sweat than whites do.

In Arctic regions, Inuits have made an interesting environmental adaptation; they sweat less than whites on their trunks and extremities but more on their faces. This adaptation allows for temperature regulation without causing perspiration and dampness of their clothes, which would decrease their ability to insulate against severe cold weather and would pose a serious threat to their survival.

There are several skin conditions found among Blacks:

1. Keloids—scars that form at the site of a wound and grow beyond the normal boundaries of the wound (see p. 235)
2. Areas of either postinflammatory hypopigmentation or hyperpigmentation that appear as dark or light spots
3. Pseudofolliculitis—"razor bumps" or "ingrown hairs" caused by shaving too closely with an electric razor or straight razor
4. Melasma—the "mask of pregnancy," a patchy tan to dark brown discoloration of the face

Perhaps one of the most obvious and widely variable racial differences occurs with the hair. The hair of Blacks varies widely in texture. It is very fragile and ranges from long and straight to short, spiraled, thick, and kinky. The hair and scalp have a natural tendency to be dry and require daily combing, gentle brushing, and the application of oil. Hair care products designed to care specifically for kinky hair should be available in clinical settings. In comparison, people of Asian backgrounds generally have straight, silky hair.

Hair condition is significant in diagnosing and treating certain disease states. For example, hair texture becomes dry, brittle, and lusterless with inadequate nutrition. The hair of Black children with severe malnutrition (e.g., marasmus) frequently changes not only in texture but also in color. The child's hair often becomes less kinky and assumes a copper-red color.

SUBJECTIVE DATA

1. Past history of skin disease (allergies, hives, psoriasis, eczema)
2. Change in pigmentation
3. Change in mole (size or color)
4. Excessive dryness or moisture
5. Pruritus
6. Excessive bruising
7. Rash or lesion
8. Medications
9. Hair loss
10. Change in nails
11. Environmental or occupational hazards
12. Self-care behaviors

Examiner Asks	Rationale
1. **Past history of skin disease.** Any past skin disease or problem? • How was this treated? • Any family history of allergies or allergic skin problem? • Any known allergies to drugs, plants, animals? • Any birthmarks, tattoos?	Significant familial predisposition: allergies, hay fever, psoriasis, atopic dermatitis (eczema), acne. Identify offending allergen. Use of nonsterile equipment to apply tattoos increases risk for hepatitis C.
2. **Change in pigmentation.** Any **change in skin color** or **pigmentation?** • A generalized color change (all over), or localized?	Hypopigmentation (loss of color); hyperpigmentation (increase in color). Generalized change suggests systemic illness: pallor, jaundice, cyanosis.
3. **Change in mole.** Any **change in a mole:** color, size, shape, sudden appearance of tenderness, bleeding, itching? • Any "sores" that do not heal?	Signs suggest neoplasm in pigmented nevus. May be unaware of change in nevus on back or buttocks that he or she cannot see.
4. **Excessive dryness or moisture.** Any change in the feel of your skin: temperature, **moisture,** texture? • Any excess **dryness?** Is this seasonal or constant?	Seborrhea—oily. Xerosis—dry.
5. **Pruritus.** Any skin itching? Is this mild (prickling, tingling) or intense (intolerable)? • Does it awaken you from sleep?	Pruritus is the most common skin symptom; occurs with dry skin, aging, drug reactions, allergy, obstructive jaundice, uremia, lice.

Examiner Asks	Rationale
• Where is the itching? When did it start?	Presence or absence of pruritus helps diagnosis. Scratching causes excoriation of primary lesion.
• Any other skin pain or soreness? Where?	
6. Excessive bruising. Any excess **bruising?** Where on the body? • How did this happen? • How long have you had it?	Multiple cuts and bruises, bruises in various stages of healing, bruises above knees and elbows, and illogical explanation—consider physical abuse. Frequent falls may be due to dizziness of neurologic or cardiovascular origin. Also, frequent minor trauma may be a side effect of alcoholism or other drug abuse.
7. Rash or lesion. Any skin **rash** or **lesion**? • Onset. When did you first notice it?	Rashes are a common cause of seeking health care. A careful history is important; it may predict the type of lesion you will see in the examination and its cause.
• Location. Where did it start?	Identify the primary site—it may give clue to cause.
• Where did it spread?	Migration pattern, evolution.
• Character or quality. Describe the color. • Is it raised or flat? Any crust, odor? Does it feel tender, warm? • Duration. How long have you had it?	
• Setting. Anyone at home or work with a similar rash? Have you been camping, acquired a new pet, tried a new food, drug? Does the rash seem to come with stress?	Identify new or relevant exposure, any household or social contacts with similar symptoms.
• Alleviating and aggravating factors. What home care have you tried? Bath, lotions, heat? Do they help, or make it worse? • Associated symptoms. Any itching, fever?	Myriad over-the-counter remedies are available. People try them and seek professional help only when they do not work.
• What do you think rash/lesion means?	Assess person's perception of cause: fear of cancer, tick-borne illnesses, or sexually transmitted infections.
• Coping strategies. How has rash/lesion affected your self-care, hygiene, ability to function at work/home/socially?	Assess effectiveness of coping strategies. Chronic skin diseases may increase risk for loss of self-esteem, social isolation, and anxiety.
• Any new or increased stress in your life?	Stress can exacerbate chronic skin illness.
8. Medications. What **medications** do you take? • Prescription and over-the-counter? • Recent change?	Drugs may cause allergic skin eruption: aspirin, antibiotics, barbiturates, some tonics. Drugs may increase sunlight sensitivity and give burn response: sulfonamides, thiazide diuretics, oral hypoglycemic agents, and tetracycline. Drugs can cause hyperpigmentation: antimalarials, antineoplastic agents, hormones, metals, tetracycline.
• How long on medication?	Even after a long time on medication, a person may develop sensitivity.
9. Hair loss. Any recent **hair loss?** • A gradual or sudden onset? Symmetric? Associated with fever, illness, increased stress?	**Alopecia** is a significant loss. A full head of hair equates with vitality in many cultures. If treated as a trivial problem, the person may seek alternative, unproven methods of treatment.

Examiner Asks	Rationale
• Any unusual hair growth? • Any recent change in texture, appearance?	**Hirsutism** is shaggy or excessive hair.
10. Change in nails. Any **change in nails:** shape, color, brittleness? Do you tend to bite or chew nails?	
11. Environmental or occupational hazards. Any **environmental** or **occupational** hazards? • With your occupation, such as dyes, toxic chemicals, radiation? • How about hobbies? Do you perform any household or furniture repair work? • How much sun exposure do you get from outdoor work, leisure activities, sunbathing, tanning salons?	Majority of skin neoplasms result from occupational or environmental agents. People at risk: outdoor sports enthusiasts, farmers, sailors, outdoor workers; also creosote workers, roofers, coal workers. Unprotected sun exposure accelerates aging and produces lesions. At more risk: light-skinned people, those older than 40 years, and those regularly in sun.
• Recently been bitten by insect: bee, tick, mosquito?	Identify contactants that produce lesions or contact dermatitis.
• Any recent exposure to plants, animals in yard work, camping?	Tell people with chronic recurrent urticaria (hives) to keep diary of meals and environment to identify precipitating factors.
12. Self-care behaviors. What do you do to care for your skin, hair, nails? What cosmetics, soaps, chemicals do you use? • Clip cuticles on nails, use adhesive for false fingernails? • If you have allergies, how do you control your environment to minimize exposure? • Do you perform a skin self-examination?	Assess **self-care** and influence on self-concept—may be important with this society's media stress on high norms of beauty. Many over-the-counter remedies are costly and exacerbate skin problems.
Additional History for Infants and Children	
1. Does the child have any birthmarks?	
2. Was there any change in skin color as a newborn? • Any jaundice? Which day after birth? • Any cyanosis? What were the circumstances?	Physiologic jaundice, see p. 222.
3. Have you noted any rash or sores? What seems to bring it on? • Have you introduced a new food or formula? When? Does your child eat chocolate, cow's milk, eggs?	Generalized rash—consider allergic reaction to new food. Irritability and general fussiness may indicate the presence of pruritus.
4. Does the child have any diaper rash? How do you care for this? How do you wash diapers? How often do you change diapers? How do you clean skin?	Occlusive diapers or infrequent changing may cause rash. Infant may be allergic to certain detergent or to disposable wipes.
5. Does the child have any burns or bruises? • Where? • How did it happen?	A careful history can distinguish expected childhood bumps and bruises from any lesion that indicates child abuse or neglect: cigarette burns; excessive bruising, especially above knees or elbows; linear whip marks. With abuse, the history often will not coincide with the physical appearance and location of lesion.

Examiner Asks	Rationale
6. Has the child had any exposure to contagious skin conditions: scabies, impetigo, lice? Or to communicable diseases: measles, chickenpox, scarlet fever? Or to toxic plants: poison ivy? • Are the child's vaccinations up-to-date?	
7. Does the child have any habits or habitual movements, such as nail-biting, twisting hair, rubbing head on mattress?	
8. What steps are taken to protect the child from sun exposure? What about sunscreens and sunblocks? How do you treat a sunburn?	Excessive sun exposure, especially severe or blistering sunburns in childhood, increases risk for melanoma in later life.[9]

Additional History for the Adolescent

Examiner Asks	Rationale
1. Have you noticed any skin problems such as pimples, blackheads? • How long have you had them? • How do you treat this? • How do you feel about it?	About 70% of teens will have acne; the psychological effect is more significant than the physical effect. Self-treatment is common. Many myths surround the cause. Cause is unknown; acne is not caused by poor diet, oily complexion, or contagion.

Additional History for the Aging Adult

Examiner Asks	Rationale
1. What changes have you noticed in your skin in the past few years?	Assess impact of aging on self-concept. Normal aging changes may cause distress. Many "aging" changes are due to chronic sun damage. Most skin cancers appear in aging people, although sun damage begins decades earlier.
2. Any delay in wound healing? • Any skin itching?	Pruritus is common with aging. Consider side effects of medicine or systemic disease (e.g., liver or kidney disease, cancer, lymphoma), but senile pruritus is usually due to dry skin **(xerosis).** Exacerbated by too-frequent bathing or use of soap. Scratching with dirty, jagged fingernails produces excoriations.
3. Any other skin pain?	Some diseases, such as herpes zoster (shingles), produce more intense sensations of pain, itching in aging people. Other diseases (e.g., diabetes) may reduce pain sensation in extremities. Also, some aging people tolerate chronic pain as "part of growing old" and hesitate to "complain."
4. Any change in feet, toenails? Any bunions? Is it possible to wear shoes?	Some aging people cannot reach down to their feet to give self-care.
5. Do you fall frequently?	Multiple bruises, trauma from falls.
6. Any history of diabetes, peripheral vascular disease?	Risk for skin lesions in feet or ankles.

Examiner Asks	Rationale
7. What do you do to care for your skin?	A bland lotion is important to retain moisture in aging skin. Dermatitis may ensue from certain cosmetics, creams, ointments, and dyes applied to achieve a youthful appearance. Aging skin has a delayed inflammatory response when exposed to irritants. If the person is not alerted by warning signs (e.g., pruritus, redness), exposure may continue and dermatitis may ensue.

OBJECTIVE DATA

PREPARATION

Try to control external variables that may influence skin color and confuse your findings, both in light-skinned and in dark-skinned persons (Table 12-1).

Learn to consciously attend to skin characteristics. The danger is one of omission. You grow so accustomed to seeing the skin that you are likely to ignore it as you assess the organ systems underneath. Yet the skin holds information about the body's circulation, nutritional status, and signs of systemic diseases as well as topical data on the integument itself.

Know the person's normal skin coloring. Baseline knowledge is important to assess color or pigment changes. If this is the first time you are examining the person, ask about his or her usual skin color and about any self-monitoring practices.

The Complete Physical Examination. Although it is presented alone in this chapter, skin assessment is integrated throughout the complete examination; it is not a separate step. At the beginning of the examination, assessing the person's hands and fingernails is a nonthreatening way to accustom him or her to your touch. Most people are used to having relative strangers shake their hands or touch their arms. As you move through the examination, scrutinize the outer skin surface first before you concentrate on the underlying structures. Separate intertriginous areas (areas with skinfolds) such as under large breasts, obese abdomen, and the groin and inspect them thoroughly. These areas are dark, warm, and moist and provide the perfect conditions for irritation or infection. Last, always remove the person's socks and inspect the feet, the toenails, and the folds between the toes.

EQUIPMENT NEEDED

Strong direct lighting (natural daylight is ideal to evaluate skin characteristics, but halogen light will suffice)
Small centimeter ruler
Penlight
Gloves
Needed for special procedures:
- Wood's light (filtered ultraviolet light)
- Magnifying glass, for minute lesions

TABLE 12-1 External Variables Influencing Skin Color

Variable		Causes		Misleading Outcome
Emotions				
Fear, anger	→	Peripheral vasoconstriction	→	False pallor
Embarrassment	→	Flushing in face and neck	→	False erythema
Environment				
Hot room	→	Vasodilation	→	False erythema
Chilly or air-conditioned room	→	Vasoconstriction	→	False pallor, coolness
Cigarette smoking	→	Vasoconstriction	→	False pallor
Physical				
Prolonged elevation	→	Decreased arterial perfusion	→	Pallor, coolness
Dependent position	→	Venous pooling	→	Redness, warmth, distended veins
Immobilization, prolonged inactivity	→	Slowed circulation	→	Pallor, coolness, nail beds pale, prolonged capillary filling time

The Regional Examination. At times, your assessment will be focused on the skin alone. Help the person remove clothing, and assess the skin as one entity. Stand back at first to get an overall impression; this helps reveal distribution patterns. Then inspect lesions carefully. With a skin rash, check all areas of the body because some locations the person cannot see. You cannot rely on the history alone that the rash is limited to one location. Inspect mucous membranes, too, because some disorders have characteristic lesions here.

The skills used are inspection and palpation because some skin changes have accompanying signs that can be felt.

Normal Range of Findings	Abnormal Findings

INSPECT AND PALPATE THE SKIN

Color

General Pigmentation. Observe the skin tone. Normally it is even and consistent with genetic background. It varies from pinkish tan to ruddy dark tan or from light to dark brown and may have yellow or olive overtones. Dark-skinned people normally have areas of lighter pigmentation on the palms, nail beds, and lips (Fig. 12-3, *A*).

An acquired condition is **vitiligo,** the complete absence of melanin pigment in patchy areas of white or light skin on the face, neck, hands, feet, body folds, and around orifices (Fig. 12-3, *B*). Vitiligo can occur in all races, although dark-skinned people are more severely affected and potentially suffer a greater threat to their body image.

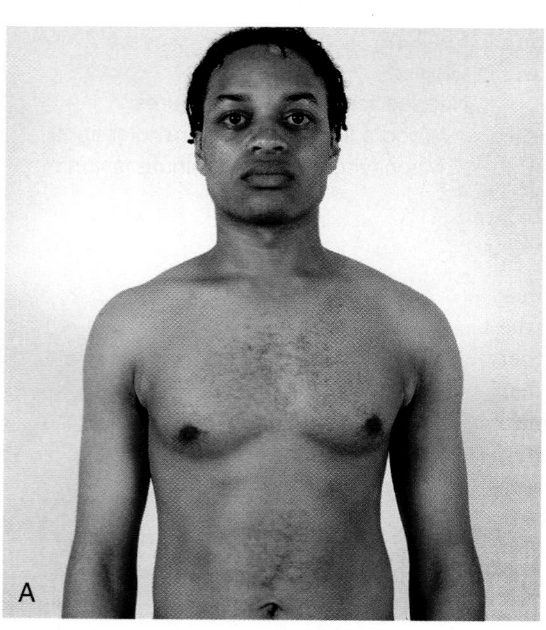

12-3 **A,** Even skin tone.

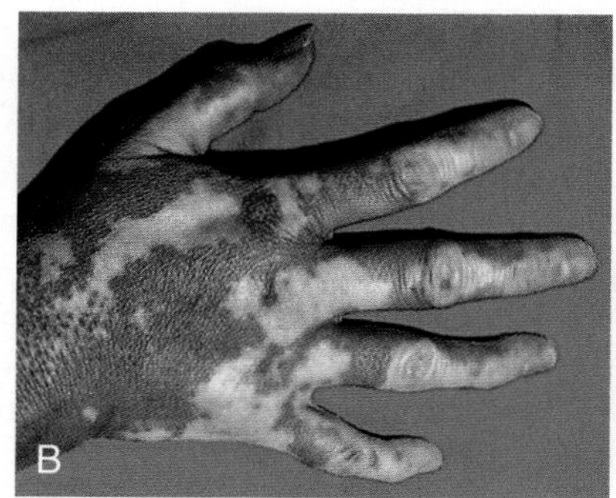

12-3 **B,** Vitiligo.

General pigmentation is darker in sun-exposed areas. Common (benign) pigmented areas also occur:

- **Freckles** (ephelides)—small, flat macules of brown melanin pigment that occur on sun-exposed skin (Fig. 12-4, *A*).
- **Mole** (nevus)—a proliferation of melanocytes, tan to brown color, flat or raised. Acquired nevi are characterized by their symmetry, small size (6 mm or less), smooth borders, and single uniform pigmentation. The **junctional nevus** (Fig. 12-4, *B*) is macular only and occurs in children and adolescents. It progresses to the **compound nevi** in young adults (Fig. 12-4, *C*) that are macular and papular. The intradermal nevus (mainly in older age) has nevus cells in only the dermis.

Danger signs: abnormal characteristics of pigmented lesions are summarized in the mnemonic **ABCDE:**

Asymmetry (*not* regularly round or oval, two halves of lesion do not look the same)

Border irregularity (notching, scalloping, ragged edges, poorly defined margins)

Color variation (areas of brown, tan, black, blue, red, white, or combination)

Normal Range of Findings

- **Birthmarks**—may be tan to brown in color.

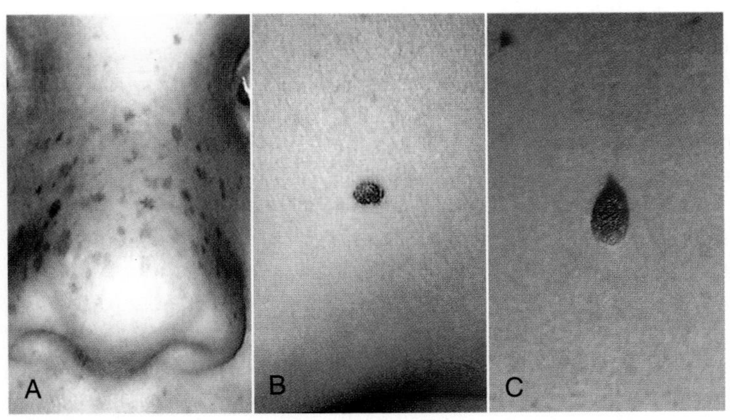

12-4 **A,** Freckles. **B,** Junctional nevus. **C,** Compound nevus.

Widespread Color Change. Note any color change over the entire body skin, such as pallor (white), erythema (red), cyanosis (blue), and jaundice (yellow). Note whether the color change is transient and expected or whether it is due to pathology.

In dark-skinned people, the amount of normal pigment may mask color changes. Lips and nail beds show some color change, but they vary with the person's skin color and may not always be accurate signs. The more reliable sites are those with the least pigmentation, such as under the tongue, the buccal mucosa, the palpebral conjunctiva, and the sclera. See Table 12-2 for specific clues to assessment.

Pallor. When the red-pink tones from the oxygenated hemoglobin in the blood are lost, the skin takes on the color of connective tissue (collagen), which is mostly white. Pallor is common in acute high-stress states, such as anxiety or fear, because of the powerful peripheral vasoconstriction from sympathetic nervous system stimulation. The skin also looks pale with vasoconstriction from exposure to cold and cigarette smoking, and in the presence of edema.

Look for pallor in dark-skinned people by the absence of the underlying red tones that normally give brown or black skin its luster. The brown-skinned individual has a more yellowish brown color, and the black-skinned person will appear ashen or gray. Generalized pallor can be observed in the mucous membranes, lips, and nail beds. The palpebral conjunctiva and nail beds are preferred sites for assessing the pallor of anemia. When inspecting the conjunctiva, lower the lid sufficiently to visualize the conjunctiva near the *outer* canthus as well as the inner canthus. The coloration is often lighter near the inner canthus.

Erythema. Erythema is an intense redness of the skin from excess blood (hyperemia) in the dilated superficial capillaries. This sign is *expected* with fever, with local inflammation, or with emotional reactions such as blushing in vascular flush areas (cheeks, neck, and upper chest).

The erythema with fever or localized inflammation has an increased skin temperature from the increased rate of blood flow. Because you cannot see

Abnormal Findings

Diameter greater than 6 mm (i.e., the size of a pencil eraser), although early melanomas may be diagnosed at a smaller size[25]

Elevation or **E**nlargement

Additional symptoms: rapidly changing lesion, a new pigmented lesion, and development of itching, burning, or bleeding in a mole. Any of these signs should raise suspicion of malignant melanoma and warrant referral.

Ashen gray color in dark skin or marked pallor in light skin occurs with anemia, shock, arterial insufficiency (see Table 12-2, Detecting Color Changes in Light and in Dark Skin, p. 229).

The pallor of impending shock presents with rapid pulse rate, oliguria, apprehension, and restlessness.

Chronic iron deficiency anemia may show "spoon" nails, with a concave shape. Fatigue, exertional dyspnea, rapid pulse, dizziness, and impaired mental function accompany most severe anemias.

Erythema occurs with polycythemia, venous stasis, carbon monoxide poisoning, and the extravascular presence of red blood cells (petechiae, ecchymosis, hematoma) (see Table 12-2 and Table 12-8, Vascular Lesions).

Normal Range of Findings	Abnormal Findings

inflammation in dark-skinned persons, it is necessary to palpate the skin for increased warmth, taut or tightly pulled surfaces that may be indicative of edema, and hardening of deep tissues or blood vessels.

Cyanosis. This is a bluish mottled color that signifies decreased perfusion; the tissues do not have enough oxygenated blood. Be aware that cyanosis can be a nonspecific sign. A person who is anemic could have hypoxemia without ever looking blue, because not enough hemoglobin is present (either oxygenated or reduced) to color the skin. On the other hand, a person with polycythemia (an increase in the number of red blood cells) looks ruddy blue at all times and may not necessarily be hypoxemic. This person just cannot fully oxygenate the massive numbers of red blood cells. Last, do not confuse cyanosis with the common and normal bluish tone on the lips of dark-skinned persons of Mediterranean origin.

Cyanosis is difficult to observe in darkly pigmented persons (see Table 12-2). Given that most conditions causing cyanosis also cause decreased oxygenation of the brain, other clinical signs—such as changes in level of consciousness and signs of respiratory distress—will be evident.

Cyanosis indicates hypoxemia and occurs with shock, heart failure, chronic bronchitis, and congenital heart disease.

Jaundice. A yellowish skin color indicates rising amounts of bilirubin in the blood. Except for physiologic jaundice in the newborn (p. 222), jaundice does not occur normally. Jaundice is *first* noted in the junction of the hard and soft palate in the mouth and in the sclera. But do not confuse scleral jaundice with the normal yellow subconjunctival fatty deposits that are common in the outer sclera of dark-skinned persons. The scleral yellow of jaundice extends up to the edge of the iris.

Jaundice occurs with hepatitis, cirrhosis, sickle-cell disease, transfusion reaction, and hemolytic disease of the newborn.

As levels of serum bilirubin rise, jaundice is evident in the skin over the rest of the body. This is best assessed in direct natural daylight. Common calluses on palms and soles often look yellow—do not interpret these as jaundice.

Light or clay-colored stools and dark golden urine often accompany jaundice in both light- and dark-skinned people.

Temperature

Note the temperature of your own hands. Then use the backs (dorsa) of your hands to palpate the person and check bilaterally. The skin should be warm, and the temperature should be equal bilaterally; warmth suggests normal circulatory status. Hands and feet may be slightly cooler in a cool environment.

Hypothermia. Generalized coolness may be induced, such as in hypothermia used for surgery or high fever. Localized coolness is expected with an immobilized extremity, as when a limb is in a cast or with an intravenous infusion.

General hypothermia accompanies central circulatory problem such as shock.

Localized hypothermia occurs in peripheral arterial insufficiency and Raynaud's disease.

Hyperthermia. Generalized hyperthermia occurs with an increased metabolic rate, such as in fever or after heavy exercise. A localized area feels hyperthermic with trauma, infection, or sunburn.

Hyperthyroidism has an increased metabolic rate, causing warm, moist skin.

Moisture

Perspiration appears normally on the face, hands, axilla, and skinfolds in response to activity, a warm environment, or anxiety. **Diaphoresis,** or profuse perspiration, accompanies an increased metabolic rate, such as occurs in heavy activity or fever.

Diaphoresis occurs with thyrotoxicosis and with stimulation of the nervous system with anxiety or pain.

Look for **dehydration** in the oral mucous membranes. Normally there is none, and the mucous membranes look smooth and moist. Be aware that dark skin may normally look dry and flaky, but this does not necessarily indicate systemic dehydration.

With dehydration, mucous membranes are dry, and lips look parched and cracked. With extreme dryness, the skin is fissured, resembling cracks in a dry lake bed.

Normal Range of Findings	Abnormal Findings

Texture

Normal skin feels smooth and firm, with an even surface.

Hyperthyroidism—skin feels smoother and softer, like velvet.

Hypothyroidism—skin feels rough, dry, and flaky.

Thickness

The epidermis is uniformly thin over most of the body, although thickened callus areas are normal on palms and soles. A callus is a circumscribed overgrowth of epidermis and is an adaptation to excessive pressure from the friction of work and weight bearing.

Very thin, shiny skin (atrophic) occurs with arterial insufficiency.

Edema

Edema is fluid accumulating in the intercellular spaces; it is not present normally. To check for edema, imprint your thumbs firmly against the ankle malleolus or the tibia. Normally the skin surface stays smooth. If your pressure leaves a dent in the skin, "pitting" edema is present. Its presence is graded on a four-point scale:

1+ Mild pitting, slight indentation, no perceptible swelling of the leg
2+ Moderate pitting, indentation subsides rapidly
3+ Deep pitting, indentation remains for a short time, leg looks swollen
4+ Very deep pitting, indentation lasts a long time, leg is very swollen

This scale is somewhat subjective; outcomes vary among examiners (see further content on grading scale in Chapter 20).

Edema masks normal skin color and obscures pathologic conditions such as jaundice or cyanosis because the fluid lies *between* the surface and the pigmented and vascular layers. It makes dark skin look lighter.

Edema is most evident in dependent parts of the body (feet, ankles, and sacral areas), where the skin looks puffy and tight. Edema makes the hair follicles more prominent, so you note a pigskin or orange-peel look (called **peau d'orange**).

Unilateral edema—consider a local or peripheral cause.

Bilateral edema or edema that is generalized over the whole body **(anasarca)**—consider a central problem such as heart failure or kidney failure.

Mobility and Turgor

Pinch up a large fold of skin on the anterior chest under the clavicle (Fig. 12-5). Mobility is the skin's ease of rising, and turgor is its ability to return to place promptly when released. This reflects the elasticity of the skin.

Mobility is decreased with edema.

Poor turgor is evident in severe dehydration or extreme weight loss; the pinched skin recedes slowly or "tents" and stands by itself.

Scleroderma, literally "hard skin," is a chronic connective tissue disorder associated with decreased mobility (see Table 13-5, p. 277).

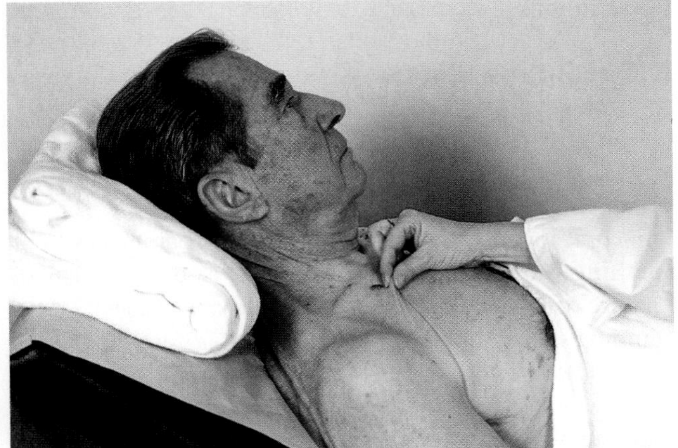

12-5

Objective Data

Normal Range of Findings

Abnormal Findings

Vascularity or Bruising

Cherry (senile) angiomas are small (1 to 5 mm), smooth, slightly raised bright red dots that commonly appear on the trunk in all adults older than 30 years (Fig. 12-6). They normally increase in size and number with aging and are not significant.

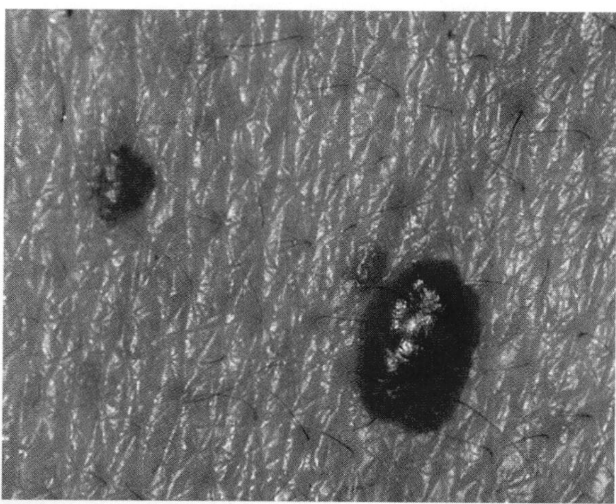

12-6 Cherry angioma.

Any bruising (contusion) should be consistent with the expected trauma of life. There are normally no venous dilations or varicosities.

Multiple bruises at different stages of healing and excessive bruises above knees or elbows raise concern about physical abuse (see Table 12-7, Lesions Caused by Trauma or Abuse).

Document the presence of any tattoos (a permanent skin design from indelible pigment) on the person's chart. Advise the person that the use of tattoo needles and tattoo parlor equipment of doubtful sterility increases the risk for hepatitis C.

Needle marks or tracks from intravenous injection of street drugs may be visible on the antecubital fossae, forearms, or on any available vein.

Lesions

If any lesions are present, note the:

1. Color.
2. Elevation: flat, raised, or pedunculated.
3. Pattern or shape: the grouping or distinctness of each lesion (e.g., annular, grouped, confluent, linear). The pattern may be characteristic of a certain disease.
4. Size, in centimeters: Use a ruler to measure. Avoid household descriptions such as "quarter size" or "pea size."
5. Location and distribution on body: Is it generalized or localized to area of a specific irritant; around jewelry, watchband, around eyes?
6. Any exudate. Note its color and any odor.

Lesions are traumatic or pathologic changes in previously normal structures. When a lesion develops on previously unaltered skin, it is **primary.** However, when a lesion changes over time or changes because of a factor such as scratching or infection, it is **secondary.** Study Table 12-3 for the shapes and Tables 12-4 and 12-5 for the characteristics of primary and secondary skin lesions. The terms used (e.g., *macule, papule*) are helpful to describe any lesion you encounter.

Note the pattern and characteristics of common skin lesions (see Table 12-10) and malignant skin lesions (Table 12-11).

Palpate lesions. Wear a glove if you anticipate contact with blood, mucosa, any body fluid, or skin lesion. Roll a nodule between the thumb and index finger to assess depth. Gently scrape a scale to see if it comes off. Note the nature of its base or whether it bleeds when the scale comes off. Note the surrounding skin temperature. However, the erythema associated with rashes is not always accompanied by noticeable increases in skin temperature.

Does the lesion blanch with pressure or stretch? Stretching the area of skin between your thumb and index finger decreases (blanches) the normal

Normal Range of Findings

underlying red tones, thus providing more contrast and brightening the macules. Red macules from dilated blood vessels *will* blanch momentarily, whereas those from extravasated blood (petechiae) do not. Blanching also helps identify a macular rash in dark-skinned people.

Use a magnifier and light for closer inspection of the lesion (Fig. 12-7). Use a Wood's light (i.e., an ultraviolet light filtered through a special glass) to detect fluorescing lesions. With the room darkened, shine the Wood's light on the area.

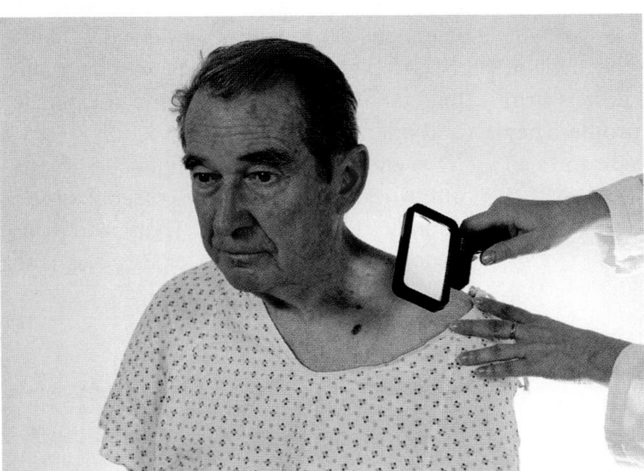

12-7

INSPECT AND PALPATE THE HAIR

Color

Hair color comes from melanin production and may vary from pale blonde to total black. Graying begins as early as the third decade of life because of reduced melanin production in the follicles. Genetic factors affect the onset of graying.

Texture

Scalp hair may be fine or thick and may look straight, curly, or kinky. It should look shiny, although this characteristic may be lost with the use of some beauty products such as dyes, rinses, or permanents.

Distribution

Fine vellus hair coats the body, whereas coarser terminal hairs grow at the eyebrows, eyelashes, and scalp. During puberty, distribution conforms to normal male and female patterns. At first, coarse curly hairs develop in the pubic area, then in the axillae, and last in the facial area in boys. In the genital area, the female pattern is an inverted triangle; the male pattern is an upright triangle with pubic hair extending up to the umbilicus. In Asians, body hair may be diminished.

Lesions

Separate the hair into sections and lift it, observing the scalp. With a history of itching, inspect the hair behind the ears and in the occipital area as well. All areas should be clean and free of any lesions or pest inhabitants. Many people normally have seborrhea (dandruff), which is indicated by loose white flakes.

Abnormal Findings

Under the Wood's light, lesions with blue-green fluorescence indicate fungal infection (e.g., tinea capitis [scalp ringworm]).

Note dull, coarse, or brittle scalp hair.

Gray, scaly, well-defined areas with broken hairs accompany tinea capitis, a ringworm infection found mostly in school-age children (see Table 12-12).

Absent or sparse genital hair suggests endocrine abnormalities.

Hirsutism—excess body hair. In females, this forms a male pattern on the face and chest and indicates endocrine abnormalities (see Table 12-12).

Head or pubic lice. Distinguish dandruff from nits (eggs) of lice, which are oval, adherent to hair shaft, and cause intense itching (see Table 12-12).

Normal Range of Findings | Abnormal Findings

INSPECT AND PALPATE THE NAILS

Shape and Contour

The nail surface is normally slightly curved or flat, and the posterior and lateral nail folds are smooth and rounded. Nail edges are smooth, rounded, and clean, suggesting adequate self-care.

Jagged nails, bitten to the quick, or traumatized nail folds suggest nervous picking habits.

Chronically dirty nails suggest poor self-care or some occupations in which it is impossible to keep them clean.

The Profile Sign. View the index finger at its profile and note the angle of the nail base; it should be about 160 degrees (Fig. 12-8). The nail base is firm to palpation. Curved nails are a variation of normal with a convex profile. They may look like clubbed nails, but notice that the angle between nail base and nail is normal (i.e., 160 degrees or less).

Clubbing of nails occurs with congenital cyanotic heart disease and neoplastic and pulmonary diseases.

In early clubbing, the angle straightens out to 180 degrees and the nail base feels spongy to palpation. Then the nail becomes convex as the digit grows (see Late Clubbing, p. 249).

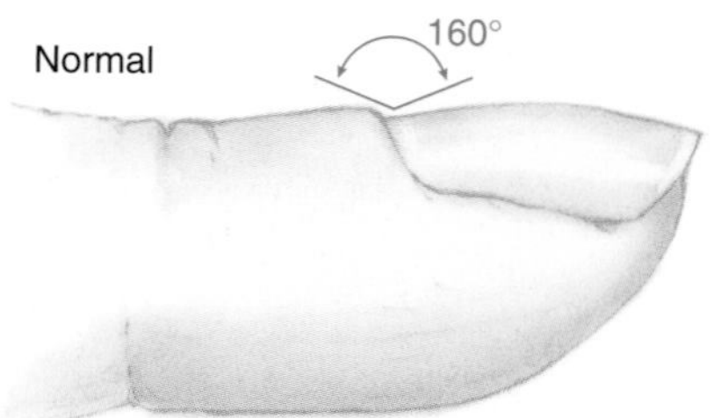

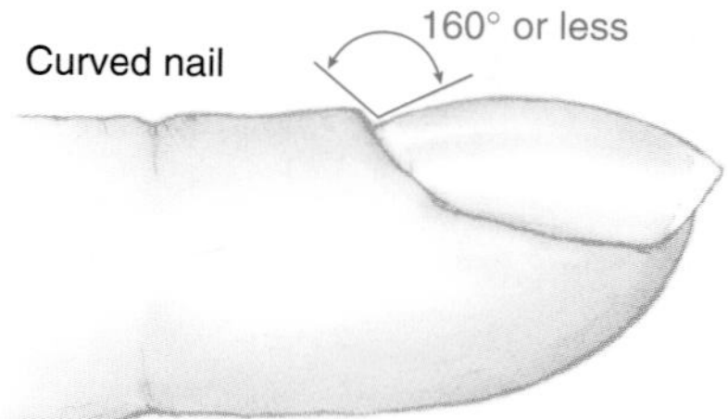

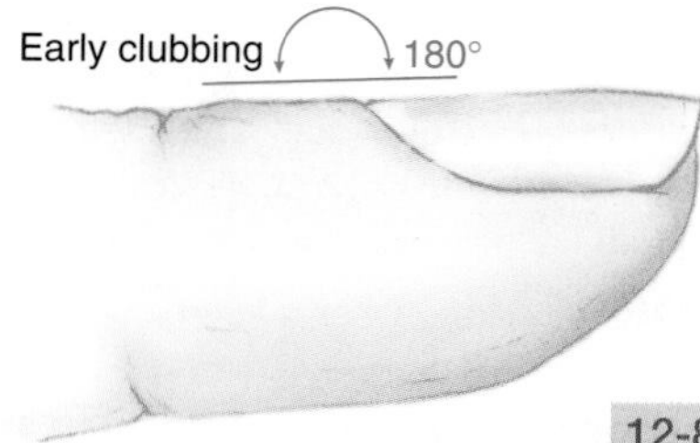

12-8

Consistency

The surface is smooth and regular, not brittle or splitting.

Pits, transverse grooves, or lines may indicate a nutrient deficiency or may accompany acute illness that disturbs nail growth (see Table 12-13, Abnormal Conditions of the Nails).

Nail thickness is uniform.

Nails are thickened and ridged with arterial insufficiency.

The nail firmly adheres to the nail bed, and the nail base is firm to palpation.

A spongy nail base accompanies clubbing.

Color

The translucent nail plate is a window to the even, pink nail bed underneath.

Cyanosis or marked pallor.

Dark-skinned people may have brown-black pigmented areas or linear bands or streaks along the nail edge (Fig. 12-9). All people normally may have white hairline linear markings from trauma or picking at the cuticle (Fig. 12-10). Note any abnormal marking in the nail beds.

Brown linear streaks (especially sudden appearance) are abnormal in light-skinned people and may indicate melanoma.

Splinter hemorrhages, transverse ridges, or Beau's lines (see Table 12-13).

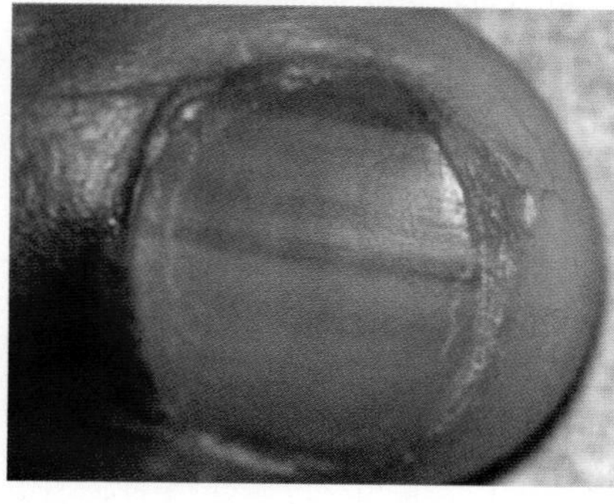

12-9 Linear pigmentation.

Normal Range of Findings

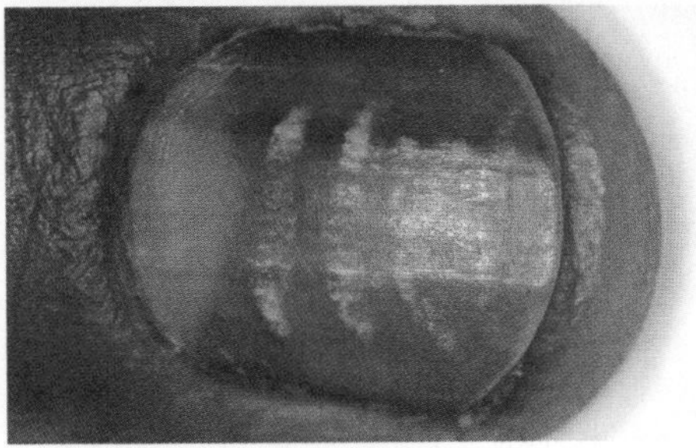

12-10 Leukonychia striata.

Capillary Refill. Depress the nail edge to blanch and then release, noting the return of color. Normally, color return is instant, or at least within a few seconds in a cold environment. This indicates the status of the peripheral circulation. A sluggish color return takes longer than 1 or 2 seconds.

Inspect the toenails. Separate the toes and note the smooth skin in between.

Abnormal Findings

Cyanotic nail beds or sluggish color return: consider cardiovascular or respiratory dysfunction.

PROMOTING HEALTH AND SELF-CARE

Teach Skin Self-Examination

Teach all adults to examine their skin once a month, using the ABCDE rule (see pp. 212-213) to raise warning signals of any suspicious lesions. Use a well-lighted room that has a full-length mirror. It helps to have a small handheld mirror. Ask a family member to search skin areas difficult to see (e.g., behind ears, back of neck, back). Follow the sequence outlined in Fig. 12-11, and report any suspicious lesions promptly to a physician or nurse.

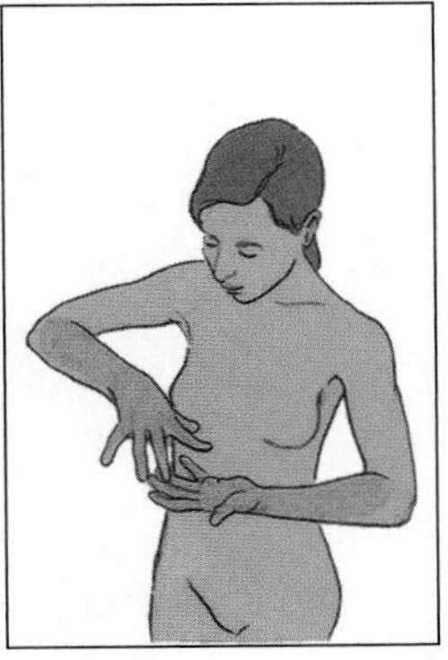

1. Undress completely. Check forearms, palms, space between fingers. Turn over hands and study the backs.

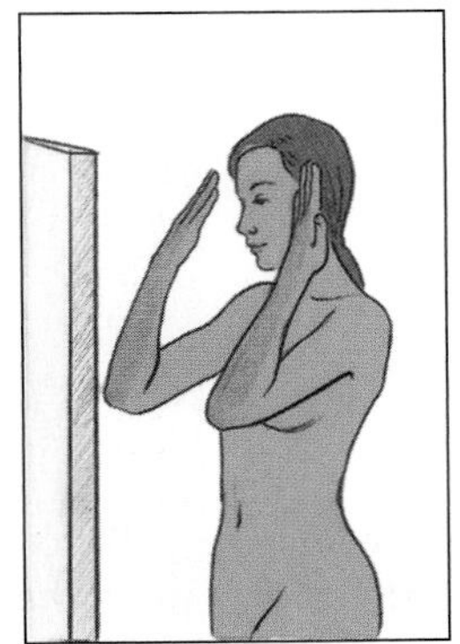

2. Face mirror; bend arms at elbow. Study arms in mirror.

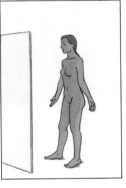

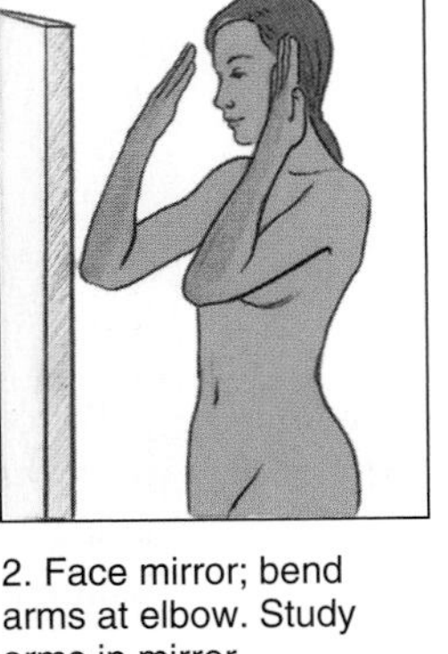

3. Face mirror and study entire front of body. Start at face, neck, torso, working down to lower legs.

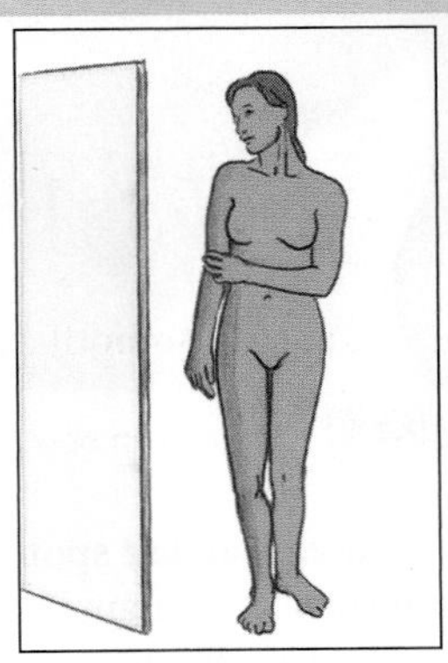

4. Pivot to right side facing mirror. Study sides of upper arms, working down to ankles. Repeat with left side.

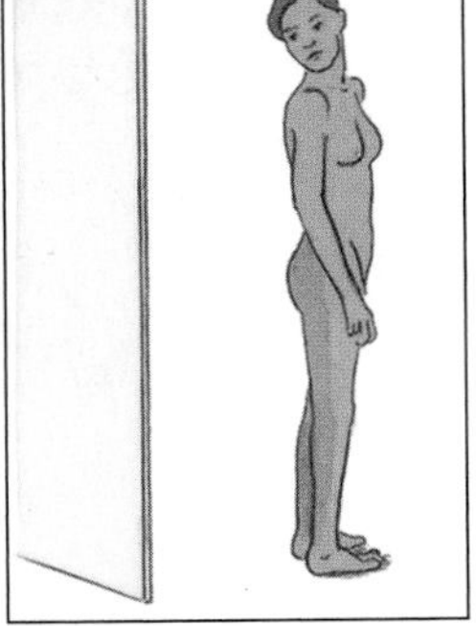

5. With back to mirror, study buttocks, thighs, lower legs.

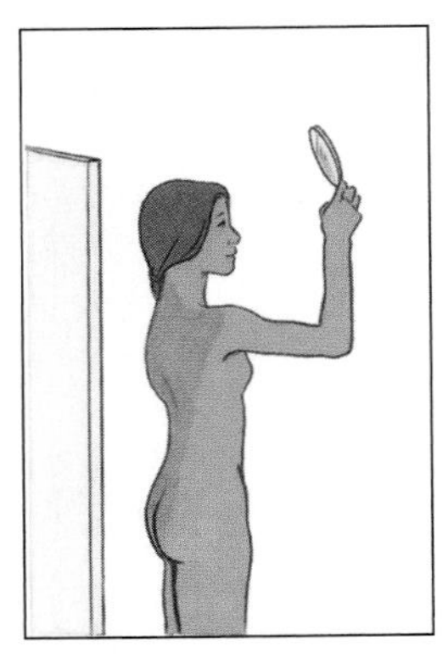

6. Use the handheld mirror to study upper back.

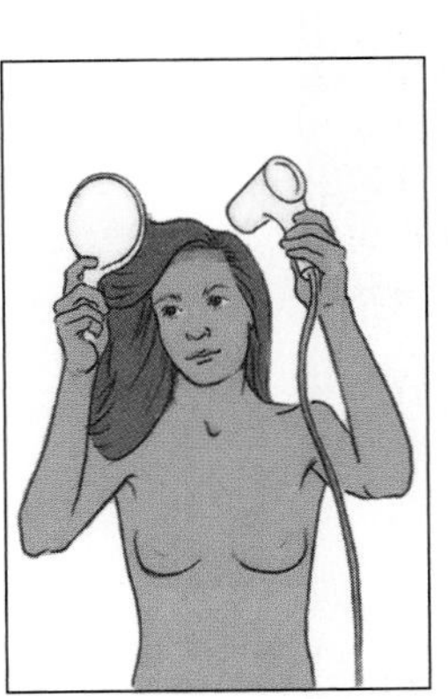

7. Use the handheld mirror to study scalp, lifting the hair. A blow-dryer on a cool setting helps to lift hair.

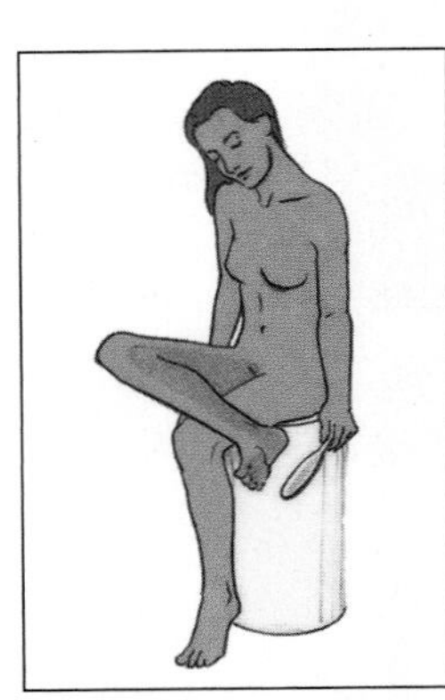

8. Sit on chair or bed. Study insides of each leg and soles of feet. Use the small mirror to help.

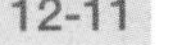

12-11 Skin self-examination.

Normal Range of Findings

Abnormal Findings

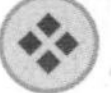

DEVELOPMENTAL COMPETENCE

Infants

Skin Color—General Pigmentation. Black newborns initially have lighter-toned skin than their parents because of a pigment function that is not yet in full production. Their full melanotic color is evident in the nail beds and scrotal folds. The **mongolian spot** is a common variation of hyperpigmentation in Black, Asian, American Indian, and Hispanic newborns (Fig. 12-12). It is a blue-black to purple macular area at the sacrum or buttocks but sometimes on the abdomen, thighs, shoulders, or arms. It is due to deep dermal melanocytes. It gradually fades during the first year. By adulthood, these spots are lighter but are frequently still visible. Mongolian spots are present in 90% of Blacks, 80% of Asians and American Indians, and 9% of whites. If you are unfamiliar with mongolian spots, be careful not to confuse them with bruises. Recognition of this normal variation is particularly important when dealing with children who might be erroneously identified as victims of child abuse.

Bruising is a common soft tissue injury that follows a rapid, traumatic, or breech birth.

Multiple bruises in various stages of healing or pattern injury suggests child abuse (see Table 12-7).

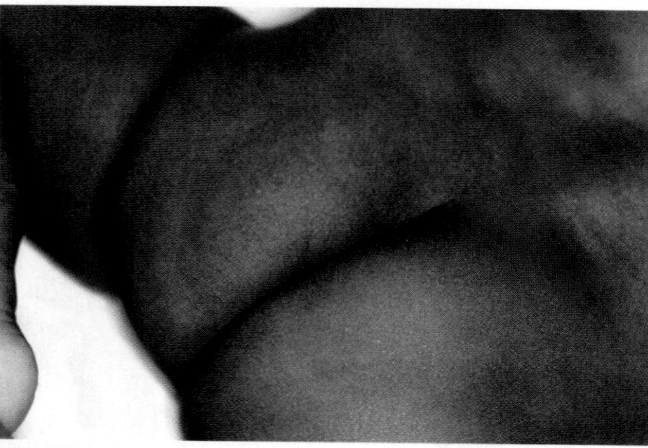

12-12 Mongolian spot.

The **café au lait spot** is a large round or oval patch of light brown pigmentation (hence, the name "coffee with milk"), which is usually present at birth (Fig. 12-13). Usually these patches are normal.

Six or more café au lait macules, each more than 1.5 cm in diameter, are diagnostic of neurofibromatosis, an inherited neurocutaneous disease.

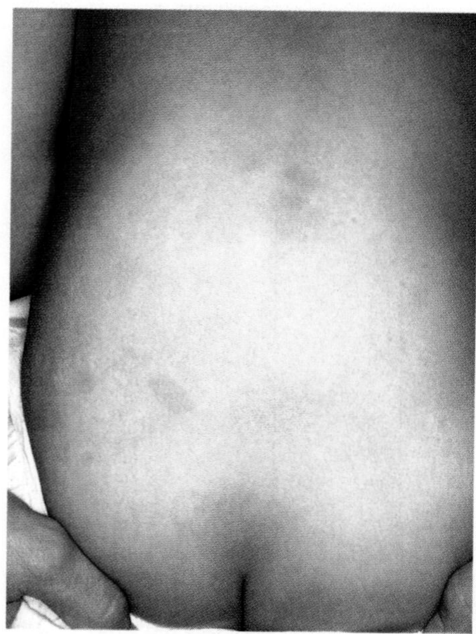

12-13 Café au lait spot.

Objective Data

Normal Range of Findings

Skin Color Change. Three erythematous states are common variations in the neonate:

1. The newborn's skin has a beefy red flush for the first 24 hours because of vasomotor instability; then the color fades to its normal color.
2. Another finding, the **harlequin color change,** occurs when the baby is in a side-lying position. The lower half of the body turns red and the upper half blanches with a distinct demarcation line down the midline. The cause is unknown, and its occurrence is transient.
3. Finally, **erythema toxicum** is a common rash that appears in the first 3 to 4 days of life. Sometimes called the "flea bite" rash or newborn rash, it consists of tiny punctate red macules and papules on the cheeks, trunk, chest, back, and buttocks (Fig. 12-14). The cause is unknown; no treatment is needed.

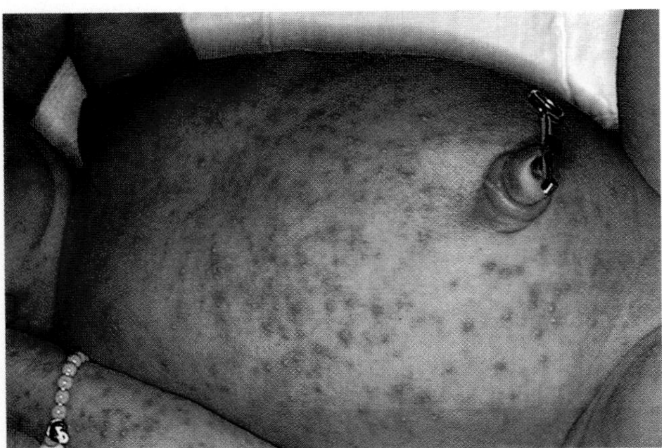

12-14 Erythema toxicum.

Two temporary cyanotic conditions may occur:

1. A newborn may have **acrocyanosis,** a bluish color around the lips, hands and fingernails, and feet and toenails. This may last for a few hours and disappear with warming.
2. **Cutis marmorata** is a transient mottling in the trunk and extremities in response to cooler room temperatures (Fig. 12-15). It forms a reticulated red or blue pattern over the skin.

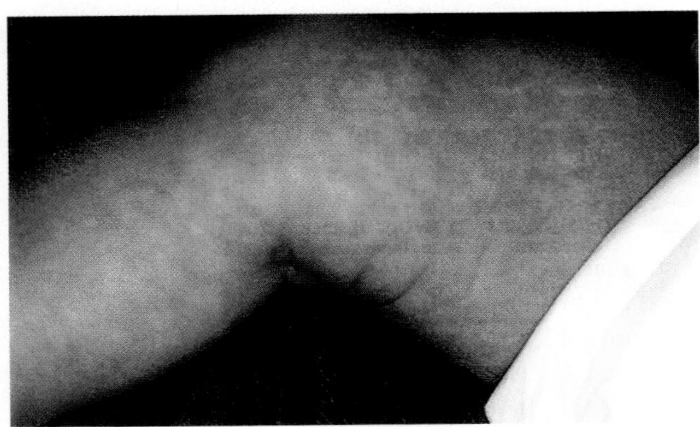

12-15 Cutis marmorata.

Abnormal Findings

Persistent generalized cyanosis indicates distress, such as cyanotic congenital heart disease.

Persistent or pronounced cutis marmorata occurs with Down syndrome or prematurity.

Green-brown discoloration of the skin, nails, and cord occurs with passing of meconium in utero, indicating fetal distress.

Normal Range of Findings

Physiologic jaundice is a common variation in about half of all newborns. A yellowing of the skin, sclera, and mucous membranes develops after the 3rd or 4th day of life because of the increased numbers of red blood cells that hemolyze after birth. The hemoglobin in the red blood cells is metabolized by the liver and spleen; its pigment is converted into bilirubin.

Carotenemia also produces a yellow-orange color in light-skinned persons but no yellowing in the sclera or mucous membranes. It comes from ingesting large amounts of foods containing carotene, a vitamin A precursor. Carotene-rich foods are popular as prepared infant foods, and the absorption of carotene is enhanced by mashing, pureeing, and cooking. The color is best seen on the palms and soles, the forehead, tip of the nose and nasolabial folds, the chin, behind the ears, and over the knuckles; it fades to normal color within 2 to 6 weeks of withdrawing carotene-rich foods from the diet.

Moisture. The vernix caseosa is the moist, white, cream cheese–like substance that covers part of the skin in all newborns. Perspiration is present after 1 month of age.

Texture. A common variation occurring in the infant is **milia** (Fig. 12-16). Milia are tiny while papules on the cheeks and forehead and across the nose and chin caused by sebum that occludes the opening of the follicles. Tell parents not to squeeze the lesions; milia resolve spontaneously within a few weeks.

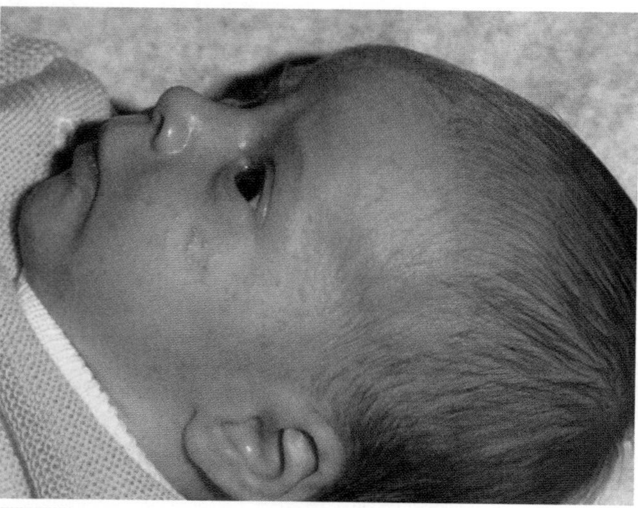

12-16 Milia.

Thickness. In the neonate, the epidermis is normally thin, but you will also note well-defined areas of subcutaneous fat. The baby's skin dimples over joints, but there is no break in the skin. Check for any defect or break in the skin, especially over the length of the spine.

Mobility and Turgor. Test mobility and turgor over the abdomen in an infant.

Vascularity or Bruising. Some vascular markings are common birthmarks in the newborn. A **storkbite** (salmon patch) is a flat, irregularly shaped red or pink patch found on the forehead, eyelid, or upper lip but most commonly at the back of the neck (nuchal area) (Fig. 12-17). It is present at birth and usually fades during the first year.

Abnormal Findings

Jaundice on the first day of life may indicate hemolytic disease. Jaundice after 2 weeks of age may indicate biliary tract obstruction.

Green-tinged vernix occurs with meconium staining.

In children, excessive sweating may accompany hypoglycemia, heart disease, or hyperthyroidism.

Lack of subcutaneous fat occurs in prematurity and malnutrition.

A red sacrococcygeal dimple occurs with a pilonidal cyst or sinus (see Table 25-1 on p. 720).

Poor turgor, or "tenting," indicates dehydration, especially combined with delayed capillary refill and tachypnea. Also occurs with malnutrition.

Port-wine stain, strawberry mark (immature hemangioma), cavernous hemangioma (see Table 12-8, Vascular Lesions).

Bruising may suggest abuse (see Table 12-7).

Normal Range of Findings	Abnormal Findings

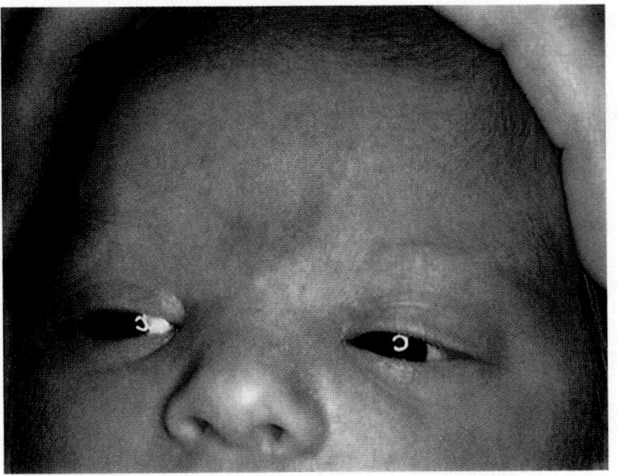

12-17 Storkbite.

Hair. A newborn's skin is covered with fine downy lanugo (Fig. 12-18), especially in a preterm infant. Dark-skinned newborns have more lanugo than lighter-skinned newborns. Scalp hair may be lost in the few weeks after birth, especially at the temples and occiput. It grows back slowly.

Scaly, crusted scalp occurs with seborrheic dermatitis, "cradle cap" (see Table 12-12).

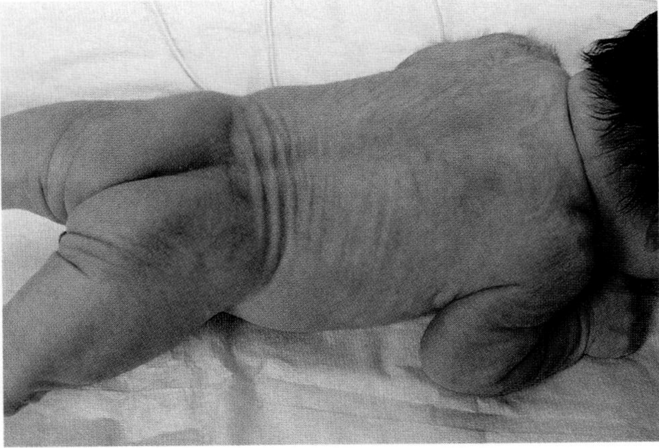

12-18 Lanugo.

Nails. A newborn's nail beds may be blue (cyanotic) for the first few hours of life; then they turn pink.

Adolescents

The increase in sebaceous gland activity creates increased oiliness and **acne.** Acne is the most common skin problem of adolescence. Almost all teens have some acne, even in the milder form of open comedones (blackheads) (Fig. 12-19, *A*) and closed comedones (whiteheads). Severe acne includes papules, pustules, and nodules (Fig. 12-19, *B*). Acne lesions usually appear on the face and sometimes on the chest, back, and shoulders. Acne may appear in children as early as 7 to 8 years of age; then the lesions increase in number and severity and peak at 14 to 16 years in girls and at 16 to 19 years in boys.

Normal Range of Findings | Abnormal Findings

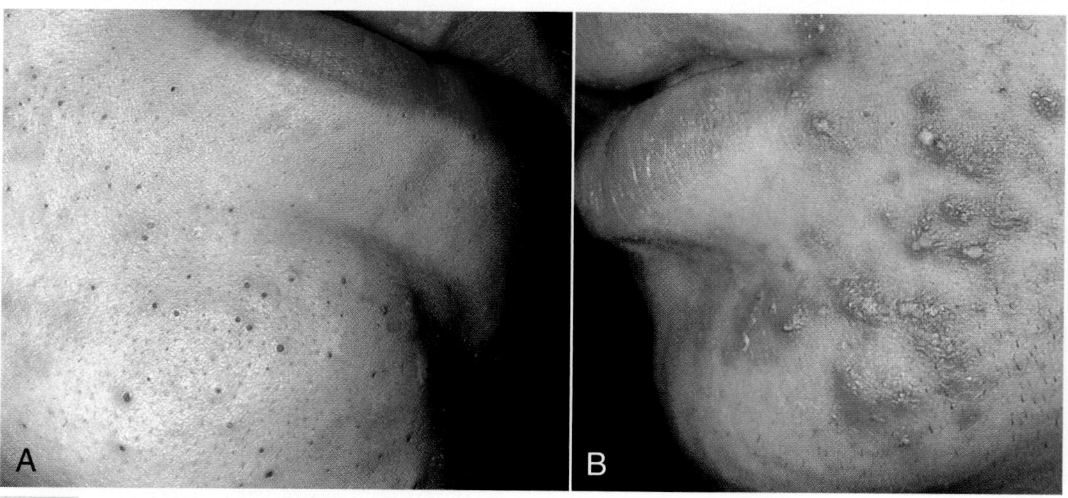

12-19 **A,** Open comedones. **B,** Severe acne.

Objective Data

The Pregnant Woman

Striae are jagged linear "stretch marks" of silver to pink color that appear during the second trimester on the abdomen, breasts, and sometimes thighs. They occur in one half of all pregnancies. They fade after delivery but do not disappear. Another skin change on the abdomen is the **linea nigra,** a brownish black line down the midline (see Fig. 29-3 on p. 807). **Chloasma** is an irregular brown patch of hyperpigmentation on the face. It may occur with pregnancy or in women taking oral contraceptive pills. Chloasma disappears after delivery or stopping the pills. **Vascular spiders** occur in two thirds of pregnancies in white women and less often in Blacks. These lesions have tiny red centers with radiating branches and occur on the face, neck, upper chest, and arms.

The Aging Adult

Skin Color and Pigmentation. Common variations of hyperpigmentation are:

Senile Lentigines. Commonly called *liver spots,* these are small, flat, brown macules (Fig. 12-20). These circumscribed areas are clusters of melanocytes that appear after extensive sun exposure. They appear on the forearms and dorsa of the hands. They are not malignant and require no treatment.

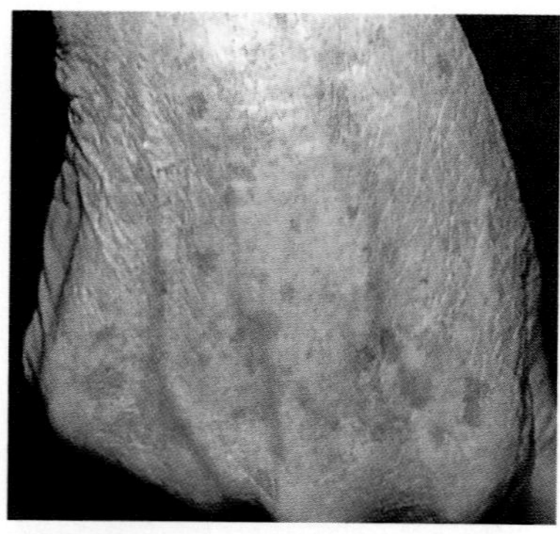

12-20 Lentigines.

Normal Range of Findings

Abnormal Findings

Keratoses. These lesions are raised, thickened areas of pigmentation that look crusted, scaly, and warty. One type, **seborrheic keratosis,** looks dark, greasy, and "stuck on" (Fig. 12-21). They develop mostly on the trunk but also on the face and hands and on unexposed as well as on sun-exposed areas. They do not become cancerous.

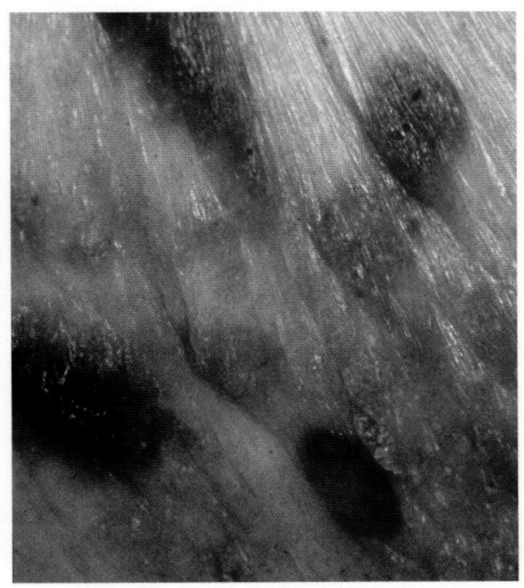

12-21 Seborrheic keratosis.

Another type, **actinic** (**senile** or **solar**) **keratosis,** is less common (Fig. 12-22). These lesions are red-tan scaly plaques that increase over the years to become raised and roughened. They may have a silvery-white scale adherent to the plaque. They occur on sun-exposed surfaces and are directly related to sun exposure. They are premalignant and may develop into squamous cell carcinoma.

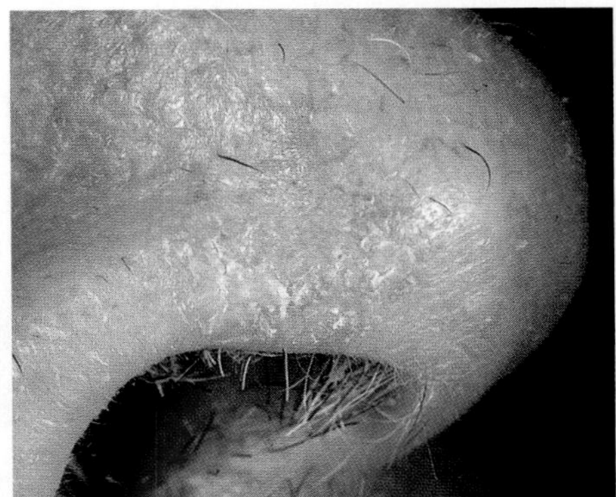

12-22 Actinic keratosis.

Moisture. Dry skin (xerosis) is common in the aging person because of a decline in the size, number, and output of the sweat glands and sebaceous glands. The skin itches and looks flaky and loose.

Texture. Common variations occurring in the aging adult are **acrochordons,** or "skin tags," which are overgrowths of normal skin that form a stalk and are polyp-like (Fig. 12-23). They occur frequently on eyelids, cheeks and neck, and axillae and trunk.

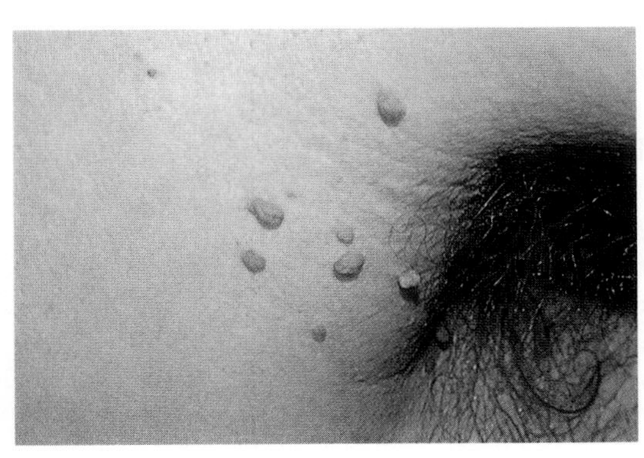

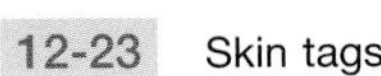

12-23 Skin tags.

Normal Range of Findings	Abnormal Findings

Sebaceous hyperplasia consists of raised yellow papules with a central depression. They are more common in men, occurring over the forehead, nose, or cheeks. They have a pebbly look (Fig. 12-24).

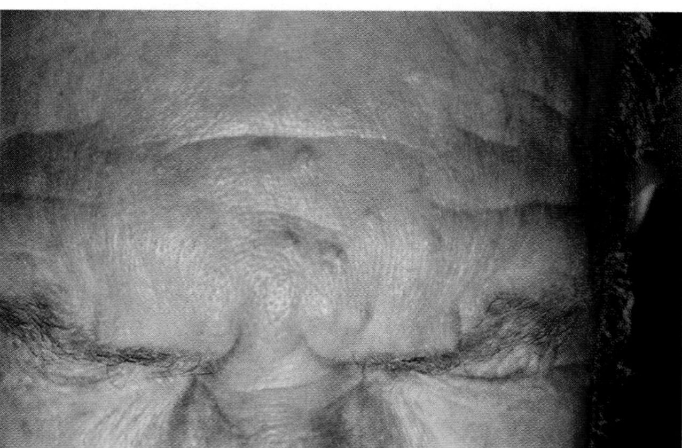

12-24 Sebaceous hyperplasia.

Thickness. With aging, the skin looks as thin as parchment and the subcutaneous fat diminishes. Thinner skin is evident over the dorsa of the hands, forearms, lower legs, dorsa of feet, and over bony prominences. The skin may feel thicker over the abdomen and chest.

Aging skin increases risk for pressure ulcer development (see Table 12-6, Pressure Ulcer [Decubitus Ulcer]).

Mobility and Turgor. The turgor is decreased (less elasticity), and the skin recedes slowly or "tents" and stands by itself (Fig. 12-25).

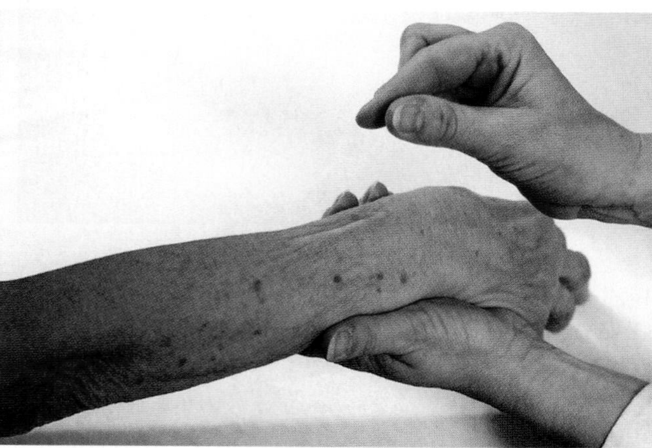

12-25

Hair. With aging, the hair growth decreases and the amount decreases in the axillae and pubic areas. After menopause, white women may develop bristly hairs on the chin or upper lip resulting from unopposed androgens. In men, coarse terminal hairs develop in the ears, nose, and eyebrows, although the beard is unchanged. Male-pattern balding, or alopecia, is a genetic trait. It is usually a gradual receding of the anterior hairline in a symmetric W shape. In men and women, scalp hair gradually turns gray because of the decrease in melanocyte function.

Nails. With aging, the nail growth rate decreases and local injuries in the nail matrix may produce longitudinal ridges. The surface may be brittle or peeling and sometimes yellowed. Toenails also are thickened and may grow misshapen, almost grotesque. The thickening may be a process of aging, or it may be due to chronic peripheral vascular disease.

Fungal infections are common in aging, with thickened, crumbling toenails and erythematous scaling on contiguous skin surfaces.

PROMOTING A HEALTHY LIFESTYLE: INDOOR TANNING AND SKIN CANCER RISK

The Dangers of Indoor Tanning

During the skin examination, health care providers have the opportunity to educate patients about the dangers of excessive ultraviolet (UV) exposure from direct sun exposure or from indoor tanning equipment, such as sun lamps, beds, or booths. Although most individuals understand the risk of direct sun exposure, they often underestimate the dangers of indoor tanning. Many feel that tanning gives you a "healthy glow"; on the contrary, the long-term use of tanning can lead to something more frightening and deadly.

Exposure to UV radiation from indoor tanning devices not only increases the risk for melanoma but also is associated with an increased risk for non-melanoma skin cancer, such as squamous cell and basal cell carcinomas. Both the International Agency for Research on Cancer (IARC), part of the World Health Organization, and the U.S. Department of Health and Human Services (HHS) have declared UV radiation, from the sun and from artificial sources, to be carcinogenic. Recently, the IARC moved tanning beds to its highest cancer-risk category alongside other cancer-causing agents, such as asbestos and cigarettes. Yet, despite these public health warnings and increasing evidence of the dangers of artificial UV radiation, more than 1 million individuals in the United States frequent tanning salons each day. The tanning industry appears to have convinced the public that indoor tanning is healthy, emphasizing that tanning produces a psychological sense of well-being and can even induce vitamin D production. Further, they claim that getting a tan before you go out into the sun can actually prevent sunburn, a known risk factor for skin cancer. "Pretanning" before a vacation or outdoor sun exposure is a particularly dangerous practice, because not only does it lead to extra UV exposure but it also appears to lead to decreased use of subsequent outdoor sun-protective precautions. At best, artificial "pretans" offer the protection equal to a sunscreen with only an SPF of 2 to 3, well under the minimum protective recommendation—SPF 15.

The "tan tax," tucked within the health care law signed by President Obama in July 2010, is a new step in the fight to discourage the use of indoor tanning beds. Similar to the idea behind taxing cigarettes, the 10% tax on the use of UV indoor tanning beds is estimated to decrease the use of indoor tanning beds while raising over $2.5 billion toward the cost of expanding health coverage. More important, it may save lives.

Resources

American Academy of Dermatology (AAD). Website: www.aad.org/.

Download an Indoor Tanning Fact Sheet. Website: www.aad.org/public/exams/screenings/documents/AAD_Indoor_Tanning_Fact_Sheet.pdf.

International Agency for Research on Cancer (IARC). Website: www.iarc.fr/.

Levine, J. A., Sorace, J. A., Spencer, J., et al. (2005). The indoor UV tanning industry: a review of skin cancer risk, health benefit claims, and regulation. *Journal of the American Academy of Dermatology*, *53*(6), 1038-1044.

The International Agency for Research on Cancer Working Group on Artificial Ultraviolet Light and Skin Cancer. (2007). The association of use of sunbeds with cutaneous malignant melanoma and other skin cancers: a systematic review. *International Journal of Cancer*, *120*(5), 1116-1122.

The Skin Cancer Foundation. Website: www.skincancer.org/.

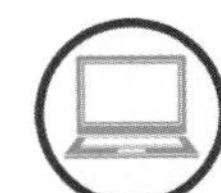

DOCUMENTATION AND CRITICAL THINKING

Sample Charting

SUBJECTIVE

No history of skin disease; no present change in pigmentation or in nevi; no pruritus, bruising, rash, or lesions. On no medications. No work-related skin hazards. Uses sun block cream when outdoors.

OBJECTIVE

Skin: Color tan-pink, even pigmentation, with no suspicious nevi. Warm to touch, dry, smooth, and even. Turgor good, no lesions.
Hair: Even distribution, thick texture, no lesions or pest inhabitants.
Nails: No clubbing or deformities. Nail beds pink with prompt capillary refill.

ASSESSMENT

Warm, dry, intact skin.

Focused Assessment: Clinical Case Study 1*

Ethan E. is a 3-year-old white male presenting with his mother, who seeks health care because of Ethan's fever, fatigue, and rash of 3 days' duration.

SUBJECTIVE

2 weeks PTA (prior to arrival)—Ethan was playing with a child who was subsequently diagnosed as having chickenpox.
3 days PTA—mother reports fever 100° to 101° F and fatigue, irritability. That evening noted "tiny blisters" on chest and back.
1 day PTA—blisters on chest changed to white with scab on top. New eruption of blisters on shoulders, thighs, face. Intense itching and scratching.

OBJECTIVE

Temp 38.0° C (100.4° F), P 110, R 24.
Skin: Generalized vesiculopustular rash covering face, trunk, upper arms, and thighs. Small vesicles on face, pustules and red-honey–colored crusts on trunk. Otherwise skin is warm and dry, turgor good.
Ears: Tympanic membranes pearl gray with landmarks intact. No discharge.
Mouth and throat: Mucosa dark pink, no lesions. Tonsils 1+, no exudate. No lymphadenopathy.
Heart: S_1, S_2 normal, not accentuated or diminished, no murmurs or extra sounds.
Lungs: Hyperresonant to percussion. Breath sounds clear, no adventitious sounds.

ASSESSMENT

Varicella
Impaired skin integrity R/T infection and scratching

Focused Assessment: Clinical Case Study 2

Myra G. is a 79-year-old white widowed retired college professor, in good health until recent hospitalization after a fall.
Problem List 1 Fractured right hip—hip replacement on 11/24

SUBJECTIVE

11/27, Aching pain in left hip (nonoperative side).

OBJECTIVE

Erosion 2 × 2 cm with surrounding erythema covering L ischium. Erosion is moist, no active bleeding. Area very warm and tender to touch.

ASSESSMENT

Pressure sore, L hip
Impaired skin integrity R/T immobility and pressure
Acute pain

*Please note that space does not allow a detailed plan for each sample clinical problem in the text. Please consult the appropriate text for current treatment plans.

ABNORMAL FINDINGS

TABLE 12-2 Detecting Color Changes in Light and in Dark Skin

	Note Appearance	
Etiology	Light Skin	Dark Skin
Pallor		
Anemia—decreased hematocrit Shock—decreased perfusion, vasoconstriction	Generalized pallor	Brown skin appears yellow-brown, dull; black skin appears ashen gray, dull; skin loses its healthy glow—check areas with least pigmentation, such as conjunctivae, mucous membranes
Local arterial insufficiency	Marked localized pallor (e.g., lower extremities, especially when elevated)	Ashen gray, dull; cool to palpation
Albinism—total absence of pigment melanin throughout the integument	Whitish pink	Tan, cream, white
Vitiligo—patchy depigmentation from destruction of melanocytes	Patchy milky white spots, often symmetric bilaterally	Same
Cyanosis		
Increased amount of unoxygenated hemoglobin Central—chronic heart and lung disease cause arterial desaturation	Dusky blue	Dark but dull, lifeless; only severe cyanosis is apparent in skin—check conjunctivae, oral mucosa, nail beds
Peripheral—exposure to cold, anxiety	Nail beds dusky	
Erythema		
Hyperemia—increased blood flow through engorged arterioles, such as in inflammation, fever, alcohol intake, blushing	Red, bright pink	Purplish tinge, but difficult to see; palpate for increased warmth with inflammation, taut skin, and hardening of deep tissues
Polycythemia—increased red blood cells, capillary stasis	Ruddy blue in face, oral mucosa, conjunctiva, hands and feet	Well concealed by pigment—check for redness in lips
Carbon monoxide poisoning	Bright cherry red in face and upper torso	Cherry red color in nail beds, lips, and oral mucosa
Venous stasis—decreased blood flow from area, engorged venules	Dusky rubor of dependent extremities; a prelude to necrosis with pressure sore	Easily masked; use palpation for warmth or edema
Jaundice		
Increased serum bilirubin, more than 2 to 3 mg/100 mL from liver inflammation or hemolytic disease, such as after severe burns, some infections	Yellow in sclera, hard palate, mucous membranes, then over skin	Check sclera for yellow near limbus; do not mistake normal yellowish fatty deposits in the periphery under the eyelids for jaundice—jaundice best noted in junction of hard and soft palate and also palms
Carotenemia—increased serum carotene from ingestion of large amounts of carotene-rich foods	Yellow-orange in forehead, palms and soles, nasolabial folds, but no yellowing in sclera or mucous membranes	Yellow-orange tinge in palms and soles

Continued

TABLE 12-2 Detecting Color Changes in Light and in Dark Skin—cont'd

	Note Appearance	
Etiology	Light Skin	Dark Skin
Uremia—renal failure causes retained urochrome pigments in the blood	Orange-green or gray overlying pallor of anemia; may also have ecchymoses and purpura	Easily masked; rely on laboratory and clinical findings
Brown-Tan		
Addison's disease—cortisol deficiency stimulates increased melanin production	Bronzed appearance, an "eternal tan," most apparent around nipples, perineum, genitalia, and pressure points (inner thighs, buttocks, elbow, axillae)	Easily masked; rely on laboratory and clinical findings
Café au lait spots—caused by increased melanin pigment in basal cell layer	Tan to light brown, irregularly shaped, oval patch with well-defined borders	

TABLE 12-3 Common Shapes and Configurations of Lesions

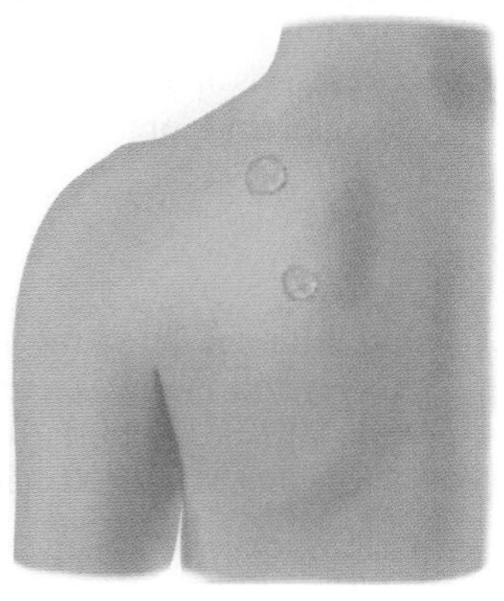

ANNULAR, or circular, begins in center and spreads to periphery (e.g., tinea corporis or ringworm, tinea versicolor, pityriasis rosea).

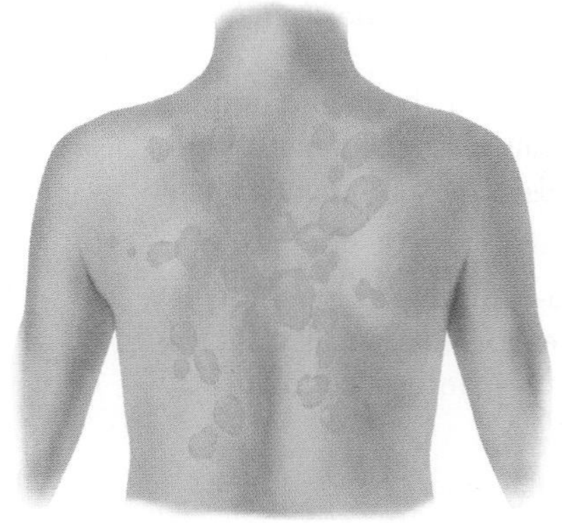

CONFLUENT, lesions run together (e.g., urticaria [hives]).

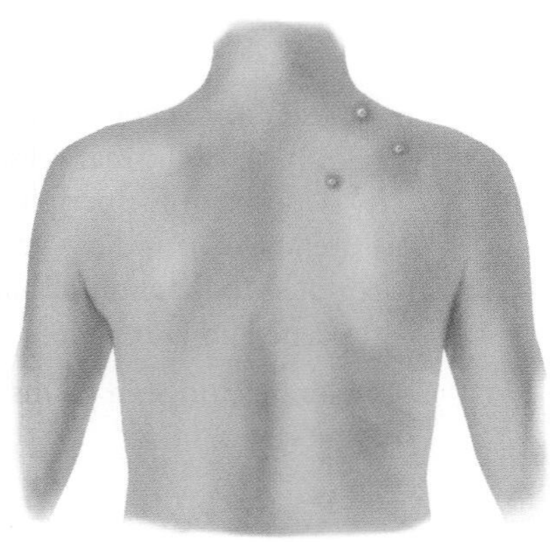

◀ **DISCRETE,** distinct, individual lesions that remain separate (e.g., acrochordon or skin tags, acne).

TABLE 12-3 Common Shapes and Configurations of Lesions—cont'd

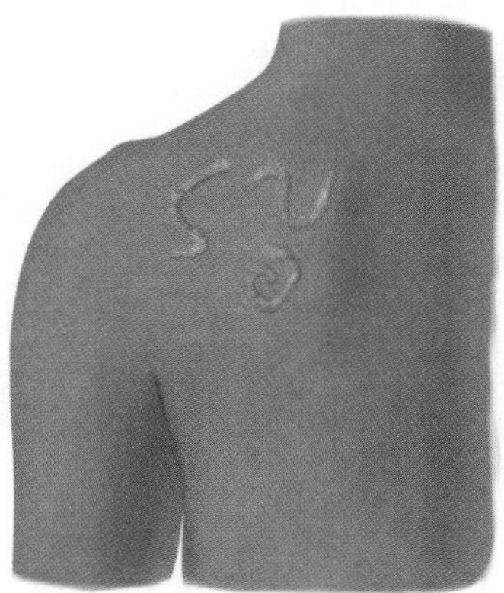

GYRATE, twisted, coiled spiral, snakelike.

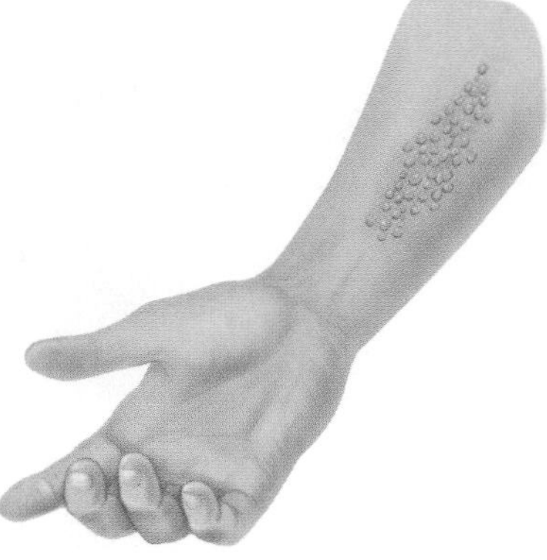

GROUPED, clusters of lesions (e.g., vesicles of contact dermatitis).

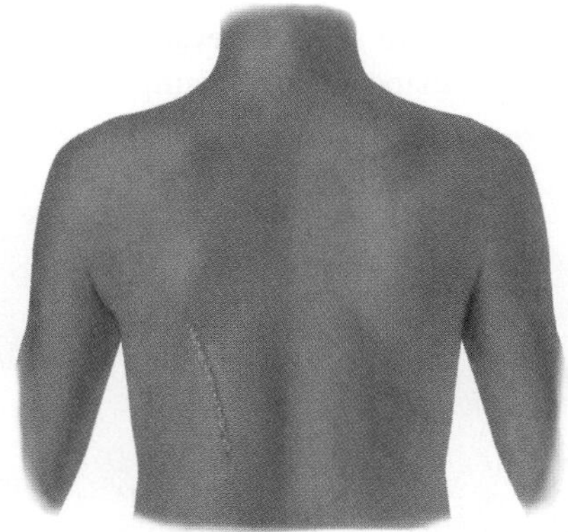

LINEAR, a scratch, streak, line, or stripe.

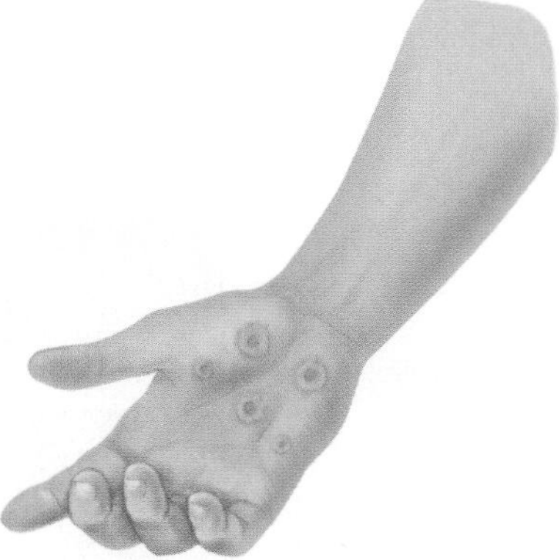

TARGET, or iris, resembles iris of eye, concentric rings of color in the lesions (e.g., erythema multiforme).

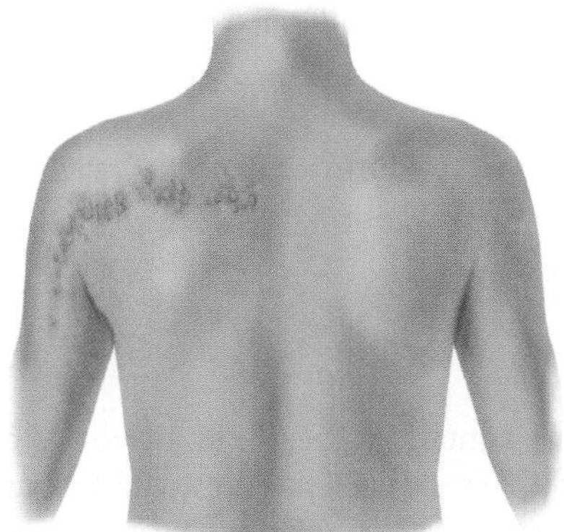

ZOSTERIFORM, linear arrangement along a unilateral nerve route (e.g., herpes zoster).

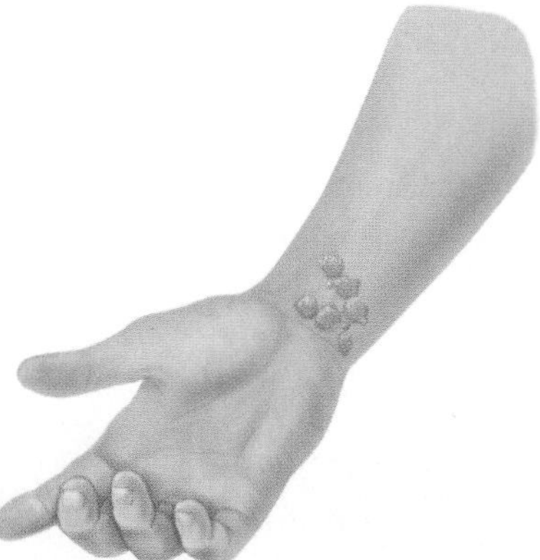

POLYCYCLIC, annular lesions grow together (e.g., lichen planus, psoriasis).

TABLE 12-4 **Primary Skin Lesions***

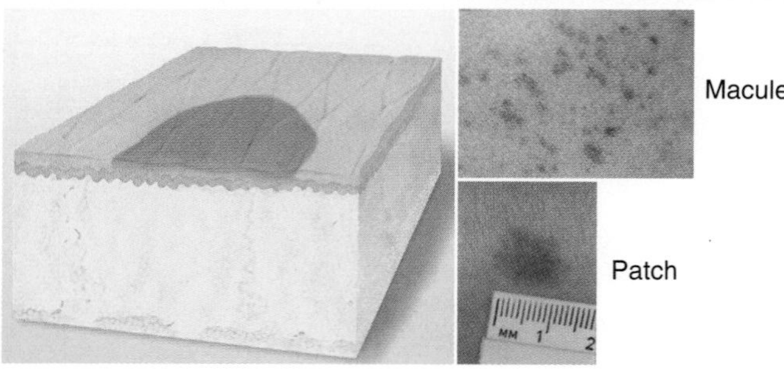

Papule
Plaque

Macule

Solely a color change, flat and circumscribed, of less than 1 cm. Examples: freckles, flat nevi, hypopigmentation, petechiae, measles, scarlet fever.

Patch

Macules that are larger than 1 cm. Examples: mongolian spot, vitiligo, café au lait spot, chloasma, measles rash.

Papule

Something you can feel (i.e., solid, elevated, circumscribed, less than 1 cm diameter) caused by superficial thickening in the epidermis. Examples: elevated nevus (mole), lichen planus, molluscum, wart (verruca).

Plaque

Papules coalesce to form surface elevation wider than 1 cm. A plateau-like, disk-shaped lesion. Examples: psoriasis, lichen planus.

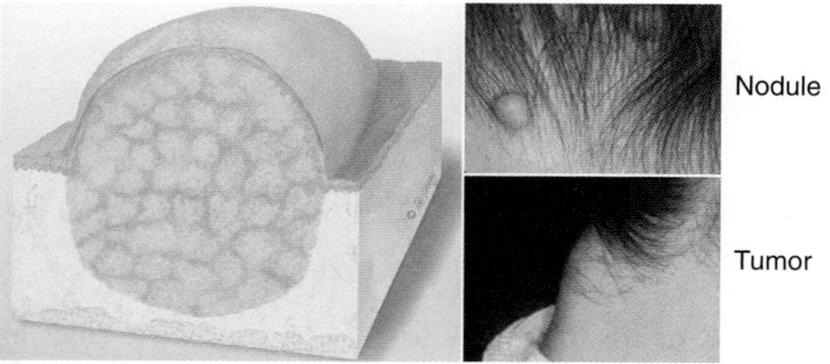

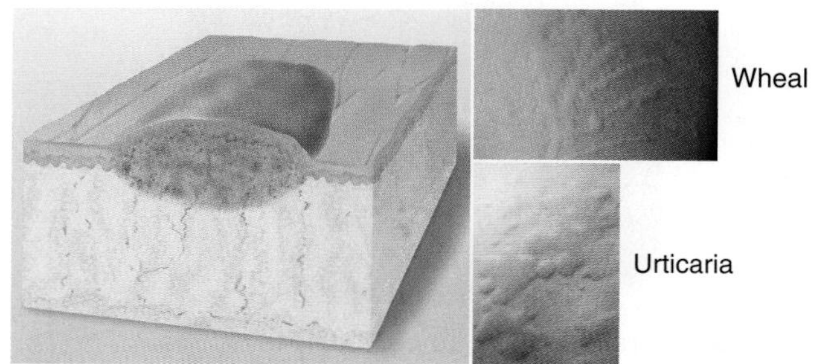

Nodule

Solid, elevated, hard or soft, larger than 1 cm. May extend deeper into dermis than papule. Examples: xanthoma, fibroma, intradermal nevi.

Tumor

Larger than a few centimeters in diameter, firm or soft, deeper into dermis; may be benign or malignant, although "tumor" implies "cancer" to most people. Examples: lipoma, hemangioma.

Wheal

Superficial, raised, transient, and erythematous; slightly irregular shape due to edema (fluid held diffusely in the tissues). Examples: mosquito bite, allergic reaction, dermographism.

Urticaria (Hives)

Wheals coalesce to form extensive reaction, intensely pruritic.

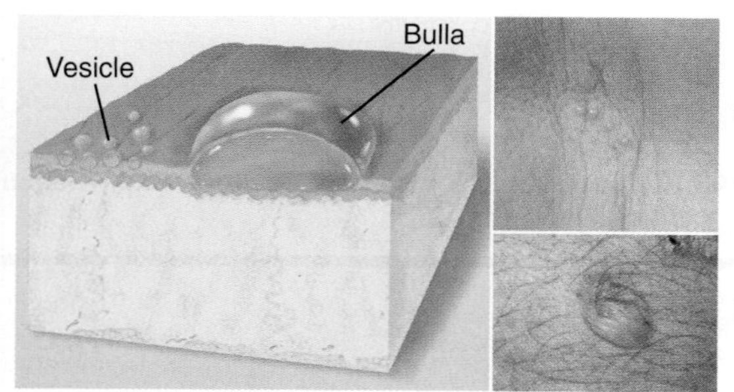

Vesicle
Bulla

◀ Vesicle

Elevated cavity containing free fluid, up to 1 cm; a "blister." Clear serum flows if wall is ruptured. Examples: herpes simplex, early varicella (chickenpox), herpes zoster (shingles), contact dermatitis.

◀ Bulla

Larger than 1 cm diameter; usually single chambered (unilocular); superficial in epidermis; it is thin walled, so it ruptures easily. Examples: friction blister, pemphigus, burns, contact dermatitis.

TABLE 12-4 Primary Skin Lesions—cont'd

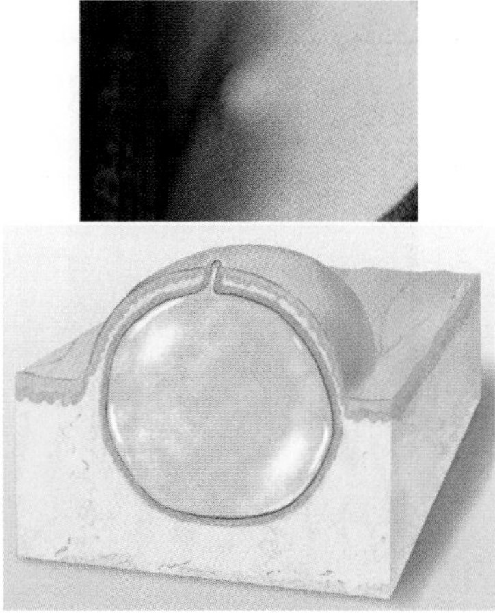

Cyst

Encapsulated fluid-filled cavity in dermis or subcutaneous layer, tensely elevating skin. Examples: sebaceous cyst, wen.

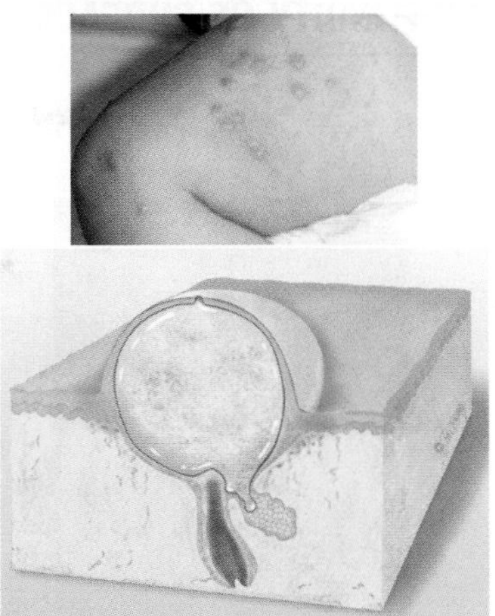

Pustule

Turbid fluid (pus) in the cavity. Circumscribed and elevated. Examples: impetigo, acne.

*The immediate result of a specific causative factor; primary lesions develop on previously unaltered skin.

TABLE 12-5 Secondary Skin Lesions*

DEBRIS ON SKIN SURFACE

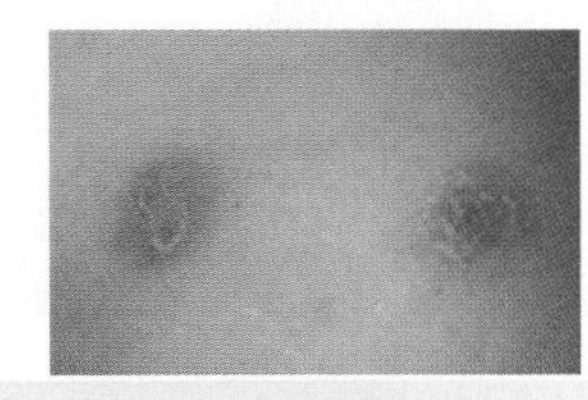

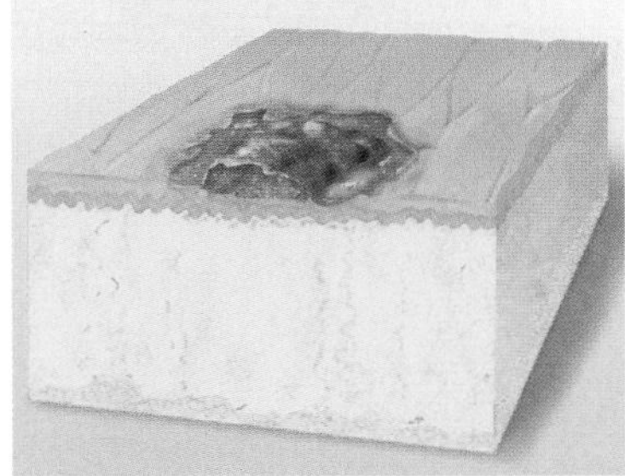

Crust

The thickened, dried-out exudate left when vesicles/pustules burst or dry up. Color can be red-brown, honey, or yellow, depending on the fluid's ingredients (blood, serum, pus). Examples: impetigo (dry, honey-colored), weeping eczematous dermatitis, scab after abrasion.

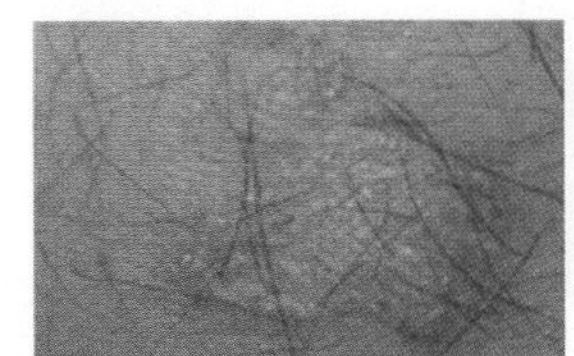

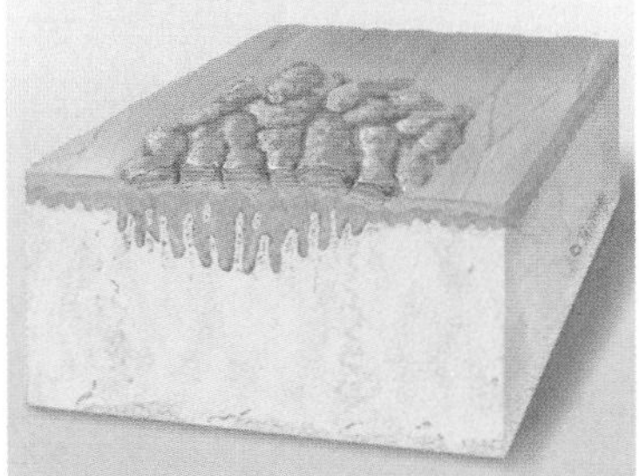

Scale

Compact, desiccated flakes of skin, dry or greasy, silvery or white, from shedding of dead excess keratin cells. Examples: after scarlet fever or drug reaction (laminated sheets), psoriasis (silver, mica-like), seborrheic dermatitis (yellow, greasy), eczema, ichthyosis (large, adherent, laminated), dry skin.

*Resulting from a change in a primary lesion from the passage of time; an evolutionary change.

Note: Combinations of primary and secondary lesions may coexist in the same person. Such combined designations may be termed *papulosquamous, maculopapular, vesiculopustular,* or *papulovesicular.*

Continued

TABLE 12-5 Secondary Skin Lesions—cont'd

BREAK IN CONTINUITY OF SURFACE

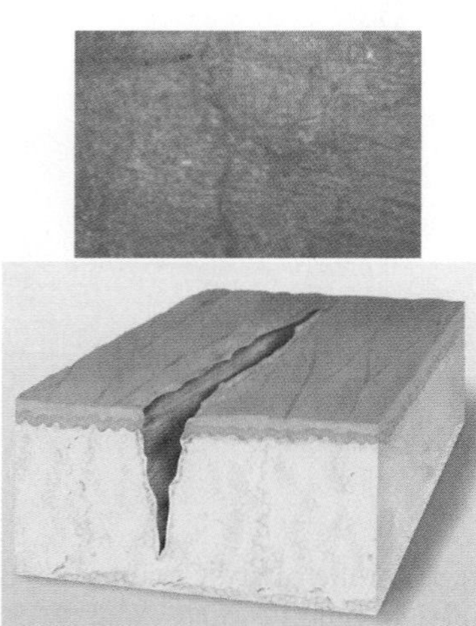

Fissure

Linear crack with abrupt edges, extends into dermis, dry or moist. Examples: cheilosis—at corners of mouth due to excess moisture; athlete's foot.

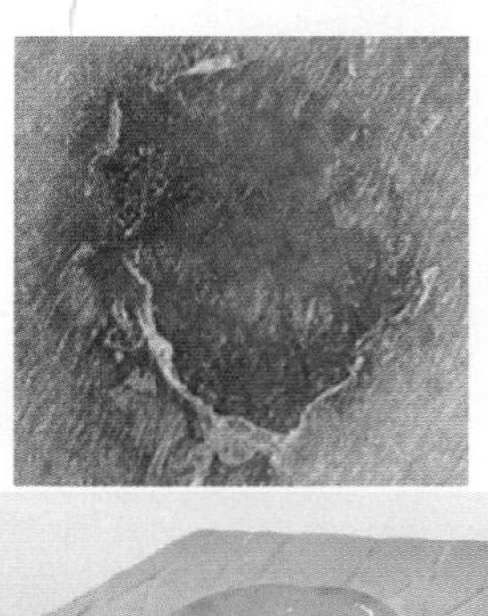

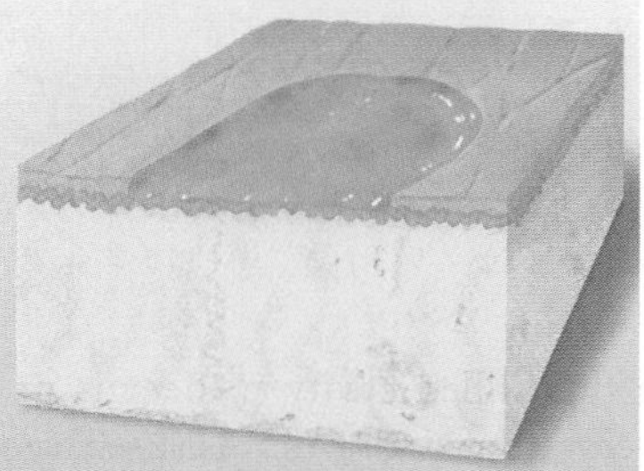

Erosion

Scooped out but shallow depression. Superficial; epidermis lost; moist but no bleeding; heals without scar because erosion does not extend into dermis.

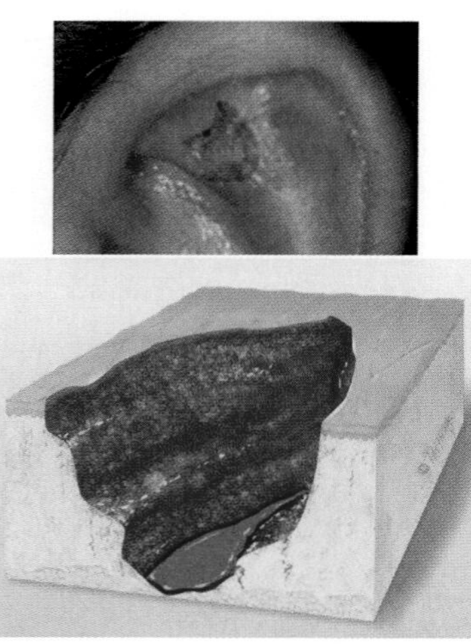

Ulcer

Deeper depression extending into dermis, irregular shape; may bleed; leaves scar when heals. Examples: stasis ulcer, pressure sore, chancre.

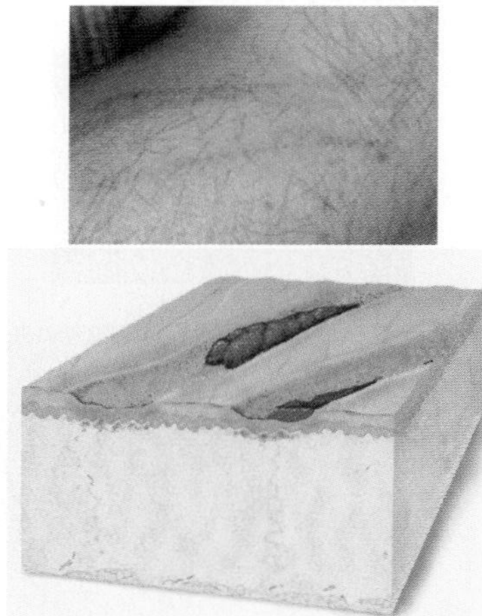

Excoriation

Self-inflicted abrasion; superficial; sometimes crusted; scratches from intense itching. Examples: insect bites, scabies, dermatitis, varicella.

TABLE 12-5 **Secondary Skin Lesions—cont'd**

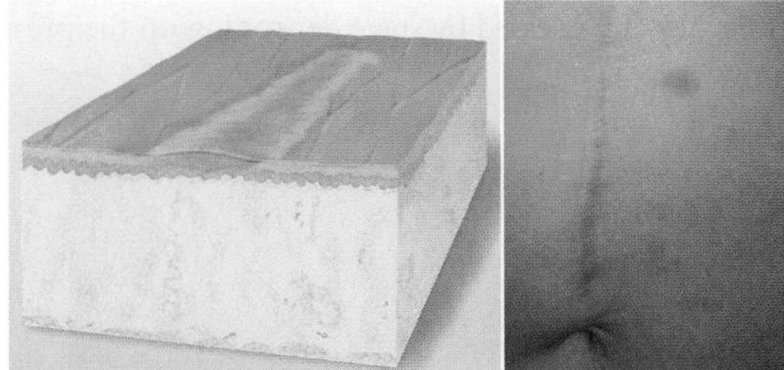

Scar

After a skin lesion is repaired, normal tissue is lost and replaced with connective tissue (collagen). This is a permanent fibrotic change. Examples: healed area of surgery or injury, acne.

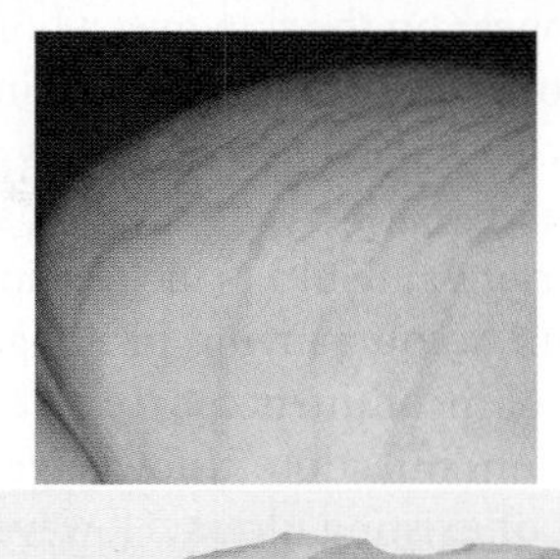

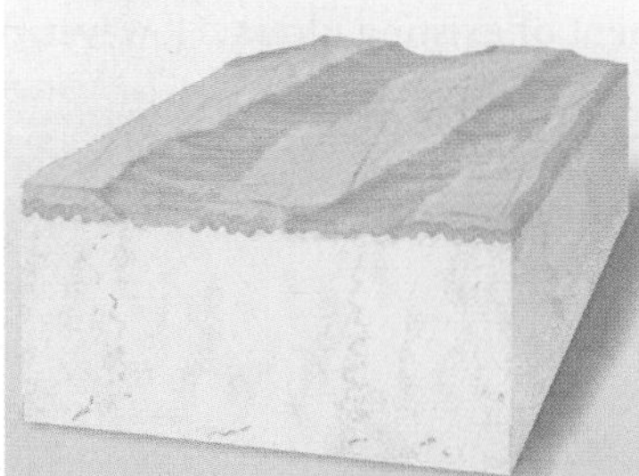

Atrophic Scar

The resulting skin level is depressed with loss of tissue; a thinning of the epidermis. Example: striae.

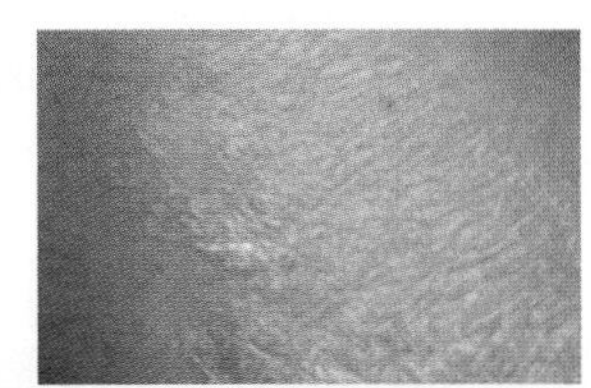

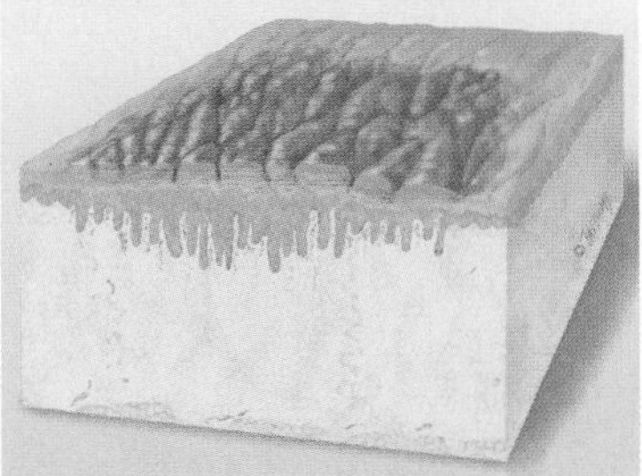

Lichenification

Prolonged, intense scratching eventually thickens the skin and produces tightly packed sets of papules; looks like surface of moss (or lichen).

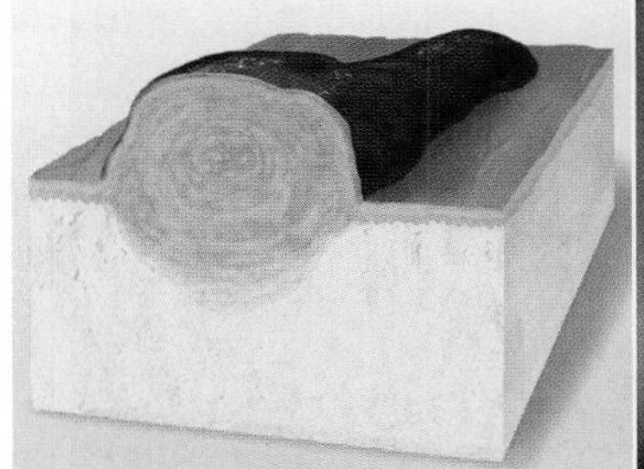

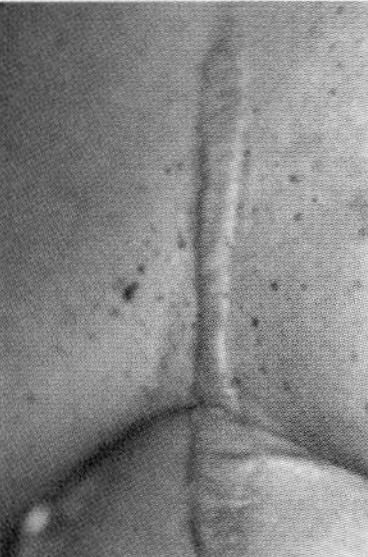

Keloid

A hypertrophic scar. The resulting skin level is elevated by excess scar tissue, which is invasive beyond the site of original injury. May increase long after healing occurs. Looks smooth, rubbery, and "clawlike" and has a higher incidence among Blacks.

TABLE 12-6 Pressure Ulcer (Decubitus Ulcer)

Pressure ulcers appear on the skin over a bony prominence when circulation is impaired. This occurs when a person is confined to bed or is immobilized. Immobilization impedes delivery of blood carrying oxygen and nutrients to the skin, and it impedes venous drainage carrying metabolic wastes away from the skin. This results in ischemia and cell death. Common sites for pressure ulcers are on the back (heel, ischium, sacrum, elbow, scapula, vertebra) or the side (ankle, knee, hip, rib, shoulder).

Risk factors for pressure ulcers include impaired mobility, thin fragile skin of aging, decreased sensory perception (so unable to respond to pain accompanying prolonged pressure), impaired level of consciousness (also unable to respond), moisture from urine or stool incontinence, excessive perspiration or wound drainage, shearing injury (being pulled down or across in bed), poor nutrition, infection. Knowledge of risk factors and prevention of pressure ulcers is far more easily accomplished than is treatment of existing ulcers. However, once pressure ulcers occur, they are assessed by stage depending on the pressure ulcer depth[15]:

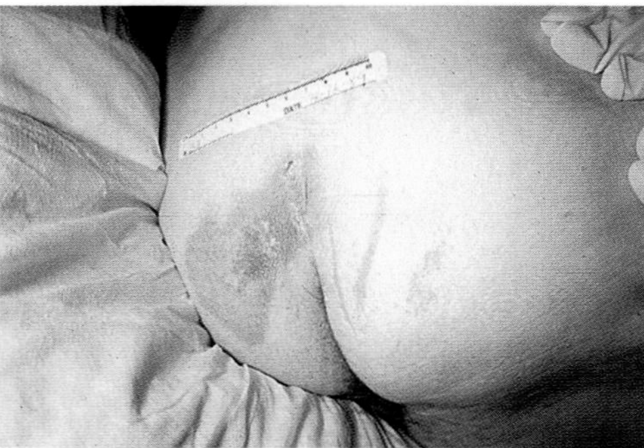

Stage I

Intact skin appears red but unbroken. Localized redness in lightly pigmented skin will not blanch (turn light with fingertip pressure). Dark skin appears darker but does not blanch.

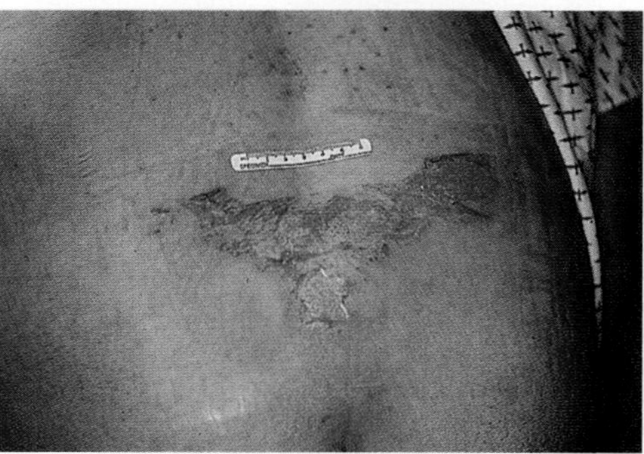

Stage II

Partial-thickness skin erosion with loss of epidermis or also the dermis. Superficial ulcer looks shallow like an abrasion or open blister with a red-pink wound bed.

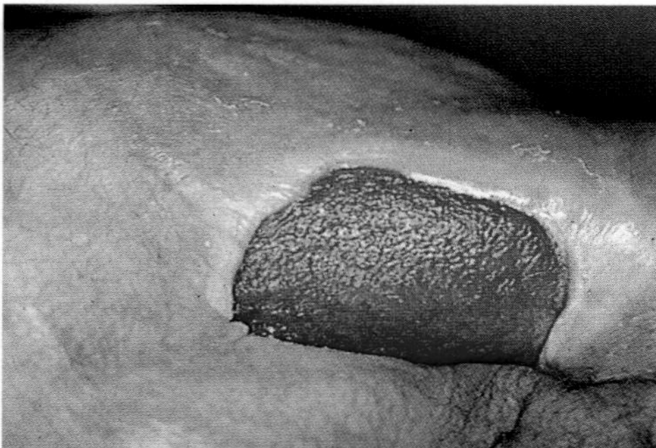

Stage III

Full-thickness pressure ulcer extending into the subcutaneous tissue and resembling a crater. May see subcutaneous fat but not muscle, bone, or tendon.

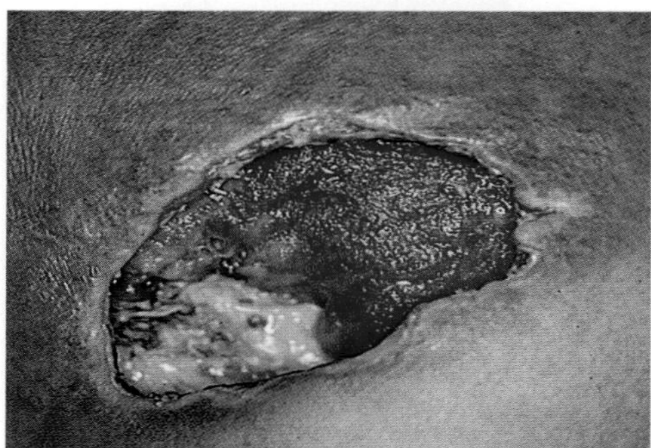

Stage IV

Full-thickness pressure ulcer involves all skin layers and extends into supporting tissue. Exposes muscle, tendon or bone, and may show slough (stringy matter attached to wound bed) or eschar (black or brown necrotic tissue).

TABLE 12-7 Lesions Caused by Trauma or Abuse

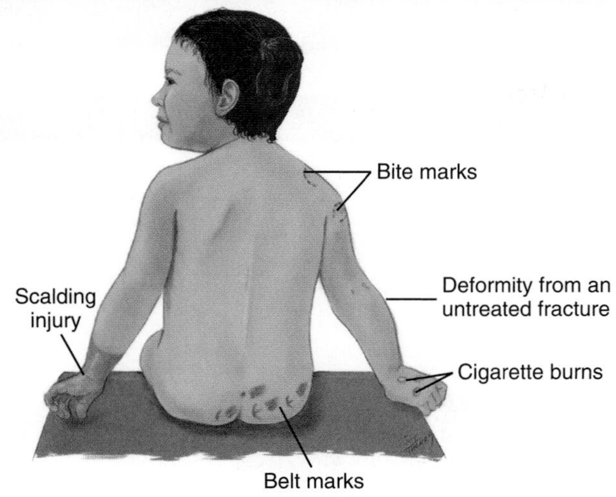

Pattern Injury

Pattern injury is a bruise or wound whose shape suggests the instrument or weapon that caused it (e.g., belt buckle, broomstick, burning cigarette, pinch marks, bite marks, or scalding-hot liquid). Inflicted scalding-water immersion burns usually have a clear border, like a glove or sock, indicating that body part was held under water intentionally. Deformity results from an untreated fracture because the bone heals out of alignment.

These physical signs suggest child abuse, together with a history that does not match the severity or type of injury, and indicate impaired or dysfunctional parent-child relationship.

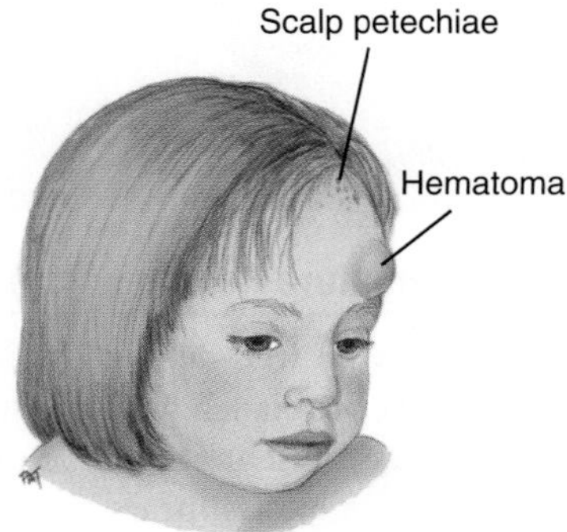

Hematoma

A hematoma is a bruise you can feel. It elevates the skin and is seen as swelling. Multiple petechiae and purpura may occur on the face when prolonged, vigorous crying or coughing raises venous pressure.

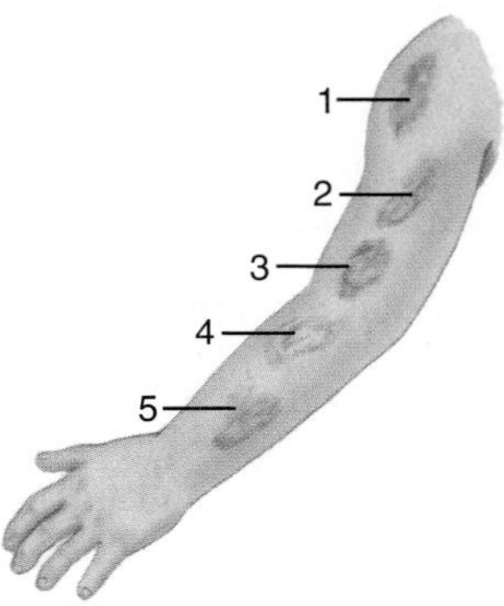

Contusion (Bruise)

A mechanical injury (e.g., a blow) results in hemorrhage into tissues. Skin is intact. Color in a light-skinned person is usually (1) red-blue or purple immediately after or within 24 hours of trauma, then generally progresses to (2) blue to purple, (3) blue-green, (4) yellow, and (5) brown to disappearing. A recent bruise in a dark-skinned person is deep, dark purple. Note that it is *not* possible to date the age of a bruise from its color. Pressure on a bruise will *not* cause it to blanch. A bruise usually occurs from trauma; also from bleeding disorders and liver dysfunction.

Note that a bruise is *different* from petechiae, ecchymosis, and purpura, because the latter three are *not* caused by blunt force trauma.[14]

ABNORMAL FINDINGS
FOR ADVANCED PRACTICE

TABLE 12-8 **Vascular Lesions**

HEMANGIOMAS

Caused by a benign proliferation of blood vessels in the dermis.

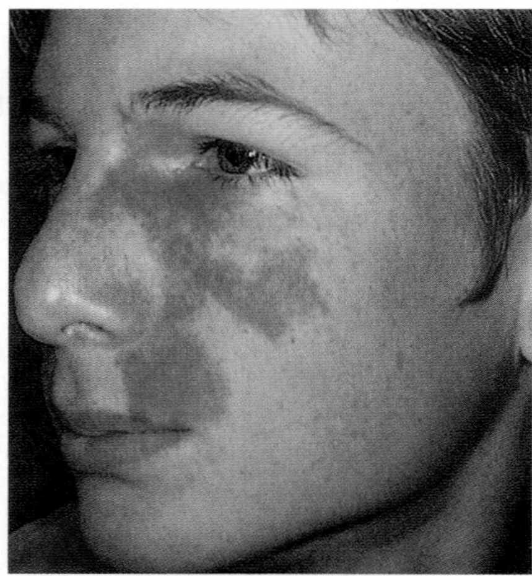

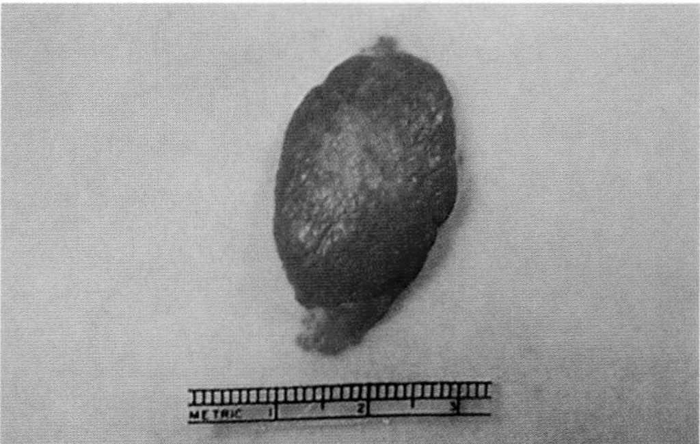

Port-Wine Stain (Nevus Flammeus)

A large, flat, macular patch covering the scalp or face, frequently along the distribution of cranial nerve V. The color is dark red, bluish, or purplish and intensifies with crying, exertion, or exposure to heat or cold. The marking consists of mature capillaries. It is present at birth and usually does not fade. The use of yellow light lasers now makes photoablation of the lesion possible, with minimal adverse effects.

Strawberry Mark (Immature Hemangioma)

A raised bright red area with well-defined borders about 2 to 3 cm in diameter. It does not blanch with pressure. It consists of immature capillaries, is present at birth or develops in the first few months, and usually disappears by age 5 to 7 years. Requires no treatment, although parental and peer pressure may prompt treatment.

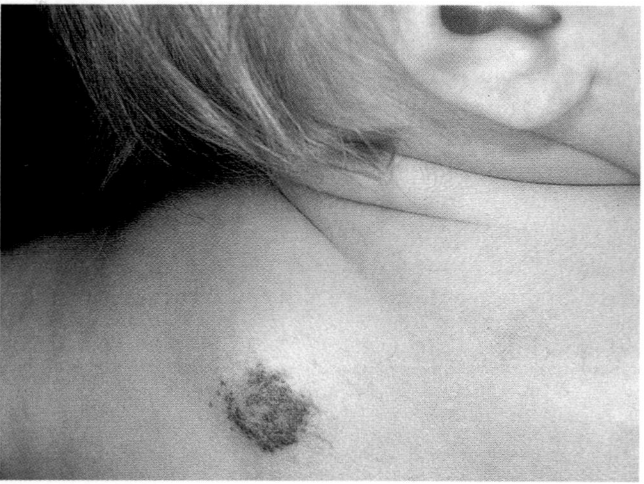

◄ **Cavernous Hemangioma (Mature)**

A reddish blue, irregularly shaped, solid and spongy mass of blood vessels. It may be present at birth, may enlarge during the first 10 to 15 months, and will not involute spontaneously.

TABLE 12-8 Vascular Lesions—cont'd

TELANGIECTASES

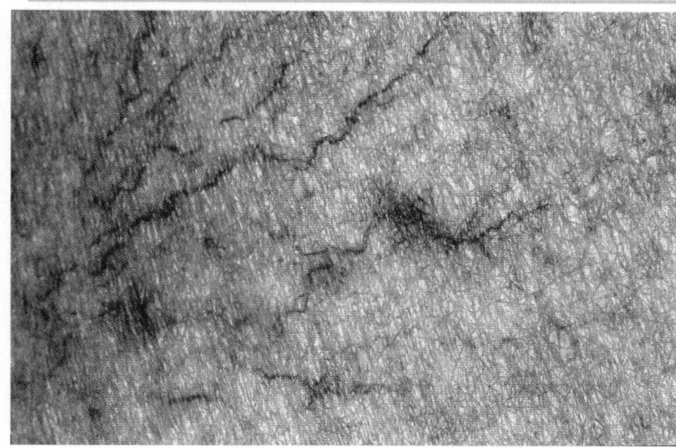

Telangiectasia

Caused by vascular dilation; permanently enlarged and dilated blood vessels that are visible on the skin surface.

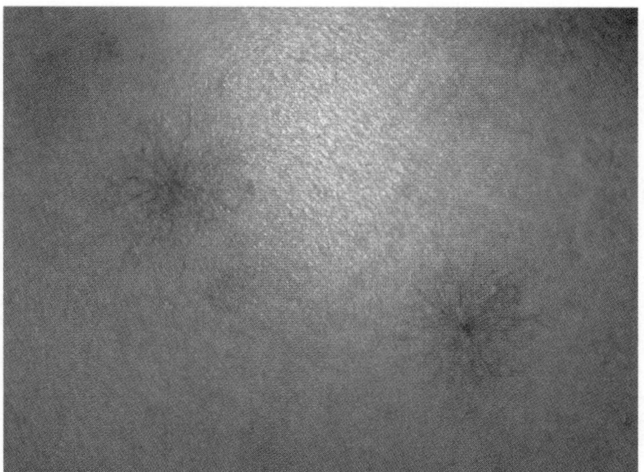

Spider or Star Angioma

A fiery red, star-shaped marking with a solid circular center. Capillary radiations extend from the central arterial body. With pressure, note a central pulsating body and blanching of extended legs. Develops on face, neck, or chest; may be associated with pregnancy, chronic liver disease, or estrogen therapy, or may be normal.

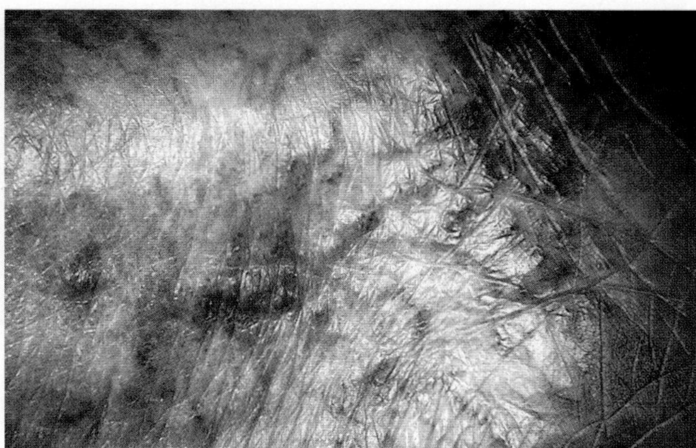

Venous Lake

A blue-purple dilation of venules and capillaries in a star-shaped, linear, or flaring pattern. Pressure causes them to empty or disappear. Located on the legs near varicose veins and also on the face, lips, ears, and chest.

Continued

TABLE 12-8 Vascular Lesions—cont'd

PURPURIC LESIONS

Caused by blood flowing out of breaks in the vessels. Red blood cells and blood pigments are deposited in the tissues (extravascular). Difficult to see in dark-skinned people.

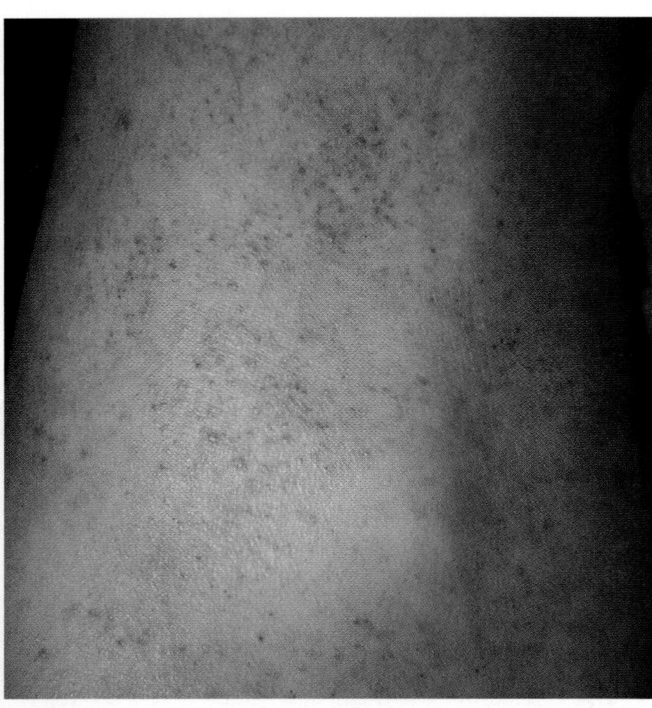

◀ Petechiae

Tiny punctate hemorrhages, 1 to 3 mm, round and discrete, dark red, purple, or brown in color. Caused by bleeding from superficial capillaries; will not blanch. May indicate abnormal clotting factors. In dark-skinned people, petechiae are best visualized in the areas of lighter melanization (e.g., the abdomen, buttocks, and volar surface of the forearm). When the skin is black or very dark brown, petechiae cannot be seen in the skin.

Most of the diseases that cause bleeding and microembolism formation—such as thrombocytopenia, subacute bacterial endocarditis, and other septicemias—are characterized by petechiae in the mucous membranes as well as on the skin. Thus you should inspect for petechiae in the mouth, particularly the buccal mucosa, and in the conjunctivae.

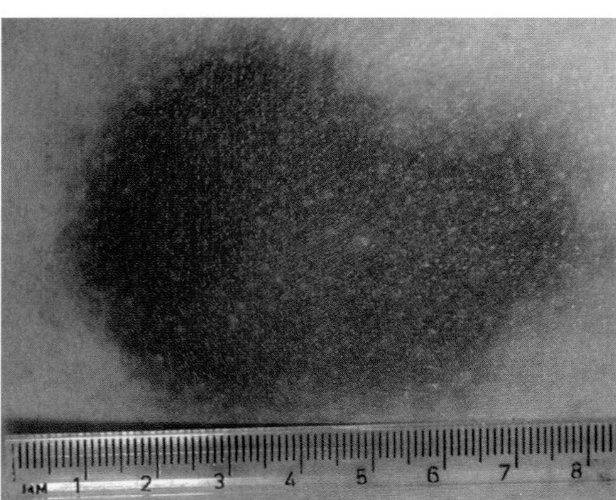

Ecchymosis

A purplish patch resulting from extravasation of blood into the skin, >3 mm in diameter.

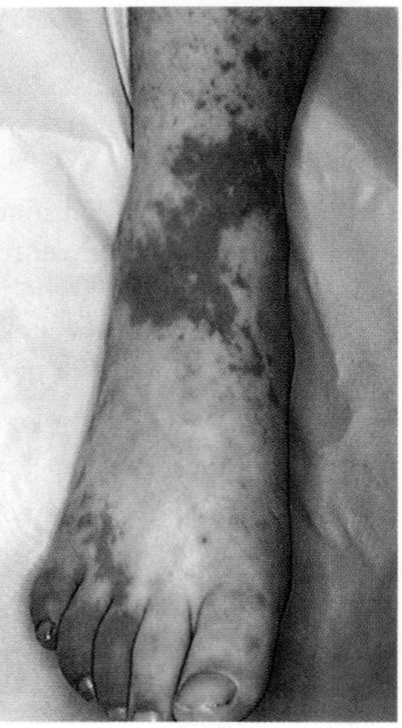

Purpura

Confluent and extensive patch of petechiae and ecchymoses, >3 mm flat, red to purple, macular hemorrhage. Seen in generalized disorders such as thrombocytopenia and scurvy. Also occurs in old age as blood leaks from capillaries in response to minor trauma and diffuses through dermis.

TABLE 12-9 **Common Skin Lesions in Children**

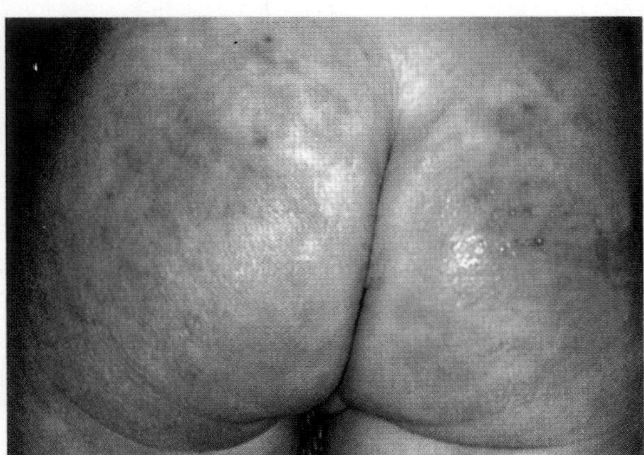

Diaper Dermatitis

Red, moist, maculopapular patch with poorly defined borders in diaper area, extending along inguinal and gluteal folds. History of infrequent diaper changes or occlusive coverings. Inflammatory disease caused by skin irritation from ammonia, heat, moisture, occlusive diapers.

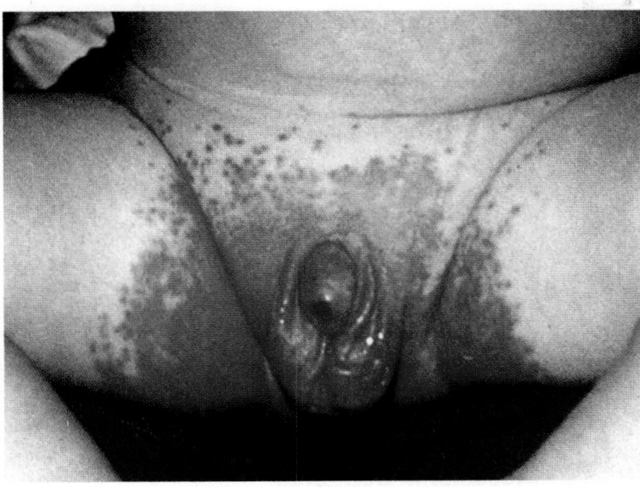

Intertrigo (Candidiasis)

Scalding red, moist patches with sharply demarcated borders, some loose scales. Usually in genital area extending along inguinal and gluteal folds. Aggravated by urine, feces, heat, and moisture, the *Candida* fungus infects the superficial skin layers.

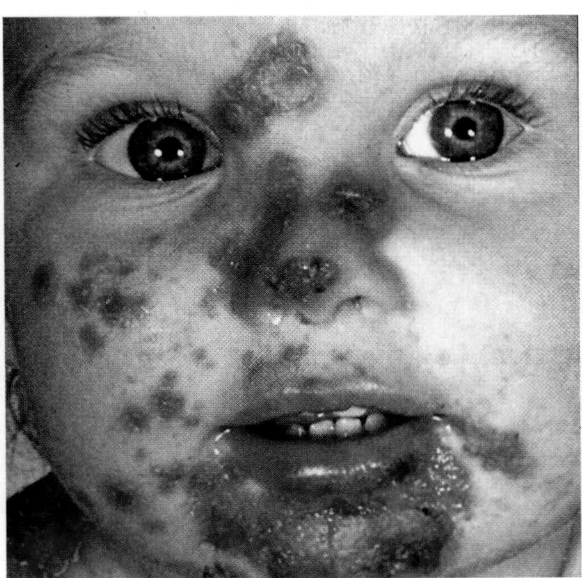

Impetigo

Moist, thin-roofed vesicles with thin, erythematous base. Rupture to form thick, honey-colored crusts. Contagious bacterial infection of skin; most common in infants and children.

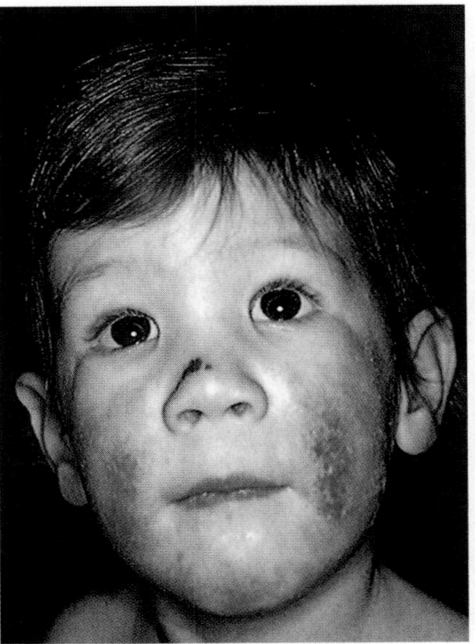

Atopic Dermatitis (Eczema)

Erythematous papules and vesicles, with weeping, oozing, and crusts. Lesions usually on scalp, forehead, cheeks, forearms and wrists, elbows, backs of knees. Paroxysmal and severe pruritus. Family history of allergies.

Continued

TABLE 12-9 **Common Skin Lesions in Children—cont'd**

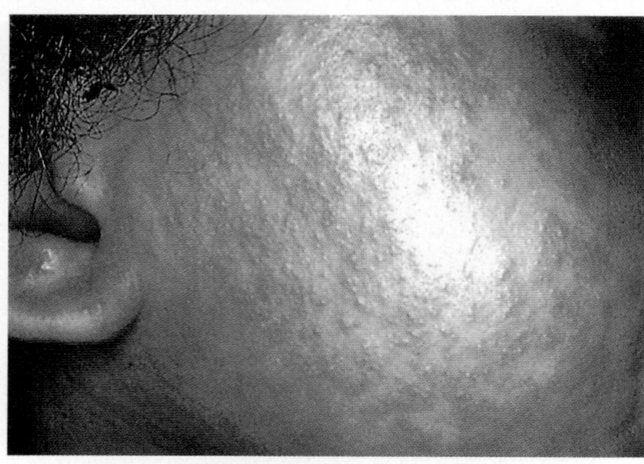

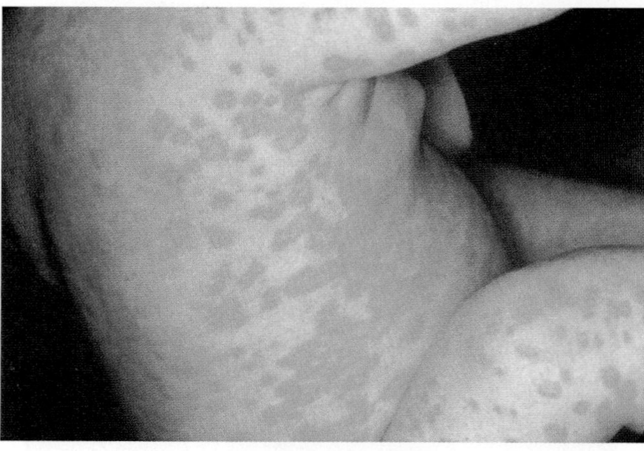

Measles (Rubeola) in Dark Skin

Measles (Rubeola) in Light Skin

Red-purple maculopapular blotchy rash in dark skin *(on left)* and in light skin *(on right)* appears on third or fourth day of illness. Rash appears first behind ears and spreads over face, then over neck, trunk, arms, and legs; looks "coppery" and does not blanch. Also characterized by Koplik spots in mouth—bluish white, red-based elevations of 1 to 3 mm (see Table 16-4, p. 378).

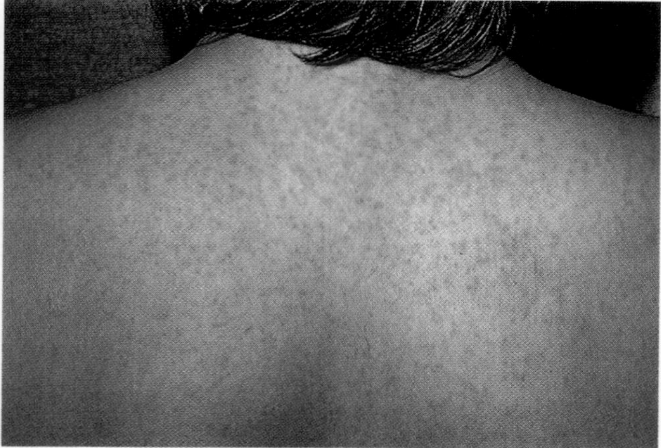

German Measles (Rubella)

Pink, papular rash (similar to measles but paler) first appears on face, then spreads. Distinguished from measles by presence of neck lymphadenopathy and absence of Koplik spots.

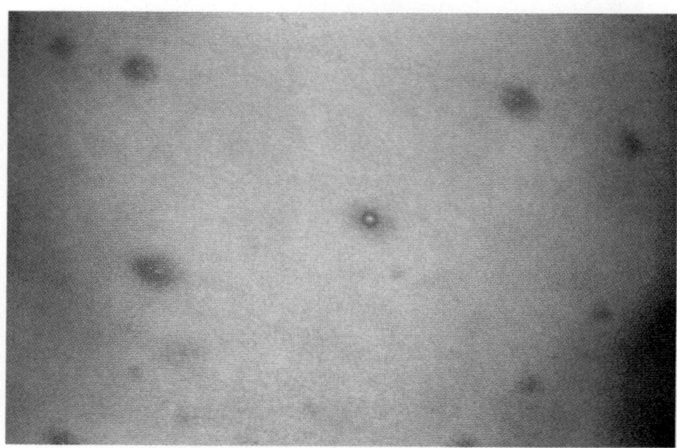

Chickenpox (Varicella)

Small, tight vesicles first appear on trunk, then spread to face, arms, and legs (not palms or soles). Shiny vesicles on an erythematous base are commonly described as the "dewdrop on a rose petal." Vesicles erupt in succeeding crops over several days, then become pustules, and then crusts. Intensely pruritic.

TABLE 12-10 Common Skin Lesions

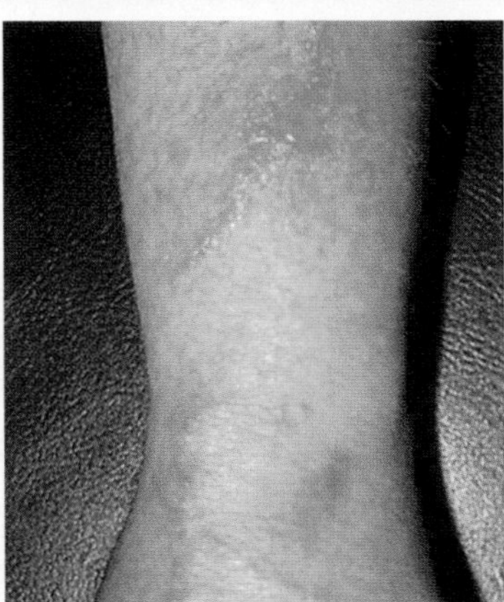

Primary Contact Dermatitis

Local inflammatory reaction to an irritant in the environment or an allergy. Characteristic location of lesions often gives clue. Often erythema shows first, followed by swelling, wheals (or urticaria), or maculopapular vesicles, scales. Frequently accompanied by intense pruritus. Example here: poison ivy.

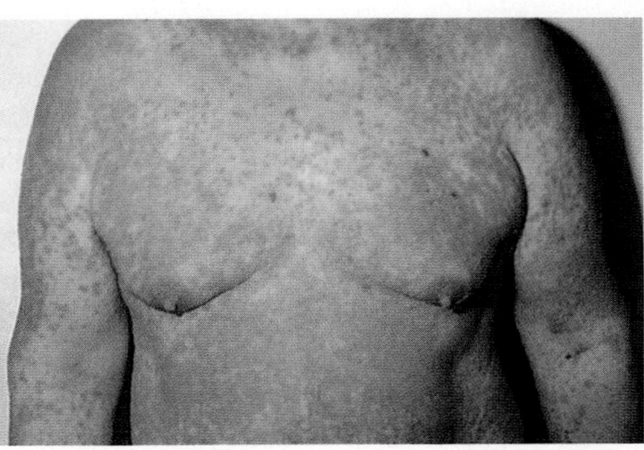

Allergic Drug Reaction

Erythematous and symmetric rash, usually generalized. Some drugs produce urticarial rash or vesicles and bullae. History of drug ingestion.

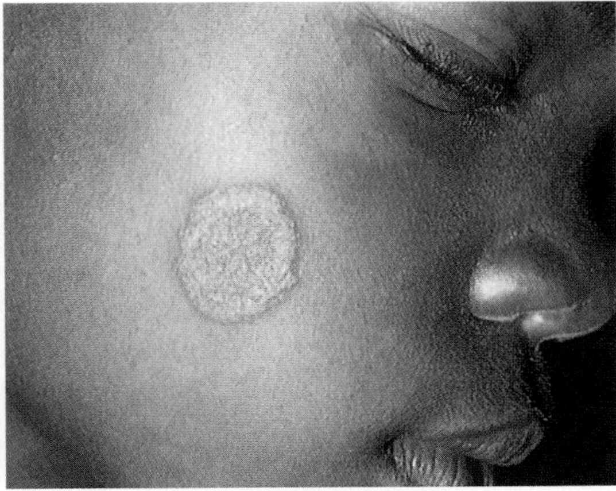

Tinea Corporis (Ringworm of the Body)

Scales—hyperpigmented in whites, depigmented in dark-skinned persons—on chest, abdomen, back of arms forming multiple circular lesions with clear centers.

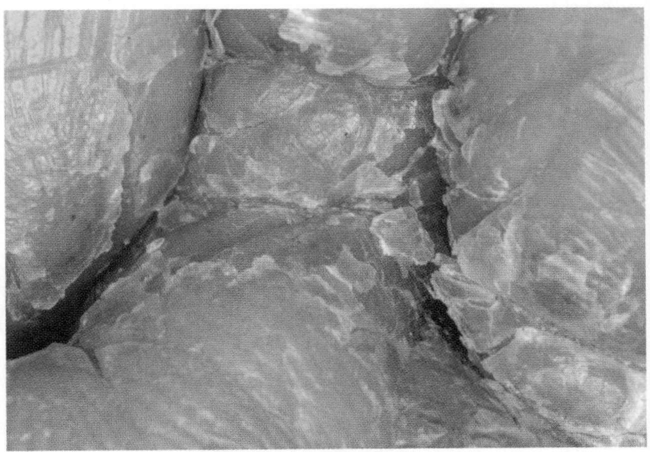

Tinea Pedis (Ringworm of the Foot)

"Athlete's foot," a fungal infection, first appears as small vesicles between toes, sides of feet, and soles and then grows scaly and hard. Found in chronically warm, moist feet: children after gymnasium activities, athletes, aging adults who cannot dry their feet well.

Continued

TABLE 12-10 **Common Skin Lesions—cont'd**

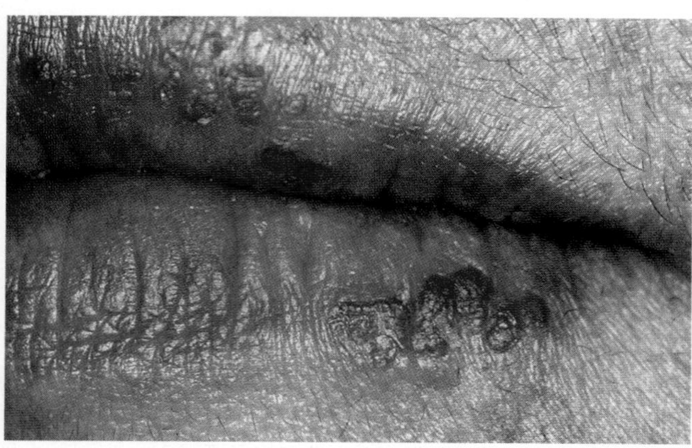

Labial Herpes Simplex (Cold Sores)

Herpes simplex virus (HSV) infection has a prodrome of skin tingling and sensitivity. Lesion then erupts with tight vesicles followed by pustules and then produces acute gingivostomatitis with many shallow, painful ulcers. Common location is upper lip, also in oral mucosa and tongue.

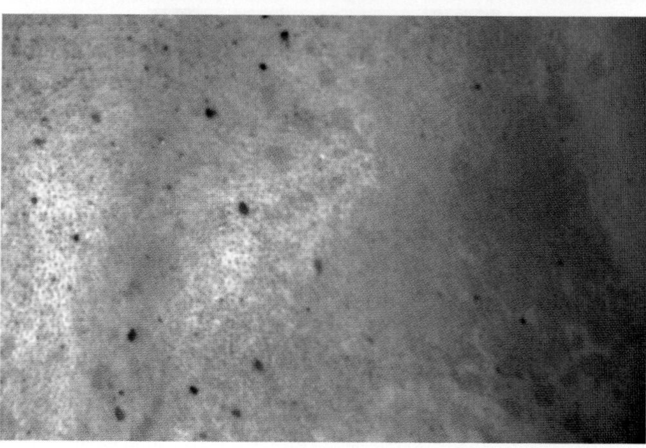

Tinea Versicolor

Fine, scaling, round patches of pink, tan, or white that (hence the name) do not tan in sunlight, caused by a superficial fungal infection. Usual distribution is on neck, trunk, and upper arms—a short-sleeved turtleneck sweater area. Most common in otherwise healthy young adults. Responds to oral antifungal medication.

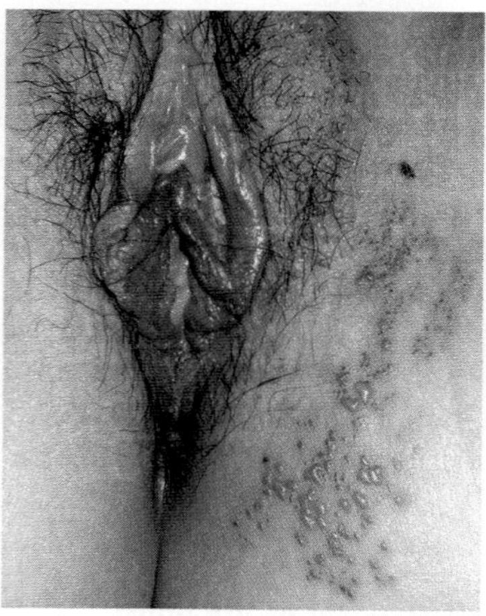

Herpes Zoster (Shingles)

Small, grouped vesicles emerge along route of cutaneous sensory nerve, then pustules, then crusts. Caused by the varicella zoster virus (VZV), a reactivation of the dormant virus of chickenpox. Acute appearance, unilateral, does not cross midline. Commonly on trunk, can be anywhere. If on ophthalmic branch of cranial nerve V, it poses risk to eye. Most common in adults older than 50 years. Pain is often severe and long lasting in aging adults, called *postherpetic neuralgia.*

NOTE: Be observant! The photo above is not genital herpes. This is herpes zoster with a linear lesion on only one side.

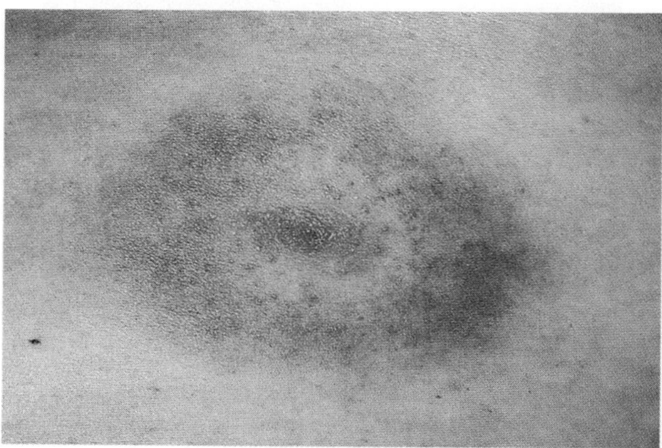

Erythema Migrans of Lyme Disease

Lyme disease (LD) is not fatal but may have serious arthritic, cardiac, or neurologic sequelae. It is caused by a spirochete bacterium carried by the black or dark brown deer tick. Deer ticks are common in the Northeast, upper Midwest, and California (with cases occurring in people who spend time outdoors) in May through September.

The first stage (early localized LD) has the distinctive bull's eye, red macular or papular rash (shown above) in 50% of cases. The rash radiates from the site of the tick bite (5 cm or larger), with some central clearing, and is usually located in axillae, midriff, inguina, or behind knees, with regional lymphadenopathy. Rash fades in 4 weeks; untreated individual then may have disseminated disease with fatigue, anorexia, fever, chills, joint or muscle aches. Antibiotic treatment shortens symptoms and decreases risk for sequelae.

TABLE 12-10 Common Skin Lesions—cont'd

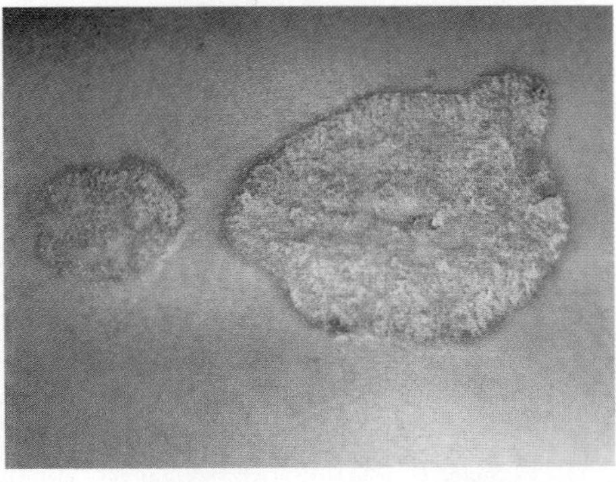

Psoriasis

Scaly, erythematous patch, with silvery scales on top. Usually on scalp, outside of elbows and knees, low back, and anogenital area.

TABLE 12-11 Malignant Skin Lesions

The link between ultraviolet (UV) radiation and skin cancer is well known; the UV radiation in sunlight promotes all three forms of skin cancer shown below. More than half a person's lifetime sun damage occurs before adulthood.[4]

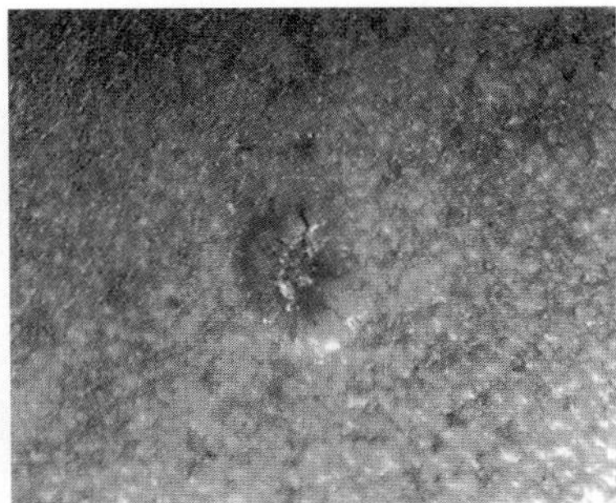

Basal Cell Carcinoma

Usually starts as a skin-colored papule (may be deeply pigmented) with a pearly translucent top and overlying telangiectasia (broken blood vessel). Then develops rounded, pearly borders with central red ulcer, or looks like large open pore with central yellowing. Most common form of skin cancer; slow but inexorable growth. Basal cell cancers occur on sun-exposed areas of face, ears, scalp, shoulders.

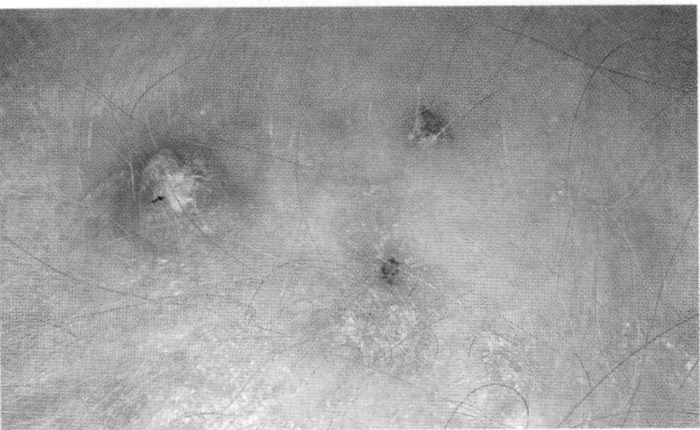

Squamous Cell Carcinoma

Squamous cell cancers arise from actinic keratoses or de novo. Erythematous scaly patch with sharp margins, 1 cm or more. Develops central ulcer and surrounding erythema. Usually on hands or head, areas exposed to UV radiation; above, on habitually sun-exposed bald scalp. Less common than basal cell carcinoma but grows rapidly.

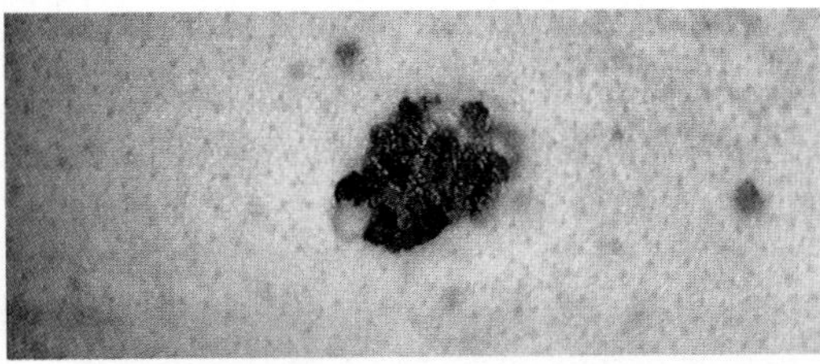

Malignant Melanoma

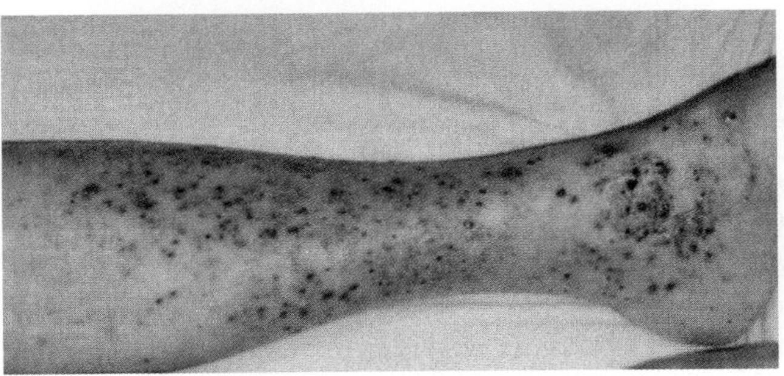

Metastatic Malignant Melanoma

Half of these lesions arise from preexisting nevi. Usually brown; can be tan, black, pink-red, purple, or mixed pigmentation. Often irregular or notched borders. May have scaling, flaking, oozing texture. Common locations are on the trunk and back in men and women, on the legs in women, and on the palms, soles of feet, and nails in Blacks.

TABLE 12-12 Abnormal Conditions of Hair

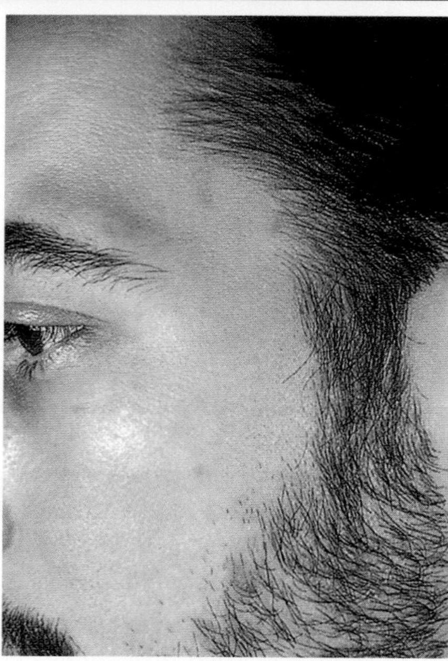

AIDS-related Kaposi Sarcoma: Patch Stage

Kaposi sarcoma (KS) is a vascular tumor and is the most common tumor in HIV-infected persons. Considered an AIDS-defining illness, KS can occur at any stage of HIV infection. Here, multiple patch-stage early lesions are faint pink on the temple and beard area. They easily could be mistaken for bruises or nevi and be ignored.

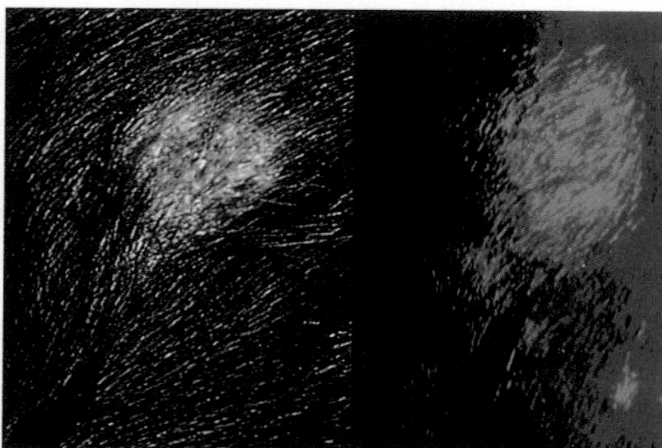

Tinea Capitis (Scalp Ringworm)

Rounded, patchy hair loss on scalp, leaving broken-off hairs, pustules, and scales on skin. Caused by fungal infection; lesions may fluoresce blue-green under Wood's light. Usually seen in children and farmers; highly contagious, may be transmitted by another person, by domestic animals, or from soil.

Traumatic Alopecia: Traction Alopecia ▶

Linear or oval patch of hair loss along hair line, a part, or scattered distribution; caused by trauma from hair rollers, tight braiding, tight ponytail, barrettes.

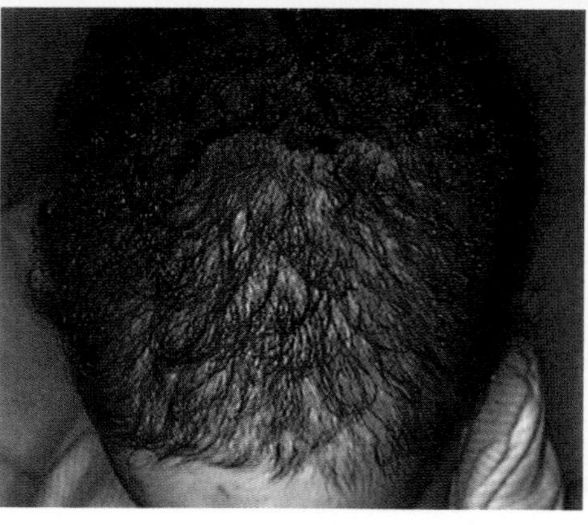

Toxic Alopecia

Patchy, asymmetric balding that accompanies severe illness or use of chemotherapy where growing hairs are lost and resting hairs are spared. Regrowth occurs after illness or discontinuation of toxin.

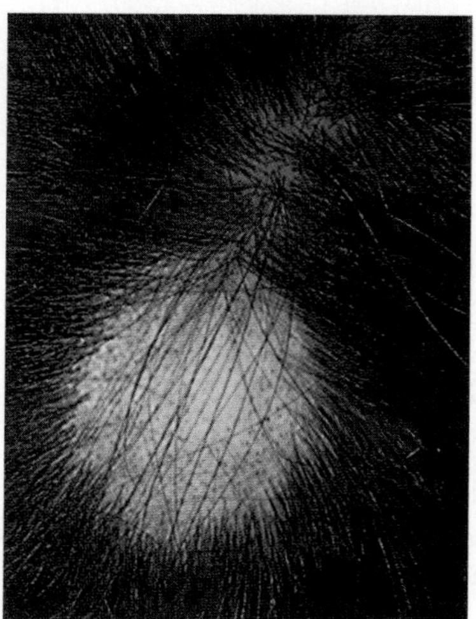

Alopecia Areata

Sudden appearance of a sharply circumscribed, round or oval balding patch, usually with smooth, soft, hairless skin underneath. Unknown cause; when limited to a few patches, person usually has complete regrowth.

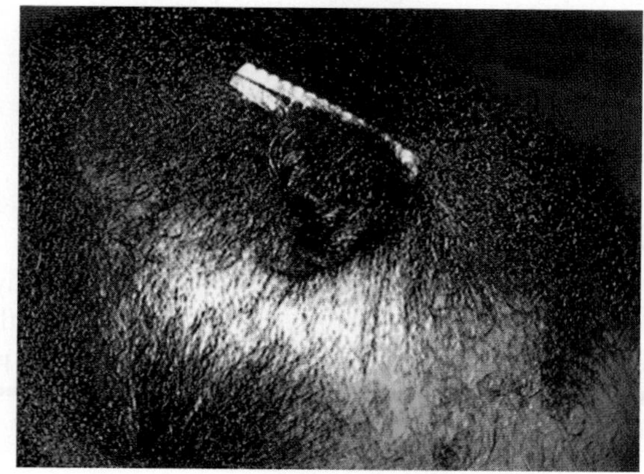

TABLE 12-12 Abnormal Conditions of Hair—cont'd

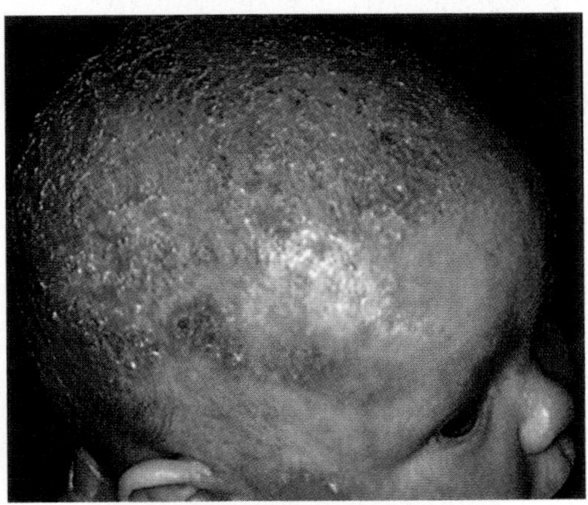

Seborrheic Dermatitis (Cradle Cap)

Thick, yellow to white, greasy, adherent scales with mild erythema on scalp and forehead; very common in early infancy. Resembles eczema lesions except cradle cap is distinguished by absence of pruritus, "greasy" yellow-pink lesions, and negative family history of allergy.

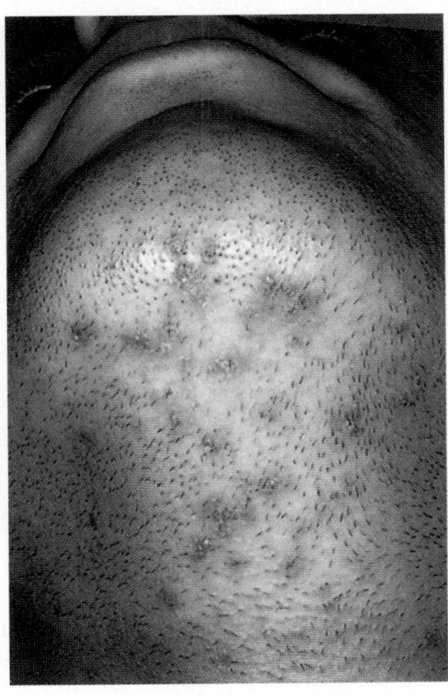

Folliculitis

Superficial infection of hair follicles. Multiple pustules, "whiteheads," with hair visible at center and erythematous base. Usually on arms, legs, face, and buttocks.

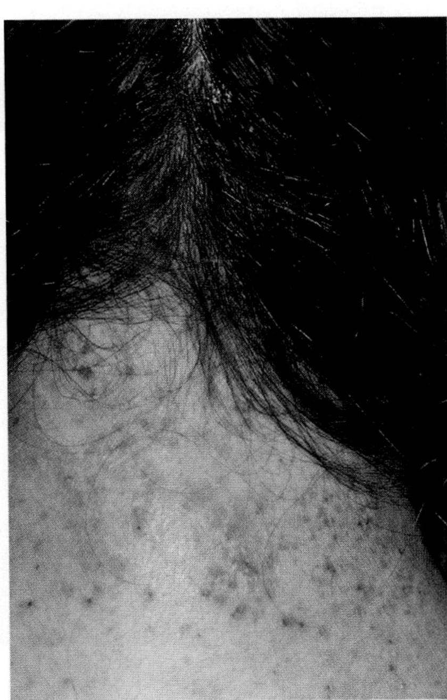

Pediculosis Capitis (Head Lice)

History includes intense itching of the scalp, especially the occiput. The nits (eggs) of lice are easier to see in the occipital area and around the ears, appearing as 2- to 3-mm oval translucent bodies, adherent to the hair shafts. Common among school-age children. Over-the-counter pediculicide shampoos are available; however, nit removal by daily combing of wet hair with a fine-tooth metal comb is especially important.

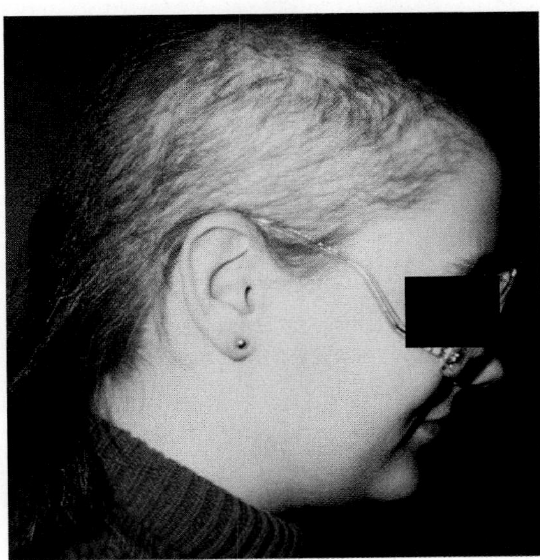

Trichotillomania

Traumatic self-induced hair loss usually the result of compulsive twisting or plucking. Forms irregularly shaped patch, with broken-off, stublike hairs of varying lengths; person is never completely bald. Occurs as child rubs or twists area absently while falling asleep, reading, or watching television. In adults, it can be a serious problem and is usually a sign of a personality disorder.

Continued

TABLE 12-12 Abnormal Conditions of Hair—cont'd

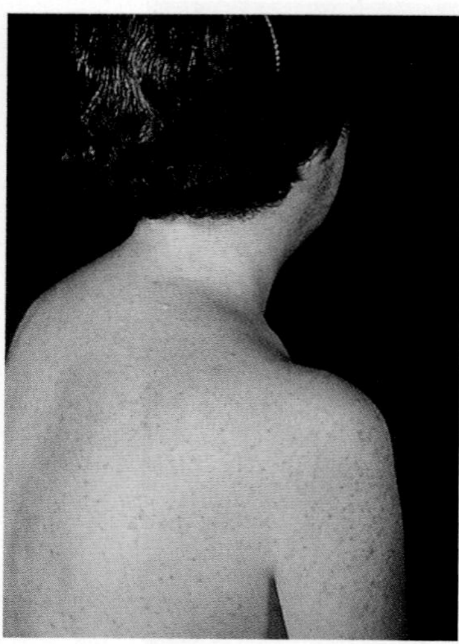

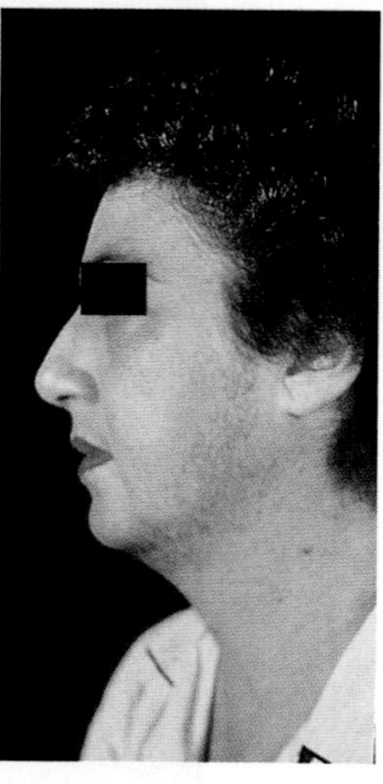

Hirsutism

Excess body hair in females forming a male sexual pattern (upper lip, face, chest, abdomen, arms, legs); caused by endocrine or metabolic dysfunction or occasionally idiopathic.

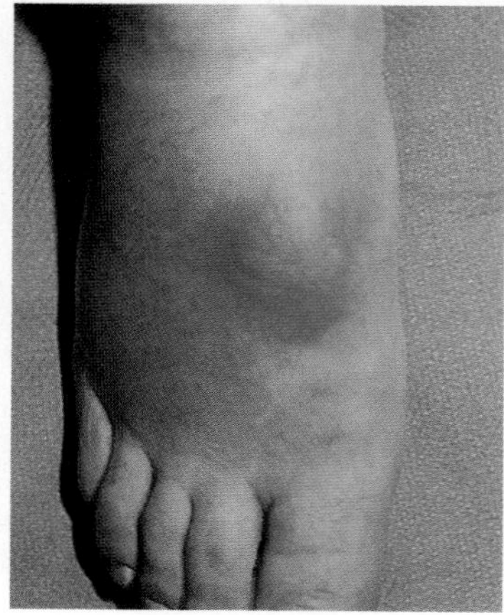

Furuncle and Abscess

Red, swollen, hard, tender, pus-filled lesion caused by acute, localized bacterial (usually staphylococcal) infection; usually on back of neck, buttocks, occasionally on wrists or ankles. Furuncles are due to infected hair follicles, whereas abscesses are due to traumatic introduction of bacteria into the skin. Abscesses are usually larger and deeper than furuncles.

TABLE 12-13 Abnormal Conditions of the Nails

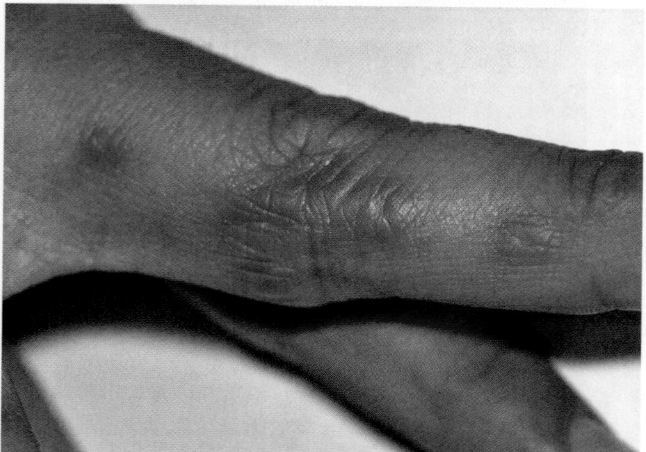

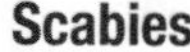

Scabies

An intensely pruritic contagion caused by the scabies mite. Mites form a linear or curved elevated burrow on the fingers, web spaces of hands, and wrists. Other family members are usually infected. The patient cannot stop scratching.[10]

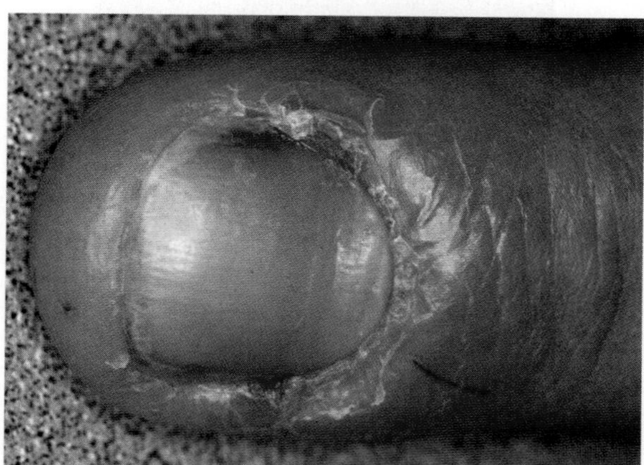

Paronychia

Red, swollen, tender inflammation of the nail folds. Acute paronychia is usually a bacterial infection; chronic paronychia is most often a fungal infection from a break in the cuticle in those who perform "wet" work.

TABLE 12-13 Abnormal Conditions of the Nails—cont'd

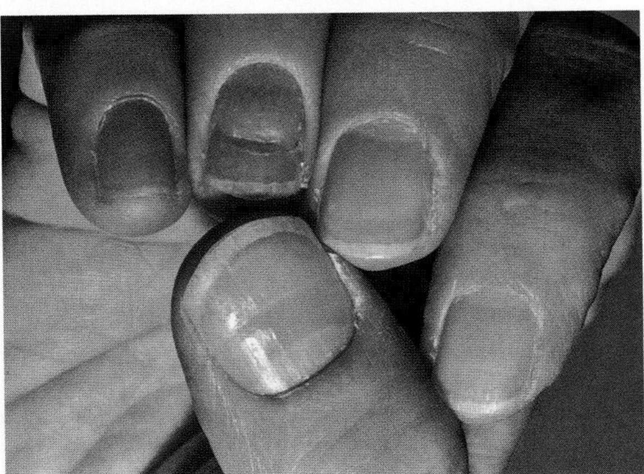

Beau's Line

Transverse furrow or groove. A depression across the nail that extends down to the nail bed. Occurs with any trauma that temporarily impairs nail formation, such as acute illness, toxic reaction, or local trauma. Dent appears first at the cuticle and moves forward as nail grows.

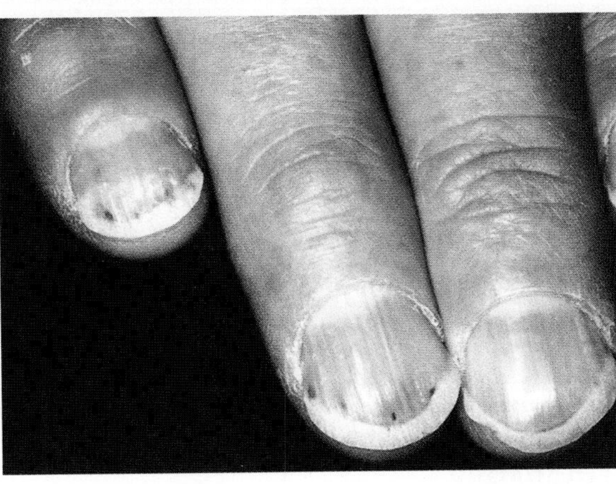

Splinter Hemorrhages

Red-brown linear streaks, embolic lesions, occur with subacute bacterial endocarditis; also may occur with minor trauma.

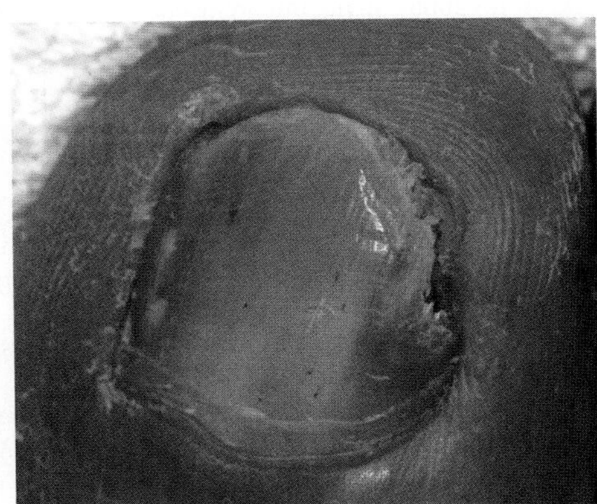

Onycholysis

This is a slow, persistent fungal infection of fingernails and, more often, toenails, common in older adults. Fungus causes change in color (green where nail plate separated from bed), texture, thickness, with nail crumbling or breaking, and loosening of the nail plate, usually beginning at the distal edge and progressing proximally.

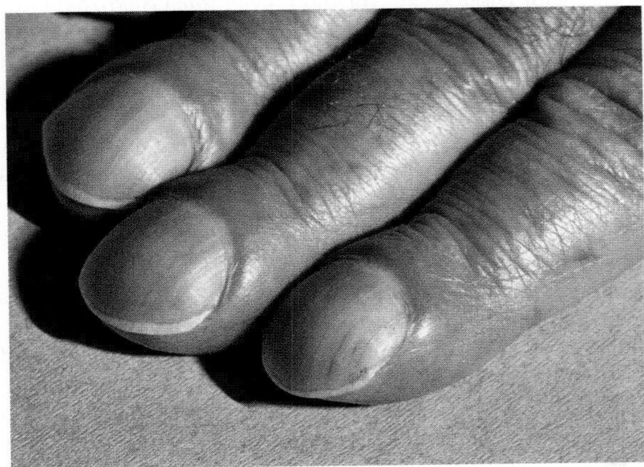

Late Clubbing

Inner edge of nail elevates; nail bed angle is greater than 180 degrees. Distal phalanx looks rounder and wider. Recent research links clubbing with the physiology of platelet production.[21] Diseases that disrupt normal pulmonary circulation (chronic lung inflammation, bronchial tumors, heart defects with right-to-left shunts) cause fragmented platelets to become trapped in the fingertip vasculature, releasing platelet-derived growth factor and promoting growth of vessels, which shows as clubbing. Clubbing usually develops slowly over years; if the primary disease is treated, clubbing can reverse.

Reprinted from the Clinical Slide Collection on the Rheumatic Diseases, © 1991, 1995, 1997. Used by permission of the American College of Rheumatology.

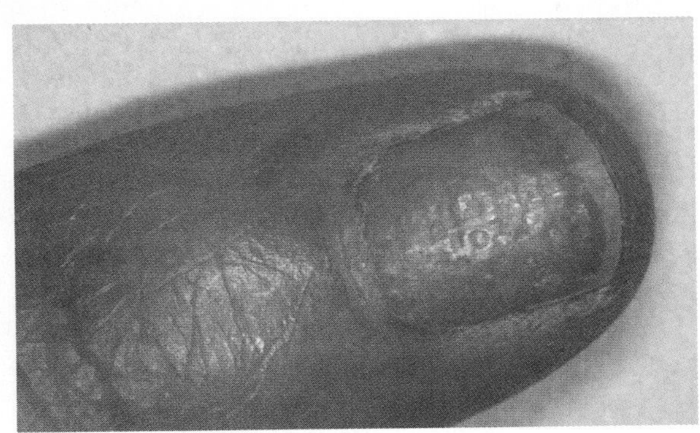

◀ Pitting

Sharply defined pitting and crumbling of the nails with distal detachment often occurs with psoriasis.

Continued

TABLE 12-13 Abnormal Conditions of the Nails—cont'd

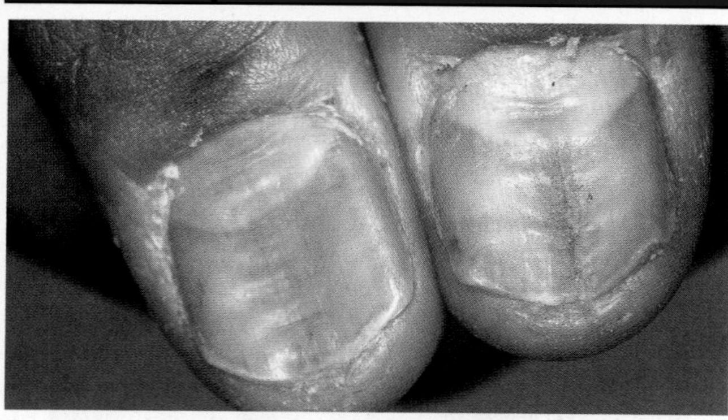

◀ **Habit-Tic Dystrophy**

Depression down middle of nail or multiple horizontal ridges, caused by continuous picking of cuticle by another finger of same hand, which causes injury to nail base and nail matrix.

BIBLIOGRAPHY

1. American Cancer Society (ACS). (2009). *Skin cancer*. Retrieved September 20, 2009, from www.cancer.org/downloads/PRO/SkinCancer.pdf.
2. Arora, A., & Attwood, J. (2009). Common skin cancers and their precursors. *Surgical Clinics of North America, 89*(3), 703-712.
3. Borfitz, J. M. (2009). Commonly missed dermatologic conditions. *Nurse Practitioner, 34*(10), 35-45.
4. Centers for Disease Control and Prevention. (2006). *Skin cancer*. Retrieved September 20, 2009, from www.cdc.gov/healthyyouth/skincancer/guidelines/summary.htm.
5. Christopher, G. F., & Meires, J. (2008). Treating acute onset of psoriasis. *Nurse Practitioner, 33*(7), 7-10.
6. Drugge, J. M., & Allen, P. J. (2008). A nurse practitioner's guide to the management of herpes simplex virus-1 in children. *Pediatric Nursing, 34*(4), 310-318.
7. Emond, R. T., Welsby, P., & Rowland, H. (2003). *Colour atlas of infectious diseases* (4th ed.). St. Louis: Mosby.
8. Friedman-Kien, A. E. (1996). *Color atlas of AIDS* (2nd ed.). Philadelphia: Saunders.
9. Gordon, R. M. (2009). Skin cancer: more than skin deep. *The Nurse Practitioner, 34*(4), 21-28.
10. Habif, T. P., Campbell, J. L., Jr., Chapman, M. S., et al. (2005). *Skin disease: diagnosis and treatment* (2nd ed.). St. Louis: Mosby.
11. Holzberg, M. (2006). Common nail disorders. *Dermatologic Clinics, 24*(3), 349-354.
12. Howard, J., & Loiselle, J. (2006). A clinician's guide to safe and effective tick removal. *Contemporary Pediatrics, 23*(5), 36-42.
13. Marks, J. G., & Miller, J. (2006). *Lookingbill and Marks' principles of dermatology* (4th ed.). Philadelphia: Saunders.
14. Nash, K. R., & Sheridan, D. J. (2009). Can one accurately date a bruise? State of the science. *Journal of Forensic Nursing, 5*, 31-37.
15. National Pressure Ulcer Advisory Panel (NPUAP). (2007). *Pressure ulcer stages revised by NPUAP*. Retrieved September 20, 2009, from www.npaup.org/pr2.htm.
16. Pandya, K. A., & Radke, F. (2009). Benign skin lesions: lipomas, epidermal inclusion cysts, muscle and nerve biopsies. *Surgical Clinics of North America, 89*(3), 677-687.
17. Rhoads, J. (2009). Managing bites and stings. *Nurse Practitioner, 34*(8), 37-43.
18. Roebuck, H. L. (2006). Acne: intervene early. *Nurse Practitioner, 31*(10), 24-45.
19. Roebuck, H., & Siegel, M. (2006). The ABCs of melanoma recognition. *Nurse Practitioner, 31*(6), 11-13.
20. Spector, R. E. (2004). *Cultural diversity in health and illness*. Upper Saddle River, NJ: Prentice Hall.
21. Spicknall, K. E., Zirwas, M. J., & English, J. C. (2005). Clubbing: an update on diagnosis, differential diagnosis, pathophysiology, and clinical relevance. *Journal of the American Academy of Dermatology, 52*, 1020-1028.
22. Stanger, C. B. (2009). Actinic keratosis: do the numbers add up? *Nurse Practitioner, 34*(2), 36-39.
23. Sullivan, J. R., & Shear, N. H. (2002). Drug eruptions and other adverse drug effects in aged skin. *Clinics in Geriatric Medicine, 18*(1), 21-42.
24. Trent, J., & Kirsner, R. (2004). Cutaneous manifestations of HIV: a primer. *Advances in Skin & Wound Care, 17*(3), 116-129.
25. U.S. Preventive Services Task Force (USPSTF). (2008). *Skin cancer screening: guide to clinical preventive services*. Retrieved September 20, 2009, from www.ahrq.gov/clinic/prevenix.htm.
26. Wilson, D. D. (2007). Herpes zoster: prevention, diagnosis, and treatment. *Nurse Practitioner, 32*(9), 19-25.
27. Wolff, T., Tai, E., & Miller, T. (2009). Screening for skin cancer: an update of the evidence for the U.S. Preventive Services Task Force. *Annals of Internal Medicine, 150*(3), 194-198.

Summary Checklist: Skin, Hair, and Nails Examination

For a PDA-downloadable version, go to http://evolve.elsevier.com/Jarvis/.

1. **Inspect the skin:**
   - Color
   - General pigmentation
   - Areas of hypopigmentation or hyperpigmentation
   - Abnormal color changes
2. **Palpate the skin:**
   - Temperature
   - Moisture
   - Texture
   - Thickness
   - Edema
   - Mobility and turgor
   - Hygiene
   - Vascularity or bruising
3. **Note any lesions:**
   - Color
   - Shape and configuration
   - Size
   - Location and distribution on body
4. **Inspect and palpate the hair:**
   - Texture
   - Distribution
   - Any scalp lesions
5. **Inspect and palpate the nails:**
   - Shape and contour
   - Consistency
   - Color
6. **Teach skin self-examination**

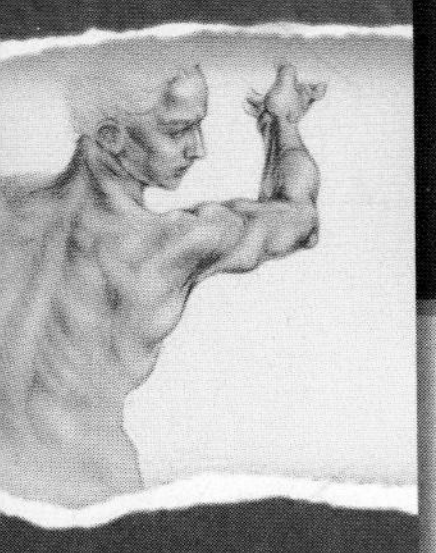

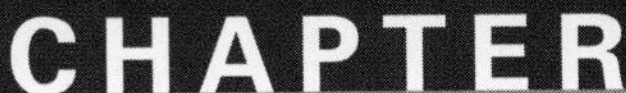

CHAPTER

13

Head, Face, and Neck, Including Regional Lymphatics

evolve WEBSITE

http://evolve.elsevier.com/Jarvis/

- Animations
- Audio Key Points
- Bedside Assessment Summary Checklist
- Case Study
  Pain Behind Ear
- NCLEX Review Questions
- Physical Examination Summary Checklist
- Video—Assessment
  Head and Face
  Neck

OUTLINE

Structure and Function, 251

The Head
The Neck
Lymphatics

Subjective Data, 256

Health History Questions

Objective Data, 259

The Head
The Neck

Documentation and Critical Thinking, 268

Abnormal Findings, 270

STRUCTURE AND FUNCTION

THE HEAD

The **skull** is a rigid bony box that protects the brain and special sense organs, and it includes the bones of the cranium and the face (Fig. 13-1). Note the location of these **cranial bones:** frontal, parietal, occipital, and temporal. Use these names to describe any of your clinical findings in the corresponding areas.

The adjacent cranial bones unite at meshed immovable joints called the **sutures.** The bones are not firmly joined at birth; this allows for the mobility and change in shape needed for the birth process. The sutures gradually ossify during early childhood. The **coronal** suture *crowns* the head from ear to ear at the union of the frontal and parietal bones. The **sagittal** suture *separates* the head lengthwise between the two parietal bones. The **lambdoid** suture separates the parietal bones crosswise from the occipital bone.

The 14 **facial bones** also articulate at sutures (note the nasal bone, zygomatic bone, and maxilla), except for the mandible (the lower jaw). It moves up, down, and sideways from the temporomandibular joint, which is anterior to each ear.

The cranium is supported by the cervical vertebra: C1, the "atlas"; C2, the "axis"; and down to C7. The C7 vertebra has a long spinous process that is palpable when the head is flexed. Feel this useful landmark, the **vertebra prominens,** on your own neck.

The human **face** has myriad appearances and a large array of facial expressions that reflect mood. The expressions are formed by the facial muscles (Fig. 13-2), which are mediated

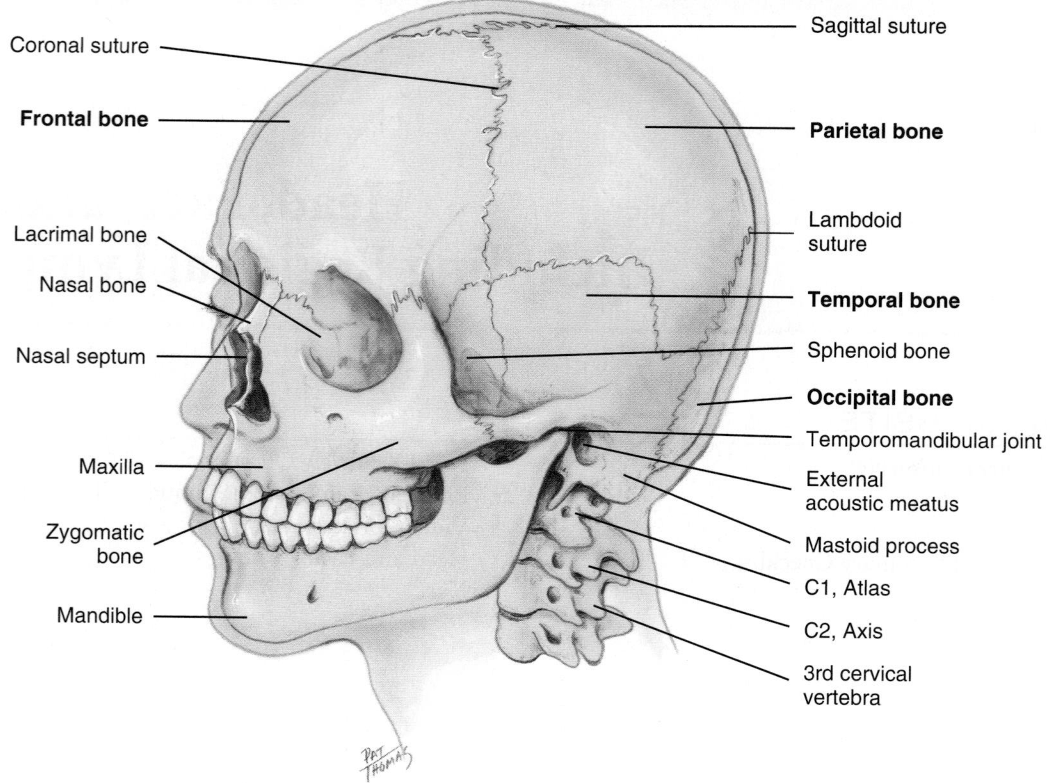
Coronal suture
Sagittal suture
Frontal bone
Parietal bone
Lacrimal bone
Lambdoid suture
Nasal bone
Temporal bone
Nasal septum
Sphenoid bone
Occipital bone
Temporomandibular joint
Maxilla
External acoustic meatus
Zygomatic bone
Mastoid process
C1, Atlas
Mandible
C2, Axis
3rd cervical vertebra
PAT THOMAS

13-1

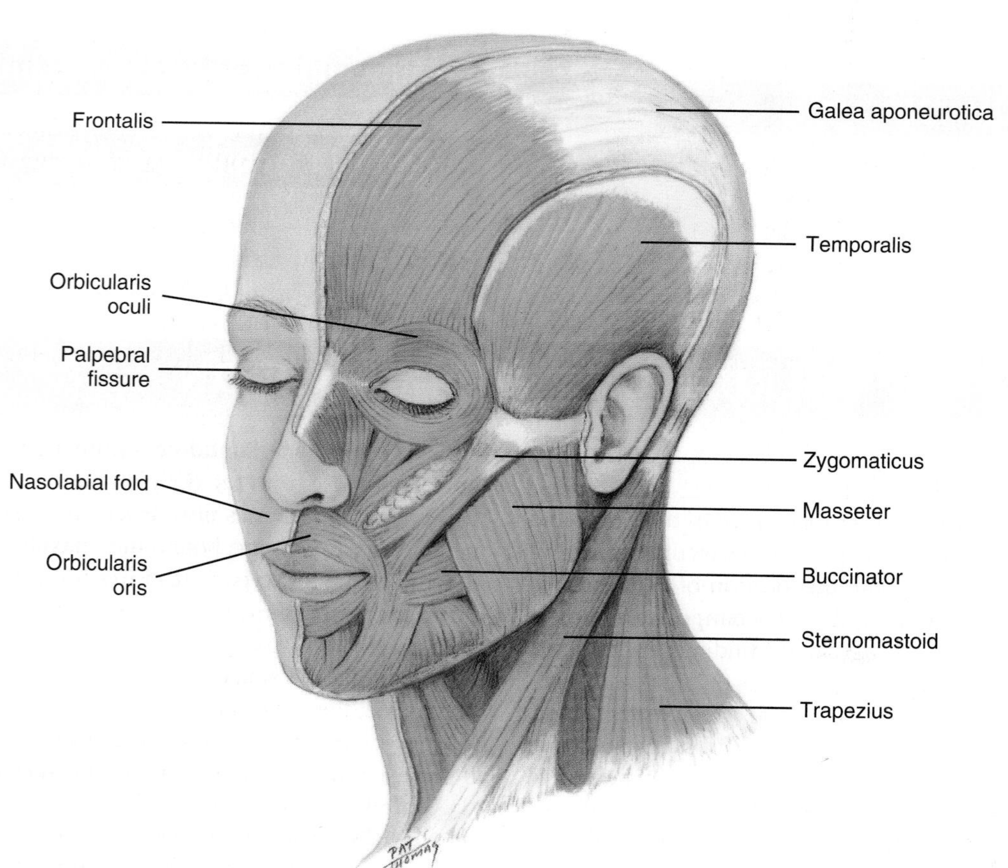
Frontalis
Galea aponeurotica
Temporalis
Orbicularis oculi
Palpebral fissure
Zygomaticus
Nasolabial fold
Masseter
Orbicularis oris
Buccinator
Sternomastoid
Trapezius
PAT THOMAS

13-2 Facial muscles.

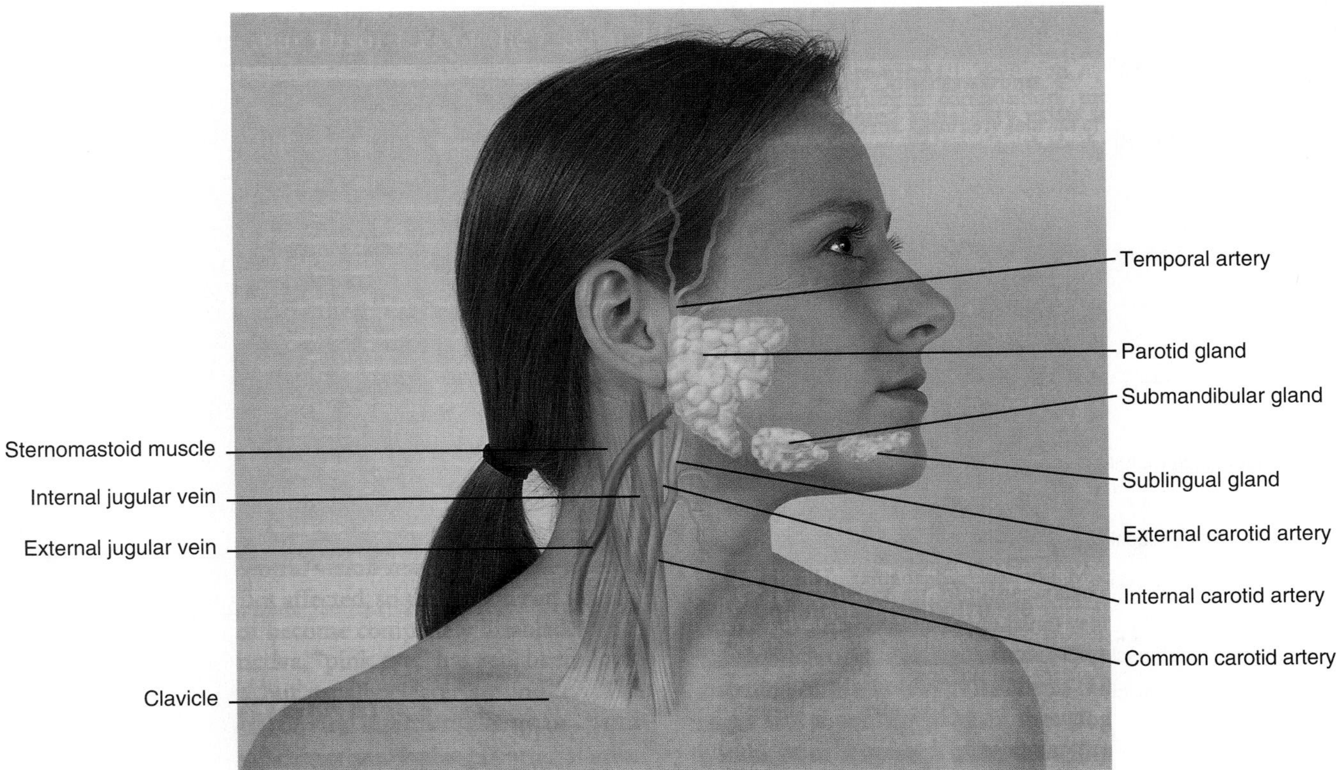

13-3

by cranial nerve VII, the facial nerve. Facial muscle function is symmetric bilaterally, except for an occasional quirk or wry expression.

Facial structures also are symmetric; the eyebrows, eyes, ears, nose, and mouth appear about the same on both sides. The palpebral fissures—the openings between the eyelids—are equal bilaterally. Also, the nasolabial folds, the creases extending from the nose to each corner of the mouth, should look symmetric. Facial sensations of pain or touch are mediated by the three sensory branches of cranial nerve V, the trigeminal nerve. (Testing for sensory function is described in Chapter 23.)

Two pairs of **salivary glands** are accessible to examination on the face (Fig. 13-3). The **parotid** glands are in the cheeks over the mandible, anterior to and below the ear. They are the largest of the salivary glands but are not normally palpable. The **submandibular** glands are beneath the mandible at the angle of the jaw. A third pair, the **sublingual** glands, lie in the floor of the mouth. (Salivary gland function follows in Chapter 16.) The **temporal artery** lies superior to the temporalis muscle; its pulsation is palpable anterior to the ear.

THE NECK

The **neck** is delimited by the base of the skull and inferior border of the mandible above, and by the manubrium sterni, the clavicle, the first rib, and the first thoracic vertebra below. Think of the neck as a *conduit* for the passage of many structures, which are lying in close proximity: blood vessels, muscles, nerves, lymphatics, and viscera of the respiratory and digestive systems. Blood vessels include the common and internal carotid arteries and their associated veins (see Fig. 13-3). The internal carotid branches off the common carotid and runs inward and upward to supply the brain; the external carotid supplies the face, salivary glands, and superficial temporal area. The carotid artery and internal jugular vein lie beneath the sternomastoid muscle. The external jugular vein runs diagonally across the sternomastoid muscle. (See assessment of the neck vessels beginning on p. 470 in Chapter 19.)

The major **neck muscles** are the **sternomastoid** and the **trapezius** (Fig. 13-4); they are innervated by cranial nerve XI, the spinal accessory. The sternomastoid muscle arises from the sternum and the clavicle and extends diagonally across the neck to the mastoid process behind the ear. It accomplishes head rotation and head flexion. The two trapezius muscles on the upper back arise from the occipital bone and the vertebrae and extend fanning out to the scapula and clavicle. The trapezius muscles move the shoulders and extend and turn the head.

The sternomastoid muscle divides each side of the neck into two triangles. The **anterior triangle** lies in front, between the sternomastoid and the midline of the body, with its base up along the lower border of the mandible and its apex down at the suprasternal notch. The **posterior triangle** is behind the sternomastoid muscle, with the trapezius muscle on the

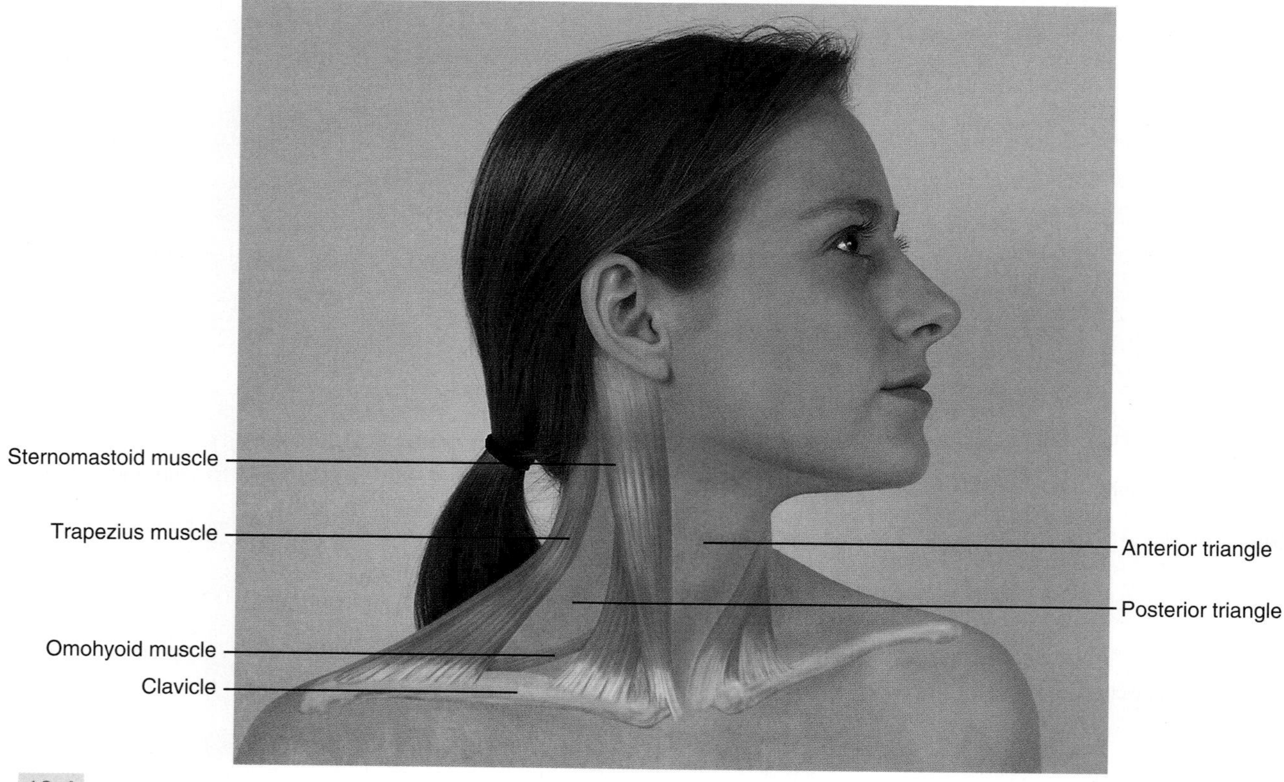

13-4

other side and with its base along the clavicle below. It contains the posterior belly of the omohyoid muscle. These triangles are helpful guidelines when describing findings in the neck.

The **thyroid gland** is an important endocrine gland with a rich blood supply. It straddles the trachea in the middle of the neck (Fig. 13-5). This highly vascular endocrine gland synthesizes and secretes thyroxine (T_4) and triiodothyronine (T_3), hormones that stimulate the rate of cellular metabolism. The gland has two lobes, both conical in shape, each curving posteriorly between the trachea and the sternomastoid muscle. The lobes are connected in the middle by a thin isthmus lying over the second and third tracheal rings.

Just above the thyroid isthmus, within about 1 cm, is the **cricoid** cartilage or upper tracheal ring. The **thyroid** cartilage is above that, with a small, palpable notch in its upper edge.

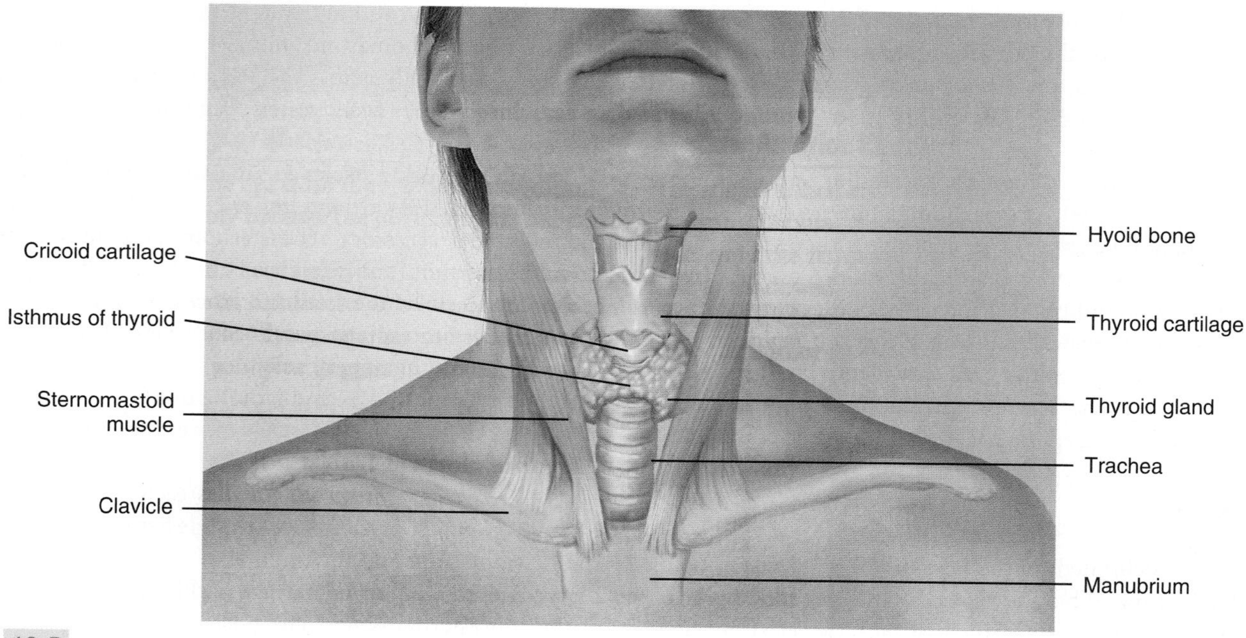

13-5

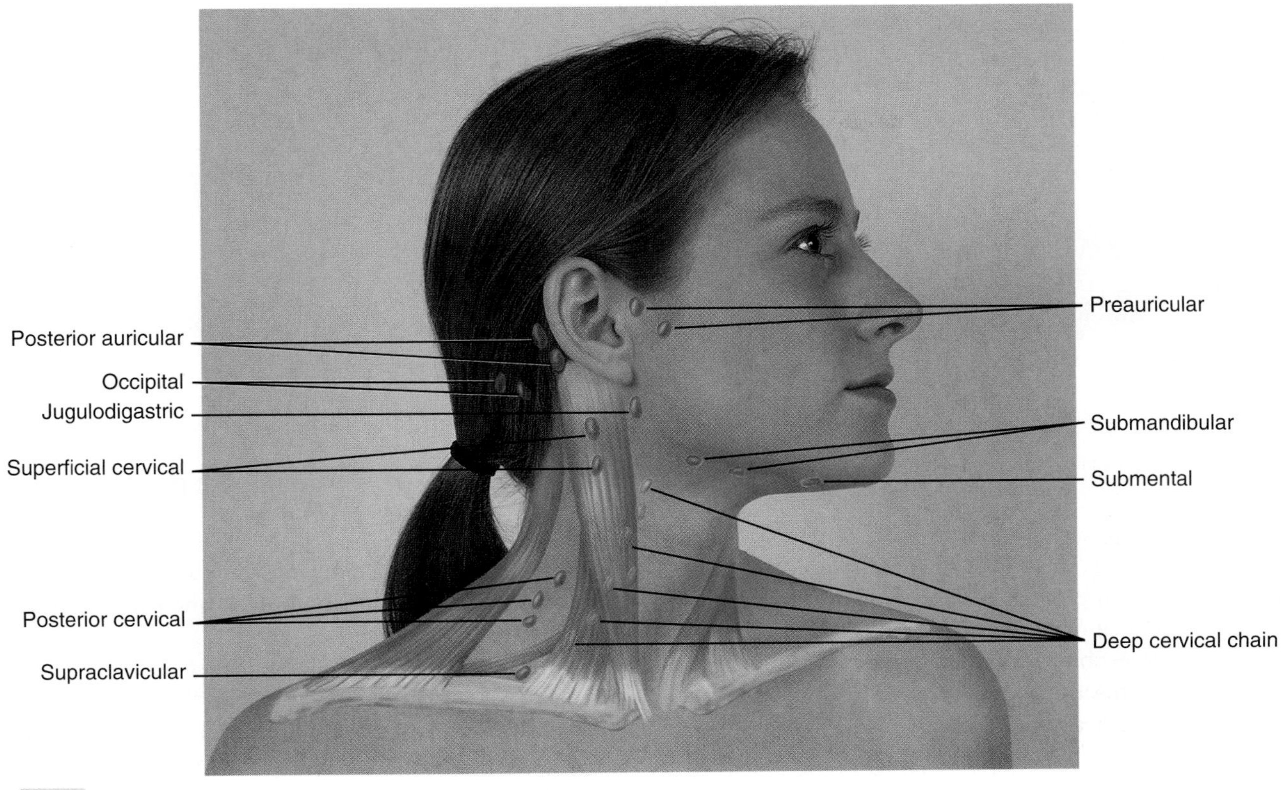

13-6

This is the prominent "Adam's apple" in males. The highest is the **hyoid** bone, palpated high in the neck at the level of the floor of the mouth.

LYMPHATICS

The lymphatic system is developed more fully in Chapter 20, p. 502. However, the head and neck have a rich supply of **lymph nodes** (Fig. 13-6). Although sources differ as to their nomenclature, one commonly used system is given here. Note that their labels correspond to adjacent structures.

- *Preauricular,* in front of the ear
- *Posterior auricular* (mastoid), superficial to the mastoid process
- *Occipital,* at the base of the skull
- *Submental,* midline, behind the tip of the mandible
- *Submandibular,* halfway between the angle and the tip of the mandible
- *Jugulodigastric,* under the angle of the mandible
- *Superficial cervical,* overlying the sternomastoid muscle
- *Deep cervical,* deep under the sternomastoid muscle
- *Posterior cervical,* in the posterior triangle along the edge of the trapezius muscle
- *Supraclavicular,* just above and behind the clavicle, at the sternomastoid muscle

You also should be familiar with the direction of the **drainage patterns** of the lymph nodes (Fig. 13-7). When nodes are abnormal, check the area they drain for the source of the problem. Explore the area proximal (upstream) to the location of the abnormal node.

The lymphatic system is an extensive vessel system, which is separate from the cardiovascular system and is phylogenetically older. The lymphatics are a major part of the immune system, whose job it is to detect and eliminate foreign substances from the body. The vessels allow the flow of clear, watery fluid (lymph) from the tissue spaces into the circulation. Lymph nodes are small, oval clusters of lymphatic tissue that are set at intervals along the lymph vessels

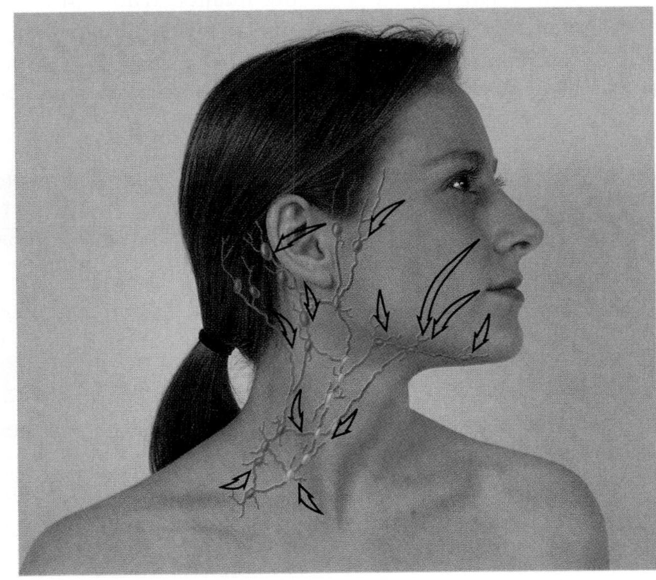

13-7

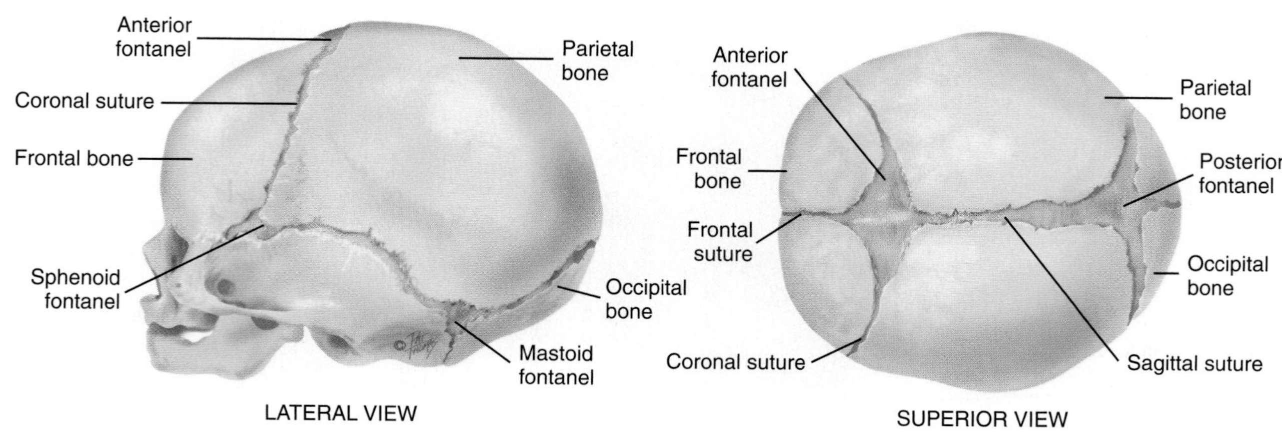

13-8 BONES OF THE NEONATAL SKULL

like beads on a string. The nodes filter the lymph and engulf pathogens, preventing potentially harmful substances from entering the circulation. Nodes are located throughout the body but are accessible to examination only in four areas: head and neck, arms, axillae, and inguinal region. The greatest supply is in the head and neck.

DEVELOPMENTAL COMPETENCE

Infants and Children

The bones of the neonatal skull are separated by sutures and by **fontanels,** the spaces where the sutures intersect (Fig. 13-8). These membrane-covered "soft spots" allow for growth of the brain during the 1st year. They gradually ossify; the triangle-shaped posterior fontanel is closed by 1 to 2 months, and the diamond-shaped anterior fontanel closes between 9 months and 2 years.

During the fetal period, head growth predominates. Head size is greater than chest circumference at birth. The head size grows during childhood, reaching 90% of its final size when the child is 6 years old. But during infancy, trunk growth predominates so that head size changes in proportion to body height. Facial bones grow at varying rates, especially nasal and jaw bones. In the toddler, the mandible and maxilla are small and the nasal bridge is low, so that the whole face seems small compared with the skull.

Lymphoid tissue is well developed at birth and grows to adult size when the child is 6 years old. The child's lymphatic tissue continues to grow rapidly until age 10 or 11 years, actually exceeding its adult size before puberty. Then the lymphatic tissue slowly atrophies.

In adolescence, facial hair appears on boys, first above the lip, then on cheeks and below the lip, and last on the chin. A noticeable enlargement of the thyroid cartilage occurs, and with it, the voice deepens.

The Pregnant Woman

The thyroid gland enlarges slightly during pregnancy as a result of hyperplasia of the tissue and increased vascularity.

The Aging Adult

The facial bones and orbits appear more prominent, and the facial skin sags as a result of decreased elasticity, decreased subcutaneous fat, and decreased moisture in the skin. The lower face may look smaller if teeth have been lost.

SUBJECTIVE DATA

1. Headache
2. Head injury
3. Dizziness
4. Neck pain, limitation of motion
5. Lumps or swelling
6. History of head or neck surgery

Examiner Asks	Rationale
1. Headache. Any unusually frequent or unusually severe **headaches?** • Onset. When did *this kind* of headache start? • Gradual, over hours, or a day? • Or, suddenly, over minutes, or less than 1 hour?	This is a more meaningful question than "Do you ever have headaches?" because most people have had at least one headache. Because many conditions have a headache as a symptom, a detailed history is important.

Examiner Asks	Rationale
• Ever had *this kind* of headache before?	A red flag is a severe headache in an adult or child who has never had it before.
• Location. Where do you feel it: frontal, temporal, behind your eyes, like a band around the head, in the sinus area, or in the occipital area?	Tension headaches tend to be occipital, frontal, or with bandlike tightness; migraines (vascular) tend to be supraorbital, retro-orbital, or frontotemporal; cluster headaches (vascular) produce pain around the eye, temple, forehead, cheek.
• Is pain localized on one side, or all over?	Unilateral or bilateral (e.g., with cluster headaches, pain is always unilateral and always on the same side of the head).
• Character. Throbbing (pounding, shooting) or aching (viselike, constant pressure, dull)?	Character is typically viselike with tension headache, throbbing with migraine or temporal arteritis.
• Is it mild, moderate, or severe?	Pain is often severe with migraine, or excruciating with cluster headache.
• Course and duration. What time of day do the headaches occur: morning, evening, awaken you from sleep? How long do they last? Hours, days? Have you noted any daily headaches, or several within a time period?	Migraines occur about twice per month, each lasting 1 to 3 days; cluster headaches occur once or twice per day, each lasting ½ to 2 hours for 1 to 2 months, and remission may last for months or years.
• Precipitating factors. What brings it on: activity or exercise, work environment, emotional upset, anxiety, alcohol? (Also note signs of depression.)	Alcohol ingestion and daytime napping typically precipitate cluster headaches, whereas alcohol, letdown after stress, menstruation, and eating chocolate or cheese precipitate migraines.
• Associated factors. Any relation to other symptoms: any nausea and vomiting? (Note which came first, headache or nausea.) Any vision changes, pain with bright lights, neck pain or stiffness, fever, weakness, moodiness, stomach problems?	Nausea, vomiting, and visual disturbances are associated with migraines; eye reddening and tearing, eyelid drooping, rhinorrhea, and nasal congestion are associated with cluster headaches; anxiety and stress are associated with tension headaches; nuchal rigidity and fever are associated with meningitis or encephalitis.
• Do you have any other illness?	Hypertension, fever, hypothyroidism, and vasculitis produce headaches.
• Do you take any medications?	Oral contraceptives, bronchodilators, alcohol, nitrates, carbon monoxide inhalation produce headaches.
• What makes it worse: movement, coughing, straining, exercise?	
• Pattern. Any family history of headache? What is the frequency of your headaches: once a week? Are your headaches occurring closer together? Are they getting worse? Or are they getting better? (For females) When do they occur in relation to your menstrual periods?	Migraines are associated with family history of migraine. See Table 13-1, Primary Headaches, p. 270.
• Effort to treat. What seems to help: going to sleep, medications, positions, rubbing the area?	With migraines, people lie down to feel better, whereas with cluster headaches they need to move—even to pace the floor—to feel better.
• Coping strategies. How have these headaches affected your self-care or your ability to function at work, home, and socially?	
2. Head injury. Any **head injury** or blow to your head? • Onset. When? Please describe exactly what happened. • Setting. Any hazardous conditions? Were you wearing a helmet or hard hat?	

Subjective Data

Examiner Asks	Rationale
• How about yourself just before injury: dizzy, light-headed, had a blackout, had a seizure? Lose consciousness and then fall? (Note which came first.) Knocked unconscious? Or did you fall and lose consciousness a few minutes later?	Loss of consciousness *before* a fall may have a cardiac cause (e.g., heart block).
• Any history of illness (e.g., heart trouble, diabetes, epilepsy)?	
• Location. Exactly where did you hit your head?	
• Duration. How long were you unconscious? Any symptoms afterward—headache, vomiting, projectile vomiting? Any change in level of consciousness *after* injury: dazed or sleepy?	A change in level of consciousness is most important in evaluating a neurologic deficit.
• Associated symptoms. Any pain in the head or the neck, vision change, discharge from ear or nose—is it bloody or watery? Are you able to move all extremities? Any tremors, staggered walk, numbness and tingling?	
• Pattern. Symptoms become worse, better, unchanged since injury?	
• Effort to treat. Emergency department or hospitalized? Any medications?	
3. Dizziness. Experienced any **dizziness?** (Determine exactly what the person means by dizziness.) Was it a feeling of light-headedness or of falling? Or was it a spinning sensation?	Dizziness is a light-headed, swimming sensation, feeling of falling. True **vertigo** is true rotational spinning from neurologic disease (labyrinthine-vestibular apparatus, vestibular nuclei in brainstem). When vertigo is *objective,* the person feels like the room spins. When vertigo is *subjective,* the perception is that the person spins.
• Onset. Abrupt or gradual? After a change in position, such as sudden standing?	
• Associated factors. Any nausea and vomiting, pallor, immobility, decreased hearing acuity, or tinnitus along with the dizziness?	
4. Neck pain. Any neck pain?	
• Onset. How did the pain start: injury, automobile accident, after lifting, from a fall? Or with fever? Or did it have a gradual onset?	Acute onset of neck stiffness with headache and fever occurs with meningeal inflammation.
• Location. Does pain radiate? To the shoulders, arms?	
• Associated symptoms. Any **limitations to range of motion** (ROM), numbness or tingling in shoulders, arms, or hands?	
• Precipitating factors. What movements cause pain? Do you need to lift or bend at work or home?	
• Does stress seem to bring it on?	
• Coping strategies. Able to do your work, to sleep?	Pain creates a vicious circle. Tension increases pain and disability, which produces more anxiety.
5. Lumps or swelling. Any **lumps or swelling** in the neck? Any recent infection? Any tenderness?	Tenderness suggests acute infection.
For a lump that persists, how long have you had it? Has it changed in size?	A persistent lump arouses suspicion of malignancy. For people older than 40 years, suspect malignancy until proven otherwise.
• Any history of prior irradiation of head, neck, upper chest?	Increased risk for salivary and thyroid tumors.
• Any difficulty swallowing?	**Dysphagia.**
• Do you smoke? For how long? How many packs a day? Do you chew tobacco?	Smoking and chewing tobacco increase risk for oral and respiratory cancer.

Examiner Asks	Rationale
• When was your last alcohol drink? How much alcohol do you drink a day? • Ever had a thyroid problem? Overfunctioning or underfunctioning? How was it treated: surgery, irradiation, any medication?	Smoking and large alcohol consumption together increase the risk for cancer.
6. **History of head or neck surgery.** Ever had surgery of the head or neck? For what condition? When did the surgery occur? How do you feel about results?	Surgery for head and neck cancer often is disfiguring and increases risk for body image disturbance.
Additional History for Infants and Children	
1. Did the mother use alcohol or street drugs during pregnancy? How often? How much was used per episode?	Alcohol increases the risk for fetal alcohol syndrome, with distinctive facial features (see Table 13-4, Pediatric Facial Abnormalities, p. 274). Cocaine use causes neurologic, developmental, and emotional problems.
2. Was delivery vaginal or by cesarean section? Any difficulty? Use of forceps?	Forceps may increase the risk for caput succedaneum, cephalhematoma, and Bell's palsy.
3. What were you told about the baby's growth? Was it on schedule? Did the head seem to grow and fontanels close on schedule? At what age (in months) did the baby achieve head control?	
Additional History for the Aging Adult	
1. If dizziness is a problem, how does this affect your daily activities? Are you able to drive safely, maneuver about the house safely? 2. If neck pain is a problem, how does this affect your daily activities? Are you able to drive, perform at work, do housework, sleep, look down when using stairs?	Assess self-care. Assess potential for injury.

OBJECTIVE DATA

Normal Range of Findings	Abnormal Findings
THE HEAD	
Inspect and Palpate the Skull	
Size and Shape	
Note the general size and shape. **Normocephalic** is the term that denotes a round symmetric skull that is appropriately related to body size. Be aware that "normal" includes a wide range of sizes.	Deformities: microcephaly, abnormally small head; macrocephaly, abnormally large head (hydrocephaly, acromegaly, Paget's disease), see Table 13-2, Abnormalities in Head Size and Contour, p. 271.
To assess shape, place your fingers in the person's hair and palpate the scalp. The skull normally feels symmetric and smooth. Cranial bones that have normal protrusions are the forehead, the side of each parietal bone, the occipital bone, and the mastoid process behind each ear. There is no tenderness to palpation.	Note lumps, depressions, or abnormal protrusions.

Normal Range of Findings	Abnormal Findings

Temporal Area

Palpate the temporal artery above the zygomatic (cheek) bone between the eye and top of the ear.

The artery looks tortuous, feels hardened and tender with temporal arteritis.

The temporomandibular joint is just below the temporal artery and anterior to the tragus. Palpate the joint as the person opens the mouth, and note normally smooth movement with no limitation or tenderness.

Crepitation, limited ROM, or tenderness.

Inspect the Face

Facial Structures

Inspect the face, noting the facial expression and its appropriateness to behavior or reported mood. Anxiety is common in the hospitalized or ill person.

Hostility or aggression.

Tense, rigid muscles may indicate anxiety or pain; a flat affect may indicate depression.

Although the shape of facial structures may vary somewhat among races, they always should be symmetric. Note symmetry of eyebrows, palpebral fissures, nasolabial folds, and sides of the mouth.

Marked asymmetry with central brain lesion (e.g., stroke) or with peripheral cranial nerve VII damage (Bell's palsy). See Table 13-5, Abnormal Facies with Chronic Illnesses.

Note any abnormal facial structures (coarse facial features, exophthalmos, changes in skin color or pigmentation) or any abnormal swelling. Also note any involuntary movements (tics) in the facial muscles. Normally none occur.

Edema in the face occurs first around the eyes (periorbital) and the cheeks where the subcutaneous tissue is relatively loose.

Note grinding of jaws, tics, fasciculations, or excessive blinking.

THE NECK

Inspect and Palpate the Neck

Symmetry

Head position is centered in the midline, and the accessory neck muscles should be symmetric. The head should be held erect and still.

Head tilt occurs with muscle spasm. Rigid head and neck occur with arthritis.

Range of Motion (ROM)

Note any limitation of movement during active motion. Ask the person to touch the chin to the chest, to turn the head to the right and left, to try to touch each ear to the shoulder (without elevating shoulders), and to extend the head backward. When the neck is supple, motion is smooth and controlled.

Note pain at any particular movement.

Note ratchety or limited movement from cervical arthritis or inflammation of neck muscles. The arthritic neck is rigid; the person turns at the shoulders rather than at the neck.

Test muscle strength and the status of cranial nerve XI by trying to resist the person's movements with your hands as the person shrugs the shoulders and turns the head to each side.

As the person moves the head, note enlargement of the salivary glands and lymph glands. Normally no enlargement is present. Note a swollen parotid gland when the head is extended; look for swelling below the angle of the jaw. Also, note thyroid gland enlargement. Normally none is present.

Thyroid enlargement may be a unilateral lump, or it may be diffuse and look like a doughnut lying across the lower neck (see Table 13-3, Swellings on the Head or Neck).

Also note any obvious pulsations. The carotid artery runs medial to the sternomastoid muscle, and it creates a brisk localized pulsation just below the angle of the jaw. Normally, there are no other pulsations while the person is in the sitting position (see Chapter 19).

Lymph Nodes

Using a gentle circular motion of your fingerpads, palpate the lymph nodes (Fig. 13-9). (Normally the salivary glands are not palpable. When symptoms warrant,

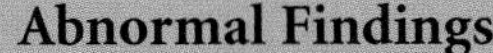

Normal Range of Findings

check for parotid tenderness by palpating in a line from the outer corner of the eye to the lobule of the ear.) Beginning with the preauricular lymph nodes in front of the ear, palpate the 10 groups of lymph nodes in a routine order. Many nodes are closely packed, so you must be systematic and thorough in your examination. Once you establish your sequence, do not vary or you may miss some small nodes.

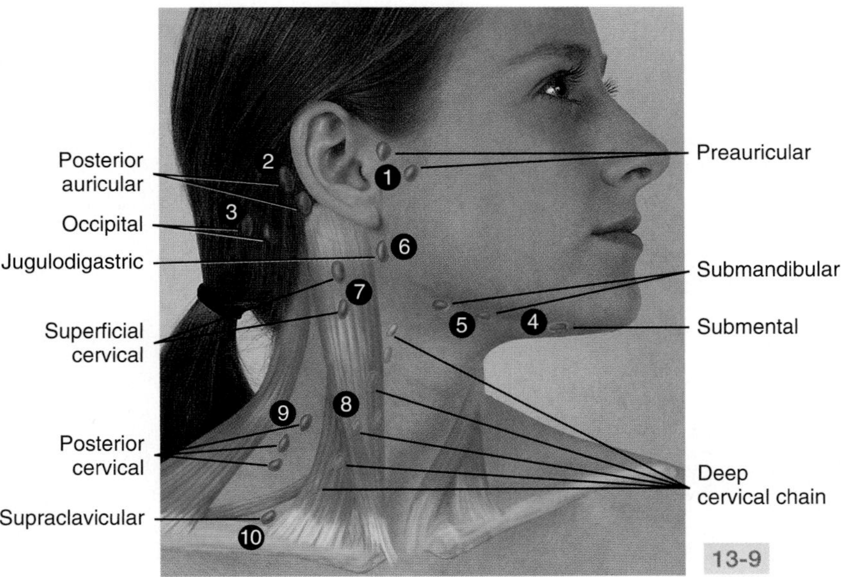

13-9

Use gentle pressure because strong pressure could push the nodes into the neck muscles. It is usually most efficient to palpate with both hands, comparing the two sides symmetrically. However, the submental gland under the tip of the chin is easier to explore with one hand. When you palpate with one hand, use your other hand to position the person's head. For the deep cervical chain, tip the person's head toward the side being examined to relax the ipsilateral muscle (Fig. 13-10). Then you can press your fingers under the muscle. Search for the supraclavicular node by having the person hunch the shoulders and elbows forward (Fig. 13-11); this relaxes the skin. The inferior belly of the omohyoid muscle crosses the posterior triangle here; do not mistake it for a lymph node.

Abnormal Findings

The parotid is swollen with mumps (see Table 13-3).

Parotid enlargement has been found with AIDS.

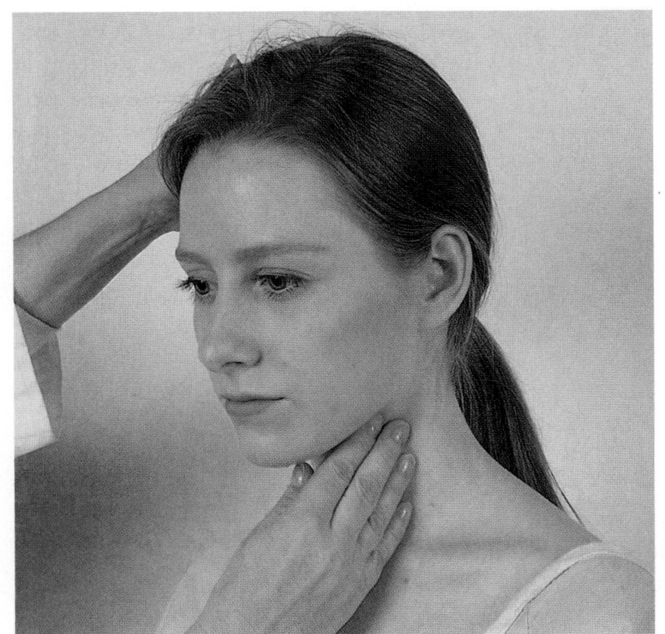

13-10

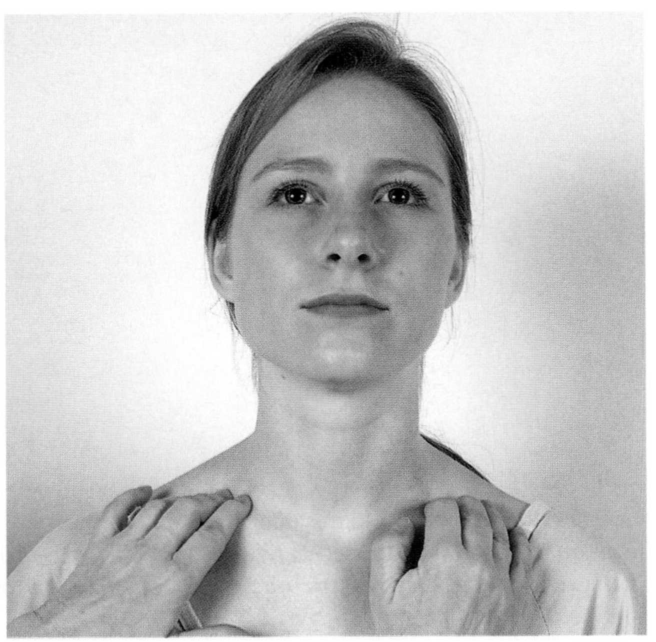

13-11

Normal Range of Findings

If any nodes are palpable, note their location, size, shape, delimitation (discrete or matted together), mobility, consistency, and tenderness. Cervical nodes often are palpable in healthy persons, although this palpability decreases with age (Fig. 13-12). Normal nodes feel movable, discrete, soft, and nontender.

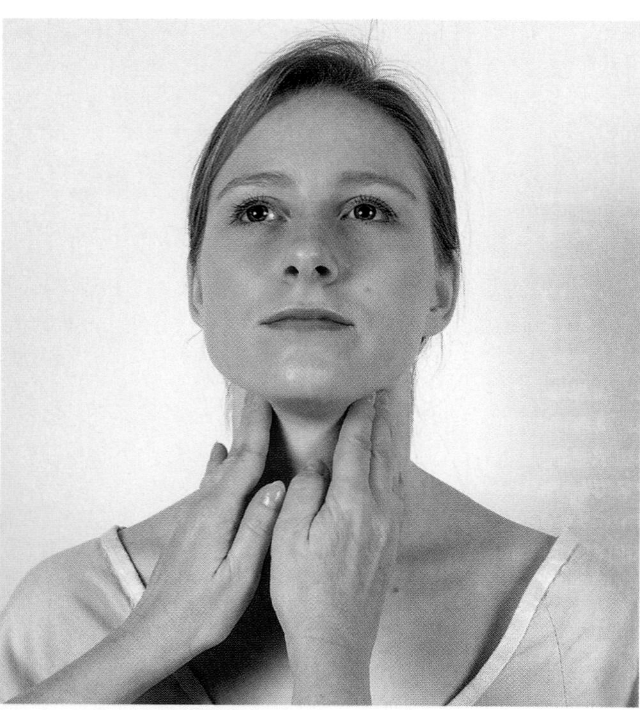

13-12

If nodes are enlarged or tender, check the area they drain for the source of the problem. For example, those in the upper cervical or submandibular area often relate to inflammation or a neoplasm in the head and neck. Follow up on or refer your findings. An enlarged lymph node, particularly when you cannot find the source of the problem, deserves prompt attention.

Trachea

Normally, the trachea is midline; palpate for any tracheal shift. Place your index finger on the trachea in the sternal notch, and slip it off to each side (Fig. 13-13). The space should be symmetric on both sides. Note any deviation from the midline.

Abnormal Findings

Lymphadenopathy is enlargement of the lymph nodes (>1 cm) from infection, allergy, or neoplasm.

The following criteria are common clues but are not definitive in all cases:

- Acute infection—acute onset, <14 days' duration, nodes are bilateral, enlarged, warm, tender, and firm but freely movable.
- Chronic inflammation (e.g., in tuberculosis the nodes are clumped).
- Cancerous nodes are hard, >3 cm, unilateral, nontender, matted, and fixed.
- Nodes with HIV infection are enlarged, firm, nontender, and mobile. Occipital node enlargement is common with HIV infection.
- A single enlarged, nontender, hard, left supraclavicular node (Virchow's node) may indicate neoplasm in thorax or abdomen.
- Painless, rubbery, discrete nodes that gradually appear occur with Hodgkin's lymphoma.

Normal Range of Findings

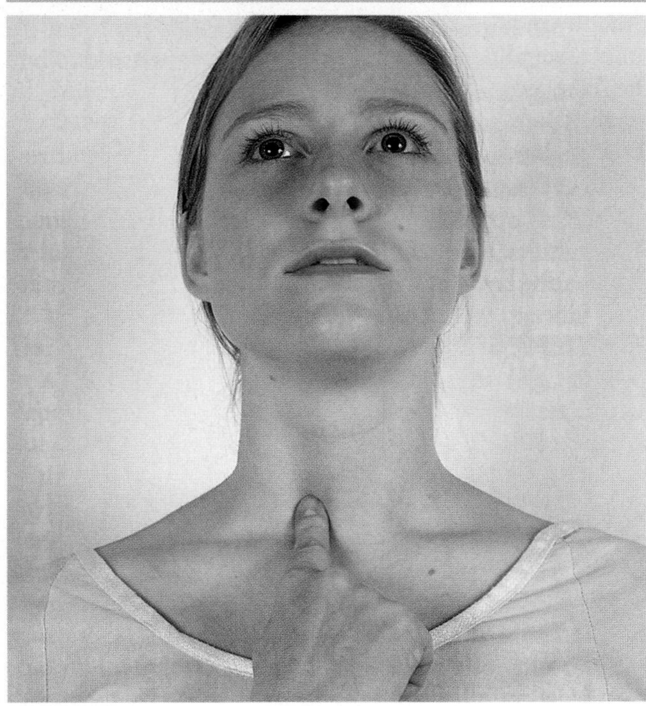

13-13

Thyroid Gland

The thyroid gland is difficult to palpate; arrange your setting to maximize your likelihood of success. Position a standing lamp to shine tangentially across the neck to highlight any possible swelling. Supply the person with a glass of water, and first inspect the neck as the person takes a sip and swallows. Thyroid tissue moves up with a swallow.

Posterior Approach. To palpate, move behind the person (Fig. 13-14, *A*). Ask the person to sit up very straight and then to bend the head slightly forward and to the right. This will relax the neck muscles on the right side. Use the fingers of your left hand to push the trachea slightly to the right.

Then curve your right fingers between the trachea and the sternomastoid muscle, retracting it slightly, and ask the person to take a sip of water. The thyroid moves up under your fingers with the trachea and larynx as the person swallows. Reverse the procedure for the left side.

Usually you cannot palpate the normal adult thyroid. If the person has a long, thin neck, you sometimes will feel the isthmus over the tracheal rings. The lateral lobes usually are not palpable; check them for enlargement, consistency, symmetry, and the presence of nodules.

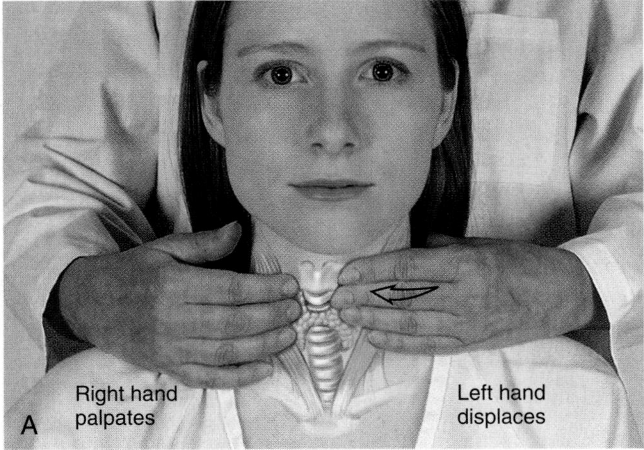

13-14, A

Abnormal Findings

Conditions of tracheal shift:

- The trachea is *pushed to the unaffected* (or healthy) side with an aortic aneurysm, a tumor, unilateral thyroid lobe enlargement, and pneumothorax.
- The trachea is *pulled toward the affected* (diseased) side with large atelectasis, pleural adhesions, or fibrosis.
- Tracheal tug is a rhythmic downward pull that is synchronous with systole and that occurs with aortic arch aneurysm.

Look for diffuse enlargement or a nodular lump.

Abnormalities: enlarged lobes that are easily palpated before swallowing or are tender to palpation (see large goiter in Fig. 13-14, *B*) ; or the presence of nodules or lumps. See Table 13-3, p. 272.

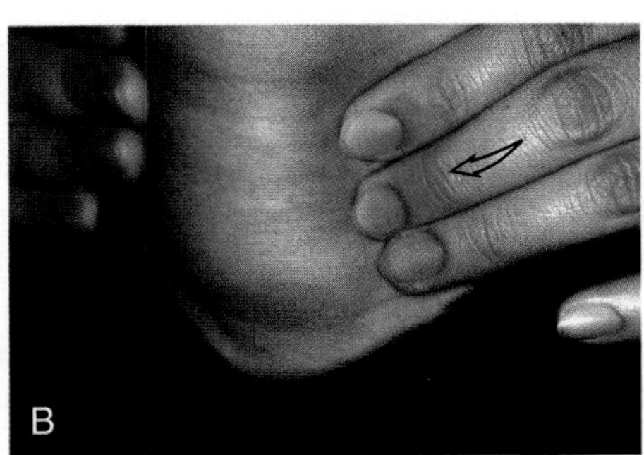

13-14, B

Objective Data

Normal Range of Findings	Abnormal Findings

Anterior Approach. This is an alternate method of palpating the thyroid, but it is more awkward to perform, especially for a beginning examiner. Stand facing the person. Ask him or her to tip the head forward and to the right. Use your right thumb to displace the trachea slightly to the person's right. Hook your left thumb and fingers around the sternomastoid muscle. Feel for lobe enlargement as the person swallows (Fig. 13-15).

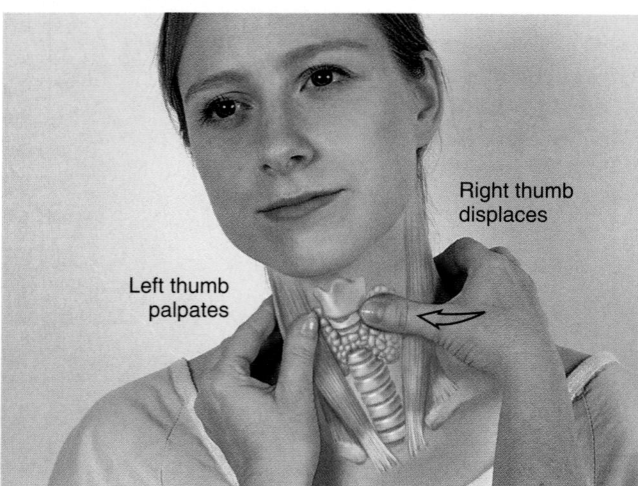

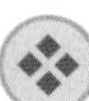
13-15

Auscultate the Thyroid

If the thyroid gland is enlarged, auscultate it for the presence of a **bruit.** This is a soft, pulsatile, whooshing, blowing sound heard best with the bell of the stethoscope. The bruit is not present normally.

A bruit occurs with accelerated or turbulent blood flow, indicating hyperplasia of the thyroid (e.g., hyperthyroidism).

DEVELOPMENTAL COMPETENCE

Infants and Children

Skull

Measure an infant's **head size** with measuring tape at each visit up to age 2 years, then yearly up to age 6 years. (Measurement of head circumference is presented in detail in Chapter 9.)

Note an abnormal increase in head size or failure to grow.

The newborn's head measures about 32 to 38 cm (average around 34 cm) and is 2 cm larger than chest circumference. At age 2 years, both measurements are the same. During childhood, the chest circumference grows to exceed head circumference by 5 to 7 cm.

Microcephalic—head size below norms for age. Macrocephalic—an enlarged head or rapidly increasing in size (e.g., hydrocephalus [increased cerebrospinal fluid]).

Observe the infant's head from all angles, not just the front. The contour should be symmetric. Some racial variation occurs in normal head shapes; Nordic children tend to have long heads, and Asian children have broad heads.

Frontal bulges, or "bossing," occur with prematurity or rickets.

Two common variations in the newborn cause the shape of the skull to look markedly asymmetric. A **caput succedaneum** is edematous swelling and ecchymosis of the presenting part of the head caused by birth trauma (Fig. 13-16). It feels soft, and it may extend across suture lines. It gradually resolves during the first few days of life and needs no treatment.

Normal Range of Findings	Abnormal Findings

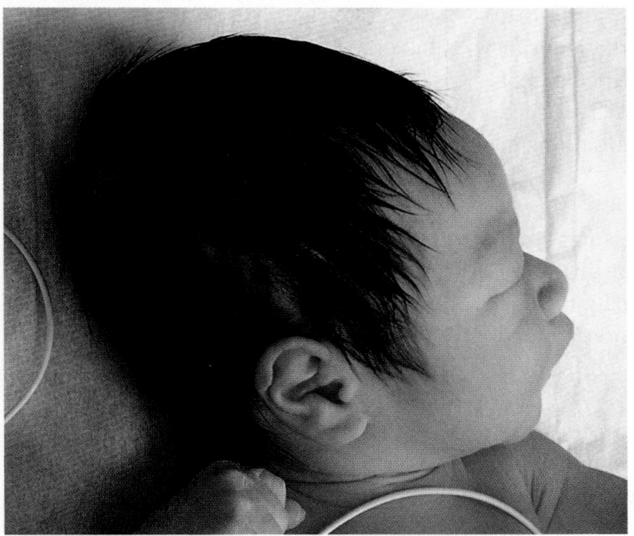

13-16 Caput succedaneum.

A **cephalhematoma** is a subperiosteal hemorrhage, which is also a result of birth trauma (Fig. 13-17, *A*). It is soft, fluctuant, and well defined over one cranial bone because the periosteum (i.e., the covering over each bone) holds the bleeding in place. It appears several hours after birth and gradually increases in size. No discoloration is present, but it looks bizarre, so parents need reassurance that it will be reabsorbed during the first few weeks of life without treatment. Rarely, a large hematoma may persist to 3 months.

An infant with cephalhematoma is at greater risk for jaundice as the red blood cells within the hematoma are broken down and reabsorbed (Fig. 13-17, *B*).

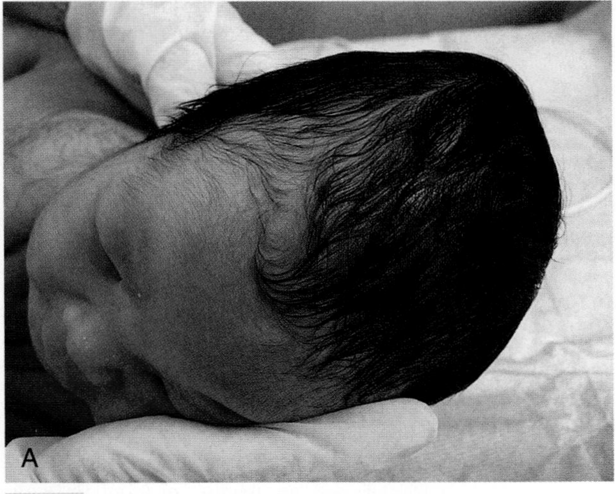

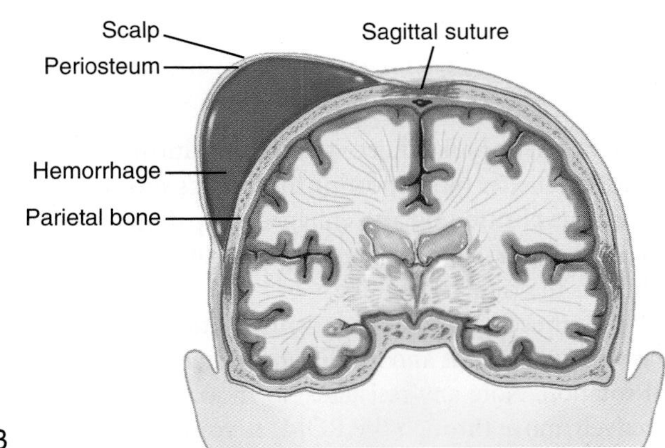

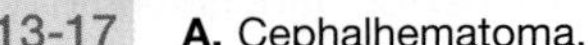

13-17 **A,** Cephalhematoma.

As you palpate the newborn's head, the suture lines feel like ridges. By 5 to 6 months, they are smooth and not palpable.

A newborn's head may feel asymmetric and the involved ridges more prominent due to *molding* of the cranial bones during engagement and passage through the birth canal. Molding is overriding of the cranial bones; usually, the parietal bone overrides the frontal or occipital bone. Reassure parents that this lasts only a few days or a week. Babies delivered by cesarean section are noted for their evenly round heads. Also, some asymmetry may occur if an infant continually sleeps in one position; this is a flattening of the dependent cranial bone, usually the occiput.

Sutures palpable when the child is older than 6 months.

Marked asymmetry, as in *craniosynostosis,* a severe deformity caused by premature closure of the sutures. Premature closing of the suture results in a long, narrow head.

Flattening also occurs with rickets or mental retardation.

Normal Range of Findings	Abnormal Findings
Gently palpate the skull and **fontanels** while the infant is calm and somewhat in a sitting position (crying, lying down, or vomiting may cause the anterior fontanel to look full and bulging). The skull should feel smooth and fused except at the fontanels. The fontanels feel firm, slightly concave, and well defined against the edges of the cranial bones. You may see slight arterial pulsations in the anterior fontanel.	A true tense or bulging fontanel occurs with acute increased intracranial pressure. Depressed and sunken fontanels occur with dehydration or malnutrition. Marked pulsations occur with increased intracranial pressure.
The posterior fontanel may not be palpable at birth. If it is, it measures 1 cm and closes by 1 to 2 months. The anterior fontanel may be small at birth and enlarge to 2.5 cm × 2.5 cm. A large diameter of 4 to 5 cm occasionally may be normal under 6 months. A small fontanel usually is normal. The anterior fontanel closes between 9 months and 2 years. Early closure may be insignificant if head growth proceeds normally.	Delayed closure or larger-than-normal fontanel size occurs with hydrocephalus, Down syndrome, hypothyroidism, or rickets. A small fontanel is a sign of microcephaly, as is early closure.
Note the infant's **head posture** and **head control.** The infant can turn the head side to side by 2 weeks and shows the **tonic neck reflex** when supine and the head is turned to one side (extension of same arm and leg, flexion of opposite arm and leg). The tonic neck reflex disappears between 3 and 4 months, and then the head is maintained in the midline. Head control is achieved by 4 months, when the baby can hold the head erect and steady when pulled to a vertical position. (See Chapters 22 and 23 for further details.)	Tonic neck reflex beyond 5 months may indicate brain damage. In children, head tilt occurs with habit spasm, poor vision, and brain tumor. Head lag after 4 months may indicate mental or motor retardation.
Face	
Check **facial features** for symmetry, appearance, and presence of swelling. Note symmetry of wrinkling when the infant cries or smiles (e.g., both sides of the lips rise and both sides of forehead wrinkle). Children love to comply when you ask them to "make a face." Normally, no swelling is evident. Parotid gland enlargement is seen best when the child sits and looks up at the ceiling; the swelling appears below the angle of the jaw.	Unilateral immobility indicates nerve damage (central or peripheral) (e.g., note angle of mouth droop on paralyzed side). Some facies are characteristic of congenital abnormalities or chronic allergy. See Table 13-4, Pediatric Facial Abnormalities, and Table 13-5.
Neck	
An infant's neck looks short; it lengthens during the first 3 to 4 years. You can see the neck better by supporting the infant's shoulders and tilting the head back a little. This positioning also enhances palpation of the trachea, which is buried deep in the neck. Feel for the row of cartilaginous rings in the midline or just slightly to the right of midline.	A short neck or webbing (loose fanlike folds) may indicate congenital abnormality (e.g., Down or Turner syndrome), or it may occur alone.
Assess muscle development with gentle passive ROM. Cradle the infant's head with your hands and turn it side to side and test forward flexion, extension, and rotation. Note any resistance to movement, especially flexion. Ask a child to actively move through the ROM, as you would an adult.	Head tilt and limited ROM occur with torticollis (wryneck) or from sternomastoid muscle injury during birth or a congenital defect. Resistance to flexion (nuchal rigidity) and pain on flexion indicate meningeal irritation or meningitis.
During infancy, cervical lymph nodes are not palpable normally. But a child's lymph nodes are—they feel more prominent than an adult's until after puberty, when lymphoid tissue begins to atrophy. Palpable nodes less than 3 mm are normal. They may be up to 1 cm in size in the cervical and inguinal areas but are discrete, move easily, and are nontender. Children have a higher incidence of infection, so you will expect a greater incidence of inflammatory adenopathy. No other mass should occur in the neck. The thyroid gland is difficult to palpate in an infant because of the short, thick neck. The child's thyroid may be palpable normally.	Cervical nodes >1 cm are considered enlarged. Thyroglossal duct cyst—cystic lump high up in midline, freely movable, and rises up when swallowing. Supraclavicular nodes enlarge with Hodgkin's disease.

Normal Range of Findings	Abnormal Findings

Special Procedures

Percussion. With an infant, you may directly percuss with your plexor finger against the head surface. This yields a resonant or "cracked pot" sound, which is normal before closure of the fontanels.

The sound occurs with hydrocephalus from separation of cranial sutures (Macewen's sign).

Auscultation. Bruits are common in the skull in children younger than 4 or 5 years or in children with anemia. They are systolic or continuous and are heard over the temporal area.

After 5 years of age, bruits indicate increased intracranial pressure, aneurysm, or arteriovenous shunt.

The Pregnant Woman

During the second trimester, chloasma may show on the face. This is a blotchy, hyperpigmented area over the cheeks and forehead that fades after delivery. The thyroid gland may be palpable normally during pregnancy.

The Aging Adult

The temporal arteries may look twisted and prominent. In some aging adults, a mild rhythmic tremor of the head may be normal. **Senile tremors** are benign and include head nodding (as if saying yes or no) and tongue protrusion. If some teeth have been lost, the lower face looks unusually small, with the mouth sunken in.

The neck may show an increased anterior cervical (concave or inward) curve when the head and jaw are extended forward to compensate for kyphosis of the spine. During the examination, direct the aging person to perform ROM slowly; he or she may experience dizziness with side movements. An aging person may have prolapse of the submandibular glands, which could be mistaken for a tumor. But drooping submandibular glands will feel soft and be present bilaterally.

Objective Data

PROMOTING A HEALTHY LIFESTYLE: BRAIN INJURY PREVENTION

Use Your Head. Wear a Helmet.

Helmets are designed to protect the brain from injury and trauma by absorbing the impact energy in a collision or fall. Different types of helmets are available, depending on the specific type(s) of impact associated with a particular sport or activity. So, the first step is pick the right helmet for the right sport or activity, because they are not interchangeable. The second step is to make sure that the helmet is safe by looking for a U.S. Consumer Product Safety Commission (CPSC) sticker or label. The final step is to make sure it fits. The helmet should not move in any direction when adjusted properly and the chinstrap needs to be securely buckled to be effective. Wearing a properly fitted bicycle helmet can reduce an individual's risk for head injury by 85% and reduce the risk for brain injury by 88%. A proper fit is as important as wearing the correct helmet. This is particularly important for children.

Not all sports or activities require helmets. In fact, there are certain activities for which an individual, especially a child, should not wear a helmet. In these situations, a helmet's chinstrap might get caught and pose a risk for strangulation. Further, the helmet itself may also pose an entrapment hazard or risk.

Children and adults should wear a sport- or activity-specific helmet when participating in the following sports or recreational activities:

- Alpine sports, including skiing, snowboarding, and snowmobiling
- ATV riding and Go-karting
- Baseball and softball
- Bicycling
- Football
- Horseback riding
- Ice hockey
- Lacrosse
- Roller and in-line skating
- Rock climbing
- Scooter riding and segways
- Skateboarding

Resources

The CPSC is the primary contact for safety and recalls of helmets. It also has a helpful brochure entitled *Which Helmet for Which Activity?,* which is available at www.cpsc.gov/cpscpub/pubs/349.pdf.

The Bicycle Helmet Safety Institute (BHSI) is another good resource for bicycle helmets. It is also helpful for other types of helmets and protective headgear for special needs and developmental disabilities. It can be accessed as follows:

- Other helmets. Website: http://bhsi.org/other.htm.
- Protective headgear for special needs and developmental disabilities. Website: http://bhsi.org/special.htm.

DOCUMENTATION AND CRITICAL THINKING

Sample Charting

SUBJECTIVE

Denies any unusually frequent or severe headache; no history of head injury, dizziness, or syncope; no neck pain, limitation of motion, lumps, or swelling.

OBJECTIVE

Head: Normocephalic, no lumps, no lesions, no tenderness, no trauma.

Face: Symmetric, no drooping, no weakness, no involuntary movements.

Neck: Supple with full ROM, no pain. Symmetric, no cervical lymphadenopathy or masses. Trachea midline, thyroid not palpable. No bruits.

ASSESSMENT

Normocephalic, atraumatic, and symmetric head and neck.

Focused Assessment: Clinical Case Study 1

Frank V. is a 57-year-old insurance executive who is in his fourth postoperative day after a transurethral resection of the prostate gland. He also has chronic hypertension, managed by oral hydrochlorothiazide, exercise, and a low-salt diet.

SUBJECTIVE

Complaining of dizziness, a light-headed feeling that occurred on standing and cleared on sitting. No previous episodes of dizziness. Denies palpitations, nausea, or vomiting. States urine pink-tinged as it was yesterday, with no red blood. No pain meds today. On second day of same antihypertensive medication he took before surgery.

OBJECTIVE

BP 142/88 RA sitting, 94/58 RA standing. Pulse 94 sitting and standing, regular rhythm, no skipped beats. Temp 37° C. Color tannish-pink, no pallor, skin warm and dry.

Neuro: Alert and oriented to person, place, and time. Speech clear and fluent. Moving all extremities, no weakness. No nystagmus, no ataxia, past pointing normal. Romberg's sign negative (normal). Intake/output in balance. Urine faint pink-tinged, no clots.

Lab: Hct 45, serum chemistries normal.

ASSESSMENT

Orthostatic hypotension

Risk for injury R/T orthostatic hypotension

Focused Assessment: Clinical Case Study 2

Mara is a 19-year-old single white female college student with a history of good health and no chronic illnesses; she enters the outpatient clinic today looking anxious, stating, "I think I've had a stroke!"

SUBJECTIVE

One day PTA—first noticed at dinner at college cafeteria when joking with friends, started to stick out tongue and roll tongue and could not do it, right side of tongue was not working. Mara left room to look in mirror and became scared; when smiled, noticed right side was not working. Tried to pucker lips, could not. Could not whistle, could not raise eyebrow. "I looked like a Vulcan." No other movement disorder below neck. Mild pain behind right ear with buzzing in ear. Able to sleep last night, but roommate said Mara's right eyelid did not close completely during sleep.

Today—still no movement on complete right side of face. Feeling self-conscious in class and during conversations with friends. Now has taste aversion, fluids with high water content taste especially bitter. No hearing loss.

OBJECTIVE

T 37° C, P 64, R 14, B/P 108/78.

Forehead appears smooth and immobile on right, unable to wrinkle right side. Unable to close right eye, Bell's phenomenon present when attempts to close (right eyeball rolls upward), right palpebral fissure appears wider. No corneal reflex on right. Unable to whistle or puff right cheek. Absent nasolabial fold on right. Mouth droops on right, sags on right when tries to smile. Slight drooling. Left side of face responds appropriately to all these movements. Superficial sensation intact.

Rest of musculoskeletal system intact: able to hold balance while standing, able to walk, walk heel-to-toe, do knee bend on each knee. Arm strength and ROM intact.

ASSESSMENT

Right-sided facial paralysis, consistent with Bell's palsy
Disturbed body image R/T effects of loss of facial function
Risk for deficient fluid volume R/T taste aversion and dietary alteration
Risk for sensory deficit, visual impairment, R/T effects of neurologic impairment

ABNORMAL FINDINGS

TABLE 13-1 Primary Headaches—Compare and Contrast

	Tension	Migraine	Cluster
Location	Usually both sides, across the frontal, temporal, and/or occipital region of head: forehead, sides, and back of head	Commonly one-sided but may occur on both sides Pain is often behind the eyes, the temples, or forehead	Always one-sided Often behind or around the eye, temple, forehead, cheek
Character	Bandlike tightness, viselike Non-throbbing	Throbbing, pulsating	Continuous, burning, piercing, excruciating
Duration	Gradual onset, lasts 30 minutes to days	Rapid onset, peaks 1-2 hr, lasts 4 hr to 72 hr, sometimes longer	Abrupt onset, peaks in minutes, lasts 45-90 min
Quantity and severity	Diffuse, dull, aching pain Mild to moderate pain	Moderate to severe pain	Can occur multiple times a day, in "clusters" Severe stabbing pain
Timing	Situational, in response to overwork, posture	About 2/month, lasts 1-3 days	1-2/day, each lasting ½ to 2 hr, for 1 to 2 months; then remission for months or years
Aggravating symptoms or triggers	Stress, anxiety, depression, poor posture	Hormonal fluctuations (premenstrual) Foods (e.g., alcohol, caffeine, MSG, nitrates, chocolate, cheese) Letdown after stress Changes in sleep pattern Sensory stimuli (e.g., flashing lights or perfumes) Changes in weather Physical activity	Exacerbated by alcohol, stress, wind or heat exposure
Associated symptoms	Fatigue, anxiety, stress Sensation of a band tightening around head, of being gripped like a vice Sometimes photophobia or phonophobia	Often preceded by an aura (visual changes such as blind spots or flashes of light, tingling in an arm or leg, vertigo) Nausea, vomiting, photophobia, abdominal pain Family history of migraine	Nasal congestion or runny nose, watery or reddened eye, eyelid drooping, miosis, feelings of agitation
Relieving factors, efforts to treat	Rest, massaging muscles in area, NSAID	Lie down, darken room, use eyeshade, sleep, take NSAID or narcotic when severe	Need to move, pace the floor

NSAID, Nonsteroidal anti-inflammatory drug.

TABLE 13-2 Abnormalities in Head Size and Contour

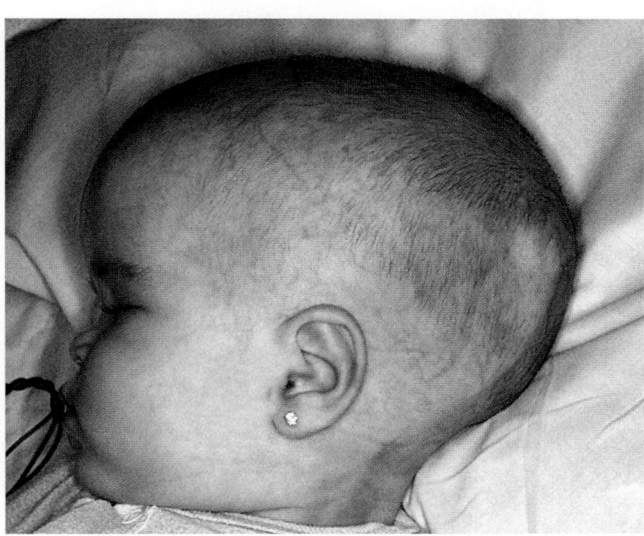

Hydrocephalus

Obstruction of drainage of cerebrospinal fluid results in excessive accumulation, increasing intracranial pressure, and enlargement of the head. The face looks small compared with the enlarged cranium. The increasing pressure also produces dilated scalp veins, frontal bossing, and downcast or "setting sun" eyes (sclera visible above iris). The cranial bones thin, sutures separate, and percussion yields a "cracked pot" sound (Macewen's sign).

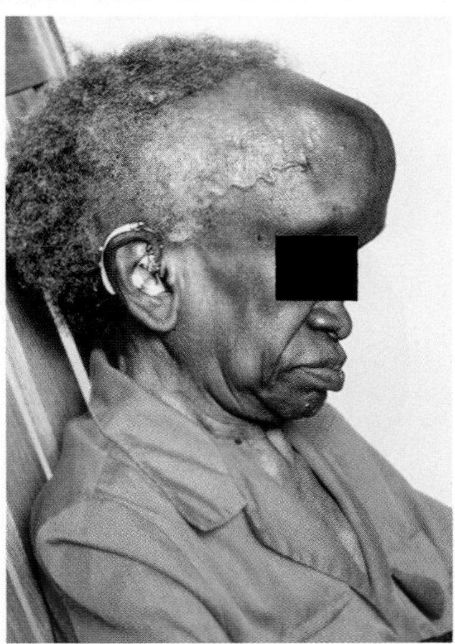

Paget's Disease of Bone (Osteitis Deformans)

A skeletal disease of increased bone resorption and formation, which softens, thickens, and deforms bone. It affects 10% of those older than 80 years and occurs more often in males. The disease is characterized by bowed long bones, sudden fractures, frontal bossing, and enlarging skull bones that form an acorn-shaped cranium. Enlarging skull bones press on cranial nerves, causing symptoms of headache, vertigo, tinnitus, progressive deafness, and optic atrophy and compression of the spinal cord.

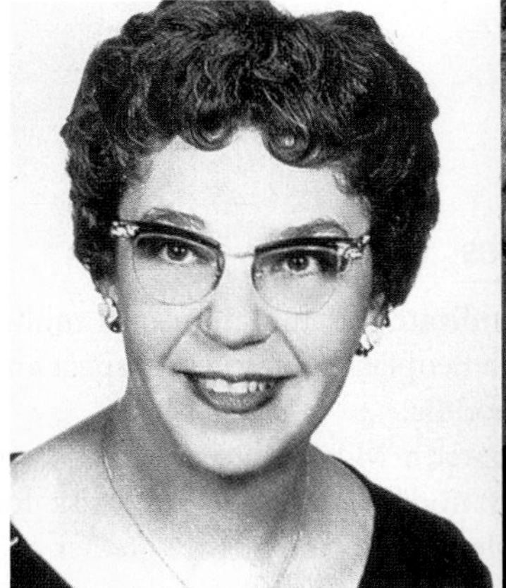

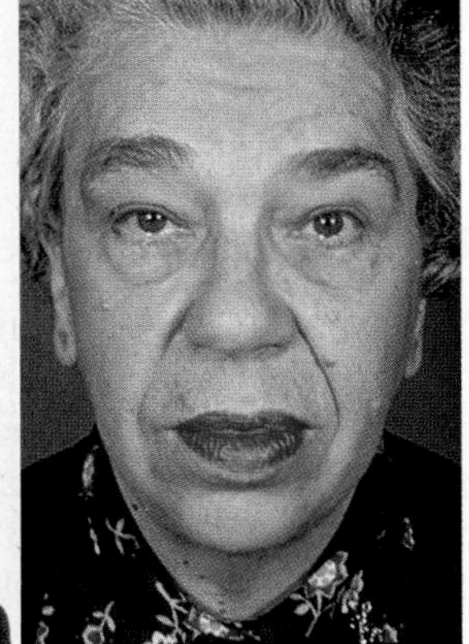

Acromegaly

Excessive secretion of growth hormone from the pituitary gland after puberty creates an enlarged skull and thickened cranial bones. Note the elongated head, massive face, prominent nose and lower jaw, heavy eyebrow ridge, and coarse facial features, especially when compared with the same woman's face on the left pictured several years before she had a pituitary tumor.

Abnormal Findings

TABLE 13-3 Swellings on the Head or Neck

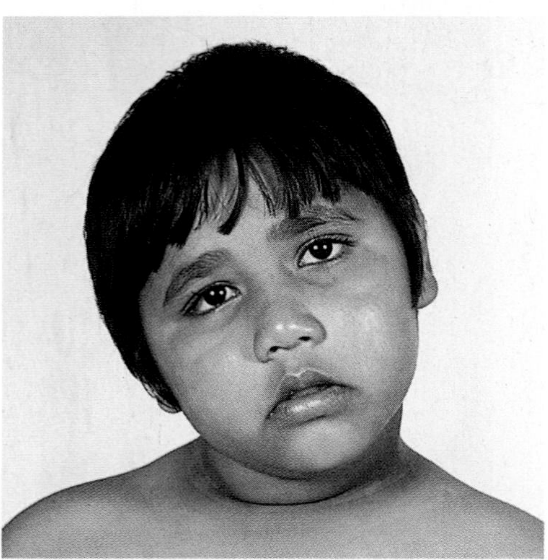

Torticollis (Wryneck)

A hematoma in one sternomastoid muscle, probably injured by intrauterine malposition, results in head tilt to one side and limited neck ROM to the opposite side. You will feel a firm, discrete, nontender mass in mid-muscle on the involved side. This requires treatment, or the muscle becomes fibrotic and permanently shortened with permanent limitation of ROM, asymmetry of head and face, and visual problems from a non-horizontal position of the eyes.

Goiter

A chronic enlargement of the thyroid gland that occurs in some regions of the world where the soil is low in iodine. Not due to a neoplasm.

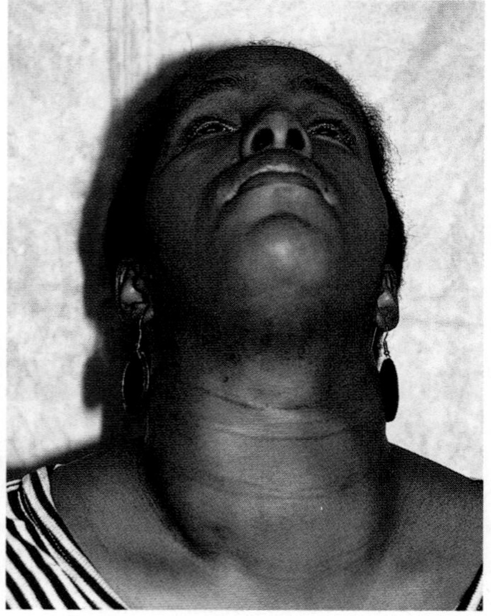

◀ Thyroid—Multiple Nodules

Multiple nodules usually indicate inflammation or a multinodular goiter rather than a neoplasm. However, suspect any rapidly enlarging or firm nodule.

Single Nodule (not illustrated): Most solitary nodules are benign, although a solitary nodule poses a greater risk for malignancy than do multiple nodules and poses a greater risk in a young person. Suspect any painless, rapidly growing nodule, especially the appearance of a single nodule in a young person. Cancerous nodules tend to be hard and are fixed to surrounding structures.

TABLE 13-3 Swellings on the Head or Neck—cont'd

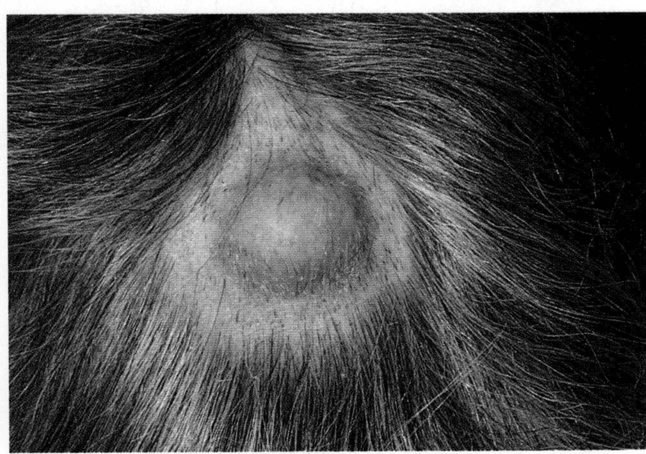

Pilar Cyst (Wen)

Smooth, firm, fluctuant swelling on the scalp that contains sebum and keratin. Tense pressure of the contents causes overlying skin to be shiny and taut. It is a benign growth.

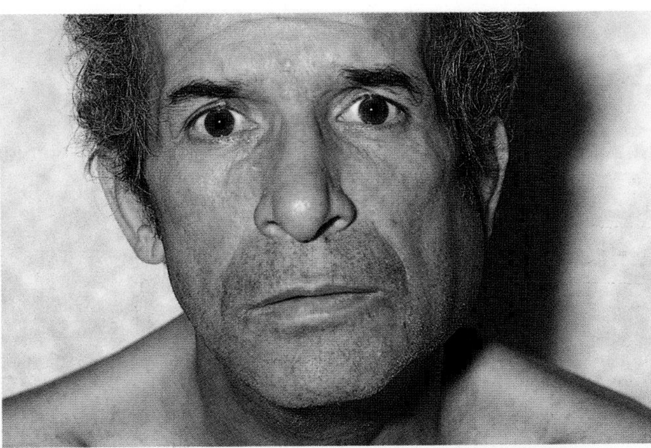

Parotid Gland Enlargement

Rapid painful inflammation of the parotid occurs with mumps. Parotid swelling also occurs with blockage of a duct, abscess, or tumor. Note swelling anterior to lower ear lobe. Stensen duct obstruction can occur in aging adults dehydrated from diuretics or anticholinergics.

TABLE 13-4 Pediatric Facial Abnormalities

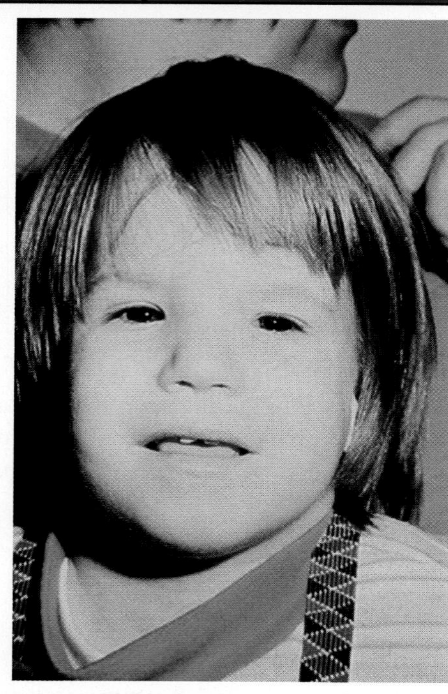

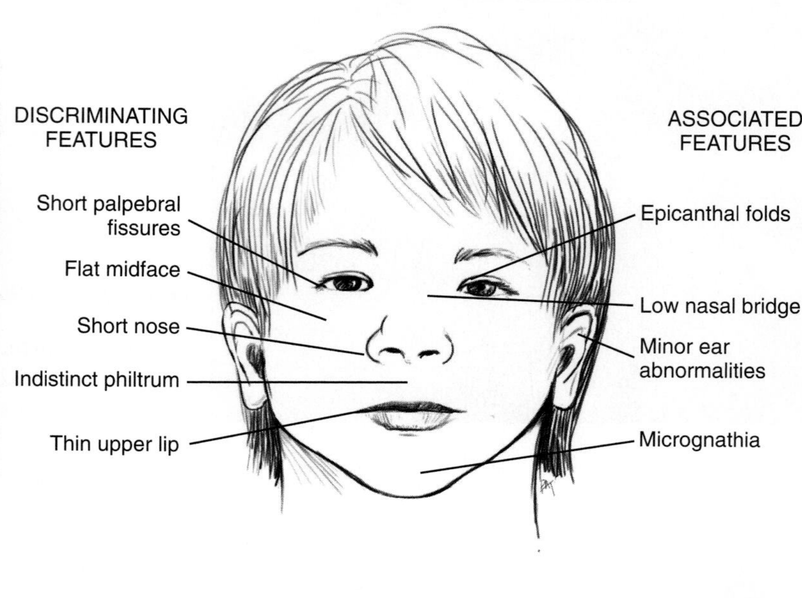

Fetal Alcohol Syndrome

A pregnant woman who abuses alcohol is at great risk for producing a baby with a wide range of growth and developmental abnormalities. Facial malformations may be recognizable at birth. Characteristic facies include narrow palpebral fissures, epicanthal folds, and midfacial hypoplasia.

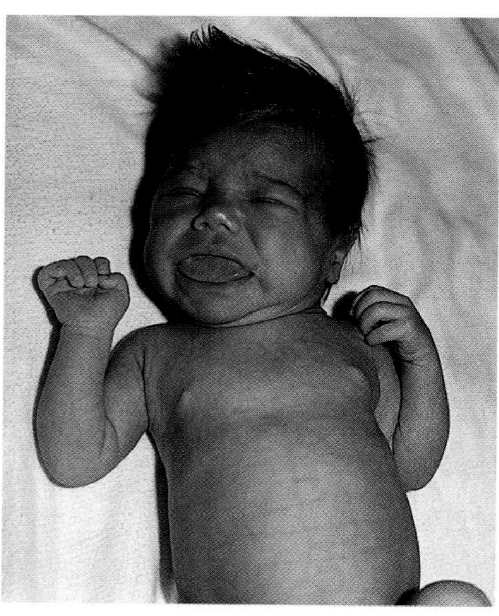

Congenital Hypothyroidism

Thyroid deficiency at an early age produces impaired growth and neurologic deficit. Without neonatal screening, characteristic facies develop by 3 to 6 months of age: low hairline, hirsute forehead, swollen eyelids, narrow palpebral fissures, widely spaced eyes, depressed nasal bridge, puffy face, thick tongue protruding through an open mouth, and a dull expression. Head size is normal, but the anterior and posterior fontanels are wide open.

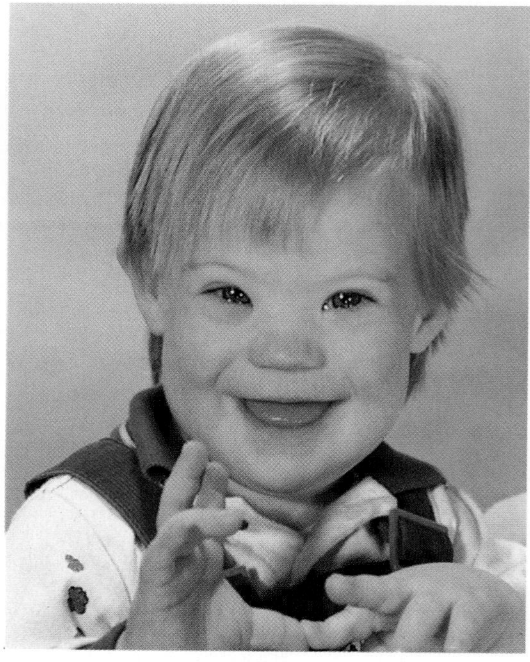

Down Syndrome

Chromosomal aberration (trisomy 21). Head and face characteristics may include upslanting eyes with inner epicanthal folds; flat nasal bridge; small, broad, flat nose; protruding, thick tongue; ear dysplasia; short, broad neck with webbing; and small hands with single palmar crease.

TABLE 13-4 Pediatric Facial Abnormalities—cont'd

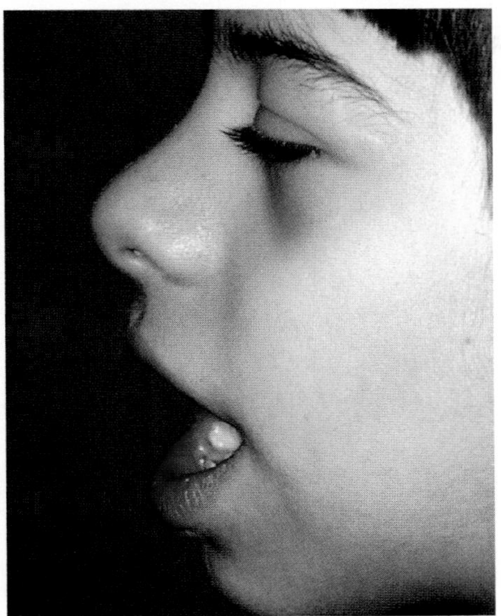

Atopic (Allergic) Facies

Children with chronic allergies such as atopic dermatitis often develop characteristic facial features. These include exhausted face, blue shadows below the eyes ("allergic shiners") from sluggish venous return, a double or single crease on the lower eyelids (Morgan's lines), central facial pallor, and open-mouth breathing (allergic gaping). The open-mouth breathing can lead to malocclusion of the teeth and malformed jaw because the child's bones are still forming.

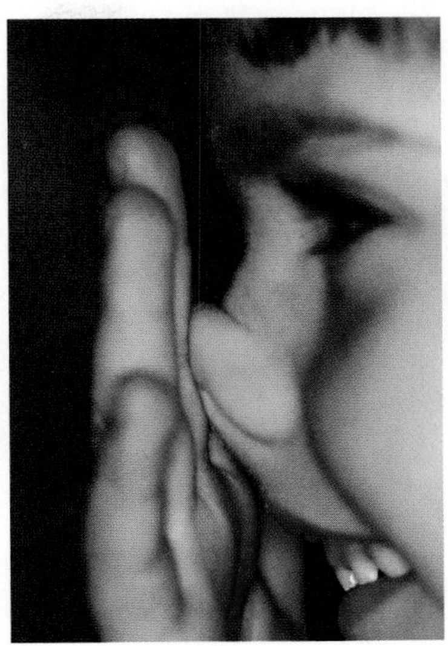

Allergic Salute and Crease

The transverse line on the nose is also a feature of chronic allergies. It is formed when the child chronically uses the hand to push the nose up and back (the "allergic salute") to relieve itching and to free swollen turbinates, which allows air passage.

TABLE 13-5 Abnormal Facies with Chronic Illnesses

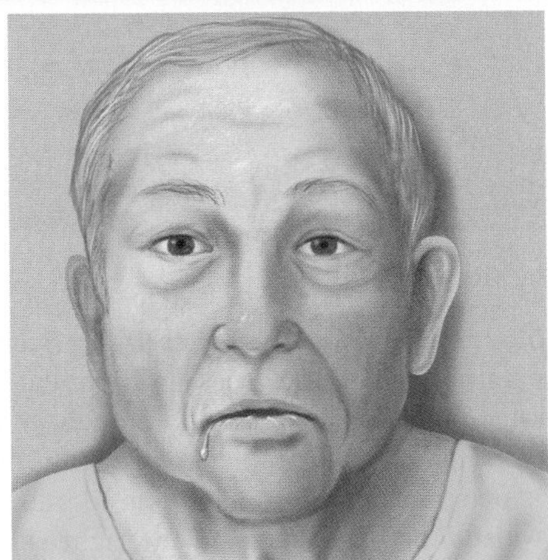

Parkinson Syndrome

A deficiency of the neurotransmitter *dopamine* and degeneration of the basal ganglia in the brain. The immobility of features produces a face that is flat and expressionless, "mask-like," with elevated eyebrows, staring gaze, oily skin, and drooling.

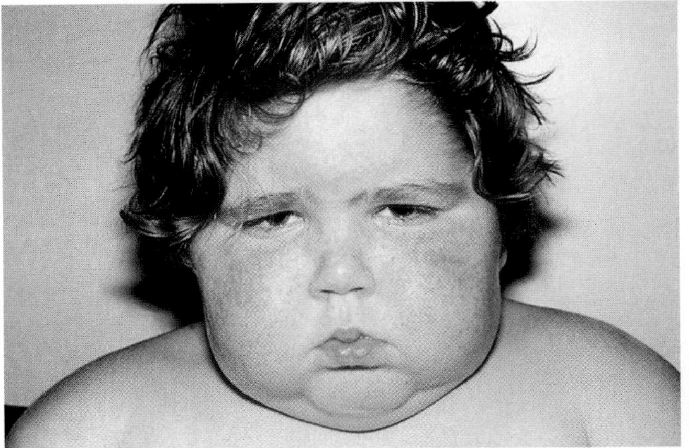

Cushing Syndrome

With excessive secretion of corticotropin hormone (ACTH) and chronic steroid use, the person develops a plethoric, rounded, "moonlike" face; prominent jowls; red cheeks; hirsutism on the upper lip, lower cheeks, and chin; and acneiform rash on the chest.

Continued

TABLE 13-5 Abnormal Facies with Chronic Illnesses—cont'd

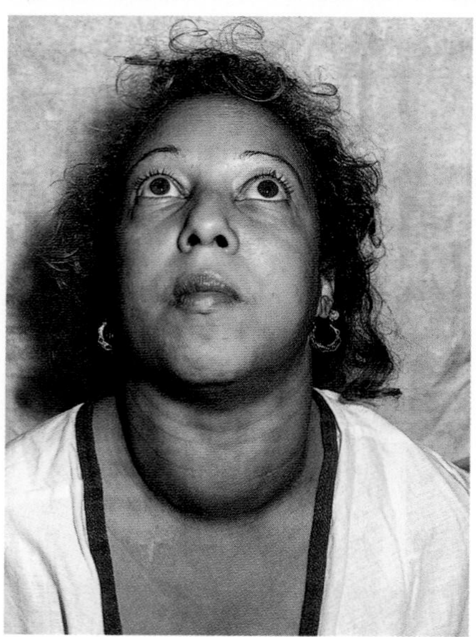

Hyperthyroidism

Goiter is an increase in the size of the thyroid gland and occurs with hyperthyroidism, Hashimoto's thyroiditis, and hypothyroidism. Graves' disease (shown here) is the most common cause of hyperthyroidism, manifested by goiter and exophthalmos (bulging eyeballs). Symptoms include nervousness, fatigue, weight loss, muscle cramps, and heat intolerance; signs include tachycardia, shortness of breath, excessive sweating, fine muscle tremor, thin silky hair and skin, infrequent blinking, and a staring appearance.

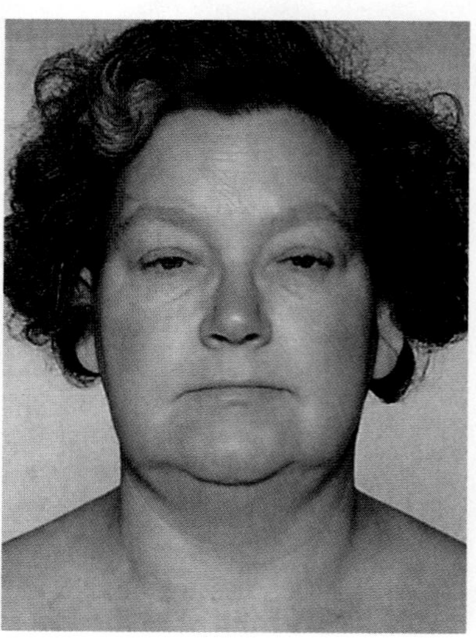

Myxedema (Hypothyroidism)

A deficiency of thyroid hormone, when severe, causes a nonpitting edema or myxedema. Note puffy, edematous face, especially around eyes (periorbital edema), coarse facial features, dry skin, and dry, coarse hair and eyebrows.

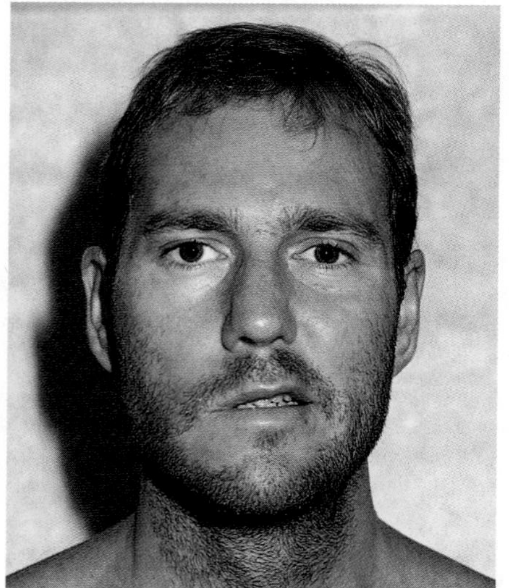

◀ Bell's Palsy (Right Side)

A **lower motor neuron** lesion **(peripheral),** producing cranial nerve VII paralysis, which is almost always unilateral. It has a rapid onset, and its cause is currently thought to be herpes simplex virus (HSV). Note complete paralysis of one half of the face; the person cannot wrinkle forehead, raise eyebrow, close eye, whistle, or show teeth on the right side. Usually presents with smooth forehead, wide palpebral fissure, flat nasolabial fold, drooling, and pain behind the ear.

TABLE 13-5 **Abnormal Facies with Chronic Illnesses—cont'd**

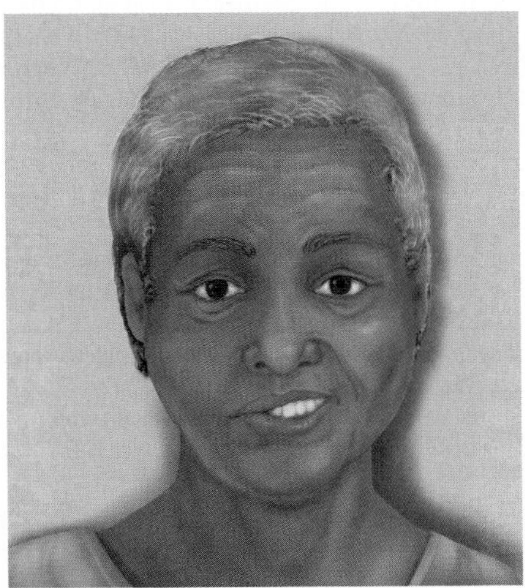

◀ Stroke or Cerebrovascular Accident

An **upper motor neuron** lesion **(central).** A stroke (or brain attack) is an acute neurologic deficit caused by an obstruction of a cerebral vessel, as in atherosclerosis, or a rupture in a cerebral vessel. If you suspect a stroke, ask if the person can smile. Note paralysis of the lower facial muscles, but also note that the upper half of face is not affected because of the intact nerve from the unaffected hemisphere. The person is still able to wrinkle the forehead and close the eyes.

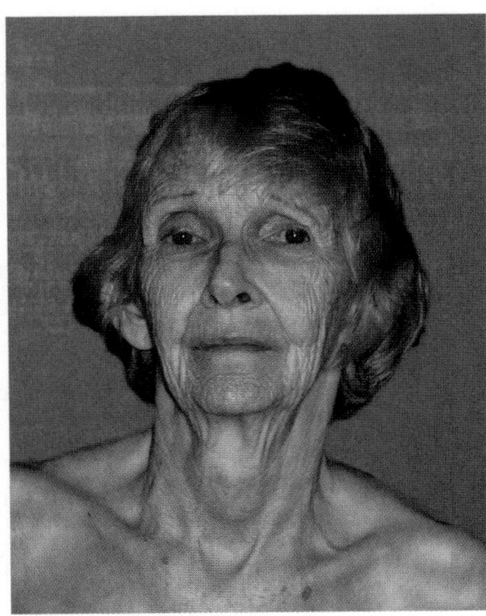

Cachectic Appearance

Accompanies chronic wasting diseases such as cancer, dehydration, and starvation. Features include sunken eyes; hollow cheeks; and exhausted, defeated expression.

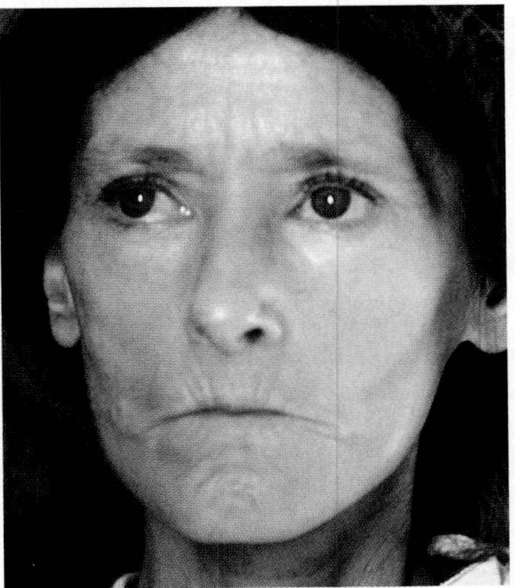

Scleroderma

Literally, "hard skin," this rare connective tissue disease is characterized by chronic hardening and shrinking degenerative changes in the skin, blood vessels, synovium, and skeletal muscles. Changes can occur in the skin, heart, esophagus, kidney, lung. Characteristic facies: hard, shiny skin on forehead and cheeks; thin, pursed lips with radial furrowing; absent skinfolds; muscle atrophy on face and neck; absence of expression.

Reprinted from the Clinical Slide Collection on the Rheumatic Diseases. © 1991, 1995, 1997. Used by permission of the American College of Rheumatology.

BIBLIOGRAPHY

1. Buse, D. C., Rupnow, M. F. T., & Lipton, R. B. (2009). Assessing and managing all aspects of migraine: migraine attacks, migraine-related functional impairment, common comorbidities, and quality of life. *Mayo Clinic Proceedings, 84*(5), 422-435.
2. Chan, Y. (2009). Differential diagnosis of dizziness. *Current Opinion in Otolaryngology & Head and Neck Surgery, 17*(3), 200-203.
3. Chen, L. Y., Benditt, D. G., & Shen, W. (2008). Management of syncope in adults: an update. *Mayo Clinic Proceedings, 83*(11), 1280-1293.
4. Davenport, R. (2008). The bare essentials: headache. *Practical Neurology, 8*(5), 335-343.
5. Fleener, V., & Holloway, B. (2004). Migraines: not just an adult problem. *The Nurse Practitioner, 29*(11), 27-40.
6. Foley, A. L. (2009). The "Grand Slam" triage assessment. *Journal of Emergency Nursing, 35*(1), 76-77.
7. Gladstein, J. (2009). Controlling pain: understanding headache pain in children. *Nursing, 39*(7), 57-58.
8. Joslin, N. (2004). Early identification key to scleroderma treatment. *The Nurse Practitioner, 29*(7), 24-41.

8a. Kapustin, J. F. (August 2010). Hypothyroidism: an evidence-based approach to a complex disorder. *The Nurse Practitioner, 35*(8):45-53.

9. Koch, J., & Alverson, E. (2003). Lymphadenopathy: a case study in clinical decision-making. *The American Journal for Nurse Practitioners, 7*(4), 21-32.
10. Lipton, R. B. (2009). Tracing transformation: chronic migraine classification, progression, and epidemiology. *Neurology, 72*(Suppl. 5), S3-S7.
11. Lipton, R. B., Bigal, M. E., Steiner, T. J., et al. (2004). Classification of primary headaches. *Neurology, 63*(3), 427-435.
12. Mistry, N., Wass, J., & Turner, M. R. (2009). When to consider thyroid dysfunction in the neurology clinic. *Practical Neurology, 9*(3), 145-156.
13. Morris, P. S. (2009). Upper respiratory tract infections (including otitis media). *Pediatric Clinics of North America, 56*(1), 101-117.

13a. National Stroke Association. (2009). What is Stroke? Retrieved December 10, 2009, from www.stroke.org/site/PageServer?pagename=STROKE.

14. Roodman, G. (2003). Recent developments in Paget's disease. *Advanced Studies in Medicine, 3*(5), 286-292.
15. Tan, M. P., & Parry, S. W. (2008). Vasovagal syncope in the older patient. *Journal of the American College of Cardiology, 51*, 599-606.
16. Tepper, S. J., Zatochill, M., Szeto, M., Sheftell, F., Tepper, D. E., & Bigal, M. (2008). Development of a simple menstrual migraine screening tool for obstetric and gynecology clinics: the menstrual migraine assessment tool. *Headache, 48*(10), 1419-1425.
17. Thyroid troubles: subtle symptoms with age. (2008). *Mayo Clinic Health Letter, 26*(5), 4-5.
18. Uneri, A., & Polat, S. (2007). Vertigo, dizziness, and imbalance in the elderly. *The Journal of Laryngology and Otology, 122*(5), 466-469.
19. Weeks, B. (2005). Graves' disease: the importance of early diagnosis. *The Nurse Practitioner, 30*(11), 34-47.

Summary Checklist: Head, Face, and Neck, Including Regional Lymphatics Examination

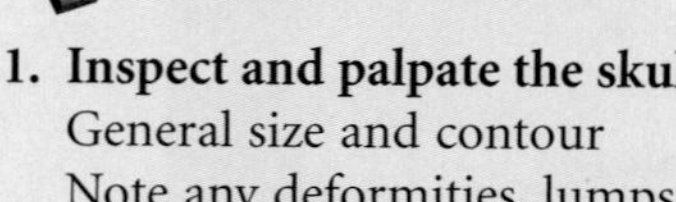

For a PDA-downloadable version, go to http://evolve.elsevier.com/Jarvis/.

1. Inspect and palpate the skull
General size and contour
Note any deformities, lumps, tenderness
Palpate temporal artery, temporomandibular joint

2. Inspect the face
Facial expression
Symmetry of movement (cranial nerve VII)
Any involuntary movements, edema, lesions

3. Inspect and palpate the neck
Active ROM
Enlargement of salivary glands, lymph nodes, thyroid gland
Position of the trachea

4. Auscultate the thyroid (if enlarged) for bruit

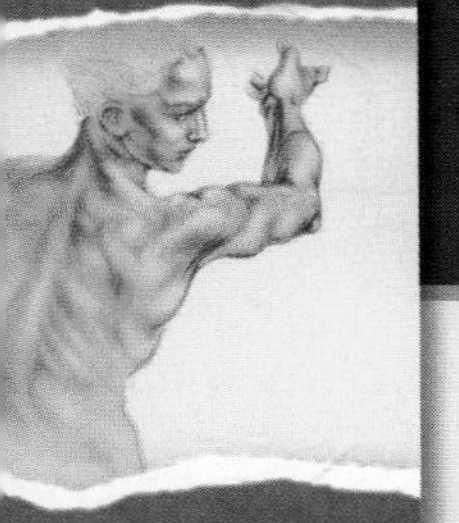

CHAPTER 14

Eyes

evolve WEBSITE

http://evolve.elsevier.com/Jarvis/

- Animations
- Audio Key Points
- Bedside Assessment Summary Checklist
- Health Promotion Guide
  Glaucoma
- NCLEX Review Questions
- Physical Examination Summary Checklist
- Video—Assessment
  Eyes

OUTLINE

Structure and Function, 279

External Anatomy
Internal Anatomy
Visual Pathways and Visual Fields
Visual Reflexes

Subjective Data, 285

Health History Questions

Objective Data, 287

Preparation
Central Visual Acuity
Visual Fields
Extraocular Muscle Function
External Ocular Structures
Anterior Eyeball Structures
The Ocular Fundus

Documentation and Critical Thinking, 309

Abnormal Findings, 311

Abnormal Findings for Advanced Practice, 316

STRUCTURE AND FUNCTION

EXTERNAL ANATOMY

The eye is the sensory organ of vision. Humans are very visual beings. More than half the neocortex is involved with processing visual information.

Because this sense is so important to humans, the eye is well protected by the bony orbital cavity, surrounded with a cushion of fat. The **eyelids** are like two movable shades that further protect the eye from injury, strong light, and dust. The upper eyelid is the larger and more mobile one. The eyelashes are short hairs in double or triple rows that curve outward from the lid margins, filtering out dust and dirt.

The **palpebral fissure** is the elliptical open space between the eyelids (Fig. 14-1). When closed, the lid margins approximate completely. When open, the upper lid covers part of the iris. The lower lid margin is just at the **limbus,** the border between the cornea and sclera. The **canthus** is the corner of the eye, the angle where the lids meet. At the inner canthus, the **caruncle** is a small, fleshy mass containing sebaceous glands.

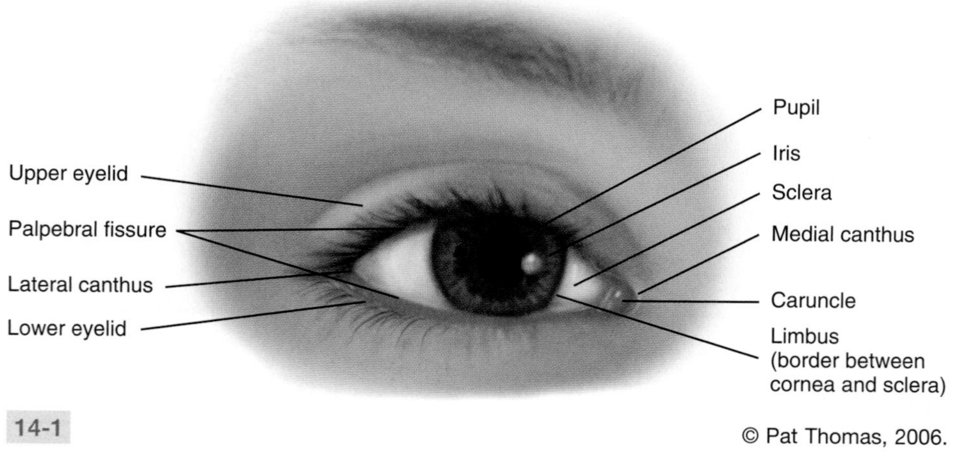

14-1

Within the upper lid, **tarsal plates** are strips of connective tissue that give it shape (Fig. 14-2). The tarsal plates contain the **meibomian glands,** modified sebaceous glands that secrete an oily lubricating material onto the lids. This stops the tears from overflowing and helps form an airtight seal when the lids are closed.

The exposed part of the eye has a transparent protective covering, the **conjunctiva.** The conjunctiva is a thin mucous membrane folded like an envelope between the eyelids and the eyeball. The *palpebral* conjunctiva lines the lids and is clear, with many small blood vessels. It forms a deep recess and then folds back over the eye. The *bulbar* conjunctiva overlays the eyeball, with the white sclera showing through. At the limbus, the conjunctiva merges with the cornea. The cornea covers and protects the iris and pupil.

The **lacrimal apparatus** provides constant irrigation to keep the conjunctiva and cornea moist and lubricated (Fig. 14-3). The lacrimal gland, in the upper outer corner over the eye, secretes tears. The tears wash across the eye and are drawn up evenly as the lid blinks. The tears drain into the **puncta,** visible on the upper and lower lids at the inner canthus. The tears then drain into the nasolacrimal sac, through the one-half-inch-long nasolacrimal duct, and empty into the inferior meatus inside the nose. A tiny fold of mucous membrane prevents air from being forced up the nasolacrimal duct when the nose is blown.

Extraocular Muscles. Six muscles attach the eyeball to its orbit (Fig. 14-4, *A*) and serve to direct the eye to points of the person's interest. These extraocular muscles give the eye both straight and rotary movement. The four straight, or *rectus,* muscles are the superior, inferior, lateral, and medial

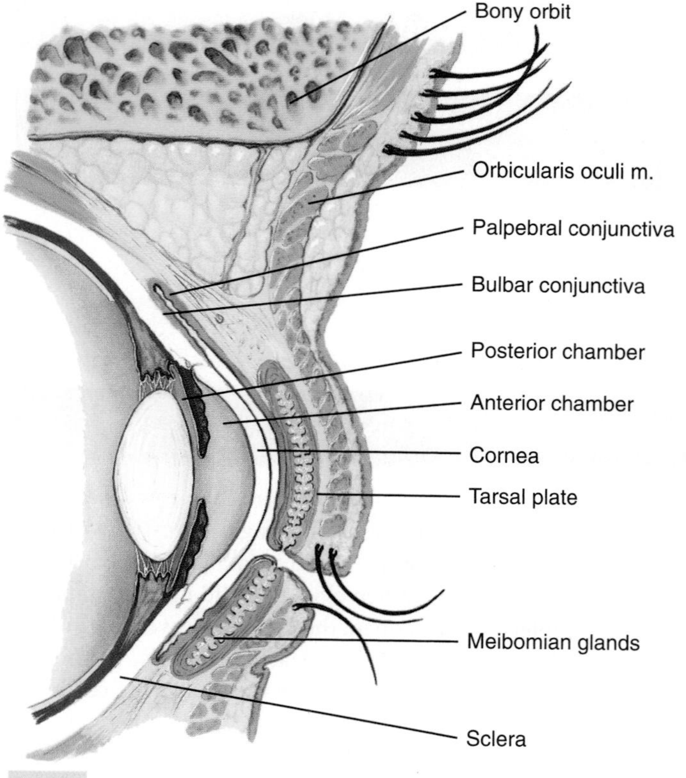

14-2

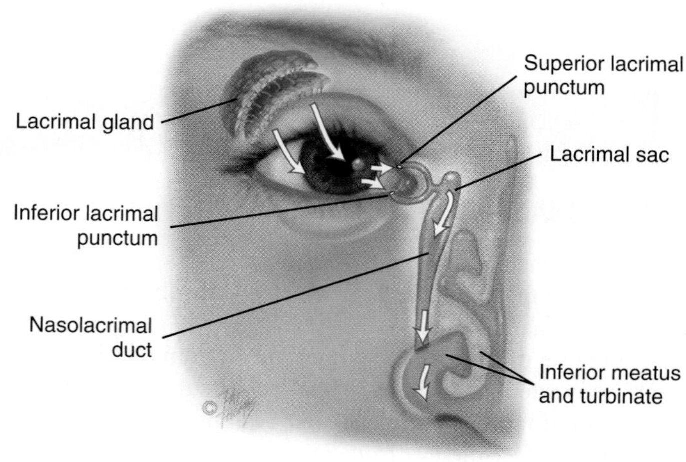

14-3 Lacrimal apparatus.

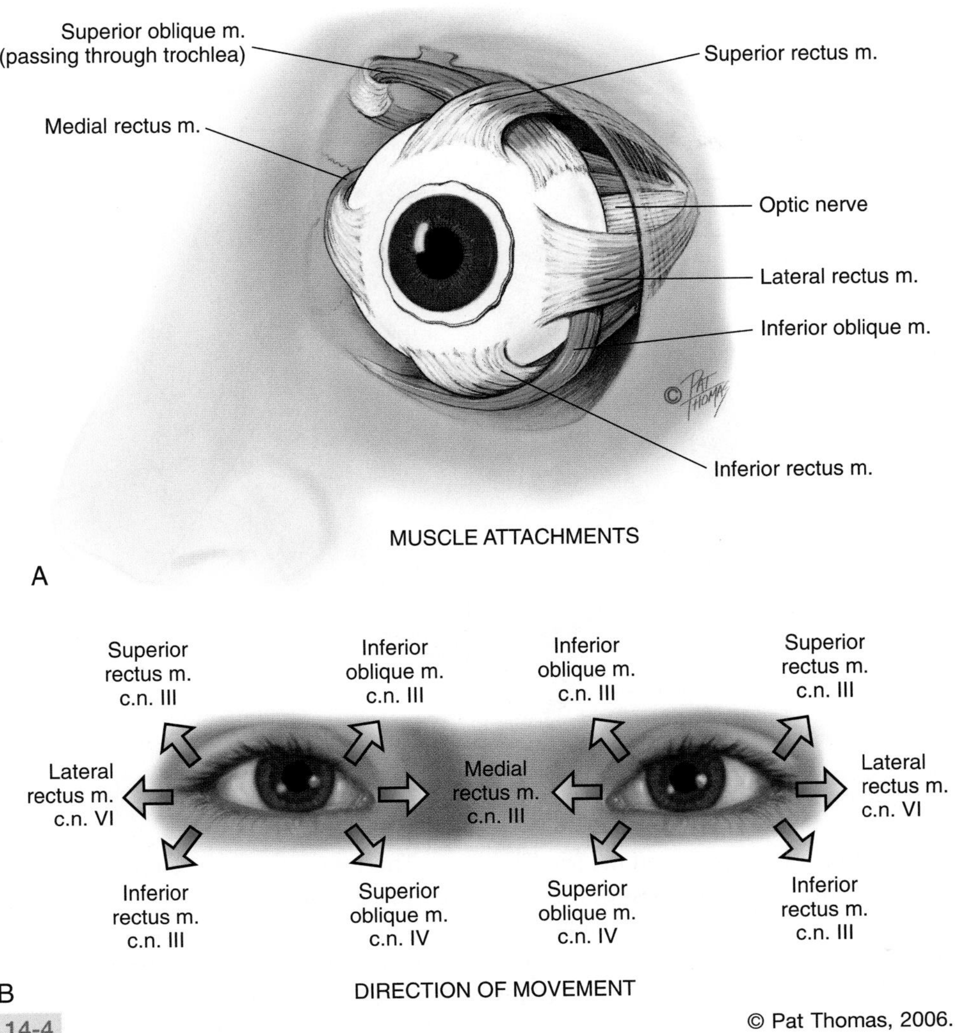

14-4

rectus muscles. The two slanting, or *oblique,* muscles are the superior and inferior muscles.

Each muscle is coordinated, or yoked, with one in the other eye. This ensures that when the two eyes move, their axes always remain parallel (called *conjugate movement*). Parallel axes are important because the human brain can tolerate seeing only one image. Although some animals can perceive two different pictures through each eye, human beings have a binocular, single-image visual system. This occurs because our eyes move as a pair. For example, the two yoked muscles that allow looking to the far right are the right lateral rectus and the left medial rectus.

Movement of the **extraocular muscles** (Fig. 14-4, *B*) is stimulated by three **cranial nerves.** Cranial nerve VI, the abducens nerve, innervates the lateral rectus muscle (which abducts the eye); cranial nerve IV, the trochlear nerve, innervates the superior oblique muscle; and cranial nerve III, the oculomotor nerve, innervates all the rest—the superior, inferior, and medial rectus and the inferior oblique muscles. Note that the superior oblique muscle is located on the superior aspect of the eyeball, but when it contracts, it enables the person to look downward and inward.

INTERNAL ANATOMY

The eye is a sphere composed of three concentric coats: (1) the outer fibrous **sclera,** (2) the middle vascular **choroid,** and (3) the inner nervous **retina** (Fig. 14-5). Inside the retina is the transparent vitreous body. The only parts accessible to examination are the sclera anteriorly and the retina through the ophthalmoscope.

The Outer Layer. The **sclera** is a tough, protective, white covering. It is continuous anteriorly with the smooth, transparent cornea, which covers the iris and pupil. The cornea is part of the refracting media of the eye, bending incoming light rays so that they will be focused on the inner retina.

The **cornea** is very sensitive to touch; contact with a wisp of cotton stimulates a blink in both eyes, called the *corneal reflex.* The trigeminal nerve (cranial nerve V) carries the afferent sensation into the brain, and the facial nerve (cranial nerve VII) carries the efferent message that stimulates the blink.

The Middle Layer. The **choroid** has dark pigmentation to prevent light from reflecting internally and is heavily vascularized to deliver blood to the retina. Anteriorly, the

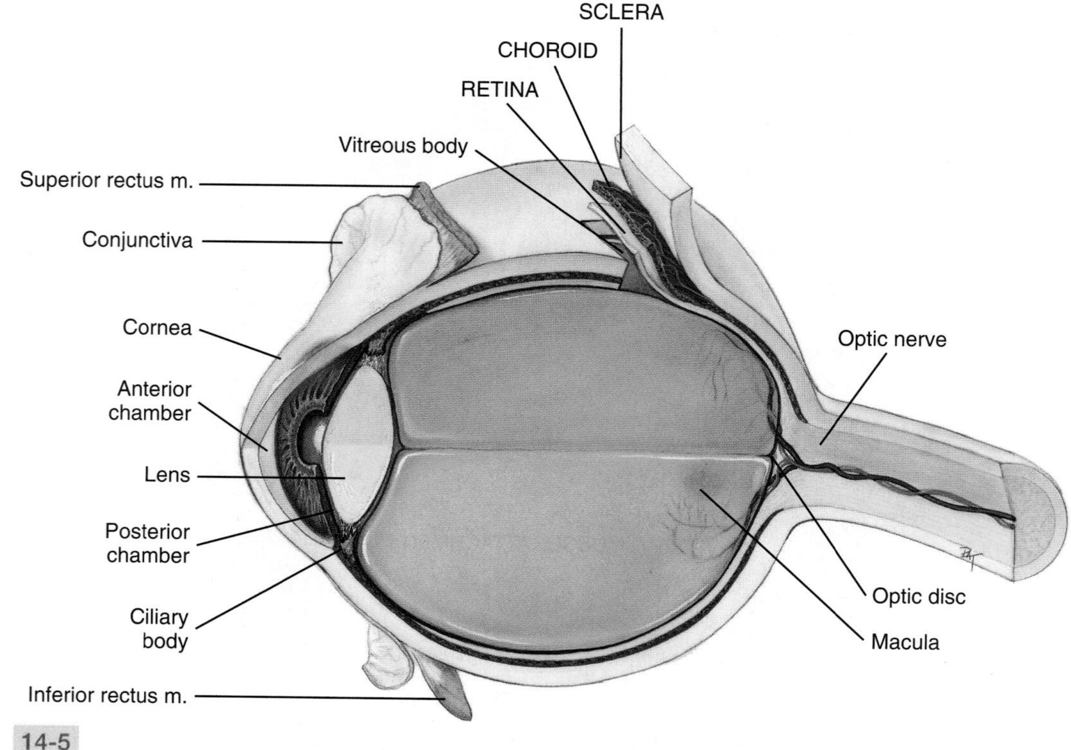

14-5

choroid is continuous with the ciliary body and the iris. The muscles of the ciliary body control the thickness of the lens. The iris functions as a diaphragm, varying the opening at its center, the pupil. This controls the amount of light admitted into the retina. The muscle fibers of the iris contract the pupil in bright light and to accommodate for near vision; they dilate the pupil in dim light and accommodate for far vision. The color of the iris varies from person to person.

The **pupil** is round and regular. Its size is determined by a balance between the parasympathetic and sympathetic chains of the autonomic nervous system. Stimulation of the parasympathetic branch, through cranial nerve III, causes constriction of the pupil. Stimulation of the sympathetic branch dilates the pupil and elevates the eyelid. As mentioned earlier, the pupil size also reacts to the amount of ambient light and to accommodation, or focusing an object on the retina.

The **lens** is a biconvex disc located just posterior to the pupil. The transparent lens serves as a refracting medium, keeping a viewed object in continual focus on the retina. Its thickness is controlled by the ciliary body; the lens bulges for focusing on near objects and flattens for far objects.

The **anterior chamber** is posterior to the cornea and in front of the iris and lens. The **posterior chamber** lies behind the iris to the sides of the lens. These contain the clear, watery aqueous humor that is produced continually by the ciliary body. The continuous flow of fluid serves to deliver nutrients to the surrounding tissues and to drain metabolic wastes. Intraocular pressure is determined by a balance between the amount of aqueous produced and resistance to its outflow at the angle of the anterior chamber.

The Inner Layer. The **retina** is the visual receptive layer of the eye in which light waves are changed into nerve impulses. The retina surrounds the soft, gelatinous vitreous humor. The retinal structures viewed through the ophthalmoscope are the optic disc, the retinal vessels, the general background, and the macula (Fig. 14-6).

The **optic disc** (or optic papilla) is the area in which fibers from the retina converge to form the optic nerve. Located toward the nasal side of the retina, it has these characteristics: a color that varies from creamy yellow-orange to pink; a round or oval shape; margins that are distinct and sharply demarcated, especially on the temporal side; and a physiologic cup, the smaller circular area inside the disc where the blood vessels exit and enter.

The **retinal vessels** normally include a paired artery and vein extending to each quadrant, growing progressively smaller in caliber as they reach the periphery. The arteries appear brighter red and narrower than the veins, and the arteries have a thin sliver of light on them (the arterial light reflex). The general background of the fundus varies in color, depending on the person's skin color. The **macula** is located on the temporal side of the fundus. It is a slightly darker pigmented region surrounding the **fovea centralis,** the area of sharpest and keenest vision. The macula receives and transduces light from the center of the visual field.

VISUAL PATHWAYS AND VISUAL FIELDS

Objects reflect light. The light rays are refracted through the transparent media (cornea, aqueous humor, lens, and vitreous body) and strike the retina. The retina transforms the

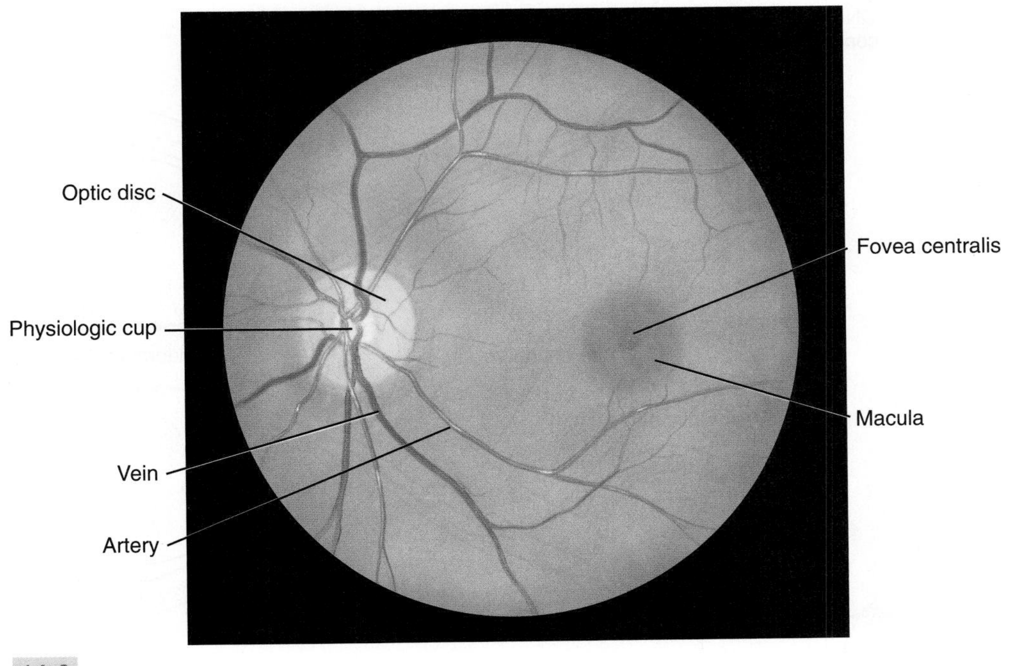

14-6

light stimulus into nerve impulses that are conducted through the optic nerve and the optic tract to the visual cortex of the occipital lobe.

The image formed on the retina is upside down and reversed from its actual appearance in the outside world (Fig. 14-7). That is, an object in the upper temporal visual field of the right eye reflects its image onto the lower nasal area of the retina. All retinal fibers collect to form the optic nerve, but they maintain this same spatial arrangement, with nasal fibers running medially and temporal fibers running laterally.

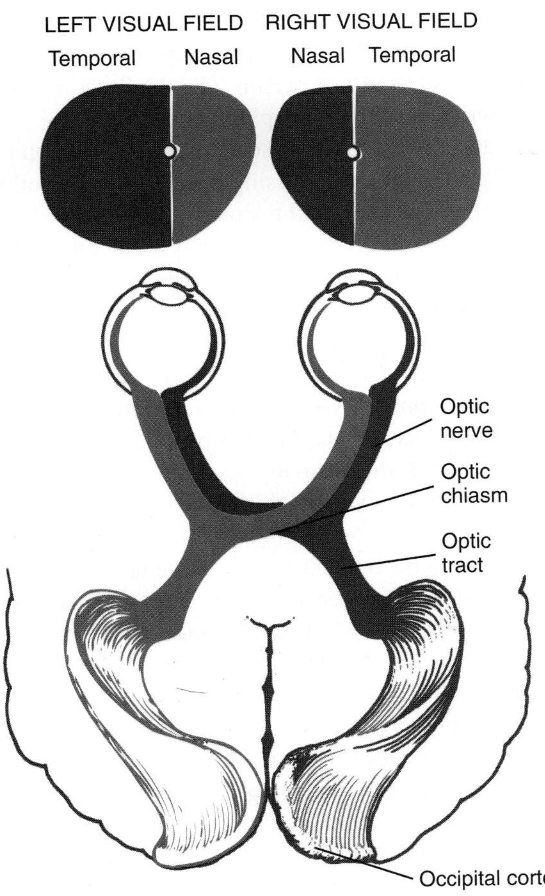

14-7 Visual pathways (viewed from above).

At the optic chiasm, nasal fibers (from both temporal visual fields) cross over. The left optic tract now has fibers from the left half of each retina, and the right optic tract contains fibers only from the right. Thus the right side of the brain looks at the left side of the world.

VISUAL REFLEXES

Pupillary Light Reflex. The pupillary light reflex is the normal constriction of the pupils when bright light shines on the retina (Fig. 14-8). It is a subcortical reflex arc (i.e., a person has no conscious control over it); the sensory afferent link is cranial nerve II (the optic nerve), and the motor efferent path is cranial III (the oculomotor nerve).

When one eye is exposed to bright light, a *direct light reflex* occurs (constriction of that pupil) as well as a *consensual light reflex* (simultaneous constriction of the other pupil). This happens because the optic nerve carries the sensory afferent message in and then synapses with both sides of the brain. For example, consider the light reflex in a person who is blind in one eye. Stimulation of the normal eye produces both a direct and a consensual light reflex. Stimulation of the blind eye causes no response because the sensory afferent in cranial nerve II is destroyed.

Fixation. This is a reflex direction of the eye toward an object attracting a person's attention. The image is fixed in the center of the visual field, the fovea centralis. This consists of very rapid ocular movements to put the target back on the fovea and somewhat slower (smooth pursuit) movements to

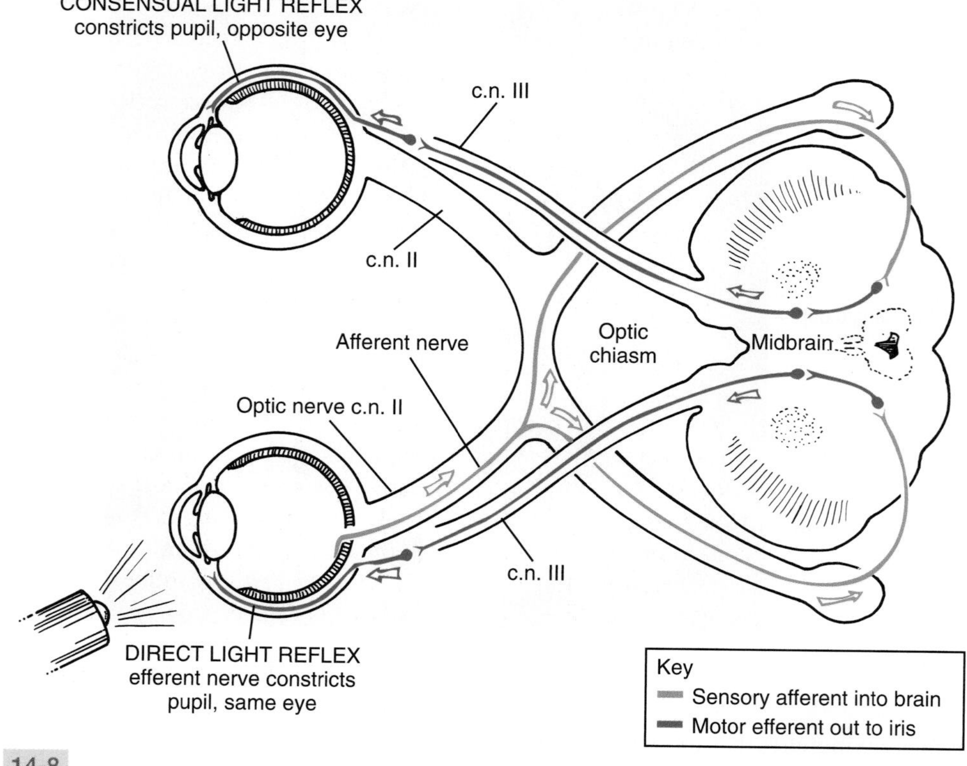

14-8

track the target and keep its image on the fovea. These ocular movements are impaired by drugs, alcohol, fatigue, and inattention.

Accommodation. This is adaptation of the eye for near vision. It is accomplished by increasing the curvature of the lens through movement of the ciliary muscles. Although the lens cannot be observed directly, the components of accommodation that can be observed are convergence (motion toward) of the axes of the eyeballs and pupillary constriction.

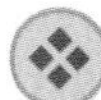

DEVELOPMENTAL COMPETENCE

Infants and Children

At birth, eye function is limited, but it matures fully during the early years. Peripheral vision is intact in the newborn infant. The macula, the area of keenest vision, is absent at birth but is developing by 4 months and is mature by 8 months. Eye movements may be poorly coordinated at birth. By 3 to 4 months of age, the infant establishes binocularity and can fixate on a single image with both eyes simultaneously. Most neonates (80%) are born farsighted; this gradually decreases after 7 to 8 years of age.

In structure, the eyeball reaches adult size by 8 years. At birth, the iris shows little pigment and the pupils are small. The lens is nearly spherical at birth, growing flatter throughout life. Its consistency changes from that of soft plastic at birth to rigid glass in old age.

The Aging Adult

Changes in eye structure contribute greatly to the distinct facial changes of the aging person. The skin loses its elasticity, causing wrinkling and drooping; fat tissues and muscles atrophy; and the external eye structures appear as on p. 306. Lacrimal glands involute, causing decreased tear production and a feeling of dryness and burning.

On the globe itself, the cornea may show an infiltration of degenerative lipid material around the limbus (see discussion of *arcus senilis,* p. 307). Pupil size decreases. The lens loses elasticity, becoming hard and glasslike. This glasslike quality decreases the lens's ability to change shape to accommodate for near vision; this condition is termed **presbyopia.** By 40 years of age, 50% of people have presbyopia.[6] By 70 years of age, the normally transparent fibers of the lens begin to thicken and yellow; this is the beginning of a senile cataract.

Inside the globe, floaters appear in the vitreous as a result of debris that accumulates because the vitreous is not renewed as continuously as the aqueous humor. Visual acuity may diminish gradually after 50 years of age, and even more so after 70 years. Near vision is commonly affected because of the decreased power of accommodation in the lens (presbyopia). In the early 40s, a person may have blurred vision and difficulty reading. Also, the aging person needs more light to see because of a decreased adaptation to darkness, and this condition may affect the function of night driving.

In older adults, the most common causes of decreased visual functioning are:

1. Cataract formation, or lens opacity, resulting from a clumping of proteins in the lens. Some cataract formation should be expected by age 70 years. Studies indicate that 46% of people ages 75 to 85 years have cataracts.[9]
2. Glaucoma, or increased intraocular pressure. The incidence increases with age to 7.2% at ages 75 to 85 years, affecting men at higher rates than women.[9] Chronic open-angle glaucoma is the most common type; it involves a gradual loss of peripheral vision.
3. Macular degeneration, or the breakdown of cells in the macula of the retina. Loss of central vision, the area of clearest vision, is the most common cause of blindness. It affects 28% of those ages 75 to 85 years, with women affected more often than men.[9] With this, the person is unable to read fine print, sew, or do fine work and may have difficulty distinguishing faces. Depending on how much the lifestyle is oriented around activities requiring close work, loss of central vision may cause great distress. Peripheral vision is not affected, so the person can manage self-care and will not become completely disabled.

CULTURE AND GENETICS

Racial differences are evident in the palpebral fissures. Persons of Asian origin are often identified by their characteristic eyes, whereas the presence of narrowed palpebral fissures in non-Asian individuals may be diagnostic of a serious congenital anomaly, *Down syndrome.*

Culturally based variability exists in the color of the iris and in retinal pigmentation, with darker irides having darker retinas behind them. Individuals with light retinas generally have better night vision but can have pain in an environment that has too much light.

Racial Variations in Disease. Primary open-angle glaucoma affects Blacks three to six times more often than whites and is six times more likely to cause blindness in Blacks than in whites.[6] Reasons for this are not known.

The percent of adults 18 years of age and older reporting visual limitations and trouble seeing with glasses in 2006 was the highest, 16.7%, among American Indians and Alaska natives; African Americans 10.4%; and whites 9.5%. Poverty is also an extenuating factor in this problem; 26.4% of the population living within poverty levels report this.[15]

The prevalence of blindness also has racial and ethnic variations. In whites older than 40 years, the leading cause of blindness is age-related macular degeneration (54%), followed by cataracts (9%).[5] In Blacks older than 40 years, cataracts and open-angle glaucoma together cause 60% of blindness. In Hispanics older than 40 years, the leading cause of blindness is open-angle glaucoma.

SUBJECTIVE DATA

1. Vision difficulty (decreased acuity, blurring, blind spots)
2. Pain
3. Strabismus, diplopia
4. Redness, swelling
5. Watering, discharge
6. History of ocular problems
7. Glaucoma
8. Use of glasses or contact lenses
9. Self-care behaviors

Examiner Asks	Rationale
1. **Vision difficulty.** Any **difficulty seeing** or any blurring? Any blind spots? Come on suddenly, or progress slowly? In one eye or both? • Constant, or does it come and go? • Do objects appear out of focus, or does it feel like a clouding over objects? Does it feel like "grayness" of vision?	
• Do spots move in front of your eyes? One or many? In one or both eyes?	Floaters are common with myopia or after middle age due to condensed vitreous fibers. Usually not significant, but acute onset of floaters ("shade" or "cobwebs") occurs with retinal detachment.
• Any halos/rainbows around objects? Or rings around lights?	Halos around lights occur with acute narrow-angle glaucoma.
• Any blind spot? Does it move as you shift your gaze? Any loss of peripheral vision?	**Scotoma,** a blind spot surrounded by an area of normal or decreased vision, occurs with glaucoma, with optic nerve disorders.
• Any night blindness?	Night blindness occurs with optic atrophy, glaucoma, or vitamin A deficiency.

Examiner Asks	Rationale
2. **Pain.** Any **eye pain?** Please describe. • Come on suddenly?	*Sudden onset* of eye symptoms (pain, floaters, blind spot, loss of peripheral vision) is an emergency. Refer immediately.
• Quality—a burning or itching? Or sharp, stabbing pain? Pain with bright light? • A foreign body sensation? Or deep aching? Or headache in brow area?	Quality is valuable in diagnosis. **Photophobia** is the inability to tolerate light. Note: Some common eye diseases cause no pain (e.g., cataract, glaucoma).
3. **Strabismus, diplopia.** Any history of crossed eyes? Now or in the past? Does this occur with eye fatigue? • Ever see double? Constant, or does it come and go? In one eye or both?	Strabismus is a deviation in the axis of the eye. **Diplopia** is the perception of two images of a single object.
4. **Redness, swelling.** Any **redness** or **swelling** in the eyes? • Any infections? Now or in the past? When do these occur? In a particular time of year?	
5. **Watering, discharge.** Any **watering** or excessive tearing?	Lacrimation (tearing) and epiphora (excessive tearing) are due to irritants or obstruction in drainage of tears.
• Any **discharge?** Any matter in the eyes? Is it hard to open your eyes in the morning? What color is the discharge? • How do you remove matter from your eyes?	Purulent discharge is thick and yellow. Crusts form at night. Assess hygiene practices and knowledge of cross-contamination.
6. **Past history of ocular problems.** Any **history** of injury or surgery to eye? Or any history of allergies?	Allergens cause irritation of conjunctiva or cornea (e.g., makeup, contact lens solution).
7. **Glaucoma.** Ever been tested for **glaucoma?** Results? • Any family history of glaucoma?	Glaucoma is characterized by increased intraocular pressure.
8. **Use of glasses or contact lenses.** Do you wear **glasses** or **contact lenses?** How do they work for you? • Last time your prescription was checked? Was it changed? • If you wear contact lenses, are there any problems such as pain, photophobia, watering, or swelling? • How do you care for contacts? How long do you wear them? How do you clean them? Do you remove them for certain activities?	Assess self-care behaviors.
9. **Self-care behaviors.** Last vision test? Ever tested for color vision? • Any environmental conditions at home or at work that may affect your eyes? For example, flying sparks, metal bits, smoke, dust, chemical fumes? If so, do you wear goggles to protect your eyes?	Self-care behaviors for eyes and vision. Work-related eye disease (e.g., an auto mechanic with a foreign body from metal working or radiation damage from welding).
10. What medications are you taking? Systemic or topical? Do you take any medication specifically for the eyes?	Some medications affect the eyes (e.g., prednisone may cause cataracts or increased intraocular pressure).
11. If you have experienced a vision loss, how do you cope? Do you have books with large print, books on audio tape or CD, braille? • Do you maintain your living environment the same? • Do you sometimes fear complete loss of vision?	A constant spatial layout eases navigation through the home.

Examiner Asks	Rationale
Additional History for Infants and Children	
1. Any vaginal infections in the mother at time of delivery?	Genital herpes and gonorrhea vaginitis have ocular sequelae for the newborn.
2. Considering age of child, which developmental milestones of vision have you (parent) noted?	The parent is most often the one to detect vision problems.
3. Does the child have routine vision testing at school?	
4. Are you (parent) aware of safety measures to protect child's eyes from trauma? Do you inspect toys? • Have you taught the child safe care of sharp objects and how to carry and how to use them?	
Additional History for the Aging Adult	
1. Have you noticed any visual difficulty with climbing stairs or driving? Any problem with night vision?	Any loss of depth perception or central vision.
2. When was the last time you were tested for glaucoma? • Any aching pain around eyes? Any loss of peripheral vision? • If you have glaucoma, how do you manage your eyedrops?	Compliance may be a problem if symptoms are absent. Assess ability to administer eyedrops.
3. Is there a history of cataracts? Any loss or progressive blurring of vision?	
4. Do your eyes ever feel dry? Burning? What do you do for this?	Decreased tear production may occur with aging.
5. Any decrease in usual activities, such as reading or sewing?	Macular degeneration causes a loss in central vision acuity.

Objective Data

OBJECTIVE DATA

PREPARATION

Position the person standing for vision screening; then sitting up with the head at your eye level.

EQUIPMENT NEEDED

Snellen eye chart
Handheld visual screener
Opaque card or occluder
Penlight
Applicator stick
Ophthalmoscope

Normal Range of Findings	Abnormal Findings

TEST CENTRAL VISUAL ACUITY

Snellen Eye Chart

The Snellen alphabet chart is the most commonly used and accurate measure of visual acuity. It has lines of letters arranged in decreasing size.

Place the Snellen alphabet chart in a well-lit spot at eye level. Position the person on a mark exactly 20 feet from the chart. Hand over an opaque card with which to shield one eye at a time during the test; inadvertent peeking may result

Normal Range of Findings	Abnormal Findings

when shielding the eye with the person's own fingers (Fig. 14-9). If the person wears glasses or contact lenses, leave them on. Remove only reading glasses because they will blur distance vision. Ask the person to read through the chart to the smallest line of letters possible. Encourage trying the next smallest line also. (Note: Use a Snellen picture chart for people who cannot read letters. See p. 303.)

Note hesitancy, squinting, leaning forward, misreading letters.

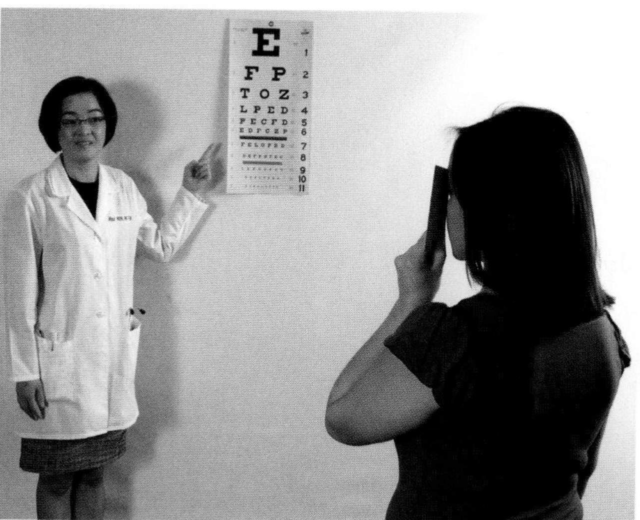

14-9

Record the result using the numeric fraction at the end of the last successful line read. Indicate whether the person missed any letters or if corrective lenses were worn—for example, "Right 20/30 − 1, with glasses." That is, the right eye scored 20/30, missing one letter.

Normal visual acuity is 20/20. Contrary to some people's impression, the numeric fraction is *not* a percentage of normal vision. Instead, the top number (numerator) indicates the distance the person is standing from the chart, and the denominator gives the distance at which a normal eye could have read that particular line. Thus "20/30" means, "You can read at 20 feet what the normal eye can see from 30 feet away."

The larger the denominator, the poorer the vision. If vision is poorer than 20/30, refer to an ophthalmologist or optometrist. Impaired vision may be due to refractive error, opacity in the media (cornea, lens, vitreous), or disorder in the retina or optic pathway.

If the person is unable to see even the largest letters, shorten the distance to the chart until it is seen and record that distance (e.g., "10/200"). If visual acuity is even lower, assess whether the person can count your fingers when they are spread in front of the eyes or distinguish light perception from your penlight.

Near Vision

For people older than 40 years or for those who report increasing difficulty reading, test near vision with a handheld vision screener with various sizes of print (e.g., a Jaeger card) (Fig. 14-10). Hold the card in good light about 35 cm (14 inches) from the eye—this distance equals the print size on the 20-foot chart. Test each eye separately, with glasses on. A normal result is "14/14" in each eye, read without hesitancy and without moving the card closer or farther away. When no vision screening card is available, ask the person to read from a magazine or newspaper.

Presbyopia, the decrease in power of accommodation with aging, is suggested when the person moves the card farther away.

Normal Range of Findings

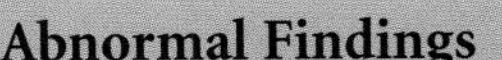

Abnormal Findings

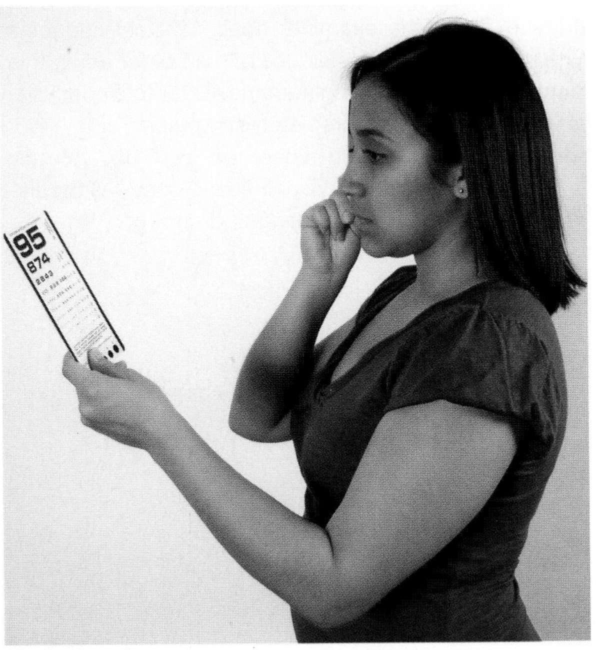

14-10

TEST VISUAL FIELDS

Confrontation Test

This is a gross measure of peripheral vision. It compares the person's peripheral vision with your own, assuming yours is normal. Position yourself at eye level with the person, about 2 feet away. Direct the person to cover one eye with an opaque card, and with the other eye to look straight at you. Cover your own eye opposite to the person's covered one. You are testing the uncovered eye. Hold a pencil or your flicking finger as a target midline between you and slowly advance it in from the periphery in several directions (Fig. 14-11, *A* and *B*).

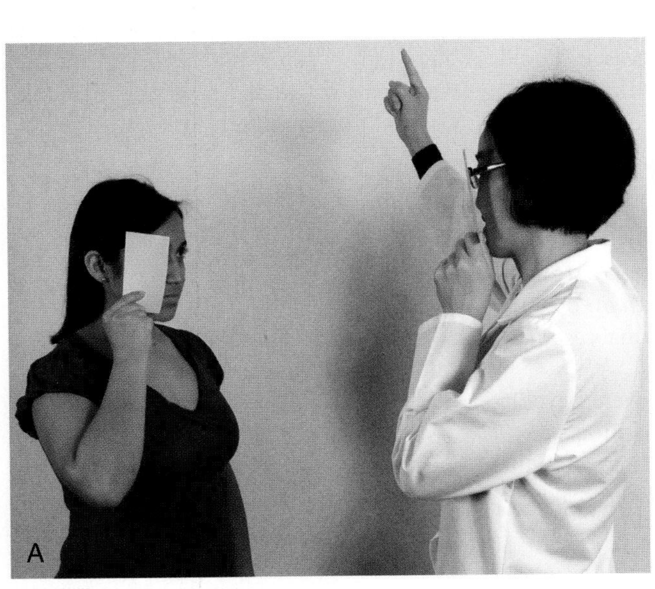

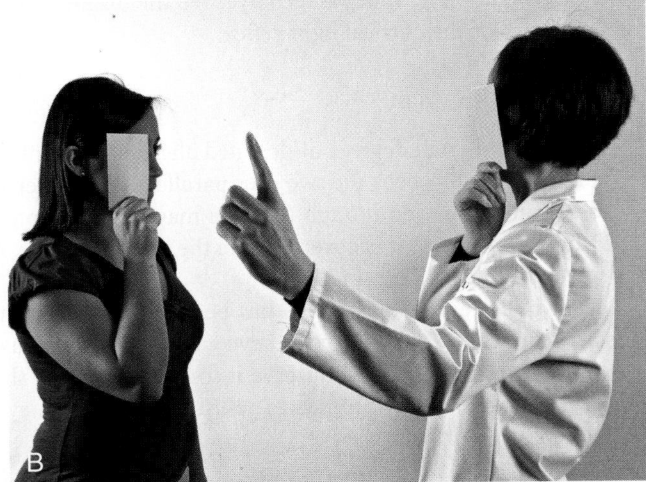

14-11

Normal Range of Findings

Ask the person to say "now" as the target is first seen; this should be just as you see the object also. (This works with all but the temporal visual field, with which you would need a 6-foot arm to avoid being seen initially! With the temporal direction, start the object somewhat behind the person.) Estimate the angle between the anteroposterior axis of the eye and the peripheral axis where the object is first seen. Normal results are about 50 degrees upward, 90 degrees temporally, 70 degrees down, and 60 degrees nasally (Fig. 14-12).

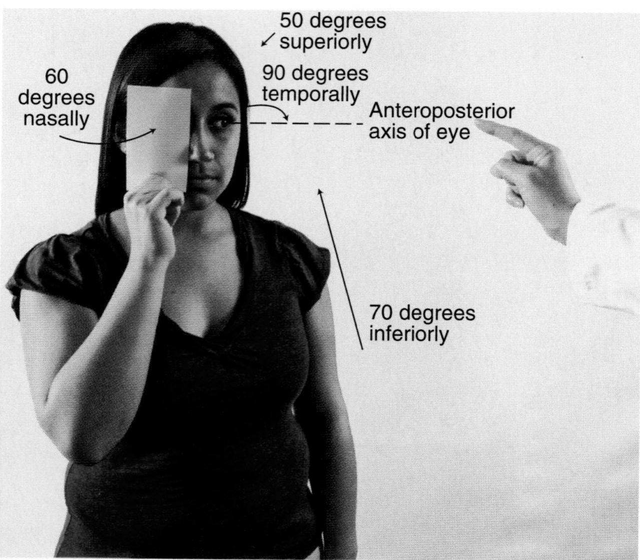

14-12 Range of peripheral vision.

Abnormal Findings

If the person is unable to see the object as the examiner does, the test suggests peripheral field loss. In an older adult, this screens for glaucoma. Refer to a specialist for more precise testing (see Table 14-5, Visual Field Loss, on p. 316). Acutely diminished visual fields occur with diseases of the retina and stroke.

INSPECT EXTRAOCULAR MUSCLE FUNCTION

Corneal Light Reflex (The Hirschberg Test)

Assess the parallel alignment of the eye axes by shining a light toward the person's eyes. Direct the person to stare straight ahead as you hold the light about 30 cm (12 inches) away. Note the reflection of the light on the corneas; it should be in exactly the same spot on each eye. See the bright white dots in Fig. 14-30 for symmetry of the corneal light reflex.

Asymmetry of the light reflex indicates deviation in alignment from eye muscle weakness or paralysis. If you see this, perform the cover test.

Cover Test

This test detects small degrees of deviated alignment by interrupting the fusion reflex that normally keeps the two eyes parallel. Ask the person to stare straight ahead at your nose even though the gaze may be interrupted. With an opaque card, cover one eye. As it is covered, note the uncovered eye. A normal response is a steady fixed gaze (Fig. 14-13, *A*).

If the eye jumps to fixate on the designated point, it was out of alignment before.

Meanwhile, the macular image has been suppressed on the covered eye. If muscle weakness exists, the covered eye will drift into a relaxed position.

Now uncover the eye and observe it for movement. It should stare straight ahead (Fig. 14-13, *B*). If it jumps to re-establish fixation, eye muscle weakness exists. Repeat with the other eye.

A **phoria** is a mild weakness noted only when fusion is blocked. **Tropia** is more severe—a constant malalignment of the eyes (see Table 14-1, Extraocular Muscle Dysfunction, on p. 311).

Normal Range of Findings | Abnormal Findings

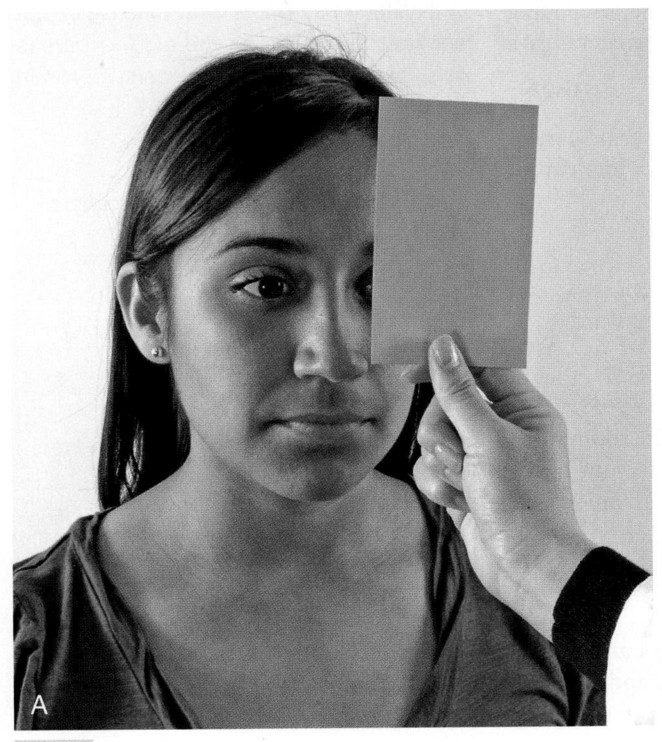

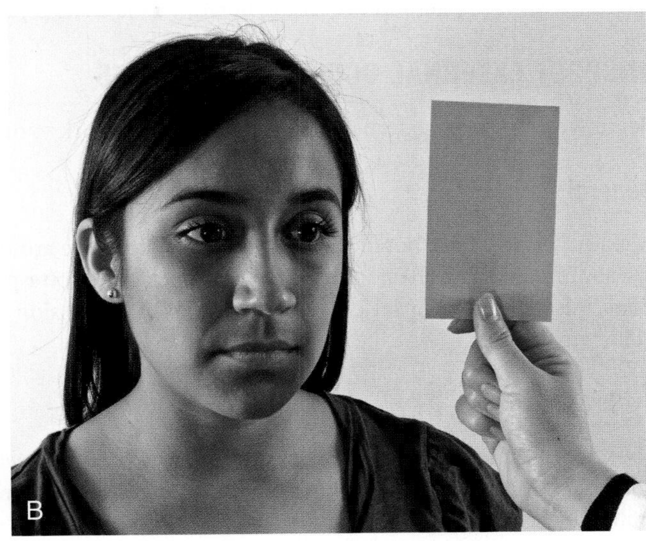

14-13

Diagnostic Positions Test

Leading the eyes through the six cardinal positions of gaze will elicit any muscle weakness during movement (Fig. 14-14). Ask the person to hold the head steady and to follow the movement of your finger, pen, or penlight only with the eyes. Hold the target back about 12 inches so the person can focus on it comfortably, and move it to each of the six positions, hold it momentarily, then back to center. Progress clockwise. A normal response is parallel tracking of the object with both eyes.

Eye movement is not parallel. Failure to follow in a certain direction indicates weakness of an extraocular muscle (EOM) or dysfunction of cranial nerve innervating it.

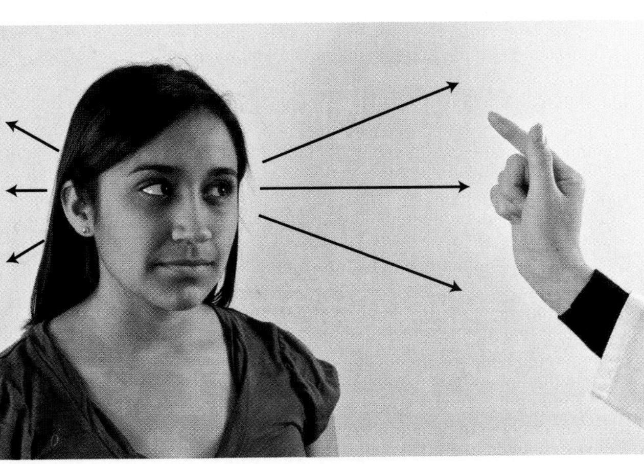

14-14 Diagnostic positions test.

Normal Range of Findings	Abnormal Findings

In addition to parallel movement, note any **nystagmus**—a fine, oscillating movement best seen around the iris. Mild nystagmus at an extreme lateral gaze is normal; nystagmus at any other position is not.

Nystagmus occurs with disease of the semicircular canals in the ears, a paretic eye muscle, multiple sclerosis, or brain lesions.

Finally, note that the upper eyelid continues to overlap the superior part of the iris, even during downward movement. You should not see a white rim of sclera between the lid and the iris. If noted, this is termed "lid lag."

Lid lag occurs with hyperthyroidism.

INSPECT EXTERNAL OCULAR STRUCTURES

Begin with the most external points, and logically work your way inward.

General

Already you will have noted the person's ability to move around the room, with vision functioning well enough to avoid obstacles and to respond to your directions. Also note the facial expression; a relaxed expression accompanies adequate vision.

Groping with hands.

Squinting or craning forward.

Eyebrows

Look for symmetry between the two eyes. Normally the eyebrows are present bilaterally, move symmetrically as the facial expression changes, and have no scaling or lesions (Fig. 14-15).

Unequal or absent movement with nerve damage.

Scaling with seborrhea.

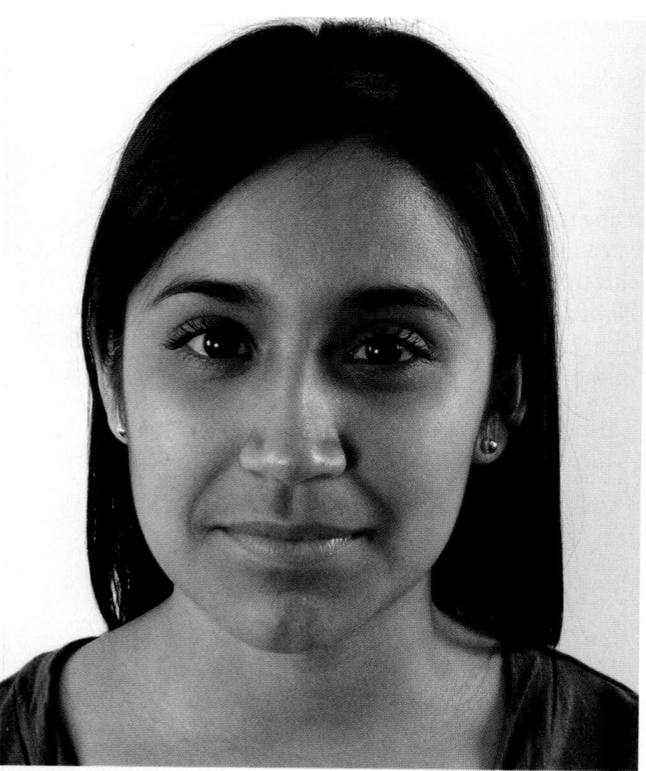

14-15

Eyelids and Lashes

The upper lids normally overlap the superior part of the iris and approximate completely with the lower lids when closed. The skin is intact without redness, swelling, discharge, or lesions.

Lid lag with hyperthyroidism.

Incomplete closure creates risk for corneal damage.

Objective Data

Normal Range of Findings

The palpebral fissures are horizontal in non-Asians, whereas Asians normally have an upward slant.

Note that the eyelashes are evenly distributed along the lid margins and curve outward.

Eyeballs

The eyeballs are aligned normally in their sockets with no protrusion or sunken appearance. African Americans normally may have a slight protrusion of the eyeball beyond the supraorbital ridge.

Conjunctiva and Sclera

Ask the person to look up. Using your thumbs, slide the lower lids down along the bony orbital rim. Take care not to push against the eyeball. Inspect the exposed area (Fig. 14-16). The eyeball looks moist and glossy. Numerous small blood vessels normally show through the transparent conjunctiva. Otherwise, the conjunctivae are clear and show the normal color of the structure below—pink over the lower lids and white over the sclera. Note any color change, swelling, or lesions.

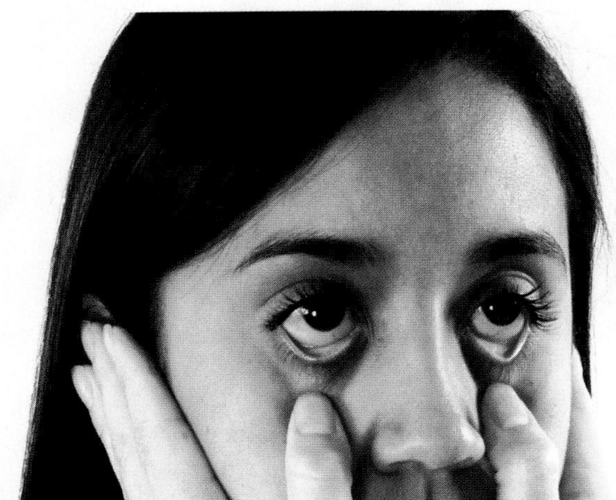

14-16

The sclera is china white, although African Americans occasionally have a gray-blue or "muddy" color to the sclera. Also in dark-skinned people, you normally may see small brown macules (like freckles) on the sclera, which should not be confused with foreign bodies or petechiae. Last, African Americans may have yellowish fatty deposits beneath the lids away from the cornea. Do not confuse these yellow spots with the overall scleral yellowing that accompanies jaundice.

Abnormal Findings

Ptosis, drooping of upper lid.

Periorbital edema, lesions (see Tables 14-2 and 14-3).

Ectropion and entropion (see Table 14-2, Abnormalities in the Eyelids, p. 313).

Exophthalmos (protruding eyes) and enophthalmos (sunken eyes) (see Table 14-2).

General reddening (see Table 14-6, Vascular Disorders).

Cyanosis of the lower lids.

Pallor near the outer canthus of the lower lid may indicate anemia (the inner canthus normally contains less pigment).

Scleral icterus is an even yellowing of the sclera extending up to the cornea, indicating jaundice.

Tenderness, foreign body, discharge, or lesions.

Normal Range of Findings | Abnormal Findings

Eversion of the Upper Lid

This maneuver is not part of the normal examination, but it is useful when you must inspect the conjunctiva of the upper lid, as with eye pain or suspicion of a foreign body. Most people are apprehensive of any eye manipulation. Enhance their cooperation by using a calm and gentle, yet deliberate, approach.

1. Ask the person to keep both eyes open and look down. This relaxes the eyelid, whereas closing it would tense the orbicularis muscle.
2. Slide the upper lid up along the bony orbit to lift up the eyelashes.
3. Grasp the lashes between your thumb and forefinger and gently pull down and outward.
4. With your other hand, place the tip of an applicator stick on the upper lid above the level of the internal tarsal plates (Fig. 14-17, *A*).
5. Gently push down with the stick as you lift the lashes up. This uses the edge of the tarsal plate as a fulcrum and flips the lid inside out. Take special care not to push in on the eyeball.
6. Secure the everted position by holding the lashes against the bony orbital rim (Fig. 14-17, *B*).

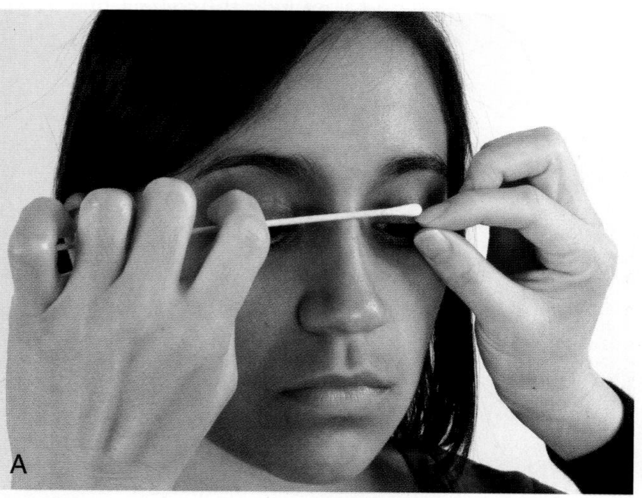

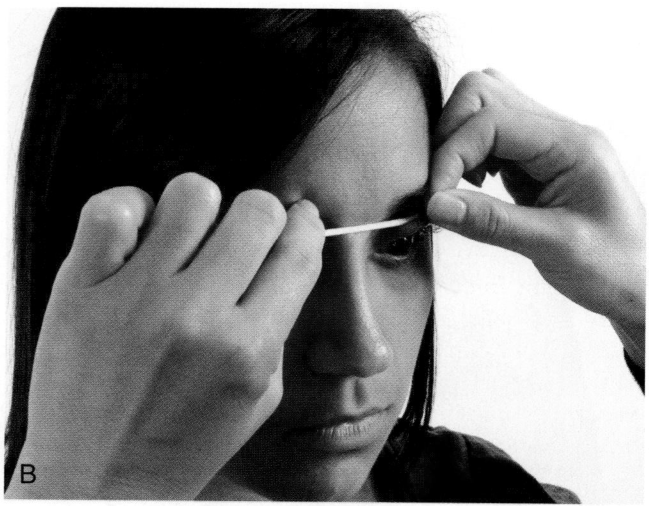

14-17

7. Inspect for any color change, swelling, lesion, or foreign body.
8. To return to normal position, gently pull the lashes outward as the person looks up.

Lacrimal Apparatus

Ask the person to look down. With your thumbs, slide the outer part of the upper lid up along the bony orbit to expose under the lid. Inspect for any redness or swelling.

Swelling of the lacrimal gland may show as a visible bulge in the outer part of the upper lid.

Normally the puncta drain the tears into the lacrimal sac. Presence of excessive tearing may indicate blockage of the nasolacrimal duct. Check this by pressing the index finger against the sac, just inside the lower orbital rim, not against the side of the nose (Fig. 14-18). Pressure will slightly evert the lower lid, but there should be no other response to pressure.

Puncta red, swollen, tender to pressure.

Watch for any regurgitation of fluid out of the puncta, which confirms duct blockage.

Normal Range of Findings	Abnormal Findings

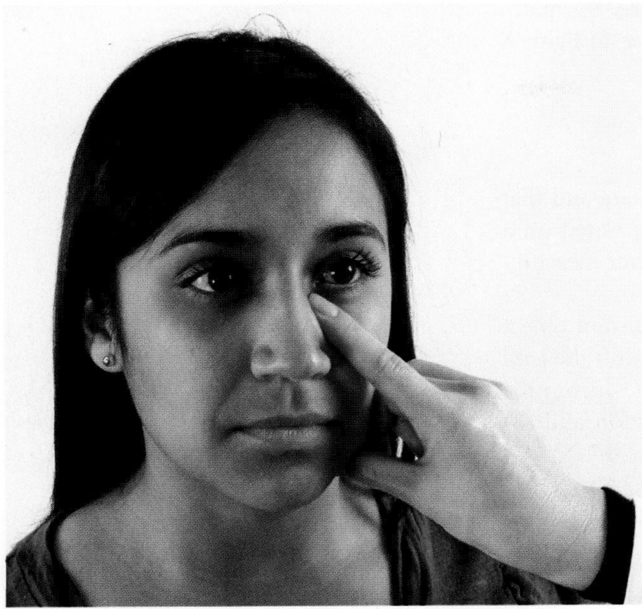

14-18

INSPECT ANTERIOR EYEBALL STRUCTURES

Cornea and Lens

Shine a light from the side across the cornea, and check for smoothness and clarity. This oblique view highlights any abnormal irregularities in the corneal surface. There should be no opacities (cloudiness) in the cornea, the anterior chamber, or the lens behind the pupil. Do not confuse an **arcus senilis** with an opacity. The arcus senilis is a normal finding in aging persons and is illustrated on p. 307.

A corneal abrasion causes irregular ridges in reflected light, producing a shattered look to light rays (see Table 14-7, Abnormalities on the Cornea and Iris).

Iris and Pupil

The iris normally appears flat, with a round regular shape and even coloration. Note the size, shape, and equality of the pupils. Normally the pupils appear round, regular, and of equal size in both eyes. In the adult, resting size is from 3 to 5 mm. A small number of people (5%) normally have pupils of two different sizes, which is termed **anisocoria.**

Irregular shape.

Although they may be normal, all unequal-size pupils call for a consideration of central nervous system injury.

To test the **pupillary light reflex,** darken the room and ask the person to gaze into the distance. (This dilates the pupils.) Advance a light in from the side* and note the response. Normally you will see (1) constriction of the same-sided pupil (a *direct light reflex*) and (2) simultaneous constriction of the other pupil (a *consensual light reflex*).

Dilated pupils.

Dilated and fixed pupils.

Constricted pupils.

Unequal or no response to light (see Table 14-4, Abnormalities in the Pupil).

In the acute care setting, gauge the pupil size in millimeters, both before and after the light reflex. Recording the pupil size in millimeters is more accurate when many nurses and physicians care for the same person or when small

*Always advance the light in from the *side* to test the light reflex. If you advance from the front, the pupils will constrict to accommodate for near vision. Thus you do not know what the pure response to the light would have been.

Normal Range of Findings	Abnormal Findings
changes may be significant signs of increasing intracranial pressure. Normally, the resting size is 3, 4, or 5 mm and decreases equally in response to light. A normal response is recorded as: $$R\frac{3}{1} = \frac{3}{1}L$$ This indicates that both pupils measure 3 mm in the resting state and that both constrict to 1 mm in response to light. A graduated scale printed on a handheld vision screener or taped onto a tongue blade facilitates your measurement (see Fig. 23-58 in Chapter 23). Test for **accommodation** by asking the person to focus on a distant object (Fig. 14-19). This process dilates the pupils. Then have the person shift the gaze to a near object, such as your finger held about 7 to 8 cm (3 inches) from the person's nose. A normal response includes (1) pupillary constriction and (2) convergence of the axes of the eyes.	Absence of constriction or convergence. Asymmetric response.

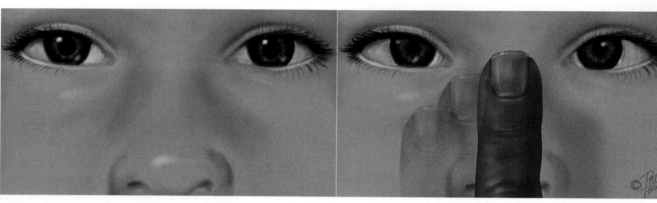

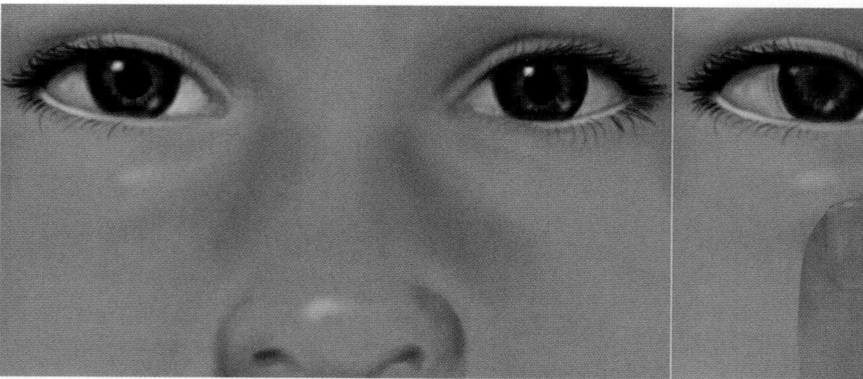
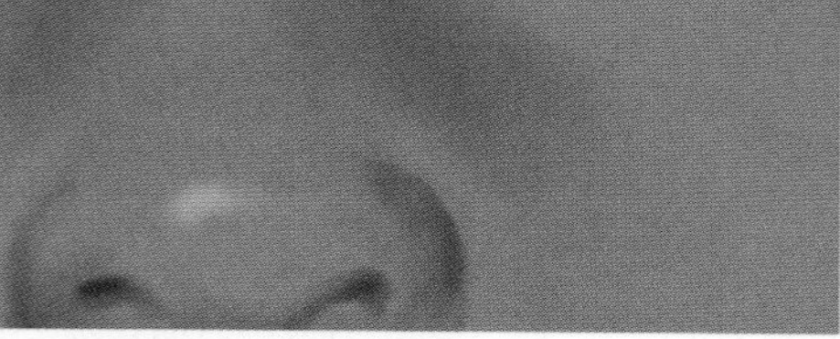

Far vision - pupils dilate

Near vision - pupils constrict

14-19

Record the normal response to all these maneuvers as PERRLA, or **P**upils **E**qual, **R**ound, **R**eact to **L**ight, and **A**ccommodation.

INSPECT THE OCULAR FUNDUS

The ophthalmoscope enlarges your view of the eye so that you can inspect the **media** (anterior chamber, lens, vitreous) and the **ocular fundus** (the internal surface of the retina). It accomplishes this by directing a beam of light through the pupil to illuminate the inner structures. Thus using the ophthalmoscope is like peering through a keyhole (the pupil) into an interesting room beyond.

The ophthalmoscope should function as an appendage of your own eye. This takes some practice. Practice holding the instrument and focusing at objects around the room before you approach a "real" person. Hold the ophthalmoscope right up to your eye, braced firmly against the cheek and brow. Extend your index finger onto the lens selector dial so that you can refocus as needed during the procedure without taking your head away from the ophthalmoscope to look. Now look about the room, moving your head and the instrument together as one unit. Keep both your eyes open; just view the field through the ophthalmoscope.

Normal Range of Findings

Abnormal Findings

Recall that the ophthalmoscope contains a set of lenses that control the focus (Fig. 14-20). The unit of strength of each lens is the *diopter.* The black numbers indicate a positive diopter; they focus on objects nearer in space to the ophthalmoscope. The red numbers show a negative diopter and are for focusing on objects farther away.

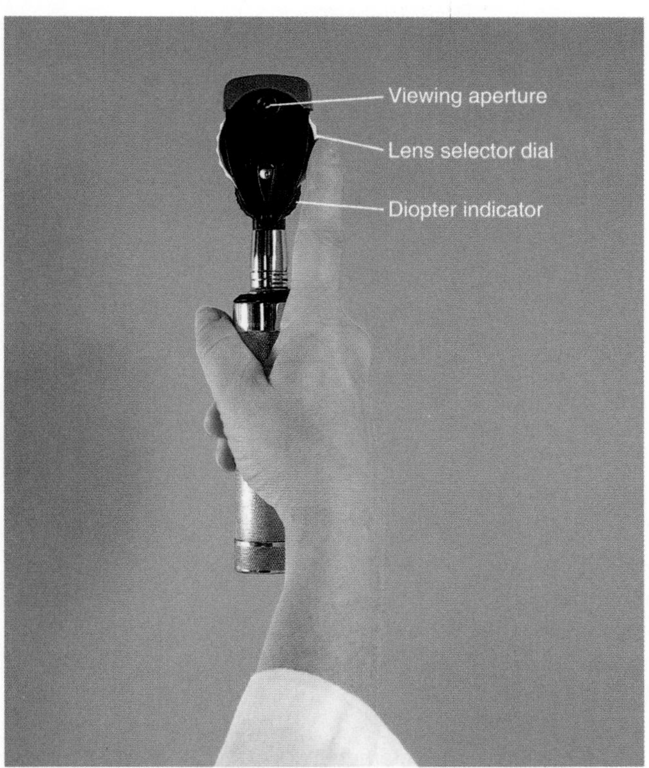

14-20

To examine a person, darken the room to help dilate the pupils. (Dilating eyedrops are not needed during a screening examination. When indicated, they dilate the pupils for a wider look at the fundus background and macular area. Eyedrops are used only when glaucoma can be completely ruled out, because dilating the pupils in the presence of glaucoma can precipitate an acute episode.)

Remove your eyeglasses and those of the other person; they obstruct close movement and you can compensate for their correction by using the diopter setting. Contact lenses may be left in; they pose no problem as long as they are clean.

Select the large round aperture with the white light for the routine examination. If the pupils are small, use the smaller white light. (Although the instrument has other shape and colored apertures, these are rarely used in a screening examination.) The light must have maximum brightness; replace old or dim batteries.

Tell the person, "Please keep looking at that light switch (or mark) on the wall across the room, even though my head will get in the way." Staring at a distant fixed object helps to dilate the pupils and to hold the retinal structures still.

Normal Range of Findings

Match sides with the person. That is, hold the ophthalmoscope in your *right* hand up to your *right* eye to view the person's *right* eye. You must do this to avoid bumping noses during the procedure. Place your free hand on the person's shoulder or forehead (Fig. 14-21, *A*). This helps orient you in space, because once you have the ophthalmoscope in position, you only have a very narrow range of vision. Also, your thumb can anchor the upper lid and help prevent blinking.

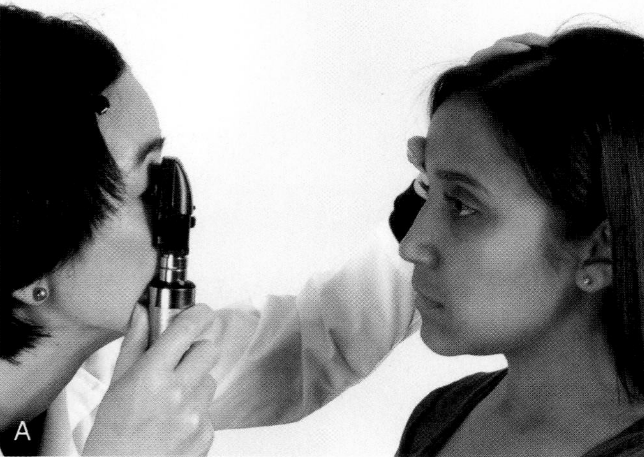

14-21, A

Begin about 25 cm (10 inches) away from the person at an angle about 15 degrees lateral to the person's line of vision. Note the red glow filling the person's pupil. This is the **red reflex,** caused by the reflection of your ophthalmoscope light off the inner retina. Keep sight of the red reflex, and steadily move closer to the eye. If you lose the red reflex, the light has wandered off the pupil and onto the iris or sclera. Adjust your angle to find it again.

As you advance, adjust the lens to +6 and note any opacities in the media. These appear as dark shadows or black dots interrupting the red reflex. Normally, none are present. Progress toward the person until your foreheads almost touch (Fig. 14-21, *B*).

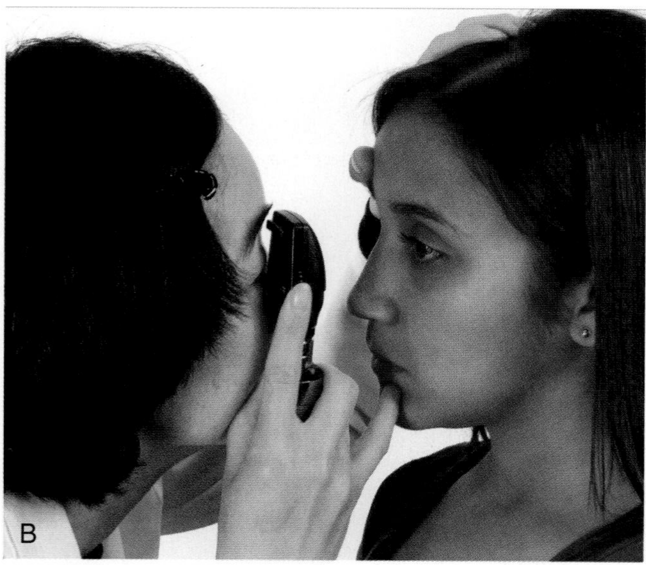

14-21, B

Abnormal Findings

Cataracts appear as opaque black areas against the red reflex (see Table 14-8, Opacities in the Lens).

Normal Range of Findings

Adjust the diopter setting to bring the ocular fundus into sharp focus. If you and the person have normal vision, this should be at 0. Moving the diopters compensates for nearsightedness or farsightedness. Use the red lenses for nearsighted eyes and the black for farsighted eyes (Fig. 14-22).

Abnormal Findings

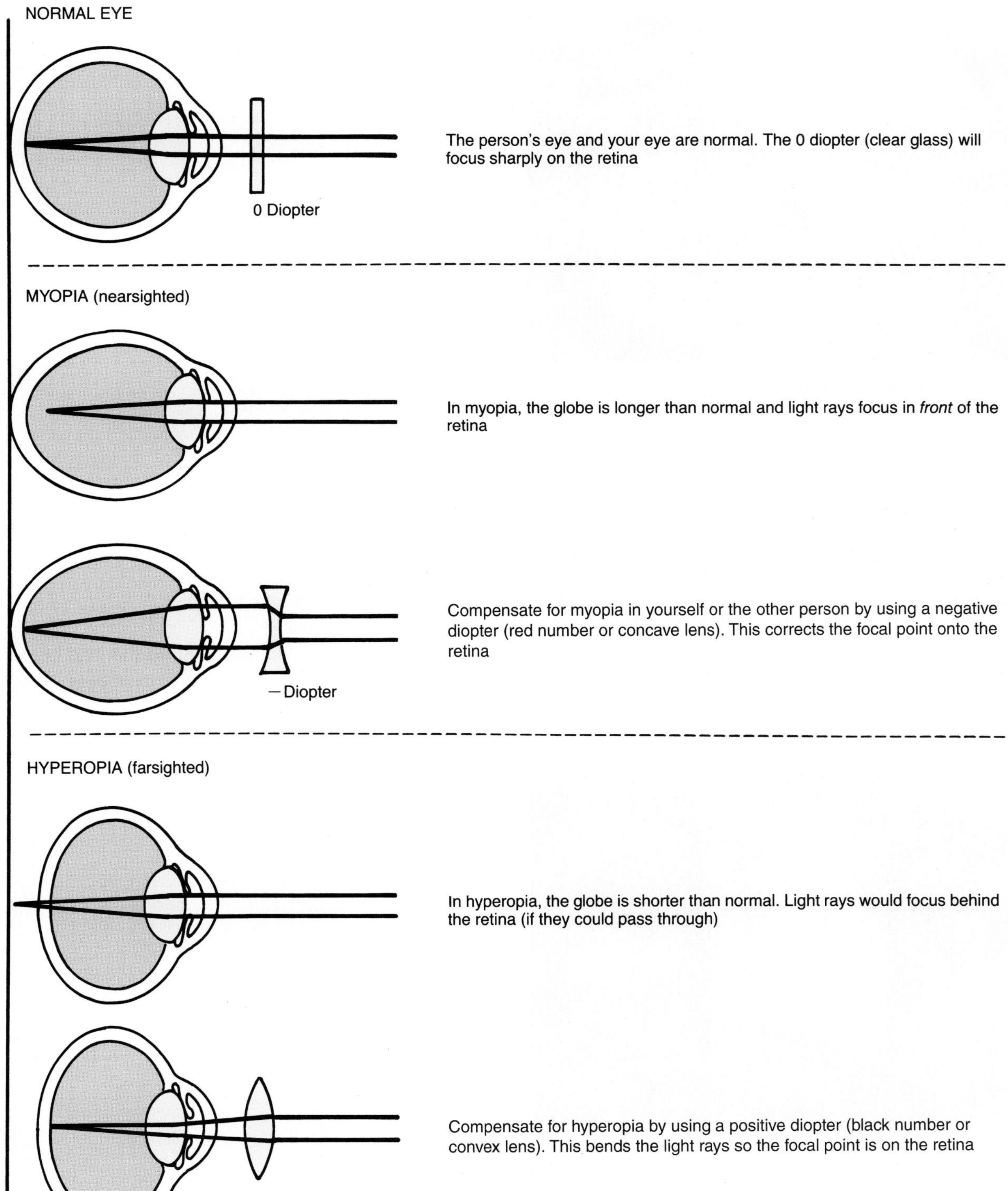

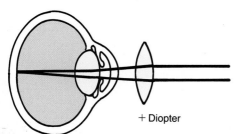

NORMAL EYE
0 Diopter
The person's eye and your eye are normal. The 0 diopter (clear glass) will focus sharply on the retina
MYOPIA (nearsighted)
In myopia, the globe is longer than normal and light rays focus in *front* of the retina

Compensate for myopia in yourself or the other person by using a negative diopter (red number or concave lens). This corrects the focal point onto the retina
HYPEROPIA (farsighted)
In hyperopia, the globe is shorter than normal. Light rays would focus behind the retina (if they could pass through)

Compensate for hyperopia by using a positive diopter (black number or convex lens). This bends the light rays so the focal point is on the retina

14-22

Objective Data

Normal Range of Findings	Abnormal Findings

Moving in on the 15-degree lateral line should bring your view just to the optic disc. If the disc is not in sight, track a blood vessel as it grows larger and it will lead you to the disc. Systematically inspect the structures in the ocular fundus: (1) optic disc, (2) retinal vessels, (3) general background, and (4) macula (Fig. 14-23). (Note the illustration here shows a large area of the fundus. Your actual view through the ophthalmoscope is much smaller—slightly larger than 1 disc diameter.)

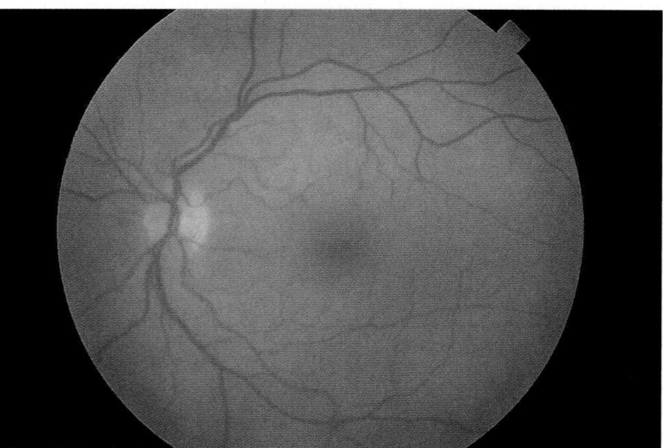

14-23 Normal ocular fundus.

Optic Disc

The most prominent landmark is the optic disc, located on the nasal side of the retina. Explore these characteristics:

Characteristic	Normal Range of Findings	Abnormal Findings
1. **Color**	Creamy yellow-orange to pink.	Pallor. Hyperemia.
2. **Shape**	Round or oval.	Irregular shape.
3. **Margins**	Distinct and sharply demarcated, although the nasal edge may be slightly fuzzy.	Blurred margins.
4. **Cup-disc ratio**	Distinctness varies. When visible, physiologic cup is a brighter yellow-white than rest of the disc. Its width is not more than one-half the disc diameter (Fig. 14-24).	Cup extending to the disc border (see Table 14-9, Abnormalities in the Optic Disc).

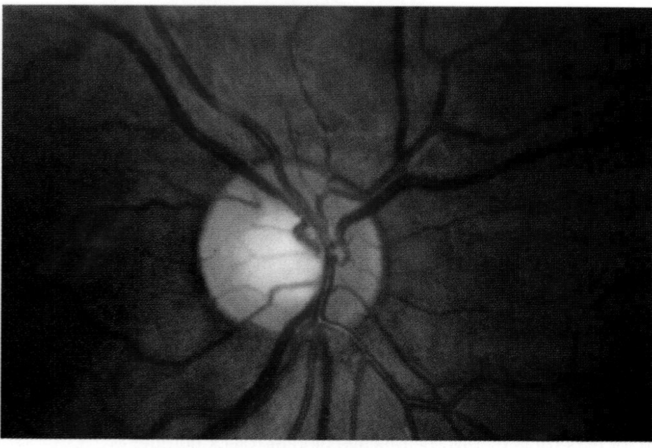

14-24 Normal optic disc.

Two normal variations may ring around the disc margins. A **scleral crescent** is a gray-white, new-moon shape. It occurs when pigment is absent in the choroid layer and you are looking directly at the sclera. A **pigment crescent** is black; it is due to accumulation of pigment in the choroid.

Normal Range of Findings

Abnormal Findings

The diameter of the disc, or DD, is a standard of measure for other fundus structures (see Fig. 14-25). To describe a finding, note its clock-face position as well as its relationship to the disc in size and distance (e.g., "… macula at 3:00, 2 DD from the disc").

Retinal Vessels

This is the only place in the body where you can view blood vessels directly. Many systemic diseases that affect the vascular system show signs in the retinal vessels. Follow a paired artery and vein out to the periphery in the four quadrants (see Fig. 14-23), noting these points:

	Normal Range of Findings	Abnormal Findings
1. **Number**	A paired artery and vein pass to each quadrant. Vessels look straighter at the nasal side.	Absence of major vessels.
2. **Color**	Arteries are brighter red than veins. Also, they have the arterial light reflex, with a thin stripe of light down the middle.	
3. **A:V ratio**	The ratio comparing the artery-to-vein width is 2:3 or 4:5.	Arteries too constricted. Veins dilated.
4. **Caliber**	Arteries and veins show a regular decrease in caliber as they extend to the periphery.	Focal constriction. Neovascularization (proliferation of new vessels).
5. **A-V (arteriovenous) crossing**	An artery and vein may cross paths. This is not significant if within 2 DD of disc and if no sign of interruption in blood flow is seen. There should be no indenting or displacing of vessel.	Crossings more than 2 DD away from disc. Nicking or pinching of underlying vessel. Vessel engorged peripheral to crossing (see Table 14-10).
6. **Tortuosity**	Mild vessel twisting when present in both eyes is usually congenital and not significant.	Extreme tortuosity or marked asymmetry in two eyes.
7. **Pulsations**	Present in veins near disc as their drainage meets the intermittent pressure of arterial systole. (Often hard to see.)	Absent pulsations.

General Background of the Fundus

The color normally varies from light red to dark brown-red, generally corresponding with the person's skin color. Your view of the fundus should be clear; no lesions should obstruct the retinal structures.

Abnormal lesions: hemorrhages, exudates, microaneurysms.

Macula

The macula is 1 DD in size and located 2 DD temporal to the disc (Fig. 14-25). Inspect this area last in the funduscopic examination. A bright light on this area of central vision causes some watering and discomfort and pupillary constriction. Note that the normal color of the area is somewhat darker than the rest of the fundus but is even and homogeneous. Clumped pigment may occur with aging.

Clumped pigment occurs with trauma or retinal detachment.

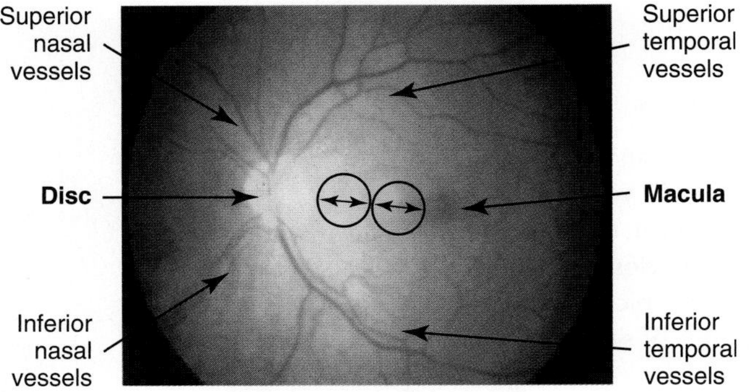

14-25

Normal Range of Findings	Abnormal Findings
Within the macula, you may note the foveal light reflex. This is a tiny white glistening dot reflecting your ophthalmoscope light.	Hemorrhage or exudate in the macula occurs with senile macular degeneration.

DEVELOPMENTAL COMPETENCE

Infants and Children

The eye examination is often deferred at birth because of transient edema of the lids from birth trauma or from the instillation of silver nitrate at birth. The eyes should be examined within a few days and at every well-child visit thereafter.

Visual Acuity. The child's age determines the screening measures used. With a newborn, test visual reflexes and attending behaviors. Test **light perception** using the blink reflex; the neonate blinks in response to bright light (Fig. 14-26). Also, the pupillary light reflex shows that the pupils constrict in response to light. These reflexes indicate that the lower portion of the visual apparatus is intact. But you cannot infer that the infant can *see;* that requires later observation to show that the brain has received images and can interpret them.

Absent blinking.

Absent pupillary light reflex, especially after 3 weeks, indicates blindness.

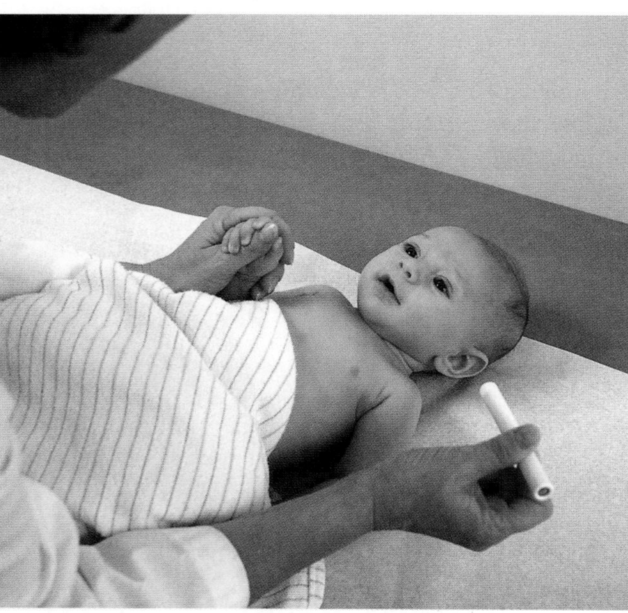

14-26

As you introduce an object to the infant's line of vision, note these attending behaviors:

Birth to 2 weeks—Refusal to reopen eyes after exposure to bright light; increasing alertness to object; infant may fixate on an object.
By 2 to 4 weeks—Infant can fixate on an object.
By 1 month—Infant can fixate and follow a light or bright toy.
By 3 to 4 months—Infant can fixate, follow, and reach for the toy.
By 6 to 10 months—Infant can fixate and follow the toy in all directions.

The Allen test (picture cards) screens children from $2\frac{1}{2}$ years to 2 years and 11 months of age and is even reliable with cooperative toddlers as young as 2 years. The test contains seven cards of familiar objects (birthday cake, teddy bear, tree, house, car, telephone, and horse and rider). First, show the pictures up close to the child to make sure the child can identify them. Then, present each picture at a distance of 15 feet. Results are normal if the child can name three of seven cards within three to five trials.

Normal Range of Findings

Use a picture chart or the Snellen E chart for the preschooler from 3 to 6 years of age. The E chart shows the capital letter E in varying sizes pointing in different directions. The child points his or her fingers in the direction the "table legs" are pointing. By 7 to 8 years of age, when the child is familiar with reading letters, begin to use the standard Snellen alphabet chart. Normally a child achieves 20/20 acuity by 6 to 7 years of age (Fig. 14-27).

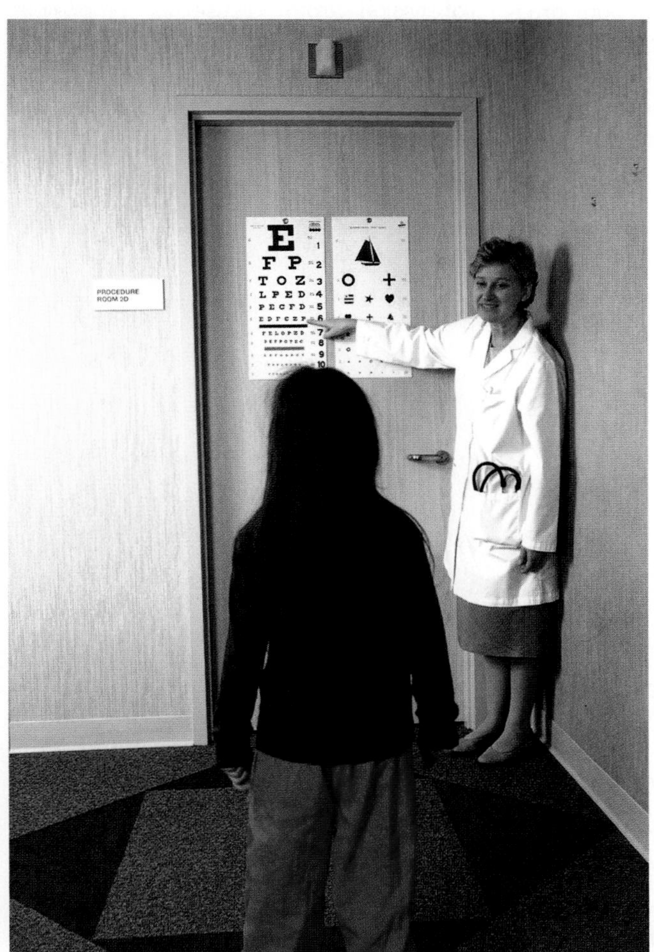

14-27

Visual Fields. Assess peripheral vision with the confrontation test in children older than 3 years when the preschooler is able to stay in position. As with the adult, the child should see the moving target at the same time your normal eyes do. Often a young child forgets to say "now" or "stop" as the moving object is seen. Rather, note the instant the child's eyes deviate or head shifts position to gaze at the moving object. Match this nearly automatic response with your own sighting.

Color Vision. Color blindness is an inherited recessive X-linked trait affecting about 8% of white males and 4% of Black males. It is rare in females (0.4%). "Color deficient" is a more accurate term, because the condition is relative and not disabling. Often, it is just a social inconvenience, although it may affect the person's ability to discern traffic lights or it may affect school performance in which color is a learning tool.

Test only boys for color vision, once between the ages of 4 and 8 years. Use Ishihara's test, a series of polychromatic cards. Each card has a pattern of dots printed against a background of many colored dots. Ask the child to identify each pattern. A boy with normal color vision can see each pattern. A color-blind person cannot see the letter against the field color.

Abnormal Findings

The National Society for Prevention of Blindness states these criteria for referral:

1. Age 3 years—vision 20/50 or less in either eye.
2. Age 4 years and older—20/40 or less in either eye.
3. Difference between two eyes is one line or more.
4. Child shows other signs of vision impairment, regardless of acuity.

Screen two separate times before referral.

Normal Range of Findings

Extraocular Muscle Function. Testing for **strabismus** (squint, crossed eye) is an important screening measure during early childhood. Strabismus causes disconjugate vision because one eye deviates off the fixation point. To avoid diplopia or unclear images, the brain begins to suppress data from the weak eye (a suppression scotoma). Then visual acuity in this otherwise normal eye begins to deteriorate from disuse. Early recognition and treatment are essential to restore binocular vision. Diagnosis after 6 years of age has a poor prognosis. Test malalignment by the corneal light reflex and the cover test.

Check the **corneal light reflex** by shining a light toward the child's eyes. The light should be reflected at exactly the same spot in the two corneas (Fig. 14-28). Some asymmetry (where one light falls off center) under 6 months of age is normal.

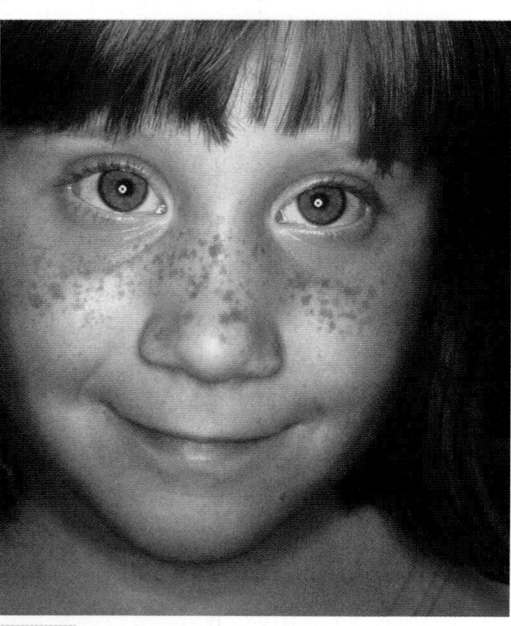

14-28

Perform the **cover test** on all children as described on p. 290. Some examiners omit the opaque card and place a hand on the child's head. The examiner's thumb extends down and blocks vision over the eye without actually touching the eye. One can use a familiar character puppet to attract the child's attention. The normal results are the same as those listed in the adult section.

Function of the extraocular muscles during movement can be assessed during the early weeks by the child's following a brightly colored toy as a target. An older infant can sit on the parent's lap as you move the toy in all directions. After 2 years of age, direct the child's gaze through the six cardinal positions of gaze. You may stabilize the child's chin with your hand to prevent him or her from moving the entire head.

External Eye Structures. Inspect the ocular structures as described in the earlier section. A neonate usually holds the eyes tightly shut. Do not attempt to pry them open; that just increases contraction of the orbicularis oculi muscle. Hold the newborn supine and gently lower the head; the eyes will open. Also, the eyes will open when you hold the infant at arm's length and slowly turn the infant in one direction (Fig. 14-29). In addition to inspecting the ocular structures, this also tests the vestibular function reflex. That is, the baby's eyes will look in the same direction as the body is being turned. When the turning stops, the eyes will shift to the opposite direction after a few quick beats of nystagmus. Also termed "doll's eyes," this reflex disappears by 2 months of age.

Abnormal Findings

Untreated strabismus can lead to permanent visual damage. The resulting loss of vision from disuse is amblyopia exanopsia.

Asymmetry in the corneal light reflex after 6 months is abnormal and must be referred.

Normal Range of Findings	Abnormal Findings

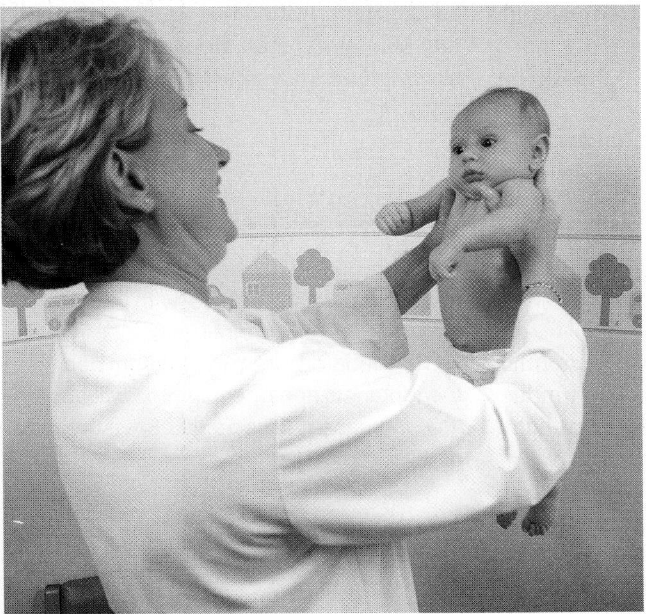

14-29

Eyelids and Lashes. Normally the upper lids overlie the superior part of the iris. In newborns, the *setting-sun sign* is common. The eyes appear to deviate down, and you see a white rim of sclera over the iris. It may show as you rapidly change the neonate from a sitting to a supine position.

The setting-sun sign also occurs with hydrocephalus as the globes protrude.

Blank sunken eyes accompany malnutrition, dehydration, and a severe illness.

Many infants have an *epicanthal fold,* an excess skinfold extending over the inner corner of the eye, partly or totally overlapping the inner canthus. It occurs frequently in Asian children and in 20% of whites. In non-Asians, it disappears as the child grows, usually by 10 years of age. While they are present, epicanthal folds give a false appearance of malalignment, termed **pseudostrabismus** (Fig. 14-30). Yet the corneal light reflex is normal.

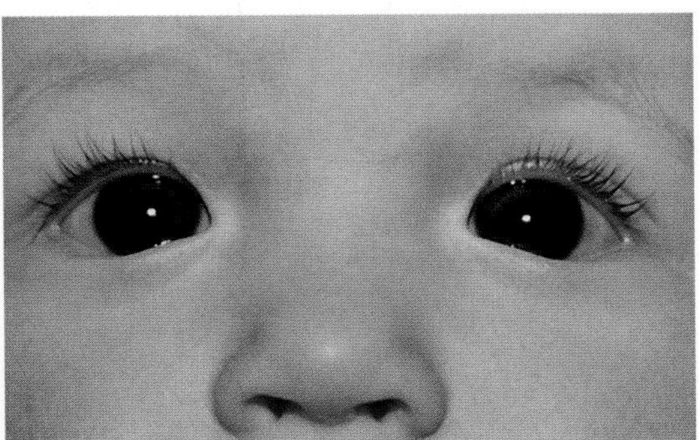

14-30 Pseudostrabismus.

Asian infants normally have an upward slant of the palpebral fissures. Entropion, a turning inward of the eyelid, is found normally in some Asian children. If the lashes do not abrade the corneas, it is not significant.

An upward lateral slope together with epicanthal folds and hypertelorism (large spacing between eyes) occurs with Down syndrome.

Conjunctiva and Sclera. A newborn may have a transient chemical conjunctivitis from the instillation of silver nitrate. This appears within 1 hour and lasts not more than 24 hours after birth. The sclera should be white and clear, although it may have a blue tint as a result of thinness at birth. The lacrimal glands are not functional at birth.

Ophthalmia neonatorum (conjunctivitis of the newborn) is a purulent discharge caused by a chemical irritant or a bacterial or viral agent from the birth canal.

Iris and Pupils. The iris normally is blue or slate gray in light-skinned newborns and brown in dark-skinned infants. By 6 to 9 months, the permanent color is differentiated. Brushfield's spots, or white specks around the edge of the iris, occasionally may be normal.

Absence of iris color occurs with albinism.

Brushfield's spots usually suggest Down syndrome.

Normal Range of Findings

A searching nystagmus is common just after birth. The pupils are small but constrict to light.

Abnormal Findings

Constant nystagmus, prolonged setting-sun sign, marked strabismus, and slow lateral movements suggest vision loss.

The Ocular Fundus. The amount of data gathered during the funduscopic examination depends on the child's ability to hold the eyes still and on your ability to glean as much data as possible in a brief period of time.

A complete funduscopic examination is difficult to perform on an infant, but at least check the red reflex when the infant fixates at the bright light for a few seconds. Note any interruption.

An interruption in the red reflex indicates an opacity in the cornea or lens. An absent red reflex occurs with congenital cataracts or retinal disorders.

Perform a funduscopic examination on an infant between 2 and 6 months of age. Position the infant (up to 18 months) lying on the table. The fundus appears pale, and the vessels are not fully developed. There is no foveal light reflection because the macula area will not be mature until 1 year.

Papilledema is rare in the infant because the fontanels and open sutures will absorb any increased intracranial pressure if it occurs.

Inspect the fundus of the young child and school-age child as described in the preceding section on the adult. Allow the child to handle the equipment. Explain why you are darkening the room and that you will leave a small light on. Assure the child that the procedure will not hurt. Direct the young child to look at an appealing picture, perhaps a toy or an animal, during the examination.

The Aging Adult

Visual Acuity. Perform the same examination as described in the adult section. Central acuity may decrease, particularly after 70 years of age. Peripheral vision may be diminished.

In older adults, an increased risk of falls and fractures occurs with a distance visual acuity of 20/25 or greater.[19]

Ocular Structures. The eyebrows may show a loss of the outer one third to one half of hair because of a decrease in hair follicles. The remaining brow hair is coarse (Fig. 14-31). As a result of atrophy of elastic tissues, the skin around the eyes may show wrinkles or crow's feet. The upper lid may be so elongated as to rest on the lashes, resulting in a pseudoptosis.

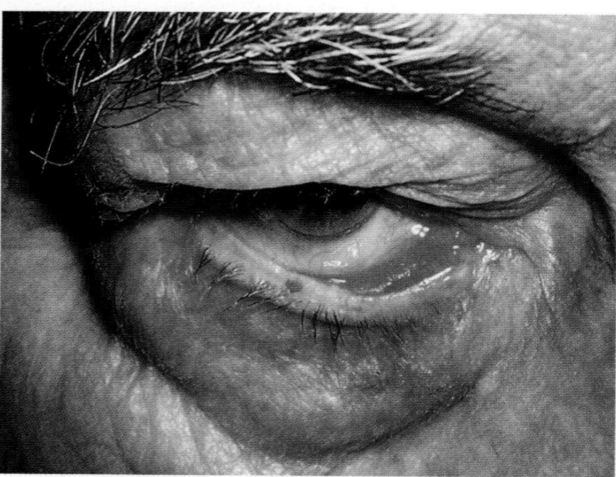

14-31 Pseudoptosis.

The eyes may appear sunken from atrophy of the orbital fat. Also, the orbital fat may herniate, causing bulging at the lower lids and inner third of the upper lids.

Ectropion (lower lid dropping away) and entropion (lower lid turning in) (see Table 14-2).

The lacrimal apparatus may decrease tear production, causing the eyes to look dry and lusterless and the person to report a burning sensation. **Pingueculae** commonly show on the sclera (Fig. 14-32). These yellowish, elevated nodules are due to a thickening of the bulbar conjunctiva from prolonged exposure to sun, wind, and dust. Pingueculae appear at the 3 and 9 o'clock positions—first on the nasal side and then on the temporal side.

Distinguish pinguecula from the abnormal **pterygium,** also an opacity on the bulbar conjunctiva, but one that grows over the cornea (see Table 14-7).

Normal Range of Findings	Abnormal Findings

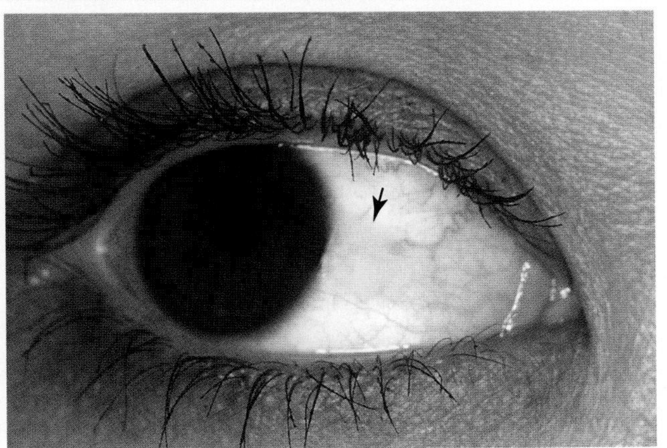

14-32 Pinguecula.

The cornea may look cloudy with age. An **arcus senilis** is commonly seen around the cornea (Fig. 14-33). This is a gray-white arc or circle around the limbus; it is due to deposition of lipid material. As more lipid accumulates, the cornea may look thickened and raised, but the arcus has no effect on vision.

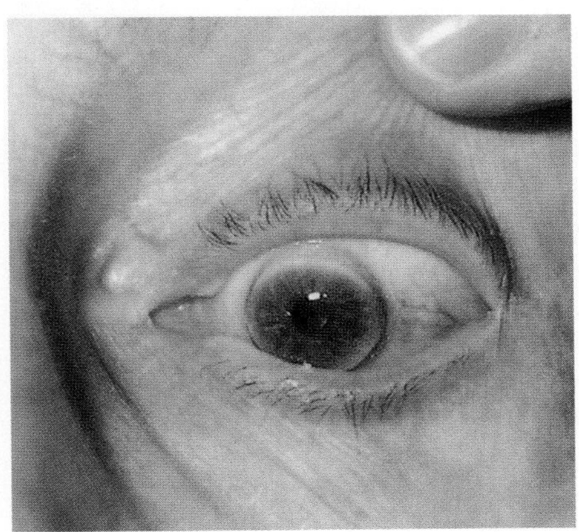

14-33 Arcus senilis.

Xanthelasma are soft, raised yellow plaques occurring on the lids at the inner canthus (Fig. 14-34). They commonly occur around the fifth decade of life and more frequently in women. They occur with both high and normal blood levels of cholesterol and have no pathologic significance.

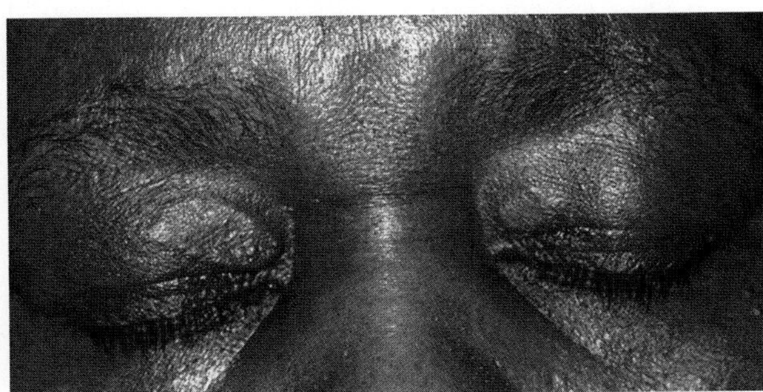

14-34 Xanthelasma.

Pupils are small in old age, and the pupillary light reflex may be slowed. The lens loses transparency and looks opaque.

The Ocular Fundus. Retinal structures generally have less shine. The blood vessels look paler, narrower, and attenuated. Arterioles appear paler and straighter, with a narrower light reflex. More arteriovenous crossing defects occur.

Normal Range of Findings

A normal development on the retinal surface is **drusen,** or benign degenerative hyaline deposits (Fig. 14-35). They are small, round, yellow dots that are scattered haphazardly on the retina. Although they do not occur in a pattern, they are usually symmetrically placed in the two eyes. They have no effect on vision.

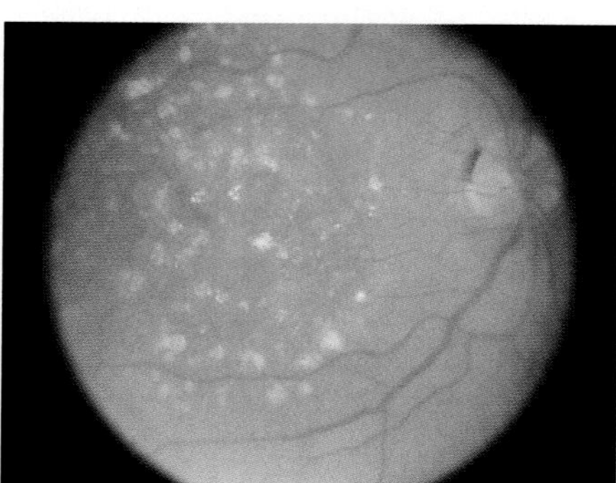

14-35 Drusen.

Abnormal Findings

Drusen are easily confused with the abnormal finding *hard exudates,* which occur with a more circular or linear pattern (see Table 14-10, p. 321). Also, drusen in the macular area occur with macular degeneration.

PROMOTING A HEALTHY LIFESTYLE: SCREENING FOR GLAUCOMA

Preventing Irreversible Blindness

According to the National Eye Institute (NEI), the National Institutes of Health (NIH) lead agency for vision research, glaucoma is a leading cause of blindness in the United States. Glaucoma is a condition that involves optic nerve damage and visual field changes. The risk of glaucoma increases with age but can occur in anyone in any age-group. There is no cure, but medication, laser trabeculoplasty, and/or surgery can slow or prevent further vision loss. Unfortunately, treatments do not improve sight already lost from glaucoma. Therefore early detection is critical to stopping progression of the disease.

There are many forms of glaucoma, but most fall into one of two categories: open-angle (more common) or closed-angle glaucoma. In *open-angle glaucoma,* the drainage canals of the eye gradually become clogged. The entrance to these drainage canals is clear (open) and working correctly, but the clogging occurs further inside the canals. There is a slow buildup of intraocular pressure (IOP) as fluids continue to be produced at normal rates. The process is gradual, painless, and causes no early symptoms. Vision loss begins with the peripheral vision, and this often goes unnoticed because the individual learns to compensate intuitively by turning the head. As the condition progresses, the field of peripheral vision decreases until eventually the individual cannot see anything on either side (tunnel vision).

In *closed-angle glaucoma*, the drainage canals are blocked or covered over by the outer edge of the iris when the pupil enlarges too much or too quickly. This blockage most often occurs suddenly (acute) but can develop slowly (chronic). Acute closed-angle glaucoma involves an abrupt onset of symptoms, including eye pain, headaches, nausea and/or vomiting, blurred or sudden loss of vision, and rainbow-colored halos around lights, especially at night. If left untreated, an individual can lose vision within 2 to 3 hours.

The American Academy of Ophthalmology (AAO) recommends screening for glaucoma as part of a comprehensive eye exam starting at 29 years of age. Subsequent screening schedules depend on individual risk factors, which include:

1. Age over 60 years (over 40 years for African Americans)
2. African American ethnicity or heritage
3. Increased intraocular pressure (IOP)
4. Family history of glaucoma
5. Steroid use
6. History of blunt eye injury (often sports-related)
7. Hypertension
8. Decreased central corneal thickness less than 0.5 mm
9. Severe myopia (nearsightedness)
10. Diabetes

Because glaucoma does not produce symptoms in its early stages, early and ongoing comprehensive eye exams are extremely important and should include the following:

1. Visual acuity test—to assess overall vision
2. Visual field test—to identify decreased peripheral vision
3. Dilated eye examination—to examine the retina and optic nerve
4. Tonometry—to measure the pressure inside the eye
5. Pachymetry— to measure the thickness of the cornea

EyeSmart™—Know your Risk, Save your Sight is a public awareness campaign sponsored by the American Academy of Ophthalmology (AAO) to empower individuals to take charge of their eye health. The aim of the campaign is to address and correct information gaps by educating the public. Health care providers can access patient-friendly information sheets on various eye diseases or refer the public to their website and resources.

Resources

Glaucoma Research Foundation: http://www.glaucoma.org/

American Academy of Ophthalmology (AAO): http://www.aao.org/aao/

Eye Smart™ Information Sheet on Glaucoma: http://www.geteyesmart.org/eyesmart/diseases/glaucoma.cfm

National Eye Institute (NEI Health Information) Facts about Glaucoma: http://www.nei.nih.gov/health/glaucoma/glaucoma_facts.asp

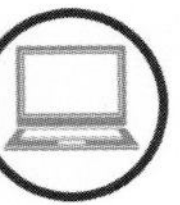

DOCUMENTATION AND CRITICAL THINKING

Sample Charting

SUBJECTIVE

Vision reported "good" with no recent change. No eye pain, no inflammation, no discharge, no lesions. Wears no corrective lenses, vision last tested 1 year PTA, test for glaucoma at that time was normal.

OBJECTIVE

Snellen chart—Right 20/20, Left 20/20 −1. Fields normal by confrontation. Corneal light reflex symmetric bilaterally. Diagnostic positions test shows EOMs intact. Brows and lashes present. No ptosis. Conjunctiva clear. Sclera white. No lesions. PERRLA.

Fundi—Red reflex present bilaterally. Discs flat with sharp margins. Vessels present in all quadrants without crossing defects. Retinal background has even color with no hemorrhages or exudates. Macula has even color.

ASSESSMENT

Healthy vision function
Healthy eye structures

Focused Assessment: Clinical Case Study 1

Emma K. is a 34-year-old married, white female homemaker brought to the emergency department by police after a reported domestic quarrel.

SUBJECTIVE

States husband struck her about the face and eyes with his fists about 1 hour PTA. "I ruined the dinner again. I can't do anything right." Pain in left cheek and both eyes felt immediately and continues. Alarmed at "bright red blood on eyeball." No bleeding from eye area or cheek. Vision intact just after trauma. Now reports difficulty opening lids.

OBJECTIVE

Sitting quietly and hunched over, hands over eyes. Voice tired and flat. L cheek swollen and discolored, no laceration. Lids edematous and discolored both eyes. No skin laceration. L lid swollen almost shut. L eye—round 1-mm bright red patch over lateral aspect of globe. No active bleeding out of eye, iris intact, anterior chamber clear. R eye—conjunctiva clear, sclera white, cornea and iris intact, anterior chamber clear. PERRLA. Pupils R 4/1 = 4/1 L. Vision 14/14 both eyes by Jaeger card.

ASSESSMENT

Ecchymoses L cheek and both eyes
Subconjunctival hemorrhage L eye
Pain R/T inflammation
Chronic low self-esteem R/T effects of domestic violence

Focused Assessment: Clinical Case Study 2

Sam T. is a 63-year-old married, white male postal carrier admitted to the medical center for surgery for suspected brain tumor. After postanesthesia recovery, Sam T. is admitted to the neurology ICU, awake, lethargic with slowed but correct verbal responses, oriented × 3, moving all four extremities, vital signs stable. Pupils R 4/2 = 4/2 L with sluggish response. Assessments are made q 15 minutes.

SUBJECTIVE

No response now to verbal stimuli.

OBJECTIVE

Semicomatose—no response to verbal stimuli, does withdraw R arm and leg purposefully to painful stimuli. No movement L arm or leg. Pupils R 5/5 ≠ L 4/2. Vitals remain stable as noted on graphic sheet.

ASSESSMENT

Unilateral dilated and fixed R pupil
Clouding of consciousness
Focal motor deficit—no movement L side
Ineffective tissue perfusion R/T interruption of cerebral flow

Focused Assessment: Clinical Case Study 3

Trung Q. is a 4-year-old male born in Southeast Asia who arrived in this country 1 month PTA. Lives with parents, 2 siblings. Speaks only native language; here with uncle, who acts as interpreter.

SUBJECTIVE

Seeks care because RN in church sponsoring family noted "crossed eyes." Uncle states vision seemed normal to parents. Plays with toys and manipulates small objects without difficulty. Identifies objects in picture books; does not read.

OBJECTIVE

With uncle interpreting directions for test to Trung, vision by Snellen E chart—Right 20/30, Left 20/50 −1. Fields seem intact by confrontation—jerks head to gaze at object entering field.

EOMs: Asymmetric corneal light reflex with outward deviation L eye. Cover test—as R eye covered, L eye jerks to fixate, R eye steady when uncovered. As L eye covered, R eye holds steady gaze, L eye jerks to fixate as uncovered. Diagnostic positions—able to gaze in six positions, although L eye obviously malaligned at extreme medial gaze.

Eye structures: Brows and lashes present and normal bilaterally. Upward palpebral slant, epicanthal folds bilaterally—consistent with racial heritage. Conjunctiva clear, sclera white, iris intact, PERRLA.

Fundi: Discs flat with sharp margins. Observed vessels normal. Unable to see in all four quadrants or to see macular area.

ASSESSMENT

L exotropia
Abnormal vision in L eye
Disturbed visual sensory perception R/T effects of neurologic impairment

Focused Assessment: Clinical Case Study 4

Vera K. is an 87-year-old widowed, Black female homemaker living independently who is admitted to hospital for observation and adjustment of digitalis medication. Cardiac status has been stable during hospital stay.

SUBJECTIVE

Reports desire to monitor own medication at home but fears problems because of blurred vision. First noted distant vision blurred 5 years ago but near vision seemed to improve at that time. "I started to read better without my glasses!" Since then, blurring at distant vision has increased, near vision now blurred also.

Able to navigate home environment without difficulty. Fixes simple meals with cold foods. Receives hot meal from "Meals on Wheels" at lunch. Enjoys TV, though it looks somewhat blurred. Unable to write letters, sew, or read paper, which she regrets.

OBJECTIVE

Vision by Jaeger card Right 20/200, Left 20/400 −1, with glasses on. Fields intact by confrontation. EOMs intact. Brow hair absent lateral third. Upper lids have folds of redundant skin, but lids do not droop. Lower lids and lashes intact. Xanthelasma present both inner canthi. Conjunctiva clear, sclera white, iris intact, L pupil looks cloudy, PERRLA, pupils R 3/2 = 3/2 L.

Fundi: Red reflex has central dark spot both eyes. Discs flat, with sharp margins. Observed vessels normal. Unable to see in all four quadrants or macular area because of small pupils.

ASSESSMENT

Central opacity, both eyes
Central visual acuity deficit, both eyes
Deficient diversional activity R/T poor vision

ABNORMAL FINDINGS

TABLE 14-1 Extraocular Muscle Dysfunction

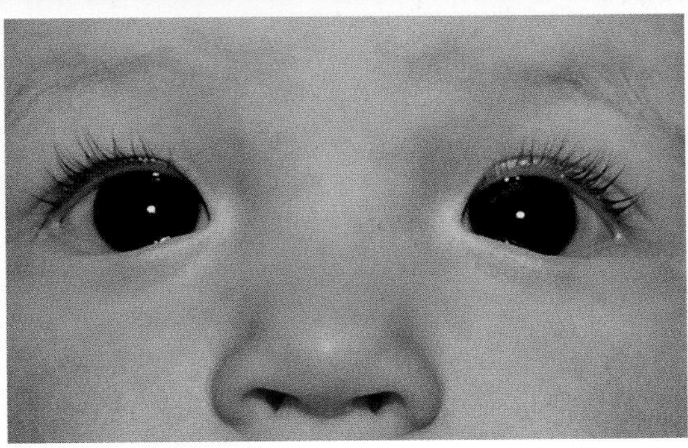

A, Pseudostrabismus.

Symmetric Corneal Light Reflex

A. **Pseudostrabismus** has the appearance of strabismus because of epicanthic fold but is normal for a young child.

Asymmetric Corneal Light Reflex

Strabismus is true disparity of the eye axes. This constant malalignment is also termed *tropia* and is likely to cause amblyopia.

B. Esotropia—inward turning of the eye.
C. Exotropia—outward turning of the eyes.

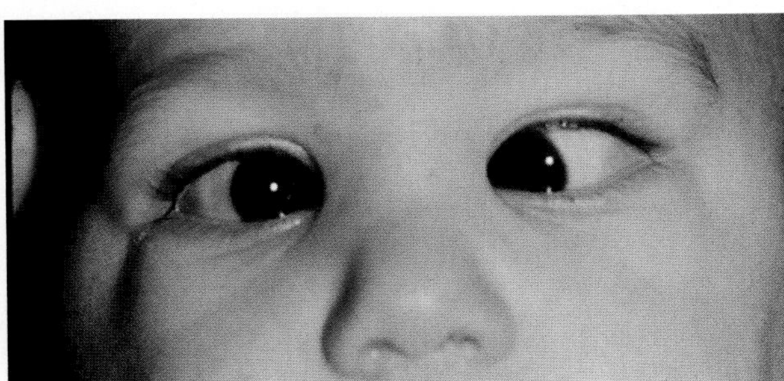

B, Left esotropia.

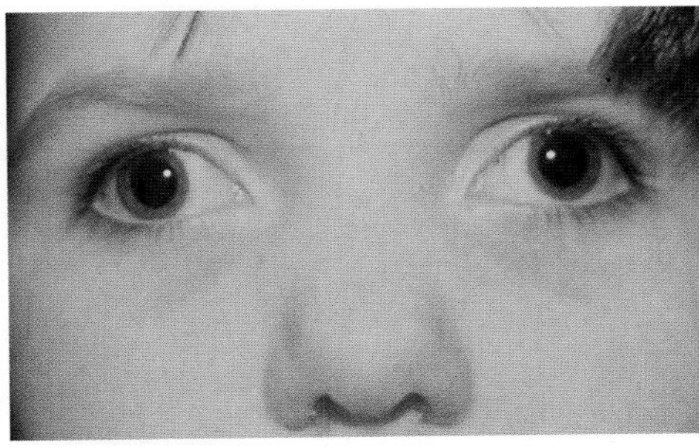

C, Exotropia.

Cover Test

D. Uncovered eye—If it jumps to fixate on designated point, it was out of alignment before (i.e., when you cover the stronger eye [D1], the weaker eye now tries to fixate [D2]).

Phoria—mild weakness, apparent only with the cover test and less likely to cause amblyopia than a tropia but still possible.

E. Covered eye—If this is the weaker eye, once macular image is suppressed, it will drift to relaxed position (E1).

As eye is uncovered—If it jumps to reestablish fixation (E2), weakness exists.

Esophoria—nasal (inward) drift.

Exophoria—temporal (outward) drift.

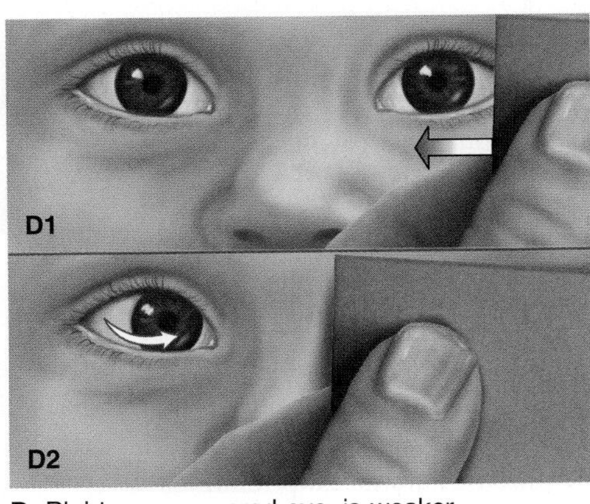

D, Right, or uncovered eye, is weaker.

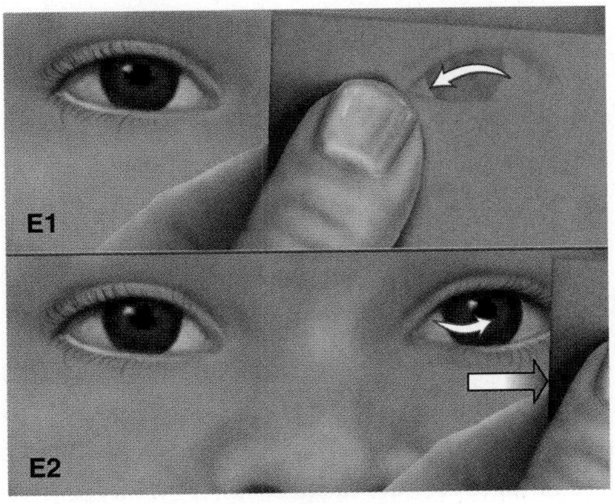

E, Left, or covered eye, is weaker.

Continued

TABLE 14-1 Extraocular Muscle Dysfunction—cont'd

Diagnostic Positions Test

(Paralysis apparent during movement through six cardinal positions of gaze.)

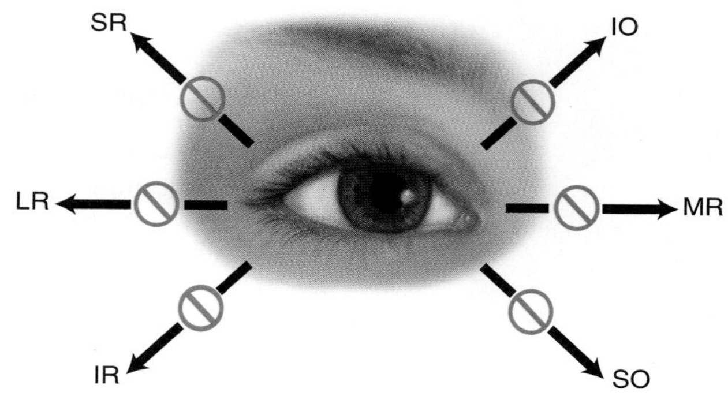

If eye will not turn:	Indicates paralysis in:	or cranial nerve
Straight nasal	Medial rectus	III
Up and nasal	Inferior oblique	III
Up and temporal	Superior rectus	III
Straight temporal	Lateral rectus	VI
Down and temporal	Inferior rectus	III
Down and nasal	Superior oblique	IV

TABLE 14-2 Abnormalities in the Eyelids

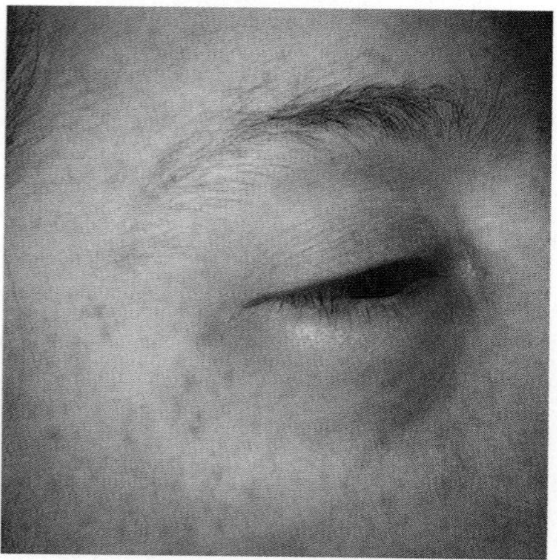

Periorbital Edema

Lids are swollen and puffy. Lid tissues are loosely connected so excess fluid is easily apparent. This occurs with local infections; crying; and systemic conditions such as congestive heart failure, renal failure, allergy, hypothyroidism (myxedema).

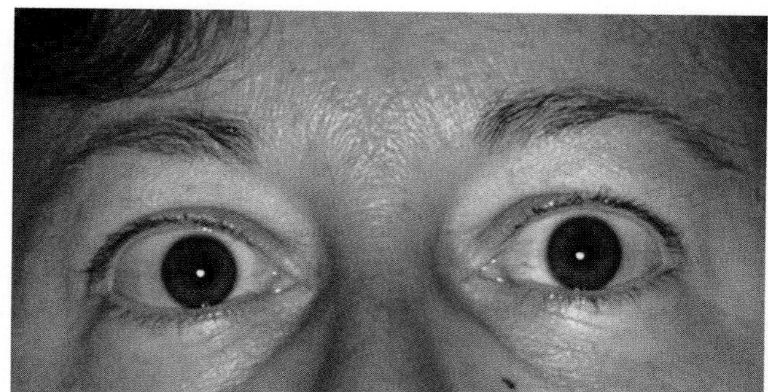

Exophthalmos (Protruding Eyes)

Exophthalmos is a forward displacement of the eyeballs and widened palpebral fissures. Note "lid lag," in which the upper lid rests well above the limbus and white sclera is visible. Acquired bilateral exophthalmos is associated with thyrotoxicosis.

TABLE 14-2 Abnormalities in the Eyelids—cont'd

Enophthalmos (Sunken Eyes) (not illustrated)

A look of narrowed palpebral fissures shows with enophthalmos, in which the eyeballs are recessed. Bilateral enophthalmos is caused by loss of fat in the orbits and occurs with dehydration and chronic wasting illnesses. For illustration, see Cachectic Appearance in Table 13-4, p. 277.

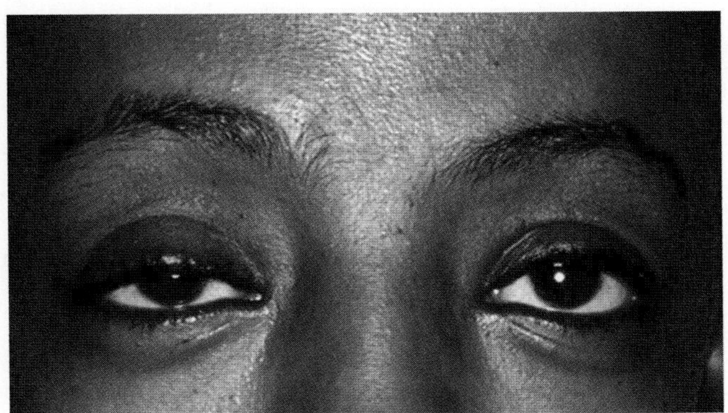

Ptosis (Drooping Upper Lid)

Ptosis occurs from neuromuscular weakness (e.g., myasthenia gravis with bilateral fatigue as the day progresses), oculomotor cranial nerve III damage, or sympathetic nerve damage (e.g., Horner's syndrome) or congenital as in this example. It is a positional defect that gives the person a sleepy appearance and impairs vision.

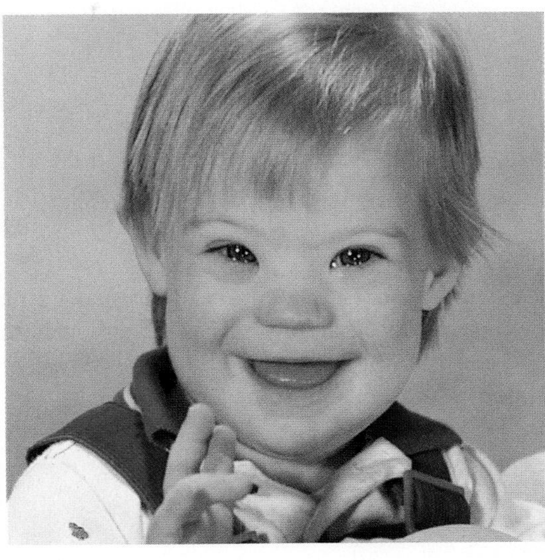

Upward Palpebral Slant

Although normal in many children, when combined with epicanthal folds, hypertelorism (large spacing between the eyes), and Brushfield spots (light-colored areas in outer iris), indicates Down syndrome.

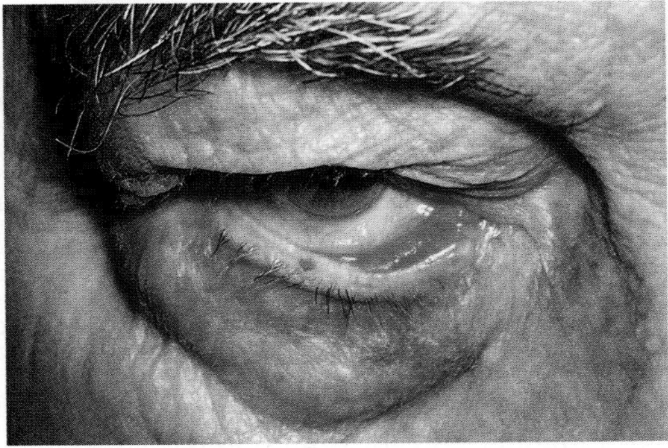

Ectropion

The lower lid is loose and rolling out, does not approximate to eyeball. Puncta cannot siphon tears effectively, so excess tearing results. The eyes feel dry and itchy because the tears do not drain correctly over the corner and toward the medial canthus. Exposed palpebral conjunctiva increases risk for inflammation. Occurs in aging as a result of atrophy of elastic and fibrous tissues but may result from trauma.

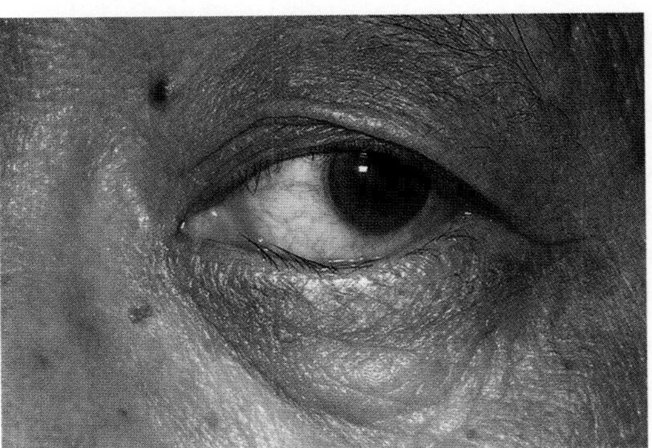

Entropion

The lower lid rolls in because of spasm of lids or scar tissue contracting. Constant rubbing of lashes may irritate cornea. The person feels a "foreign body" sensation.

TABLE 14-3 Lesions on the Eyelids

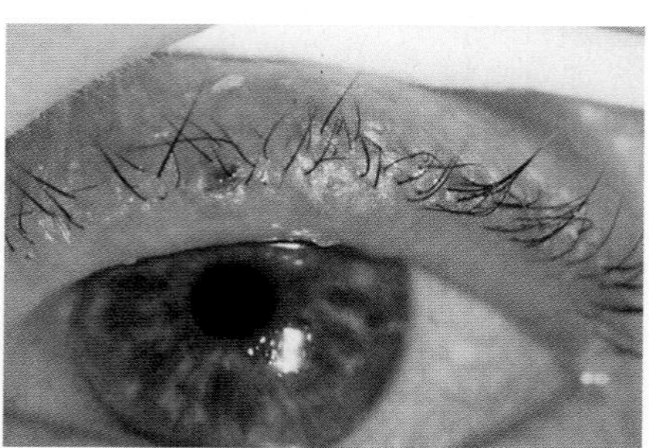

Blepharitis (Inflammation of the Eyelids)

Red, scaly, greasy flakes and thickened, crusted lid margins occur with staphylococcal infection or seborrheic dermatitis of the lid edge. Symptoms include burning, itching, tearing, foreign body sensation, and some pain.

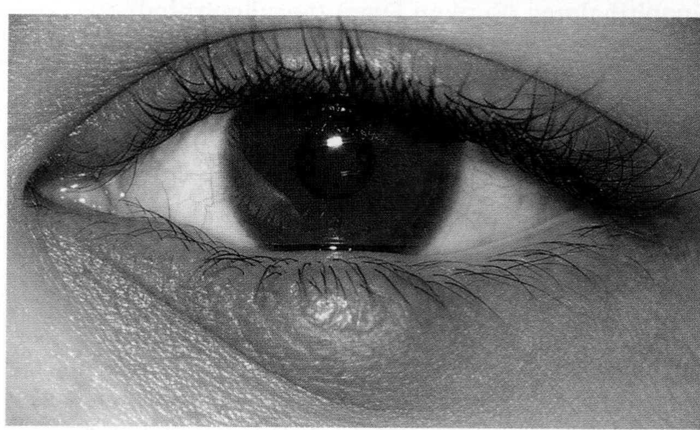

Chalazion

A beady nodule protruding on the lid, chalazion is an infection or retention cyst of a meibomian gland. It is a nontender, firm, discrete swelling with freely movable skin overlying the nodule. If it becomes inflamed, it points inside and not on lid margin (in contrast with stye).

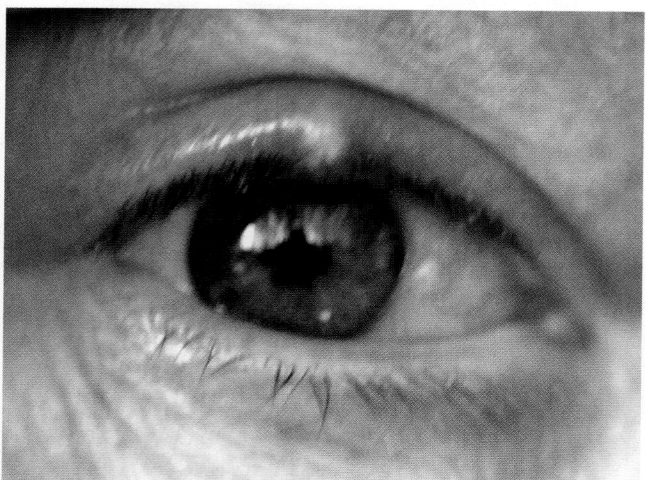

Hordeolum (Stye)

Hordeolum is a localized staphylococcal infection of the hair follicles at the lid margin. It is painful, red, and swollen—a pustule at the lid margin. Rubbing the eyes can cause cross-contamination and development of another stye.

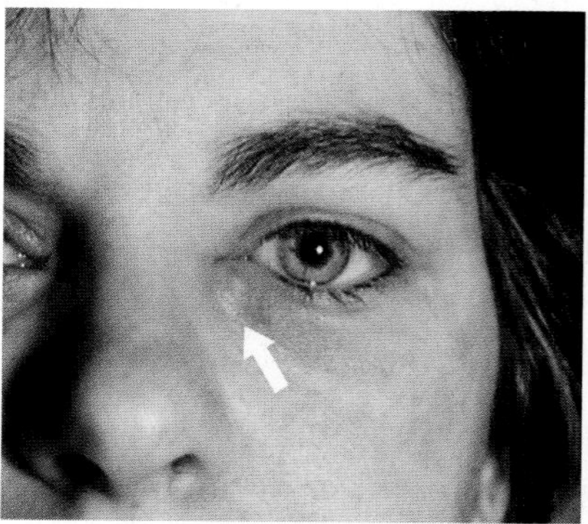

Dacryocystitis (Inflammation of the Lacrimal Sac)

Dacryocystitis is infection and blockage of sac and duct. Pain, warmth, redness, and swelling occur below the inner canthus toward nose. Tearing is present. Pressure on sac yields purulent discharge from puncta.

Dacryoadenitis is an infection of the lacrimal gland (not illustrated). Pain, swelling, and redness occur in the outer third of the upper lid. It occurs with mumps, measles, and infectious mononucleosis or from trauma.

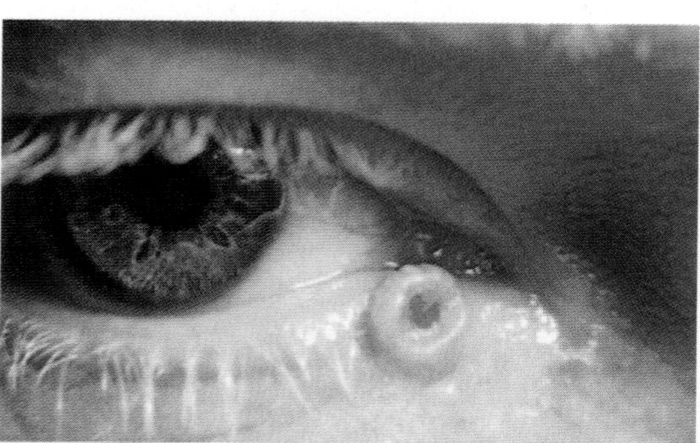

◀ Basal Cell Carcinoma

Carcinoma is rare, but it occurs most often on the lower lid and medial canthus. It looks like a papule with an ulcerated center. Note the rolled-out pearly edges. Metastasis is rare but should be referred for removal.

TABLE 14-4 Abnormalities in the Pupil

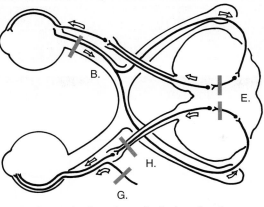

Red lines indicate the location of a lesion that interrupts the transmission of information.

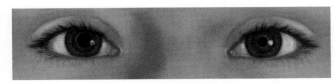

A. Unequal Pupil Size—Anisocoria

Although this exists normally in 5% of the population, consider central nervous system disease.

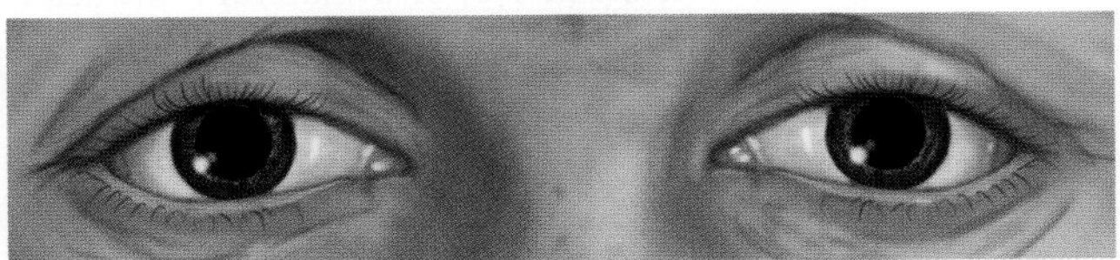

C. Dilated and Fixed Pupils—Mydriasis

Enlarged pupils occur with stimulation of the sympathetic nervous system, reaction to sympathomimetic drugs, use of dilating drops, acute glaucoma, or past or recent trauma. Also, they herald central nervous system injury, circulatory arrest, or deep anesthesia.

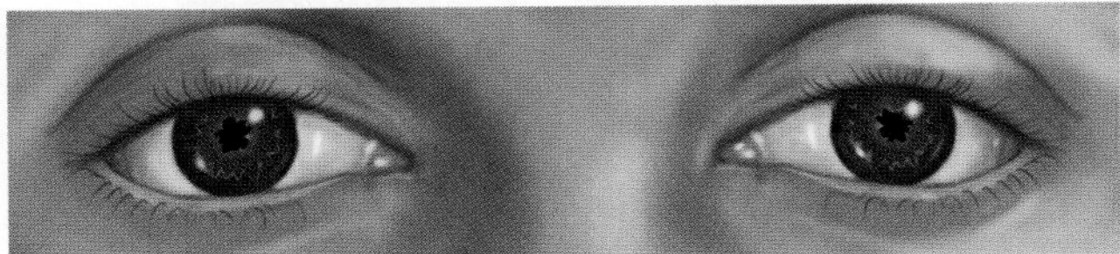

E. Argyll Robertson Pupil

No reaction to light, pupil does constrict with accommodation. Small and irregular bilaterally. Argyll Robertson pupil occurs with central nervous system syphilis, brain tumor, meningitis, and chronic alcoholism.

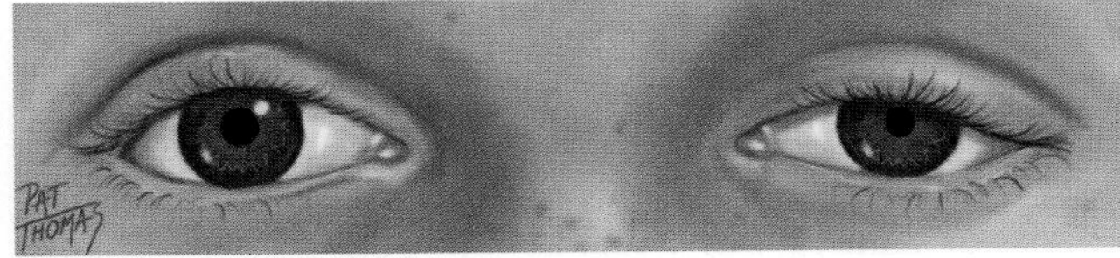

G. Horner's Syndrome

Unilateral, small, regular pupil does react to light and accommodation. Occurs with Horner's syndrome, a lesion of the sympathetic nerve. Also, note ptosis and absence of sweat (anhidrosis) on same side.

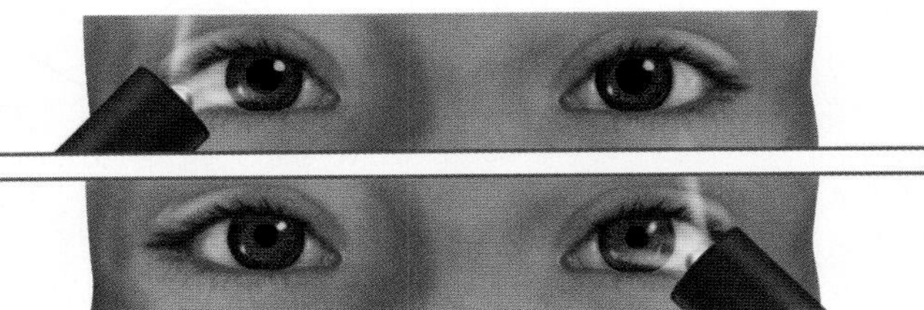

B. Monocular Blindness

When light is directed to the blind eye, no response occurs in either eye. When light is directed to the normal eye, both pupils constrict (direct and consensual response to light) as long as the oculomotor nerve is intact.

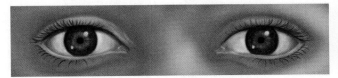

D. Constricted and Fixed Pupils—Miosis

Miosis occurs with the use of pilocarpine drops for glaucoma treatment, the use of narcotics, with iritis, and with brain damage of pons.

F. Tonic Pupil (Adie's Pupil)

Sluggish reaction to light and accommodation. Tonic pupil is usually unilateral, a large regular pupil that does react, but sluggishly after long latent time. No pathologic significance.

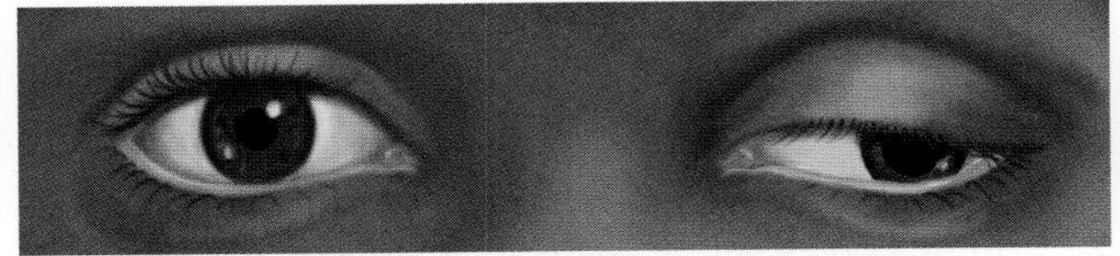

H. Cranial Nerve III Damage

Unilateral dilated pupil with no reaction to light or accommodation, occurs with oculomotor nerve damage. May also have ptosis with eye deviating down and laterally.

ABNORMAL FINDINGS
FOR ADVANCED PRACTICE

TABLE 14-5 Visual Field Loss

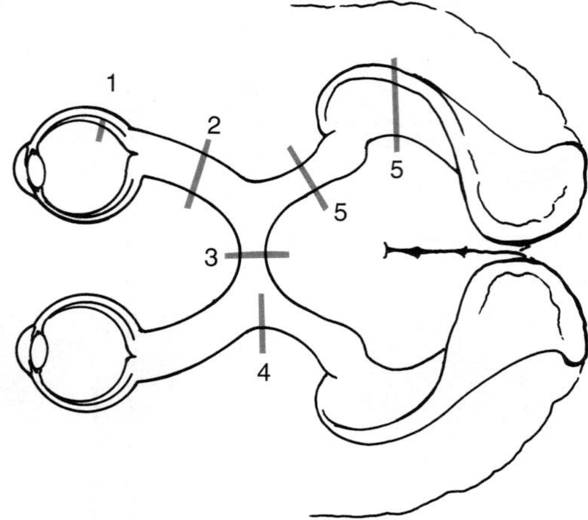

Red lines indicate the location of a lesion that interrupts the transmission of information.

1. Retinal damage
   - Macula—central blind area (e.g., diabetes):

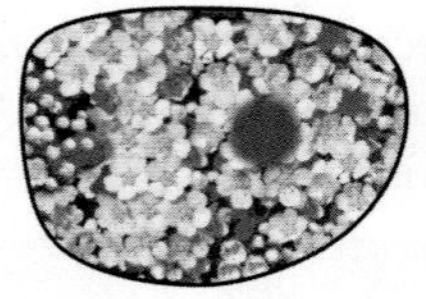
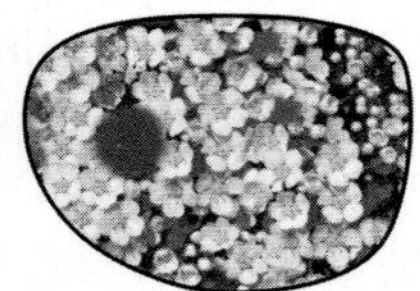

   - Localized damage—blind spot (scotoma) corresponding to particular area:

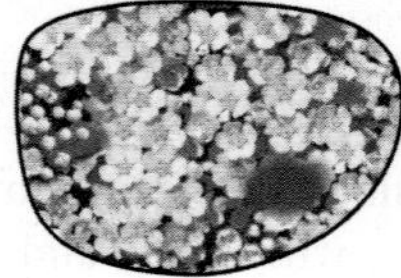
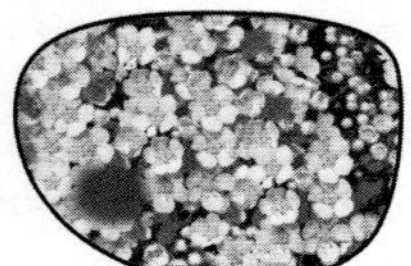

   - Increasing intraocular pressure—decrease in peripheral vision (e.g., glaucoma). Starts with paracentral scotoma in early stage:

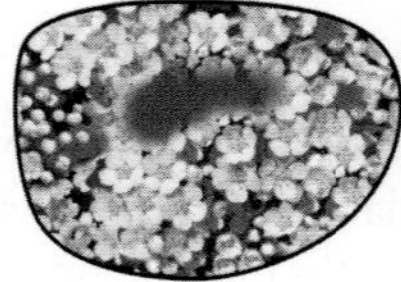
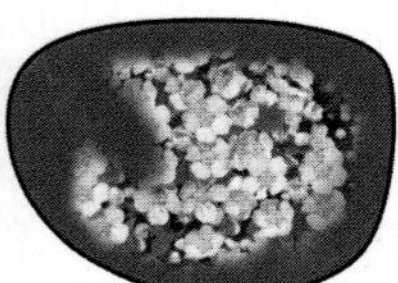

   - Retinal detachment—a shadow or diminished vision in one quadrant or one half of visual field:

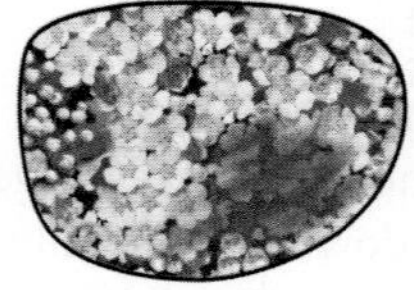
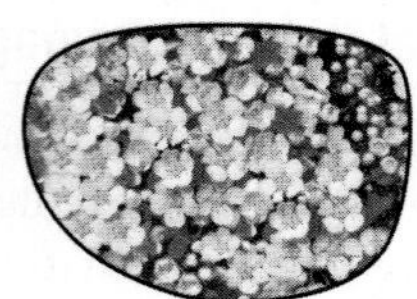

2. Lesion in globe or optic nerve
   Injury here yields one blind eye, or unilateral blindness:

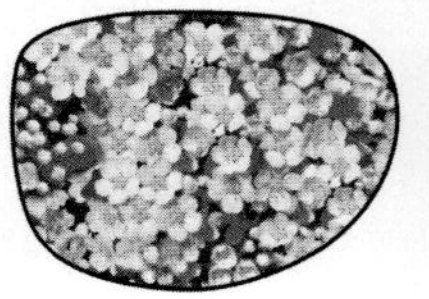

3. Lesion at optic chiasm (e.g., pituitary tumor)—injury to crossing fibers only yields a loss of nasal part of each retina and a loss of both temporal visual fields.
   Bitemporal (heteronymous) hemianopsia:

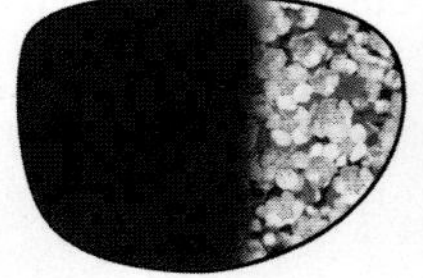
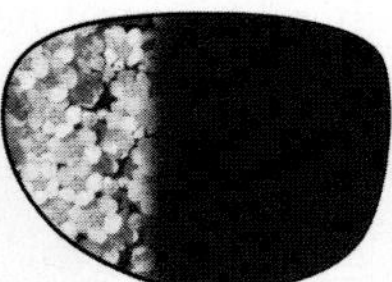

4. Lesion of outer uncrossed fibers at optic chiasm (e.g., aneurysm of left internal carotid artery exerts pressure on uncrossed fibers). Injury yields left nasal hemianopsia:

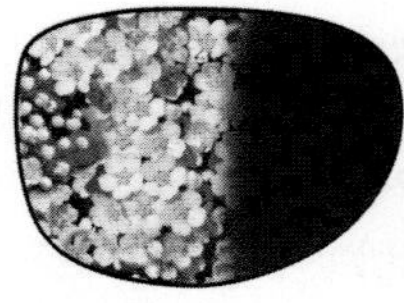
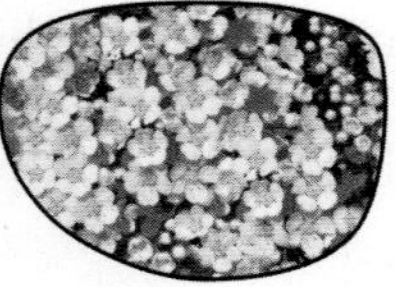

5. Lesion R optic tract or R optic radiation
   Visual field loss in R nasal and L temporal fields
   Loss of same half of visual field in both eyes is homonymous hemianopsia:

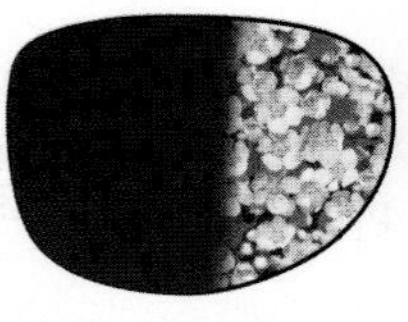
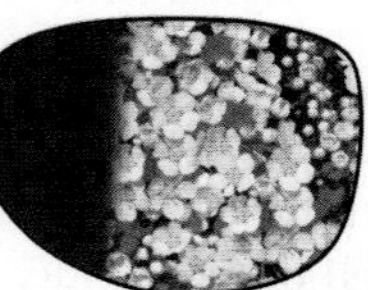

TABLE 14-6 Vascular Disorders of the External Eye

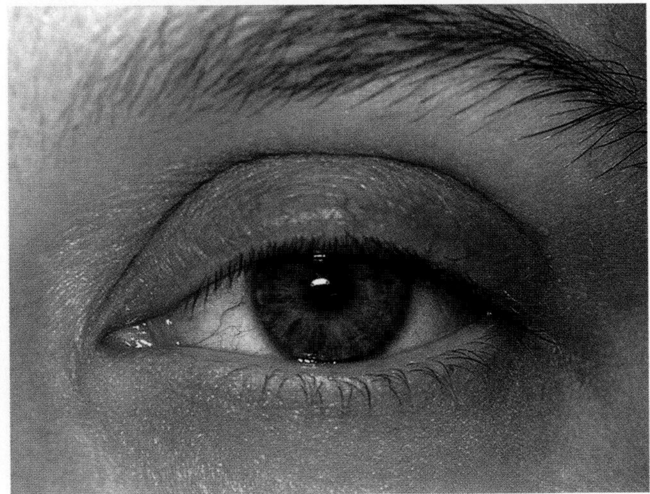

Conjunctivitis

Infection of the conjunctiva, "pink eye," has red, beefy-looking vessels at periphery but usually clearer around iris. This is common from bacterial or viral infection, allergy, or chemical irritation. Purulent discharge accompanies bacterial infection. Preauricular lymph node is often swollen and painful, with a history of upper respiratory infection. Symptoms include itching, burning, foreign body sensation, and eyelids stuck together on awakening.

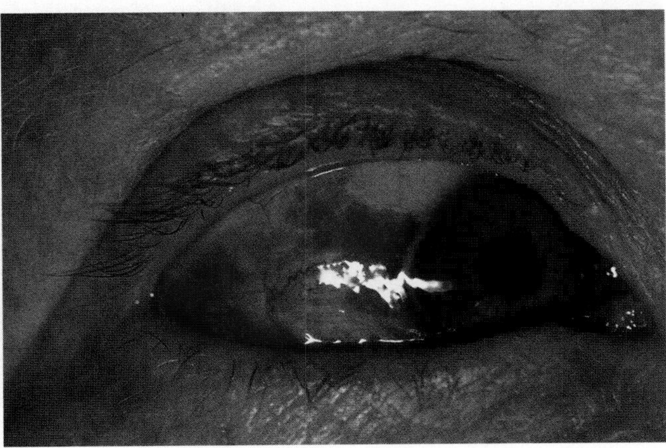

Subconjunctival Hemorrhage

A red patch on the sclera, subconjunctival hemorrhage looks alarming but is usually not serious. The red patch has sharp edges like a spot of paint, although here it is extensive. It occurs from increased intraocular pressure from coughing, vomiting, weight lifting, labor during childbirth, straining at stool, or trauma.

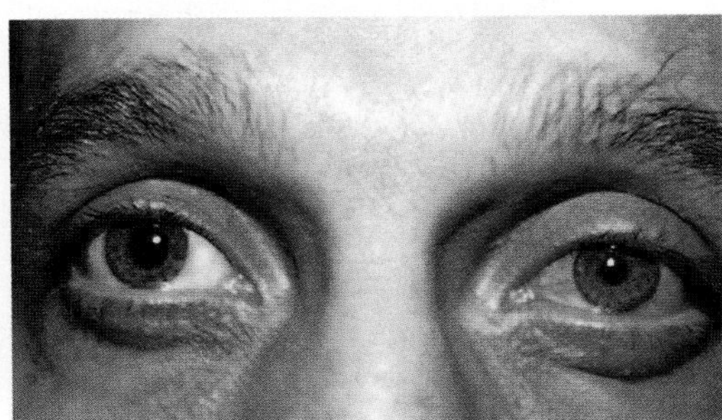

Iritis (Circumcorneal Redness)

Deep, dull red halo around the iris and cornea. Note that redness is around iris, in contrast with conjunctivitis, in which redness is more prominent at the periphery. Pupil shape may be irregular from swelling of iris. Person also has marked photophobia, constricted pupil, blurred vision, and throbbing pain. Warrants immediate referral.

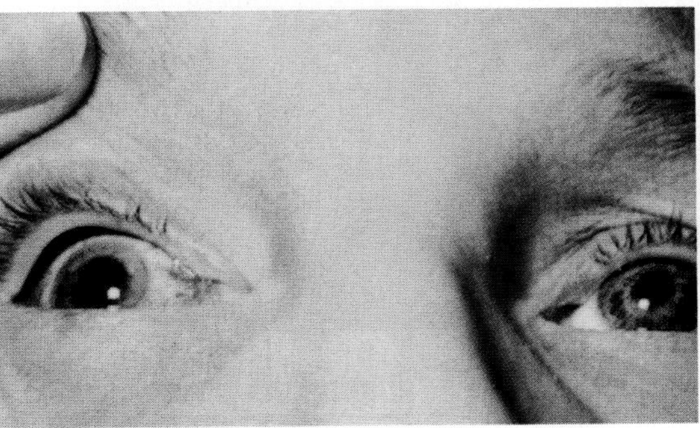

Acute Glaucoma

Acute narrow-angle glaucoma shows a circumcorneal redness around the iris, with a dilated pupil. Pupil is oval, dilated; cornea looks "steamy"; and anterior chamber is shallow. Acute glaucoma occurs with sudden increase in intraocular pressure from blocked outflow from anterior chamber. The person experiences a sudden clouding of vision, sudden eye pain, and halos around lights. This requires emergency treatment to avoid permanent vision loss.

TABLE 14-7 Abnormalities on the Cornea and Iris

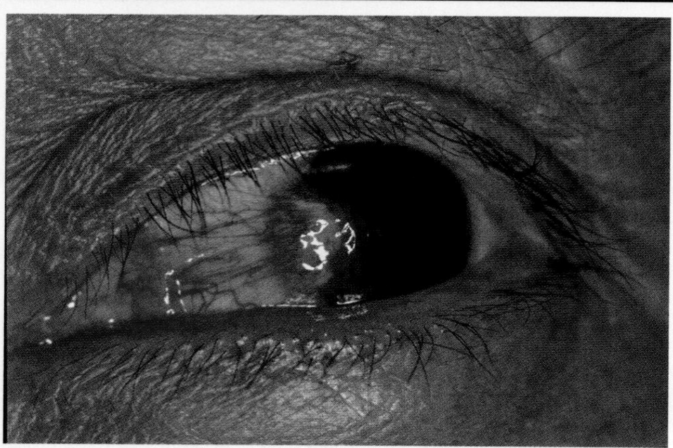

Pterygium

A triangular opaque wing of bulbar conjunctiva overgrows toward the center of the cornea. It looks membranous, translucent, and yellow to white, usually invades from nasal side, and may obstruct vision as it covers pupil. Occurs usually from chronic exposure to hot, dry, sandy climate, which stimulates the growth of a pinguecula (see p. 307) into a pterygium.

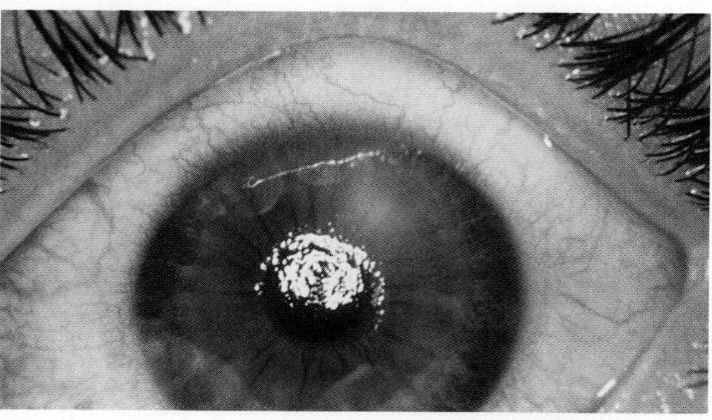

Corneal Abrasion

This is the most common result of a blunt eye injury, but irregular ridges usually visible only when fluorescein stain reveals yellow-green branching. Top layer of corneal epithelium removed, from scratches or poorly fitting or overworn contact lenses. Because the area is rich in nerve endings, the person feels intense pain, a foreign body sensation, and lacrimation, redness, and photophobia.

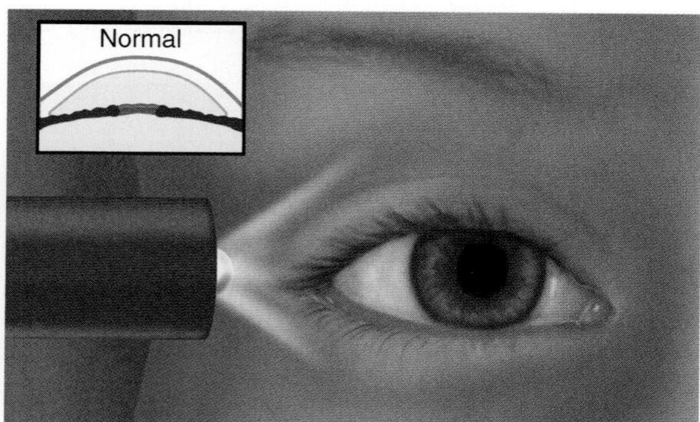

Normal Anterior Chamber (for Contrast)

A light directed across the eye from the temporal side illuminates the entire iris evenly because the normal iris is flat and creates no shadow.

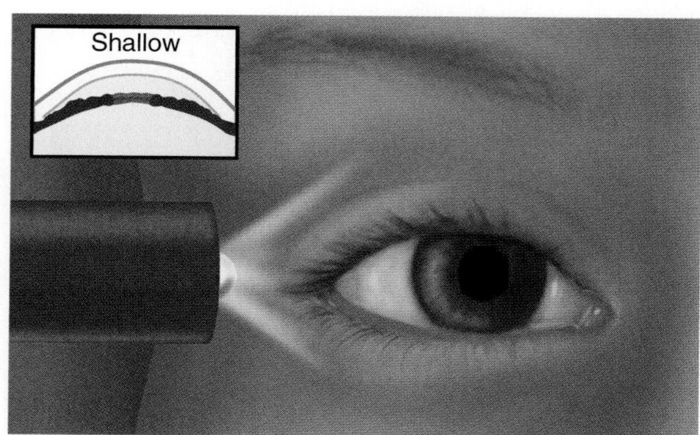

Shallow Anterior Chamber

The iris is pushed anteriorly because of increased intraocular pressure. Because direct light is received from the temporal side, only the temporal part of iris is illuminated; the nasal side is shadowed, the "shadow sign." This may be a sign of acute angle-closure glaucoma; the iris looks bulging because aqueous humor cannot circulate.

TABLE 14-7 **Abnormalities on the Cornea and Iris—cont'd**

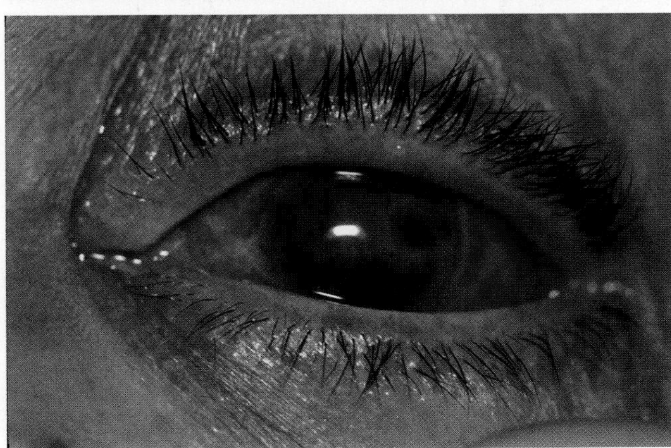

Hyphema

Blood in anterior chamber is a serious result of herpes zoster infection. Also occurs with blunt trauma (a fist or a baseball) or spontaneous hemorrhage. Suspect scleral rupture or major intraocular trauma. Note that gravity settles blood.

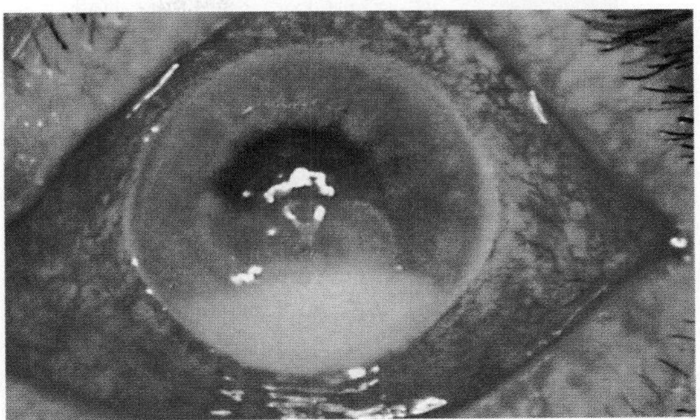

Hypopyon

Purulent matter in anterior chamber occurs with iritis and with inflammation in the anterior chamber.

TABLE 14-8 **Opacities in the Lens**

Senile Cataracts

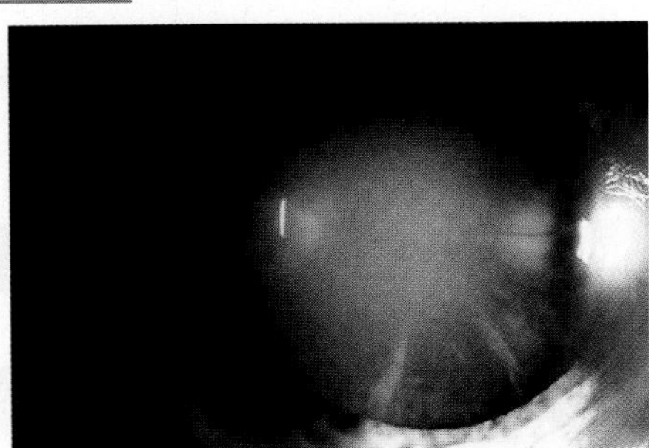

Central Gray Opacity—Nuclear Cataract

Nuclear cataract shows as an opaque gray surrounded by black background as it forms in the center of lens nucleus. Through the ophthalmoscope, it looks like a black center against the red reflex. It begins after age 40 years and develops slowly, gradually obstructing vision.

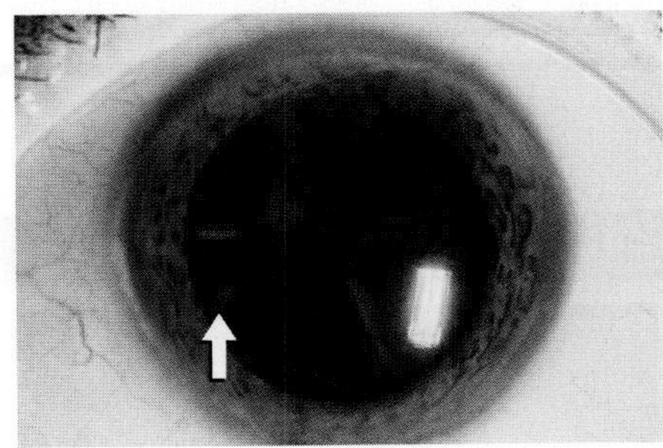

Star-Shaped Opacity—Cortical Cataract

Cortical cataract shows as asymmetric, radial, white spokes with black center. Through ophthalmoscope, black spokes are evident against the red reflex. This forms in outer cortex of lens, progressing faster than nuclear cataract.

TABLE 14-9 Abnormalities in the Optic Disc

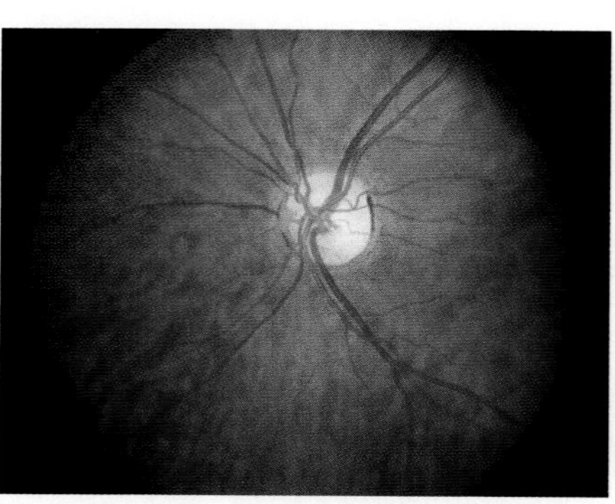

Optic Atrophy (Disc Pallor)

Optic atrophy is a white or gray color of the disc as a result of partial or complete death of the optic nerve. This results in decreased visual acuity, decreased color vision, and decreased contrast sensitivity.

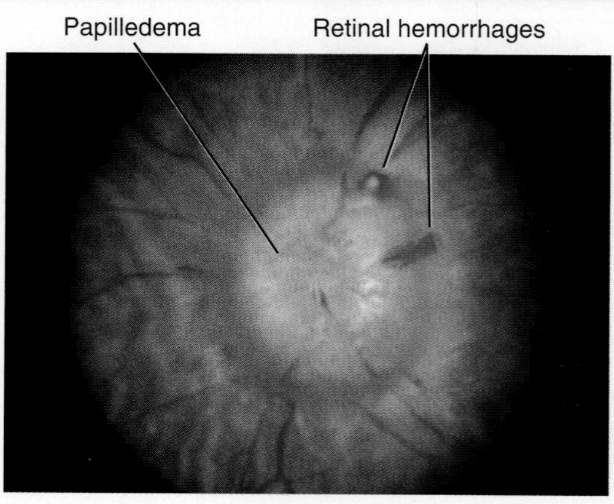

Papilledema (Choked Disc)

Increased intracranial pressure causes venous stasis in the globe, showing redness, congestion, and elevation of the disc; blurred margins; hemorrhages; and absent venous pulsations. This is a serious sign of intracranial pressure, usually caused by a space-occupying mass (e.g., a brain tumor or hematoma). Visual acuity is not affected.

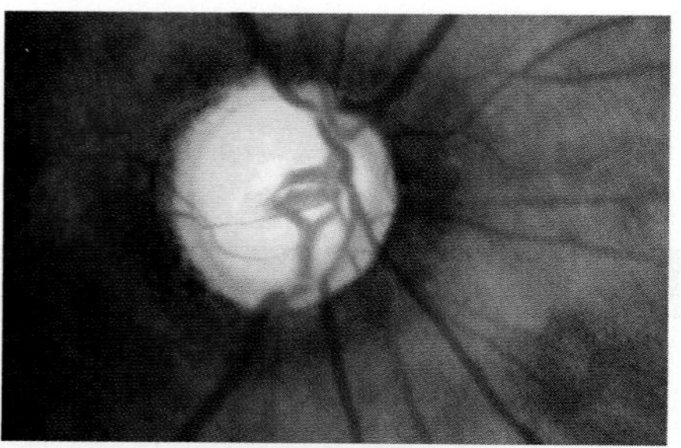

Excessive Cup-Disc Ratio

With primary open-angle glaucoma, the increased intraocular pressure decreases blood supply to retinal structures. The physiologic cup enlarges to more than half of the disc diameter, vessels appear to plunge over edge of cup, and the vessels are displaced nasally. This is asymptomatic, although the person may have decreased vision or visual field defects in the late stages of glaucoma.

TABLE 14-10 Abnormalities in Retinal Vessels and Background

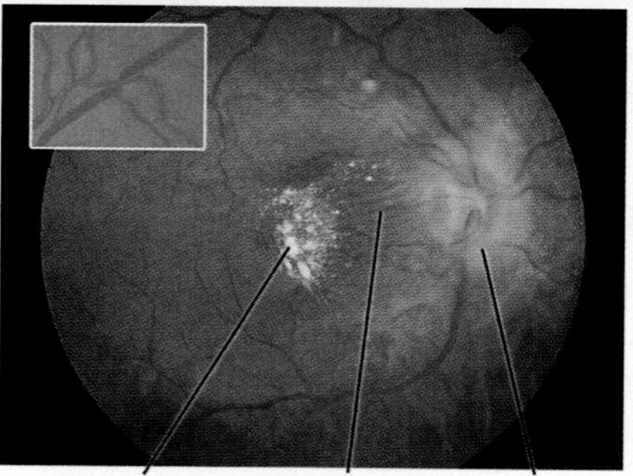

Arteriovenous Crossing (Nicking)

Inset shows arteriovenous crossing with interruption of blood flow. When vein is occluded, it dilates distal to crossing. This person also has disc edema and hard exudates in a macular star pattern that occur with acutely elevated (malignant) hypertension. With hypertension, the arteriole wall thickens and becomes opaque so that no blood is seen inside it (silverwire arteries).

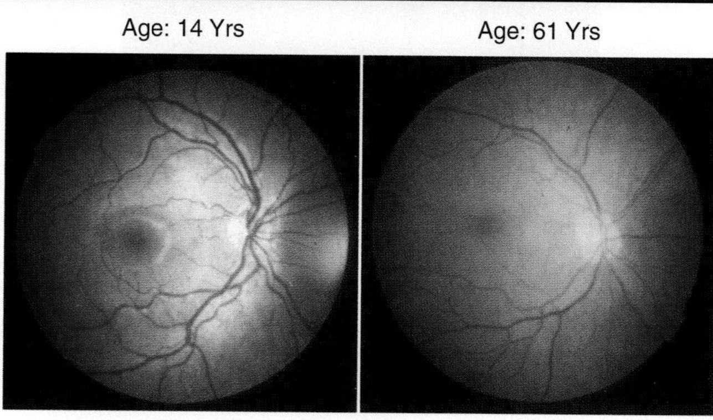

Narrowed (Attenuated) Arteries

This is a generalized decrease in arteriole diameter. The light reflex also narrows. It occurs with severe hypertension (shown above on the right) and with occlusion of the central retinal artery and retinitis pigmentosa.

Abnormal Findings

TABLE 14-10 Abnormalities in Retinal Vessels and Background—cont'd

Diabetic Retinopathy

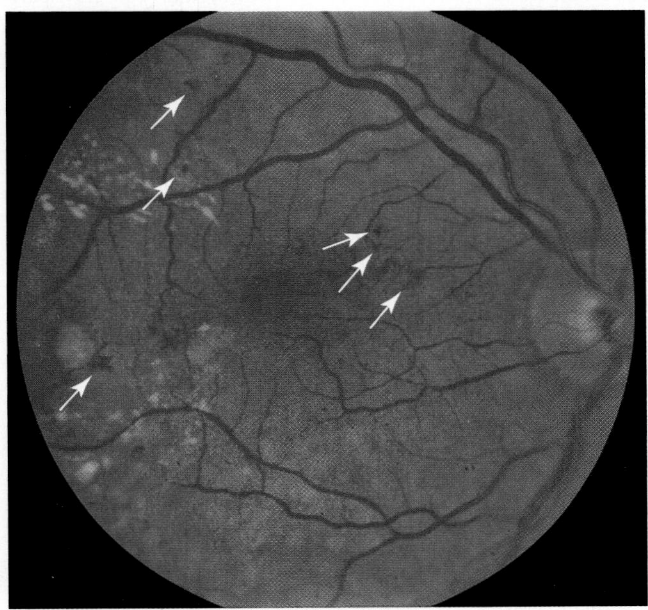

Microaneurysms

Microaneurysms are round punctate red dots that are localized dilations of a small vessel. Their edges are smooth and discrete. The vessel itself is too small to view with the ophthalmoscope; only the isolated red dots are seen. This occurs with diabetes.

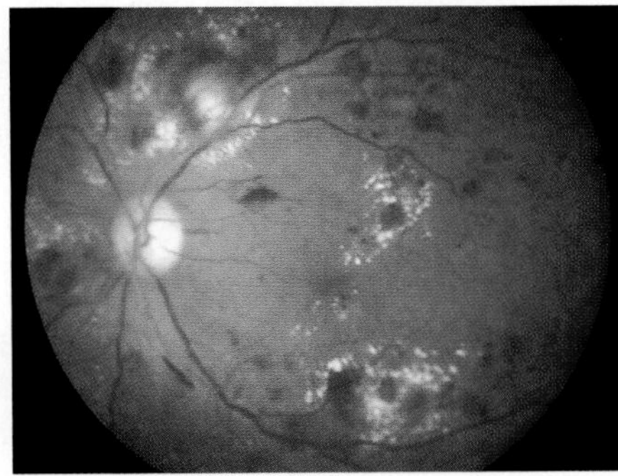

Intraretinal Hemorrhages

Dot-shaped hemorrhages are deep intraretinal hemorrhages that look splattered on. They may be distinguished from microaneurysms by the blurred irregular edges. Flame-shaped hemorrhages are superficial retinal hemorrhages that look linear and spindle shaped. They occur with hypertension.

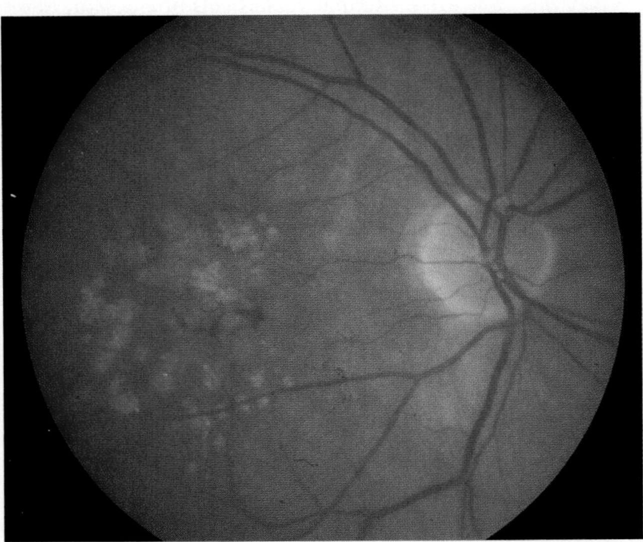

Exudates

Soft exudates or "cotton wool" areas look like fluffy gray-white cumulus clouds. They are arteriolar microinfarctions that envelop and obscure the vessels. They occur with diabetes, hypertension, subacute bacterial endocarditis, lupus, and papilledema of any cause. Hard exudates are numerous small yellow-white spots, having distinct edges and a smooth, solid-looking surface. They often form a circular pattern, clustered around a venous microinfarction. They also may form a linear or star pattern. (This is in contrast with drusen, which have a scattered haphazard location [see Fig. 14-35].)

BIBLIOGRAPHY

1. Anderson, J., Shuey, N. H., & Wall, M. (2009). Rapid confrontation screening for peripheral visual field defects and extinction. *Clinical and Experimental Optometry, 92*(1), 45-48.
2. Bakes, K., & Cadnapaphornchai, L. (2005). Clinical assessment of vision loss. *Emergency Medicine, 37*, 14-24.
3. Bloomgarden, Z. T. (2007). Screening for and managing diabetic retinopathy: current approaches. *American Journal of Health-System Pharmacy, 64*(12), S8-S14.
4. Brown, G. (Ed.) (2005). Retinal, vitreous and macular disorders. *Current Opinion in Ophthalmology, 16*, 139-229.
5. Congdon, N., et al. (2004). Growing older, seeing less. *Archives of Ophthalmology, 122*, 477-485.
6. Friedman, N. J., Kaiser, P. K., & Pineda, R. (2009). *The Massachusetts Eye and Ear Infirmary illustrated manual of ophthalmology* (3rd ed.). Philadelphia: Saunders.
7. Gillig, P. M., & Sanders, R. D. (2009). Cranial nerve II: vision. *Psychiatry, 6*(9), 32-37.
8. Hammersmith, K. (Ed.) (2005). Corneal and external disorders. *Current Opinion in Ophthalmology, 16*, 231-250.
9. Kane, R. T., Ouslander, J. G., & Abrass, I. B. (2009). *Essentials of clinical geriatrics* (6th ed.). New York: McGraw-Hill.
10. Khare, G. D., Symons, R. C., & Do, D. V. (2008). Common ophthalmic emergencies. *International Journal of Clinical Practice, 62*(11), 1176-1784.
11. Koch, J., & Sikes, K. (2009). Getting the red out: primary angle-closure glaucoma. *Nurse Practitioner, 34*(5), 6-9.
12. Kowing, D., & Kester, E. (2007). Keep an eye out for glaucoma. *Nurse Practitioner, 32*(7), 18-23.
13. Levine, N. (2008). Asymptomatic lesions on eyelids. *Geriatrics, 63*(8), 31.
14. McLaughlin, C., & Levin, A. (2006). The red reflex. *Pediatric Emergency Care, 22*, 137-140.
15. National Center for Health Statistics. (2009). *Health, United States, 2009 with chartbook on trends in the health of Americans*, Hyattsville, Md. Accessed February 1, 2010, from www.cdc.gov/nchs/hus/htm.
16. Nsiah-Kumi, P., Ortmeier, S. R., & Brown, A. E. (2009). Disparities in diabetic retinopathy screening and disease for racial and ethnic minority populations. *Journal of the National Medical Association, 101*(5), 430-437.
17. Pham, T. T., & Perry, J. D. (2007). Floppy eyelid syndrome. *Current Opinion in Ophthalmology, 18*(5), 430-433.
18. Robinett, D. A., & Kahn, J. H. (2007). The physical examination of the eye. *Emergency Medicine Clinics of North America, 26*(1), 1-16.
19. Rowe, S., & MacLean, C. H. (2007). Quality indicators for the care of vision impairment in vulnerable elders. *American Geriatrics Society, 55*(Suppl 2), S450-S456.
20. Saligan, L., & Yeh, S. (2008). Seeing red: guiding the management of ocular hyperemia. *Nurse Practitioner, 33*(6), 13-20.
21. Sharts-Hopko, N. C., & Glynn-Milley, C. (2009). Primary open-angle glaucoma. *American Journal of Nursing, 109*(2), 40-48.
22. Smith, S. C. (2008). Aging and vision. *Journal of American Ophthalmic Registered Nurses, 33*(1), 16-22.
23. Smith, S. C. (2008). Basic ocular anatomy. *Journal of American Registered Nurses, 33*(3), 19-23.
24. Tingley, D. (2010). Vision screening essentials: screening today for eye disorders in the pediatric patient. *Pediatrics in Review, 28*(2), 53-61.
25. Wagner, H., Fink, B. A., & Zadnik, K. (2008). Sex- and gender-based differences in healthy and diseased eyes. *American Optometric Association, 79*(11), 636-652.
26. Whiteside, M., Wallhagen, M., & Pettengill, E. (2006). Sensory impairment in older adults. Part 2. Vision loss. *American Journal of Nursing, 106*, 52-62.
27. Zucker, J. L. (2009). The eyelids: some common disorders seen in everyday practice. *Geriatrics, 64*(4), 14-16, 19, 28.

Summary Checklist: Eye Exam

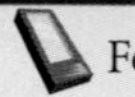
For a PDA-downloadable version, go to http://evolve.elsevier.com/Jarvis/.

1. **Test visual acuity**
   Snellen eye chart
   Near vision (those older than 40 years or those having difficulty reading)
2. **Test visual fields—confrontation test**
3. **Inspect extraocular muscle function**
   Corneal light reflex (Hirschberg test)
   Cover test
   Diagnostic positions test
4. **Inspect external eye structures**
   General
   Eyebrows
   Eyelids and lashes
   Eyeball alignment
   Conjunctiva and sclera
   Lacrimal apparatus
5. **Inspect anterior eyeball structures**
   Cornea and lens
   Iris and pupil
      Size, shape, and equality
      Pupillary light reflex
      Accommodation
6. **Inspect the ocular fundus**
   Optic disc (color, shape, margins, cup-disc ratio)
   Retinal vessels (number, color, artery-vein [A:V] ratio, caliber, arteriovenous crossings, tortuosity, pulsations)
   General background (color, integrity)
   Macula

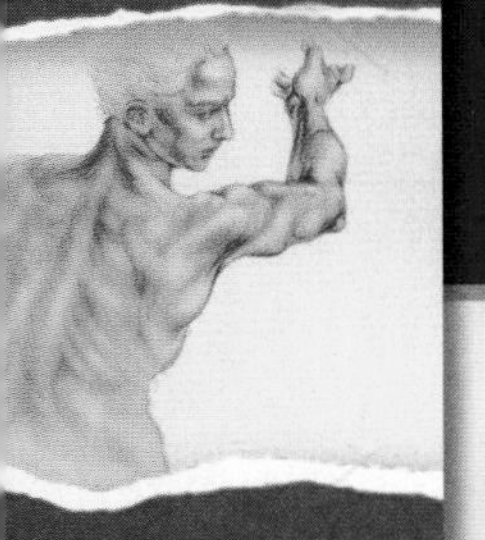

CHAPTER 15

Ears

evolve WEBSITE

http://evolve.elsevier.com/Jarvis/

- Animations
- Audio Key Points
- Bedside Assessment Summary Checklist
- Case Study
  Hearing Deficit
- NCLEX Review Questions
- Physical Examination Summary Checklist
- Quick Assessment for Common Conditions
  Otitis Media
- Video—Assessment
  Ears

OUTLINE

Structure and Function, 323

External Ear
Middle Ear
Inner Ear
Hearing

Subjective Data, 327

Health History Questions

Objective Data, 330

Preparation
The External Ear
The Otoscopic Examination
Hearing Acuity
The Vestibular Apparatus

Documentation and Critical Thinking, 338

Abnormal Findings, 341

Abnormal Findings for Advanced Practice, 344

STRUCTURE AND FUNCTION

The ear is the sensory organ for hearing and maintaining equilibrium. The ear has three parts: the external ear, the middle ear, and the inner ear. The external ear is called the **auricle** or **pinna** and consists of movable cartilage and skin (Fig. 15-1). Note the landmarks of the auricle, and use these terms to describe your findings. The mastoid process, the bony prominence behind the lobule, is not part of the ear but is an important landmark.

EXTERNAL EAR

The external ear has a characteristic shape and serves to funnel sound waves into its opening, the **external auditory canal** (Fig. 15-2). The canal is a cul-de-sac 2.5 to 3 cm long in the adult and terminates at the eardrum, or tympanic

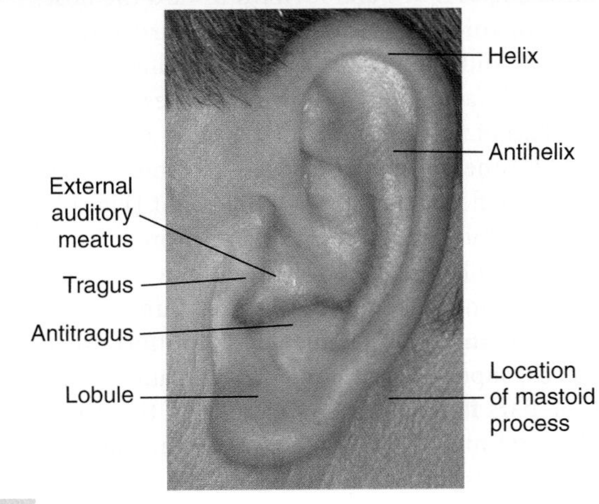

15-1

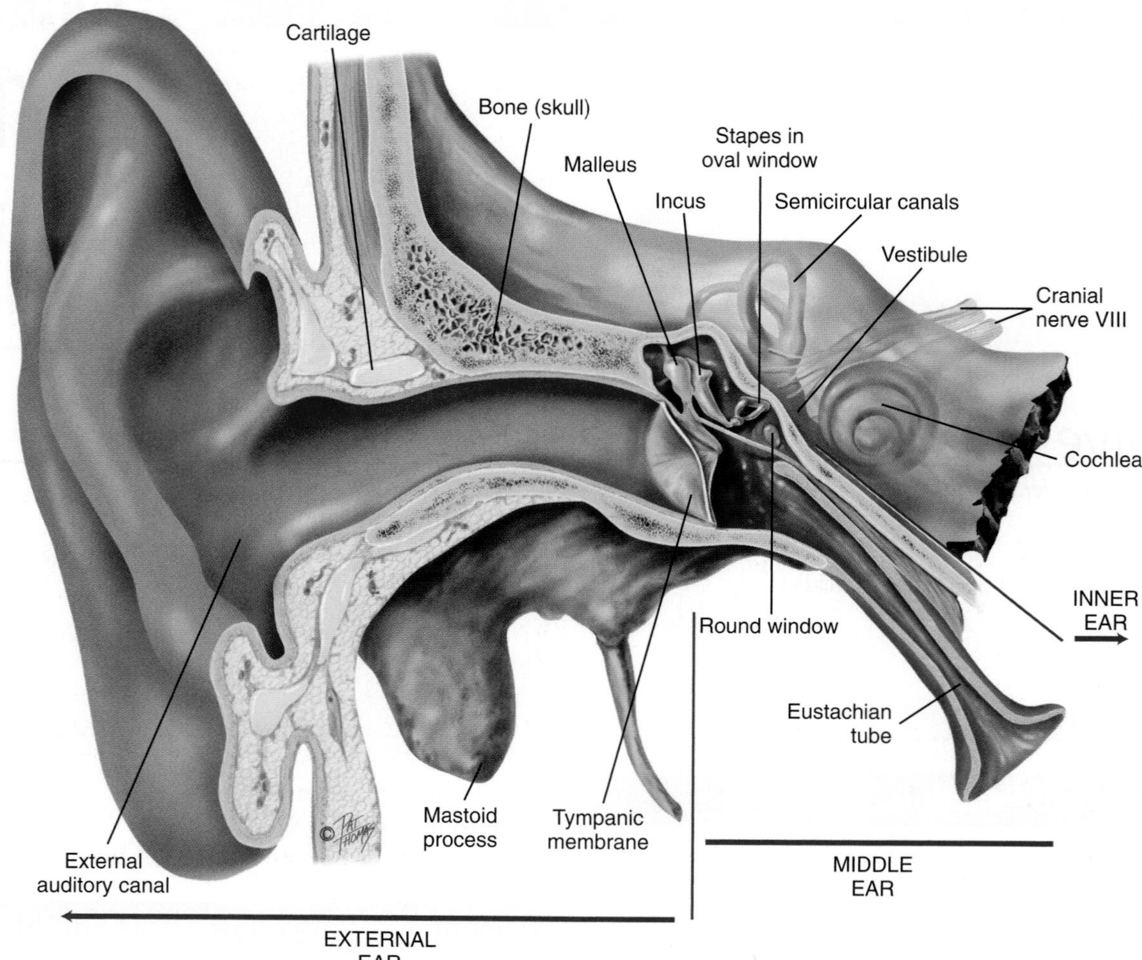

15-2

© Pat Thomas, 2010.

membrane. The canal is lined with glands that secrete cerumen, a yellow, waxy material that lubricates and protects the ear. The wax forms a sticky barrier that helps keep foreign bodies from entering and reaching the sensitive tympanic membrane. Cerumen migrates out to the meatus by the movements of chewing and talking.

The outer one third of the canal is cartilage; the inner two thirds consists of bone covered by thin, sensitive skin. The canal has a slight S-curve in the adult. The outer one third curves up and toward the back of the head, whereas the inner two thirds angles down and forward toward the nose.

The **tympanic membrane (TM),** or **eardrum,** separates the external and the middle ear and is tilted obliquely to the ear canal, facing downward and somewhat forward. It is a translucent membrane with a pearly gray color and a prominent cone of light in the anteroinferior quadrant, which is the reflection of the otoscope light (Fig. 15-3). The drum is oval and slightly concave, pulled in at its center by one of the middle ear ossicles, the **malleus.** The parts of the malleus show through the translucent drum; these are the **umbo,** the **manubrium** (handle), and the **short process.** The small, slack, superior section of the tympanic membrane is called the **pars flaccida.** The remainder of the drum, which is thicker and more taut, is the **pars tensa.** The **annulus** is the outer fibrous rim of the drum.

Lymphatic drainage of the external ear flows to the parotid, mastoid, and superficial cervical nodes.

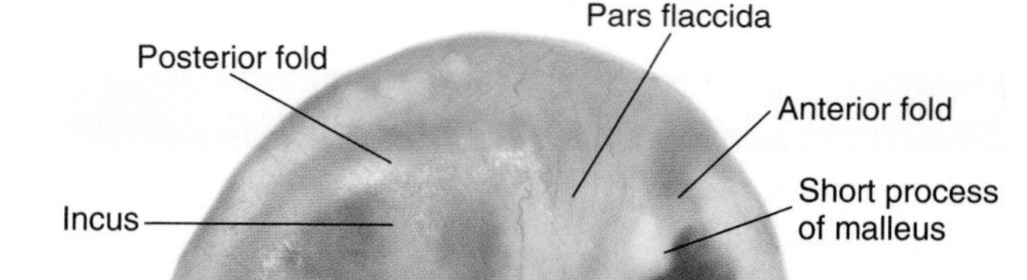
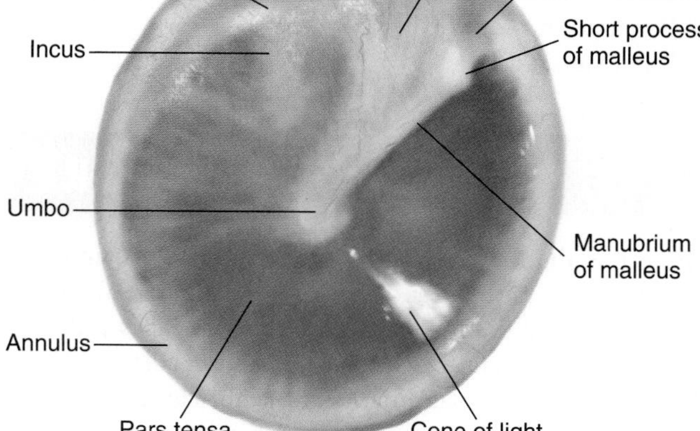

15-3

MIDDLE EAR

The middle ear is a tiny air-filled cavity inside the temporal bone (see Fig. 15-2). It contains tiny ear bones, or auditory ossicles: the **malleus, incus,** and **stapes.** The middle ear has several openings. Its opening to the outer ear is covered by the tympanic membrane. The openings to the inner ear are the oval window at the end of the stapes and the round window. Another opening is the **eustachian tube,** which connects the middle ear with the nasopharynx and allows passage of air. The tube is normally closed, but it opens with swallowing or yawning.

The middle ear has three functions: (1) it conducts sound vibrations from the outer ear to the central hearing apparatus in the inner ear; (2) it protects the inner ear by reducing the amplitude of loud sounds; and (3) its eustachian tube allows equalization of air pressure on each side of the tympanic membrane so that the membrane does not rupture (e.g., during altitude changes in an airplane).

INNER EAR

The inner ear is embedded in bone. It contains the **bony labyrinth,** which holds the sensory organs for equilibrium and hearing. Within the bony labyrinth, the **vestibule** and the **semicircular canals** compose the vestibular apparatus and the **cochlea** (Latin for "snail shell") contains the central hearing apparatus. Although the inner ear is not accessible to direct examination, you can assess its functions.

HEARING

The function of hearing involves the auditory system at three levels: peripheral, brainstem, and cerebral cortex. At the peripheral level, the ear transmits sound and converts its vibrations into electrical impulses, which can be analyzed by the brain. For example, you hear an alarm bell ringing in the hall. Its sound waves travel instantly to your ears. The *amplitude* is how loud the alarm is; its *frequency* is the pitch (in this case, high) or the number of cycles per second. The sound waves produce vibrations on your tympanic membrane. These vibrations are carried by the middle ear ossicles to your oval window. Then the sound waves travel through your cochlea, which is coiled like a snail's shell, and are dissipated against the round window. Along the way, the **basilar membrane** vibrates at a point specific to the frequency of the sound. In this case, the alarm's high frequency stimulates the basilar membrane at its base near the stapes (Fig. 15-4). The numerous fibers along the basilar membrane are the receptor hair cells of the **organ of Corti,** the sensory organ of hearing. As the hair cells bend, they mediate the vibrations into electric impulses. The electrical impulses are conducted by the auditory portion of cranial nerve VIII to the brainstem.

The function at the brainstem level is *binaural interaction,* which permits locating the direction of a sound in space as well as identifying the sound. How does this work? Each ear is actually one half of the total sensory organ. The ears are located on each side of a movable head. The cranial nerve VIII from each ear sends signals to both sides of the brainstem. Areas in the brainstem are sensitive to differences in intensity and timing of the messages from the two ears, depending on the way the head is turned.

Finally, the function of the cortex is to interpret the meaning of the sound and begin the appropriate response.

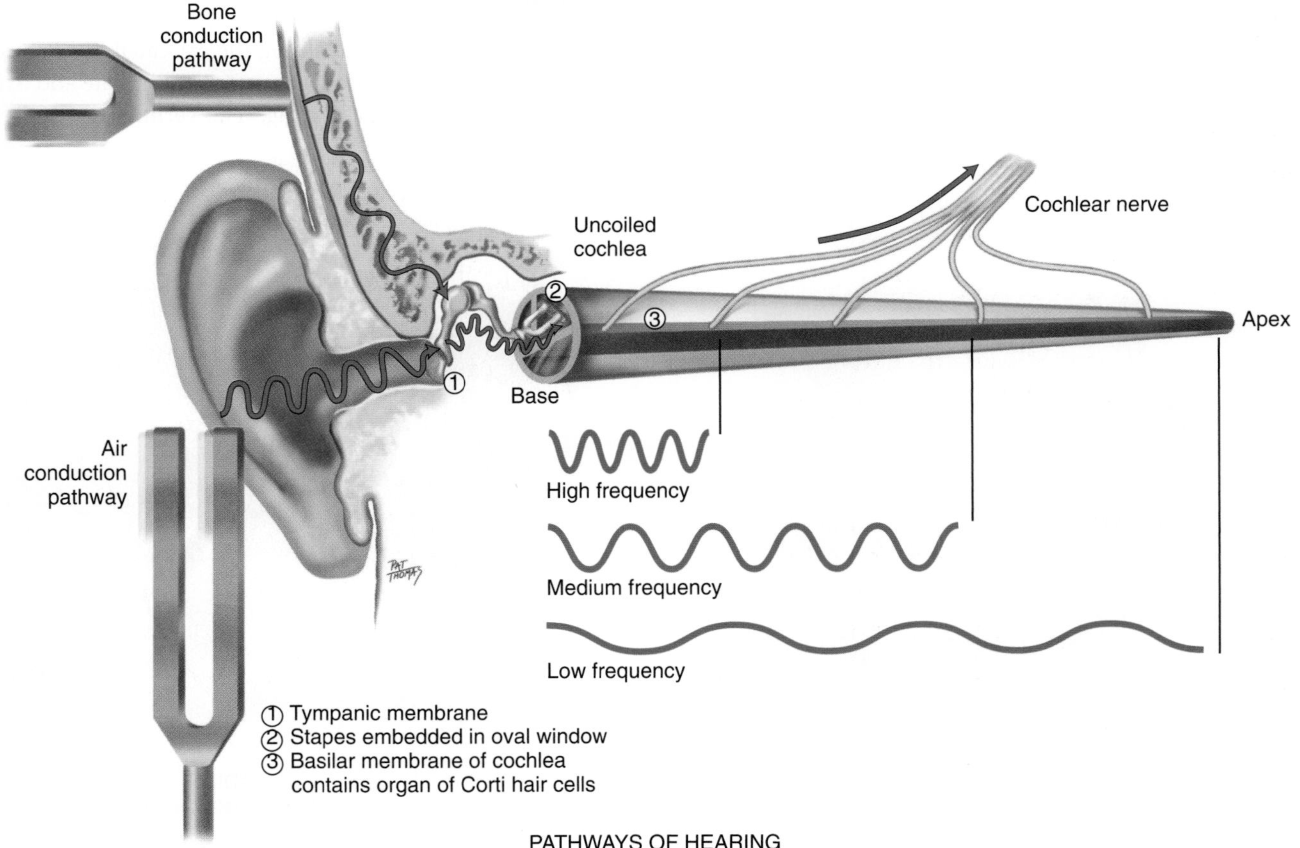

15-4 PATHWAYS OF HEARING

All this happens in the split second it takes you to react to the alarm.

Pathways of Hearing. The normal pathway of hearing is air conduction (AC), described earlier; it is the most efficient. An alternate route of hearing is by bone conduction (BC). Here, the bones of the skull vibrate. These vibrations are transmitted directly to the inner ear and to cranial nerve VIII.

Hearing Loss. Anything that obstructs the transmission of sound impairs hearing. A **conductive** hearing loss involves a mechanical dysfunction of the external or middle ear. It is a partial loss because the person is able to hear if the sound amplitude is increased enough to reach normal nerve elements in the inner ear. Conductive hearing loss may be caused by impacted cerumen, foreign bodies, a perforated tympanic membrane, pus or serum in the middle ear, and otosclerosis (a decrease in mobility of the ossicles).

Sensorineural (or perceptive) loss signifies pathology of the inner ear, cranial nerve VIII, or the auditory areas of the cerebral cortex. A simple increase in amplitude may not enable the person to understand words. Sensorineural hearing loss may be caused by *presbycusis,* a gradual nerve degeneration that occurs with aging, and by ototoxic drugs, which affect the hair cells in the cochlea. A **mixed** loss is a combination of conductive and sensorineural types in the same ear.

Equilibrium. The labyrinth in the inner ear constantly feeds information to your brain about your body's position in space. It works like a plumb line to determine verticality or depth. The ear's plumb lines register the angle of your head in relation to gravity. If the labyrinth ever becomes inflamed, it feeds the wrong information to the brain, creating a staggering gait and a strong, spinning, whirling sensation called *vertigo.*

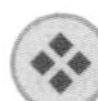

DEVELOPMENTAL COMPETENCE

Infants and Children

The inner ear starts to develop early in the fifth week of gestation. In early development, the ear is posteriorly rotated and low set; later it ascends to its normal placement around eye level. If maternal rubella infection occurs during the first trimester, it can damage the organ of Corti and impair hearing.

The infant's eustachian tube is relatively shorter and wider and its position is more horizontal than the adult's, so it is easier for pathogens from the nasopharynx to migrate through to the middle ear (Fig. 15-5). The lumen is surrounded by lymphoid tissue, which increases during childhood; thus the lumen is easily occluded. These factors place the infant at greater risk for middle ear infections than the adult.

The infant's and the young child's ear canal is shorter and has a slope opposite to that of the adult's (see Fig. 15-13 on p. 336).

The Adult

Otosclerosis is a common cause of conductive hearing loss in young adults between the ages of 20 and 40 years. It is a gradual hardening that causes the footplate of the stapes to become fixed in the oval window, impeding the transmission of sound and causing progressive deafness.

The Aging Adult

In the aging person, cilia lining the ear canal become coarse and stiff. This may cause cerumen to accumulate and oxidize, which greatly reduces hearing. The cerumen itself is drier

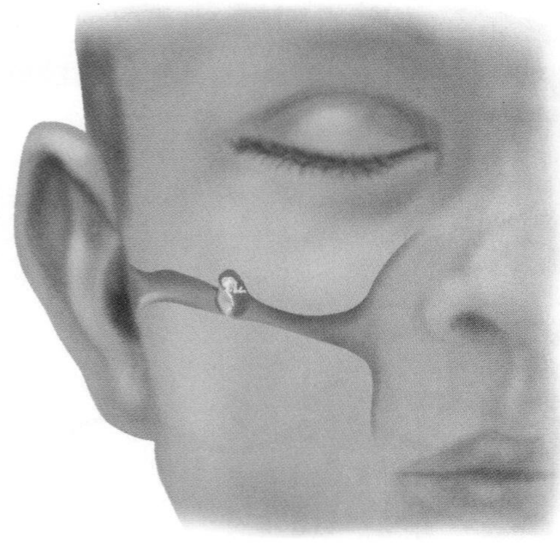

INFANT
Horizontal eustachian tube

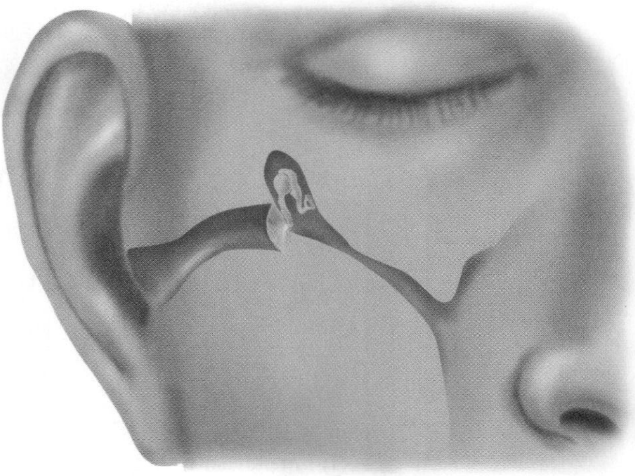

ADULT
Sloped eustachian tube

15-5

because of atrophy of the apocrine glands. Also, a life history of frequent ear infections may result in scarring on the drum.

Impacted cerumen is common in aging adults (up to 57%) and in other at-risk groups (e.g., institutionalized and mentally disabled) who may underreport the associated hearing loss. Cerumen impaction also blocks conduction in those wearing hearing aids and accounts for 70% of the malfunction in hearing aids returned to the manufacturer.[12] Cerumen should be removed when it leads to conductive hearing loss or interferes with full assessment of the ear. Ceruminolytics are wax-softening agents that expedite removal with electric or manual irrigators. After removal, those persons with hearing loss have shown improvement by 5 to 36 dB.[12]

A person living in a noise-polluted area (e.g., near an airport or a busy highway) has a greater risk for hearing loss. But **presbycusis** is a type of hearing loss that occurs with 60% of those older than 65 years, even in people living in a quiet environment. It is a gradual sensorineural loss caused by nerve degeneration in the inner ear that slowly progresses after the fifth decade.[13] The person first notices a high-frequency tone loss; it is harder to hear consonants than vowels. Much speech information is lost, and words sound garbled. The ability to localize sound is impaired also. This communication dysfunction is accentuated when unfavorable background noise is present (e.g., with music, with dishes clattering, or at a large, noisy party).

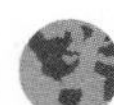

CULTURE AND GENETICS

Otitis media, or OM (middle ear infection), occurs because of obstruction of the eustachian tube or passage of nasopharyngeal secretions into the middle ear. Otitis media is one of the most common illnesses in children. It is so common that 90% of all children younger than 2 years have had at least one episode of OM.[17] The incidence and severity are increased in indigenous children from North America, Australia, New Zealand, and Northern Europe, although genetic factors have not been determined. Rather, the most important cause is environmental; children in high-risk groups usually have multiple pathogens, and the total bacterial load is high.[16]

Predisposing factors for OM include absence of breastfeeding in the first 3 months of age, exposure to tobacco smoke, daycare attendance, male gender, pacifier use, seasonality (fall and winter), and underlying diseases.[17] Feeding by bottle in the supine position increases risk because the effects of gravity and sucking draw the nasopharyngeal contents directly into the middle ear. Urge parents to breastfeed whenever possible. But when bottle-feeding, do not prop the bottle or let the baby take a bottle to bed.

The most important side effect of acute otitis media is the persistence of fluid in the middle ear after treatment. This middle ear effusion can impair hearing, placing the child at risk for delayed cognitive development.

Genetic variations. Cerumen is genetically determined to be of two major types: (1) dry cerumen, which is gray and flaky and frequently forms a thin mass in the ear canal; and (2) wet cerumen, which is honey brown to dark brown and moist. Chromosome 16 holds one gene trait determining the wet or dry phenotype.[19] The wet cerumen phenotype occurs more often in Caucasians and African Americans, whereas the dry cerumen is more frequent in Asians and American Indians.[11] The presence and composition of cerumen are not related to poor hygiene. Take caution to avoid mistaking the flaky, dry cerumen for eczematous lesions.

SUBJECTIVE DATA

1. Earaches
2. Infections
3. Discharge
4. Hearing loss
5. Environmental noise
6. Tinnitus
7. Vertigo
8. Self-care behaviors

Examiner Asks	Rationale
1. Earache. Any **earache** or other pain in ears? • Location—feel close to the surface or deep in the head? • Does it hurt when you push on the ear? • Character—dull, aching or sharp, stabbing? Constant or come and go? Is it affected by changing position of head?	**Otalgia** may be directly due to ear disease or may be referred pain from a problem in teeth or oropharynx.
• Any accompanying cold symptoms or sore throat? Any problems with sinuses or teeth?	Virus/bacteria from upper respiratory infection may migrate up the eustachian tube to involve the middle ear.
• Ever been hit on the ear or on the side of the head or had any sport injury? Ever had any trauma from a foreign body?	Trauma may rupture the tympanic membrane (TM).
• What have you tried to relieve pain?	Assess effect of coping strategies.

Examiner Asks	Rationale
2. **Infections.** Any ear **infections?** As an adult, or in childhood? • How frequent were they? How were they treated?	A history of chronic ear problems suggests possible sequelae.
3. **Discharge.** Any **discharge** from your ears? • Does it look like pus, or is it bloody? • Any odor to the discharge? • Any relationship between the discharge and the ear pain?	**Otorrhea** suggests infected canal or perforated eardrum, such as: *External otitis*—purulent, sanguineous, or watery discharge. *Acute otitis media with perforation*—purulent discharge. *Cholesteatoma*—dirty yellow/gray discharge, foul odor. Typically with perforation—ear pain occurs first, stops with a popping sensation, then drainage occurs.
4. **Hearing loss.** Ever had any trouble hearing? • Onset—did the loss come on slowly or all at once?	**Presbycusis** is gradual onset over years, whereas a trauma hearing loss is often sudden. Refer any sudden loss in one or both ears *not* associated with upper respiratory infection (URI).
• Character—has all your hearing decreased, or just on hearing certain sounds? • In what situations do you notice the loss: conversations, using the telephone, listening to TV, at a party?	Loss shows with competition from background noise, as at a party.
• Do people seem to shout at you?	*Recruitment*—a marked loss when speech is at low intensity, but sound actually becomes painful when speaker repeats in a loud voice.
• Do ordinary sounds seem hollow, as if you are hearing in a barrel or under water? • Recently traveled by airplane? • Any family history of hearing loss? • Effort to treat—any hearing aid or other device? Anything to help hearing?	Character of hearing loss when cerumen expands and becomes impacted, as after swimming or showering.
• Coping strategies—how does the loss affect your daily life? Any job problem? Feel embarrassed? Frustrated? How do your family, friends react?	Hearing loss can cause social isolation and lessen pleasure of leisure activities.

Note to examiner—during history, note these clues from normal conversation that indicate possible hearing loss.

1. Person lip reading or watching your face and lips closely rather than your eyes
2. Frowning or straining forward to hear
3. Posturing of head to catch sounds with better ear
4. Misunderstands your questions or frequently asks you to repeat
5. Acts irritable or shows startle reflex when you raise your voice (recruitment)
6. Person's speech sounds garbled, possibly vowel sounds distorted
7. Inappropriately loud voice
8. Flat, monotonous tone of voice

Examiner Asks	Rationale
5. **Environmental noise.** Any loud noises at home or on the job? For example, do you live in a noise-polluted area, near an airport or busy traffic area? Now or in the past? • Are you near other noises such as heavy machinery, loud persistent music, gunshots while hunting?	Old trauma to hearing initially goes unnoticed but results in further decibel loss in later years.

Examiner Asks	Rationale
• Coping strategies—any steps to protect your ears, such as headphones or ear plugs?	
6. Tinnitus. Ever felt ringing, crackling, or buzzing in your ears? When did this occur?	**Tinnitus** originates within the person; it accompanies some hearing or ear disorders.
• Seem louder at night?	Tinnitus seems louder with no competition from environment noise.
• Are you taking any medications?	Many medications have ototoxic sequelae: aspirin, aminoglycosides (streptomycin, gentamicin, kanamycin, neomycin), ethacrynic acid, furosemide, indomethacin, naproxen, quinine, vancomycin.
7. Vertigo. Ever felt **vertigo;** that is, the room spinning around or yourself spinning? (Vertigo is a true twirling motion.)	True rotational spinning occurs with dysfunction of labyrinth. **Objective vertigo**—feels like room spins. **Subjective vertigo**—person feels like he or she spins.
• Ever felt dizzy, like you are not quite steady, like falling or losing your balance? Giddy, light-headed?	Distinguish true vertigo from dizziness or light-headedness.
8. Self-care behaviors. How do you clean your ears?	Assess potential trauma from invasive instruments. Cotton-tipped applicators can impact cerumen, causing hearing loss.
• Last time you had your hearing checked? • If a hearing loss was noted, did you obtain a hearing aid? How long have you had it? Do you wear it? How does it work? Any trouble with upkeep, cleaning, changing batteries?	Prescribe frequency of hearing assessment according to person's age or risk factors.

Additional History for Infants and Children

Examiner Asks	Rationale
1. Ear infections. At what age was the child's first episode? How many ear infections in the past 6 months? How many total? How were these treated? • Has the child had any surgery, such as insertion of ear tubes or removal of tonsils? • Are infections increasing in frequency, in severity, or staying the same?	A first episode that occurs within 3 months of life increases risk for recurrent OM. Recurrent OM is 3 episodes in past 3 months or 4 within past year.[4]
• Does anyone in the home smoke cigarettes?	Passive and gestational smoke are risk factors for OM.[15]
• Does your child receive childcare outside your home? In a daycare center or someone else's home? How many children in the group care?	Daycare attendance and bottle-feeding (as opposed to breastfeeding) are risk factors for OM.
2. Does the child seem to be hearing well? • Have you noticed that the infant startles with loud noise? Did the infant babble around 6 months? Does he or she talk? At what age did talking start? Was the speech intelligible? • Ever had the child's hearing tested? If there was a hearing loss, did it follow any diseases in the child, or in the mother during pregnancy? (NOTE: It is important to catch any problem early, because a child with hearing loss is at risk for delayed speech and social development and learning deficit.)	Children at risk for hearing deficit include those exposed to maternal rubella or to maternal ototoxic drugs in utero; premature infants; low-birth-weight infants; trauma or hypoxia at birth; and infants with congenital liver or kidney disease. In children, the incidence of meningitis, measles, mumps, otitis media, and any illness with persistent high fever may increase risk for hearing deficit.
3. Does the child tend to put objects in the ears? Is the older child or adolescent active in contact sports?	These children are at increased risk for trauma.

Subjective Data

OBJECTIVE DATA

PREPARATION

Position the adult sitting up straight with his or her head at your eye level. Occasionally the ear canal is partially filled with cerumen, which obstructs your view of the TM. If the eardrum is intact and no current infection is present, a preferred method of cleaning the adult canal is to soften the cerumen with a warmed solution of mineral oil and hydrogen peroxide. Then the canal is irrigated with warm water (body temperature) with a bulb syringe or a low-pulsatile dental irrigator (WaterPik). Direct fluid to the posterior wall. Leave space around the irrigator tip for water to escape. Do not irrigate if the history or the examination suggests perforation or infection.

EQUIPMENT NEEDED

Otoscope with bright light (fresh batteries give off white—not yellow—light).

Pneumatic bulb attachment, sometimes used with infant or young child.

Normal Range of Findings	Abnormal Findings

INSPECT AND PALPATE THE EXTERNAL EAR

Size and Shape

The ears are of equal size bilaterally with no swelling or thickening. Ears of unusual size and shape may be a normal familial trait with no clinical significance.

Microtia—ears smaller than 4 cm vertically; *macrotia*—ears larger than 10 cm.

Edema with infection or trauma.

Skin Condition

The skin color is consistent with the person's facial skin color. The skin is intact, with no lumps or lesions. On some people you may note **Darwin's tubercle,** a small, painless nodule at the helix. This is a congenital variation and is not significant (Fig 15-6).

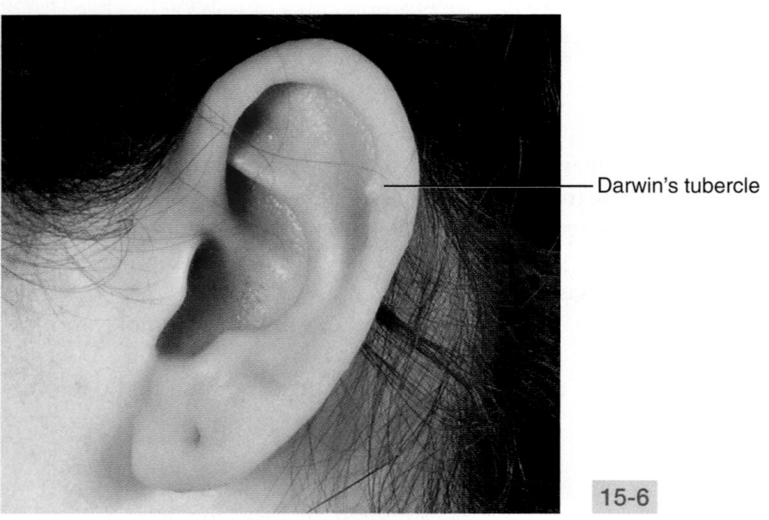

15-6

Reddened, excessively warm skin with inflammation (see Table 15-1, Abnormalities of the External Ear, p. 341).

Crusts and scaling occur with otitis externa, eczema, contact dermatitis, seborrhea.

Enlarged, tender lymph nodes in the region indicate inflammation of the pinna or mastoid process.

Red-blue discoloration with frostbite.

Tophi, sebaceous cyst, chondrodermatitis, keloid, carcinoma (see Table 15-2, Lumps and Lesions on the Ear, pp. 342-343).

Tenderness

Move the pinna and push on the tragus. They should feel firm, and movement should produce no pain. Palpating the mastoid process should also produce no pain.

Pain with movement occurs with otitis externa and furuncle.

Pain at the mastoid process may indicate mastoiditis or enlarged posterior auricular node.

The External Auditory Meatus

Note the size of the opening to direct your choice of speculum for the otoscope. No swelling, redness, or discharge should be present.

A sticky, yellow discharge accompanies otitis externa or may indicate otitis media if the drum has ruptured.

Normal Range of Findings	Abnormal Findings
Some cerumen is usually present. The color varies from gray-yellow to light brown and black, and the texture varies from moist and waxy to dry and desiccated. A large amount of cerumen obscures visualization of the canal and drum.	Impacted cerumen is a common cause of conductive hearing loss.

INSPECT WITH THE OTOSCOPE

As you inspect the external ear, note the size of the auditory meatus. Then choose the largest speculum that will fit comfortably in the ear canal and attach it to the otoscope. Tilt the person's head slightly away from you toward the opposite shoulder. This method brings the obliquely sloping eardrum into better view.

Pull the pinna up and back on an adult or older child; this helps straighten the S-shape of the canal (Fig. 15-7). (Pull the pinna down on an infant and a child younger than 3 years [see Fig. 15-13]). Hold the pinna gently but firmly. Do not release traction on the ear until you have finished the examination and the otoscope is removed.

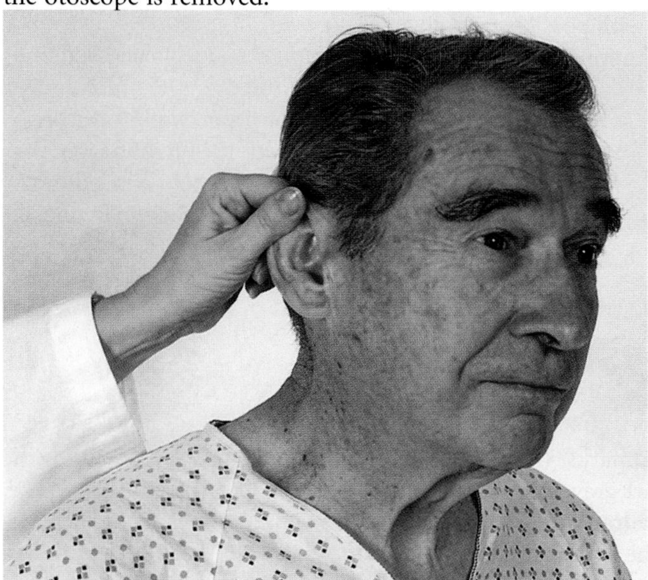

15-7

Hold the otoscope "upside down" along your fingers and have the dorsa (back) of your hand along the person's cheek braced to steady the otoscope (Fig. 15-8). This position feels awkward to you only at first. It soon will feel natural, and you will find it useful to prevent forceful insertion. Also, your stabilizing hand acts as a protecting lever if the person suddenly moves the head.

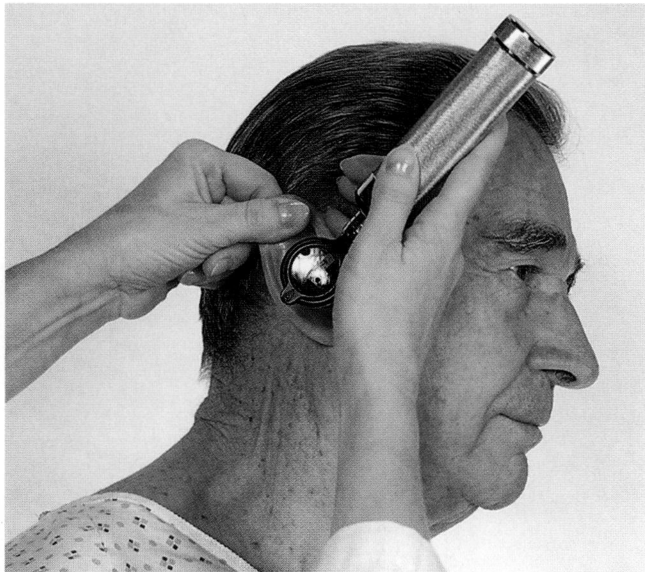

15-8

Normal Range of Findings	Abnormal Findings

Insert the speculum slowly and carefully along the axis of the canal. Watch the insertion; then put your eye up to the otoscope. Avoid touching the inner "bony" section of the canal wall, which is covered by a thin epithelial layer and is sensitive to pain. Sometimes you cannot see anything but canal wall. If so, try to reposition the person's head, apply more traction on the pinna, and re-angle the otoscope to look forward toward the person's nose.

Once it is in place, you may need to rotate the otoscope slightly to visualize the entire eardrum; do this gently. Last, perform the otoscopic examination before you test hearing; ear canals with impacted cerumen give the erroneous impression of pathologic hearing loss.

The External Canal

Note any redness and swelling, lesions, foreign bodies, or discharge. If any discharge is present, note the color and odor. (Also, clean any discharge from the speculum before examining the other ear to avoid contamination with possibly infectious material.) For a person with a hearing aid, note any irritation on the canal wall from poorly fitting ear molds.

Redness and swelling occur with otitis externa; canal may be completely closed with swelling.

Purulent otorrhea suggests otitis externa or otitis media if the drum has ruptured.

Frank blood or clear, watery drainage (cerebrospinal fluid [CSF]) after trauma suggests basal skull fracture and warrants immediate referral. CSF feels oily and is positive for glucose on TesTape.

Foreign body, polyp, furuncle, exostosis (see Table 15-3, Abnormalities in the Ear Canal).

The Tympanic Membrane

Color and Characteristics. Systematically explore its landmarks (Fig. 15-9). The normal eardrum is shiny and translucent, with a pearl gray color. The cone-shaped light reflex is prominent in the anteroinferior quadrant (at the 5 o'clock position in the right drum and the 7 o'clock position in the left drum). This is the reflection of your otoscope light. Sections of the malleus are visible through the translucent drum: the umbo, manubrium, and short process. (Infrequently, you also may see the incus behind the drum; it shows as a whitish haze in the upper posterior area.) At the periphery, the annulus looks whiter and denser.

Yellow-amber drum color occurs with otitis media with effusion (serous).

Red color with acute otitis media.

Absent or distorted landmarks.

Air/fluid level or air bubbles behind drum indicate otitis media with effusion (see Tables 15-4, Abnormal Views on Otoscopy, and 15-5, Abnormal Tympanic Membranes).

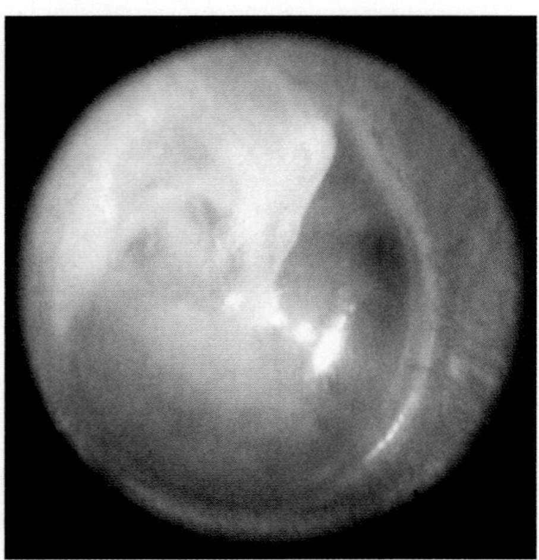

15-9 Normal tympanic membrane *(right ear)*.

Objective Data

Normal Range of Findings	Abnormal Findings
Position. The eardrum is flat, slightly pulled in at the center, and flutters when the person performs the Valsalva maneuver or holds the nose and swallows (insufflation). You may elicit these maneuvers to assess drum mobility. Avoid them with an aging person because they may disrupt equilibrium. Also avoid middle ear insufflation in a person with upper respiratory infection because it could propel infectious matter into the middle ear.	Retracted drum from vacuum in middle ear with obstructed eustachian tube. Bulging drum from increased pressure in otitis media. Drum hypomobility is an early sign of otitis media (see Table 15-5).
Integrity of Membrane. Inspect the eardrum and the entire circumference of the annulus for perforations. The normal tympanic membrane is intact. Some adults may show scarring, which is a dense white patch on the drum. This is a sequela of repeated ear infections.	Perforation shows as a dark oval area or as a larger opening on the drum. Vesicles on drum (see Table 15-5).

TEST HEARING ACUITY

Your screening for a hearing deficit begins during the history; how well does the person hear conversational speech? Also, ask the person directly if he or she thinks there is a hearing difficulty. If the answer is *yes,* perform audiometric testing or refer for audiometric testing. If the answer is *no,* screen using the whispered voice test described below.

A pure tone audiometer gives a precise quantitative measure of hearing by assessing the person's ability to hear sounds of varying frequency. This is a battery-powered, lightweight, handheld instrument that is available in most outpatient settings. With the patient sitting, prop his or her elbow on the armrest of the chair with the hand making a gentle fist.[2] Tell the patient, "You will hear faint tones of different pitches. Please raise your finger as soon as you hear the tone; then lower your finger as soon as you no longer hear the tone." Choose tones of random loudness in decibels on the audioscope. Each tone is on for 1.5 seconds and off for 1.5 seconds. Test each ear separately and record the results. An audiometer gives a precise quantitative measure of hearing by assessing the person's ability to hear sounds of varying frequency.

Whispered Voice Test

Normal Range of Findings	Abnormal Findings
Test one ear at a time while masking hearing in the other ear to prevent sound transmission around the head. This is done by placing one finger on the tragus and rapidly pushing it in and out of the auditory meatus. Shield your lips so the person cannot compensate for a hearing loss (consciously or unconsciously) by lip reading or using the "good" ear. With your head 30 to 60 cm (1 to 2 ft) from the person's ear, exhale and whisper slowly a set of 3 random numbers and letters, such as "5, B, 6." Normally, the person repeats each number/letter correctly after you say it. If the response is not correct, repeat the whispered test using a different combination of 3 numbers and letters. A passing score is correct repeating of at least 3 out of a possible 6 numbers/letters.[2] Assess the other ear using yet another set of whispered items.	The person is unable to hear whispered items. A whisper is a high-frequency sound and is used to detect high-tone loss.

Tuning Fork Tests

Tuning fork tests measure hearing by air conduction (AC) or by bone conduction (BC), in which the sound vibrates through the cranial bones to the inner ear. The AC route through the ear canal and middle ear is usually the more sensitive route. Traditionally, these tests have been taught for physical examination; yet evidence shows that both the Weber and the Rinne tuning fork tests are inaccurate and do not yield precise or reliable data.[2] Thus these tests should not be used for general screening.

Normal Range of Findings | Abnormal Findings

THE VESTIBULAR APPARATUS

The **Romberg test** assesses the ability of the vestibular apparatus in the inner ear to help maintain standing balance. Because the Romberg test also assesses intactness of the cerebellum and proprioception, it is discussed in Chapter 23 (see Fig. 23-17).

DEVELOPMENTAL COMPETENCE

Infants and Young Children

Examination of the external ear is similar to that described for the adult, with the addition of examination of position and alignment on head. Note the ear position. The top of the pinna should match an imaginary line extending from the corner of the eye to the occiput. Also, the ear should be positioned within 10 degrees of vertical (Fig. 15-10).

Low-set ears are found with trisomy 13, 18, and 21. Large prominent ears, misshapen ears, and creases on earlobes are nonspecific but occur with certain syndromes and with underlying ear structure abnormalities.

Pre-auricular skin tags may occur alone or with other facial anomalies.

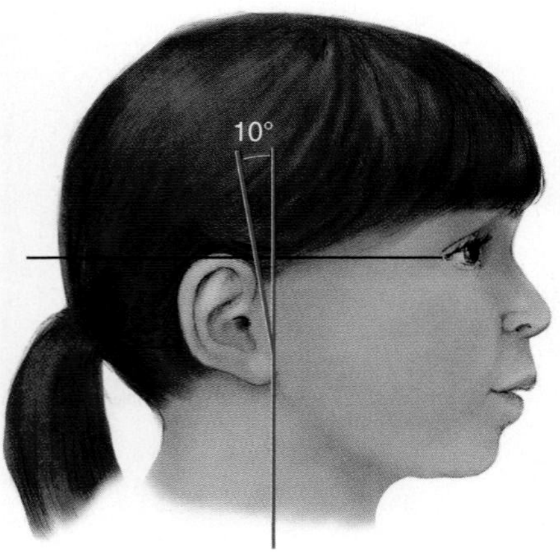

Normal alignment

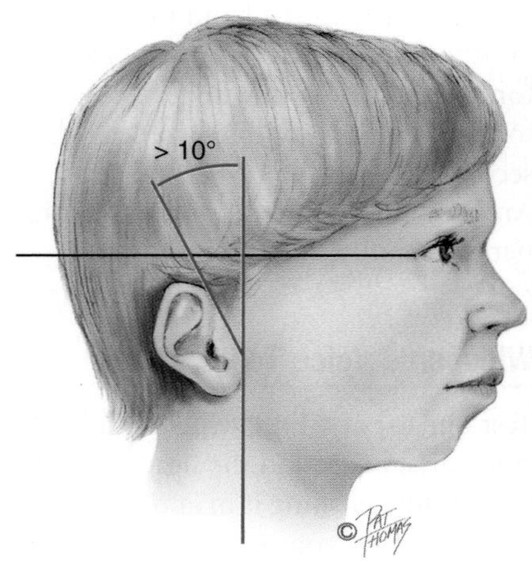

Low-set ears and deviation in alignment

15-10

Otoscopic Examination. In addition to its place in the complete examination, eardrum assessment is mandatory for any infant or child requiring care for illness or fever. For the infant or young child, the timing of the otoscopic examination is best toward the end of the complete examination. Many young children protest vigorously during this procedure no matter how well you prepare, and it is difficult to re-establish cooperation afterward. Save the otoscopic examination until last.

To help prepare the child, let him or her hold your funny-looking "flashlight." You may wish to have the child look in the parent's ear as you hold the otoscope (Fig. 15-11).

Ear pain and ear rubbing are associated with acute OM, as are a cloudy, bulging eardrum and a distinctly red eardrum.[18]

Normal Range of Findings	Abnormal Findings

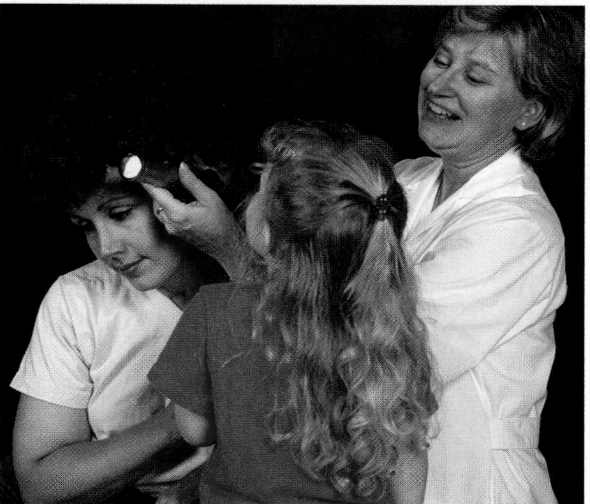

15-11

Positioning of the child is important. You need a clear view of the canal. Avoid harsh restraint, but you must protect the eardrum from injury in case of sudden head movement. Enlist the aid of a cooperative parent. Prop an infant upright against the parent's chest or shoulder, with the parent's arm around the upper part of the head (Fig. 15-12). A toddler can be held in the parent's lap with his or her arms gently secured. As you pull down on the pinna, gently push in on the child's tragus as a lead-in to inserting the speculum tip. This sometimes helps avoid the startling poke of the speculum tip.

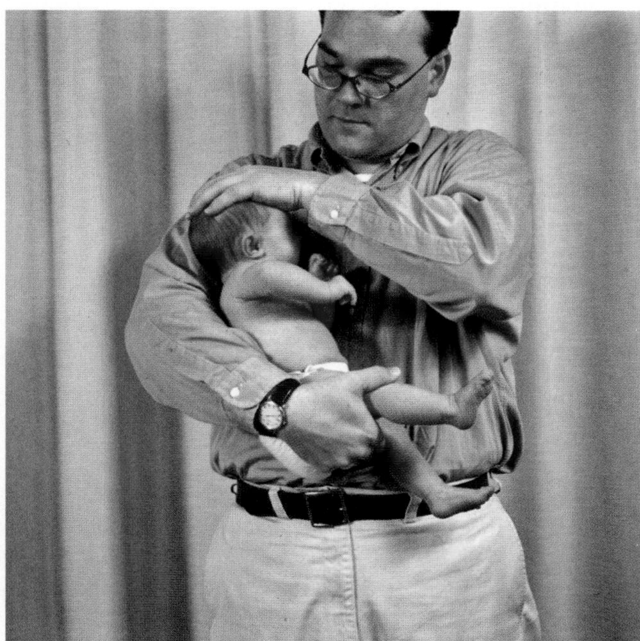

15-12

Remember to pull the pinna straight down on an infant or a child younger than 3 years. This method will match the slope of the ear canal (Fig. 15-13).

Normal Range of Findings	Abnormal Findings

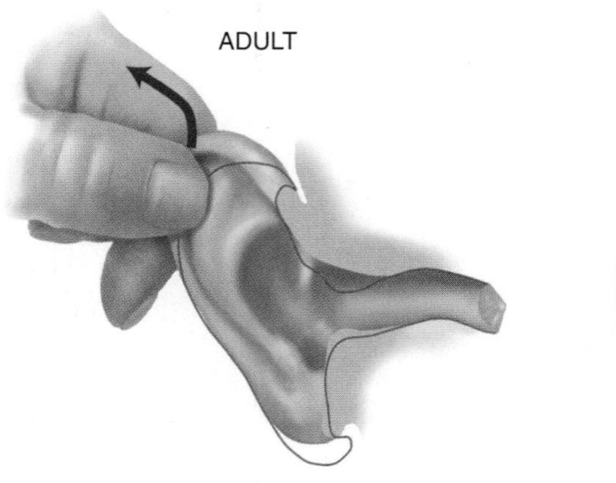

Adult—pull pinna up and back

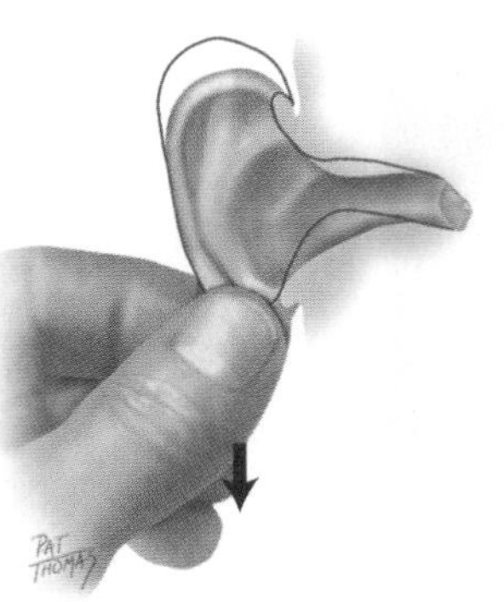

Infant/child under 3—pull pinna straight down

15-13

At birth, the patency of the ear canal is determined but the otoscopic examination is not performed because the canal is filled with amniotic fluid and vernix caseosa. After a few days, the TM is examined. During the first few days, the TM often looks thickened and opaque. It may look "injected" and have a mild redness from increased vascularity. The eardrum also looks injected in infants after crying.

Atresia—absence or closure of the ear canal.

The position of the eardrum is more horizontal in the neonate, making it more difficult to see completely and harder to differentiate from the canal wall. By 1 month of age, the drum is in the oblique (more vertical) position as in the older child and examination is a bit easier.

When examining an infant or young child, a pneumatic bulb attachment enables you to direct a light puff of air toward the drum to assess **vibratility** (Fig. 15-14). For a secure seal, choose the largest speculum that will fit in the ear canal without causing pain. A rubber tip on the end of the speculum gives a better seal. Give a small pump to the bulb (positive pressure), then release the bulb (negative pressure). Normally the tympanic membrane moves inward with a slight puff and outward with a slight release.

An abnormal response is no movement. Drum hypomobility indicates effusion or a high vacuum in the middle ear. For the newborn's first 6 weeks, drum immobility is the best indicator of middle ear infection.

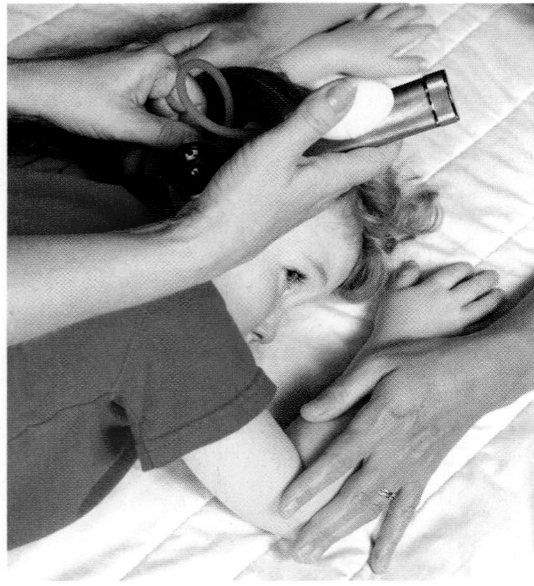

15-14

Normal Range of Findings	Abnormal Findings
Normally the TM is intact. In a child being treated for chronic otitis media, you may note the presence of a tympanostomy tube in the central part of the eardrum. This is inserted surgically to equalize pressure and drain secretions.	Chronic OM relieved by tympanostomy tubes (see Table 15-5).
Finally, although the condition is not normal, it is not uncommon to note a foreign body in a child's canal, such as a small stone or a bead.	Foreign body (see Table 15-3).

Test Hearing Acuity. Use the developmental milestones mentioned in this section to assess hearing in an infant. Also, attend to the parents' concern over the infant's inability to hear; their assessment is usually well founded.

The room should be silent and the baby contented. Make a loud, sudden noise (hand clap or squeeze toy) out of the baby's peripheral range of vision of about 30 cm (12 in). You may need to repeat a few times, but you should note these responses:

- Newborn—startle (Moro) reflex, acoustic blink reflex
- 3 to 4 months—acoustic blink reflex, infant stops movement and appears to "listen," halts sucking, quiets if crying, cries if quiet
- 6 to 8 months—infant turns head to localize sound, responds to own name
- Preschool and school-age child—child must be screened with audiometry

Absence of alerting behavior may indicate congenital deafness.

Failure to localize sound.

No intelligible speech by age 2 years.

Note that a young child may be unaware of a hearing loss because the child does not know how one "ought" to hear. Note these behavioral manifestations of hearing loss:

1. The child is inattentive in casual conversation.
2. The child reacts more to movement and facial expression than to sound.
3. The child's facial expression is strained or puzzled.
4. The child frequently asks to have statements repeated.
5. The child confuses words that sound alike.
6. The child has an accompanying speech problem: speech is monotonous or garbled; the child mispronounces or omits sounds.
7. The child appears shy and withdrawn and "lives in a world of his or her own."
8. The child frequently complains of earaches.
9. The child hears better at times when the environment is more conducive.

The Aging Adult

An aging adult may have pendulous earlobes with linear wrinkling because of loss of elasticity of the pinna. Coarse, wiry hairs may be present at the opening of the ear canal. During otoscopy, the eardrum normally may be whiter in color and more opaque, duller than in the younger adult. It also may look thickened.

A high-tone frequency hearing loss is apparent for those affected with presbycusis, the hearing loss that occurs with aging. This condition is revealed in difficulty hearing whispered words in the voice test and in difficulty hearing consonants during conversational speech. The aging adult feels that "people are mumbling" and feels isolated in family or friendship groups.

PROMOTING A HEALTHY LIFESTYLE

Earbuds and the Increasing Prevalence of Hearing Loss in Adolescents

Today, there is a growing body of evidence that suggests users of portable media players (PMP) and earbuds are at risk for noise-induced hearing loss (NIHL) (Fligor, 2009). Unlike earphones, which are placed over the ear, earbuds are placed directly in the ear canal, resulting in the sound being placed closer to the eardrum. Further, because the sound is digital, there is virtually no distortion, no matter how loud one turns up the volume. And probably most significant, because digital music players can hold thousands of songs and can play for hours without recharging, users tend to listen continuously for hours at a time. Although people know not to look directly into the sun because the intense rays will damage their eyes, they do not seem to realize that blasting their ears with increased sound intensity is going to do damage, too. There is a certain irony when you see young people donning sunglasses and earbuds. Recently, the *Journal of the American Medical Association* (JAMA) published findings indicating the prevalence of hearing loss among U.S. adolescents has increased by 30% from early findings (Shargorodsky, Curhan, Curhan, et al., 2010).

NIHL occurs slowly and can go unnoticed until it is quite extensive, so early prevention is the key. The risk for NIHL increases as sound is played louder and for longer durations. For this reason, current research proposes the 60-60 rule. The 60-60 rule recommends that individuals use their digital music players and earbuds for no more than 60 minutes a day at levels below 60% of maximum volume. Many experts are suggesting that digital music players be designed to prevent the playing of music above 90 dB, about 60% of the maximum volume (<120 dB) of the typical digital music player today. Simply put, it means dialing down the volume to a "6" or lower and taking a break at least every hour. Other ways to avoid hearing loss include using larger headphones that rest over the ear opening or noise-canceling headphones that eliminate background noise so that listeners do not have to increase the volume so high. It is often difficult to explain this to young people who abound with youthful optimism and tend to not worry about future damage. However, listening with earbuds boosts sound signals by as much as 6 to 9 dB, about the difference between the sound of a vacuum cleaner and a motorcycle.

The decibel scale is logarithmic. In other words, 40 dB is 100 times as intense as 20 dB. Normal conversation takes place around 60 dB, whereas a chainsaw typically records at 100 dB and a rock concert at 120 dB. Federal government minimum safety standards states that workers should not be exposed to noise above 90 dB for more than 8 hours and for every 5-dB increase above 90 dB, the allowed exposure time is cut in half. This means that the recommended safe duration for exposure to sound at 120 db is less than 8 minutes.

The House Ear Institute (HEI) is a nonprofit organization dedicated to advancing hearing science through research and education to improve quality of life. You can access their Facts from the HEI entitled *Teens and Noise-Induced Hearing Loss* at http://newsroom.hei.org/pr/hei/teens-and-noise-induced-hearing-loss-facts.aspx. The HEI is also the sponsor of the "It's How You Listen that Counts" campaign, which is targeted specifically at the younger generation. Information about this campaign can be found at www.earbud.org/index.html.

Resources

Fligor, B. J. (2009). Risk for noise-induced hearing loss from use of portable media players: a summary of evidence through 2008. *Perspectives on Audiology*, 5(1), 10-20.

Portnuff, C. D. F., & Fligor, B. J. (October 19, 2006). *Sound output levels of the iPod and other MP3 players: is there potential risk to hearing?* Paper presented at the NIHL in Children Conference, Cincinnati, OH.

Selvin, J. (2005). Play it loud and you may pay for it: 4 hearing loss. Website: *www.4hearingloss.com/archives/2005/09/play_it_loud_an.html.*

Shargorodsky, J. Curhan, S. G., Curhan, G. C., & Eavey, R., et al. (2010). Change in prevalence of hearing loss in U.S. adolescents. *Journal of the American Medical Association*, 304(7), 772-778.

Vogel, I., Verschuure, H., van der Ploeg, C. P., et al. (2009). Adolescents and MP3 players: too many risks, too few precautions. *Pediatrics*, 123(6), e953-e958. DOI:10.1542/peds.2008-3179.

DOCUMENTATION AND CRITICAL THINKING

Sample Charting

SUBJECTIVE

States hearing is good, no earaches, infections, discharge, hearing loss, tinnitus, or vertigo.

OBJECTIVE

Pinna: Skin intact with no masses, lesions, tenderness, or discharge.

Otoscope: External canals are clear with no redness, swelling, lesions, foreign body, or discharge. Both tympanic membranes are pearly gray in color, with light reflex and landmarks intact, no perforations.

Hearing: Responds appropriately to conversation. Whispered words heard bilaterally.

ASSESSMENT

Healthy ear structures
Hearing accurate

Focused Assessment: Clinical Case Study 1

Jamal K. is a 9-month-old Black infant who is brought to the clinic by his mother because he "feels hot and was up crying all night."

History: Jamal is the third child of Mr. and Mrs. K. Mrs. K. received regular prenatal care. Jamal was born at 37 weeks' gestation; labor and delivery were uncomplicated. Jamal weighed 3200 g at birth and was discharged 2 days after delivery. Jamal has been bottle-fed, with solids introduced at 5 months. Well-baby care has been regular; immunizations are up to date. Jamal has had two prior episodes of otitis media, no other illnesses.

Social History: Jamal lives with his family in a two-bedroom apartment over their grocery store and shares a bedroom with a 4-year-old brother and a 2-year-old brother. Mr. K. works full time in their grocery store; Mrs. K. provides childcare in her own home for her children and for her sister's two young children. Both parents smoke cigarettes, 1 to 2 packs per day.

SUBJECTIVE

1 day PTA—Mrs. K. put Jamal down for nap with a bottle of juice, as is usual for her. Jamal woke up in the middle of the nap crying furiously. Quieted somewhat when held upright but still fussy. Took juice from bottle, refused solid baby food. Temperature 38° C rectally. Crying and fussy all night. Mrs. K. has given no medications to Jamal.

OBJECTIVE

Vital signs: Temp 38.4° C (tympanic), pulse 152, resp 36, Wt. 9.2 kg (50th percentile), Ht. 29 in. (75th percentile).
General: Alert, active, crying, and fussy. Developmentally appropriate for age.
Skin: Warm and dry, no rashes or lesions.
Head: Anterior fontanel flat, 1×1.5 cm; posterior fontanel closed.
Eyes: No exudate, conjunctivae clear, sclerae white, red reflex present bilaterally.
Ears: Both tympanic membranes dull red and bulging, no light reflex, no mobility on pneumatic otoscopy.
Mouth/throat: Oral mucosa pink, no lesions or exudate, tonsils 1+.
Neck: Supple, no lymphadenopathy.
Heart: Regular rate and rhythm, no murmurs.
Lungs: Breath sounds clear and equal bilaterally, unlabored.
Abdomen: Bowel sounds present, abdomen soft, nontender.

ASSESSMENT

Acute otitis media, both ears
Pain R/T inflammation in TMs
Risk for ear infection injury R/T supine bottle-feeding, group childcare, secondhand smoke
Deficient knowledge (parents) R/T risk factors for otitis media

Focused Assessment: Clinical Case Study 2

Todd R. is a 15-year-old high school student who comes to the health center to seek care for "cough off and on all winter and earache since last night."

SUBJECTIVE

6 weeks PTA—nonproductive cough throughout day, no fever, no nasal congestion, no chest soreness. Todd's father gave him an over-the-counter decongestant, which helped, but cough continued off/on since. Does not smoke.

1 day PTA—intermittent cough continues, nasal congestion and thick white mucus. Also earache R ear, treated self with heating pad, pain unrelieved. Pain is moderate, not deep and throbbing. Says R ear feels full, "hollow headed," voices sound muffled and far away, switches telephone to L ear to talk. No sore throat, no fever, no chest congestion or soreness.

OBJECTIVE

Vital signs: T 37° C oral, P 76, BP 106/72.
Ears: L ear, canal, TM normal. R ear and canal normal, R TM retracted, with multiple air bubbles, drum color is yellow/amber. No sinus tenderness.
Nose: Turbinates bright red and swollen, mucopurulent discharge.
Throat: Not reddened, tonsils 1+.
Neck: One R anterior cervical node enlarged, firm, movable, tender. All others not palpable.
Lungs: Breath sounds clear to auscultation, resonant to percussion throughout.
Hearing: Weber lateralizes to R.

ASSESSMENT

Serous otitis media, R ear, with mild URI
Transient conductive hearing loss
Disturbed sensory perception (auditory) R/T excessive fluid in middle ear
Pain R/T middle ear pressure

Focused Assessment: Clinical Case Study 3

Emma S., 78 years old, has a medical diagnosis of angina pectoris, which has responded to nitroglycerin PRN and periods of rest between activity. She has been independent in her own home, is coping well with activity restrictions through help from neighbors and family. Now hospitalized for evaluation of acute chest pain episode; MI has been ruled out, pain diagnosed as anginal, to be released to own home with a beta-blocking medication and nitroglycerin PRN.

Just before this hospitalization, Mrs. S. received a hearing aid after evaluation by audiologist at senior center. Mrs. S. was born in Germany, immigrated to U.S. at age 5 years, considers English her primary language.

SUBJECTIVE

Since this hospitalization, feels "irritable and nervous." Relates this to worry about heart and also, "I get so mixed up in here, this room is so strange, and I just can't hear the nurses. They talk like cavemen, 'oo-i-ee-uou.'" Tried using her new hearing aid but no relief. "It just kept screeching in my ear, and it made the monitor beep so loud it drove me crazy." States no tinnitus, no vertigo.

OBJECTIVE

Ears: Pinna with elongated lobes, but no tenderness to palpation, no discharge, no masses or lesions. Both canals clear of cerumen. Both TM appear gray-white, slightly opaque and dull, although all landmarks visible. No perforation.
Hearing: Difficulty hearing room conversation. Unable to hear whispered voice bilaterally.

ASSESSMENT

Chest pain/angina pectoris
Deficient knowledge R/T lack of teaching on hearing aid
Disturbed sensory perception (auditory) R/T effects of aging
Anxiety R/T change in cardiovascular health status and inability to communicate effectively

ABNORMAL FINDINGS

TABLE 15-1 Abnormalities of the External Ear

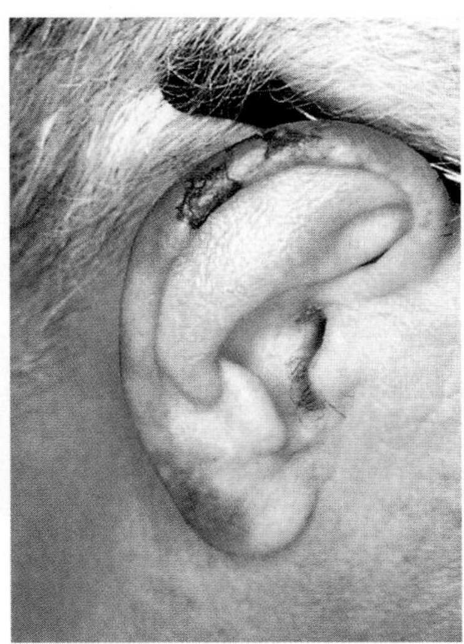

Frostbite

Reddish blue discoloration and swelling of auricle after exposure to extreme cold. Vesicles or bullae may develop, the person feels pain and tenderness, and ear necrosis may ensue.

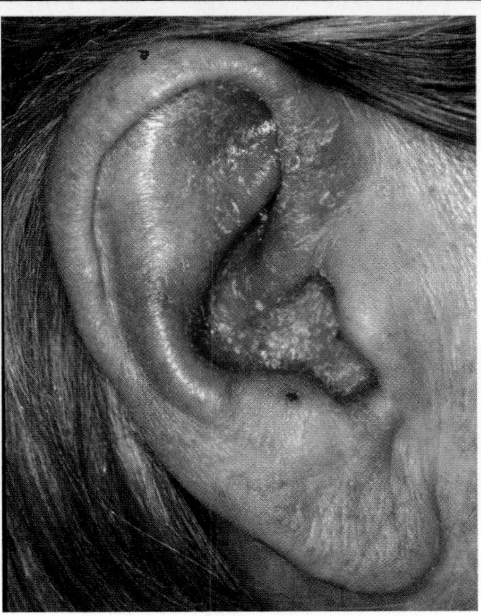

Otitis Externa (Swimmer's Ear)

An infection of the outer ear, with severe painful movement of the pinna and tragus, redness and swelling of pinna and canal, scanty purulent discharge, scaling, itching, fever, and enlarged tender regional lymph nodes. Hearing is normal or slightly diminished. More common in hot, humid weather. Swimming causes canal to become waterlogged and swell; skinfolds are set up for infection. Prevent by using rubbing alcohol or 2% acetic acid eardrops after every swim.

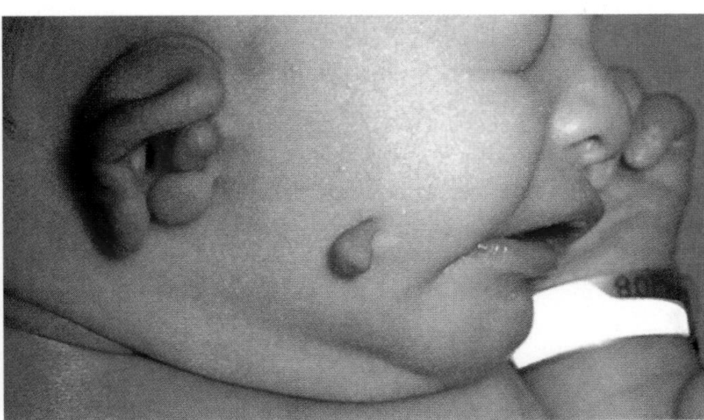

Branchial Remnant and Ear Deformity

A facial remnant or leftover of the embryologic branchial arch usually appears as a skin tag; in this case, one containing cartilage. They occur most often in the preauricular area, in front of the tragus. When bilateral, there is increased risk for renal anomalies.

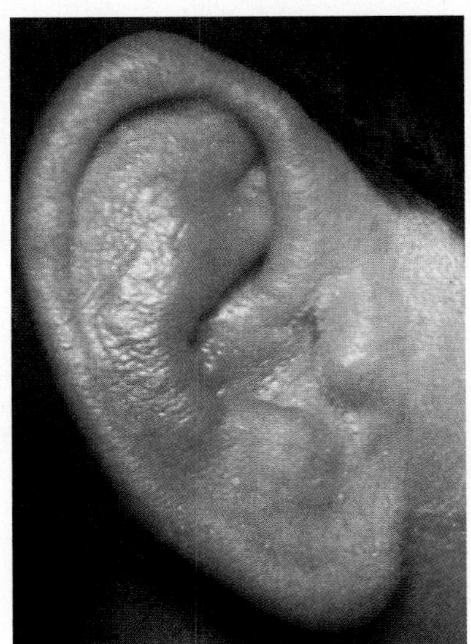

Cellulitis

Inflammation of loose, subcutaneous connective tissue. Shows as thickening and induration of auricle with distorted contours.

TABLE 15-2 Lumps and Lesions on the Ear

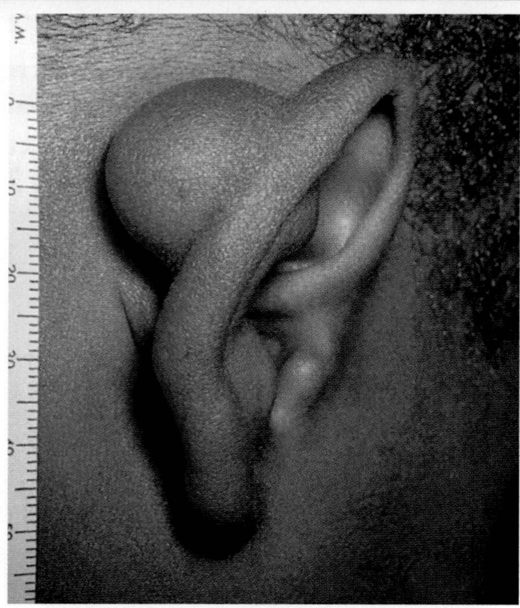

Sebaceous Cyst

Location is commonly behind lobule, in the postauricular fold. A nodule with central black punctum indicates blocked sebaceous gland. It is filled with waxy sebaceous material and is painful if it becomes infected. Often are multiple.

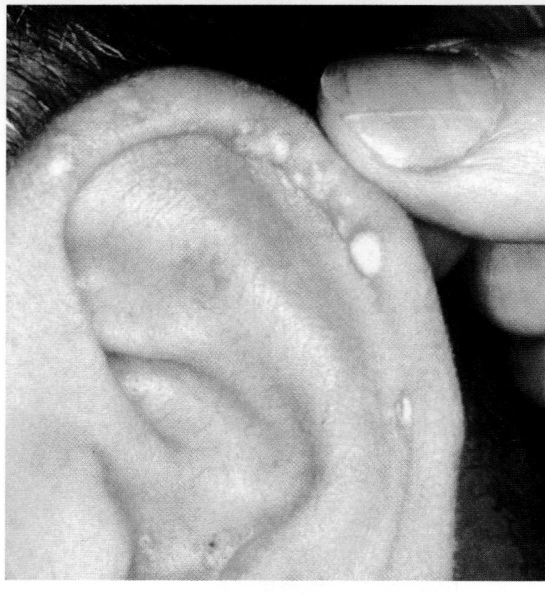

Tophi

Small, whitish yellow, hard, nontender nodules in or near helix or antihelix; contain greasy, chalky material of uric acid crystals and are a sign of gout.

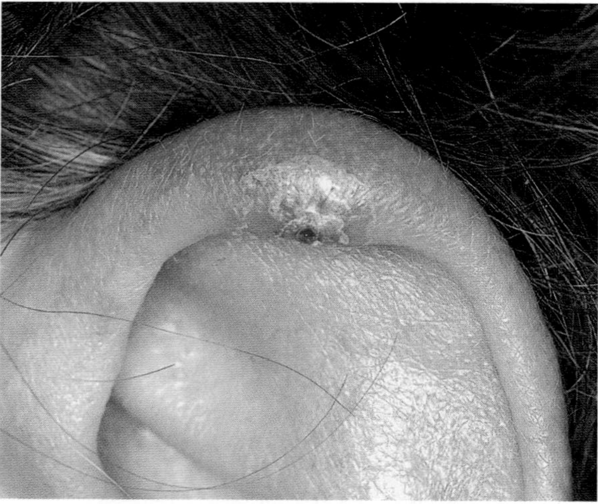

◀ Chondrodermatitis Nodularis Helicus

Painful nodules develop on the rim of the helix (where there is no cushioning subcutaneous tissue) as a result of repetitive mechanical pressure or environmental trauma (sunlight). They are small, indurated, dull red, poorly defined, and very painful.

TABLE 15-2 Lumps and Lesions on the Ear—cont'd

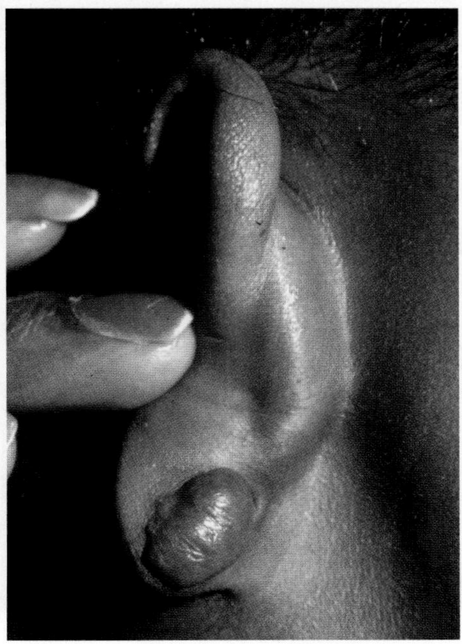

Keloid

Overgrowth of scar tissue, which invades original site of trauma. It is more common in dark-skinned people, although it also occurs in whites. In the ear it is most common at lobule at the site of a pierced ear. Overgrowth shown here is unusually large.

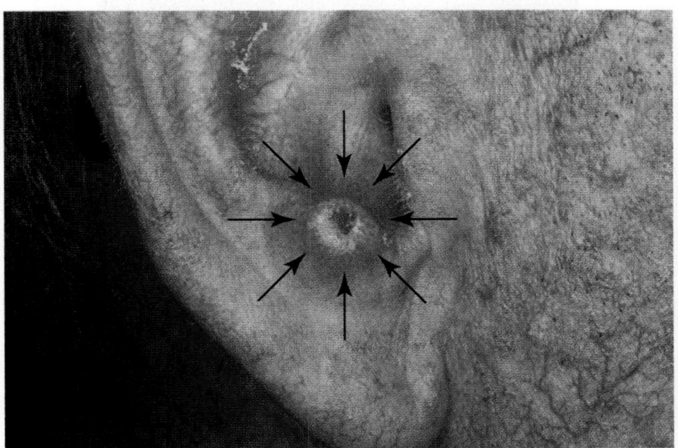

Carcinoma

Ulcerated, crusted nodule with indurated base that fails to heal. Bleeds intermittently. Must refer for biopsy. Usually occurs on the superior rim of the pinna, which has the most sun exposure. May occur also in ear canal and show chronic discharge that is either serosanguineous or bloody.

ABNORMAL FINDINGS
FOR ADVANCED PRACTICE

TABLE 15-3 Abnormalities in the Ear Canal

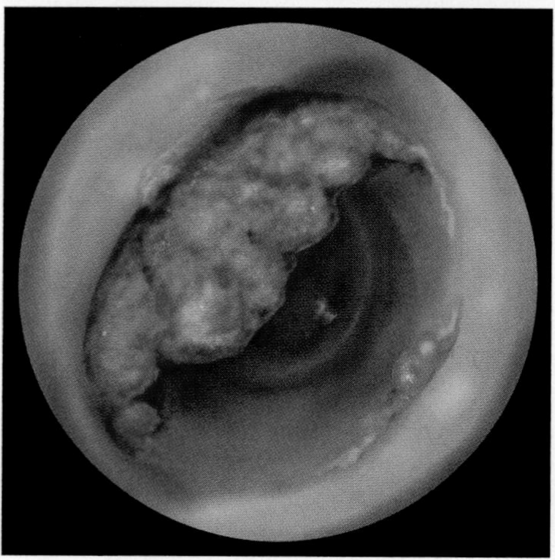

Excessive Cerumen

Excessive cerumen is produced or is impacted because of narrow, tortuous canal or poor cleaning method. May show as round ball partially obscuring drum or totally occluding canal. Even when canal is 90% to 95% blocked, hearing stays normal. But when last 5% to 10% is totally occluded (when cerumen expands after swimming or showering), person has ear fullness and sudden hearing loss.

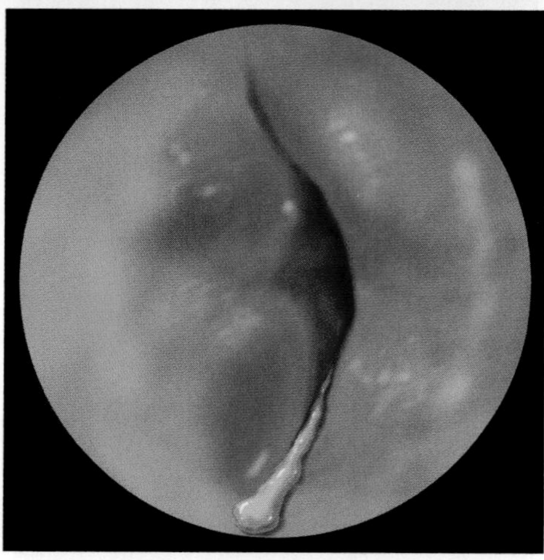

Otitis Externa

Severe swelling of canal, inflammation, tenderness. Here, canal lumen is narrowed to one-fourth normal size. (See complete description in Table 15-1.)

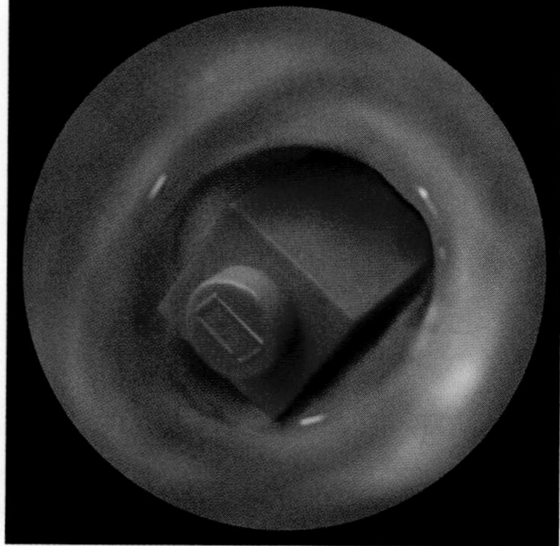

◀ Foreign Body

Usually it is children who place a foreign body in the ear (here, a toy completely occludes the canal), which is later noted on routine examination. Common objects are beans, corn, breakfast cereals, jewelry beads, small stones, sponge rubber. Cotton is most common in adults and becomes impacted from cotton-tipped applicators. A trapped live insect is uncommon but makes the person especially frantic.

TABLE 15-3 Abnormalities in the Ear Canal—cont'd

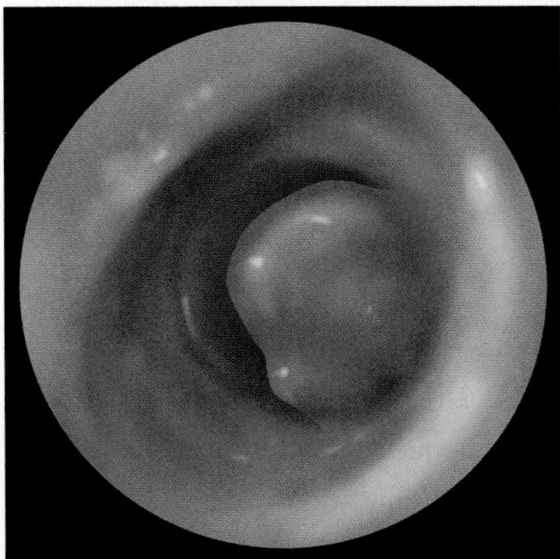

Osteoma

Single, stony hard, rounded nodule that obscures the drum; nontender; overlying skin appears normal. Attached to inner third, the bony part, of canal. Benign, but refer for removal.

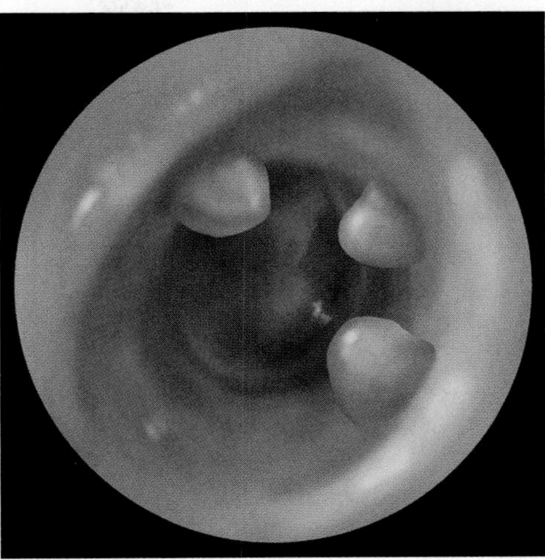

Exostosis

More common than osteoma. Small, bony hard, rounded nodules of hypertrophic bone, covered with normal epithelium. They arise near the drum but usually do not obstruct the view of the drum. They are usually multiple and bilateral. They may occur more frequently in cold-water swimmers. The condition needs no treatment, although it may cause accumulation of cerumen, which blocks the canal.

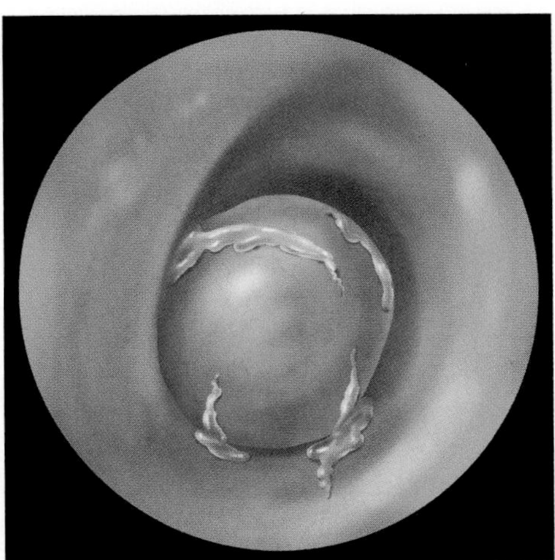

Polyp

Arises in canal from granulomatous or mucosal tissue; redder than surrounding skin and bleeds easily; bathed in foul, purulent discharge; indicates chronic ear disease. Benign, but refer for excision.

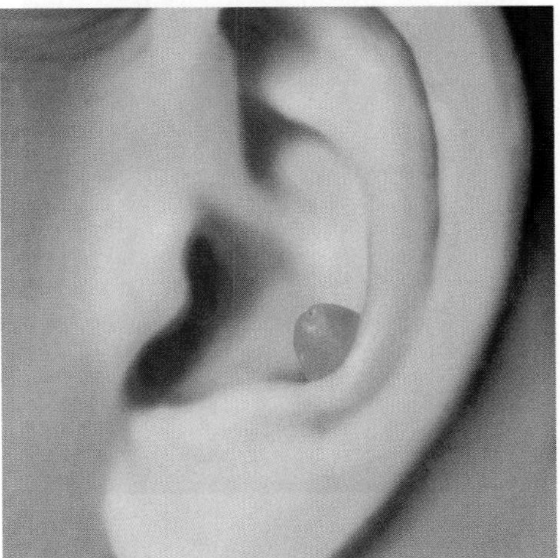

Furuncle

Exquisitely painful, reddened, infected hair follicle. It may occur on the tragus on the cartilaginous part of ear canal. Regional lymphadenopathy often accompanies a furuncle.

TABLE 15-4 Abnormal Views Seen on Otoscopy

Appearance of Eardrum	Indicates	Suggested Condition
Yellow-amber color	Serum or pus	Serous otitis media or chronic otitis media
Prominent landmarks	Retraction of drum	Negative pressure in middle ear from an obstructed eustachian tube
Air/fluid level or air bubbles	Serous fluid	Serous otitis media
Absent or distorted light reflex	Bulging of eardrum	Acute otitis media
Bright red color	Infection in middle ear	Acute purulent otitis media
Blue or dark red color	Blood behind drum	Trauma, skull fracture
Dark oval areas	Perforation	Drum rupture
White dense areas	Scarring	Sequelae of infections
Diminished or absent landmarks	Thickened drum	Chronic otitis media
Black or white dots on drum or canal	Colony of growth	Fungal infection

From Sherman, J. L., Fields, S. K. (1988). *Guide to patient evaluation* (5th ed.). New York: Medical Examination Publishing. Reprinted by permission of Elsevier Inc.

TABLE 15-5 Abnormal Tympanic Membranes

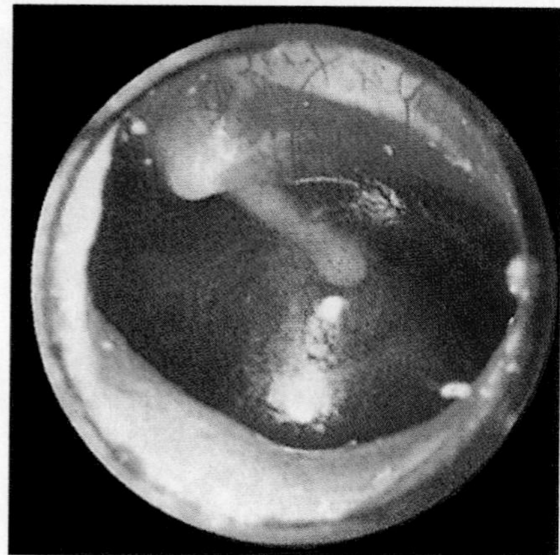

Retracted Drum

Landmarks look more prominent and well defined. Malleus handle looks shorter and more horizontal than normal. Short process is very prominent. Light reflex is absent or distorted. The drum is dull and lusterless and does not move. These signs indicate negative pressure and middle ear vacuum from obstructed eustachian tube and serous otitis media.

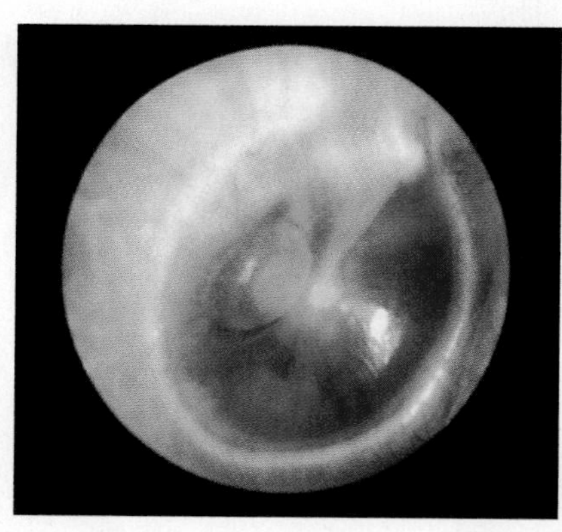

Otitis Media with Effusion (OME)

An amber-yellow drum suggests serum in middle ear that transudates to relieve negative pressure from the blocked eustachian tube. You may note an air/fluid level with fine black dividing line or air bubbles visible behind drum. Symptoms are feeling of fullness, transient hearing loss, popping sound with swallowing. Also called *serous otitis media, glue ear.*

TABLE 15-5 Abnormal Tympanic Membranes—cont'd

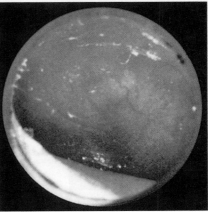

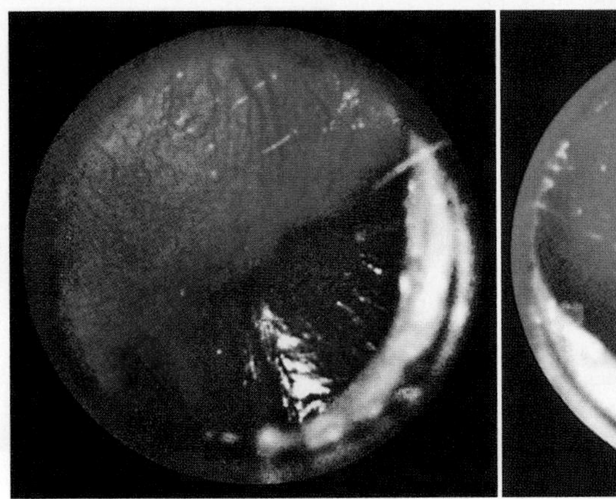

Early stage Later stage

Acute (Purulent) Otitis Media

This results when the middle ear fluid is infected. An absent light reflex from increasing middle ear pressure is an early sign. Redness and bulging are first noted in superior part of drum (pars flaccida), along with earache and fever. Then fiery red bulging of entire drum occurs along with deep throbbing pain, fever, and transient hearing loss. Pneumatic otoscopy reveals drum hypomobility.

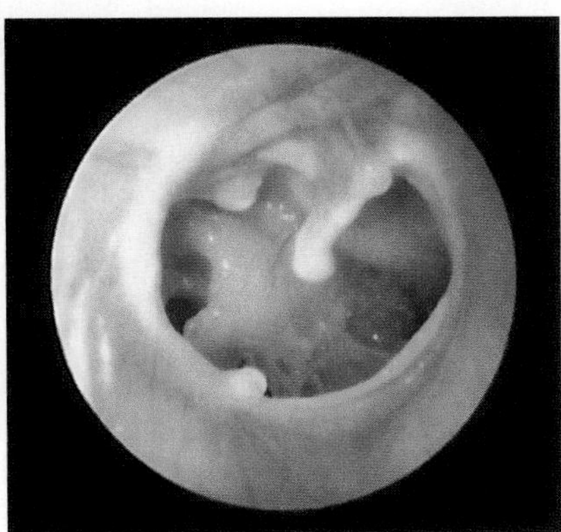

Perforation

If the acute otitis media is not treated, the drum may rupture from increased pressure. Perforations also occur from trauma (e.g., a slap on the ear). Usually the perforation appears as a round or oval darkened area on the drum, but in this photo, the perforation is very large. *Central* perforations occur in the pars tensa. *Marginal* perforations occur at the annulus. Marginal perforations are called *attic perforations* when they occur in the superior part of the drum, the pars flaccida.

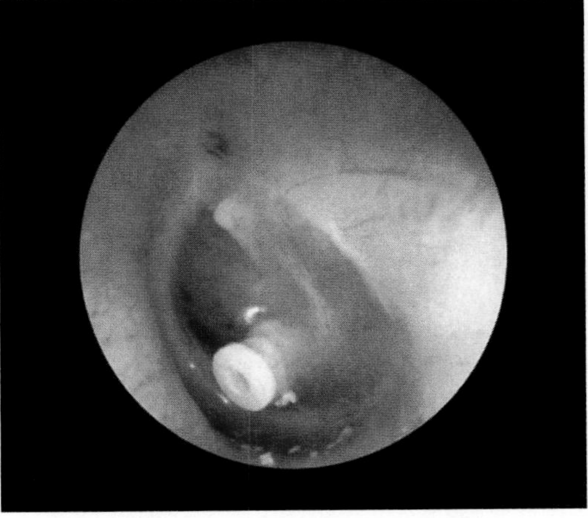

Insertion of Tympanostomy Tubes

Polyethylene tubes are inserted surgically into the eardrum to relieve middle ear pressure and promote drainage of chronic or recurrent middle ear infections. Number of acute infections tends to decrease because of improved aeration. Tubes extrude spontaneously in 12 to 18 months.

Reprinted from Fireman, P. (1995). *Atlas of allergies* (2nd ed.). St Louis: Mosby, p. 182.

Continued

TABLE 15-5 Abnormal Tympanic Membranes—cont'd

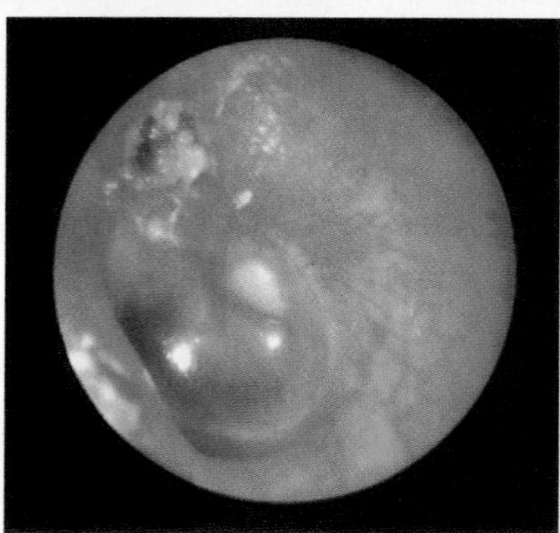

Cholesteatoma

An overgrowth of epidermal tissue in the middle ear or temporal bone may result over the years after a marginal TM perforation. It has a pearly white, cheesy appearance. Growth of cholesteatoma can erode bone and produce hearing loss. Early signs include otorrhea, unilateral conductive hearing loss, tinnitus.

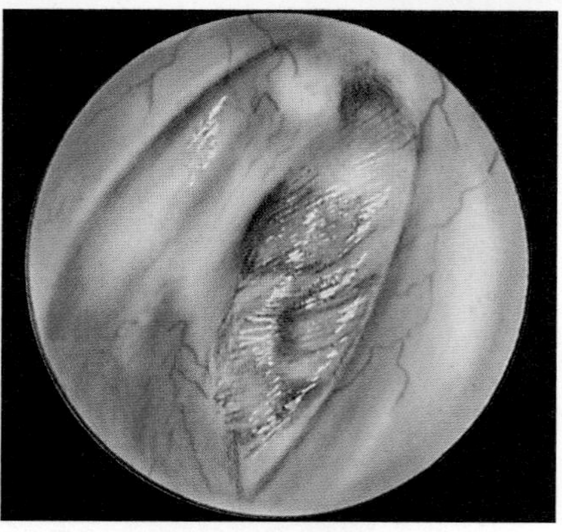

Scarred Drum

Dense white patches on the eardrum are sequelae of repeated ear infections. They do not necessarily affect hearing.

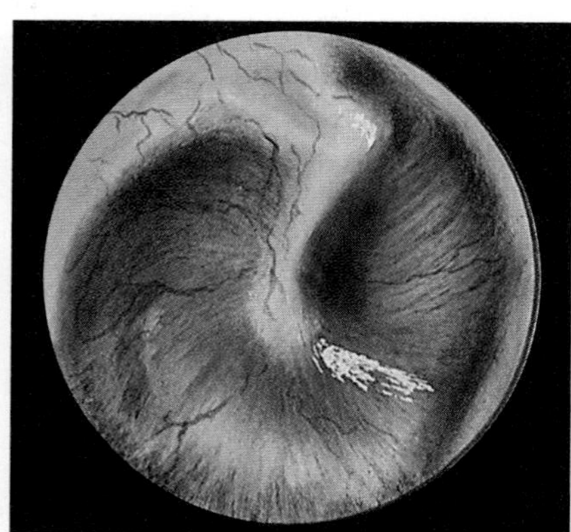

Blue Drum (Hemotympanum)

This indicates blood in the middle ear, as in trauma resulting in skull fracture.

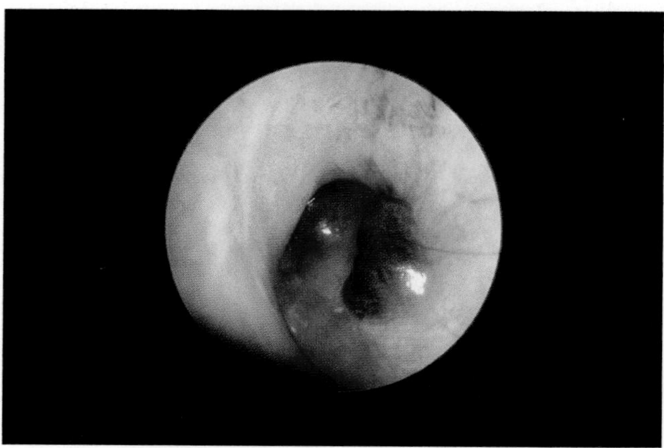

Bullous Myringitis

Small vesicles containing blood on the drum; accompany mycoplasma pneumonia and virus infections. May have blood-tinged discharge and severe otalgia.

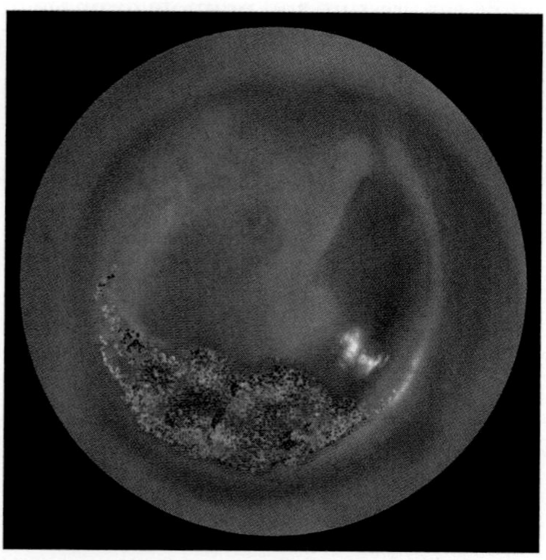

◀ Fungal Infection (Otomycosis)

Colony of black or white dots on drum or canal wall suggests a yeast or fungal infection.

BIBLIOGRAPHY

1. Askin, D. F. (2009). Physical assessment of the newborn: minor congenital anomalies. *Nursing for Women's Health, 13*(2), 140-149.
2. Bagai, A., Thavendiranathan, P., & Detsky, A. (2006). Does this patient have hearing impairment? *JAMA: Journal of the American Medical Association, 29,* 416-428.
3. Brook, I., & Gober, A. E. (2008). Recovery of potential pathogens in the nasopharynx of healthy and otitis media–prone children and their smoking and nonsmoking parents. *Annals of Otology, Rhinology, and Laryngology, 117*(10), 727-730.
4. Carlson, L. (2005). Otitis media: new information on an old disease. *Nurse Practitioner, 30,* 31-43.
5. Chantry, C., Howard, C., & Auinger, P. (2006). Full breastfeeding duration and associated decrease in respiratory tract infection in U.S. children. *Pediatrics, 117,* 425-432.
6. Daugherty, J. A. (2007). The latest buzz on tinnitus. *Nurse Practitioner, 32*(10), 42-47.
7. Ely, J. W., Hansen, M. R., & Clark, E. C. (2008). Diagnosis of ear pain. *American Family Physician, 77*(5), 621-628.
8. Feldman, H. M., & Paradise, J. L. (2009). OME and child development: rethinking management. *Contemporary Pediatrics, 26*(5), 40-47.
9. Fischer, T., Singer, A. J., & Chale, S. (2009). Observation option for acute otitis media in the emergency department. *Pediatric Emergency Care, 25*(9), 575-578.
10. Gates, G., & Mills, J. (2005). Presbycusis. *Lancet, 366,* 1111-1120.
11. Guest, J. F., Greener, M. J., Robinson, A. C., & Smith, A. F. (2004). Impacted cerumen: composition, production, epidemiology and management. *Quarterly Journal of Medicine, 97,* 477-488.
12. Holcomb, S. S. (2009). Get an earful of the new cerumen impaction guidelines. *Nurse Practitioner, 34*(4), 14-19.
13. Kane, R. L., Ouslander, J. G., & Abrass, I. E. (2009). *Essentials of clinical geriatrics* (6th ed.). New York: McGraw-Hill.
14. Kerschner, J. E. (2008). Bench and bedside advances in otitis media. *Current Opinion in Otolaryngology & Head and Neck Surgery, 16,* 543-547.
15. Lieu, J., & Feinstein, A. (2007). Effect of gestational and passive smoke exposure on ear infections in children. *Archives of Pediatrics & Adolescent Medicine, 156,* 147-154.
16. Morris, P. S., & Leach, A. J. (2009). Acute and chronic otitis media. *Pediatric Clinics of North America, 56,* 1383-1399.
17. Oncel, S. (2009). Acute otitis media in children. *Journal of Pediatric Infections, 3*(Suppl. 1), 39-42.
18. Singh, A., & Bond, B. L. (2006). Does this child have acute otitis media? *Annals of Emergency Medicine, 47, 113*-116.
19. Tomita, H., Yamada, K., Ghadami, M. et al. (2002). Mapping of the wet/dry locus to the pericentromeric regiôn of chromosome 16. *Lancet, 359(*9322), 2000-2002.
20. Wallhagen, M., Pettengill, E., & Whiteside, M. (2006). Sensory impairment in older adults. Part 1. Hearing loss. *American Journal of Nursing, 106,* 40-49.

Summary Checklist: Ear Examination

For a PDA-downloadable version, go to http://evolve.elsevier.com/Jarvis/.

1. **Inspect external ear:**
   Size and shape of auricle
   Position and alignment on head
   Note skin condition—color, lumps, lesions
   Check movement of auricle and tragus for tenderness
   Evaluate external auditory meatus—note size, swelling, redness, discharge, cerumen, lesions, foreign bodies
2. **Otoscopic examination:**
   External canal
   Cerumen, discharge, foreign bodies, lesions
   Redness or swelling of canal wall
3. **Inspect tympanic membrane:**
   Color and characteristics
   Note position (flat, bulging, retracted)
   Integrity of membrane
4. **Test hearing acuity:**
   Note behavioral response to conversational speech
   Whispered voice test

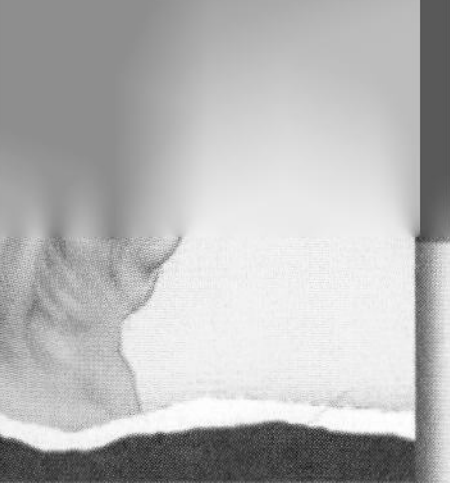

16

Nose, Mouth, and Throat

evolve WEBSITE

http://evolve.elsevier.com/Jarvis/

- Animations
- Audio Key Points
- Bedside Assessment Summary Checklist
- Health Promotion Guide
  Chewing Tobacco
- NCLEX Review Questions
- Physical Examination Summary Checklist
- Quick Assessment for Common Conditions
  Rhinovirus (Common Cold)
- Video—Assessment
  Nose, Mouth, and Throat

OUTLINE

Structure and Function, 351

Nose
Mouth
Throat

Subjective Data, 356

Health History Questions

Objective Data, 359

Preparation
The Nose
The Sinus Areas
The Mouth
The Throat

Documentation and Critical Thinking, 371

Abnormal Findings, 373

Abnormal Findings for Advanced Practice, 376

STRUCTURE AND FUNCTION

NOSE

The **nose** is the first segment of the respiratory system. It warms, moistens, and filters the inhaled air, and it is the sensory organ for smell. The external nose is shaped like a triangle with one side attached to the face (Fig. 16-1). On its leading edge, the superior part is the *bridge* and the free corner is the *tip.* The oval openings at the base of the triangle are the *nares;* just inside, each naris widens into the *vestibule.* The *columella* divides the two nares and is continuous inside

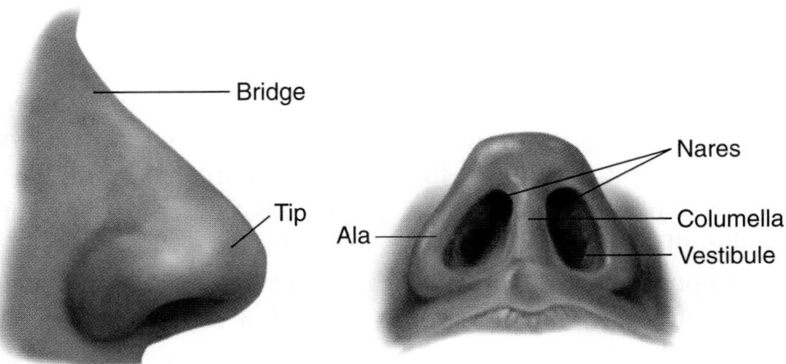

16-1 Nasal structures.

© Pat Thomas, 2006.

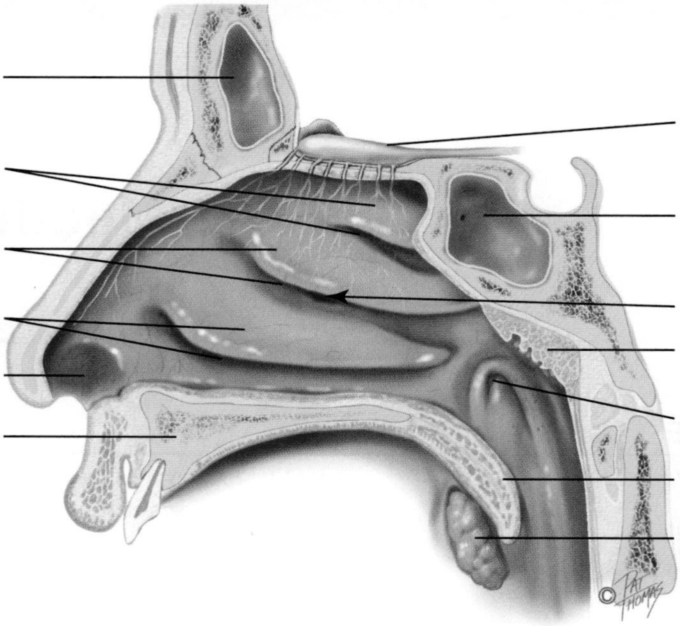

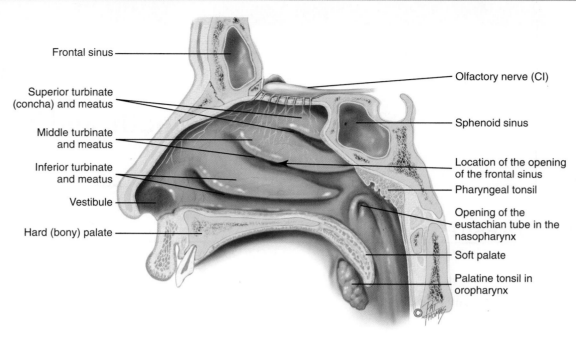

Frontal sinus
Superior turbinate (concha) and meatus
Middle turbinate and meatus
Inferior turbinate and meatus
Vestibule
Hard (bony) palate
Olfactory nerve (CI)
Sphenoid sinus
Location of the opening of the frontal sinus
Pharyngeal tonsil
Opening of the eustachian tube in the nasopharynx
Soft palate
Palatine tonsil in oropharynx

RIGHT LATERAL WALL - NASAL CAVITY

16-2

with the nasal septum. The *ala* is the lateral outside wing of the nose on either side. The upper third of the external nose is made up of bone; the rest is cartilage.

Inside, the **nasal cavity** is much larger than the external nose would indicate (Fig. 16-2). It extends back over the roof of the mouth. The anterior edge of the cavity is lined with numerous coarse nasal hairs, or vibrissae. The rest of the cavity is lined with a blanket of ciliated mucous membrane. The nasal hairs filter the coarsest matter from inhaled air, whereas the mucous blanket filters out dust and bacteria. Nasal mucosa appears redder than oral mucosa because of the rich blood supply present to warm the inhaled air.

The nasal cavity is divided medially by the **septum** into two slitlike air passages. The anterior part of the septum holds a rich vascular network, *Kiesselbach plexus,* the most common site of nosebleeds. In many people, the nasal septum is not absolutely straight and may deviate toward one passage.

The lateral walls of each nasal cavity contain three parallel bony projections—the superior, middle, and inferior **turbinates.** They increase the surface area so that more blood vessels and mucous membranes are available to warm, humidify, and filter the inhaled air. Underlying each turbinate is a cleft, the **meatus,** which is named for the turbinate above. The sinuses drain into the middle meatus, and tears from the nasolacrimal duct drain into the inferior meatus.

The olfactory receptors (hair cells) lie at the roof of the nasal cavity and in the upper one third of the septum. These receptors for smell merge into the olfactory nerve, cranial nerve I, which transmits to the temporal lobe of the brain. Although it is not necessary for human survival, the sense of smell adds to nutrition by enhancing the pleasure and taste of food.

The **paranasal sinuses** are air-filled pockets within the cranium (Fig. 16-3). They communicate with the nasal cavity and are lined with the same type of ciliated mucous membrane. They lighten the weight of the skull bones, serve as resonators for sound production, and provide mucus, which drains into the nasal cavity. The sinus openings are narrow and easily occluded, which may cause inflammation or sinusitis.

Two pairs of sinuses are accessible to examination: the **frontal** sinuses in the frontal bone above and medial to the orbits; and the **maxillary** sinuses in the maxilla (cheekbone) along the side walls of the nasal cavity. The other two sets are smaller and deeper: the **ethmoid** sinuses between the orbits; and the **sphenoid** sinuses deep within the skull in the sphenoid bone.

Only the maxillary and ethmoid sinuses are present at birth. The maxillary sinuses reach full size after all permanent teeth have erupted. The ethmoid sinuses grow rapidly between 6 and 8 years of age and after puberty. The frontal sinuses are absent at birth, are fairly well developed between 7 and 8 years of age, and reach full size after puberty. The sphenoid sinuses are minute at birth and develop after puberty.

MOUTH

The mouth is the first segment of the digestive system and an airway for the respiratory system. The **oral cavity** is a short passage bordered by the lips, palate, cheeks, and tongue. It contains the teeth and gums, tongue, and salivary glands (Fig. 16-4).

The lips are the anterior border of the oral cavity—the transition zone from the outer skin to the inner mucous membrane lining the oral cavity. The arching roof of the mouth is the palate; it is divided into two parts. The anterior

Frontal sinuses
Ethmoid sinuses
Maxillary sinus
ADULT
Ethmoid sinuses
Frontal sinus
Maxillary sinus
Sphenoid sinus
Frontal sinus
Ethmoid sinuses
Maxillary sinus
CHILD

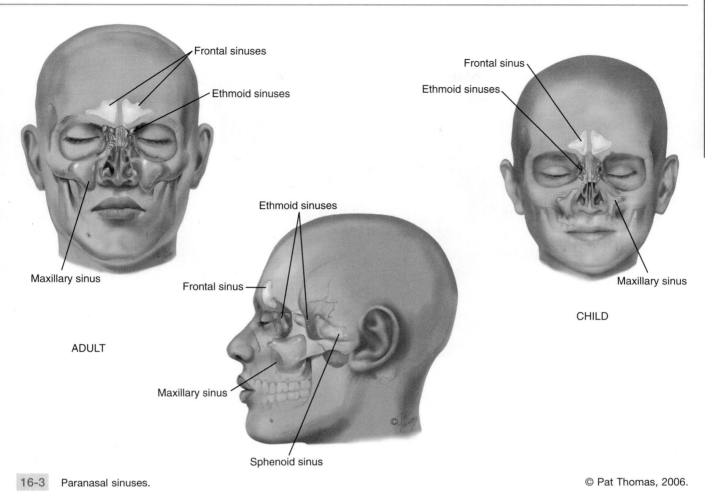

16-3 Paranasal sinuses.

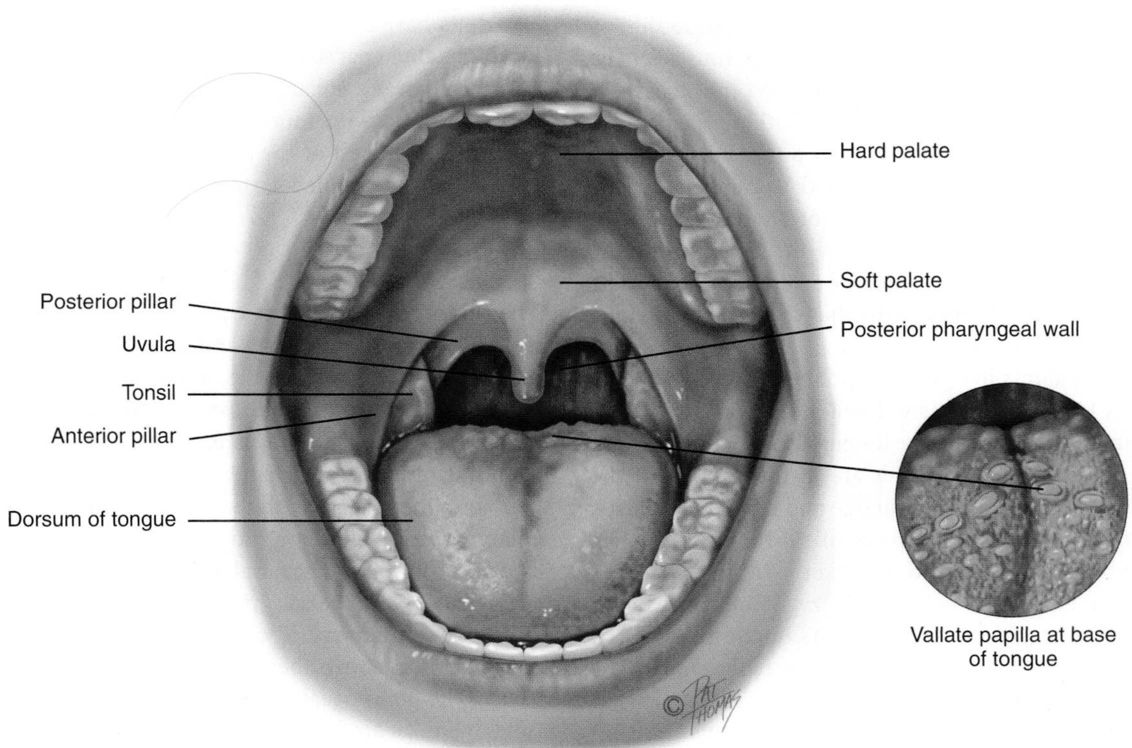

16-4

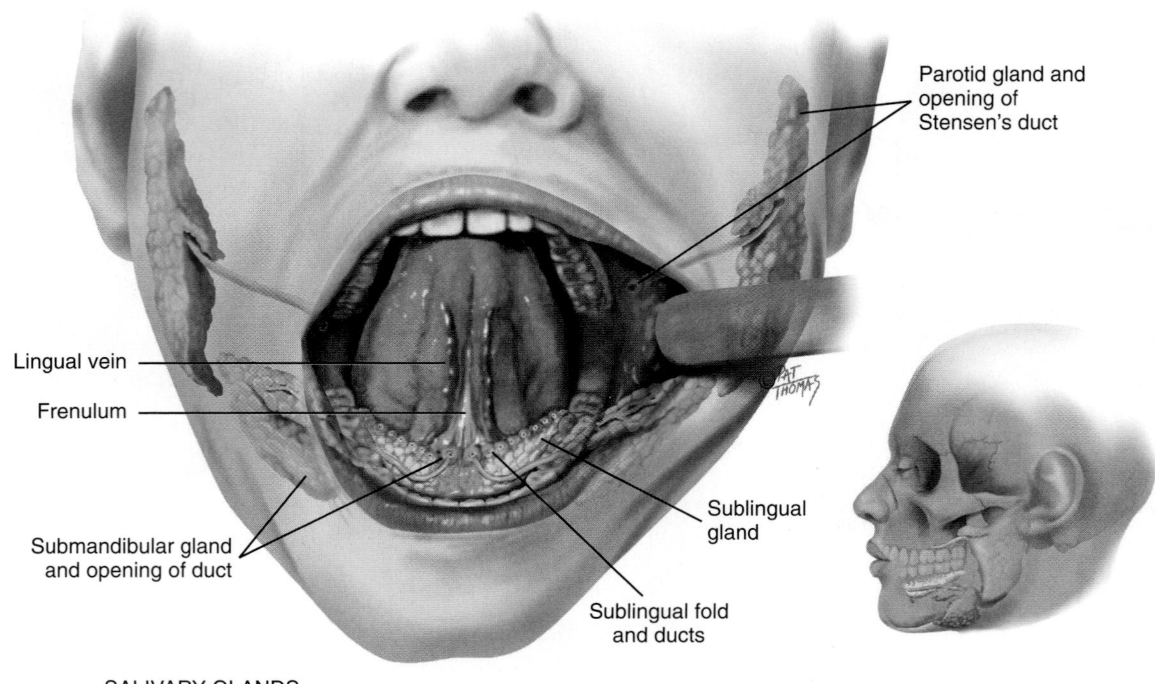

16-5

hard palate is made up of bone and is a whitish color. Posterior to this is the **soft palate,** an arch of muscle that is pinker in color and mobile. The **uvula** is the free projection hanging down from the middle of the soft palate. The cheeks are the side walls of the oral cavity.

The floor of the mouth consists of the horseshoe-shaped mandible bone, the tongue, and underlying muscles. The **tongue** is a mass of striated muscle arranged in a crosswise pattern so that it can change shape and position. The papillae are the rough, bumpy elevations on its dorsal surface. Note the larger vallate papillae in an inverted V shape across the posterior base of the tongue, and do not confuse them with abnormal growths. Underneath, the ventral surface of the tongue is smooth and shiny and has prominent veins. The **frenulum** is a midline fold of tissue that connects the tongue to the floor of the mouth.

The tongue's ability to change shape and position enhances its functions in mastication, swallowing, cleansing the teeth, and the formation of speech. The tongue also functions in taste sensation. Microscopic taste buds are in the papillae at the back and along the sides of the tongue and on the soft palate.

The mouth contains three pairs of salivary glands (Fig. 16-5). The largest, the **parotid** gland, lies within the cheeks in front of the ear extending from the zygomatic arch down to the angle of the jaw. Its duct, Stensen's duct, runs forward to open on the buccal mucosa opposite the second molar. The **submandibular** gland is the size of a walnut. It lies beneath the mandible at the angle of the jaw. Wharton's duct runs up and forward to the floor of the mouth and opens at either side of the frenulum. The smallest, the almond-shaped **sublingual** gland, lies within the floor of the mouth under the tongue. It has many small openings along the sublingual fold under the tongue.

The glands secrete saliva, the clear fluid that moistens and lubricates the food bolus, starts digestion, and cleans and protects the mucosa.

Adults have 32 **permanent** teeth—16 in each arch. Each tooth has three parts: the crown, the neck, and the root. The gums (gingivae) collar the teeth. They are thick, fibrous tissues covered with mucous membrane. The gums are different from the rest of the oral mucosa because of their pale pink color and stippled surface.

THROAT

The throat, or pharynx, is the area behind the mouth and nose. The **oropharynx** is separated from the mouth by a fold of tissue on each side, the anterior tonsillar pillar (see Fig. 16-4). Behind the folds are the **tonsils,** each a mass of lymphoid tissue. The tonsils are the same color as the surrounding mucous membrane, although they look more granular and their surface shows deep crypts. Tonsillar tissue enlarges during childhood until puberty and then involutes. The posterior pharyngeal wall is seen behind these structures. Some small blood vessels may show on it.

The **nasopharynx** is continuous with the oropharynx, although it is above the oropharynx and behind the nasal cavity. The pharyngeal tonsils (adenoids) and the eustachian tube openings are located here (see Fig. 16-2).

The oral cavity and throat have a rich lymphatic network. Review the lymph nodes and their drainage patterns in Chapter 13 and keep this in mind when evaluating the mouth.

DEVELOPMENTAL COMPETENCE

Infants and Children

In the infant, salivation starts at 3 months. The baby will drool for a few months before learning to swallow the saliva. This drooling does not herald the eruption of the first tooth, although many parents think it does.

The teeth, both sets, begin development in utero. Children have 20 **deciduous,** or temporary, teeth. These erupt between 6 months and 24 months of age. All 20 teeth should appear by 2½ years of age. The deciduous teeth are lost beginning at age 6 years through age 12 years. They are replaced by the permanent teeth, starting with the central incisors (Fig. 16-6). The permanent teeth appear earlier in girls than in boys, and they erupt earlier in Black children than in white children.

The nose develops during adolescence, along with other secondary sex characteristics. This growth starts at age 12 or 13 years, reaching full growth at age 16 years in females and age 18 years in males.

The Pregnant Woman

Nasal stuffiness and epistaxis may occur during pregnancy as a result of increased vascularity in the upper respiratory tract. Also, the gums may be hyperemic and softened and may bleed with normal toothbrushing. Contrary to superstitious folklore, pregnancy does not cause tooth decay or loss.

The Aging Adult

A gradual loss of subcutaneous fat starts during later adult years, making the nose appear more prominent in some people. The nasal hairs grow coarser and stiffer and may not filter the air as well. The hairs protrude and may cause itching and sneezing. Many older people clip these hairs, thinking them unsightly, but this practice can cause infection. The sense of smell may diminish because of a decrease in the number of olfactory nerve fibers. The decrease in the sensation of smell begins after age 60 years and continues progressively with age.

In the oral cavity, the soft tissues atrophy and the epithelium thins, especially in the cheeks and tongue. This results in loss of taste buds, with about an 80% reduction in taste functioning. Further impairments to taste include a decrease in salivary secretion that is needed to dissolve flavoring agents and the presence of upper dentures that cover secondary taste sites.

Atrophic tissues ulcerate easily, which increases risk for infections such as oral moniliasis. The risk for malignant oral lesions also increases.

Many dental changes occur with aging. The tooth surface is abraded. The gums begin to recede, and the teeth begin to erode at the gum line. A smooth V-shaped cavity forms around the neck of the tooth, exposing the nerve and making the tooth hypersensitive. Some tooth loss may occur from bone resorption (osteoporosis), which decreases the inner

UPPER DECIDUOUS	Erupt (months)	Shed (years)
Central incisor	6 to 8	6 to 7
Lateral incisior	8 to 11	8 to 9
Canine (cuspid)	16 to 20	11 to 12
First molar	10 to 16	10 to 11
Second molar	20 to 30	10 to 12

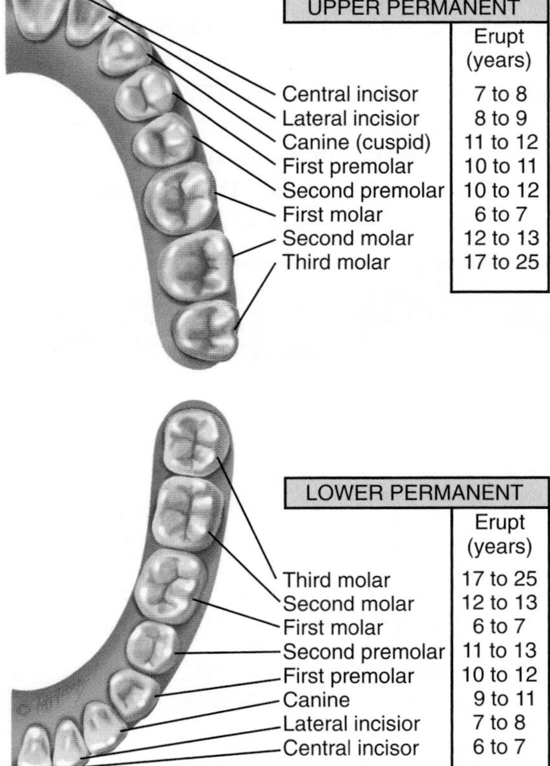

UPPER PERMANENT	Erupt (years)
Central incisor	7 to 8
Lateral incisior	8 to 9
Canine (cuspid)	11 to 12
First premolar	10 to 11
Second premolar	10 to 12
First molar	6 to 7
Second molar	12 to 13
Third molar	17 to 25

LOWER DECIDUOUS	Erupt (months)	Shed (years)
Second molar	20 to 30	11 to 13
First molar	10 to 16	10 to 12
Canine	16 to 20	9 to 11
Lateral incisior	7 to 10	7 to 8
Central incisor	5 to 7	5 to 6

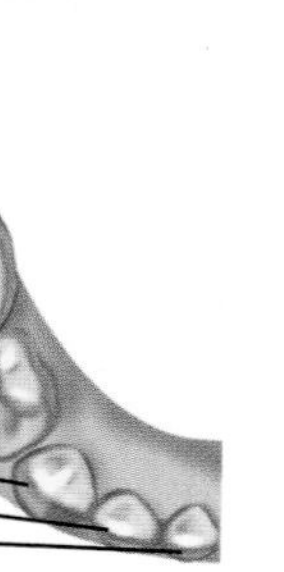

LOWER PERMANENT	Erupt (years)
Third molar	17 to 25
Second molar	12 to 13
First molar	6 to 7
Second premolar	11 to 13
First premolar	10 to 12
Canine	9 to 11
Lateral incisior	7 to 8
Central incisor	6 to 7

DECIDUOUS AND PERMANENT TEETH

16-6

tooth structure and its outer support. Natural tooth loss is exacerbated by years of inadequate dental care, decay, poor oral hygiene, and tobacco use.

If tooth loss occurs, the remaining teeth drift, causing **malocclusion.** The stress of chewing with malocclusing teeth causes further problems: (1) further tooth loss; (2) muscle imbalance from a mandible and maxilla now out of alignment, which produces muscle spasms, tenderness of muscles of mastication, and chronic headaches; and (3) stress on the temporomandibular joint, leading to osteoarthritis, pain, and inability to fully open the mouth.

A diminished sense of taste and smell decreases the aging person's interest in food and may contribute to malnutrition. Saliva production decreases; saliva acts as a solvent for food flavors and helps move food around the mouth. Decreased saliva also reduces the mouth's self-cleaning property. The major cause of decreased saliva flow is not the aging process itself but, rather, the use of medications that have anticholinergic effects. More than 250 medications have a side effect of dry mouth.

The absence of some teeth and trouble with mastication encourage the older person to eat soft foods (usually high in carbohydrates) and to decrease meat and fresh vegetable intake. This produces a risk for nutritional deficit for protein, vitamins, and minerals.

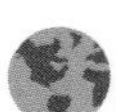

CULTURE AND GENETICS

Bifid uvula, a condition in which the uvula is split either completely or partially, occurs in 18% of some American Indian groups and in 10% of Asians. The occurrence in whites and Blacks is rare. **Cleft lip** and **cleft palate** are most common in Asian-American newborns (1/800) and American Indians, less common in Caucasians (1/1000), and least common among African Americans (1/1200).[28] Both genetic and environmental factors contribute to the emergence of **torus palatinus,** a benign bony ridge running in the middle of the hard palate (see Fig. 16-17). The prevalence of torus palatinus and torus mandibularis is higher in Asians than in Caucasians[14] and is higher in women than in men.[4] **Leukoedema** is a milky, bluish-white, opaque appearance of the buccal mucosa. It occurs more often in darkly pigmented persons and is seen most often in African Americans.[3] The incidence of natal teeth (baby born with teeth) is rare, about 1:2000 to 1:3500 live births, but is more common among American Indian infants.[18]

Throughout life, whites have more tooth decay than Blacks. The differences in tooth decay between Blacks and whites occur because Blacks have harder and denser tooth enamel, which makes their teeth less susceptible to the organisms that cause caries.

The incidence of tooth loss and edentulism has decreased substantially in the United States over the past several decades because of fluoridation, improved dental treatment, and better personal care. Although the overall prevalence of edentulism has dropped to 10.5% of the population, significant variations remain among subgroups in the population. Blacks, Hispanics, American Indians, and Alaska Natives have the poorest oral health of all racial and ethnic groups in the United States.

In the United States, the incidence and mortality rates for oral and pharyngeal cancer have declined since the mid-1980s. However, some racial disparity persists. The incidence rate was 20% higher for African-American men than for white men, while the difference between women was small. The mortality rates were 82% higher for African-American men compared with white men, but rates were similar for African-American and white women.[19] The disparity in survival rate may be attributed to racial differences in stage at diagnosis, age, gender, socioeconomic status, and treatment received.

In 2007, 62.7% of adults ages 18 to 64 years visited a dentist. Some racial disparity exists: for whites, it was 64.2%; for African Americans, 55%; and for Hispanics, 48.9%. The percentage of adults who had untreated caries between 2001 and 2004 was 26.8%. By origin, the breakdown was 21.5% for whites; 42.9% for African Americans; and 40.1% for Hispanics.[21] Poverty and access to care are factors in this disparity.

SUBJECTIVE DATA

Nose

1. Discharge
2. Frequent colds (upper respiratory infections)
3. Sinus pain
4. Trauma
5. Epistaxis (nosebleeds)
6. Allergies
7. Altered smell

Mouth and Throat

1. Sores or lesions
2. Sore throat
3. Bleeding gums
4. Toothache
5. Hoarseness
6. Dysphagia
7. Altered taste
8. Smoking, alcohol consumption
9. Self-care behaviors
   Dental care pattern
   Dentures or appliances

Examiner Asks	Rationale
Nose	
1. Discharge. Any **nasal discharge** or runny nose? Continuous? • Is the discharge watery, purulent, mucoid, bloody?	**Rhinorrhea** occurs with colds, allergies, sinus infection, trauma.

Examiner Asks	Rationale
2. **Frequent colds.** Any unusually frequent or severe colds (upper respiratory infections)? How often do these occur?	Most people have occasional colds; thus asking this more precise question yields more meaningful data.
3. **Sinus pain.** Any **sinus pain** or sinusitis? How is this treated? • Do you have chronic postnasal drip?	
4. **Trauma.** Ever had any **trauma** or a blow to the nose? • Can you breathe through your nose? Are both sides obstructed or one?	Trauma may cause deviated septum, which may cause nares to be obstructed.
5. **Epistaxis (nosebleeds).** Any nosebleeds? How often? • How much bleeding—a teaspoonful or does it pour out? • Color of the blood—red or brown? Clots? • From one nostril or both? • Aggravated by nose-picking or scratching? • How do you treat the nosebleeds? Are they difficult to stop?	**Epistaxis** occurs with trauma, vigorous nose blowing, foreign body. Person should sit up with head tilted forward, pinch nose between thumb and forefinger for 5 to 15 minutes.
6. **Allergies.** Any **allergies** or hay fever? To what are you allergic (e.g., pollen, dust, pets)? • How was this determined? • What type of environment makes it worse? Can you avoid exposure? • Use inhalers, nasal spray, nose drops? How often? Which type? • How long have you used this?	"Seasonal" rhinitis if due to pollen; "perennial" if allergen is dust. Misuse of over-the-counter nasal medications irritates the mucosa, causing rebound swelling, a common problem.
7. **Altered smell.** Experienced any change in sense of smell?	Sense of smell diminishes with cigarette smoking, chronic allergies, aging.

Mouth and Throat

Examiner Asks	Rationale
1. **Sores or lesions.** Noticed any **sores** or **lesions** in the mouth, tongue, or gums? • How long have you had it? Ever had this lesion before? • Is it single or multiple? • Does it seem to be associated with stress, season change, food? • How have you treated the sore? Applied any local medication?	History helps determine whether oral lesions have infectious, traumatic, immunologic, or malignant etiology.
2. **Sore throat.** How about **sore throats?** How frequently do you get them? Have a sore throat now? When did it start? • Is it associated with cough, fever, fatigue, decreased appetite, headache, postnasal drip, or hoarseness? • Is it worse when arising? What is the humidity level in the room where you sleep? Any dust or smoke inhaled at work? • Usually get a throat culture for the sore throats? Were any documented as streptococcal? • How have you treated this sore throat: medication, gargling? How effective are these? Have your tonsils or adenoids been taken out?	Untreated strep throat may lead to the complication of rheumatic fever.
3. **Bleeding gums.** Any **bleeding gums?** How long have you had this?	
4. **Toothache.** Any **toothache?** Do your teeth seem sensitive to hot, cold? Have you lost any teeth?	
5. **Hoarseness.** Any **hoarseness,** voice change? For how long? • Feel like having to clear your throat? Or like a "lump in your throat?" • Use your voice a lot at work, recreation? • Does the hoarseness seem associated with a cold, sore throat?	Hoarseness of the larynx has many causes: overuse of the voice, upper respiratory infection (URI), chronic inflammation, lesions, or a neoplasm.

Subjective Data

Subjective Data

Examiner Asks	Rationale
6. **Dysphagia.** Any difficulty swallowing? How long have you had it? • Feel like food gets stopped at a certain point? • Any pain with this?	**Dysphagia** occurs with pharyngitis, gastroesophageal reflux disease, stroke and other neurologic diseases, esophageal cancer.
7. **Altered taste.** Any change in sense of taste?	
8. **Smoking, alcohol consumption.** Do you smoke? Pipe or cigarettes? Smokeless tobacco? How many packs per day? For how many years?	Chronic tobacco use leads to tooth loss, coronal and root caries, and periodontal disease in older adults.
• When was your last alcohol drink? How much alcohol did you drink that time? How much alcohol do you usually drink?	Chronic tobacco use and heavy alcohol consumption highly increase risk for oral and pharyngeal cancers.
9. **Self-care behaviors.** Tell me about your daily dental care. How often do you use a toothbrush and floss?	Assess self-care behaviors for oral hygiene.
• Last dental examination? Do dental problems affect which foods you eat? • Do you have a dental appliance: braces, bridge, headgear? • Wear dentures? All the time? How long have you had this set? How do they fit?	Periodic dental screening is necessary to note caries.
• Any sores or irritation on the palate or gums? • Any problems with talking—do the dentures whistle or drop? Can you chew all foods with them? How do you clean them?	Lesions may arise from ill-fitting dentures, or the presence of dentures may mask the eruption of new lesions.

Additional History for Infants and Children

Examiner Asks	Rationale
1. Does the child have any mouth infections or sores, such as thrush or canker sores? How frequently do these occur?	
2. Does the child have frequent sore throat or tonsillitis? How often? How are these treated? Have they ever been documented as streptococcal infections?	
3. Did the child's teeth erupt about on time?	Eruption is delayed with Down syndrome, cretinism, rickets.
• Do the teeth seem straight to you?	Malocclusion.
• Is the child using a bottle? How often during the day? Does the child go to sleep with a bottle at night?	Prolonged bottle use increases risk for tooth decay and middle ear infections.
• Have you noticed any thumb sucking after the child's secondary teeth came in?	Prolonged thumb sucking (after age 6 to 7 years) may affect occlusion.
• Have you noticed the child grinding his or her teeth? Does this happen at night?	Bruxism usually occurs in sleep, from dental problems, nervous tension.
4. **Self-care behaviors.** How are the child's dental habits? Use a toothbrush regularly? How often does the child see a dentist? • Do you use fluoridated water or fluoride supplement?	Evaluate child's self-care. Early self-care has best compliance.

Additional History for the Aging Adult

Examiner Asks	Rationale
1. Any dryness in the mouth? Are you taking any medications? (Note prescribed and over-the-counter medications.)	**Xerostomia** (dry mouth) is a side effect of many drugs: antidepressants, anticholinergics, antispasmodics, antihypertensives, antipsychotics, bronchodilators.
2. Have you lost any teeth? Can you chew all types of food?	Note a decrease in eating meat, fresh vegetables, and cleansing foods such as apples.

Examiner Asks	Rationale
3. Are you able to care for your own teeth or dentures?	Self-care may be decreased by physical disability (arthritis), vision loss, confusion, or depression.
4. Noticed a change in your sense of taste or smell?	Some people add extra salt and sugar to enhance food when taste begins to wane. Also, diminished smell may decrease the person's ability to detect food spoilage, natural gas leaks, or smoke from a fire.

OBJECTIVE DATA

PREPARATION

Position the person sitting up straight with his or her head at your eye level. If the person wears dentures, offer a paper towel and ask the person to remove them.

EQUIPMENT NEEDED

Otoscope with short, wide-tipped nasal speculum attachment
Penlight
Two tongue blades
Cotton gauze pad (4 × 4 inches)
Gloves

Normal Range of Findings | **Abnormal Findings**

INSPECT AND PALPATE THE NOSE

External Nose

Normally, the nose is symmetric, in the midline, and in proportion to other facial features (Fig. 16-7). Inspect for any deformity, asymmetry, inflammation, or skin lesions. If an injury is reported or suspected, palpate gently for any pain or break in contour.

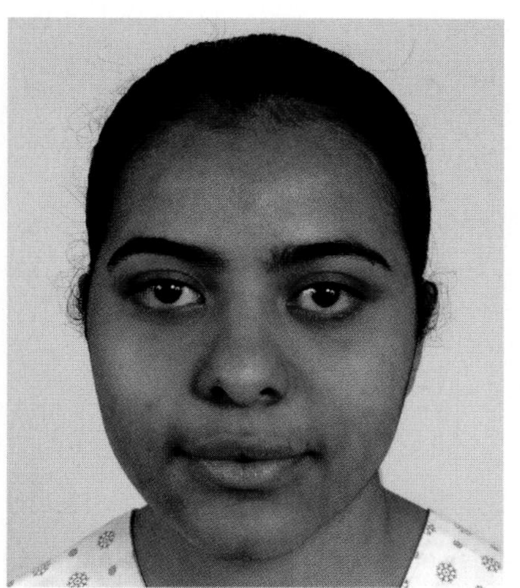

16-7

Test the patency of the nostrils by pushing each nasal wing shut with your finger while asking the person to sniff inward through the other naris. This reveals any obstruction, which later is explored using the nasal speculum. The sense of smell, mediated by cranial nerve I, is not tested in a routine examination. The procedure for assessing smell is presented with cranial nerve testing in Chapter 23.

Absence of sniff indicates obstruction (e.g., common cold, nasal polyps, rhinitis).

Normal Range of Findings	Abnormal Findings

Nasal Cavity

Attach the short wide-tipped speculum to the otoscope head and insert this combined apparatus into the nasal vestibule, avoiding pressure on the nasal septum. Gently lift up the tip of the nose with your finger before inserting.

View each nasal cavity with the person's head erect and then with the head tilted back. Inspect the nasal mucosa, noting its normal red color and smooth, moist surface (Fig. 16-8). Note any swelling, discharge, bleeding, or foreign body.

Rhinitis—nasal mucosa is swollen and bright red with URI.

Discharge is common with rhinitis and sinusitis, varying from watery and copious to thick, purulent, and green-yellow.

With chronic allergy, mucosa looks swollen, boggy, pale, and gray.

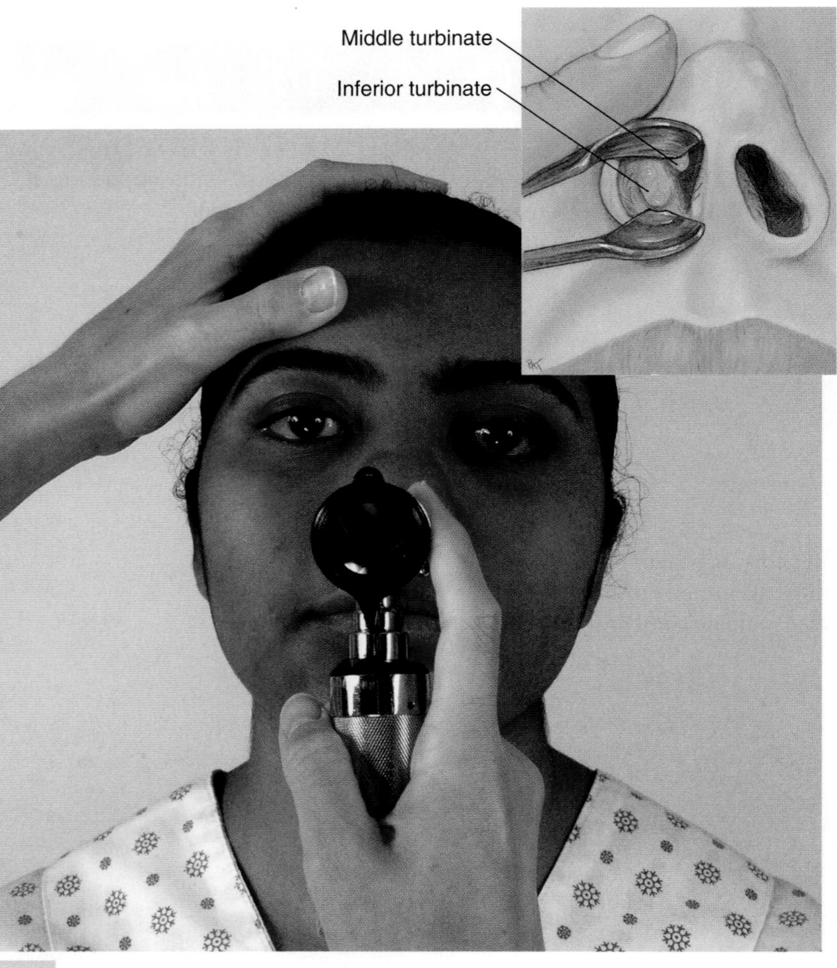

16-8

Observe the nasal septum for deviation (Fig. 16-9). A deviated septum is common and is not significant unless air flow is obstructed. (If present in a hospitalized patient, document the deviated septum in the event that the person needs nasal suctioning or a nasogastric tube.) Also note any perforation or bleeding in the septum.

A deviated septum looks like a hump or shelf in one nasal cavity.

Perforation is seen as a spot of light from a penlight shining in the other naris and occurs with cocaine use.

Epistaxis commonly comes from anterior septum (see Table 16-1, Abnormalities of the Nose, p. 373).

Normal Range of Findings | **Abnormal Findings**

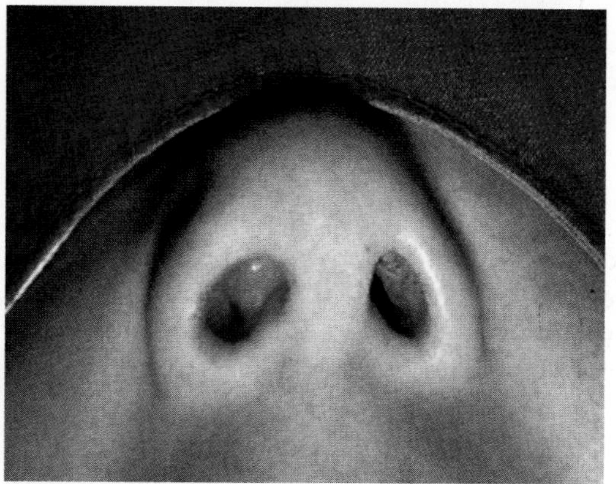

16-9 Deviated septum.

Inspect the turbinates (the bony ridges curving down from the lateral walls). The superior turbinate will not be in your view, but the middle and inferior turbinates appear the same light red color as the nasal mucosa. Note any swelling but do not try to push the speculum past it. Turbinates are quite vascular and tender if touched.

Note any polyps (benign growths that accompany chronic allergy), and distinguish them from the normal turbinates.

Polyps are smooth, pale gray, avascular, mobile, nontender (see Table 16-1).

PALPATE THE SINUS AREAS

Using your thumbs, press the frontal sinuses by pressing up and under the eyebrows (Fig. 16-10, *A*) and over the maxillary sinuses below the cheekbones (Fig. 16-10, *B*). Take care not to press directly on the eyeballs.

The person should feel firm pressure but no pain.

Sinus areas are tender to palpation in persons with chronic allergies and acute infection (sinusitis).

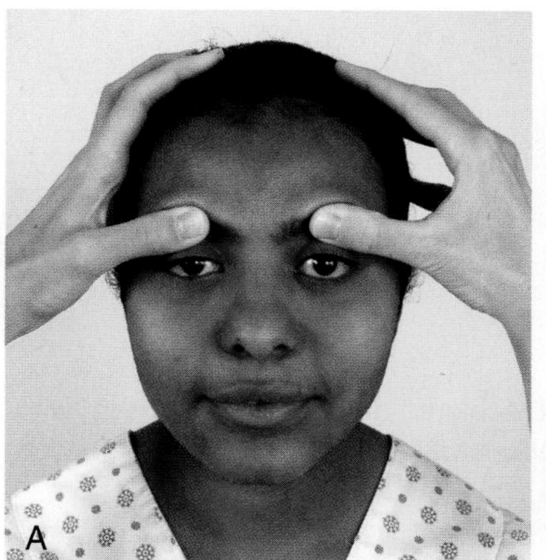

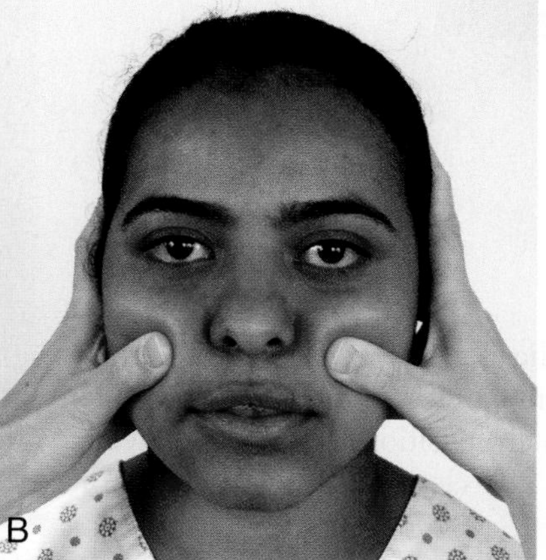

16-10

Transillumination

There is no evidence to support the practice of transillumination of the frontal or maxillary sinuses when you suspect sinus inflammation.[10] The diagnosis requires distinct differences in the illumination of one of the sinus pair. Thus the technique would not help in chronic sinusitis that has diffuse swelling of all sinus mucosa. Although there is more fluid collection with acute sinusitis, the asymmetry of light illumination still is not valid because many healthy sinuses normally will not transilluminate.

Normal Range of Findings

INSPECT THE MOUTH

Begin with anterior structures and move posteriorly. Use a tongue blade to retract structures and a bright light for optimal visualization.

Lips

Inspect the lips for color, moisture, cracking, or lesions. Retract the lips and note their inner surface as well (Fig. 16-11). All racial groups have lips that are deeper or pinker than facial skin. However, some African Americans normally may have bluish lips and a dark line on the gingival margin.

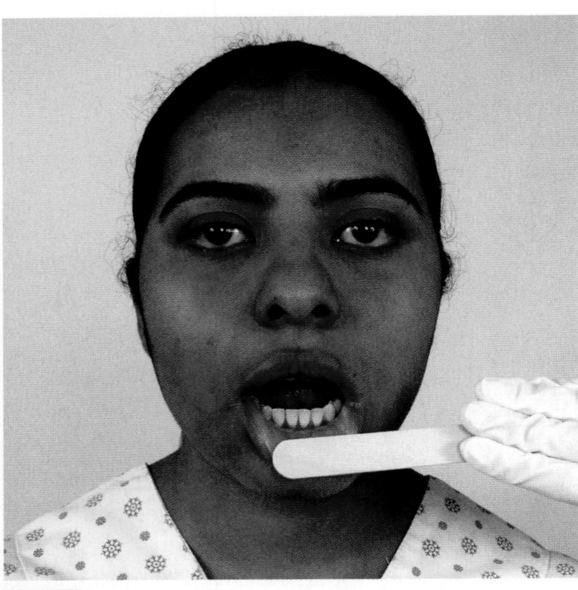

16-11

Teeth and Gums

The condition of the teeth is an index of the person's general health. Your examination should not replace the regular dental examination, but you should note any diseased, absent, loose, or abnormally positioned teeth. The teeth normally look white, straight, evenly spaced, and clean and free of debris or decay.

Compare the number of teeth with the number expected for the person's age. Ask the person to bite as if chewing something and note alignment of upper and lower jaw. Normal occlusion in the back is the upper teeth resting directly on the lowers; in the front, the upper incisors slightly override the lower incisors.

Normally, the gums look pink or coral with a stippled (dotted) surface. The gum margins at the teeth are tight and well defined (Fig. 16-12). Check for swelling; retraction of gingival margins; and spongy, bleeding, or discolored gums. Some African Americans normally may have a dark melanotic line along the gingival margin.

Abnormal Findings

In light-skinned people: circumoral pallor occurs with shock and anemia; cyanosis with hypoxemia and chilling; cherry red lips with carbon monoxide poisoning, acidosis from aspirin poisoning, or ketoacidosis.

Cheilitis (perlèche)—cracking at the corners.

Herpes simplex, other lesions (see Table 16-2, Abnormalities of the Lips, p. 375).

Discolored teeth appear brown with excessive fluoride use, yellow with tobacco use.

Grinding down of tooth surface; plaque—soft debris; caries—decay.

Malocclusion (poor biting relationship), protrusion of upper or lower incisors (see Table 16-3).

Gingival hyperplasia (see Table 16-3), crevices between teeth and gums, pockets of debris.

Gums bleed with slight pressure, indicating gingivitis.

Dark line on gingival margins occurs with lead and bismuth poisoning.

Normal Range of Findings	Abnormal Findings

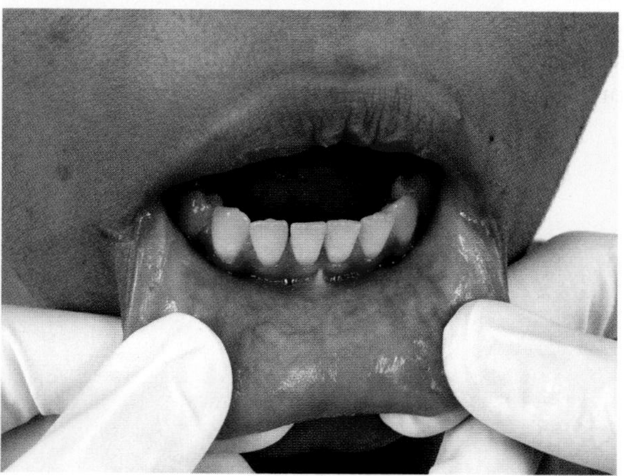

16-12

Tongue

Check the tongue for color, surface characteristics, and moisture. The color is pink and even. The dorsal surface is normally roughened from the papillae. A thin white coating may be present (Fig. 16-13). Ask the person to touch the tongue to the roof of the mouth. Its ventral surface looks smooth and glistening and shows veins. Saliva is present.

Beefy red, swollen tongue. Smooth glossy areas (see Table 16-5).

Enlarged tongue occurs with mental retardation, hypothyroidism, acromegaly; a small tongue accompanies malnutrition.

Dry mouth occurs with dehydration, fever; tongue has deep vertical fissures.

Saliva is decreased when taking anticholinergic and other medications.

Excess saliva and drooling occur with gingivostomatitis and neurologic dysfunction.

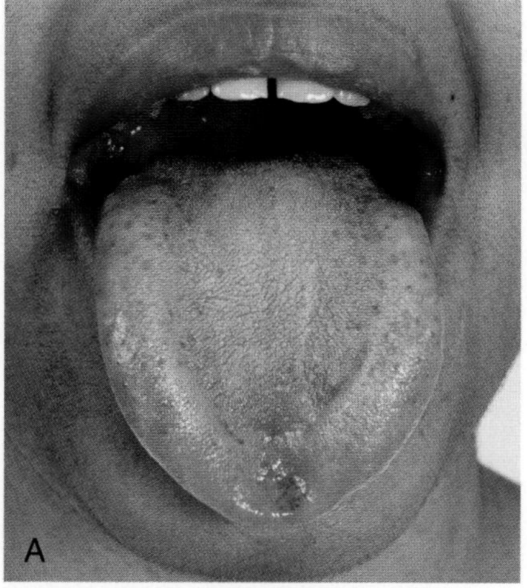

A

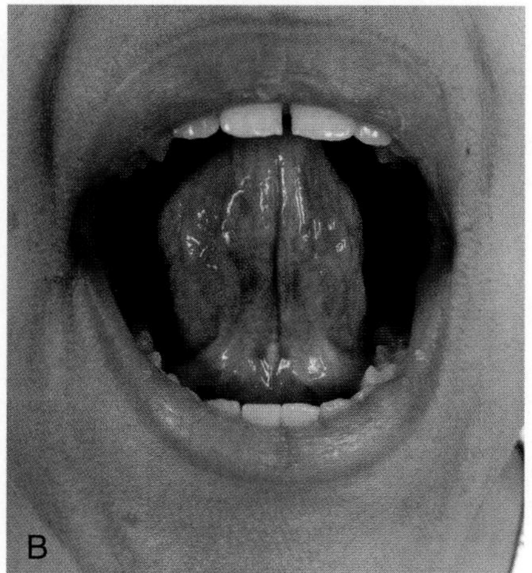

B

16-13

Normal Range of Findings

With a glove,* hold the tongue with a cotton gauze pad for traction and swing the tongue out and to each side (Fig. 16-14). Inspect for any white patches or lesions—normally none are present. If any occur, palpate these lesions for induration.

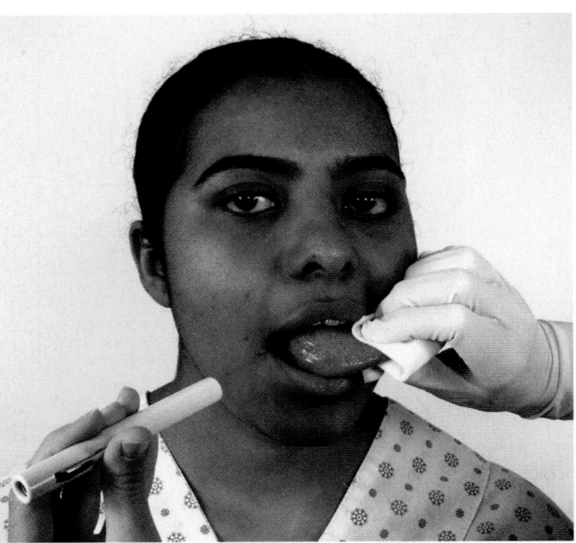

16-14

Inspect carefully the entire U-shaped area under the tongue behind the teeth. Oral malignancies are most likely to develop here. Note any white patches, nodules, or ulcerations. If lesions are present or with any person older than 50 years or with a positive history of smoking or alcohol use, use your gloved hand to palpate the area. Place your other hand under the jaw to stabilize the tissue and to "capture" any abnormality (Fig. 16-15). Note any induration.

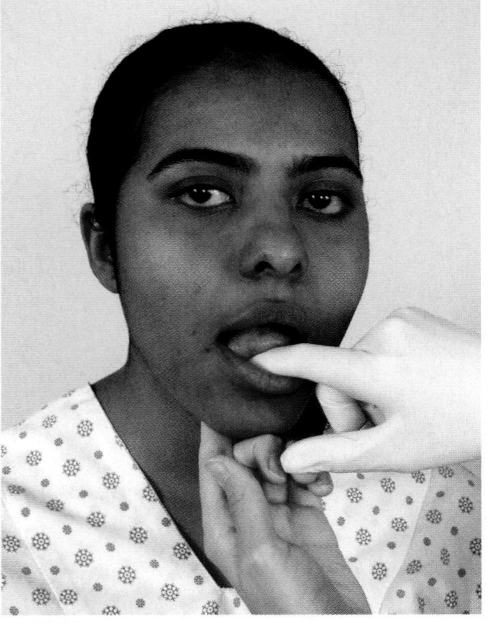

16-15

*Always wear gloves to examine mucous membranes. This follows Standard Precautions to prevent the spread of possible communicable disease.

Abnormal Findings

Any lesion or ulcer persisting for more than 2 weeks must be investigated.

An indurated area may be a mass or lymphadenopathy, and it must be investigated.

Normal Range of Findings

Buccal Mucosa

Hold the cheek open with a wooden tongue blade, and check the buccal mucosa for color, nodules, or lesions. It looks pink, smooth, and moist, although patchy hyperpigmentation is common and normal in dark-skinned people.

An expected finding is **Stensen's duct,** the opening of the parotid salivary gland. It looks like a small dimple opposite the upper second molar. You also may see a raised occlusion line on the buccal mucosa parallel with the level the teeth meet. This is caused by the teeth closing against the cheek.

A larger patch also may be present along the buccal mucosa. This is **leukoedema,** a benign, milky, bluish white, opaque area, more common in Blacks and East Indians. When it is mild, the patch disappears as you stretch the cheeks. It is always bilateral. With age, it looks grayish white and thickened. The cause is unknown. Do not mistake leukoedema for oral infections such as candidiasis (thrush).

Fordyce granules are small, isolated white or yellow papules on the mucosa of cheek, tongue, and lips (Fig. 16-16). These little sebaceous cysts are painless and not significant.

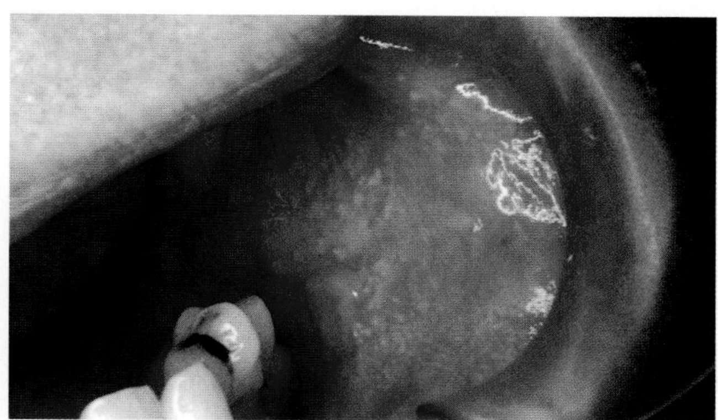

16-16 Fordyce granules.

Palate

Shine your light up to the roof of the mouth. The more anterior hard palate is white with irregular transverse rugae. The posterior soft palate is pinker, smooth, and upwardly movable. A normal variation is a nodular bony ridge down the middle of the hard palate, a **torus palatinus** (Fig. 16-17). This benign growth arises after puberty and is a more common finding in American Indians, Inuits, and Asians.

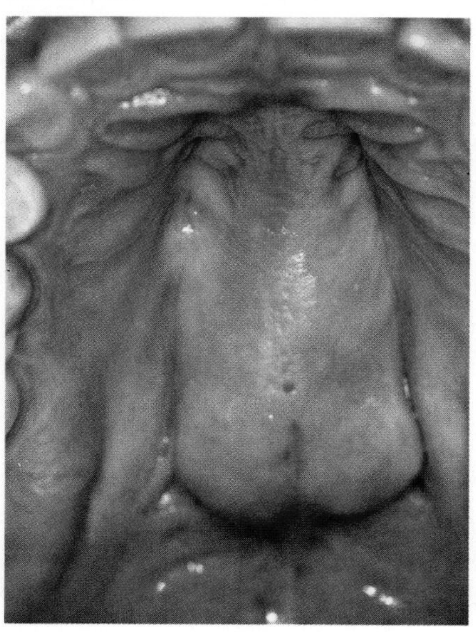

16-17 Torus palatinus.

Abnormal Findings

Dappled brown patches are present with Addison's disease (chronic adrenal insufficiency).

Orifice of Stensen's duct looks red with mumps.

Koplik spots—early prodromal (early warning) sign of measles.

Candida infection will usually rub off, leaving a clear or raw denuded surface.

The chalky white raised patch of **leukoplakia** is abnormal (see Table 16-4, Abnormalities of the Buccal Mucosa).

The hard palate appears yellow with jaundice. In Blacks with jaundice, it may look yellow, muddy yellow, or green-brown.

Oral Kaposi sarcoma is the most common early lesion in people with AIDS (see Table 16-6).

Normal Range of Findings

Observe the uvula; it normally looks like a fleshy pendant hanging in the midline (Fig. 16-18). Ask the person to say "ahhh" and note the soft palate and uvula rise in the midline. This tests one function of cranial nerve X, the vagus nerve.

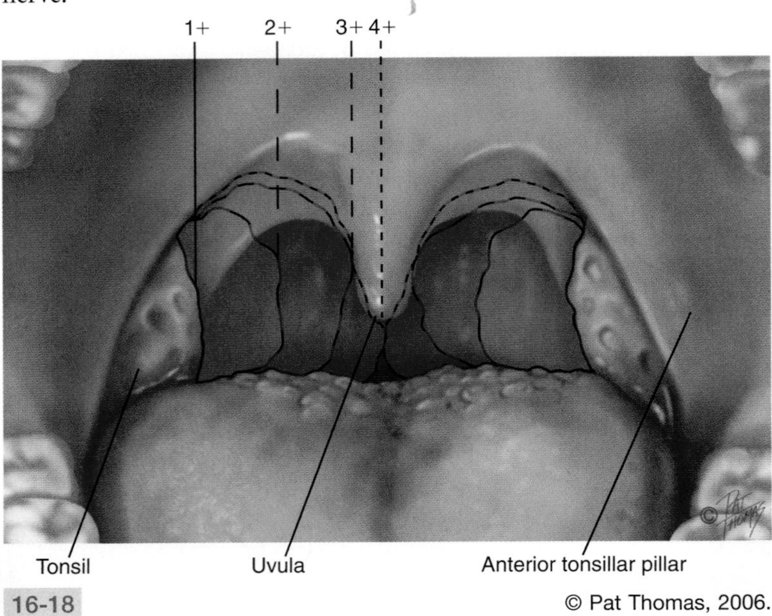

16-18 © Pat Thomas, 2006.

INSPECT THE THROAT

With your light, observe the oval, rough-surfaced **tonsils** behind the anterior tonsillar pillar (see Fig. 16-18). Their color is the same pink as the oral mucosa, and their surface is peppered with indentations, or crypts. In some people, the crypts collect small plugs of whitish cellular debris. This does not indicate infection. However, there should be no exudate on the tonsils. Tonsils are graded in size as follows:

1+ Visible
2+ Halfway between tonsillar pillars and uvula
3+ Touching the uvula
4+ Touching each other

You may normally see 1+ or 2+ tonsils in healthy people, especially in children, because lymphoid tissue is proportionately enlarged until puberty.

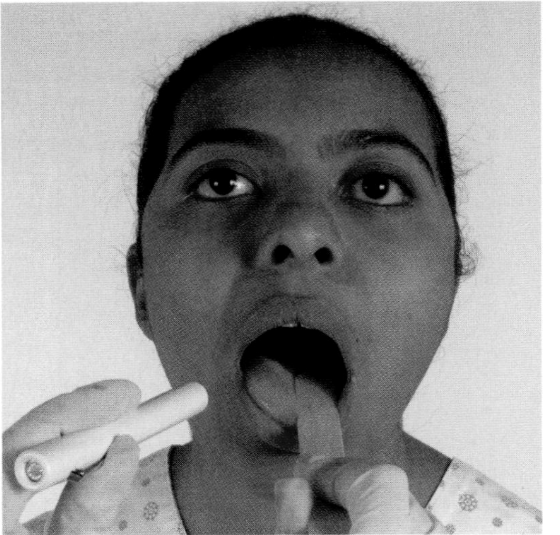

16-19

Abnormal Findings

A *bifid* uvula looks like it is split in two; more common in American Indians (see Table 16-6).

Any deviation to the side or absent movement indicates nerve damage, which also occurs with poliomyelitis and diphtheria.

With an acute infection, tonsils are bright red and swollen and may have exudate or large white spots.

A white membrane covering the tonsils may accompany infectious mononucleosis, leukemia, and diphtheria.

Tonsils are enlarged to 2+, 3+, or 4+ with an acute infection.

Normal Range of Findings

Enlarge your view of the posterior pharyngeal wall by depressing the tongue with a tongue blade (Fig. 16-19). Push down halfway back on the tongue; if you push on its tip, the tongue will hump up in back. Press slightly off center to avoid eliciting the gag reflex. You can help the person whose gag reflex is easily triggered by offering a tongue blade to depress his or her own tongue. (Some people can lower their own tongue so the tongue blade is not needed.) Scan the posterior wall for color, exudate, and lesions. When finished, discard the tongue blade.

Although usually it is not done in the screening examination, touching the posterior wall with the tongue blade elicits the gag reflex. This tests cranial nerves IX and X, the glossopharyngeal and vagus.

Test cranial nerve XII, the hypoglossal nerve, by asking the person to stick out the tongue. It should protrude in the midline. Children enjoy this request! Note any tremor, loss of movement, or deviation to the side.

During the examination, notice any breath odor, *halitosis.* This is common and usually has a local cause, such as poor oral hygiene, consumption of odoriferous foods, alcohol consumption, heavy smoking, or dental infection. Occasionally it may indicate a systemic disease.

Abnormal Findings

With cranial nerve XII damage, the tongue deviates *toward* the paralyzed side.

A fine tremor of the tongue occurs with hyperthyroidism; a coarse tremor occurs with cerebral palsy and alcoholism.

Diabetic ketoacidosis has a sweet, fruity breath odor; this acetone smell also occurs in children with malnutrition or dehydration. Others are an ammonia breath odor with uremia; a musty odor with liver disease; a foul, fetid odor with dental or respiratory infections; an alcohol odor with alcohol ingestion or chemicals; a mouselike smell of the breath with diphtheria.

DEVELOPMENTAL COMPETENCE

Infants and Children

Because the oral examination is intrusive for the infant or young child, the timing is best toward the end of the complete examination, along with the ear examination. But if any crying episodes occur earlier, seize the opportunity to examine the open mouth and oropharynx.

As with the ear examination, let the parent help position the child. Place the infant supine on the examining table, with the arms restrained (Fig. 16-20). The older infant and toddler may be held on the parent's lap with one of the parent's hands holding the arms down and the other hand securing the child's head against the parent's chest.

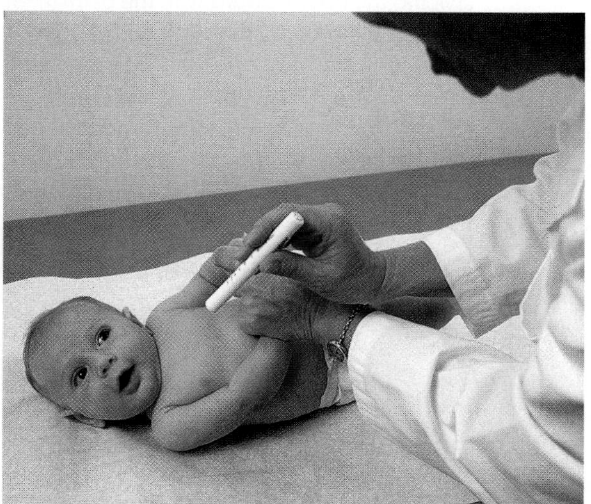

16-20

Normal Range of Findings	Abnormal Findings

Use a game to help prepare the young child. Encourage the preschool child to use a tongue blade to look into a puppet's mouth. Or place a mirror so that the child can look into the mouth while you do. The school-age child is usually cooperative and loves to show off missing or new teeth (Fig. 16-21).

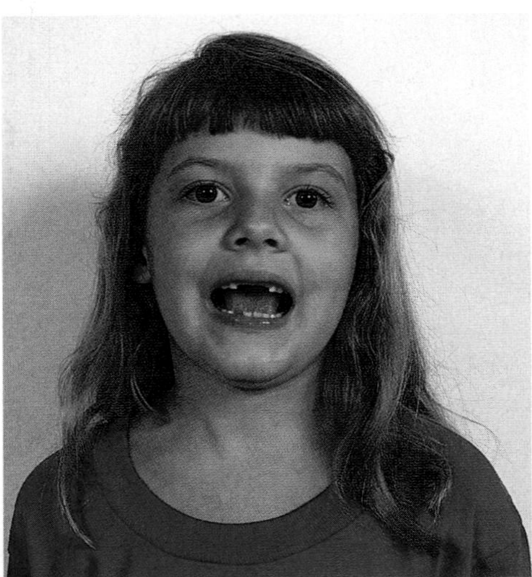

16-21

Be discriminating in your use of the tongue blade. It may be necessary for a full view of oral structures, but it produces a strong gag reflex in the infant. You may avoid the tongue blade completely with a cooperative preschooler and school-age child. Try asking the young child to "Open your mouth as big as a lion," "Can you stick out your WHOLE TONGUE?" and to move the tongue in different directions. To enlarge your view of the oropharynx, ask the child to stick out the tongue and "pant like a dog."

At some point, you will encounter an uncooperative young child who clenches the teeth and refuses to open the mouth. If all your other efforts have failed, slide the tongue blade along the buccal mucosa and turn it between the back teeth. Push down to depress the tongue. This stimulates the gag reflex, and the child opens the mouth wide for a few seconds. You will have a *brief* look at the throat. Make the most of it.

Nose. The newborn may have milia across the nose. The nasal bridge may be flat in Black and Asian children. There should be no nasal flaring or narrowing with breathing.

Nasal flaring in the infant indicates respiratory distress.

A transverse ridge across the nose occurs in a child with chronic allergy from wiping the nose upward with the palm (see Table 13-4 on p. 275). Nasal narrowing on inhalation is seen with chronic nasal obstruction and mouth breathing.

It is essential to determine the patency of the nares in the immediate newborn period because most newborns are obligate nose breathers. Nares blocked with amniotic fluid are suctioned gently with a bulb syringe. If obstruction is suspected, a small-lumen (5 to 10 Fr) catheter is passed down each naris to confirm patency.

Inability to pass catheter through nasal cavity indicates choanal atresia, which needs immediate intervention (see Table 16-1 on p. 373).

Avoid the nasal speculum when examining the infant and young child. Instead, gently push up the tip of the nose with your thumb while using your other hand to shine the light into the naris. With a toddler, be alert for the possible foreign body lodged in the nasal cavity (see Table 16-1).

Only in children older than 8 years do you need to palpate the sinus areas. In younger children, sinus areas are too small for palpation.

Mouth and Throat. A normal finding in infants is the **sucking tubercle,** a small pad in the middle of the upper lip from friction of breastfeeding or bottle-feeding. Note the number of teeth and whether it is appropriate for the child's age. Also note pattern of eruption, position, condition, and hygiene. Use this

No teeth by age 1 year.

Discolored teeth appear yellow or

Normal Range of Findings

guide for children younger than 2 years: the child's age in months minus the number 6 should equal the expected number of deciduous teeth. Normally, all 20 deciduous teeth are in by 2½ years. Saliva is present after 3 months of age and shows in excess with teething children.

Mobility should allow the tongue to extend at least as far as the alveolar ridge.

Note any bruising or laceration on the buccal mucosa or gums of the infant or young child.

On the palate, **Epstein pearls** are a normal finding in newborns and infants (Fig. 16-22). They are small, whitish, glistening, pearly papules along the median raphe of the hard palate and on the gums, where they look like teeth. They are small retention cysts and disappear in the first few weeks.

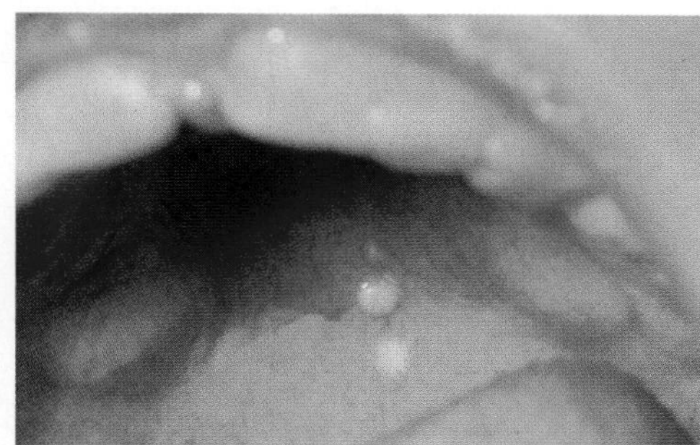

16-22 Epstein pearls.

Bednar aphthae are traumatic areas or ulcers on the posterior hard palate on either side of the midline. They result from abrasions while sucking.

The tonsils are not visible in the newborn. They gradually enlarge during childhood, remaining proportionately larger until puberty. Tonsils appear still larger if the infant is crying or gagging. Normally the newborn can produce a strong, lusty cry.

Insert your gloved finger into the baby's mouth and palpate the hard and soft palate as the baby sucks. The sucking reflex can be elicited in infants up to 12 months old.

As teeth begin to erupt in the older infant and child, check age at eruption, sequence, and condition. Teeth should emerge straight up or down from the gums, and enamel could be clear white and smooth. Lift the upper lip to check for dental caries (tooth decay); normally there are none.

The Pregnant Woman

Gum hypertrophy (surface looks smooth and stippling disappears) may occur normally at puberty or during pregnancy (pregnancy gingivitis) (Fig. 16-23).

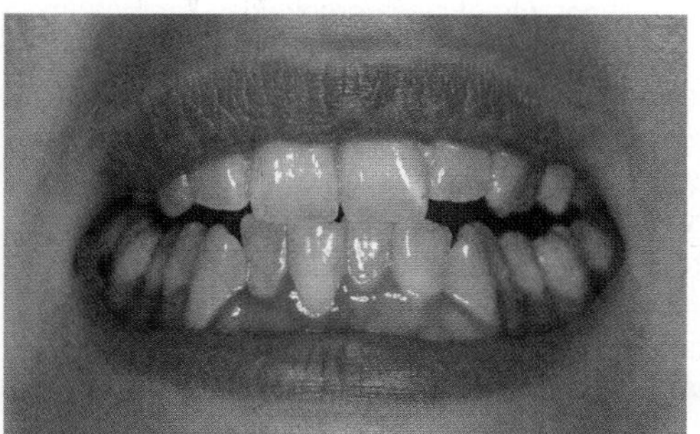

16-23 Early gingivitis.

Abnormal Findings

yellow-brown with infants taking tetracycline or whose mothers took the drug during the last trimester; appear green or black with excessive iron ingestion, although this reverses when the iron is stopped.

Malocclusion: upper or lower dental arches are out of alignment.

Ankyloglossia, a short lingual frenulum, can limit protrusion and impair speech development (see Table 16-5).

Trauma may indicate child abuse from forced feeding of bottle or spoon.

A high-arched palate is usually normal in the newborn, but a very narrow or high arch also occurs with Turner's syndrome, Ehlers-Danlos syndrome, Marfan's syndrome, and Treacher Collins syndrome or develops in the mouth-breather in chronic allergies.

Nursing bottle caries are brown discolorations on upper front teeth (see photo in Table 16-3).

Normal Range of Findings	Abnormal Findings

The Aging Adult

The nose may appear more prominent on the face from a loss of subcutaneous fat. In the edentulous person, the mouth and lips fold in, giving a "purse-string" appearance. The teeth may look slightly yellowed, although the color is uniform. Yellowing results from the dentin visible through worn enamel. The surface of the incisors may show vertical cracks from a lifetime of exposure to extreme temperatures. The teeth may look longer as the gum margins recede (Fig. 16-24).

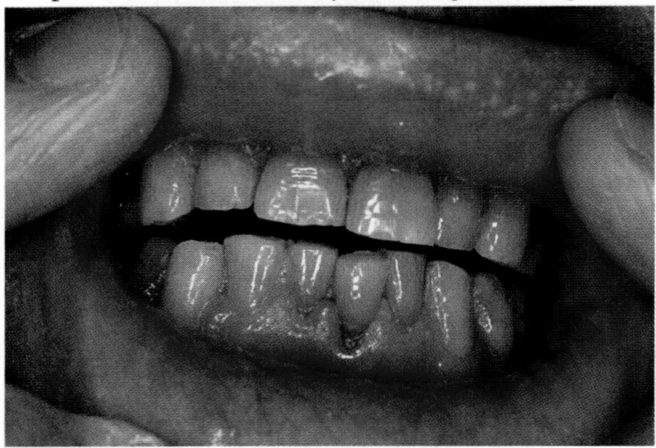

16-24 Receded gums.

The surfaces look worn down or abraded. Old dental work deteriorates, especially at the gum margins. The teeth loosen with bone resorption and may move with palpation.

The tongue looks smoother as a result of papillary atrophy. The aging adult's buccal mucosa is thinned and may look shinier, as though it were "varnished."

PROMOTING A HEALTHY LIFESTYLE: SMOKELESS TOBACCO AND CANCER RISK

Smokeless Does Not Mean Harmless!

Smokeless tobacco (SL-T) carries significant health risks, including cancers, fatal myocardial infarcts and stroke, dental decay, hypertension, and decreased sperm counts and sterility. Of particular concern is that using SL-T carries an even greater risk for oral cavity cancers than does smoking.

The types of SL-T commonly used in the United States include chewing tobacco and snuff. *Chewing tobacco* comes as loose leaf, plug, or twist and, just as the name implies, is chewed. *Snuff* is finely ground tobacco and comes dry, moist, or in packaged sachets, like tea bags. Dry snuff can be sniffed through the nose. However, most snuff users put a "pinch" or "dip" between their gingival and buccal mucosa, suck on the tobacco, and spit out the juices, which gives rise to the term *spitting tobacco.* Holding one pinch of SL-T in the mouth ("dipping") for 30 minutes delivers as much nicotine as three cigarettes.

SL-T use is higher in young white and American-Indian/Alaskan-Native males. There is also increased use of SL-T in sports, primarily baseball, and young men often say that they start because they see their idols or heroes participating. About 35% of major league baseball players use SL-T, but at least 50% of these users also report that they are trying to quit. In 1990, major league baseball issued a report on the hazards of SL-T and started efforts to help players to not start and help others to quit. In 1991, minor league baseball banned the use of SL-T at the rookie level and in 1993 extended the ban throughout all minor leagues. In 1994, the National Collegiate Athletic Association banned the use of all tobacco products, including SL-T.

Pain is rarely an early symptom of oral cancer, which is why a thorough examination of the mouth is important. Early signs of oral cancer to look for include:

- A sore that does not seem to heal
- A smooth or leathery white patch or lump
- A prolonged sore throat or feeling that something is in the throat
- Difficulty chewing
- Restricted movement of the tongue or jaw

Resources

The National Institute of Dental and Craniofacial Research has developed a booklet directed at young men who want to quit using spit tobacco. *Smokeless Tobacco: A Guide for Quitting* can be downloaded from www.nidcr.nih.gov/NR/rdonlyres/DF314871-B0A6-4171-B831-C472F543C154/0/SpitTobacco.pdf.

The Office on Smoking and Health is the lead Centers for Disease Control and Prevention agency for comprehensive tobacco prevention and control. It has a number of resources, including *Smokeless Tobacco Facts* at www.cdc.gov/tobacco/data_statistics/fact_sheets/smokeless/smokeless_facts/index.htm.

Other resource sites include the National Cancer Institute's *Smokeless Tobacco: Just the Facts!* available at http://dccps.nci.nih.gov/tcrb/less_facts.html. For patients, Oral Health America has developed NSTEP®, which focuses primarily on preventing young people from starting to use SL-T and helping current users quit. Information about NSTEP® can be found at http://oralhealthamerica.org/programs/nstep%C2%AE.

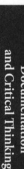

DOCUMENTATION AND CRITICAL THINKING

Sample Charting

SUBJECTIVE

Nose: No history of discharge, sinus problems, obstruction, epistaxis, or allergy. Colds 1-2/yr, mild. Fractured nose during high school sports, treated by MD.

Mouth and Throat: No pain, lesions, bleeding gums, toothache, dysphagia, or hoarseness. Occasional sore throat with colds. Tonsillectomy, age 8. Smokes cigarettes 1 PPD × 9 years. Alcohol-1-2 drinks socially, about 2×/month. Visits dentist annually, dental hygienist 2×/year, flosses daily. No dental appliance.

OBJECTIVE

Nose: Symmetric, no deformity or skin lesions. Nares patent. Mucosa pink; no discharge, lesions, or polyps; no septal deviation or perforation. Sinuses—no tenderness to palpation.

Mouth: Can clench teeth. Mucosa and gingivae pink, no masses or lesions. Teeth are all present, straight, and in good repair. Tongue smooth, pink, no lesions, protrudes in midline, no tremor.

Throat: Mucosa pink, no lesions or exudate. Uvula rises in midline on phonation. Tonsils out. Gag reflex present.

ASSESSMENT

Structures intact and appear healthy

Focused Assessment: Clinical Case Study 1

Brad D., a 34-year-old electrician, seeks care for "sore throat for 2 days."

SUBJECTIVE

2 days PTA—experienced sudden onset of sore throat, swollen glands, fever 101° F, occasional shaking chills, extreme fatigue.

Today—symptoms remain. Cough productive of yellow sputum. Treated self with aspirin for minimal relief. Unable to eat past 2 days because "throat on fire." Taking adequate fluids, on bedrest. Not aware of exposure to other sick persons. Does not smoke.

OBJECTIVE

Ears: Tympanic membranes pearl gray with landmarks intact.
Nose: No discharge. Mucosa pink, no swelling.
Mouth: Mucosa and gingivae pink, no lesions.
Throat: Tonsils 3+. Pharyngeal wall bright red with yellow-white exudate, exudate also on tonsils.
Neck: Enlarged anterior cervical nodes bilaterally, painful to palpation. No other lymph adenopathy.
Chest: Resonant to percussion throughout. Breath sounds clear anterior and posterior. No adventitious sounds.

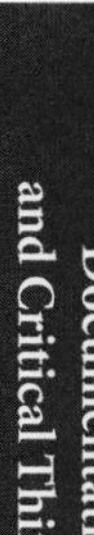

ASSESSMENT

Pharyngitis
Pain R/T inflammation
Imbalanced nutrition: less than body requirements R/T dysphagia

Focused Assessment: Clinical Case Study 2

Calvin W., a 53-year-old white businessman, is in the hospital awaiting coronary bypass surgery for coronary artery disease. He is allergic to dust and animal hair. As part of a preoperative teaching plan for coughing and deep breathing, a respiratory assessment is performed.

SUBJECTIVE

States understanding of reason for admission to hospital and extent of coronary artery disease. Unaware of details of surgical procedure and postoperative care. Interested: "I do better when I know what I'm dealing with." History of exertional angina after walking one short block or climbing one flight of stairs, treats self with nitroglycerin. Does not smoke. Chronic watery nasal discharge, "comes and goes, but present most of time."

OBJECTIVE

Nose: Only R naris patent. Mucosa gray and boggy bilaterally. L naris has mobile, gray, nontender mass, obstructing view of turbinates and rest of nasal cavity.

Mouth and Throat: Mucosa pink, no lesions. Uvula midline, rises on phonation. Tonsils absent. No lumps or lesions on palpation.

Chest: Thorax symmetric; AP < transverse diameter; respirations 18/min, effortless. Resonant to percussion. Breath sounds are clear. No adventitious sounds.

ASSESSMENT

L nasal mass, possibly polyp
Deficient knowledge for surgery and expected postop course R/T lack of exposure

Focused Assessment: Clinical Case Study 3

Esther V. is a 61-year-old professor who has been admitted to the hospital for chemotherapy for carcinoma of the breast. This is her 5th day in the hospital. An oral assessment is performed when she complains of "soreness and a white coating" in the mouth.

SUBJECTIVE

Felt soreness on tongue and cheeks during night. Now pain persists, and E.V. can see a "white coating" on tongue and cheeks. "I'm worried. Is this more cancer?"

OBJECTIVE

E.V. generally appears restless and overly aware.
Oral mucosa pink. Large white, cheesy patches covering most of dorsal surface of tongue and buccal mucosa. Will scrape off with tongue blade, revealing red eroded area beneath.
Bleeds with slight contact. Posterior pharyngeal wall pink, no lesions. Patches are soft to palpation. No palpable lymph nodes.

ASSESSMENT

Oral lesion, appears as candidiasis
Impaired oral mucous membrane R/T effects of chemotherapy
Pain R/T infectious process
Anxiety R/T threat to health status

ABNORMAL FINDINGS

TABLE 16-1 Abnormalities of the Nose

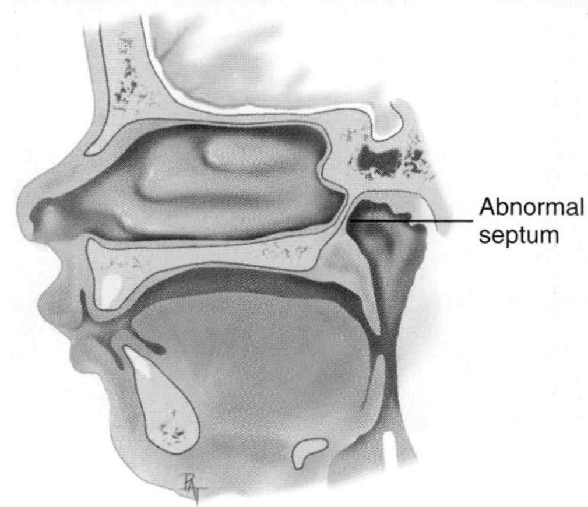

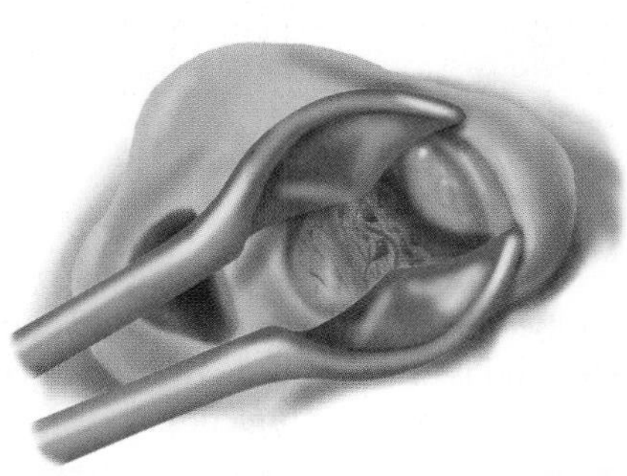

Choanal Atresia

A bony or membranous septum between the nasal cavity and the pharynx of the newborn. When the condition is bilateral, it requires the immediate insertion of an oral airway to prevent asphyxia because most newborns are obligate nose breathers. When the condition is unilateral, the infant may be asymptomatic until the onset of the first respiratory infection.

Epistaxis

The most common site of a nosebleed is Kiesselbach plexus in the anterior septum. It may be spontaneous from a local cause or a sign of underlying illness. Causes include nose picking, forceful coughing or sneezing, fracture, foreign body, rhinitis, heavy exertion, or a coagulation disorder. Bleeding from the anterior septum is easily controlled and rarely severe. A posterior hemorrhage is less common (<10%) but is more profuse, harder to manage, and more serious.

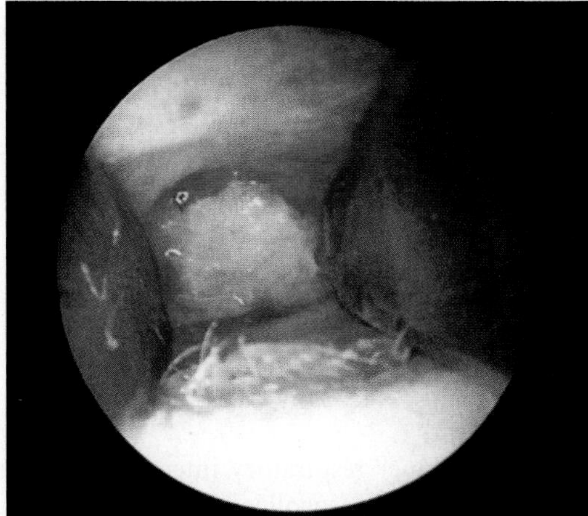

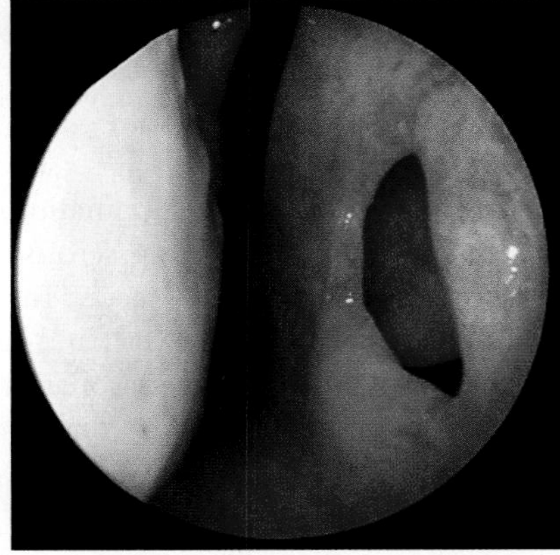

Foreign Body

Children particularly are apt to put an object up the nose (here, yellow plastic foam), producing unilateral mucopurulent drainage and foul odor. Because some risk for aspiration exists, removal should be prompt. A further problem comes from impaction from a small button battery from an electronic device (watch, video game). Once occluding the nostril, the battery can release voltage or chemicals that cause burns, necrosis, or perforation.

Perforated Septum

A hole in the septum, usually in the cartilaginous part, may be caused by snorting cocaine, chronic infection, trauma from continual picking of crusts, or nasal surgery. It is seen directly or as a spot of light when the penlight is directed into the other naris.

Continued

TABLE 16-1 Abnormalities of the Nose—cont'd

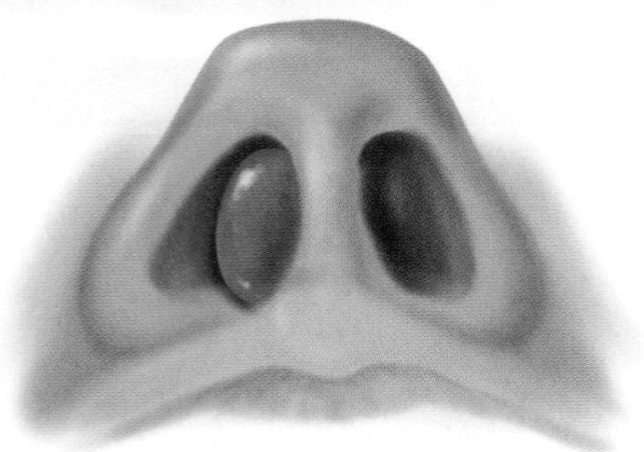

Furuncle

A small boil located in the skin or mucous membrane; appears red and swollen and is quite painful. Avoid any manipulation or trauma that may spread the infection.

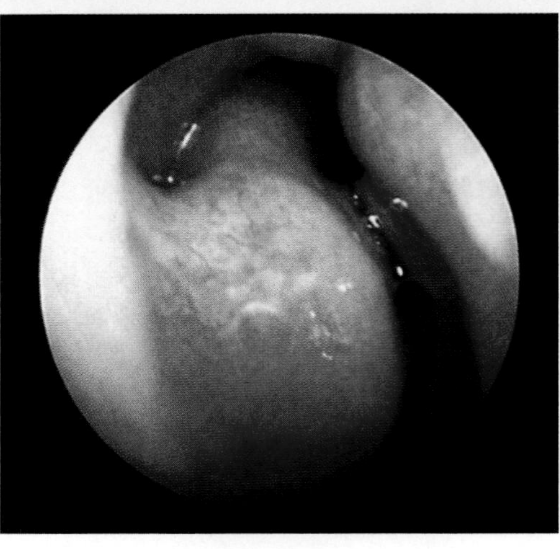

Acute Rhinitis

The first sign is a clear, watery discharge, rhinorrhea, which later becomes purulent. This is accompanied by sneezing and swollen mucosa, which causes nasal obstruction. Turbinates are dark red and swollen.

Reprinted from Fireman P. (1995). *Atlas of allergies* (2nd ed.). St Louis, Mosby, by permission of the publisher.

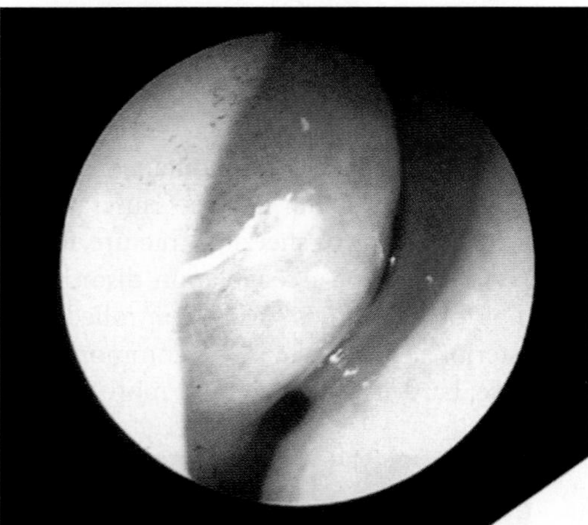

Allergic Rhinitis

Rhinorrhea, itching of nose and eyes, lacrimation, nasal congestion, and sneezing are present. Note serous edema and swelling of turbinates to fill the air space. Turbinates are usually pale (although may appear violet), and their surface looks smooth and glistening. May be seasonal or perennial, depending on allergen. Individual has a strong family history of seasonal allergies.

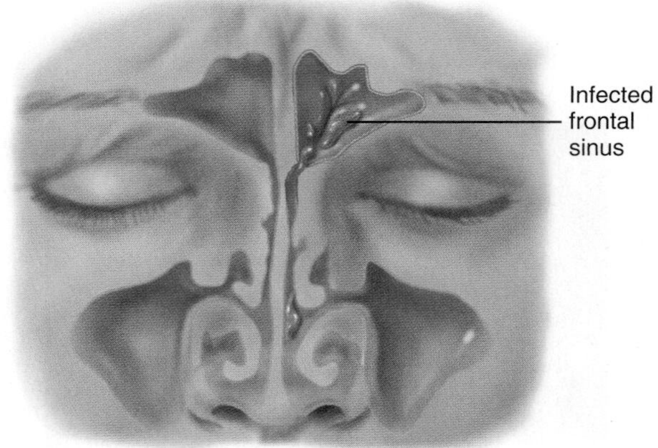

Sinusitis

Facial pain, after upper respiratory infection. Signs include red, swollen nasal mucosa; swollen turbinates; and purulent discharge. Person also has fever, chills, malaise. With maxillary sinusitis, dull, throbbing pain occurs in cheeks and teeth on the same side, and pain with palpation is present. With frontal sinusitis, pain is above the supraorbital ridge.

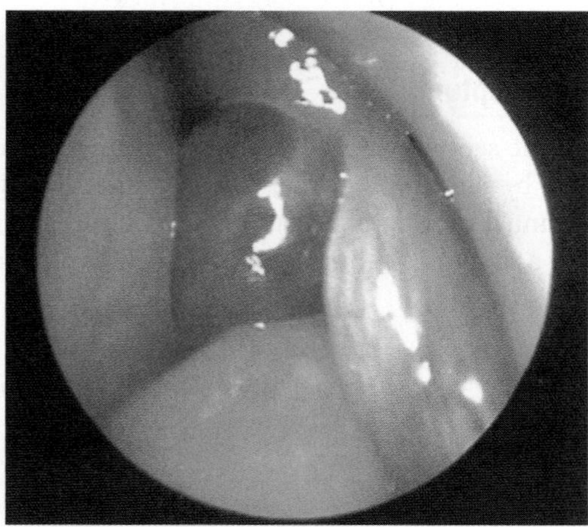

◀ Nasal Polyps

Smooth, pale gray nodules, which are overgrowths of mucosa, most commonly caused by chronic allergic rhinitis. May be stalked. A common site is protrusion from the middle meatus. Often multiple, they are mobile and nontender in contrast to turbinates. They may obstruct air passageways as they get larger. Symptoms include the absence of a sense of smell and a "valve that moves" in the nose as the person breathes.

TABLE 16-2 Abnormalities of the Lips

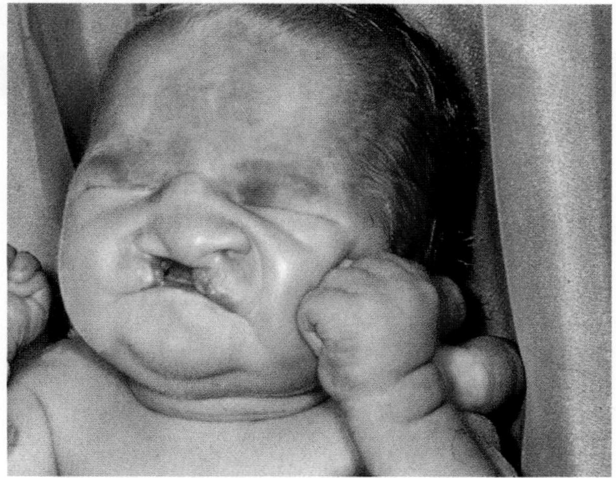

Cleft Lip

Maxillofacial clefts are the most common congenital deformities of the head and neck. The incidence varies among racial groups, being highest in American Indians and in Asians and lowest in Blacks. Early treatment preserves the functions of speech and language formation and deglutition (swallowing).

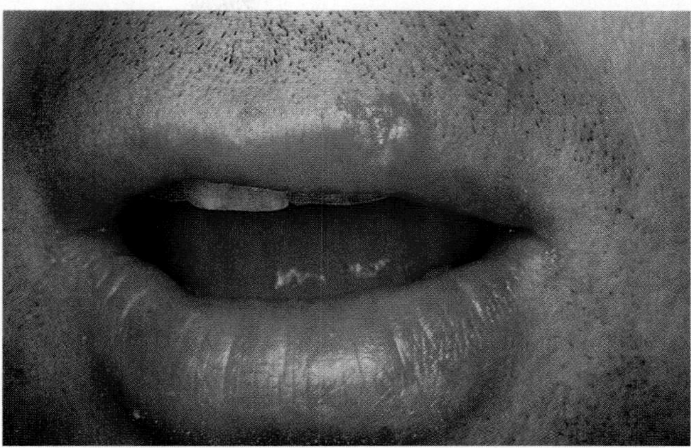

Herpes Simplex 1

The cold sores are groups of clear vesicles with a surrounding indurated erythematous base. These evolve into pustules, which rupture, weep, and crust and heal in 4 to 10 days. The most likely site is the lip-skin junction; infection often recurs in same site. Caused by the herpes simplex virus (HSV-1), the lesion is highly contagious and is spread by direct contact. Recurrent herpes infections may be precipitated by sunlight, fever, colds, and allergy. It is a very common lesion, affecting 50% of adults.

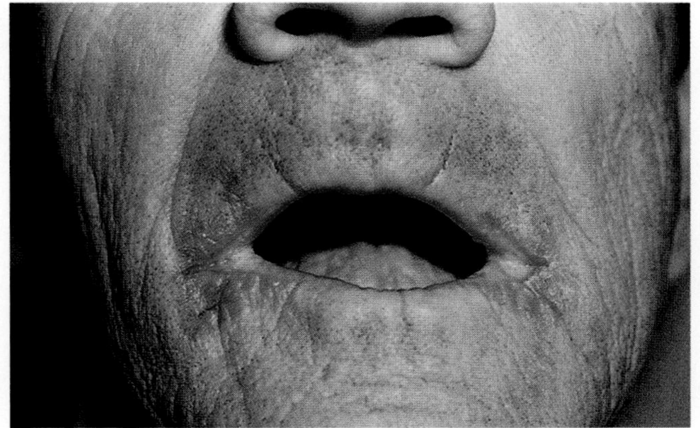

Angular Cheilitis (Stomatitis, Perlèche)

Erythema, scaling, shallow and painful fissures at the corners of the mouth occur with excess salivation and *Candida* infection. It is often seen in edentulous persons and in those with poorly fitting dentures causing folding in of corners of mouth, creating a warm, moist environment favoring growth of yeast.

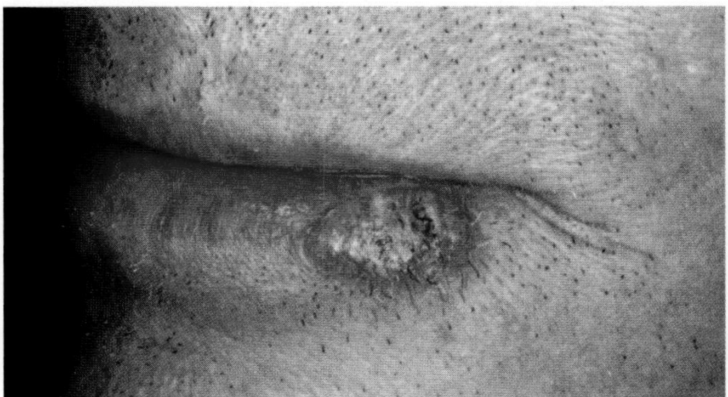

Carcinoma

The initial lesion is round and indurated, and then it becomes crusted and ulcerated with an elevated border. The majority occur between the outer and middle thirds of lip. Any lesion that is still unhealed after 2 weeks should be referred.

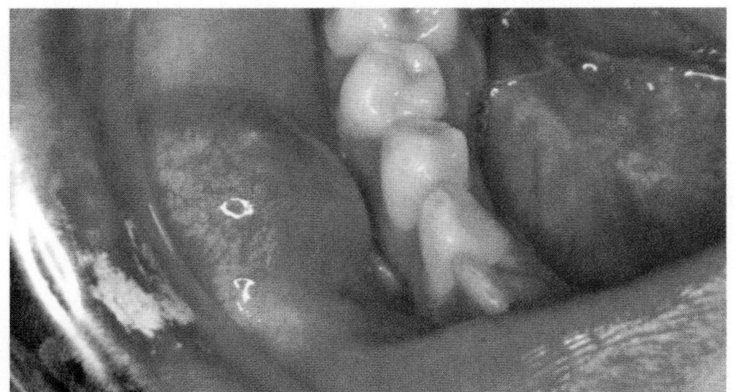

◀ Retention "Cyst" (Mucocele)

A round, well-defined, translucent nodule that may be very small or up to 1 to 2 cm. It is a pocket of mucus that forms when a duct of a minor salivary gland ruptures. The benign lesion also may occur on the buccal mucosa, on the floor of the mouth, or under the tip of the tongue.

ABNORMAL FINDINGS FOR ADVANCED PRACTICE

TABLE 16-3 Abnormalities of the Teeth and Gums

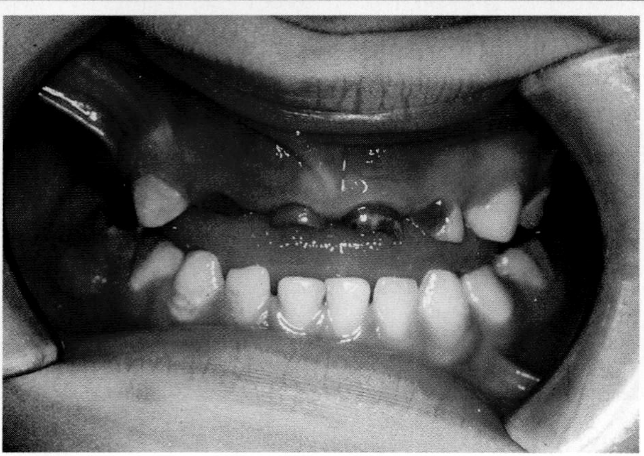

Baby Bottle Tooth Decay

Destruction of numerous deciduous teeth may occur in older infants and toddlers who take a bottle of milk, juice, or sweetened drink to bed and prolong bottle-feeding past the age of 1 year. Liquid pools around the upper front teeth. Mouth bacteria act on carbohydrates in the liquid, especially sucrose, forming metabolic acids. Acids break down tooth enamel and destroy its protein.

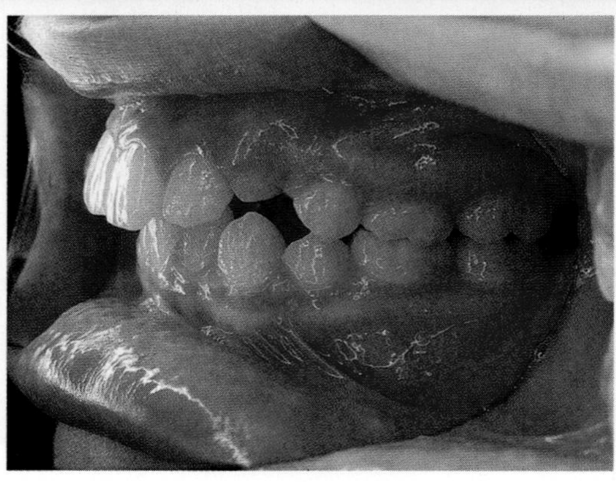

Malocclusion

Upper or lower dental arches are not in alignment and incisors protrude from developmental problem of mandible or maxilla or incompatibility between jaw size and tooth size. The condition increases risk for facial deformity, negative body image, chewing problems, or speech dysfluency.

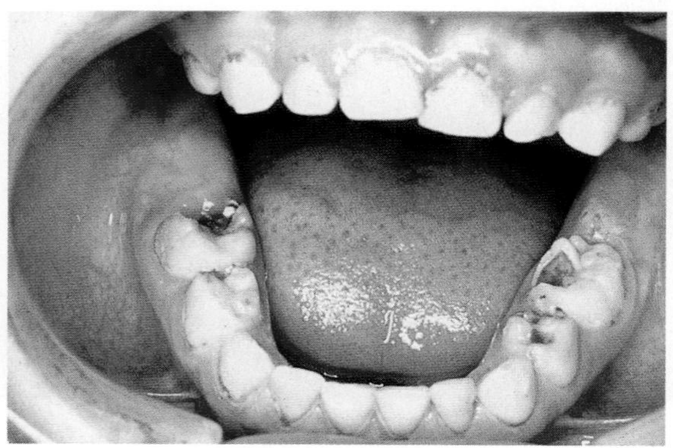

Dental Caries

Progressive destruction of tooth. Decay initially looks chalky white. Later, it turns brown or black and forms a cavity. Early decay is apparent only on x-ray study. Susceptible sites are tooth surfaces where food debris, bacterial plaque, and saliva collect.

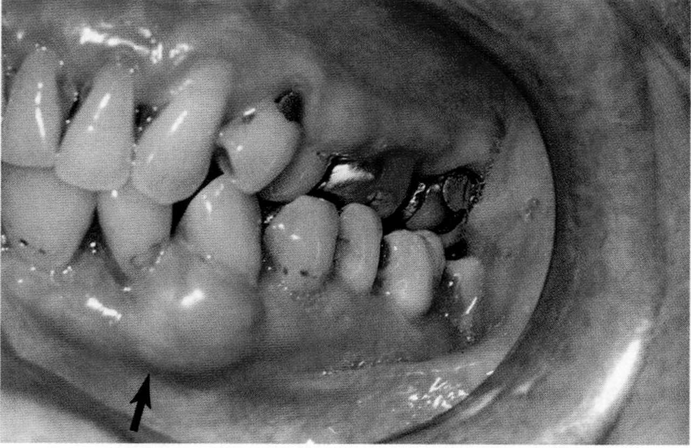

Epulis

A nontender, fibrous nodule of the gum, seen emerging between the teeth; an inflammatory response to injury or hemorrhage.

TABLE 16-3 Abnormalities of the Teeth and Gums—cont'd

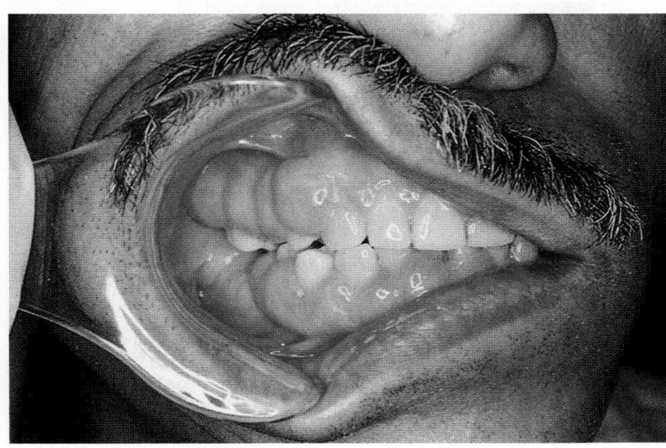

Gingival Hyperplasia

Painless enlargement of the gums, sometimes overreaching the teeth. This occurs with puberty, pregnancy, and leukemia and with long therapeutic use of phenytoin (Dilantin).

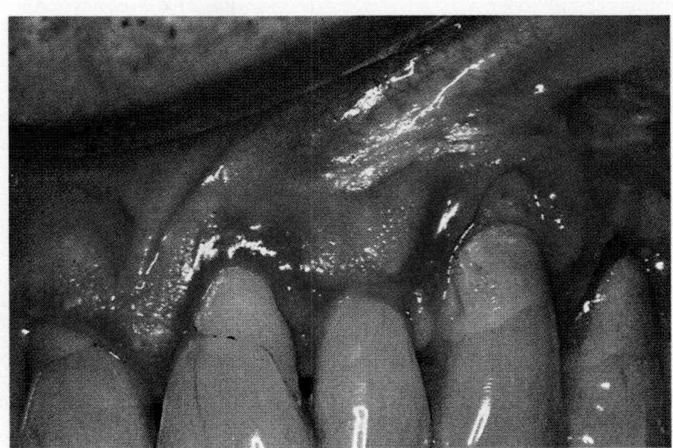

Gingivitis

Gum margins are red and swollen and bleed easily. This case is severe; gingival tissue has desquamated, exposing roots of teeth. Inflammation is usually due to poor dental hygiene or vitamin C deficiency. The condition may occur in pregnancy and puberty because of changing hormonal balance.

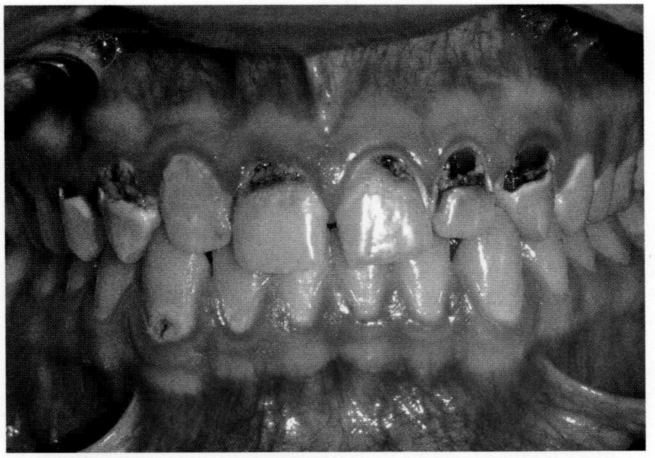

Meth Mouth

Illicit methamphetamine abuse (crystal meth, meth ice) leads to extensive dental caries, gingivitis, tooth cracking, and edentulism. Methamphetamine causes vasoconstriction and decreased saliva, and its use increases the urge to consume sugars and starches and to give up oral hygiene. Absence of the buffering saliva leads to increased acidity in the mouth, and the increased plaque encourages bacterial growth. These conditions and the presence of carbohydrates set up an oral environment prone to caries, cracking of enamel, and the damage seen here.

From Neville, B. W., Damm, D. D., Allen, C. M., et al. (2009). *Oral and maxillofacial pathology* (3rd ed.). St Louis, Saunders.

TABLE 16-4 Abnormalities of the Buccal Mucosa

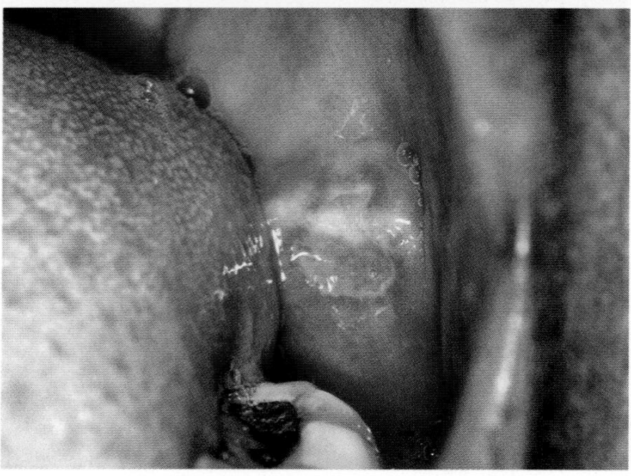

Aphthous Ulcers

A "canker sore" is a vesicle at first and then a small, round, "punched-out" ulcer with a white base surrounded by a red halo. It is quite painful and lasts for 1 to 2 weeks. The cause is unknown, although it is associated with stress, fatigue, and food allergy. It is common, affecting 20% to 60% of the population.

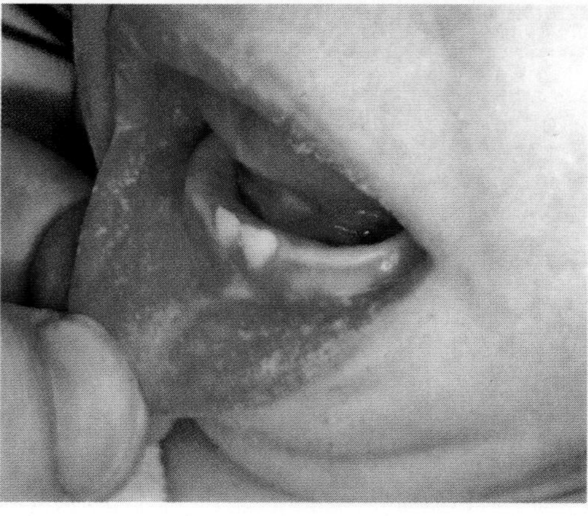

Koplik Spots

Small blue-white spots with irregular red halo scattered over mucosa opposite the molars. An early sign, and pathognomonic, of measles.

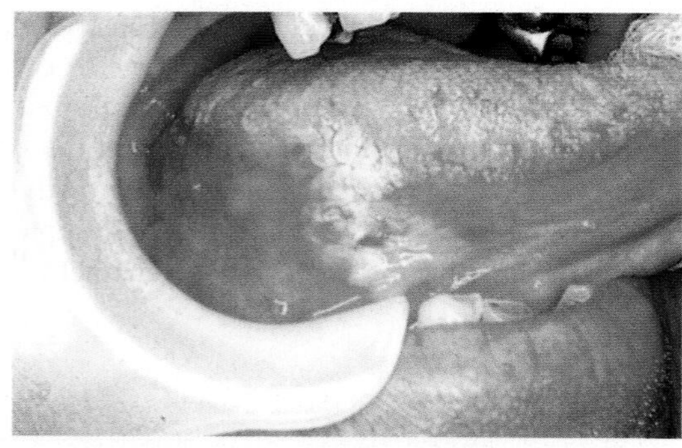

Leukoplakia

Chalky white, thick, raised patch with well-defined borders. The lesion is firmly attached and does not scrape off. It may occur on the lateral edges of tongue. It is due to chronic irritation and occurs more frequently with heavy smoking and heavy alcohol use. Lesions are precancerous, and the person should be referred. (Here, the lesion is associated with squamous carcinoma.)

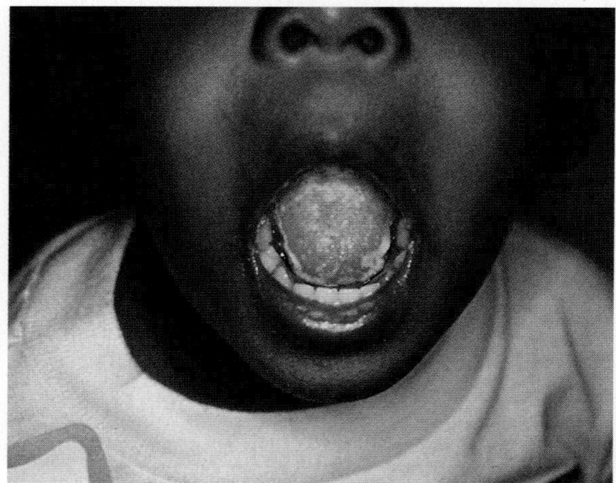

Candidiasis or Monilial Infection

A white, cheesy, curdlike patch on the buccal mucosa and tongue. It scrapes off, leaving a raw, red surface that bleeds easily. Termed "thrush" in the newborn. It is an opportunistic infection that occurs after the use of antibiotics and corticosteroids and in immunosuppressed persons.

TABLE 16-4 **Abnormalities of the Buccal Mucosa—cont'd**

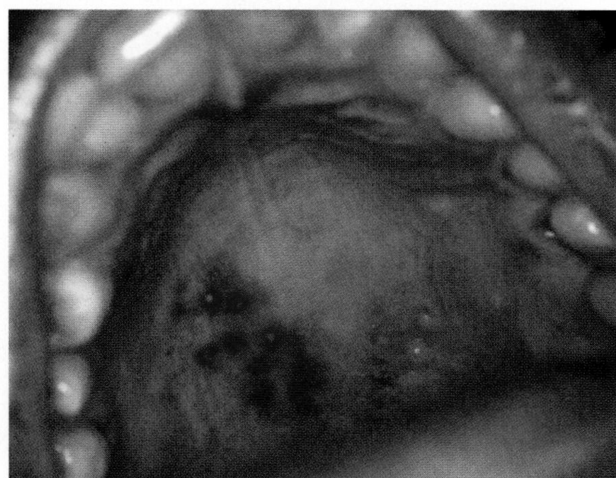

Herpes Simplex 1

Herpes infection on the hard palate (see discussion in Table 16-2).

TABLE 16-5 **Abnormalities of the Tongue**

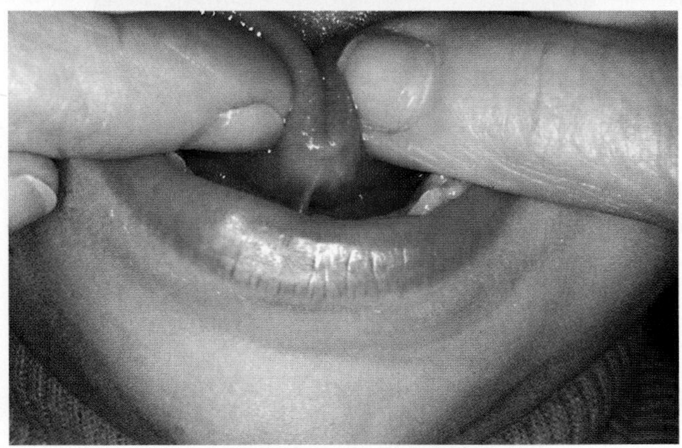

Ankyloglossia

(Tongue-tie.) A short lingual frenulum, here fixing the tongue tip to the floor of the mouth and gums. This limits mobility and will affect speech (pronunciation of *a, d, n*) if the tongue tip cannot be elevated to the alveolar ridge. A congenital defect.

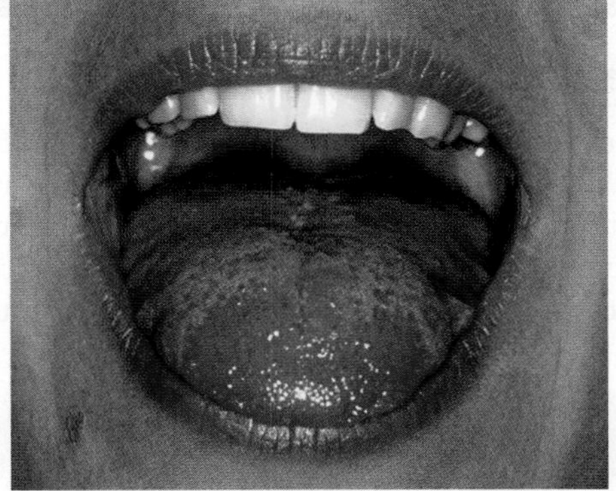

Geographic Tongue (Migratory Glossitis)

Pattern of normal coating interspersed with bright red, shiny, circular bald areas with raised pearly borders. Pattern resembles a map and changes in a few days. Not significant, and its cause is not known.

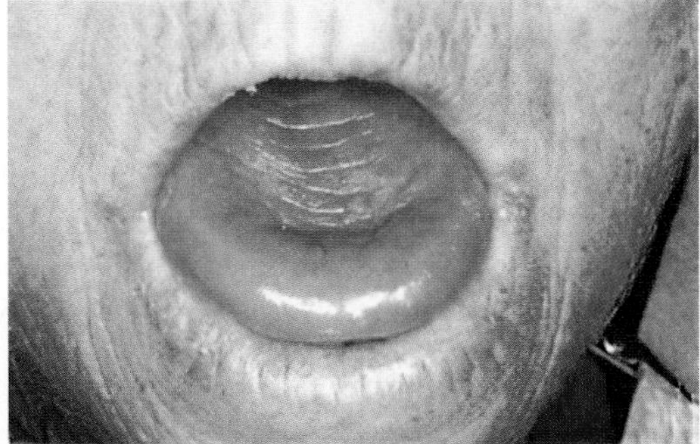

Smooth, Glossy Tongue (Atrophic Glossitis)

The surface is slick and shiny; the mucosa thins and looks red from decreased papillae. Accompanied by dryness of tongue and burning. Occurs with vitamin B_{12} deficiency (pernicious anemia), folic acid deficiency, and iron deficiency anemia. Here, also note angular cheilitis.

Continued

TABLE 16-5 Abnormalities of the Tongue—cont'd

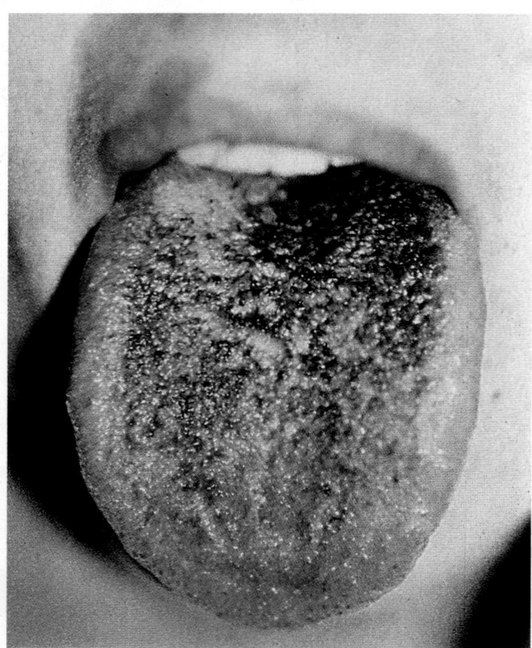

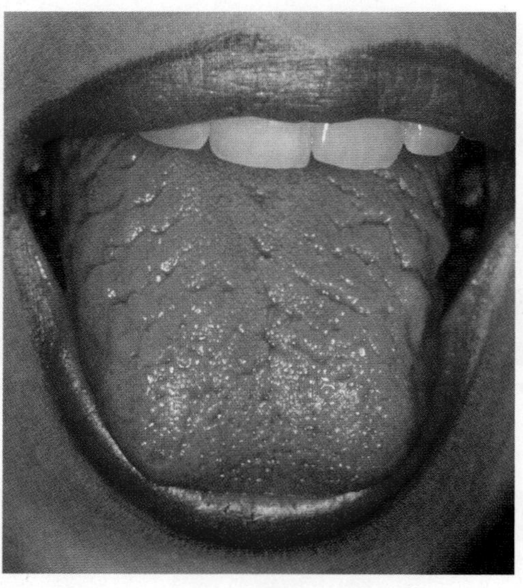

Black Hairy Tongue

This is not really hair but, rather, the elongation of filiform papillae and painless overgrowth of mycelial threads of fungus infection on the tongue. Color varies from black-brown to yellow. It occurs after use of antibiotics, which inhibit normal bacteria and allow proliferation of fungus.

Fissured or Scrotal Tongue

Deep furrows divide the papillae into small irregular rows. The condition occurs in 5% of the general population and in Down syndrome. The incidence increases with age. (Vertical, or longitudinal, fissures also occur with dehydration because of reduced volume of the tongue.)

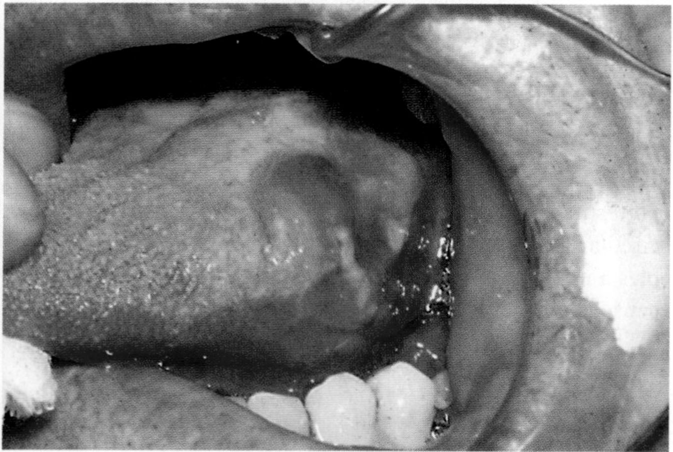

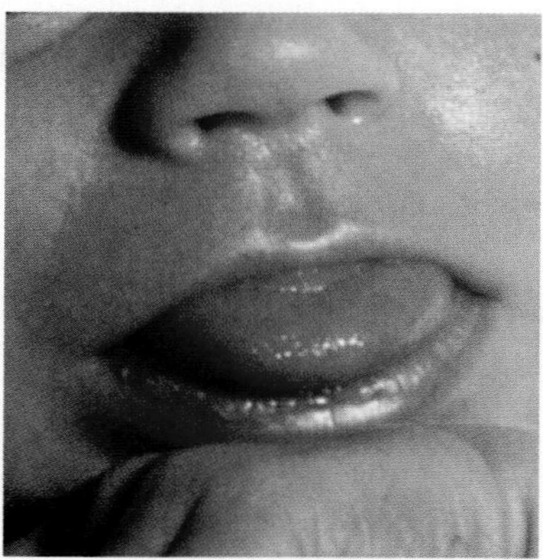

Carcinoma

An ulcer with rolled edges; indurated. Occurs particularly at sides, base, and under the tongue. When it is in the floor of mouth, it may cause painful movement or limited movement of tongue. Risk for early metastasis is present because of rich lymphatic drainage. Heavy smoking and heavy alcohol use place persons at greater risk.

Enlarged Tongue (Macroglossia)

The tongue is enlarged and may protrude from mouth. The condition is not painful but may impair speech development. Here, it occurs with Down syndrome; it also occurs with cretinism, myxedema, acromegaly. Also, a transient swelling occurs with local infections.

TABLE 16-6 Abnormalities of the Oropharynx

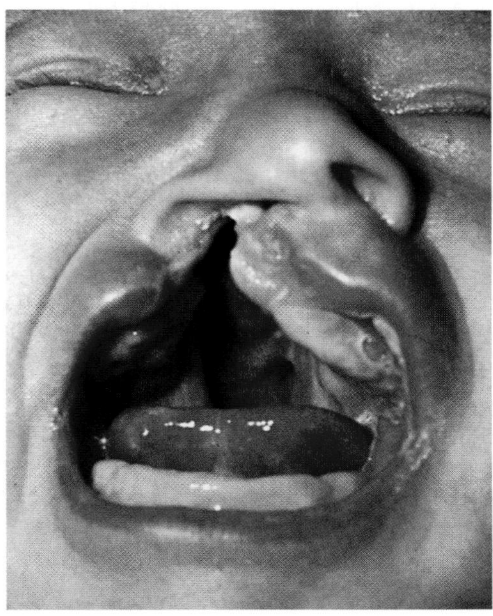

Cleft Palate

A congenital defect, the failure of fusion of the maxillary processes. Wide variation occurs in the extent of cleft formation, from upper lip only, palate only, uvula only, to cleft of the nostril and the hard and soft palates.

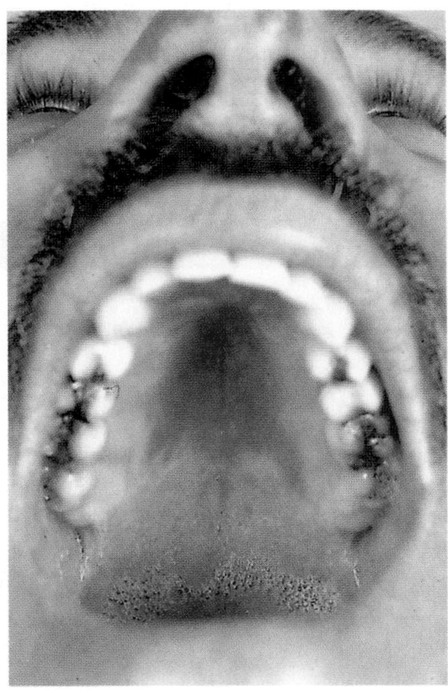

Oral Kaposi Sarcoma

Bruiselike, dark red or violet, confluent macule, usually on the hard palate, may be on soft palate or gingival margin. Oral lesions may be among the earliest lesions to develop with AIDS.

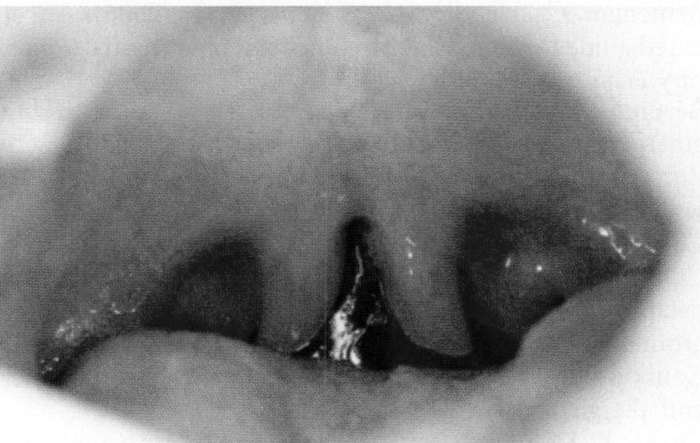

Bifid Uvula

The uvula looks partly severed. May indicate a submucous cleft palate, which feels like a notch at the junction of the hard and soft palates. The submucous cleft palate may affect speech development because it prevents necessary air trapping. The incidence of bifid uvula varies among racial groups: it is common in American Indians, uncommon in whites, and rare in Blacks.

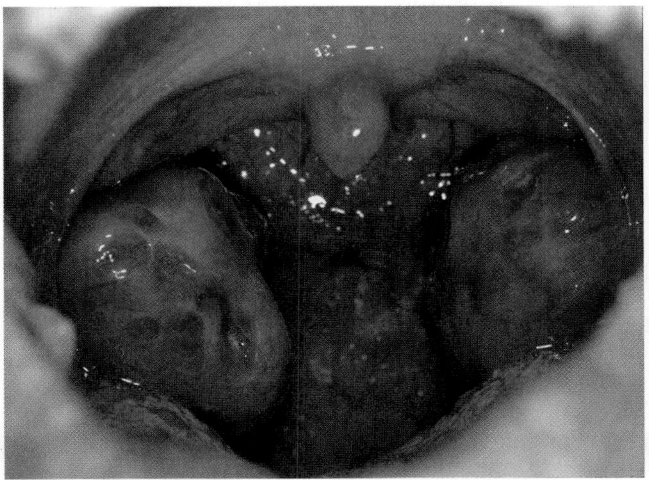

Acute Tonsillitis and Pharyngitis

Bright red throat; swollen tonsils; white or yellow exudate on tonsils and pharynx; swollen uvula; and enlarged, tender anterior cervical and tonsillar nodes. Accompanied by severe sore throat, painful swallowing, fever >101° F of sudden onset.

Evidence-based practice recommends using the criteria listed above to determine when to seek further testing.[29] A rapid antigen test or standard throat culture will then diagnose streptococcal pharyngitis and limit antibiotic therapy to those who test positive. If untreated, group A beta-hemolytic streptococcal pharyngitis may lead to glomerulonephritis and rheumatic fever. This is a serious complex illness characterized by fever, malaise, swollen joints, rash, and scarring on the heart valves.

BIBLIOGRAPHY

1. Armengol, C., Hendley, O., & Schlager, T. (2006). An office-based guide to diagnosing streptococcal pharyngitis. *Contemporary Pediatrics, 23*, 64-70.
2. Bernius, M., & Perlin, D. (2006). Pediatric ear, nose, and throat emergencies. *Pediatric Clinics of North America, 53*, 195-214.
3. Burkhart, N. (2008). *Leukoedema.* Retrieved April 25, 2010, from www.rdhmag.com/display_article/346087/56/none/none/Colum/Leukoedema.
4. Chohayeb, A. A., & Volpe, A. R. (2001). Occurrence of torus palatinus and mandibularis among women of different ethnic groups. *American Journal of Dentistry, 14*(5), 278-280.
5. Conboy-Ellis, K., & Braker-Shaver, S. (2007). Intranasal steroids and allergic rhinitis. *Nurse Practitioner, 32*(4), 44-49.
6. Curtis, E. K. (2006). Meth mouth: a review of methamphetamine use and its oral manifestations. *General Dentistry, 54*(2), 125-129.
7. da Silva, C. M., Ramos, M. M., deCarvalho Carrara, C. F., et al. (2008). Oral characteristics of newborns. *Journal of Dentistry for Children, 75*(1), 4-6.
8. Eisenstadt, E. S. (2010). Dysphagia and aspiration pneumonia in older adults. *Journal of the American Academy of Nurse Practitioners, 22*, 17-22.
9. Foster, E. (2008). Uncovering sleep apnea misconceptions. *Nurse Practitioner, 33*(6), 23-28.
10. Godley, F. A. (1992). Chronic sinusitis: an update. *American Family Physician, 45*(5), 2190-2199.
11. Gonsalves, W. C., Wrightson, A. S., Henry, R. G., et al. (2008). Common oral conditions in older persons. *American Family Physician, 78*(7), 845-852.
12. Holcomb, S. S. (2008). Diagnosing rhinosinusitis: know your guidelines. *Nurse Practitioner, 33*(11), 6-9.
13. Hoyle, C. (2009). Make your strep diagnosis spot on. *Nurse Practitioner, 34*(10), 47-52.
14. Jainkittivong, A., & Langlais, R. P. (2000). Buccal and palatal exostoses: prevalence and concurrence with tori. *Oral Surgery, Oral Medicine, and Oral Pathology, 90*(1), 48-53.
15. Kamienski, M. (2007). When sore throat gets serious. *American Journal of Nursing, 107*(10), 35-38.
16. Kane, R. L., Ouslander, J. G., & Abrass, I. E. (2009). *Essentials of clinical geriatrics* (6th ed.). New York: McGraw-Hill.
17. Lafreniere, D., & Mann, N. (2009). Anosmia: loss of smell in the elderly. *Otolaryngologic Clinics of North America, 42*(1), 123-131.
18. Leung, A. K. C., & Robson, W. L. M. (2006). Natal teeth: a review. *Journal of the National Medical Association, 98*(2), 226-228.
19. Morse, D. E., & Kerr, A. R. (2006). Disparities in oral and pharyngeal cancer incidence: mortality and survival among Black and White Americans. *Journal of the American Dental Association, 137*, 203-212.
20. Myers, N. E., Compliment, J. M., Post, J. C., et al. (2006). Tonsilloliths: a common finding in pediatric patients. *The Nurse Practitioner, 31*, 53-54.
21. National Center for Health Statistics. (2009). *Health, United States, 2009 with chartbook on trends in the health of Americans* (USDHHS Publication No. 2009-1232). Hyattsville, MD: Author.
22. Palmer, J. L., & Metheny, N. A. (2008). Preventing aspiration in older adults with dysphagia. *American Journal of Nursing, 108*(2), 40-48.
23. Parthasarathy, P., & Ritamarie, J. (2008). Identification of childhood caries. *Nurse Practitioner, 33*(9), 41-48.
24. Petersen, P. E. (2009). Oral cancer prevention and control: the approach of the World Health Organization. *Oral Oncology, 45*, 454-460.
25. Regan, E. N. (2008). Diagnosing rhinitis: viral and allergic characteristics. *Nurse Practitioner, 33*(9), 20-26.
26. Sieracki, R. L., Voelz, L. M., Johannik, T. M., et al. (2009). Development and implementation of an oral care protocol for patients with cancer. *Clinical Journal of Oncology Nursing, 13*(6), 718-722.
27. Stockdell, R., & Amella, E. J. (2008). The Edinburgh Feeding Evaluation in Dementia Scale. *The American Journal of Nursing, 108*(8), 46-54.
28. U.S. Department of Health & Human Services, The Office of Minority Health. (2009). *Cleft lip/palate more prevalent in Asians.* Retrieved April 25, 2010, from http://minorityhealth.hhs.gov/templates/content.aspx?ID=7590&lvl=3&lv1ID=287.
29. Wagner, F. P., & Mathiason, M. A. (2008). Using Centor criteria to diagnose streptococcal pharyngitis. *Nurse Practitioner, 33*(9), 10-12.

Summary Checklist: Nose, Mouth, and Throat Examination

 For a PDA-downloadable version, go to http://evolve.elsevier.com/Jarvis/.

Nose

1. **Inspect external nose for symmetry, any deformity, or lesions**
2. **Palpation—test patency of each nostril**
3. **Inspect with nasal speculum:**
   - Color and integrity of nasal mucosa
   - Septum—note any deviation, perforation, or bleeding
   - Turbinates—note color, any exudate, swelling, or polyps
4. **Palpate the sinus areas—note any tenderness**

Mouth and Throat

1. **Inspect with penlight:**
   - Lips, teeth and gums, tongue, buccal mucosa—note color; whether structures are intact; any lesions
   - Palate and uvula—note integrity and mobility as person phonates
   - Grade tonsils
   - Pharyngeal wall—note color, any exudate, or lesions
2. **Palpation:**
   - When indicated in adults, bimanual palpation of mouth
   - With the neonate, palpate for integrity of palate and to assess sucking reflex

17

Breasts and Regional Lymphatics

evolve WEBSITE

http://evolve.elsevier.com/Jarvis/

- Animations
- Audio Key Points
- Bedside Assessment Summary Checklist
- Case Study
  Breast Lumps
  Post-Mastectomy
- Health Promotion Guide
  Breast Cancer
- NCLEX Review Questions
- Physical Examination Summary Checklist
- Video—Assessment
  Breasts

OUTLINE

Structure and Function, 383

Surface Anatomy
Internal Anatomy
Lymphatics
The Male Breast

Subjective Data, 389

Health History Questions

Objective Data, 392

Preparation
The Breasts
The Axillae
Breast Palpation
Breast Self-Examination
The Male Breast

Documentation and Critical Thinking, 402

Abnormal Findings, 404

Abnormal Findings for Advanced Practice, 407

STRUCTURE AND FUNCTION

The breasts, or mammary glands, are present in both females and males, although in men they are rudimentary throughout life. The female breasts are accessory reproductive organs whose function is to produce milk for nourishing the newborn.

SURFACE ANATOMY

The **breasts** lie anterior to the pectoralis major and serratus anterior muscles (Fig. 17-1). The breasts are located between the second and sixth ribs, extending from the side of the sternum to the midaxillary line. The superior lateral corner of breast tissue, called the axillary **tail of Spence,** projects up and laterally into the axilla.

The **nipple** is just below the center of the breast. It is rough, round, and usually protuberant; its surface looks wrinkled and indented with tiny milk duct openings. The **areola** surrounds the nipple for a 1- to 2-cm radius. In the areola are small elevated sebaceous glands, called *Montgomery's glands.* These secrete a protective lipid material during lactation. The areola also has smooth muscle fibers that cause nipple erection when stimulated. Both the nipple and areola are more darkly pigmented than the rest of the breast surface; the color varies from pink to brown depending on the person's skin color and parity (condition of giving birth).

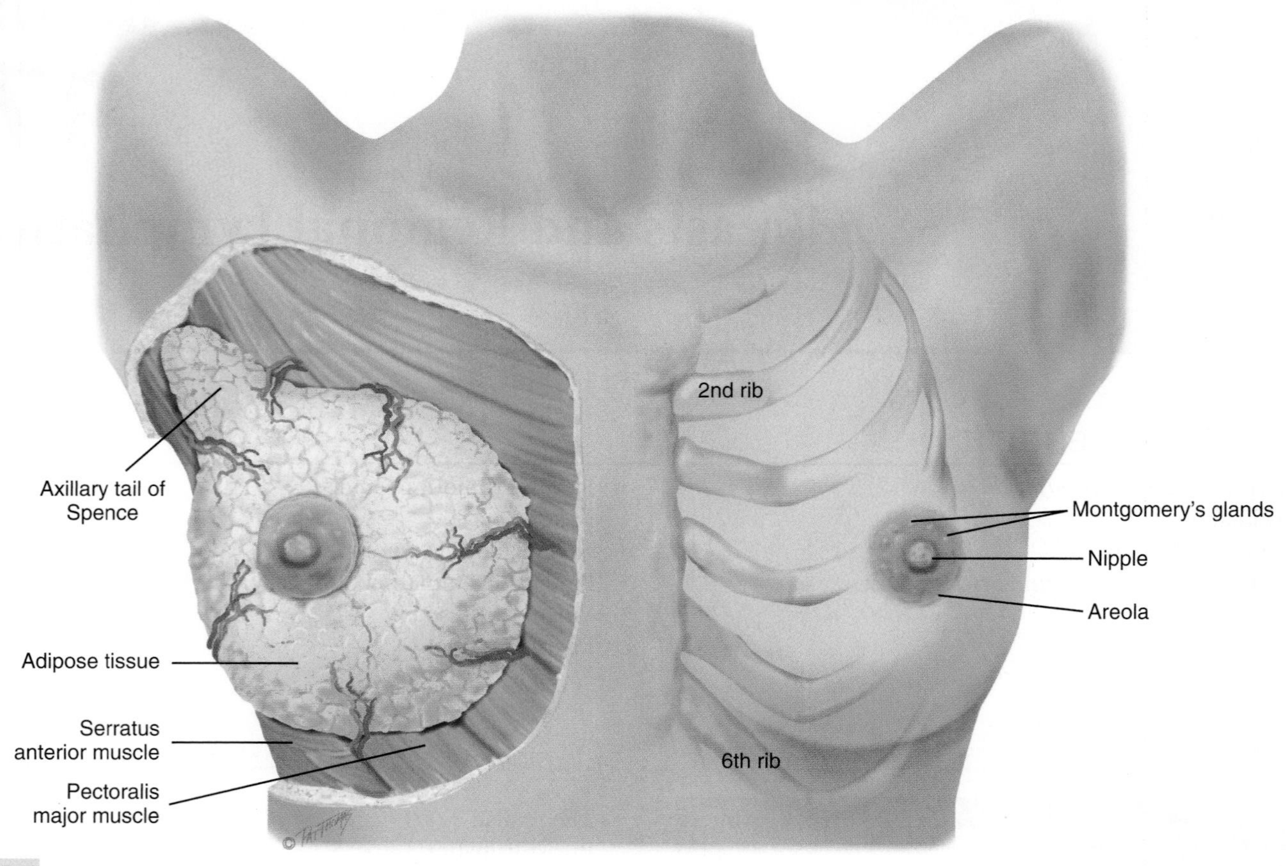

17-1

© Pat Thomas, 2010.

INTERNAL ANATOMY

The breast is composed of (1) glandular tissue, (2) fibrous tissue including the suspensory ligaments, and (3) adipose tissue (Fig. 17-2). The **glandular tissue** contains 15 to 20 lobes radiating from the nipple, and these are composed of lobules. Within each lobule are clusters of alveoli that produce milk. Each lobe empties into a lactiferous duct. The 15 to 20 lactiferous ducts form a collecting duct system converging toward the nipple. There, the ducts form ampullae, or lactiferous sinuses, behind the nipple, which are reservoirs for storing milk.

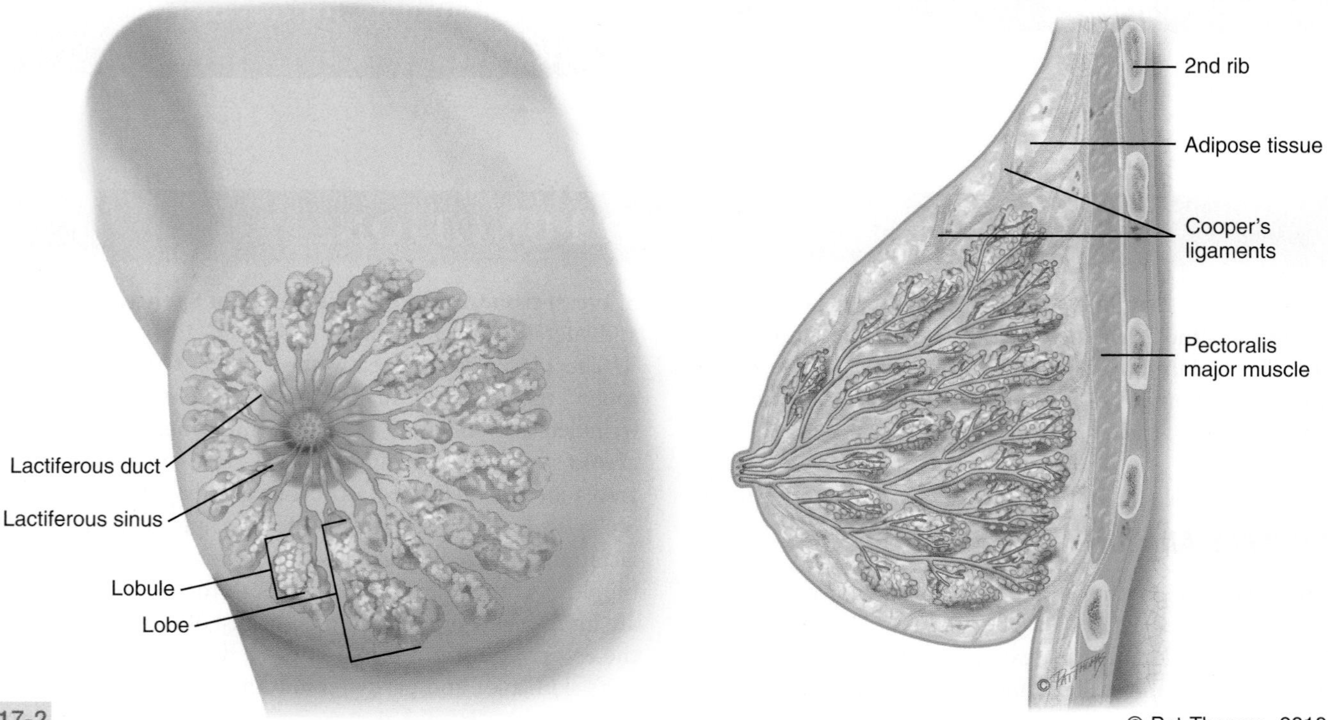

17-2

© Pat Thomas, 2010.

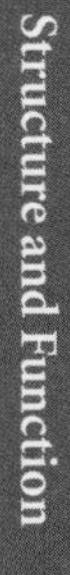

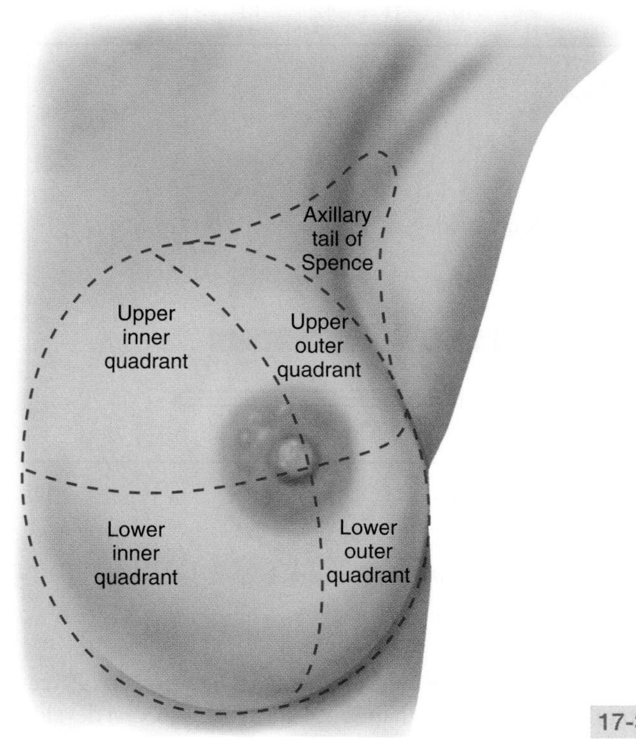

17-3

The suspensory ligaments, or **Cooper's ligaments,** are fibrous bands extending vertically from the surface to attach on chest wall muscles. These support the breast tissue. They become contracted in cancer of the breast, producing pits or dimples in the overlying skin.

The lobes are embedded in **adipose tissue.** These layers of subcutaneous and retromammary fat actually provide most of the bulk of the breast. The relative proportion of glandular, fibrous, and fatty tissue varies depending on age, cycle, pregnancy, lactation, and general nutritional state.

The breast may be divided into four quadrants by imaginary horizontal and vertical lines intersecting at the nipple (Fig. 17-3). This makes a convenient map to describe clinical findings. In the upper outer quadrant, note the axillary **tail of Spence,** the cone-shaped breast tissue that projects up into the axilla, close to the pectoral group of axillary lymph nodes. The upper outer quadrant is the site of most breast tumors.

LYMPHATICS

The breast has extensive lymphatic drainage. Most of the lymph, more than 75%, drains into the ipsilateral (same side) axillary nodes. Four groups of axillary nodes are present (Fig. 17-4):

1. **Central axillary nodes**—high up in the middle of the axilla, over the ribs and serratus anterior muscle. These receive lymph from the other three groups of nodes.
2. **Pectoral** (anterior)—along the lateral edge of the pectoralis major muscle, just inside the anterior axillary fold.
3. **Subscapular** (posterior)—along the lateral edge of the scapula, deep in the posterior axillary fold.
4. **Lateral**—along the humerus, inside the upper arm.

From the central axillary nodes, drainage flows up to the infraclavicular and supraclavicular nodes.

A smaller amount of lymphatic drainage does not take these channels but, instead, flows directly up to the infraclavicular group, deep into the chest, or into the abdomen, or directly across to the opposite breast.

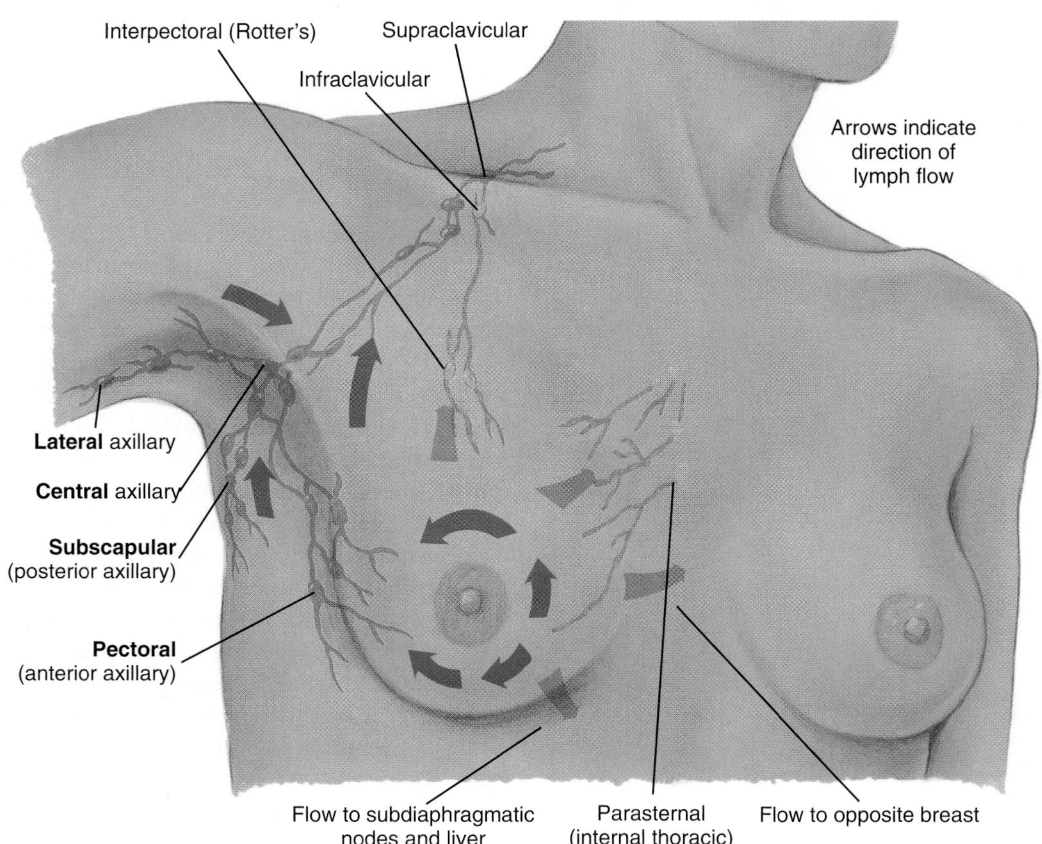

17-4

DEVELOPMENTAL COMPETENCE

During embryonic life, ventral epidermal ridges, or "milk lines," are present and curve down from the axilla to the groin bilaterally (Fig. 17-5). The breast develops along the ridge over the thorax, and the rest of the ridge usually atrophies. Occasionally a **supernumerary nipple** (i.e., an extra nipple) persists and is visible somewhere along the track of the mammary ridge (see Fig. 17-8).

At birth, the only breast structures present are the lactiferous ducts within the nipple. No alveoli have developed. Little change occurs until puberty.

The Adolescent

At puberty, the estrogen hormones stimulate breast changes. The breasts enlarge, mostly as a result of extensive fat deposition. The duct system also grows and branches, and masses of small, solid cells develop at the duct endings. These are potential alveoli.

A 1997 study of 17,077 girls in the United States ages 3 through 12 years indicates that puberty is occurring earlier than classically used norms.[14] The onset of breast development occurred at an average (mean) age between 8 and 9 years for African-American girls and by 10 years for white girls. Occasionally, one breast may grow faster than the other, producing a temporary asymmetry. This may cause some distress; reassurance is necessary. Tenderness is common also. Although the age of onset varies widely, the five stages of breast development follow this classic description of sexual maturity rating, or **Tanner staging** (Table 17-1).

Full development from stage 2 to stage 5 takes an average of 3 years, although the range is 1.5 to 6 years. During this time, pubic hair develops, and axillary hair appears 2 years after the onset of pubic hair. The beginning of breast development precedes **menarche** (beginning of menstruation) by about 2 years. Menarche occurs in breast development stage 3 or 4, usually just after the peak of the adolescent growth spurt around age 12 years. Note the relationship of these events (Fig. 17-6). This aids in assessing the development of adolescent girls and increases their knowledge about their own development.

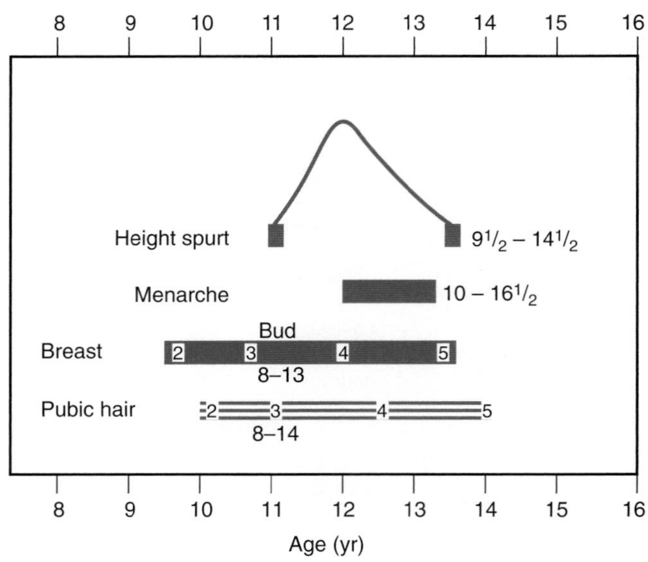

17-6 Relationship of puberty events in girls.

Breasts of the nonpregnant woman change with the ebb and flow of hormones during the monthly menstrual cycle. Nodularity increases from midcycle up to menstruation. During the 3 to 4 days before menstruation, the breasts feel full, tight, heavy, and occasionally sore. The breast volume is smallest on days 4 to 7 of the menstrual cycle.

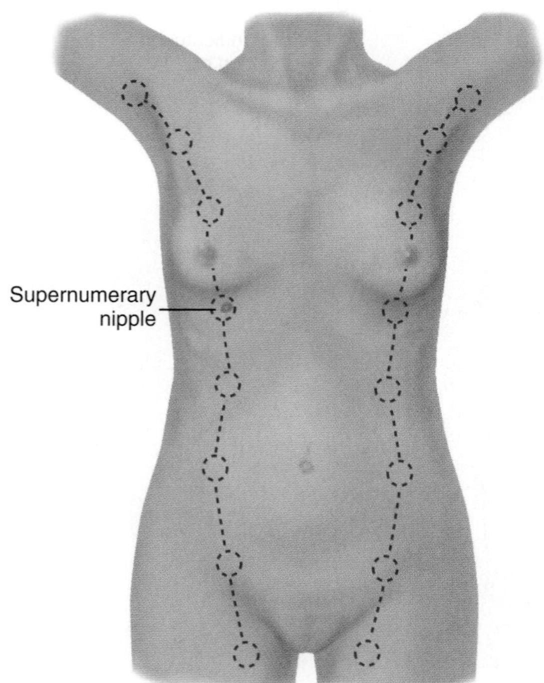

17-5

The Pregnant Woman

During pregnancy, breast changes start during the second month and are an early sign of pregnancy for most women. Pregnancy stimulates the expansion of the ductal system and supporting fatty tissue as well as development of the true secretory alveoli. Thus the breasts enlarge and feel more nodular. The nipples are larger, darker, and more erectile. The areolae become larger and grow a darker brown as pregnancy progresses, and the tubercles become more prominent. (The brown color fades after lactation, but the areolae never return to the original color.) A venous pattern is prominent over the skin surface (see Fig. 29-4 on p. 808).

After the fourth month, **colostrum** may be expressed. This thick, yellow fluid is the precursor for milk, containing the same amount of protein and lactose but practically no fat. The breasts produce colostrum for the first few days after delivery. It is rich with antibodies that protect the newborn against infection, so breastfeeding is important. Milk production (lactation) begins 1 to 3 days postpartum. The whitish color is from emulsified fat and calcium caseinate.

TABLE 17-1 Sexual Maturity Rating in Girls

Stage

1 **Preadolescent:** Only a small elevated nipple

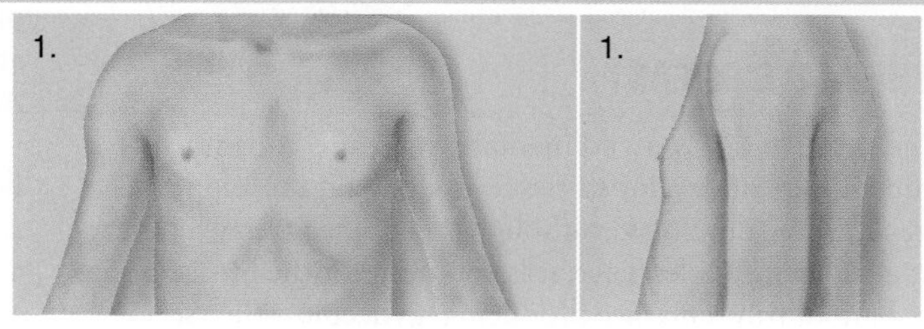

2 **Breast bud stage:** A small mound of breast and nipple develops; the areola widens

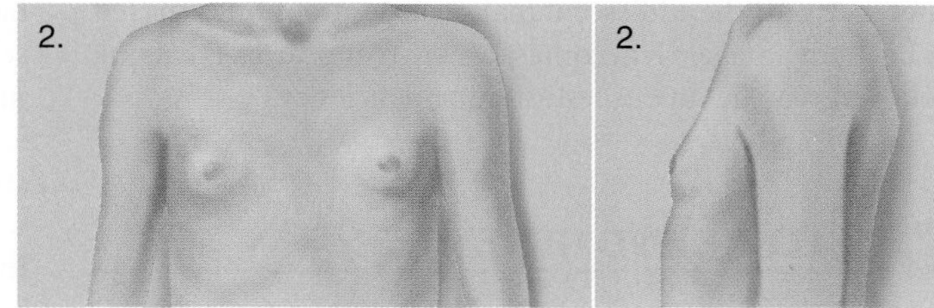

3 The breast and areola enlarge; the nipple is flush with the breast surface

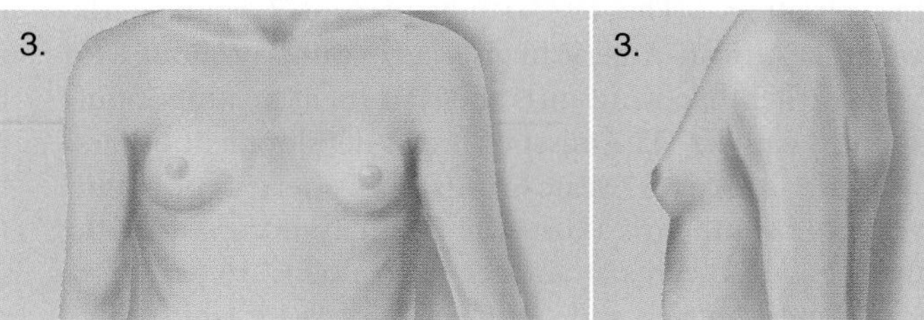

4 The areola and nipple form a secondary mound over the breast

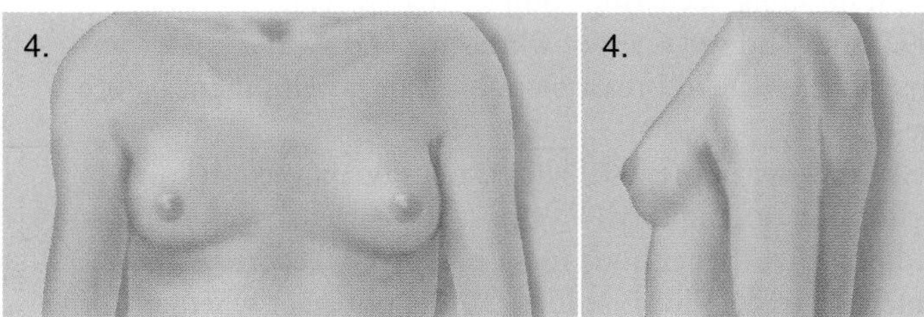

5 **Mature breast:** Only the nipple protrudes; the areola is flush with the breast contour (the areola may continue as a secondary mound in some normal women)

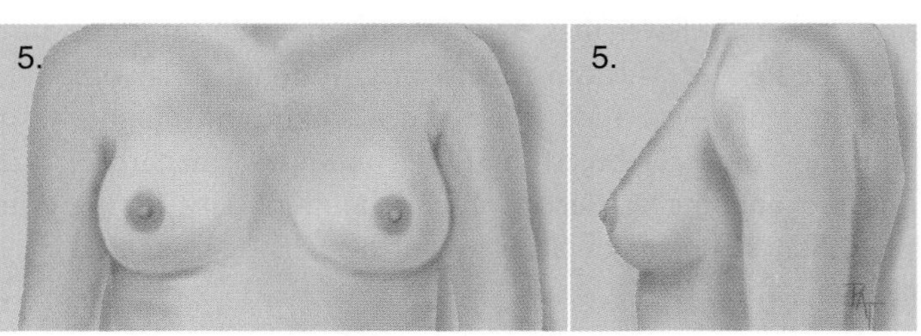

The Aging Woman

After menopause, ovarian secretion of estrogen and progesterone decreases, which causes the breast glandular tissue to atrophy. This is replaced with fibrous connective tissue. The fat envelope atrophies also, beginning in the middle years and becoming marked in the eighth and ninth decades. These changes decrease breast size and elasticity so the breasts droop and sag, looking flattened and flabby. Drooping is accentuated by the kyphosis in some older women.

The decreased breast size makes inner structures more prominent. A breast lump may have been present for years but is suddenly palpable. Around the nipple, the lactiferous ducts are more palpable and feel firm and stringy because of fibrosis and calcification. The axillary hair decreases.

THE MALE BREAST

The male breast is a rudimentary structure consisting of a thin disk of undeveloped tissue underlying the nipple. The areola is well developed, although the nipple is relatively very small. During adolescence, it is common for the breast tissue to temporarily enlarge, producing **gynecomastia** (see Fig. 17-21). This condition is usually temporary, but reassurance is necessary for the adolescent male, whose attention is riveted on his body image. Gynecomastia may reappear in the aging male and may be due to testosterone deficiency.

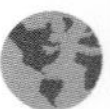

CULTURE AND GENETICS

The timing of puberty is influenced by genetic and environmental factors, with genetics determining about 50% to 80% of the variation.[13] The 1997 study of 17,077 young girls showed that African-American girls begin puberty about 1 to 1.5 years earlier than white girls and start menstruating about 8.5 months earlier.[14] The onset of breast development occurs at an average age of 8.87 years for African-American girls and 10 years for white girls (Hispanic ethnicity occurs in both groups). Menses begins at an average age of 12.16 years for African-American girls and at almost 13 years for white girls. For over 50 years, precocious puberty had been defined as breast budding occurring younger than 8 years; however, the 1997 study showed 6.5% of white girls and 27.2% of African-American girls had breast or pubic hair development before age 8 years.[14]

As to environmental factors, obesity may contribute to early onset of puberty, as girls with early onset of breast budding have higher body mass index (BMI) scores than age-matched girls without budding.[14] It is not clear whether this correlation applies among different racial and ethnic groups.[33] Among girls with normal BMIs, signs of puberty occurred before 8 years in fewer than 5% of white girls, 12% of Black girls, and 19% of Mexican-American girls.[28] But girls with overweight or obese BMI levels had a significantly higher occurrence of early breast budding and early menarche. Thus the ongoing epidemic of childhood obesity in the United States is a major determinant of early-age pubertal milestones.[28]

Breast Cancer

The genetic contribution to breast cancer involves specific gene mutations at the BRCA1 and BRCA2 locations. Women with these mutations are at increased risk for breast and ovarian cancer.

White women have a higher incidence of breast cancer than African-American women starting at age 45 years. In contrast, African-American women have a higher incidence before age 45 years and they are more likely to die of their disease at every age.[4] Women from Asian-American, Hispanic, and American-Indian groups have a lower incidence and death rates from breast cancer than whites and African Americans have.

The disparity in death rates may be due, in part, to insufficient use of screening measures and lack of access to health care. The good news is that, in the United States, the percentage of women ages 40 years and older who report having had a mammogram in the past 2 years increased from 29% in 1987 to 70% in 2000. However, women least likely to have had a recent mammogram include those with less than a high school education, with no health insurance, or who are recent immigrants.[4] Data are inconsistent regarding African-American and white women's utilization of mammograms; some studies report higher rates among African Americans, and some report lower rates.[10] Somewhat fewer Hispanic women than white women (42.3% vs. 44.6%) report adhering to screening mammography guidelines, and Hispanic women were more likely than white women to have never had a mammogram in their lifetime. Low-income women have multiple barriers to screening mammography, including lack of insurance coverage, lack of access to care, not having a regular health care provider, and lack of comprehensive breast cancer knowledge, not merely screening awareness.[2] Culturally sensitive interventions aimed at increasing screening measures must occur if we are to serve all women.

Regarding spread of disease, African-American women were significantly more likely to be diagnosed with regional or distant breast cancer (compared with local) than were white women.[5] African-American women had lower 5-year survival rates, which is due, in part, to underuse of mammography, taking longer time to medical consultation after a diagnosis of breast cancer, less likely to receive surgical removal of their tumors, noncompliance with planned therapy, and incomplete adherence to treatment regimens.[5]

Diet is another environmental factor in breast cancer risk, noted because breast cancer incidence varies among countries. One study of a large French postmenopausal cohort examined two dietary patterns: (1) "alcohol/Western" (meat products, French fries, appetizers, rice/pasta, potatoes, pizza, pies, canned fish, eggs, alcohol, cakes, mayonnaise, butter/cream); and (2) "healthy/Mediterranean" (vegetables, fruits, seafood, olive oil, sunflower oil). The first pattern had a positive association with breast cancer risk, especially with estrogen or progesterone receptor positive tumors. Other diet studies have found that only alcohol intake, being overweight, and weight gain have shown consistent and positive associations with breast cancer risk.[21] Premenopausal African-American women had lower cancer risk when following a "prudent" diet (whole grains, vegetables, fruit, fish), especially those with a BMI below 25. Although the evidence is not consistent to generate preventive diet guidelines for all women, some subgroups of women may benefit from a prudent diet.

SUBJECTIVE DATA

Breast

1. Pain
2. Lump
3. Discharge
4. Rash
5. Swelling
6. Trauma
7. History of breast disease
8. Surgery
9. Self-care behaviors
   Perform breast self-examination
   Last mammogram

Axilla

1. Tenderness, lump, or swelling
2. Rash

In Western culture, the female breasts signify more than their primary purpose of lactation. Women are surrounded by messages that feminine norms of beauty and desirability are enhanced by and depend on the size of the breasts and their appearance. Women leaders have tried to refocus this attitude, stressing women's self-worth as individual human beings, not as stereotyped sexual objects. The intense cultural emphasis is slow to change, and the breasts still are crucial to a woman's self-concept and her perception of her femininity. Matters pertaining to the breast affect the body image and generate deep emotional responses.

This emotionality may take strong forms that you observe as you discuss the woman's history. One woman may be acutely embarrassed talking about her breasts, as evidenced by lack of eye contact, minimal response, nervous gestures, or inappropriate humor. Another woman may talk wryly and disparagingly about the size or development of her breasts. A young adolescent is acutely aware of her own development in relation to her peers. Or, a woman who has found a breast lump may come to you with fear, high anxiety, and even panic. Although many breast lumps are benign, women initially assume the worst possible outcome—cancer, disfigurement, and death. While you are collecting the subjective data, tune in to cues for these behaviors that call for a straightforward and reasoned attitude.

Examiner Asks	Rationale
Breast	
1. Pain. Any **pain** or tenderness in the breasts? When did you first notice it? • Where is the pain? Localized or all over? • Is the painful spot sore to touch? Do you feel a burning or pulling sensation?	**Mastalgia** occurs with trauma, inflammation, infection, and benign breast disease.
• Is the pain cyclic? Any relation to your menstrual period?	Cyclic pain is common with normal breasts, oral contraceptives, and benign breast (fibrocystic) disease.
• Is the pain brought on by strenuous activity, especially involving one arm; a change in activity; manipulation during sex; part of underwire bra; exercise?	Is pain related to specific cause?
2. Lump. Ever noticed a **lump** or **thickening** in the breast? Where? • When did you first notice it? Changed at all since then? • Does the lump have any relation to your menstrual period? • Noticed any change in the overlying skin: redness, warmth, dimpling, swelling?	Carefully explore the presence of any lump. A lump present for many years and exhibiting no change may not be serious but still should be explored. Approach any recent change or new lump with suspicion.
3. Discharge. Any **discharge** from the nipple? • When did you first notice this? • What color is the discharge? • Consistency—thick or runny? • Odor?	**Galactorrhea.** Note medications that may cause clear nipple discharge: oral contraceptives, phenothiazines, diuretics, digitalis, steroids, methyldopa, calcium channel blockers.

Examiner Asks	Rationale
	Bloody or blood-tinged discharge always is significant. Any discharge with a lump is significant.
4. Rash. Any **rash** on the breast? • When did you first notice this? • Where did it start? On the nipple, areola, or surrounding skin?	Paget's disease starts with a small crust on the nipple apex and then spreads to areola (see Table 17-6, Abnormal Nipple Discharge, p. 407). Eczema or other dermatitis rarely starts at the nipple unless it is due to breastfeeding. It usually starts on the areola or surrounding skin and then spreads to the nipple.
5. Swelling. Any **swelling** in the breasts? In one spot or all over? • Related to your menstrual period, pregnancy, or breastfeeding? • Any change in bra size?	
6. Trauma. Any **trauma** or injury to the breasts? • Did it result in any swelling, lump, or break in skin?	A lump from an injury is due to local hematoma or edema and resolves shortly. Or, trauma may cause a woman to feel the breast and find a lump that really was there before.
7. History of breast disease. Any history of breast disease yourself? • What type? How was this diagnosed? • When did this occur? • How is it being treated?	Past breast cancer increases the risk for recurrent cancer (see Table 17-2 on p. 391). The presence of benign breast disease makes the breasts harder to examine; the general lumpiness conceals a new lump.
• Any breast cancer in your family? Who? Sister, mother, maternal grandmother, maternal aunts, daughter? How about your father's side? • At what age did this relative have breast cancer?	Breast cancer occurring before menopause in certain family members increases risk for this woman (see Table 17-2).
8. Surgery. Ever had **surgery** on the breasts? Was this a biopsy? What were the biopsy results? • Mastectomy? Mammoplasty—augmentation or reduction?	
9. Self-care behaviors. • Have you ever been taught **breast self-examination?** • **(If so)** How often do you perform it? What helps you remember? That is an excellent way to be in charge of your own health. I would like you to show me your technique after we do your examination. • **(If not)** This will be an excellent way that you can take charge of your own health. You can make breast self-examination a very routine health habit, just like brushing your teeth. I will teach you the technique after we do your examination. • Ever had **mammography,** a screening x-ray examination of the breasts? When was the last x-ray? • The American Cancer Society recommends that women ages 20 to 39 years should perform BSE and have a CBE every 3 years; women ages 40 years and older should perform BSE, with an annual mammogram and an annual CBE conducted close to the same time.[4]	Awareness that breast self-examination (BSE), clinical breast examination (CBE), and mammograms are complementary screening measures. With good BSE practice, a woman knows how her breasts normally feel and can detect any change more easily. Mammography can reveal cancers too small to be detected by the woman or by the most experienced examiner. However, interval lumps may become palpable between mammograms.

Examiner Asks	Rationale

Axilla

1. **Tenderness, lump, or swelling.** Any **tenderness** or **lump** in the underarm area?
   - Where? When did you first notice this?

Breast tissue extends up into the axilla. Also, the axilla contains many lymph nodes.

2. **Rash.** Any axillary **rash?** Please describe it.
   - Seem to be a reaction to deodorant?

Additional History for the Preadolescent

1. Have you noticed your breasts changing?
   - How long has this been happening?
2. Many girls notice other changes in their bodies, too, that come with growing up. What have you noticed?
   - What do you think about all this?

Developing breasts are the most obvious sign of puberty and the focus of attention for most girls, especially in comparison with peers. Assess each girl's perception of her own development, and provide teaching and reassurance as indicated.

Additional History for the Pregnant Woman

1. Have you noticed any enlargement or fullness in the breasts?
   - Is there any tenderness or tingling?

Breast changes are expected and normal during pregnancy. Assess the woman's knowledge, and provide reassurance.

   - Do you have a history of inverted nipples?

Inverted nipples may need special care in preparation for breastfeeding.

2. Are you planning to breastfeed your baby?

Breastfeeding alone for 6 months provides the perfect food and antibodies for the baby, decreases risk for ear infections, promotes bonding, and provides relaxation.

Additional History for the Menopausal Woman

1. Have you noticed any change in the breast contour, size, or firmness? (Note: Change may not be as apparent to obese woman or to the woman whose earlier pregnancies already have produced breast changes.)

Decreased estrogen level causes decreased firmness. Rapid decrease in estrogen level causes actual shrinkage.

Risk Factor Profile for Breast Cancer

Breast cancer is the second major cause of death from cancer in women. However, early detection and improved treatment have increased survival rates. The 5-year survival rate for localized breast cancer has increased from 78% in the 1940s to 98% today. If the cancer has spread regionally, the survival rate is 84%.[4] Note the risk factors listed in Table 17-2.

The best way to detect a person's risk for breast cancer is by asking the right history questions. Table 17-2 highlights risk factors for breast cancer, and from these, you can fashion your questions. Be aware that most breast cancers occur in women with no identifiable risk factors except gender and age. Just because a woman does not report the cited risk factors does not mean that you or she should fail to consider breast cancer seriously.

TABLE 17-2 Breast Cancer Risk Factors

Risk Factors That Cannot Be Changed	Lifestyle-Related Risk Factors
Female gender, age >50 years	Nulliparity or first child after age 30 years
Personal history of breast cancer	Recent oral contraceptive use
Mutation of BRCA1 and BRCA2 genes	Never breastfed a child
First-degree relative with breast cancer (mother, sister, daughter)	Recent and long-term use of estrogen and progestin
High breast tissue density	Alcohol intake of ≥1 drink daily
Biopsy-confirmed atypical hyperplasia	Obesity (especially after menopause) and high-fat diet
High-dose radiation to chest	Physical inactivity
Early menarche (<12 years) or late menopause (>55 years)	

Data adapted from American Cancer Society, 2010.

Subjective Data

OBJECTIVE DATA

PREPARATION

The woman is sitting up facing the examiner. Use a short gown, open at the back, and lift it up to the woman's shoulders during inspection. During palpation when the woman is supine, cover one breast with the gown while examining the other. Be aware that many women are embarrassed to have their breasts examined; use a sensitive but matter-of-fact approach.

After your examination, be prepared to teach the woman breast self-examination.

EQUIPMENT NEEDED

Small pillow
Ruler marked in centimeters
Pamphlet or teaching aid for BSE

Normal Range of Findings	Abnormal Findings

INSPECT THE BREASTS

General Appearance

Note symmetry of size and shape (Fig. 17-7). It is common to have a slight asymmetry in size; often the left breast is slightly larger than the right.

A sudden increase in the size of one breast signifies inflammation or new growth.

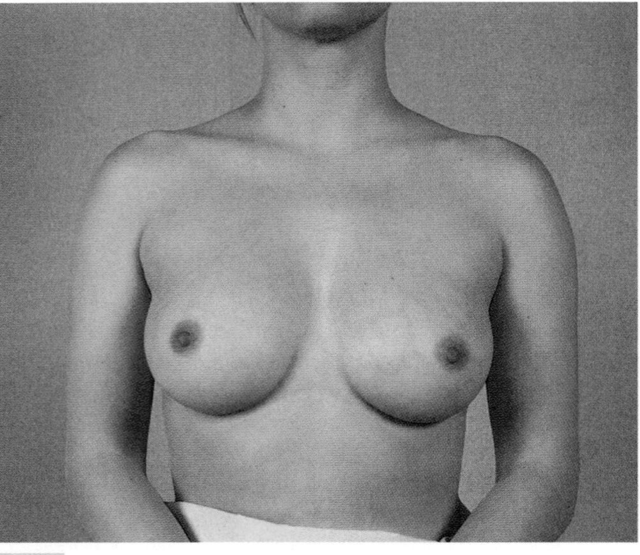

17-7

Skin

The skin normally is smooth and of even color. Note any localized areas of redness, bulging, or dimpling. Also, note any skin lesions or focal vascular pattern. A fine blue vascular network is visible normally during pregnancy. Pale linear striae, or stretch marks, often follow pregnancy.

Normally, no edema is present. Edema exaggerates the hair follicles, giving a "pigskin" or "orange-peel" look (also called *peau d'orange*).

Hyperpigmentation.

Redness and heat with inflammation.

Unilateral dilated superficial veins in a nonpregnant woman.

Edema (see Table 17-3, Signs of Retraction and Inflammation in the Breast, p. 404).

Lymphatic Drainage Areas

Observe the axillary and supraclavicular regions. Note any bulging, discoloration, or edema.

Objective Data

Normal Range of Findings	Abnormal Findings

Nipple

The nipples should be symmetrically placed on the same plane on the two breasts. Nipples usually protrude, although some are flat and some are inverted. They tend to stay in their original condition. Distinguish a recently retracted nipple from one that has been inverted for many years or since puberty. Normal nipple inversion may be unilateral or bilateral and usually can be pulled out (i.e., it is not fixed).

Abnormal: Deviation in pointing (see Table 17-3).

Abnormal: Recent nipple retraction signifies acquired disease (see Table 17-3).

Note any dry scaling, any fissure or ulceration, and bleeding or other discharge.

Abnormal: Explore any discharge, especially in the presence of a breast mass.

A **supernumerary nipple** is a normal and common variation (Fig. 17-8). An extra nipple along the embryonic "milk line" on the thorax or abdomen is a congenital finding. Usually, it is 5 to 6 cm below the breast near the midline and has no associated glandular tissue. It looks like a mole, although a close look reveals a tiny nipple and areola. It is not significant; merely distinguish it from a mole.

Abnormal: Rarely, additional glandular tissue, called a *supernumerary breast,* is present.

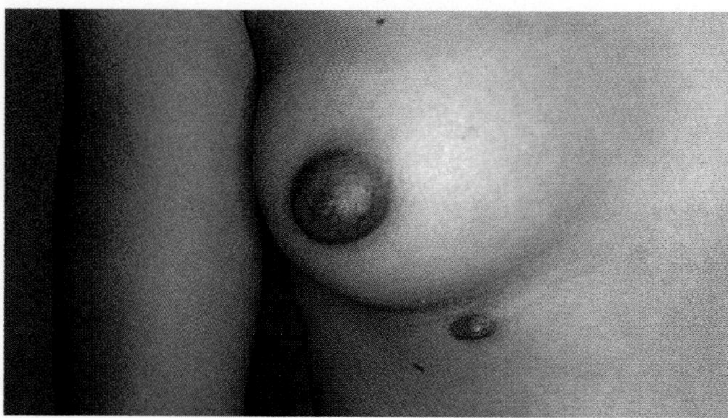

17-8 Supernumerary nipple and areolar complex.

Maneuvers to Screen for Retraction

Direct the woman to change position while you check the breasts for skin retraction signs. First ask her to lift her arms slowly over her head. Both breasts should move up symmetrically (Fig. 17-9).

Abnormal: Retraction signs are due to fibrosis in the breast tissue, usually caused by growing neoplasms. The fibrosis shortens with time, causing contrasting signs with the normally loose breast tissue.

Abnormal: Note a lag in the movement of one breast.

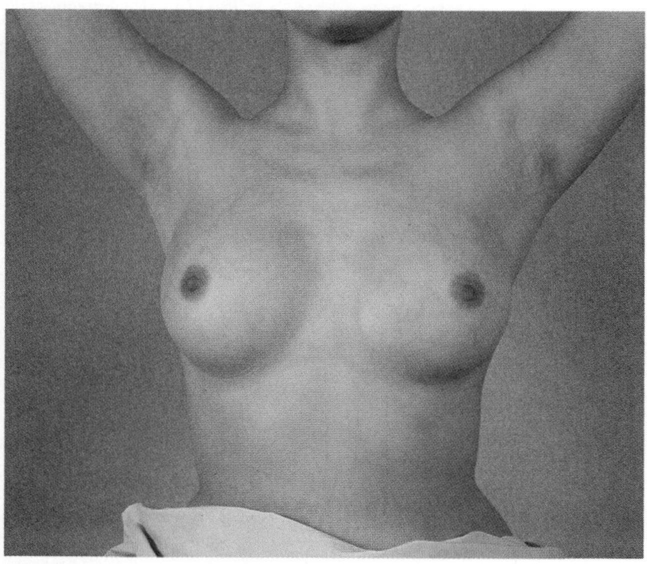

17-9 Retraction maneuver.

Normal Range of Findings

Next ask her to push her hands onto her hips (Fig. 17-10) and to push her two palms together (Fig. 17-11). These maneuvers contract the pectoralis major muscle. A slight lifting of both breasts will occur.

Abnormal Findings

Note a dimpling or a pucker, which indicates skin retraction (see Table 17-3).

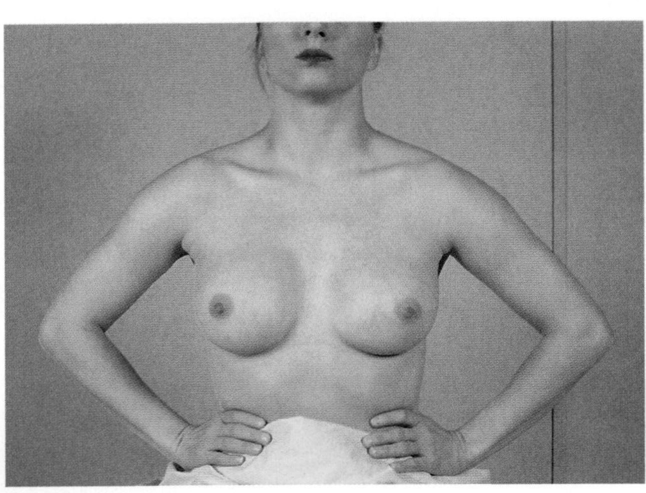

17-10

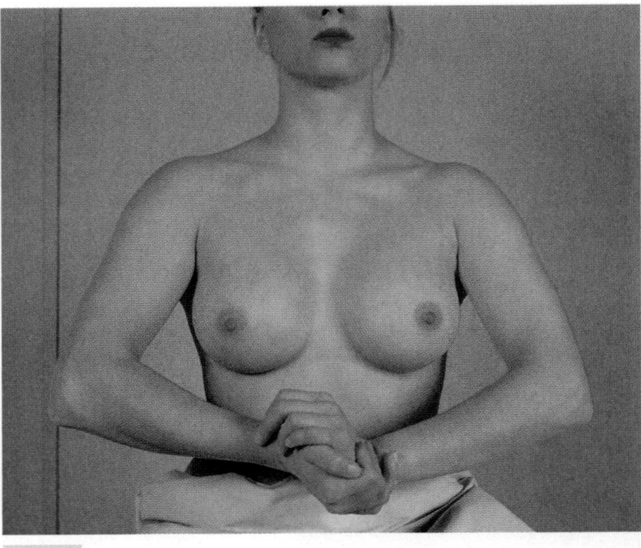

17-11

Ask the woman with large pendulous breasts to lean forward while you support her forearms. Note the symmetric free-forward movement of both breasts (Fig. 17-12).

Note fixation to chest wall or skin retraction (see Table 17-3).

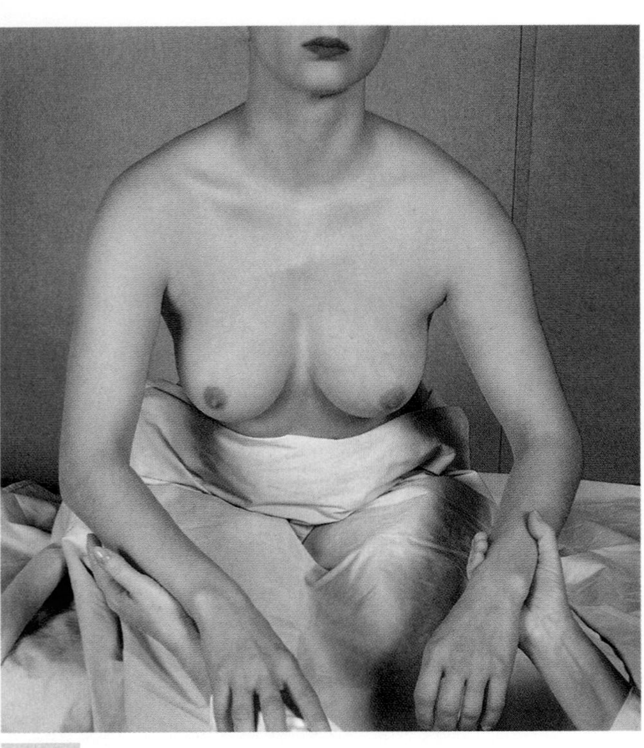

17-12

Normal Range of Findings	Abnormal Findings

INSPECT AND PALPATE THE AXILLAE

Examine the axillae while the woman is sitting. Inspect the skin, noting any rash or infection. Lift the woman's arm and support it yourself, so that her muscles are loose and relaxed. Use your right hand to palpate the left axilla (Fig. 17-13). Reach your fingers high into the axilla. Move them firmly down in four directions: (1) down the chest wall in a line from the middle of the axilla, (2) along the anterior border of the axilla, (3) along the posterior border, and (4) along the inner aspect of the upper arm. Move the woman's arm through range-of-motion to increase the surface area you can reach.

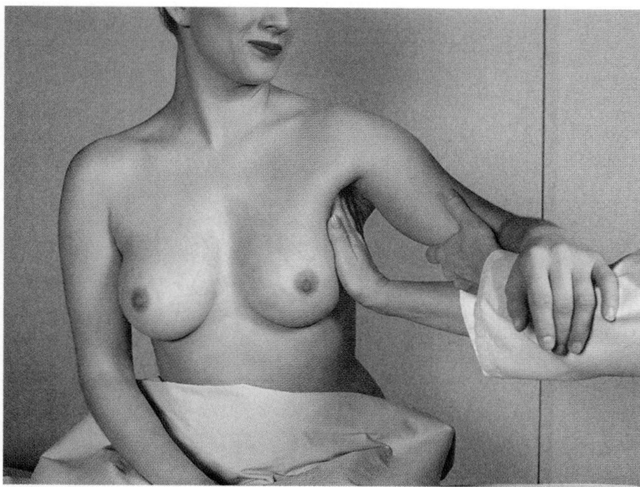

17-13

Usually nodes are not palpable, although you may feel a small, soft, nontender node in the central group. Expect some tenderness when palpating high in the axilla. Note any enlarged and tender lymph nodes.

Nodes enlarge with any local infection of the breast, arm, or hand and with breast cancer metastases.

PALPATE THE BREASTS

Help the woman to a supine position. Tuck a small pad under the side to be palpated and raise her arm over her head. These maneuvers will flatten the breast tissue and displace it medially. Any significant lumps will then feel more distinct (Fig. 17-14). For pendulous breasts, to distribute the tissue medially across the chest wall, ask the woman to rotate her hips opposite to the side you are palpating.

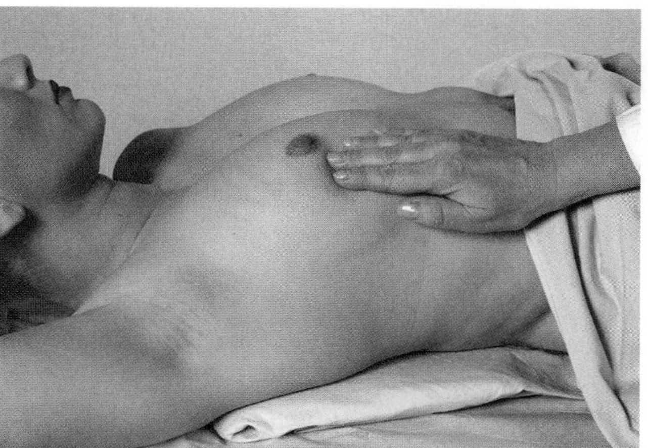

17-14

Normal Range of Findings

Abnormal Findings

Use the pads of your first three fingers and make a gentle rotary motion on the breast. Vary your pressure so you are palpating light, medium, and deep tissue in each location. The vertical strip pattern (Fig. 17-15, *A*) currently is recommended as the best way to detect a breast mass, but two other patterns are in common use: from the nipple palpating out to the periphery as if following spokes on a wheel (Fig. 17-15, *B*; and palpating in concentric circles out to the periphery (Fig. 17-15, *C*).

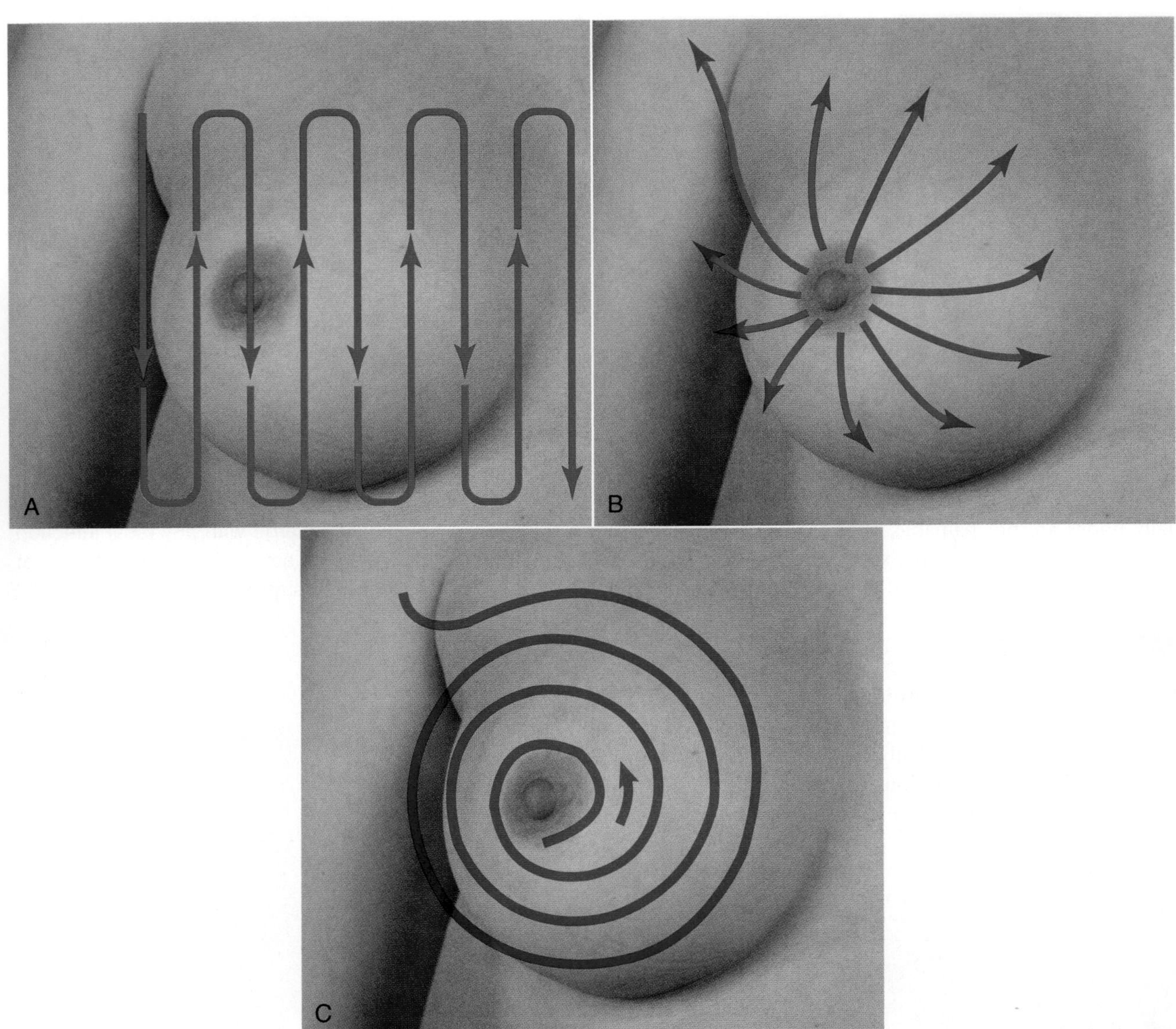

17-15 **A,** Vertical strip pattern of palpation. **B,** Spokes-on-a-wheel pattern of palpation. **C,** Concentric circles pattern of palpation.

For the vertical strip pattern, start high in the axilla and palpate down just lateral to the breast. Proceed in overlapping vertical lines ending at the sternal edge. In every pattern, take care to palpate every square inch of the breast and to examine the tail of Spence high into the axilla. Be consistent and thorough in your approach to each woman.

Normal Range of Findings	Abnormal Findings
In nulliparous women, normal breast tissue feels firm, smooth, and elastic. After pregnancy, the tissue feels softer and looser. Premenstrual engorgement is normal from increasing progesterone. This consists of a slight enlargement, a tenderness to palpation, and a generalized nodularity; the lobes feel prominent and their margins more distinct.	Heat, redness, and swelling in nonlactating and non-postpartum breasts indicate inflammation.
Also, normally you may feel a firm transverse ridge of compressed tissue in the lower quadrants. This is the **inframammary ridge,** and it is especially noticeable in large breasts. Do not confuse it with an abnormal lump.	
After palpating over the four breast quadrants, palpate the nipple (Fig. 17-16). Note any induration or subareolar mass. With your thumb and forefinger, gently depress the nipple tissue into the well behind the areola. The tissue should move inward easily. If the woman reports spontaneous nipple discharge, press the areola inward with your index finger—repeat from a few different directions. If any discharge appears, note its color and consistency.	Except in pregnancy and lactation, discharge is abnormal (see Table 17-6). Note the number of discharge droplets and the quadrant(s) producing them. Blot the discharge on a white gauze pad to ascertain its color. Test any abnormal discharge for the presence of blood.

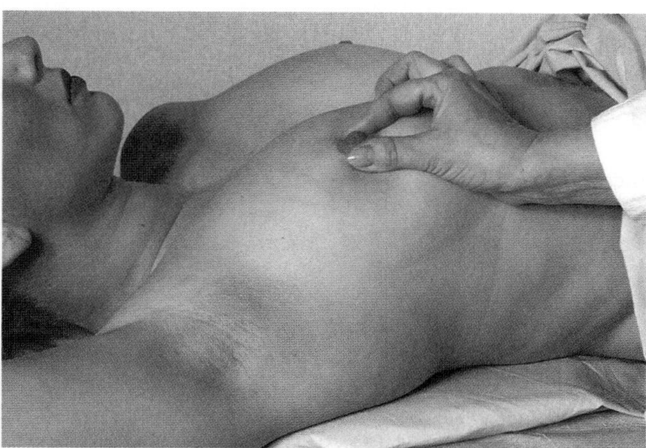

17-16

For the woman with large pendulous breasts, you may palpate by using a bimanual technique (Fig. 17-17). The woman is in a sitting position, leaning forward. Support the inferior part of the breast with one hand. Use your other hand to palpate the breast tissue against your supporting hand.

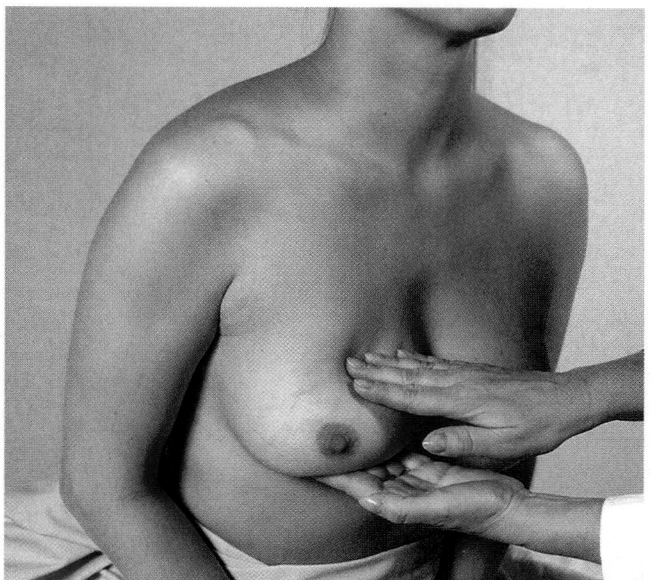

17-17

Normal Range of Findings

If the woman mentions a breast lump that she has discovered herself, examine the unaffected breast first to learn a baseline of normal consistency for this woman. If you do feel a lump or mass, note these characteristics (Fig. 17-18):

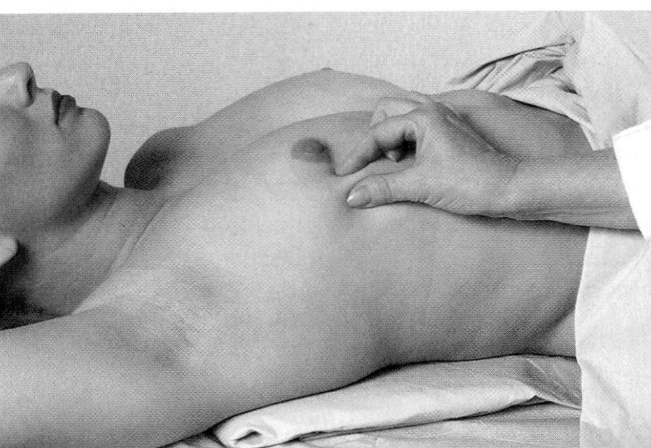

17-18

1. **Location**—Using the breast as a clock face, describe the distance in centimeters from the nipple (e.g., "7:00, 2 cm from the nipple"). Or diagram the breast in the woman's record and mark in the location of the lump.
2. **Size**—Judge in centimeters in three dimensions: width × length × thickness.
3. **Shape**—State whether the lump is oval, round, lobulated, or indistinct.
4. **Consistency**—State whether the lump is soft, firm, or hard.
5. **Movable**—Is the lump freely movable, or is it fixed when you try to slide it over the chest wall?
6. **Distinctness**—Is the lump solitary or multiple?
7. **Nipple**—Is it displaced or retracted?
8. **Note the skin over the lump**—Is it erythematous, dimpled, or retracted?
9. **Tenderness**—Is the lump tender to palpation?
10. **Lymphadenopathy**—Are any regional lymph nodes palpable?

Premenopausal women at midcycle often have tissue edema and mastalgia (pain) that make it hard to detect a lesion. If your findings are in question, consider asking this woman to return for a follow-up examination the first week after her menses when hormone levels are lower and edema is not present.

TEACH BREAST SELF-EXAMINATION

Finish your own assessment first, and then teach self-examination. You need to focus your skill and concentration on the examination, and you may be diverted by teaching at the same time. The same is true for the woman. She waits to hear that your examination of her affirms that she is healthy. Once reassured, she can relax about the findings and concentrate on your teaching.

Help each woman establish a regular schedule of self-care. The best time to conduct BSE is right after the menstrual period, or the 4th through 7th day of the menstrual cycle, when the breasts are the smallest and least congested. Advise the pregnant or menopausal woman who is not having menstrual periods to select a familiar date to examine her breasts each month—for example, her birth date or the day the rent is due.

Stress that self-examination will familiarize the woman with her own breasts and their normal variation. Emphasize the absence of lumps (not the presence of them). However, do encourage her to report any unusual finding promptly.

Abnormal Findings

See Table 17-4, Breast Lump, and Table 17-5, Differentiating Breast Lumps, for a description of common breast lumps with these characteristics.

Normal Range of Findings	Abnormal Findings

While teaching, focus on the positive aspects of BSE. Avoid citing frightening mortality statistics about breast cancer. This may generate excessive fear and denial that actually obstruct a woman's self-care action. Rather, be selective in your choice of factual material: (1) the majority of women will never get breast cancer; (2) the great majority of breast lumps are benign; and (3) early detection of breast cancer is important—if the cancer is not invasive, the survival rate is 98%.

Keep your teaching simple! The simpler the plan, the more likely the person is to comply. Describe the correct technique and rationale and the expected findings to note as the woman inspects her own breasts (Fig. 17-19). Teach the woman to do this in front of a mirror while she is disrobed to the waist. At home, she can start palpation in the shower, where soap and water assist palpation. Then palpation should be performed while lying supine. Encourage the woman to palpate her own breasts while you are there to monitor her technique. Use the return demonstration to assess her technique and understanding of the procedure.

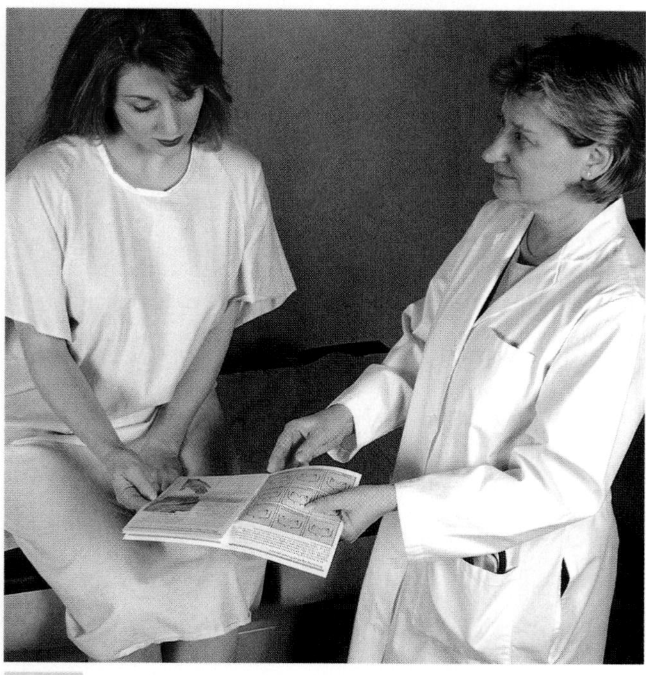

17-19

Many examiners use a simulated breast model so that the woman can palpate a "lump." Pamphlets are helpful reinforcers; give the woman two pamphlets to take home, and encourage her to give one to a relative or friend. This may promote discussion, which is reinforcing.

Current evidence is inconclusive on the effectiveness of detection procedures of BSE and CBE.[18] Concern exists that these procedures may result in more benign biopsies and create anxiety.[8,32] However, the value of early detection of breast cancer is clear. While screening mammography is available for many groups of women in developed countries, BSE is available to virtually all women. BSE is valuable to women who are younger or older than the ages recommended for screening mammography or who have barriers to access mammography. BSE is cheap, noninvasive, can be accomplished without visits to expert professionals, and enhances self-care action.

Normal Range of Findings | Abnormal Findings

THE MALE BREAST

Your examination of the male breast can be abbreviated, but do not omit it. Combine the breast examination with that of the anterior thorax. Inspect the chest wall, noting the skin surface and any lumps or swelling. Palpate the nipple area for any lump or tissue enlargement (Fig. 17-20). It should feel even, with no nodules. Palpate the axillary lymph nodes.

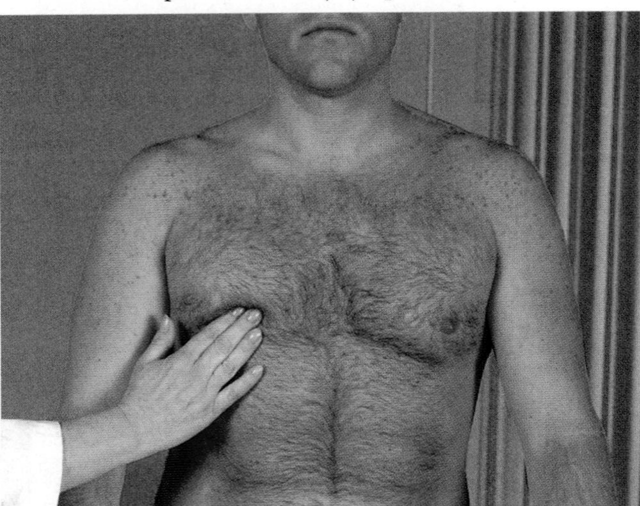

17-20

The normal male breast has a flat disk of undeveloped breast tissue beneath the nipple. **Gynecomastia** is a benign growth of this breast tissue, making it distinguishable from the other tissues in the chest wall (Fig. 17-21). It feels like a smooth, firm, movable disk. This occurs normally during puberty. It can be unilateral or bilateral and is temporary. The adolescent is acutely aware of his body image. Reassure him that this change is normal, common, and temporary.

Gynecomastia also occurs with use of anabolic steroids, some medications, and some disease states. See Table 17-8, Abnormalities in the Male Breast.

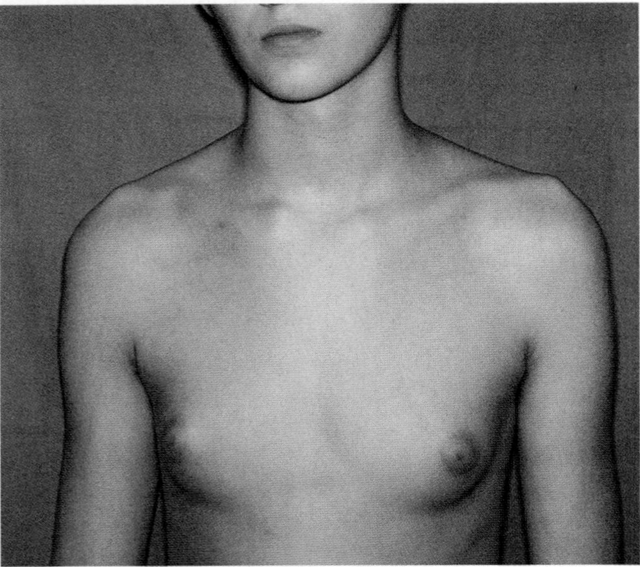

17-21 Adolescent gynecomastia.

DEVELOPMENTAL COMPETENCE

Infants and Children

In the neonate, the breasts may be enlarged and visible due to maternal estrogen crossing the placenta. They may secrete a clear or white fluid, called "witch's milk." This is not significant and is resolved within a few days to a few weeks.

Normal Range of Findings	Abnormal Findings

Note the position of the nipples on the prepubertal child. They should be symmetric, just lateral to the midclavicular line, between the fourth and fifth ribs. The nipple is flat, and the areola is darker pigmented.

Premature thelarche is early breast development with no other hormone-dependent signs (pubic hair, menses).

The Adolescent

Adolescent breast development begins on an average between 8 and 10 years of age. Expect some asymmetry during growth. Record the stage of development using Tanner's staging described on p. 386. Use the chart to teach the adolescent normal developmental stages and to assure her of her own normal progress.

Note precocious development before age 8 years. It is usually normal but also occurs with thyroid dysfunction, stilbestrol ingestion, or ovarian or adrenal tumor.

Note delayed development with hormonal failure, anorexia nervosa, or severe malnutrition.

You should consider BMI (derived from weight and height) when evaluating breast budding before age 8 years. With normal BMI levels, breast budding before age 8 is premature in non-Hispanic white girls but may be normal in 7-year-old Black and Mexican-American girls.[28] Note that it is difficult to distinguish breast budding from excess adipose tissue.

With maturing adolescents, palpate the breasts as you would with the adult. The breasts normally feel firm and uniform. Note any mass.

At this age, a mass is almost always a benign fibroadenoma or a cyst (see Table 17-4).

Teach BSE now, so that the technique will become a natural, comfortable habit by the time the girl becomes an adult and will be at higher risk.

The Pregnant Woman

A delicate blue vascular pattern is visible over the breasts. The breasts increase in size, as do the nipples. Jagged linear stretch marks, or striae, may develop if the breasts have a large increase. The nipples also become darker and more erectile. The areolae widen; grow darker; and contain the small, scattered, elevated Montgomery's glands. On palpation, the breasts feel more nodular, and thick yellow colostrum can be expressed after the first trimester.

The Lactating Woman

Colostrum changes to milk production around the 3rd postpartum day. At this time, the breasts may become engorged, appearing enlarged, reddened, and shiny and feeling warm and hard. Frequent nursing helps drain the ducts and sinuses and stimulate milk production. Nipple soreness is normal, appearing around the 20th nursing, lasting 24 to 48 hours, and then disappearing rapidly. The nipples may look red and irritated. They may even crack but will heal rapidly if kept dry and exposed to air. Again, frequent nursings are the best treatment for nipple soreness.

One section of the breast surface appearing red and tender indicates a plugged duct (see Table 17-7).

The Aging Woman

Increasing age is the primary risk factor for developing breast cancer, so a yearly CBE is important. On inspection, the breasts look pendulous, flattened, and sagging. Nipples may be retracted but can be pulled outward. On palpation, the breasts feel more granular and the terminal ducts around the nipple feel more prominent and stringy. Thickening of the inframammary ridge at the lower breast is normal, and it feels more prominent with age.

Because atrophy causes shrinkage of normal glandular tissue, cancer detection is somewhat easier. Any palpable lump that cannot be positively identified as a normal structure should be referred.

Reinforce the value of the breast self-examination. Women older than 50 years have an increased risk for breast cancer. Older women may have problems with arthritis, limited range of motion, or decreased vision that may inhibit self-care. Suggest aids to the self-examination; for example, talcum powder helps fingers glide over skin.

PROMOTING A HEALTHY LIFESTYLE: ASSESSING BREAST CANCER RISK

Breast Cancer Risk Screening Tool

During a breast examination, there is an opportunity to review the individual's breast self-examination technique and inquire about scheduled mammogram surveillance. It is also an opportunity to assess the individual's breast cancer risk, including family history.

The use of breast cancer risk assessment tools in the clinical setting has the potential to improve health substantially by reducing breast cancer incidence through cancer prevention and by more effective early detection programs for high-risk individuals. The *Gail Model* is widely used for calculating an individual's risk estimate for breast cancer. This model takes into account identified risk factors, including current age, age at menarche, age at first live birth, and family history of breast cancer in first-degree relatives. It calculates a 5-year and a 30-year or lifetime risk estimate for each individual. It is easy to complete, and many computer-based data programs are available to clinicians. However, the Gail Model may underestimate the breast cancer risk in the subgroup of women with family cancer histories suggestive of hereditary breast cancer syndromes, such as BRCA1 and BRCA2. For information about hereditary breast cancer syndromes, go to the National Cancer Institute (NCI) website at www.cancer.gov/cancertopics/pdq/genetics/breast-and-ovarian/healthprofessional.

The *Pedigree Assessment Tool (PAT)* (Hoskins et al., 2006) was developed to identify this subgroup of women with family cancer histories suggesting hereditary breast cancer syndromes. The PAT can be used along with the Gail Model to screen for breast cancer risk in primary care. The PAT score is calculated by adding the points assigned to every family member, including second- and third-degree relatives, with a breast or ovarian cancer diagnosis. Additional points are calculated for the presence of male breast cancer, bilateral disease, the occurrence of both breast and ovarian cancer, Ashkenazi Jewish heritage, and for the age (before age 50 or 50 years and older) at diagnosis. A separate score is calculated for an individual's maternal and paternal family history. The higher of the two scores is used. The specific inclusion of both sides of a women's family is important, because many women often disregard or overlook paternal lineage altogether when thinking about or reporting family history of breast cancer. A PAT score of 8 or higher is considered high risk for hereditary breast cancer syndrome. All women in this category should consider genetic counseling to discuss the current options for cancer risk-reduction and increased breast cancer surveillance. A PAT score less than 8 does not mean the woman is not low risk but just that DNA testing for BRCA mutations or other hereditary breast cancer syndromes may not be as beneficial. Information about the PAT is available at https//:myosfhealth.osfhealthcare.org/sites/OSF/BCRA/default.aspx.

In addition to the PAT and Gail Model, the NCI provides an interactive online tool, the Breast Cancer Risk Assessment Tool, to assist health care providers in estimating a woman's risk for developing breast cancer. It is available on the NCI website at www.cancer.gov/bcrisktool/.

Resources

Hoskins, K. F., Zwaagstra, A., & Ranz, M. (2006). Validation of a tool for identifying women at high risk for hereditary breast cancer in population-based screening. *Cancer, 107*, 1769-1776.

Teller, P., Hoskins, K. F., Zwaagstram, A., et al. (2010). Validation of the Pedigree Assessment Tool (PAT) in families with BRCA1 and BRCA2 mutations. *Annals of Surgical Oncology*, *17*(1), 240-246.

DOCUMENTATION AND CRITICAL THINKING

Sample Charting

FEMALE

SUBJECTIVE

States no breast pain, lump, discharge, rash, swelling, or trauma. No history of breast disease herself; does have mother with fibrocystic disease. No history of breast surgery. Never been pregnant. Performs BSE monthly.

OBJECTIVE

Inspection: Breasts symmetric. Skin smooth with even color and no rash or lesions. Arm movement shows no dimpling or retractions. No nipple discharge, no lesions.

Palpation: Breast contour and consistency firm and homogeneous. No masses or tenderness. No lymphadenopathy.

ASSESSMENT

Healthy breast structure
Has knowledge of breast self-exam

MALE

SUBJECTIVE

No pain, lump, rash, or swelling.

OBJECTIVE

No masses or tenderness. No lymphadenopathy.

Focused Assessment: Clinical Case Study 1

J.G. is a 32-year-old white female high school teacher, married, with no children. She reports good health until finding "lump in right breast 2 weeks ago."

SUBJECTIVE

2 weeks PTA—noticed lump in R breast on self-examination. Lump firm, nonmovable area "the size of a quarter," in upper outer quadrant of breast, tender on touch only. No skin changes, no nipple discharge, on no medications. Last breast exam by MD 3 months before was reported normal. Did not notice lump on previous self-exam 1 month before. No history of breast disease in self or family.

2 days PTA—saw MD, who confirmed presence of lump and recommended biopsy as outpatient. Last menstrual period 1/25 (2½ weeks PTA). States that for the past 2 days she has been so nervous that she has been unable to sleep well or to concentrate at work. "I just know it's cancer."

OBJECTIVE

Voice trembling and breathless during history. Sitting posture stiff and rigid. BP, 148/78 mm Hg; TPR, 37°-92-16.

Inspection: Breasts symmetric, nipples everted. No skin lesions, no dimpling, no retraction, no fixation.

Palpation: Left breast firm, no mass, no tenderness, no discharge. Right breast firm, with 2 cm × 2 cm × 1 cm mass at 10 o'clock position, 5 cm from the nipple. Lump is firm, oval, with smooth discrete borders, nonmovable, tender to palpation. No other mass. No discharge. No lymphadenopathy.

ASSESSMENT

Lump in R breast
Anxiety R/T threat to health status

Focused Assessment: Clinical Case Study 2

D.B. is a 62-year-old Black female bank comptroller, married, with no children. History of hypertension, managed by diuretic medication and diet. No other health problems until yearly company physical exam 3 days PTA, when MD "found a lump in my right breast."

SUBJECTIVE

3 days PTA—MD noted lump in R breast during yearly physical exam. MD did not describe lump but told D.B. it was "serious" and needed immediate biopsy. D.B. has not felt it herself. States has noted no skin changes, no nipple discharge. No previous history of breast disease. Mother died age 54 years of breast cancer, no other relative with breast disease. D.B. has had no term pregnancies; two spontaneous abortions, ages 28, 31 years. Menopause completed at age 52 years.

Aware of BSE but has never performed it. "I feel so bad. If only I had been doing it. I should have found this myself." Married 43 years. States husband supportive, but "I just can't talk to him about this. I can't even go near him now."

OBJECTIVE

Inspection: Breasts symmetric when sitting, arms down. Nipples flat. No lesions, no discharge. As lifts arms, left breast elevates, right breast stays fixed. Dimple in right breast, 9 o'clock position, apparent at rest and with muscle contraction. Leaning forward reveals left breast falls free, right breast flattens.

Palpation: Left breast feels soft and granular throughout, no mass. Right breast soft and granular, with large, stony hard mass in outer quadrant. Lump is 5 cm × 4 cm × 2 cm, at 9 o'clock position, 3 cm from nipple. Borders irregular, mass fixed to tissues, no pain with palpation.

One firm, palpable lymph node in center of right axilla. No palpable nodes on the left.

ASSESSMENT

Lump in R breast
Ineffective coping R/T effects of breast lump

ABNORMAL FINDINGS

TABLE 17-3 Signs of Retraction and Inflammation in the Breast

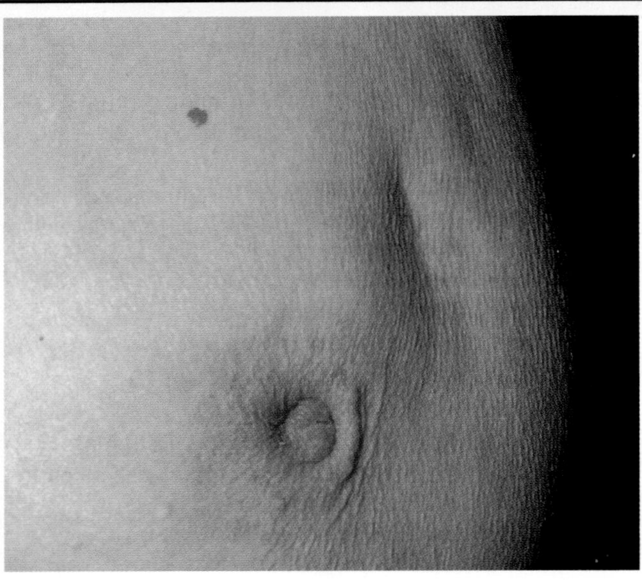

Dimpling

The shallow dimple (also called a *skin tether*) shown here is a sign of skin retraction. Cancer causes fibrosis, which contracts the suspensory ligaments. The dimple may be apparent at rest, with compression, or with lifting of the arms. Also note the distortion of the areola here as the fibrosis pulls the nipple toward it.

Nipple Retraction. The retracted nipple looks flatter and broader, like an underlying crater. A recent retraction suggests cancer, which causes fibrosis of the whole duct system and pulls in the nipple. It also may occur with benign lesions such as ectasia of the ducts. Do not confuse retraction with the normal long-standing type of nipple inversion, which has no broadening and is not fixed.

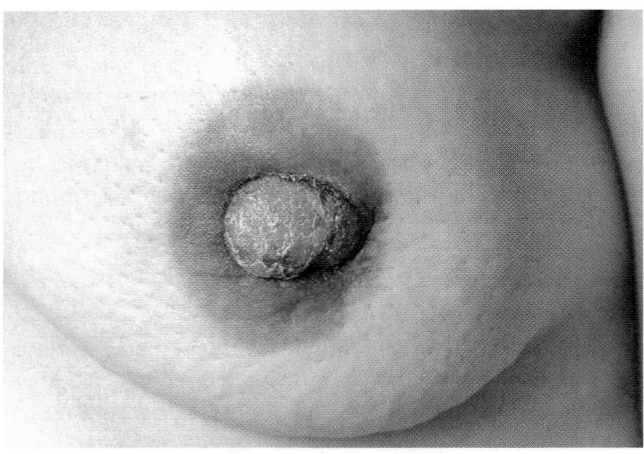

Edema (Peau d'Orange)

Lymphatic obstruction produces edema. This thickens the skin and exaggerates the hair follicles, giving a pigskin or orange-peel look. This condition suggests cancer. Edema usually begins in the skin around and beneath the areola, the most dependent area of the breast. Also note nipple infiltration here.

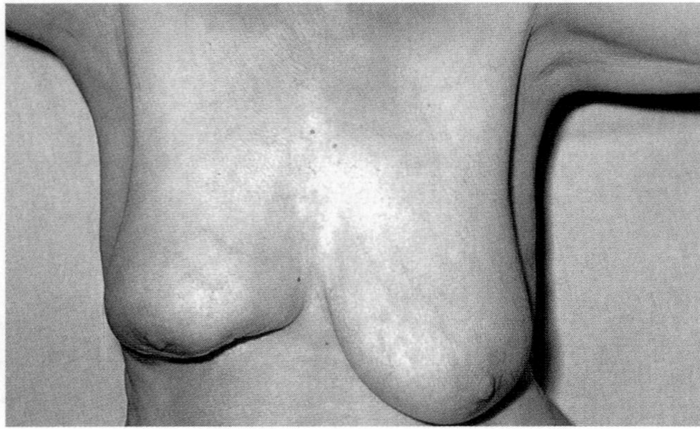

Fixation

Asymmetry, distortion, or decreased mobility with the elevated arm maneuver. As cancer becomes invasive, the fibrosis fixes the breast to the underlying pectoral muscles. Here, note the right breast is held against the chest wall.

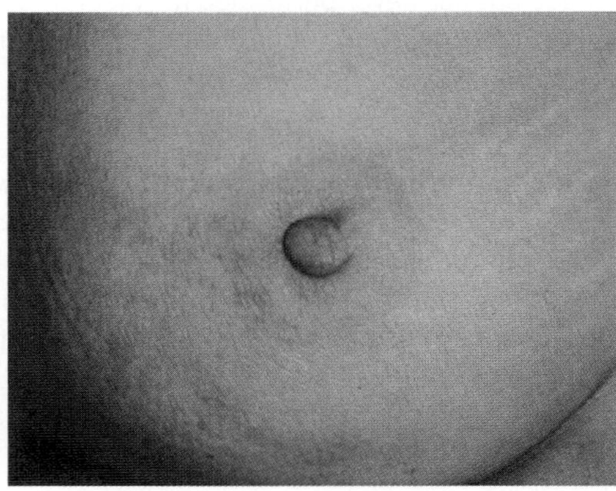

Deviation in Nipple Pointing

An underlying cancer causes fibrosis in the mammary ducts, which pulls the nipple angle toward it. Here, note the swelling behind the right nipple and the nipple tilts laterally.

TABLE 17-4 Breast Lump

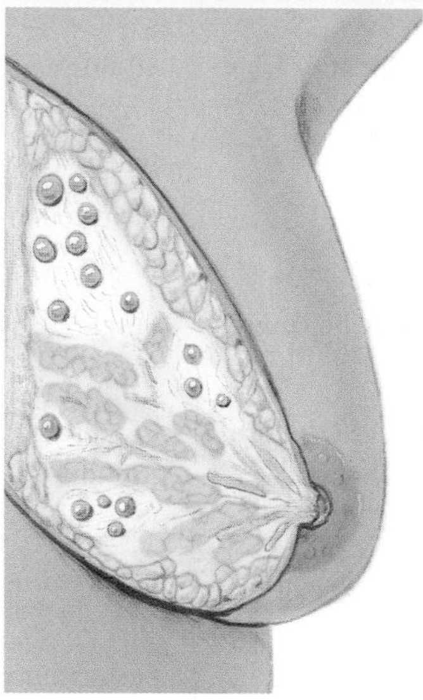

Benign Breast Disease (Formerly Fibrocystic Breast Disease)

Multiple tender masses. "Fibrocystic disease" is not accurate because, actually, six diagnostic categories exist, based on symptoms and physical findings[22]:

- Swelling and tenderness (cyclic discomfort)
- Mastalgia (severe pain, both cyclic and noncyclic)
- Nodularity (significant lumpiness, both cyclic and noncyclic)
- Dominant lumps (including cysts and fibroadenomas)
- Nipple discharge (including intraductal papilloma and duct ectasia)
- Infections and inflammations (including subareolar abscess, lactational mastitis, breast abscess, and Mondor's disease)

About 50% of all women have some form of benign breast disease. Nodularity occurs bilaterally; regular, firm nodules that are mobile, well demarcated, and feel rubbery, like small water balloons. Pain may be dull, heavy, and cyclic or just before menses as nodules enlarge. Some women have nodularity but no pain, and vice versa. Cysts are discrete, fluid-filled sacs. Dominant lumps and nipple discharge must be investigated carefully and may need biopsy to rule out cancer. Nodularity itself is not premalignant but produces difficulty in detecting other cancerous lumps.

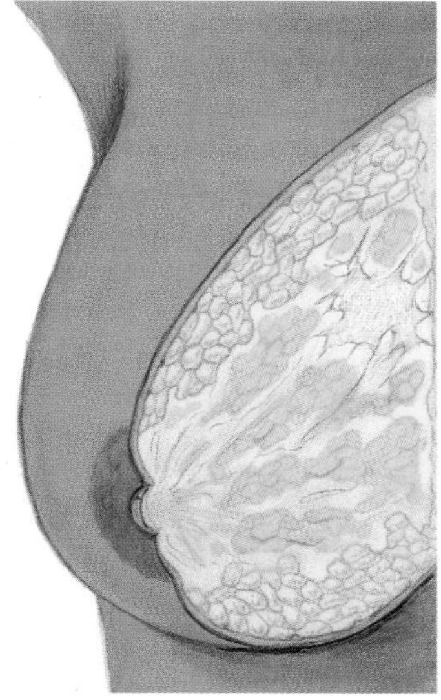

Cancer

Solitary, unilateral, nontender mass. Single focus in one area, although it may be interspersed with other nodules. Solid, hard, dense, and fixed to underlying tissues or skin as cancer becomes invasive. Borders are irregular and poorly delineated. Grows constantly. Often painless, although the person may have pain. Most common in upper outer quadrant. Usually found in women 30 to 80 years of age; increased risk in ages 40 to 44 years and in women older than 50 years. As cancer advances, signs include firm or hard irregular axillary nodes; skin dimpling; nipple retraction, elevation, and discharge.

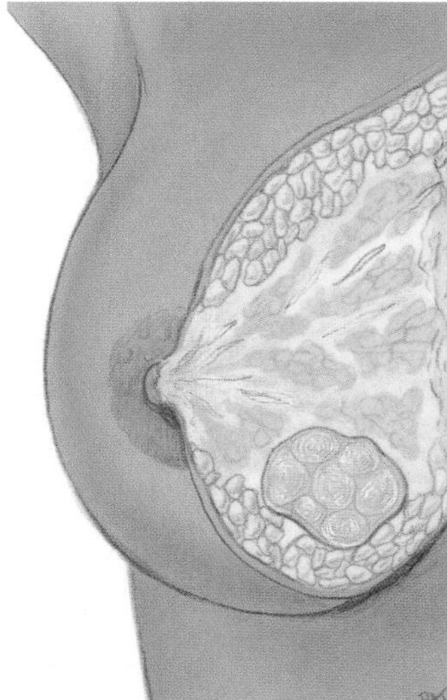

Fibroadenoma

Benign tumors, most commonly present as self-detected in late adolescence. Solitary nontender mass that is solid, firm, rubbery, and elastic. Round, oval, or lobulated; 1 to 5 cm. Freely movable, slippery, fingers slide it easily through tissue. Usually no axillary lymphadenopathy. Diagnose by triple test (palpation, ultrasound, and needle biopsy); however; adolescents with rapidly growing mass need surgical excision anyway.[15]

TABLE 17-5 Differentiating Breast Lumps

	Fibroadenoma	Benign Breast Disease	Cancer
Likely age	15-30 years, can occur up to 55 years	30-55 years, decreases after menopause	30-80 years, risk increases after 50 years
Shape	Round, lobular	Round, lobular	Irregular, star-shaped
Consistency	Usually firm, rubbery	Firm to soft, rubbery	Firm to stony hard
Demarcation	Well demarcated, clear margins	Well demarcated	Poorly defined
Number	Usually single	Usually multiple, may be single	Single
Mobility	Very mobile, slippery	Mobile	Fixed
Tenderness	Usually none	Tender, usually increases before menses, may be noncyclic	Usually none, can be tender
Skin retraction	None	None	Usually
Pattern of growth	Grows quickly and constantly	Size may increase or decrease rapidly	Grows constantly
Risk to health	None; they are benign— diagnose by ultrasound and biopsy	Benign, although general lumpiness may mask other cancerous lump	Serious, needs early treatment

ABNORMAL FINDINGS FOR ADVANCED PRACTICE

TABLE 17-6 Abnormal Nipple Discharge

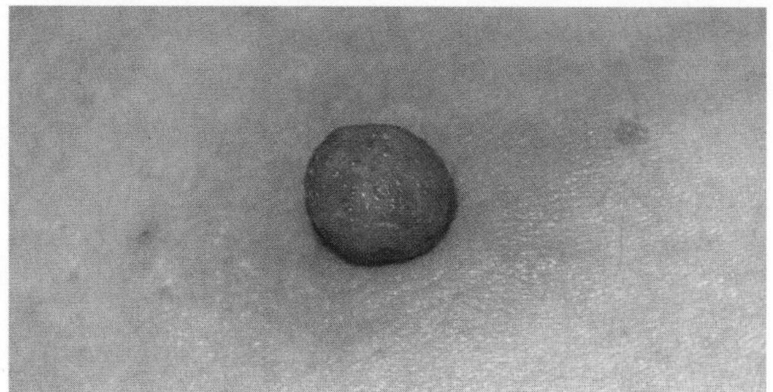

Mammary Duct Ectasia

Pastelike matter in subareolar ducts produces sticky, purulent discharge that may be white, gray, brown, green, or bloody. A light green, single duct discharge is shown here. Caused by stagnation of cellular debris and secretions in the ducts, leading to obstruction, inflammation, and infection. Occurs in women who have lactated; usually occurs in perimenopause.

Itching, burning, or drawing pain occurs around nipple. May have subareolar redness and swelling. Ducts are palpable as rubbery, twisted tubules under areola. May have palpable mass, soft or firm, poorly delineated. Not malignant, but needs biopsy.

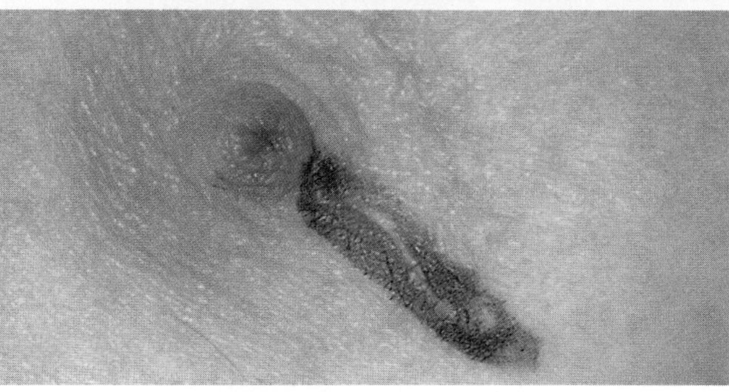

Intraductal Papilloma

Serous or serosanguineous discharge, which is spontaneous, unilateral, or from a single duct. Lesion consists of tiny tumors, 2 to 3 mm. Often there is a palpable nodule in the underlying duct (highlighted here). Papillomas affect women 40 to 60 years of age; most are benign. Refer any bloody discharge for careful evaluation, including biopsy, to rule out cancer.

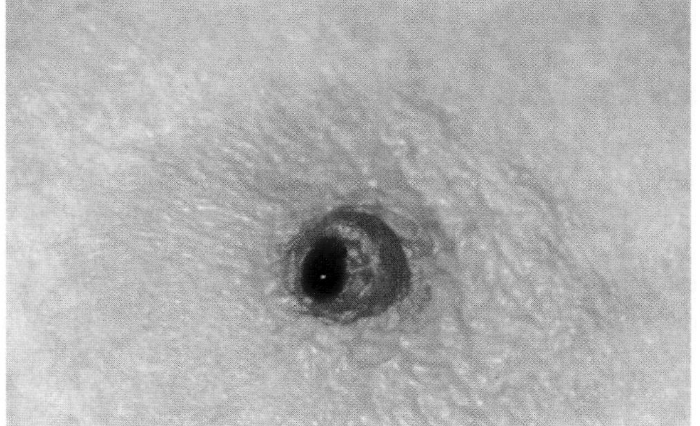

Carcinoma

Bloody nipple discharge that is unilateral and from a single duct requires further investigation. Although there was no palpable lump associated with the discharge shown here, mammography revealed a 1-cm, centrally located, ill-defined mass.

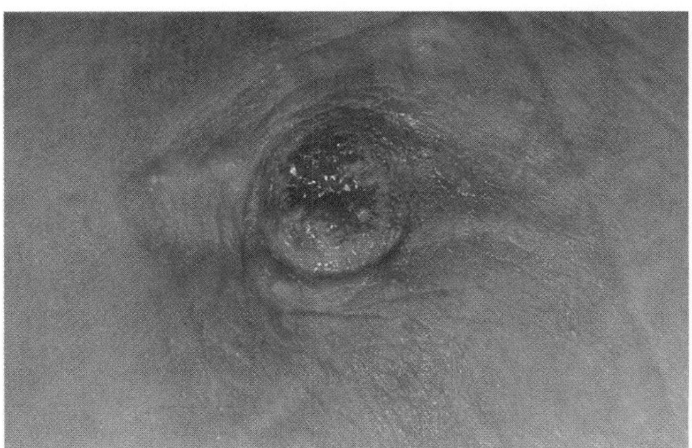

Paget's Disease (Intraductal Carcinoma)

Early lesion has unilateral, clear, yellow discharge and dry, scaling crusts, friable at nipple apex. Spreads outward to areola with erythematous halo on areola and crusted, eczematous, retracted nipple. Later lesion shows nipple reddened, excoriated, ulcerated, with bloody discharge when surface is eroded, and an erythematous plaque surrounding the nipple. Symptoms include tingling, burning, itching.

Except for the redness and occasional cracking from initial breastfeeding, any dermatitis of the nipple area must be carefully explored and referred immediately.

TABLE 17-7 Disorders Occurring During Lactation

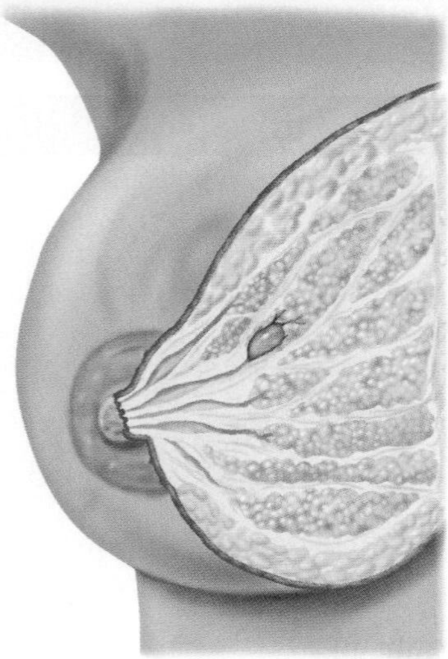

Plugged Duct

A fairly common and not serious condition. One milk duct is clogged. One section of the breast is tender; may be reddened. No infection. It is important to keep breast as empty as possible and milk flowing. The woman should nurse her baby frequently, on affected side first to ensure complete emptying, and manually express any remaining milk. A plugged duct usually resolves in less than 1 day.

Mastitis

This is uncommon; an inflammatory mass before abscess formation. Usually occurs in single quadrant. Area is red, swollen, tender, very hot, and hard, here forming outward from areola upper edge, in right breast. Also the woman has a headache, malaise, fever, chills and sweating, increased pulse, flu-like symptoms. May occur during first 4 months of lactation from infection or from stasis from plugged duct. Treat with rest, local heat to area, antibiotics, and frequent nursing to keep breast as empty as possible. Must not wean now or the breast will become engorged and the pain will increase. Mother's antibiotic not harmful to infant. Usually resolves in 2 to 3 days.

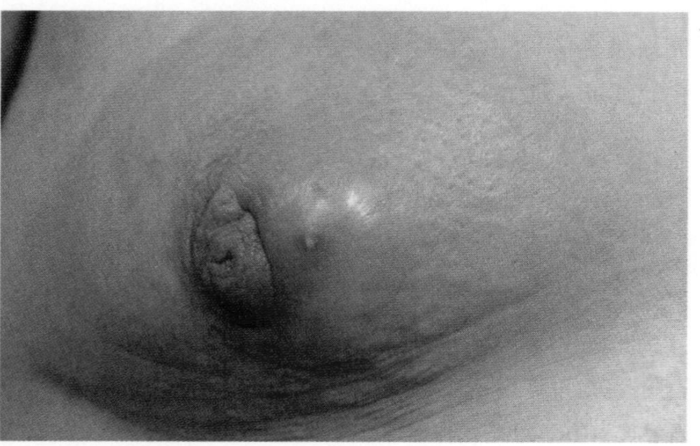

◀ Breast Abscess

A rare complication of generalized infection (e.g., mastitis) if untreated. A pocket of pus accumulates in one local area. Here, extensive nipple edema, and abscess is "pointing" at 3 o'clock position on areolar margin. Must temporarily discontinue nursing on affected breast; manually express milk and discard. Continue to nurse on unaffected side. Treat with antibiotics, surgical incision, and drainage.

TABLE 17-8 Abnormalities in the Male Breast

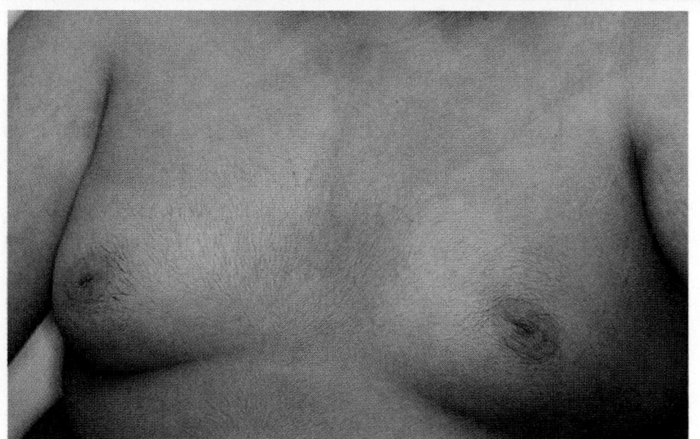

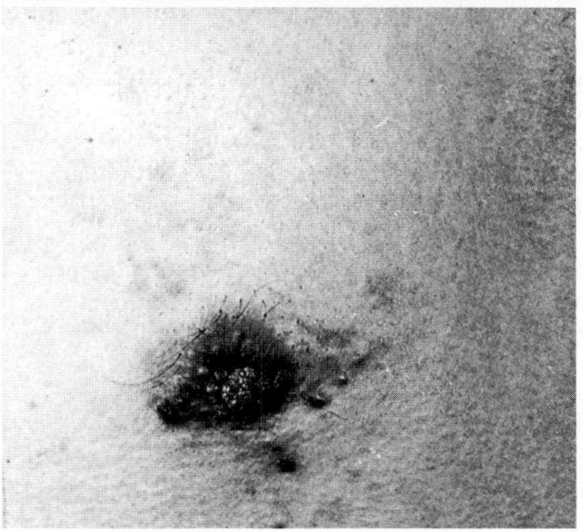

Gynecomastia

Benign enlargement of male breast that occurs when peripheral tissues convert androgen hormones to estrogens. It is a mobile disk of tissue located centrally under the nipple-areola. At puberty, it is usually mild and transient. In older men, it is bilateral, tender, and firm but not as hard as breast cancer. Gynecomastia occurs with obesity, Cushing syndrome, liver cirrhosis (because cannot metabolize estrogens), adrenal disease, hyperthyroidism, and numerous drugs: alcohol and marijuana; estrogen treatment for prostate cancer; antibiotics (metronidazole, isoniazid); digoxin, ACE inhibitors; psychoactive drugs (diazepam, tricyclic antidepressants).[16]

Male Breast Cancer

Although 1% of breast cancers occur in men, there is no standard screening mammography and it is detected by clinical symptoms. It usually presents as a painless palpable mass; hard, irregular, nontender, fixed to the area, may have nipple retraction. Nipple discharge, with or without a palpable mass, is a significant warning of early breast cancer.[25] Early spread to axillary lymph nodes occurs due to minimal breast tissue. Because of lack of screening and general awareness, men are diagnosed 10 years later than women and at later stages, with the mean age between 60 and 70 years. The stage at diagnosis is the most important indicator for survival.

BIBLIOGRAPHY

1. Agurs-Collins, T., Rosenberg, L., Makambi, K., et al. (2009). Dietary patterns and breast cancer risk in women participating in the Black Women's Health Study. *American Journal of Clinical Nutrition, 90*(3), 621-628.
2. Ahmed, N. U., Ford, J. G., Fair, A. M., et al. (2009). Breast cancer knowledge and barriers to mammography in a low-income managed care population. *Journal of Cancer Education, 24*(4), 261-266.
3. Aksglaede, L., Sørensen, K., Peterson, J. H., et al. (2009). Recent decline in age at breast development: the Copenhagen Puberty Study. *Pediatrics, 123*(5), e932-e939.
4. American Cancer Society. (2010). *Breast cancer: cancer facts and figures 2009-2010*. Atlanta: Author.
5. Baquet, C. R., Mishra, S. I., Commiskey, P., et al. (2008). Breast cancer epidemiology in blacks and whites: disparities in incidence, mortality, survival rates and histology. *Journal of the National Medical Association, 100*(5), 480-488.
6. Barron, M.A., & Fishel, R. S. (2007). Talk to your patients about breast disease. *Nurse Practitioner, 32*(10), 21-32.
7. Borrayo, E. A., Hines, L., Byers, T., et al. (2009). Characteristics associated with mammography screening among both Hispanic and non-Hispanic white women. *Journal of Women's Health, 18*(10), 1585-1594.
8. Chiarelli, A. M., Majpruz, V., Brown, P., et al. (2009). The contribution of clinical breast examination to the accuracy of breast screening. *Journal of the National Cancer Institute, 101*(18), 1236-1243.
9. Colditz, G. A., & Rosner, B. (2000). Cumulative risk of breast cancer to age 70 years according to risk factor status: data from the Nurses' Health Study. *American Journal of Epidemiology, 152*, 950-964.
10. Conway-Philips, R., & Millon-Underwood, S. (2009). Breast cancer screening behaviors of African American women: a comprehensive review, analysis, and critique of nursing research. *ABNF Journal, 20*(4), 97-101.
11. Cottet, V., Touvier, M., Fornier, A., et al. (2009). Postmenopausal breast cancer risk and dietary patterns in the E3N-EPIC Prospective Cohort Study. *American Journal of Epidemiology, 170*(10), 1257-1267.
12. DiVall, S. A., & Radovick, S. (2009). Endocrinology of female puberty. *Current Opinion in Endocrinology, Diabetes, and Obesity, 16*(1), 1-4.
13. Gajdos, Z. K. Z., Hirschhorn, J. N., & Palmert, M. (2009). What controls the timing of puberty? An update on progress from genetic investigation. *Current Opinion in Endocrinology, Diabetes, and Obesity, 16*(1), 16-24.
14. Herman-Giddens, M. E., Slora, E. J., Wasserman, R. C., et al. (1997). Secondary sexual characteristics and menses in young girls seen in office practice: a study from the Pediatric Research in Office Settings network. *Pediatrics, 99*, 505-512.
15. Jayasinghe, Y., & Simmons, P. S. (2009). Fibroadenomas in adolescence. *Current Opinion in Obstetrics & Gynecology, 21*(5), 402-406.

16. Johnson, R. E., & Murad, M. H. (2009). Gynecomastia: pathophysiology, evaluation, and management. *Mayo Clinic Proceedings, 84*(11), 1010-1015.
17. Katapodi, M. C., Dodd, M. J., Lee, K. A., et al. (2009). Underestimation of breast cancer risk: influence on screening behavior. *Oncology Nursing Forum, 36*(3), 306-314.
18. Kearney, A. J., & Murray, M. (2009). Breast cancer screening recommendations: is mammography the only answer? *Journal of Midwifery & Women's Health, 54*(5), 393-400.
19. Lee, C. H., Dershaw, D. D., Kopans, D., et al. (2010). Breast cancer screening with imaging: recommendations from the Society of Breast Imaging and the ACR on the use of mammography, breast MRI, breast ultrasound, and other technologies for the detection of clinically occult breast cancer. *Journal of the American College of Radiology, 7*(1), 18-27.
20. Lindberg, N. M., Stevens, V. J., Smith, K. S., et al. (2009). A brief intervention designed to increase breast cancer self-screening. *American Journal of Health Promotion, 23*(5), 320-323.
21. Lof, M., & Weiderpass, E. (2009). Impact of diet on breast cancer risk. *Current Opinion in Obstetrics & Gynecology, 21*(1), 80-85.
22. Love, S., & Lindsey, K. (2005). *Dr. Susan Love's breast book* (4th ed.). Cambridge, MA: Da Capo Lifelong Books.
23. Marshall, W. A., & Tanner, J. M. (1969). Variations in pattern of pubertal changes in girls. *Archives of Disease in Childhood, 44*, 291-303.
24. Mellington, T. E., & Fields, M. M. (2008). Targeting breast cancer with hormonal treatment options. *Nurse Practitioner, 33*(5), 17-22.
25. Morrogh, M., & King, T. A. (2009). The significance of nipple discharge of the male breast. *Breast Journal, 15*(6), 632-638.
26. Neal, L., Tortorelli, C. L., & Nassar, A. (2010). Clinician's guide to imaging and pathologic findings in benign breast disease. *Mayo Clinic Proceedings, 85*(3), 274-279.
27. Pierce, J. P. (2009). Diet and breast cancer prognosis: making sense of the Women's Healthy Eating and Living and Women's Intervention Nutrition Study Trials. *Current Opinion in Obstetrics & Gynecology, 21*(1), 86-91.
28. Rosenfield, R. L., Lipton, R. B., & Drum, M. L. (2009). Thelarche, pubarche, and menarche attainment in children with normal and elevated body mass index. *Pediatrics, 123*(1), 84-88.
29. Schonberg, M. (2010). Breast cancer screening: at what age to stop? *Consultant, 50*(5), 196-205.
30. Tanner, J. M. (1962). *Growth at adolescence* (2nd ed.). Oxford, UK: Blackwell Scientific.
31. Thind, A., Diamant, A., Hoq, L., et al. (2009). Method of detection of breast cancer in low-income women. *Journal of Women's Health, 18*(11), 1807-1811.
31a. Thomas, E. (October 2010). Men's awareness and knowledge of male breast cancer. *American Journal of Nursing, 110*(10): 32-42.
32. U.S. Department of Health and Human Services, Agency for Healthcare Research and Quality. (2009). *Screening for breast cancer*. Retrieved May 2010 from www.ahrq.gov/clinic/uspstf09/breastcancer/brcanrs.htm.
33. Wu, T., & Ronis, D. (2009). Correlates of recent and regular mammography screening among Asian-American women. *Journal of Advanced Nursing, 65*(11), 2434-2446.

Summary Checklist: Breasts and Regional Lymphatics Examination

For a PDA-downloadable version, go to http://evolve.elsevier.com/Jarvis/.

1. **Inspect breasts** as the woman sits, raises arms overhead, pushes hands on hips, leans forward.
2. **Inspect** the supraclavicular and infraclavicular areas.
3. **Palpate the axillae** and regional lymph nodes.
4. With woman supine, **palpate the breast tissue,** including tail of Spence, the nipples, and areolae.
5. **Teach BSE.**

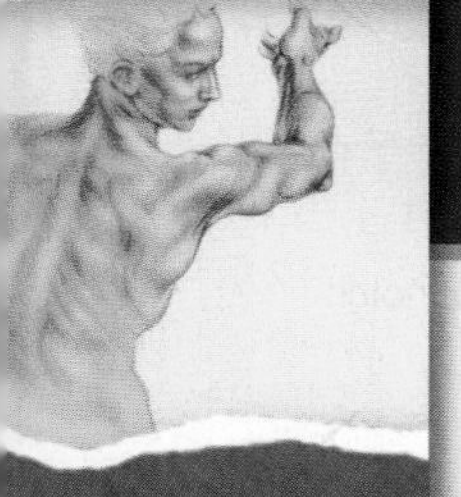

CHAPTER 18

Thorax and Lungs

evolve WEBSITE

http://evolve.elsevier.com/Jarvis/

- Animations
- Audio Key Points
- Audio—Lung Sounds
- Bedside Assessment Summary Checklist
- Case Study
  Exacerbation of COPD
  Persistent Cough
  Respiratory Assessment
  Respiratory Problems
- Health Promotion Guide
  Smoking Cessation
- NCLEX Review Questions
- Physical Examination Summary Checklist
- Quick Assessment for Common Conditions
  Asthma
  Pneumonia
- Video—Assessment
  Anterior Chest and Upper Extremities
  Posterior and Lateral Chest

OUTLINE

Structure and Function, 411

Position and Surface Landmarks
The Thoracic Cavity
Mechanics of Respiration

Subjective Data, 418

Health History Questions

Objective Data, 421

Preparation
The Posterior Chest
The Anterior Chest

Documentation and Critical Thinking, 438

Abnormal Findings, 440

Abnormal Findings for Advanced Practice, 446

STRUCTURE AND FUNCTION

POSITION AND SURFACE LANDMARKS

The **thoracic cage** is a bony structure with a conical shape, which is narrower at the top (Fig. 18-1). It is defined by the **sternum,** 12 pairs of **ribs,** and 12 thoracic **vertebrae.** Its "floor" is the **diaphragm,** a musculotendinous septum that separates the thoracic cavity from the abdomen. The first seven ribs attach directly to the sternum via their costal cartilages; ribs 8, 9, and 10 attach to the costal cartilage above, and ribs 11 and 12 are "floating," with free palpable tips. The **costochondral junctions** are the points at which the ribs join their cartilages. They are not palpable.

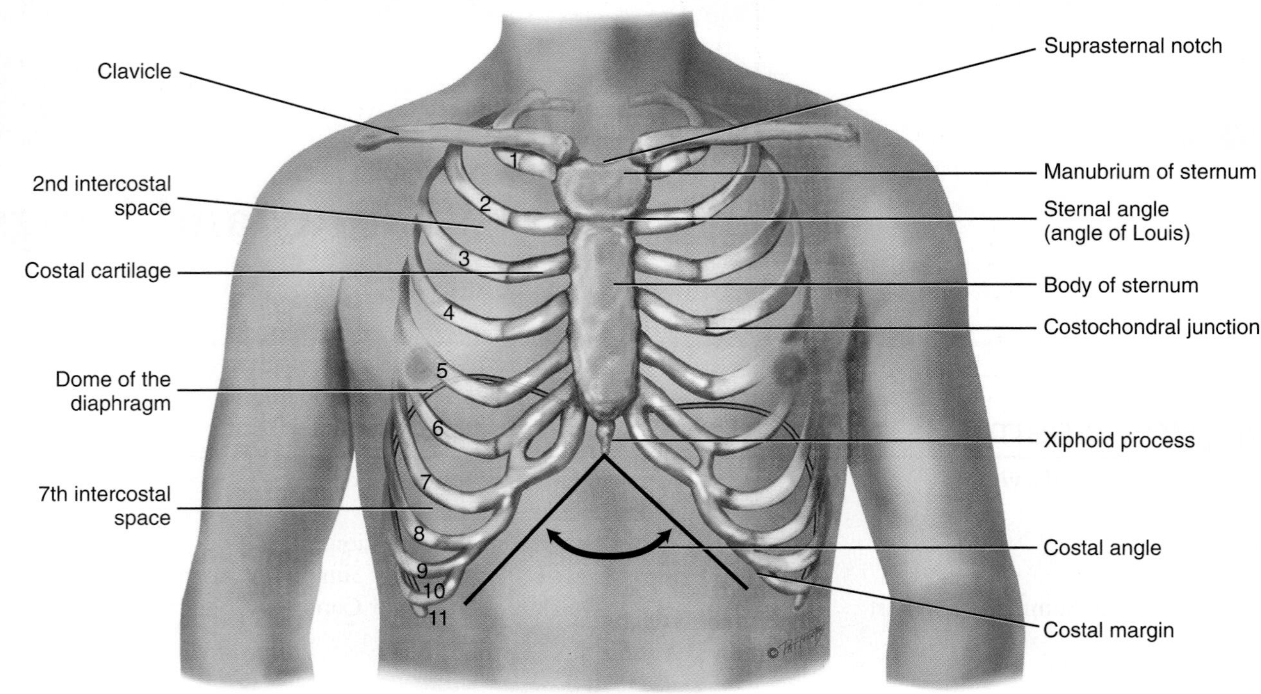

ANTERIOR THORACIC CAGE

18-1

Anterior Thoracic Landmarks

Surface landmarks on the thorax are signposts for underlying respiratory structures. Knowing landmarks will help you localize a finding and will facilitate communication of your findings to others.

Suprasternal Notch. Feel this hollow U-shaped depression just above the sternum, in between the clavicles.

Sternum. The "breastbone" has three parts—the manubrium, the body, and the xiphoid process. Walk your fingers down the manubrium a few centimeters until you feel a distinct bony ridge, the sternal angle.

Sternal Angle. Often called the "angle of Louis," this is the articulation of the manubrium and body of the sternum, and it is continuous with the second rib. The angle of Louis is a useful place to start counting ribs, which helps localize a respiratory finding horizontally. Identify the angle of Louis, palpate lightly to the second rib, and slide down to the second intercostal space. Each intercostal space is numbered by the rib above it. Continue counting down the ribs in the middle of the hemithorax, not close to the sternum where the costal cartilages lie too close together to count. You can palpate easily down to the tenth rib.

The angle of Louis also marks the site of tracheal bifurcation into the right and left main bronchi; it corresponds with the upper border of the atria of the heart, and it lies above the fourth thoracic vertebra on the back.

Costal Angle. The right and left costal margins form an angle where they meet at the xiphoid process. Usually 90 degrees or less, this angle increases when the rib cage is chronically overinflated, as in emphysema.

Posterior Thoracic Landmarks

Counting ribs and intercostal spaces on the back is a bit harder due to the muscles and soft tissue surrounding the ribs and spinal column (Fig. 18-2).

Vertebra Prominens. Start here. Flex your head and feel for the most prominent bony spur protruding at the base of the neck. This is the spinous process of C7. If two bumps seem equally prominent, the upper one is C7 and the lower one is T1.

Spinous Processes. Count down these knobs on the vertebrae, which stack together to form the spinal column. Note that the spinous processes align with their same numbered ribs only down to T4. After T4, the spinous processes angle downward from their vertebral body and overlie the vertebral body and rib below.

Inferior Border of the Scapula. The scapulae are located symmetrically in each hemithorax. The lower tip is usually at the seventh or eighth rib.

Twelfth Rib. Palpate midway between the spine and the person's side to identify its free tip.

Reference Lines

Use the reference lines to pinpoint a finding vertically on the chest. On the anterior chest, note the **midsternal** line and the

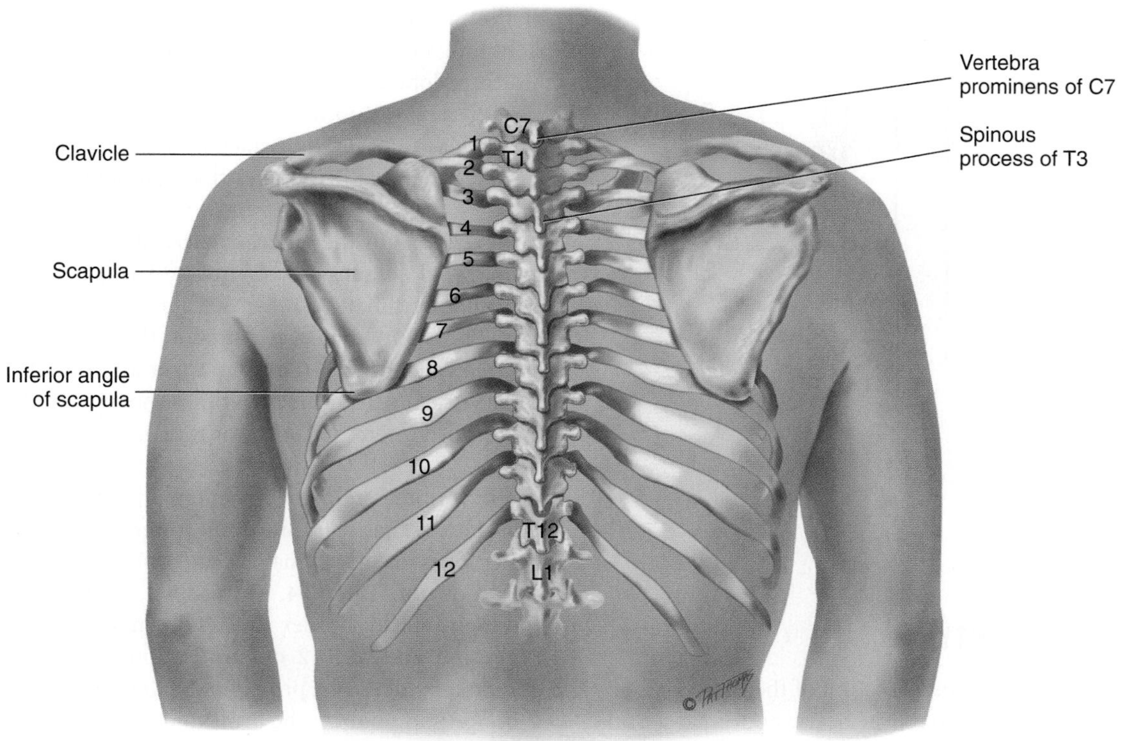

POSTERIOR THORACIC CAGE

18-2

midclavicular line. The midclavicular line bisects the center of each clavicle at a point halfway between the palpated sternoclavicular and acromioclavicular joints (Fig. 18-3).

The posterior chest wall has the **vertebral** (or midspinal) line and the **scapular** line, which extends through the inferior angle of the scapula when the arms are at the sides of the body (Fig. 18-4).

Lift up the person's arm 90 degrees, and divide the lateral chest by three lines: the **anterior axillary** line extends down from the anterior axillary fold where the pectoralis major muscle inserts; the **posterior axillary** line continues down from the posterior axillary fold where the latissimus dorsi muscle inserts; and the **midaxillary** line runs down from the apex of the axilla and lies between and parallel to the other two (Fig. 18-5).

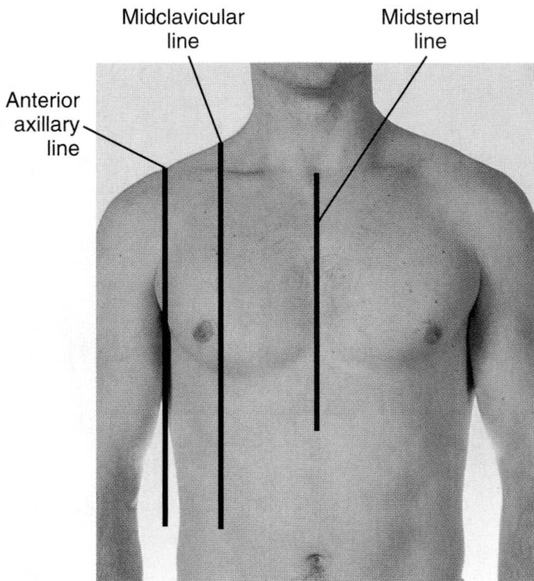

18-3

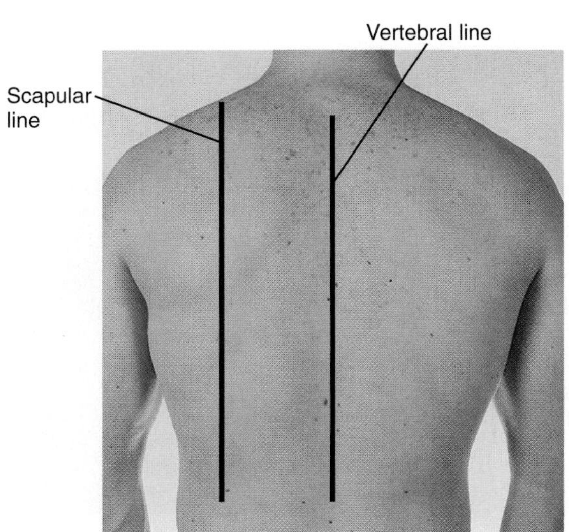

18-4

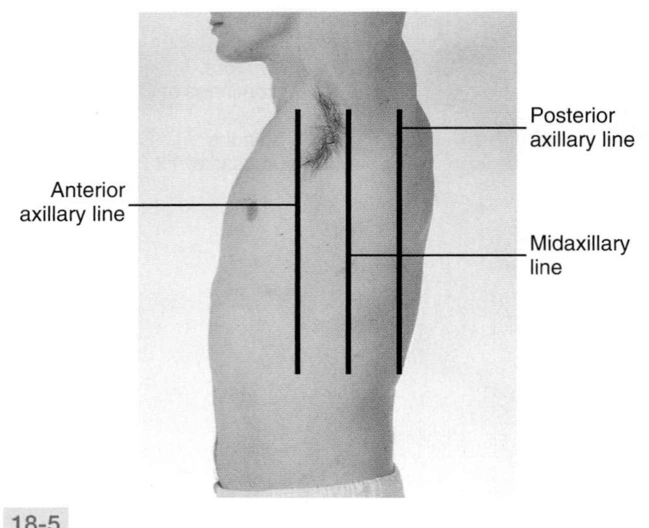

18-5

THE THORACIC CAVITY

The **mediastinum** is the middle section of the thoracic cavity containing the esophagus, trachea, heart, and great vessels. The right and left **pleural cavities,** on either side of the mediastinum, contain the lungs.

Lung Borders. In the anterior chest, the **apex,** or highest point, of lung tissue is 3 to 4 cm above the inner third of the clavicles. The **base,** or lower border, rests on the diaphragm at about the sixth rib in the midclavicular line. Laterally, lung tissue extends from the apex of the axilla down to the seventh or eighth rib. Posteriorly, the location of C7 marks the apex of lung tissue, and T10 usually corresponds to the base. Deep inspiration expands the lungs, and their lower border drops to the level of T12.

Lobes of the Lungs

The lungs are paired but not precisely symmetric structures (Fig. 18-6). The right lung is shorter than the left lung because of the underlying liver. The left lung is narrower than the right lung because the heart bulges to the left. The right lung has three lobes, and the left lung has two lobes. These lobes are not arranged in horizontal bands like dessert layers in a parfait glass. Rather, they stack in diagonal sloping segments and are separated by **fissures** that run obliquely through the chest.

Anterior. On the anterior chest, the **oblique** (the major or diagonal) fissure crosses the fifth rib in the midaxillary line and terminates at the sixth rib in the midclavicular line. The right lung also contains the **horizontal** (minor) fissure, which divides the right upper and middle lobes. This fissure extends from the fifth rib in the right midaxillary line to the third intercostal space or fourth rib at the right sternal border.

Posterior. The most remarkable point about the posterior chest is that it is almost all lower lobe (Fig. 18-7). The upper lobes occupy a smaller band of tissue from their apices at T1 down to T3 or T4. At this level, the lower lobes begin, and their inferior border reaches down to the level of T10 on expiration and to T12 on inspiration. Note that the right middle lobe does not project onto the posterior chest at all. If the person abducts the arms and places the hands on the back of the head, the division between the upper and lower lobes corresponds to the medial border of the scapulae.

Lateral. Laterally, lung tissue extends from the apex of the axilla down to the seventh or eighth rib. The right upper lobe extends from the apex of the axilla down to the horizontal fissure at the fifth rib (Fig. 18-8). The right middle lobe extends from the horizontal fissure down and forward to the sixth rib at the midclavicular line. The right lower lobe continues from the fifth rib to the eighth rib in the midaxillary line.

The left lung contains only two lobes, upper and lower (Fig. 18-9). These are seen laterally as two triangular areas separated by the oblique fissure. The left upper lobe extends from the apex of the axilla down to the fifth rib at the midaxillary line. The left lower lobe continues down to the eighth rib in the midaxillary line.

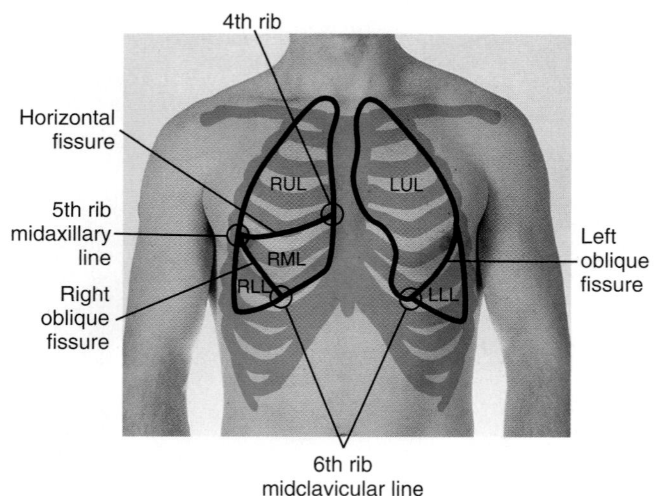

18-6

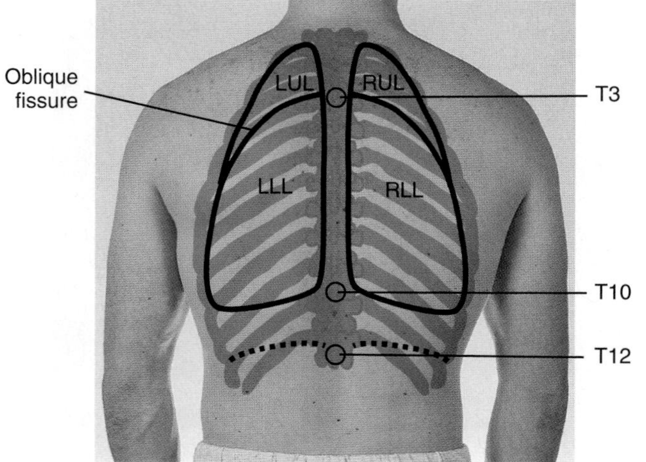

18-7

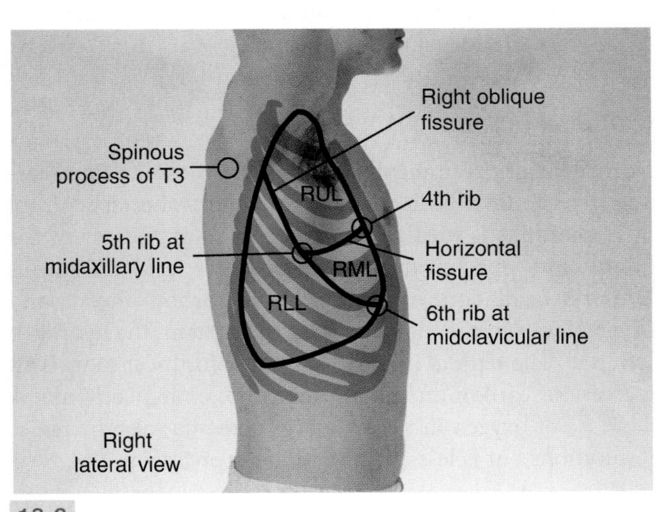

18-8

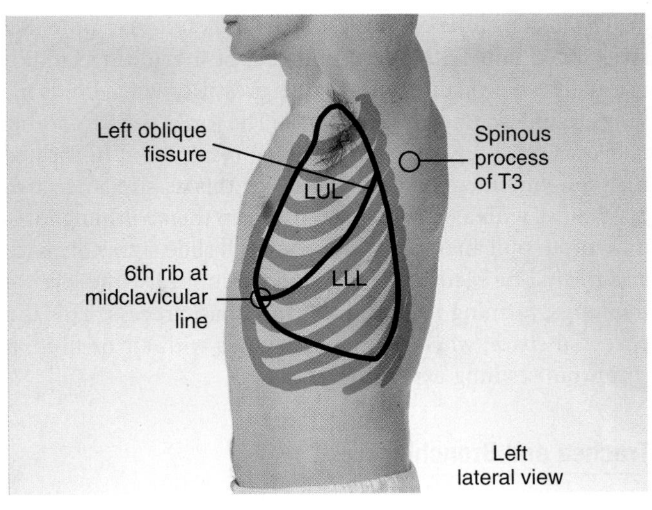

18-9

Using these landmarks, take a marker and try tracing the outline of each lobe on a willing partner. Take special note of the three points that commonly confuse beginning examiners:

1. The left lung has no middle lobe.
2. The anterior chest contains mostly upper and middle lobe with very little lower lobe.
3. The posterior chest contains almost all lower lobe.

Pleurae

The thin, slippery **pleurae** are serous membranes that form an envelope between the lungs and the chest wall (Fig. 18-10). The **visceral** pleura lines the outside of the lungs, dipping down into the fissures. It is continuous with the **parietal** pleura lining the inside of the chest wall and diaphragm.

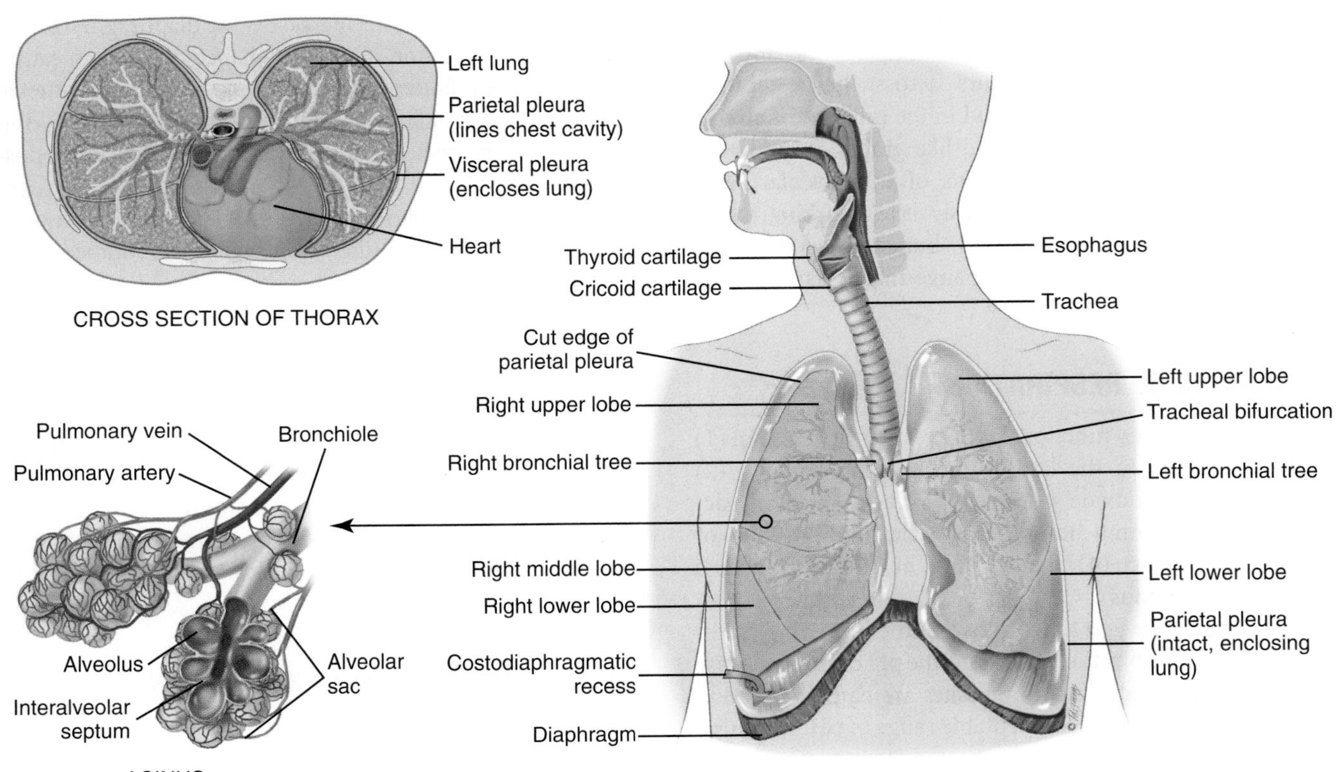

18-10

The inside of the envelope, the pleural cavity, is a potential space filled only with a few milliliters of lubricating fluid. It normally has a vacuum, or negative pressure, which holds the lungs tightly against the chest wall. The lungs slide smoothly and noiselessly up and down during respiration, lubricated by a few milliliters of fluid. Think of this as similar to two glass slides with a drop of water between them; although it is difficult to pull apart the slides, they will slide smoothly back and forth. The pleurae extend about 3 cm below the level of the lungs, forming the **costodiaphragmatic recess.** This is a potential space; when it abnormally fills with air or fluid, it compromises lung expansion.

Trachea and Bronchial Tree

The **trachea** lies anterior to the esophagus and is 10 to 11 cm long in the adult. It begins at the level of the cricoid cartilage in the neck and bifurcates just below the sternal angle into the right and left main bronchi. Posteriorly, tracheal bifurcation is at the level of T4 or T5. The right main bronchus is shorter, wider, and more vertical than the left main bronchus.

The **trachea** and **bronchi** transport gases between the environment and the lung parenchyma. They constitute the *dead space,* or space that is filled with air but is not available for gaseous exchange. This is about 150 mL in the adult. The bronchial tree also protects alveoli from small particulate matter in the inhaled air. The bronchi are lined with goblet cells, which secrete mucus that entraps the particles. The bronchi are lined with cilia, which sweep particles upward where they can be swallowed or expelled.

An **acinus** is a functional respiratory unit that consists of the bronchioles, alveolar ducts, alveolar sacs, and the alveoli. Gaseous exchange occurs across the respiratory membrane in the alveolar duct and in the millions of alveoli. Note how the alveoli are clustered like grapes around each alveolar duct. This creates millions of interalveolar septa (walls) that increase tremendously the working space available for gas exchange. This bunched arrangement creates a surface area for gas exchange that is as large as a tennis court.

MECHANICS OF RESPIRATION

There are four major functions of the respiratory system: (1) supplying oxygen to the body for energy production; (2) removing carbon dioxide as a waste product of energy reactions; (3) maintaining homeostasis (acid-base balance) of arterial blood; and (4) maintaining heat exchange (less important in humans).

By supplying oxygen to the blood and eliminating excess carbon dioxide, respiration maintains the pH or the acid-base balance of the blood. The body tissues are bathed by blood that normally has a narrow acceptable range of pH. Although a number of compensatory mechanisms regulate the pH, the lungs help maintain the balance by adjusting the level of carbon dioxide through respiration. That is, hypoventilation (slow, shallow breathing) causes carbon dioxide to build up in the blood, and hyperventilation (rapid, deep breathing) causes carbon dioxide to be blown off.

Control of Respirations

Normally, our breathing pattern changes without our awareness in response to cellular demands. This involuntary control of respirations is mediated by the respiratory center in the brainstem (pons and medulla). The major feedback loop is humoral regulation, or the change in carbon dioxide and oxygen levels in the blood and, less important, the hydrogen ion level. The *normal stimulus to breathe* for most of us is an increase of carbon dioxide in the blood, or **hypercapnia.** A decrease of oxygen in the blood (**hypoxemia**) also increases respirations but is less effective than hypercapnia.

Changing Chest Size

Respiration is the physical act of breathing; air rushes into the lungs as the chest size increases (inspiration) and is expelled from the lungs as the chest recoils (expiration). The mechanical expansion and contraction of the chest cavity alters the size of the thoracic container in two dimensions: (1) the vertical diameter lengthens or shortens, which is accomplished by downward or upward movement of the diaphragm; and (2) the anteroposterior (A-P) diameter increases or decreases, which is accomplished by elevation or depression of the ribs (Fig. 18-11).

In inspiration, increasing the size of the thoracic container creates a slightly negative pressure in relation to the atmosphere, so air rushes in to fill the partial vacuum. The major muscle responsible for this increase is the diaphragm. During inspiration, contraction of the bell-shaped diaphragm causes it to descend and flatten. This lengthens the vertical diameter. Intercostal muscles lift the sternum and elevate the ribs, making them more horizontal. This increases the anteroposterior diameter.

Expiration is primarily passive. As the diaphragm relaxes, elastic forces within the lung, chest cage, and abdomen cause it to dome up. All this squeezing creates a relatively positive pressure within the alveoli, and the air flows out.

Forced inspiration, such as that after heavy exercise or occurring pathologically with respiratory distress, commands the use of the accessory neck muscles to heave up the sternum and rib cage. These neck muscles are the sternomastoids, the scaleni, and the trapezii. In forced expiration, the abdominal muscles contract powerfully to push the abdominal viscera forcefully in and up against the diaphragm, making it dome upward and making it squeeze against the lungs.

DEVELOPMENTAL COMPETENCE

Infants and Children

During the first 5 weeks of fetal life, the primitive lung bud emerges; by 16 weeks, the conducting airways reach the same number as in the adult; at 32 weeks, **surfactant,** the complex

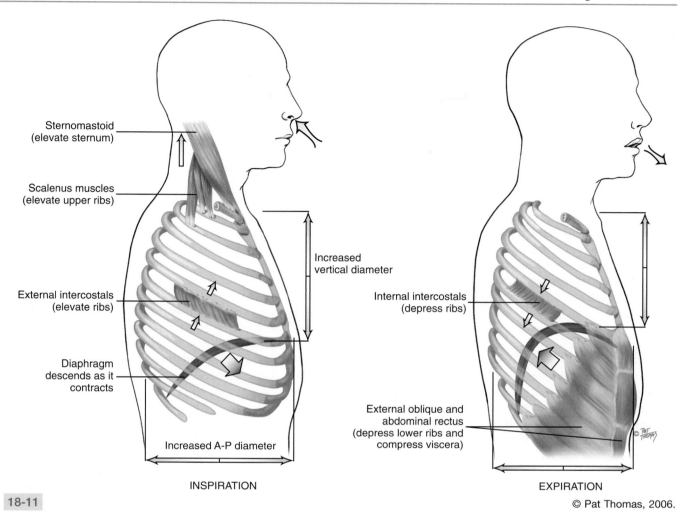

Sternomastoid (elevate sternum)

Scalenus muscles (elevate upper ribs)

External intercostals (elevate ribs)

Diaphragm descends as it contracts

Increased vertical diameter

Increased A-P diameter

INSPIRATION

Internal intercostals (depress ribs)

External oblique and abdominal rectus (depress lower ribs and compress viscera)

EXPIRATION

© Pat Thomas, 2006.

18-11

lipid substance needed for sustained inflation of the air sacs, is present in adequate amounts; and by birth, the lungs have 70 million primitive alveoli ready to start the job of respiration.

Breath is life. When the newborn inhales the first breath, the lusty cry that follows reassures straining parents that their baby is all right (Fig. 18-12). The baby's body systems all develop in utero, but the respiratory system alone does not function until birth. Birth demands its instant performance.

When the cord is cut, blood is cut off from the placenta and it gushes into the pulmonary circulation. Relatively less resistance exists in the pulmonary arteries than in the aorta, so the foramen ovale in the heart closes just after birth. (See the discussion of fetal circulation in Chapter 19.) The ductus arteriosus (linking the pulmonary artery and the aorta) contracts and closes some hours later, and pulmonary and systemic circulation are functional.

Respiratory development continues throughout childhood, with increases in diameter and length of airways and increases in size and number of alveoli, reaching the adult range of 300 million by adolescence.

The relatively smaller size and immaturity of children's pulmonary systems and the presence of parents and caregivers who smoke result in enormous vulnerability and increased risks to child health. Prenatal exposure causes chronic hypoxia and low birth weight. Also, it sensitizes the fetal brain to nicotine, which increases risk for addiction when the child is exposed to nicotine at a later age.[4] Postnatal exposure to secondhand tobacco smoke leads to sudden infant death, lower respiratory illnesses, acute and chronic otitis media, breathlessness, asthma, and adverse lung function throughout childhood.[4,14]

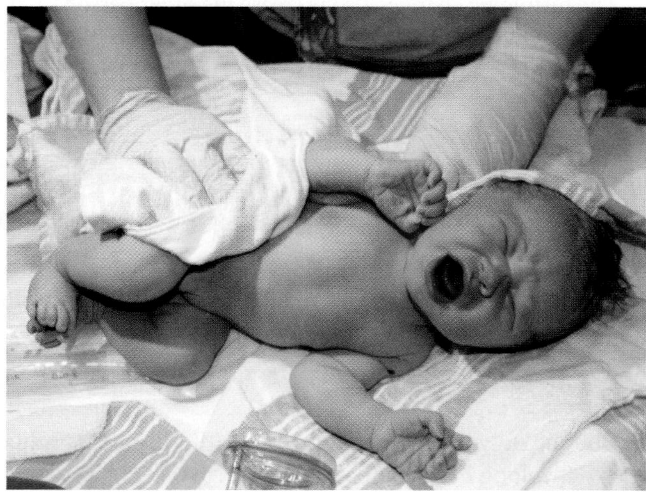

18-12

The Pregnant Woman

The enlarging uterus elevates the diaphragm 4 cm during pregnancy. This decreases the vertical diameter of the thoracic cage, but this decrease is compensated for by an increase in the horizontal diameter. The increase in estrogen level relaxes the chest cage ligaments. This allows an increase in the transverse diameter of the chest cage by 2 cm, and the costal angle widens. The total circumference of the chest cage increases by 6 cm. Although the diaphragm is elevated, it is not fixed. It moves with breathing even more during pregnancy, which results in an increase in tidal volume.[9]

The growing fetus increases the oxygen demand on the mother's body. This is met easily by the increasing tidal volume (deeper breathing). Little change occurs in the respiratory rate. An increased awareness of the need to breathe develops, even early in pregnancy, and some pregnant women may interpret this as dyspnea although, structurally, nothing is wrong.

The Aging Adult

The costal cartilages become calcified, which produces a less mobile thorax. Respiratory muscle strength declines after age 50 years and continues to decrease into the 70s. A more significant change is the decrease in elastic properties within the lungs, making them less distensible and lessening their tendency to collapse and recoil. In all, the aging lung is a more rigid structure that is harder to inflate.

These changes result in an increase in small airway closure, and that yields a *decreased vital capacity* (the maximum amount of air that a person can expel from the lungs after first filling the lungs to maximum) and an *increased residual volume* (the amount of air remaining in the lungs even after the most forceful expiration).

With aging, histologic changes (i.e., a gradual loss of intra-alveolar septa and a decreased number of alveoli) also occur, so less surface area is available for gas exchange. Also, the lung bases become less ventilated as a result of closing off of a number of airways. This increases the older person's risk for dyspnea with exertion beyond his or her usual workload.

The histologic changes also increase the older person's risk for postoperative pulmonary complications. That is, the older person has a greater risk for postoperative atelectasis and infection from a decreased ability to cough, a loss of protective airway reflexes, and increased secretions.

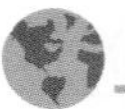

CULTURE AND GENETICS

The incidence of tuberculosis (TB) has declined in the United States; however, persons who are foreign-born and of racial/ethnic minorities have a disproportionately large burden of TB disease.[6] In 2008, the TB rates were as follows: 10 times higher in foreign-born than in U.S. born; 8 times higher among Hispanic and Blacks than among whites; and 23 times higher among Asians than among whites. These data reflect high TB rates in countries of origin for U.S. immigrants, as well as barriers to early diagnosis, prevention, and treatment adherence for latent TB infection in some minority groups.

Asthma occurs in about 5% to 12% of the U.S. population and is the most common chronic disease in childhood. Groups at increased risk include African Americans who reside in inner cities and premature or low-birth-weight infants. Asthma prevalence is highest among African-American and American Indian adults; it is lowest among Asian and Hispanic adults.[12] Regarding asthma-related problems and medical care use, African Americans, Hispanics, and especially American Indians experience more than do whites or Asians. When compared with white children, African-American and Hispanic children have more indicators of poorly controlled asthma, including more emergency department visits, more daily rescue medication use, and lower use of inhaled corticosteroids.[8] Extrinsic/allergic asthma (or pediatric onset) involves a complex interaction between genetic susceptibility (bronchial hyperresponsiveness, atopy, elevated immunoglobulin E)[23] and environmental factors (viral respiratory infections, air pollution).

Biocultural differences in the **size of the thoracic cavity** significantly influence pulmonary functioning as determined by vital capacity and forced expiratory volume. In descending order, the largest chest volumes are found in whites, Blacks, Asians, and American Indians. Even when the shorter height of Asians is considered, their chest volume remains significantly lower than that of whites and Blacks.

SUBJECTIVE DATA

1. Cough
2. Shortness of breath
3. Chest pain with breathing
4. History of respiratory infections
5. Smoking history
6. Environmental exposure
7. Self-care behaviors

Examiner Asks	Rationale
1. Cough. Do you have a **cough?** When did it start? Gradual or sudden? • How long have you had it?	Acute cough lasts less than 2 or 3 weeks; chronic cough lasts over 2 months.

Examiner Asks	Rationale
• How often do you cough? At any special time of day or just on arising? Cough wake you up at night?	Conditions with characteristic timing of cough: (1) continuous throughout day—acute illness (e.g., respiratory infection); (2) afternoon/evening—may reflect exposure to irritants at work; (3) night—postnasal drip, sinusitis; (4) early morning—chronic bronchial inflammation of smokers.
• Do you cough up any phlegm or sputum? How much? What color is it?	Chronic bronchitis presents with a history of productive cough for 3 months of the year for 2 years in a row.
• Cough up any blood? Does this look like streaks or frank blood? Does the sputum have a foul odor?	**Hemoptysis.** Some conditions have characteristic sputum production: (1) white or clear mucoid—colds, bronchitis, viral infections; (2) yellow or green—bacterial infections; (3) rust colored—tuberculosis, pneumococcal pneumonia; (4) pink, frothy—pulmonary edema, some sympathomimetic medications have a side effect of pink-tinged mucus.
• How would you describe your cough: hacking, dry, barking, hoarse, congested, bubbling?	Some conditions have a characteristic cough: mycoplasma pneumonia—hacking; early heart failure—dry; croup—barking; colds, bronchitis, pneumonia—congested.
• Does the cough seem to come with anything: activity, position (lying), fever, congestion, talking, anxiety? • Does activity make it better or worse?	
• What treatment have you tried? Prescription or over-the-counter medications, vaporizer, rest, position change?	Assess the effectiveness of coping strategies.
• Does the cough bring on anything: chest pain, ear pain? Is it tiring? Are you concerned about it?	Note severity.
2. Shortness of breath. Ever had any **shortness of breath** or hard-breathing spells? What brings it on? How severe is it? How long does it last?	Determine how much activity precipitates the shortness of breath (SOB)—state specific number of blocks walked, number of stairs.
• Is it affected by position, such as lying down?	**Orthopnea** is difficulty breathing when supine. State number of pillows needed to achieve comfort (e.g., "two-pillow orthopnea").
• Occur at any specific time of day or night?	**Paroxysmal nocturnal dyspnea** is awakening from sleep with SOB and needing to be upright to achieve comfort.
• Shortness of breath episodes associated with night sweats?	Diaphoresis.
• Or cough, chest pain, or bluish color around lips or nails? Wheezing sound?	Cyanosis signals hypoxia.
• Episodes seem to be related to food, pollen, dust, animals, season, or emotion?	Asthma attacks may be associated with a specific allergen or extreme cold, anxiety.
• What do you do in a hard-breathing attack? Take a special position, or use pursed-lip breathing? Use any oxygen, inhalers, or medications?	Assess effect of coping strategies and the need for more teaching.
• How does the shortness of breath affect your work or home activities? Getting better or worse or staying about the same?	Assess effect on activities of daily living.

Subjective Data

Subjective Data

Examiner Asks	Rationale
3. **Chest pain with breathing** Any **chest pain with breathing?** Please point to the exact location. • When did it start? Constant, or does it come and go? • Describe the pain: burning, stabbing? • Brought on by respiratory infection, coughing, or trauma? Is it associated with fever, deep breathing, unequal chest inflation? • What have you done to treat it? Medication or heat application?	Chest pain of thoracic origin occurs with muscle soreness from coughing or from inflammation of pleura overlying pneumonia. Distinguish this from chest pain of cardiac origin (see Chapter 19) or from heartburn of stomach acid.
4. **History of respiratory infections.** Any **past history** of breathing trouble or lung diseases such as bronchitis, emphysema, asthma, pneumonia?	Consider sequelae after these conditions.
• Any unusually frequent or unusually severe colds?	Because most people have had some colds, it is more meaningful to ask about excess number or severity.
• Any family history of allergies, tuberculosis, or asthma?	Assess possible risk factors.
5. **Smoking history.** Do you **smoke** cigarettes or cigars? At what age did you start? How many packs per day do you smoke now? For how long?	State number of packs per day and the number of years smoked.
• Have you ever tried to quit? What helped? Why do you think it did not work? What activities do you associate with smoking? • Live with someone who smokes?	Most people already know they should quit smoking. Instead of admonishing, assess smoking behavior, ways to modify daily smoking activities, identify triggers, how to manage withdrawal.
6. **Environmental exposure.** Are there any **environmental conditions** that may affect your breathing? Where do you work? At a factory, chemical plant, coal mine, farming, outdoors in a heavy traffic area?	Pollution exposure. Farmers may be at risk for grain inhalation, pesticide inhalation. People in the rural Midwest have a risk for histoplasmosis exposure; those in the Southwest and Mexico have a risk for coccidioidomycosis. Coal miners have a risk for pneumoconiosis. Stone cutters, miners, and potters have a risk for silicosis. Other irritants: asbestos, radon.
• Do you do anything to protect your lungs, such as wear a mask or have the ventilatory system checked at work? Do you do anything to monitor your exposure? Do you have periodic examinations, pulmonary function tests, x-ray examination?	Assess **self-care** measures.
• Do you know what specific symptoms to note that may signal breathing problems?	General symptoms: cough, shortness of breath. Some gases produce specific symptoms: carbon monoxide—dizziness, headache, fatigue; sulfur dioxide—cough, congestion.
7. **Self-care behaviors.** Last tuberculosis skin test, chest x-ray study, pneumonia vaccine or influenza immunization?	"Flu" vaccine is modified yearly; recommended for adults with chronic medical conditions, residents of nursing homes and group care, health care workers, and those who are immunosuppressed.
Additional History for Infants and Children	
1. Has the child had any frequent or very severe colds?	Limit of 4 to 6 uncomplicated upper respiratory infections per year is expected in early childhood.

Examiner Asks	Rationale
2. Is there any history of allergy in the family? • (For child younger than 2 years): At what age were new foods introduced? Was the child breastfed or bottle-fed?	Consider new foods or formula as possible allergens.
3. Does the child have a cough? Seem congested? Have noisy breathing or wheezing? (Further questions similar to those listed in the section on adults.)	Screen for onset and follow course of childhood chronic respiratory problems: asthma, bronchitis.
4. What measures have you taken to child-proof your home? Yard? Is there any possibility of the child inhaling or swallowing toxic substances? • Has anyone taught you emergency care measures in case of accidental choking or a hard-breathing spell?	Young child is at risk for accidental aspiration, poisoning, and injury. Assess knowledge level of parent and caregivers.
5. Any smokers in the home or in the car with child?	Environmental smoke increases the risk for acute and chronic ear and respiratory infections in children.[4]
Additional History for the Aging Adult	
1. Have you noticed any shortness of breath or fatigue with your daily activities?	Older adults have a less efficient respiratory system (decreased vital capacity, less surface area for gas exchange), so they have less tolerance for activity.
2. Tell me about your usual amount of physical activity.	May have reduced exercise capacity because of pulmonary function deficits. Sedentary or bedridden people are at risk for respiratory dysfunction.
3. (For those with a history of chronic obstructive pulmonary disease [COPD], lung cancer, or tuberculosis): How are you getting along each day? Any weight change in the past 3 months? How much?	Assess coping strategies.
• How about energy level? Do you tire more easily? How does your illness affect you at home? At work?	Activities may decrease because of increasing shortness of breath or pain.
4. Do you have any chest pain with breathing?	Some older adults feel pleuritic pain less intensely than younger adults.
• Any chest pain after a bout of coughing? After a fall?	Precisely localized sharp pain (points to it with one finger)—consider fractured rib or muscle injury.

Objective Data

OBJECTIVE DATA

PREPARATION

Ask the person to sit upright. Ask a man to disrobe to the waist. Ask a woman to leave the gown on and open at the back; when examining the anterior chest, lift up the gown and drape it on her shoulders rather than removing it completely. This promotes comfort by giving her the feeling of being somewhat clothed. These provisions will ensure further comfort: a warm room, a warm diaphragm endpiece, and a private examination time with no interruptions.

EQUIPMENT NEEDED

Stethoscope
Small ruler, marked in centimeters
Marking pen
Alcohol wipe

For smooth choreography in a complete examination, begin the respiratory examination just after palpating the thyroid gland when you are standing behind the person. Perform the inspection, palpation, percussion, and auscultation on the posterior and lateral thorax. Then move to face the person and repeat the four maneuvers on the anterior chest. This avoids repetitiously moving front to back around the person.

Finally, clean your stethoscope endpiece with an alcohol wipe. Because your stethoscope touches many people, it is a possible vector for both aerobic and anaerobic bacteria. Cleaning with an alcohol wipe is very effective.

Normal Range of Findings	Abnormal Findings
INSPECT THE POSTERIOR CHEST	
Thoracic Cage	
Note the **shape and configuration** of the chest wall. The spinous processes should appear in a straight line. The thorax is symmetric, in an elliptical shape, with downward sloping ribs, about 45 degrees relative to the spine. The scapulae are placed symmetrically in each hemithorax.	Skeletal deformities may limit thoracic cage excursion: scoliosis, kyphosis (see Table 18-3, Configurations of the Thorax, p. 441).
The anteroposterior diameter should be less than the transverse diameter. The ratio of anteroposterior to transverse diameter is from 1:2 to 5:7.	AP = transverse diameter, or "barrel chest." Ribs are horizontal, chest appears as if held in continuous inspiration. This occurs in chronic emphysema from hyperinflation of the lungs (see Table 18-3).
The neck muscles and trapezius muscles should be developed normally for age and occupation.	Neck muscles are hypertrophied in COPD from aiding in forced respirations.
Note the **position** the person takes to breathe. This includes a relaxed posture and the ability to support one's own weight with arms comfortably at the sides or in the lap.	People with COPD often sit in a tripod position, leaning forward with arms braced against their knees, chair, or bed. This gives them leverage so that their rectus abdominis, intercostal, and accessory neck muscles all can aid in expiration.
Assess the **skin color and condition.** Color should be consistent with person's genetic background, with allowance for sun-exposed areas on the chest and the back. No cyanosis or pallor should be present. Note any lesions. Inquire as to any change in a nevus on the back, for example, where the person may have difficulty monitoring (see Chapter 12).	Cyanosis occurs with tissue hypoxia.
PALPATE THE POSTERIOR CHEST	
Symmetric Expansion	
Confirm **symmetric chest expansion** by placing your warmed hands on the posterolateral chest wall with thumbs at the level of T9 or T10. Slide your hands medially to pinch up a small fold of skin between your thumbs (Fig. 18-13).	

Objective Data

Normal Range of Findings | Abnormal Findings

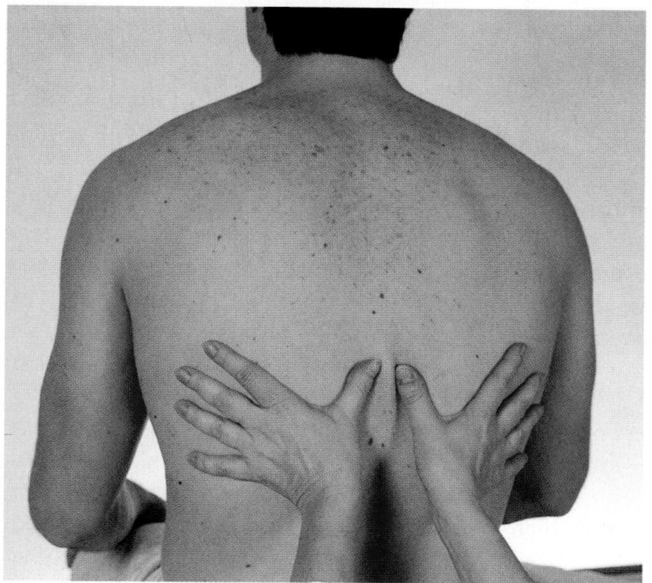

18-13

Ask the person to take a deep breath. Your hands serve as mechanical amplifiers; as the person inhales deeply, your thumbs should move apart symmetrically. Note any lag in expansion.

Unequal chest expansion occurs with marked atelectasis, lobar pneumonia, pleural effusion; with thoracic trauma, such as fractured ribs; or with pneumothorax.

Pain accompanies deep breathing when the pleurae are inflamed.

Tactile Fremitus

Assess **tactile** (or **vocal**) **fremitus.** Fremitus is a palpable vibration. Sounds generated from the larynx are transmitted through patent bronchi and through the lung parenchyma to the chest wall, where you feel them as vibrations.

Use either the palmar base (the ball) of the fingers or the ulnar edge of one hand, and touch the person's chest while he or she repeats the words "ninety-nine" or "blue moon." These are resonant phrases that generate strong vibrations. Start over the lung apices and palpate from one side to another (Fig. 18-14).

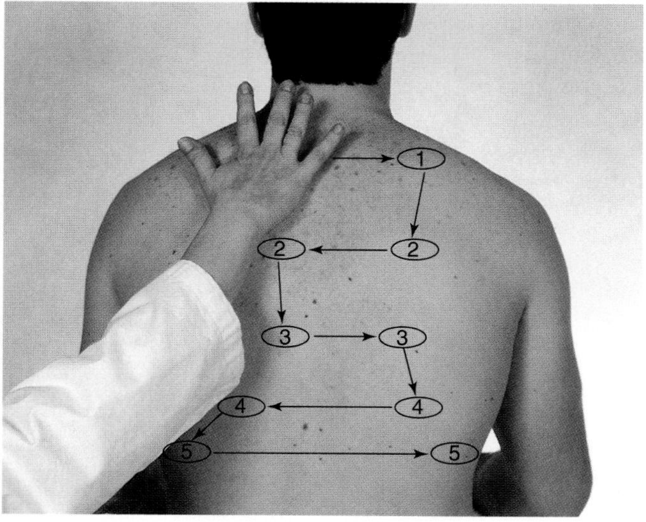

18-14

Normal Range of Findings

Fremitus varies among persons, but symmetry is most important; the vibrations should feel the same in the corresponding area on each side. However, just between the scapulae, fremitus may feel stronger on the right side than on the left side because the right side is closer to the bronchial bifurcation. Avoid palpating over the scapulae because bone damps out sound transmission.

The following factors affect the normal intensity of tactile fremitus:

- Relative location of bronchi to the chest wall.
  - Normally, fremitus is most prominent between the scapulae and around the sternum, sites where the major bronchi are closest to the chest wall. Fremitus normally decreases as you progress down because more and more tissue impedes sound transmission.
- Thickness of the chest wall.
  - Fremitus feels greater over a thin chest wall than over an obese or heavily muscular one where thick tissue damps the vibration.
- Pitch and intensity.
  - A loud, low-pitched voice generates more fremitus than a soft, high-pitched one.

Note any areas of abnormal fremitus. Sound is conducted better through a uniformly dense structure than through a porous one, which changes in shape and solidity (as does the lung tissue during normal respiration). Thus conditions that increase the density of lung tissue make a better conducting medium for sound vibrations and increase tactile fremitus.

Using the fingers, gently **palpate the entire chest wall.** This enables you to note any areas of tenderness, to note skin temperature and moisture, to detect any superficial lumps or masses, and to explore any skin lesions noted on inspection.

PERCUSS THE POSTERIOR CHEST

Lung Fields

Determine the **predominant note over the lung fields.** Start at the apices and percuss the band of normally resonant tissue across the tops of both shoulders (Fig. 18-15). Then, percussing in the interspaces, make a side-to-side comparison all the way down the lung region. Percuss at 5-cm intervals. Avoid the damping effect of the scapulae and ribs.

Abnormal Findings

Decreased fremitus occurs when anything obstructs transmission of vibrations (e.g., obstructed bronchus, pleural effusion or thickening, pneumothorax, or emphysema). Any barrier that comes between the sound and your palpating hand will decrease fremitus.

Increased fremitus occurs with compression or consolidation of lung tissue (e.g., lobar pneumonia). This is present only when the bronchus is patent and when the consolidation extends to the lung surface. Note that only gross changes increase fremitus. Small areas of early pneumonia do not significantly affect fremitus.

Rhonchal fremitus is palpable with thick bronchial secretions.

Pleural friction fremitus is palpable with inflammation of the pleura (see Table 18-5 on p. 443).

Crepitus is a coarse, crackling sensation palpable over the skin surface. It occurs in subcutaneous emphysema when air escapes from the lung and enters the subcutaneous tissue, as after open thoracic injury or surgery.

Normal Range of Findings

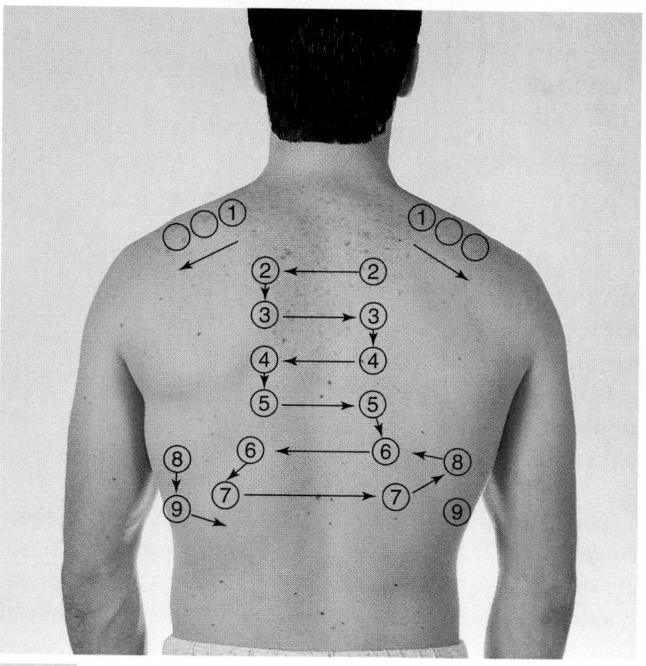

18-15 Sequence for percussion.

Resonance is the low-pitched, clear, hollow sound that predominates in healthy lung tissue in the adult (Fig. 18-16). However, resonance is a relative term and has no constant standard. The resonant note may be modified somewhat in the athlete with a heavily muscular chest wall and in the heavily obese adult in whom subcutaneous fat produces scattered dullness.

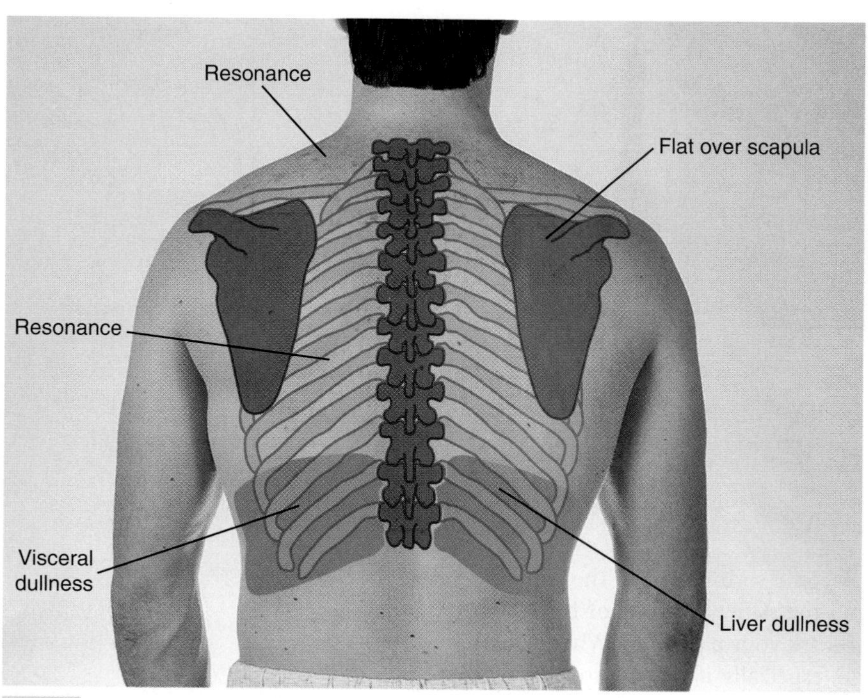

18-16 Expected percussion notes.

Abnormal Findings

Hyperresonance is a lower-pitched, booming sound found when too much air is present, such as in emphysema or pneumothorax.

A **dull** note (soft, muffled thud) signals abnormal density in the lungs, as with pneumonia, pleural effusion, atelectasis, or tumor.

Normal Range of Findings

The depth of penetration of percussion has limits. Percussion sets into motion only the outer 5 to 7 cm of tissue. It will not penetrate to reveal any change in density deeper than that. Also, an abnormal finding must be 2 to 3 cm wide to yield an abnormal percussion note. Lesions smaller than that are not detectable by percussion.

Diaphragmatic Excursion

Determine **diaphragmatic excursion** (Fig. 18-17, *A*). Percuss to map out the lower lung border, both in expiration and in inspiration. First, ask the person to "exhale and hold it" briefly while you percuss down the scapular line until the sound changes from resonant to dull on each side. This estimates the level of the diaphragm separating the lungs from the abdominal viscera. It may be somewhat higher on the right side (about 1 to 2 cm) because of the presence of the liver. Mark the spot.

Now ask the person to "take a deep breath and hold it." Continue percussing down from your first mark and mark the level where the sound changes to dull on this deep inspiration. Measure the difference. This diaphragmatic excursion should be equal bilaterally and measure about 3 to 5 cm in adults, although it may be up to 7 to 8 cm in well-conditioned people (Fig. 18-17, *B*).

Abnormal Findings

Note an abnormally high level of dullness and absence of excursion. These occur with pleural effusion (fluid in the space between the visceral and parietal pleura) or atelectasis of the lower lobes.

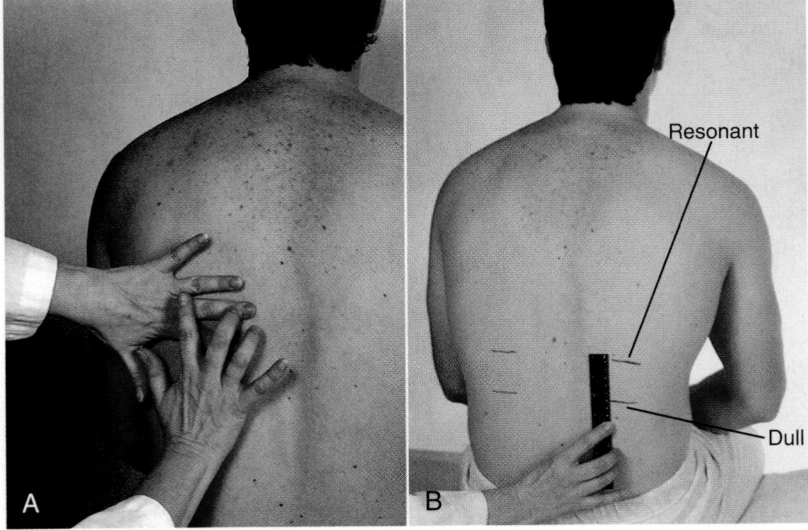

18-17

When you are a beginning examiner, you become so involved in the subtle differences of percussion notes that you extend the patient's limits of breath-holding. Always hold your own breath when you ask your patient to. When you run out of air, the other person surely has too, especially if that person has a respiratory problem.

Normal Range of Findings | **Abnormal Findings**

AUSCULTATE THE POSTERIOR CHEST

The passage of air through the tracheobronchial tree creates a characteristic set of noises that are audible through the chest wall. These noises also may be modified by obstruction within the respiratory passageways or by changes in the lung parenchyma, the pleura, or the chest wall.

Breath Sounds

Evaluate the presence and quality of **normal breath sounds.** The person is sitting, leaning forward slightly, with arms resting comfortably across the lap. Instruct the person to breathe through the mouth, a little bit deeper than usual, but to stop if he or she begins to feel dizzy. Be careful to monitor the breathing throughout the examination and offer times for the person to rest and breathe normally. The person is usually willing to comply with your instructions in an effort to please you and to be a "good patient." Watch that he or she does not hyperventilate to the point of fainting.

Clean the flat diaphragm endpiece of the stethoscope and hold it firmly on the person's chest wall. Listen to at least one full respiration in each location. Side-to-side comparison is most important.

Do not confuse background noise with lung sounds. Become familiar with these extraneous noises that may be confused with lung pathology if not recognized:

1. Examiner's breathing on stethoscope tubing
2. Stethoscope tubing bumping together
3. Patient shivering
4. Patient's hairy chest: movement of hairs under stethoscope sounds like crackles (rales)—minimize this by pressing harder or by wetting the hair with a damp cloth
5. Rustling of paper gown or paper drapes

Crackles are abnormal lung sounds (see Table 18-6, Adventitious Lung Sounds, p. 444.)

While standing behind the person, listen to the following lung areas—posterior from the apices at C7 to the bases (around T10), and laterally from the axilla down to the seventh or eighth rib. Use the sequence illustrated in Fig. 18-18.

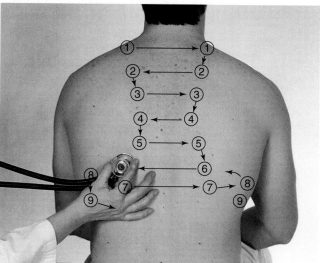

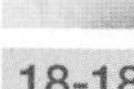

18-18

Normal Range of Findings

Continue to visualize approximate locations of the lobes of each lung so that you correlate your findings to anatomical areas. As you listen, think (1) what AM I hearing over this spot? and (2) what should I EXPECT to be hearing? You should expect to hear three types of normal breath sounds in the adult and older child: **bronchial** (sometimes called *tracheal* or *tubular*), **bronchovesicular,** and **vesicular.** Study the description of the characteristics of these normal breath sounds in Table 18-1.

Abnormal Findings

TABLE 18-1 Characteristics of Normal Breath Sounds

	Pitch	Amplitude	Duration	Quality	Normal Location
BRONCHIAL (TRACHEAL)	High	Loud	Inspiration < expiration	Harsh, hollow tubular	Trachea and larynx
BRONCHOVESICULAR	Moderate	Moderate	Inspiration = expiration	Mixed	Over major bronchi where fewer alveoli are located: posterior, between scapulae especially on right; anterior, around upper sternum in first and second intercostal spaces
VESICULAR	Low	Soft	Inspiration > expiration	Rustling, like the sound of the wind in the trees	Over peripheral lung fields where air flows through smaller bronchioles and alveoli

Note the normal location of the three types of breath sounds on the chest wall of the adult and older child (Figs. 18-19 and 18-20).

Decreased or **absent breath sounds** occur:

1. When the bronchial tree is obstructed at some point by secretions, mucus plug, or a foreign body
2. In emphysema as a result of loss of elasticity in the lung fibers and decreased force of inspired air; also, the lungs are already hyperinflated so the inhaled air does not make as much noise
3. When anything obstructs transmission of sound between the lung and your stethoscope, such as pleurisy or pleural thickening, or air (pneumothorax) or fluid (pleural effusion) in the pleural space

A silent chest means no air is moving in or out, which is an ominous sign.

Normal Range of Findings

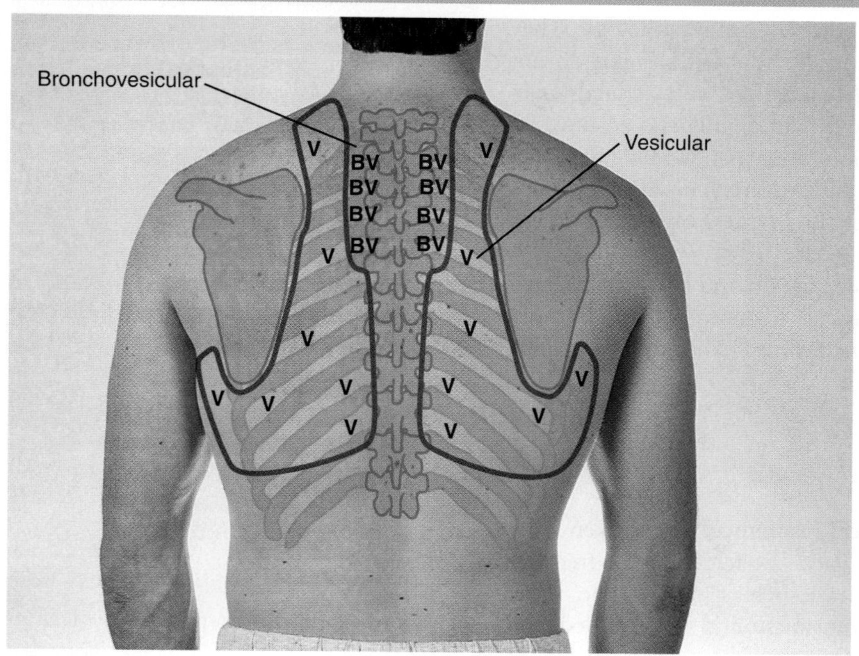

18-19

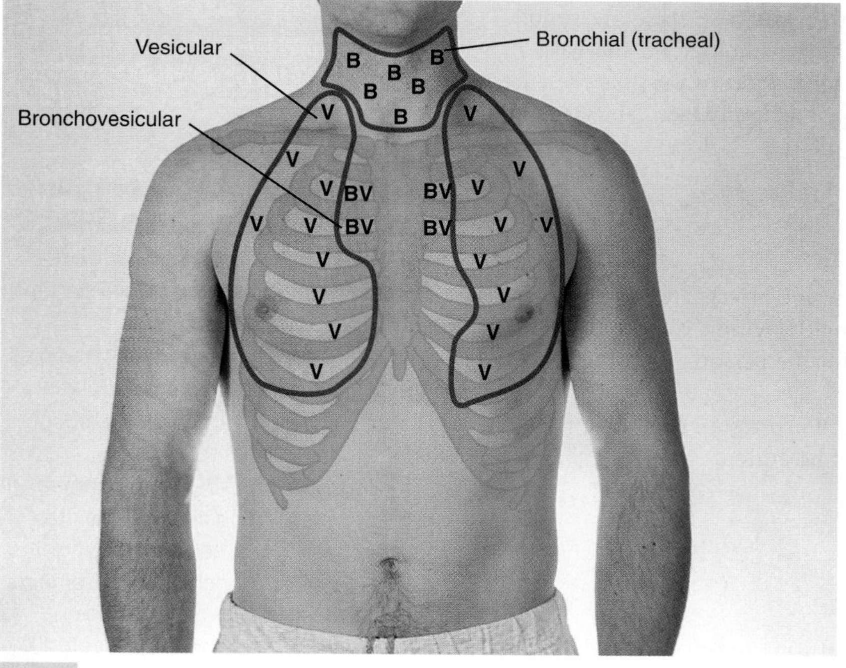

18-20

Adventitious Sounds

Note the presence of any **adventitious sounds.** These are added sounds that are *not* normally heard in the lungs. If present, they are heard as being superimposed on the breath sounds. They are caused by moving air colliding with secretions in the tracheobronchial passageways or by the popping open of previously deflated airways. Sources differ as to the classification and nomenclature of these sounds (see Table 18-6), but **crackles** (or rales) and **wheeze** (or rhonchi) are terms commonly used by most examiners.

Abnormal Findings

Increased breath sounds mean that sounds are louder than they should be (e.g., bronchial sounds are abnormal when they are heard over an abnormal location, the peripheral lung fields). They have a high-pitched, tubular quality, with a prolonged expiratory phase and a distinct pause between inspiration and expiration. They sound very close to your stethoscope, as if they were right *in* the tubing close to your ear. They occur when consolidation (e.g., pneumonia) or compression (e.g., fluid in the intrapleural space) yields a dense lung area that enhances the transmission of sound from the bronchi. When the inspired air reaches the alveoli, it hits solid lung tissue that conducts sound more efficiently to the surface.

Study Table 18-6 on pp. 444-445 for a complete description of these abnormal adventitious breath sounds.

Normal Range of Findings	Abnormal Findings

One type of adventitious sound, **atelectatic crackles,** is not pathologic. They are short, popping, crackling sounds that sound like fine crackles but do not last beyond a few breaths. When sections of alveoli are not fully aerated (as in people who are asleep or in older adults), they deflate slightly and accumulate secretions. Crackles are heard when these sections are expanded by a few deep breaths. Atelectatic crackles are heard only in the periphery, usually in dependent portions of the lungs, and disappear after the first few breaths or after a cough.

In the past, persons were asked to "take a deep breath and blow it out hard" to screen for the presence of wheezing. However, this maneuver is futile because evidence shows wheezing may occur on maximal forced exhalation in healthy people.

During normal tidal flow, high-pitched wheeze occurs with asthma.

Voice Sounds

Determine the quality of **voice sounds** or **vocal resonance.** The spoken voice can be auscultated over the chest wall just as it can be felt in tactile fremitus described earlier. Ask the person to repeat a phrase such as "ninety-nine" while you listen over the chest wall. Normal voice transmission is soft, muffled, and indistinct; you can hear sound through the stethoscope but cannot distinguish exactly what is being said. Pathology that increases lung density enhances transmission of voice sounds.

Consolidation or compression of lung tissue will enhance the voice sounds, making the words more distinct.

Eliciting the voice sounds is not done routinely. Rather, these are supplemental maneuvers performed if you suspect lung pathology on the basis of earlier data. When they are performed, you are testing for the possible presence of **bronchophony, egophony,** and **whispered pectoriloquy** (see Table 18-7 on p. 446).

INSPECT THE ANTERIOR CHEST

Note the **shape and configuration** of the chest wall. The ribs are sloping downward with symmetric interspaces. The costal angle is within 90 degrees. Development of abdominal muscles is as expected for the person's age, weight, and athletic condition.

Barrel chest has horizontal ribs and costal angle >90 degrees.

Hypertrophy of abdominal muscles occurs in chronic emphysema.

Note the person's **facial expression.** The facial expression should be relaxed and benign, indicating an unconscious effort of breathing.

Tense, strained, tired facies accompany COPD.

The person with COPD may purse the lips in a whistling position. By exhaling slowly and against a narrow opening, the pressure in the bronchial tree remains positive and fewer airways collapse.

Assess the **level of consciousness.** The level of consciousness should be alert and cooperative.

Cerebral hypoxia may be reflected by excessive drowsiness or by anxiety, restlessness, and irritability.

Note skin **color and condition.** The lips and nail beds are free of cyanosis or unusual pallor. The nails are of normal configuration. Explore any skin lesions.

Clubbing of distal phalanx occurs with chronic respiratory disease.

Cutaneous angiomas (spider nevi) associated with liver disease or portal hypertension may be evident on the chest.

Normal Range of Findings

Assess the quality of **respirations.** Normal relaxed breathing is automatic and effortless, regular and even, and produces no noise. The chest expands symmetrically with each inspiration. Note any localized lag on inspiration.

No retraction or bulging of the interspaces should occur on inspiration.

Normally, accessory muscles are not used to augment respiratory effort. However, with very heavy exercise, the accessory neck muscles (scalene, sternomastoid, trapezius) are used momentarily to enhance inspiration.

The respiratory rate is within normal limits for the person's age (see Table 9-2), and the pattern of breathing is regular. Occasional sighs normally punctuate breathing.

PALPATE THE ANTERIOR CHEST

Palpate **symmetric chest expansion.** Place your hands on the anterolateral wall with the thumbs along the costal margins and pointing toward the xiphoid process (Fig. 18-21).

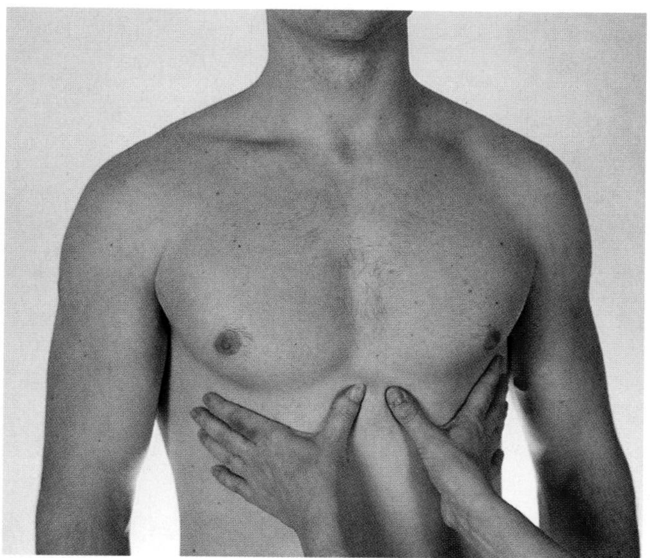

18-21

Ask the person to take a deep breath. Watch your thumbs move apart symmetrically, and note smooth chest expansion with your fingers. Any limitation in thoracic expansion is easier to detect on the anterior chest because greater range of motion exists with breathing here.

Abnormal Findings

Noisy breathing occurs with severe asthma or chronic bronchitis.

Unequal chest expansion occurs when part of the lung is obstructed or collapsed, as with pneumonia, or when guarding to avoid postoperative incisional pain or pleurisy pain.

Retraction suggests obstruction of respiratory tract or increased inspiratory effort is needed, as with atelectasis. Bulging indicates trapped air as in the forced expiration associated with emphysema or asthma.

Accessory muscles are used in acute airway obstruction and massive atelectasis.

Rectus abdominis and internal intercostal muscles are used to force expiration in COPD.

Tachypnea and hyperventilation, bradypnea and hypoventilation, periodic breathing (see Table 18-4, Respiratory Patterns, p. 442).

Abnormally wide costal angle with little inspiratory variation occurs with emphysema.

A lag in expansion occurs with atelectasis, pneumonia, and postoperative guarding.

A palpable grating sensation with breathing indicates pleural friction fremitus (see Table 18-5).

Normal Range of Findings	Abnormal Findings

Assess **tactile (vocal) fremitus.** Begin palpating over the lung apices in the supraclavicular areas (Fig. 18-22). Compare vibrations from one side to the other as the person repeats "ninety-nine." Avoid palpating over female breast tissue because breast tissue normally damps the sound.

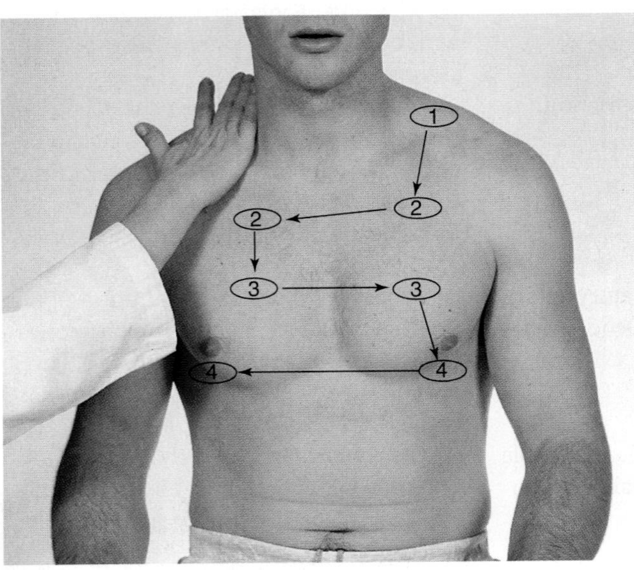

18-22 Assess tactile fremitus.

Palpate the anterior chest wall to note any tenderness (normally none is present) and to detect any superficial lumps or masses (again, normally none are present). Note skin mobility and turgor, and note skin temperature and moisture.

If any lumps are found in the breast tissue, refer the man to a specialist.

PERCUSS THE ANTERIOR CHEST

Begin percussing the apices in the supraclavicular areas. Then, percussing the interspaces and comparing one side with the other, move down the anterior chest.

Interspaces are easier to palpate on the anterior chest than on the back. Do not percuss directly over female breast tissue because this would produce a dull note. Shift the breast tissue over slightly using the edge of your stationary hand. In females with large breasts, percussion may yield little useful data. With all people, use the sequence illustrated in Fig. 18-23.

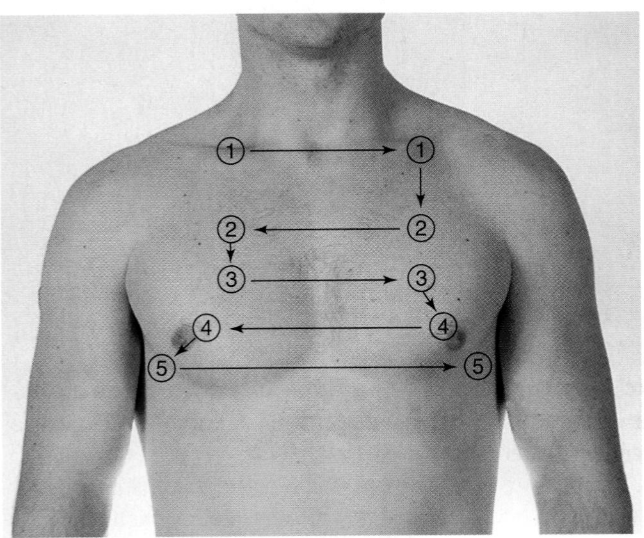

18-23 Sequence for percussion and auscultation.

Normal Range of Findings

Note the borders of cardiac dullness normally found on the anterior chest and do not confuse these with suspected lung pathology (Fig. 18-24). In the right hemithorax, the upper border of liver dullness is located in the fifth intercostal space in the right midclavicular line. On the left, tympany is evident over the gastric space.

Abnormal Findings

Lungs are hyperinflated with chronic emphysema, which results in hyperresonance where you would expect cardiac dullness.

Dullness behind the right breast occurs with right middle lobe pneumonia.

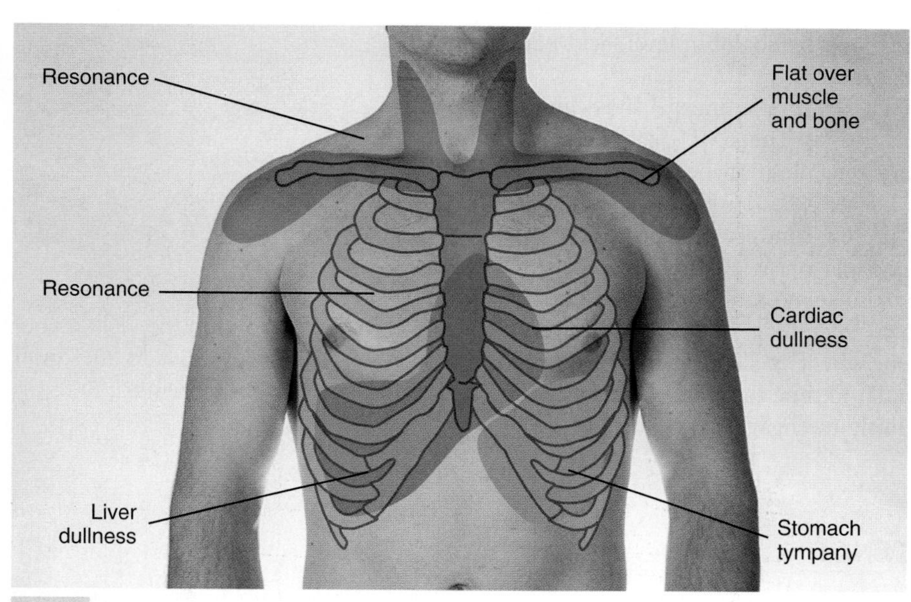

18-24 Expected percussion notes.

AUSCULTATE THE ANTERIOR CHEST

Breath Sounds

Auscultate the lung fields over the anterior chest from the apices in the supraclavicular areas down to the sixth rib. Progress from side to side as you move downward, and listen to one full respiration in each location. Use the sequence indicated for percussion. Do not place your stethoscope directly over the female breast. Displace the breast and listen directly over the chest wall.

Evaluate normal breath sounds, noting any abnormal breath sounds and any adventitious sounds. If the situation warrants, assess the voice sounds on the anterior chest.

Study Table 18-8 on pp. 447-453 for a complete description of abnormal respiratory conditions.

Measurement of Pulmonary Function Status

The **forced expiratory time** is the number of seconds it takes for the person to exhale from total lung capacity to residual volume. It is a screening measure of airflow obstruction. Although the test usually is not performed in the respiratory assessment, it is useful when you wish to screen for pulmonary function.

Ask the person to inhale the deepest breath possible and then to blow it all out hard, as quickly as possible, with the mouth open. Listen with your stethoscope over the sternum. The normal time for full expiration is 4 seconds or less.

A forced expiration of 6 seconds or more occurs with obstructive lung disease. Refer this person for more precise pulmonary function studies.

Objective Data

Normal Range of Findings

In an ambulatory care setting, a handheld **spirometer** measures lung health in chronic conditions such as asthma. Ask the patient to inhale deeply and then to exhale into the spirometer as fast as possible until the most air possible is exhaled. The *forced vital capacity (FVC)* is the total volume of air exhaled. The *forced expiratory volume in 1 second (FEV1)* is the volume exhaled in the first measured second. A normal outcome is a FEV1/FVC ratio of 75% or greater, meaning no significant obstruction of airflow is present.

The **pulse oximeter** is a noninvasive method to assess arterial oxygen saturation (Spo_2) and is described in Chapter 9. A healthy person with no lung disease and no anemia normally has an Spo_2 of 97% to 98%. However, every Spo_2 result must be evaluated in the context of the person's hemoglobin level, acid-base balance, and ventilatory status.

The **6-minute distance (6MD) walk** is a safer, simple, inexpensive, clinical measure of functional status in aging adults.[10,11] The 6MD is used as an outcome measure for people in pulmonary rehabilitation because it mirrors conditions that are used in everyday life. Locate a flat-surfaced corridor that has little foot traffic, is wide enough to permit comfortable turns, and has a controlled environment. Ensure that the person is wearing comfortable shoes, and equip him or her with a pulse oximeter to monitor oxygen saturation. Ask the person to set his or her own pace to cover as much ground as possible in 6 minutes, and assure the person it is all right to slow down or to stop to rest at any time. Use a stopwatch to time the walk. A person who walks >300 meters in 6 minutes is more likely to engage in activities of daily living.

Abnormal Findings

Mild obstruction of airflow is a FEV1/FCV ratio of 60% to 70%; moderate obstruction is a measure of 50% to 60%; severe obstruction is a ratio of less than 50%.

Ask the person to stop the walk if you measure an Spo_2 below 85% to 88% or if extreme breathlessness occurs.

Objective Data

DEVELOPMENTAL COMPETENCE

Infants and Children

To prepare, let the parent hold an infant supported against the chest or shoulder. Ignore the usual sequence of the physical examination; seize the opportunity with a sleeping infant to inspect and then to listen to lung sounds next. This way you can concentrate on the breath sounds before the baby wakes up and possibly cries. Infant crying does not have to be a problem for you, however, because it actually enhances palpation of tactile fremitus and auscultation of breath sounds.

A child may sit upright on the parent's lap. Offer the stethoscope and let the child handle it. This reduces any fear of the equipment. Promote the child's participation; school-age children usually are delighted to hear their own breath sounds when you place the stethoscope properly. While listening to breath sounds, ask the young child to take a deep breath and "blow out" your penlight while you hold the stethoscope with your other hand. Time your letting go of the penlight button so the light goes off after the child blows. Or, ask the child to "pant like a dog" while you auscultate.

Inspection. The infant has a rounded thorax with an equal AP-to-transverse chest diameter (Fig. 18-25). By age 6 years, the thorax reaches the adult ratio of 1:2 (AP-to-transverse diameter). The newborn's chest circumference is 30 to 36 cm and is 2 cm smaller than the head circumference until 2 years of age. The chest wall is thin with little musculature. The ribs and the xiphoid are prominent; you can see as well as feel the sharp tip of the xiphoid process. The thoracic cage is soft and flexible.

In newborn males and females, the breasts may look enlarged by the second or third day from maternal estrogen. Occasionally a white fluid, sometimes referred to by the slang expression "witch's milk," can be expressed. This resolves within a week.

Note a barrel shape persisting after age 6 years, which may develop with chronic asthma or cystic fibrosis.

Normal Range of Findings	Abnormal Findings

18-25 Round thorax in an infant.

In some children, "Harrison groove" occurs normally. This is a horizontal groove in the rib cage at the level of the insertion of the diaphragm, extending from the sternum to the midaxillary line.

The newborn's first respiratory assessment is part of the **Apgar scoring system** to measure the successful transition to extrauterine life (Table 18-2). The five standard parameters are scored at 1 minute and at 5 minutes after birth. A 1-minute Apgar with a total score of 7 to 10 indicates a newborn in good condition, needing only suctioning of the nose and mouth and otherwise routine care.

Harrison groove also occurs with rickets from the pull of the diaphragm on weakened ribs.

In the immediate newborn period, depressed respirations are due to maternal drugs, interruption of the uterine blood supply, or obstruction of the tracheobronchial tree with mucus or fluid.

A 1-minute Apgar score with a total score of 3 to 6 indicates a moderately depressed newborn needing more resuscitation and subsequent close observation. A score of 0 to 2 indicates a severely depressed newborn needing full resuscitation, ventilatory assistance, and subsequent intensive care.

TABLE 18-2 Apgar Scoring System

	2	1	0	
Heart rate	Over 100	Slow (below 100)	Absent	______
Respiratory effort	Good, sustained cry; regular respirations	Slow, irregular, shallow	Absent	______
Muscle tone	Active motion, spontaneous flexion	Some flexion of extremities; some resistance to extension	Limp, flaccid	______
Reflex irritability (response to catheter in nares)	Sneeze, cough, cry	Grimace, frown	No response	______
Color	Completely pink	Body pink, extremities pale	Cyanotic, pale	______
			Total score	______

Objective Data

Normal Range of Findings

The infant breathes through the nose rather than the mouth and is an obligate nose breather until 3 months. Slight flaring of the lower costal margins may occur with respirations, but normally no flaring of the nostrils and no sternal retractions or intercostal retractions occur. The diaphragm is the newborn's major respiratory muscle. Intercostal muscles are not well developed. Thus you observe the abdomen bulge with each inspiration but see little thoracic expansion.

Count the respiratory rate for 1 full minute. Normal rates for the newborn are 30 to 40 breaths per minute but may spike up to 60 per minute. Obtain the most accurate respiratory rate by counting when the infant is asleep, because infants reach rapid rates with very little excitation when awake. The respiratory pattern may be irregular when extremes in room temperature occur or with feeding or sleeping. Brief periods of apnea less than 10 to 15 seconds are common. This periodic breathing is more common in premature infants.

Palpation. Palpate symmetric chest expansion by encircling the infant's thorax with both hands. Further palpation should yield no lumps, masses, or crepitus, although you may feel the costochondral junctions in some normal infants.

Percussion. Percussion is of limited usefulness in the newborn and especially in the premature newborn because the adult's fingers are too large in relation to the tiny chest. The percussion note of hyperresonance occurs normally in the infant and young child because of the relatively thin chest wall. Anything less than hyperresonance would have the same clinical significance as dullness in the adult. If measured, diaphragmatic excursion measures about one to two rib interspaces in children.

Auscultation. Auscultation normally yields bronchovesicular breath sounds in the peripheral lung fields of the infant and young child up to age 5 to 6 years. Their relatively thin chest walls with underdeveloped musculature do not damp off the sound as do the thicker walls of adults, so breath sounds are louder and harsher.

Fine crackles are the adventitious sounds commonly heard in the immediate newborn period from opening of the airways and clearing of fluid. Because the newborn's chest wall is so thin, transmission of sounds is enhanced and sound is heard easily all over the chest, making localization of breath sounds a problem. Even bowel sounds are easily heard in the chest. Try using the smaller pediatric diaphragm endpiece, or place the bell over the infant's interspaces and not over the ribs. Use the pediatric diaphragm on an older infant or toddler (Fig. 18-26).

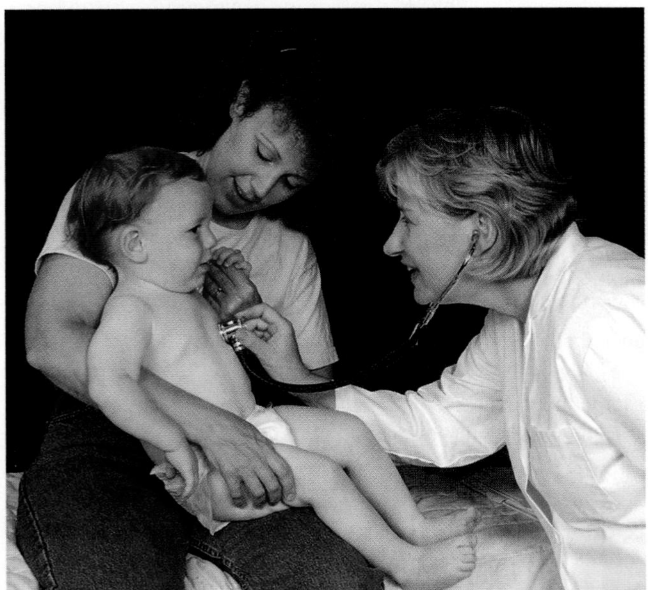

18-26

Abnormal Findings

Marked retractions of sternum and intercostal muscles indicate increased inspiratory effort, as in atelectasis, pneumonia, asthma, and acute airway obstruction.

Rapid respiratory rates accompany pneumonia, fever, pain, heart disease, and anemia.

In an infant, tachypnea of 50 to 100 per minute during sleep may be an early sign of heart failure.

Asymmetric expansion occurs with diaphragmatic hernia or pneumothorax.

Crepitus is palpable around a fractured clavicle, which may occur with difficult forceps delivery.

Diminished breath sounds occur with pneumonia, atelectasis, pleural effusion, or pneumothorax.

Persistent fine crackles that are scattered over the chest occur with pneumonia, bronchiolitis, or atelectasis.

Crackles only in upper lung fields occur with cystic fibrosis; crackles only in lower lung fields occur with heart failure.

Normal Range of Findings | **Abnormal Findings**

Expiratory wheezing occurs with lower airway obstruction (e.g., asthma or bronchiolitis). When unilateral, it may be foreign body aspiration.

Persistent peristaltic sounds with diminished breath sounds on the same side may indicate diaphragmatic hernia.

Stridor is a high-pitched inspiratory crowing sound heard without the stethoscope, occurring with upper airway obstruction (e.g., croup, foreign body aspiration, or acute epiglottitis).

The Pregnant Woman

The thoracic cage may appear wider and the costal angle may feel wider than in the nonpregnant state. Respirations may be deeper, although this can be quantified only with pulmonary function tests.

The Aging Adult

The chest cage commonly shows an increased anteroposterior diameter, giving a round barrel shape, and **kyphosis** or an outward curvature of the thoracic spine (see Table 18-3). The person compensates by holding the head extended and tilted back. You may palpate marked bony prominences because of decreased subcutaneous fat. Chest expansion may be somewhat decreased with the older person, although it still should be symmetric. The costal cartilages become calcified with aging, resulting in a less mobile thorax.

The older person may fatigue easily, especially during auscultation when deep mouth breathing is required. Take care that this person does not hyperventilate and become dizzy. Allow brief rest periods or quiet breathing. If the person does feel faint, holding the breath for a few seconds will restore equilibrium.

The Acutely Ill Person

Ask a second examiner to hold the person's arms and to support him or her in the upright position. If no one else is available, you need to roll the person from side to side, examining the uppermost half of the thorax. This obviously prevents you from comparing findings from one side to another. Also, side flexion of the trunk alters percussion findings because the ribs of the upward side may flex closer together.

PROMOTING A HEALTHY LIFESTYLE: ENVIRONMENTAL TOBACCO SMOKE (ETS)

Secondhand Smoke—There Is No Risk-Free Level of Exposure!

Secondhand smoke, also referred to as *environmental tobacco smoke (ETS),* is a mixture of sidestream *and* mainstream smoke. *Sidestream* smoke is the smoke given off at the burning end of a tobacco product, whereas *mainstream* smoke is the smoke exhaled from the individual smoking the tobacco product. Exposure to secondhand smoke, which is primarily involuntary and/or passive, increases an adult's risk for cancer and heart disease. It also increases the risk for sudden infant death syndrome (SIDS), ear infections, and asthma attacks in children. According to the National Cancer Institute (NCI), there is no safe level of exposure to secondhand smoke. Of particular note is a recent report (Crystal, 2010) indicating there is **no level of nicotine,** no matter how small, that does **not** begin to produce genetic changes at the cellular level.

Yet, despite substantial progress in tobacco control policies, many Americans continue to be exposed to secondhand smoke in their homes and workplaces. Just fewer than 60% of American children between 3 and 11 years of age, which is almost 22 million children, have been exposed to secondhand smoke, and just fewer than 30% of indoor American workers are still not covered by smoke-free workplace policies. Although levels of *cotinine*, a biomarker of secondhand smoke exposure, are falling, 43% of nonsmokers have detectable levels in their bloodstream. Cotinine levels are consistently higher in African Americans than in whites and Mexican Americans. Secondhand smoke exposure, both overall and in the home, tends to be higher for persons with lower incomes. Occupational disparities in exposure are decreasing, but African-American workers, construction workers, and blue collar workers continue to experience high levels of secondhand smoke exposure relative to others.

When workplaces across the United States initiated smoke-free policies, workplace productivity increased and absenteeism decreased. Conventional air cleaning can remove large particles but not the small particles found in secondhand smoke. Further, heating and air-conditioning systems can distribute secondhand smoke throughout a building, increasing exposure of unsuspecting individuals.

Where do you start? First, do not smoke or allow smoking in your home. Tell smokers that you do care if they smoke. Ask smokers to go outside while they smoke. Choose smoke-free worksites, daycare centers, schools, restaurants, and other places where you spend time. Help people who are trying to quit smoking. The American Lung Association is offering a new way to stop smoking through its *Freedom from Smoking* online smoking cessation clinic, which can be accessed day or night, 7 days a week, on any schedule a smoker chooses. This online clinic is available at www.ffsonline.org. Further, the Environmental Protection Agency (EPA) developed two valuable resources for families and communities: (1) the *Smoke-free Homes Community Action Kit;* and (2) a bilingual brochure entitled *Secondhand Smoke and the Health of Your Family.* Both are available to download and are listed as follows:

- *Smoke-free Homes Community Action Kit* www.epa.gov/smokefree/pdfs/community_action_kit.pdf
- *Secondhand Smoke and the Health of Your Family* www.epa.gov/smokefree/pdfs/trifold_brochure.pdf

For additional information on reducing secondhand smoke exposure, visit the Centers for Disease Control and Prevention (CDC). As part of their larger *Healthier Worksite Initiative,* they have developed an online toolkit designed to provide individuals, groups, or communities with the resources they need to take action to reduce secondhand smoke in their environment. The toolkit *Implementing a Tobacco-free Campus Initiative in Your Workplace* is available at www.cdc.gov/nccdphp/dnpao/hwi/toolkits/tobacco/index.htm.

Resources

Centers for Disease Control and Prevention (CDC). Fact sheet on secondhand smoke. Website: www.cdc.gov/tobacco/data_statistics/fact_sheets/secondhand_smoke/general_facts/.

Crystal, R. (2010). Website: www.nlm.nih.gov/medlineplus/news/fullstory_102428.html.

National Cancer Institute (NCI). Fact sheet on secondhand smoke. Website: www.cancer.gov/cancertopics/factsheet/Tobacco/ETS.

U.S. Department of Health and Human Services. (2006). The health consequences of involuntary exposure to tobacco smoke: a report of the Surgeon General. Website: www.surgeongeneral.gov/library/secondhandsmoke/.

DOCUMENTATION AND CRITICAL THINKING

Sample Charting

SUBJECTIVE

No cough, shortness of breath, or chest pain with breathing. No history of respiratory diseases. Has "one or no" colds per year. Has never smoked. Works in well-ventilated office—smoking co-workers are restricted to smoke in lounge. Last TB skin test 4 years PTA, negative. Never had chest x-ray.

OBJECTIVE

Inspection: AP < transverse diameter. Respirations 16/min, relaxed and even.

Palpation: Chest expansion symmetric. Tactile fremitus equal bilaterally. No tenderness to palpation. No lumps or lesions.

Percussion: Resonant to percussion over lung fields. Diaphragmatic excursion 5 cm and = bilaterally.
Auscultation: Vesicular breath sounds clear over lung fields. No adventitious sounds.

ASSESSMENT

Intact thoracic structures
Lung sounds clear and equal

Focused Assessment: Clinical Case Study

Thomas G. is a 58-year-old, thin, white, male traffic patrolman who appears older than stated age. Face is anxious and tense, although in no acute distress at this time. Seeks care for "increasing shortness of breath and fatigue in past couple months."

SUBJECTIVE

1 year PTA—noticed more "winded" than usual when walking >3-4 blocks. Early morning cough present daily ×10 years, but now increased sputum production to 2 T per morning, frothy white.

6 mo. PTA—had a "cold" with severe harsh coughing, productive of ½ cup thick white sputum/day. Noted midsternal chest pain (mild) with cough. Lasted 2 weeks. Treated self with humidifier and OTC cough syrup—minimal relief.

3 mo. PTA—noticed increasing SOB with less activity. Fatigue and SOB when working outside during traffic rush hours. Unable to take evening walks (usually 2-3 blocks) due to SOB and fatigue. Has 2-pillow orthopnea. Wakes 3-4 times during night.

Now—feels he is "worse and needs some help." Continues with 2-pillow orthopnea. Unable to walk >2 blocks or climb >1 flight stairs without resting. Unable to blow out birthday candles on cake last week. Morning cough productive of ¼ cup thin white sputum; cough continues sporadically during day.

No chest pain, hemoptysis, night sweats, or paroxysmal nocturnal dyspnea. No history of allergies, hospitalizations, or injuries to chest. No family history of TB, allergies, asthma, or cancer. Smokes cigarettes, 2 packs per day × 30 years. Alcohol less than one 6-pack beer/week summer months only.

OBJECTIVE

Inspection: Sitting on side of bed with arms propped on bedside table. Respirations: resting 24/min, regular, shallow with prolonged expiration; resp. ambulating 34/min. Increased use of accessory muscles, AP = transverse diameter with widening of costal angle, slightly flushed face, tense expression.

Palpation: Minimal but symmetric chest expansion. Tactile fremitus = bilaterally. No lumps, masses, or tenderness to palpation.

Percussion: Diaphragmatic excursion is 1 cm and = bilaterally. Hyperresonance over lung fields.

Auscultation: Breath sounds diminished. Expiratory wheeze throughout posterior chest, R > L. No crackles.

ASSESSMENT

Chronic and increasing SOB
Ineffective airway clearance R/T bronchial secretions and obstruction
Activity intolerance R/T imbalance between oxygen supply and demand
Insomnia R/T dyspnea and decreased mobility
Anxiety R/T change in health status

ABNORMAL FINDINGS

TABLE 18-3 Configurations of the Thorax

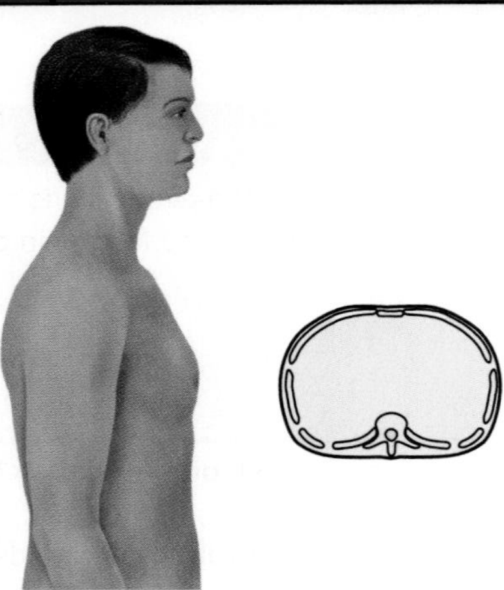

Normal Adult (for Comparison)

The thorax has an elliptical shape with an anteroposterior-to-transverse diameter of 1:2 or 5:7.

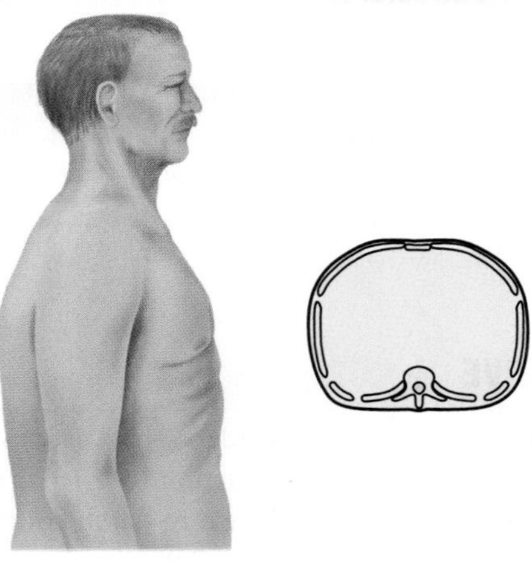

Barrel Chest

Note equal anteroposterior-to-transverse diameter and that ribs are horizontal instead of the normal downward slope. This is associated with normal aging and also with chronic emphysema and asthma as a result of hyperinflation of lungs.

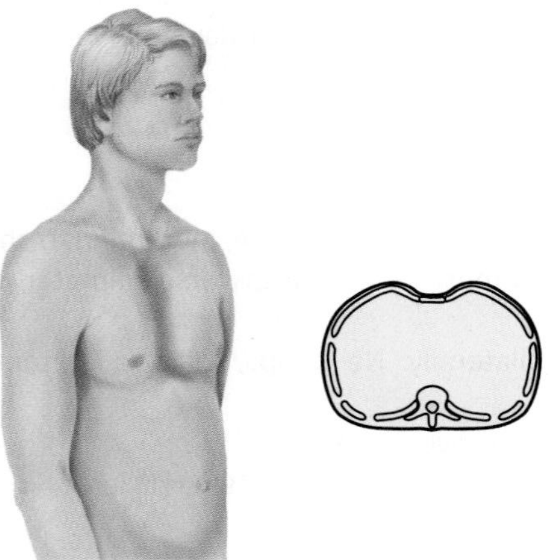

Pectus Excavatum

A markedly sunken sternum and adjacent cartilages (also called *funnel breast*). Depression begins at second intercostal space, becoming depressed most at junction of xiphoid with body of sternum. More noticeable on inspiration. Congenital, usually not symptomatic. When severe, sternal depression may cause embarrassment and a negative self-concept. Surgery may be indicated.

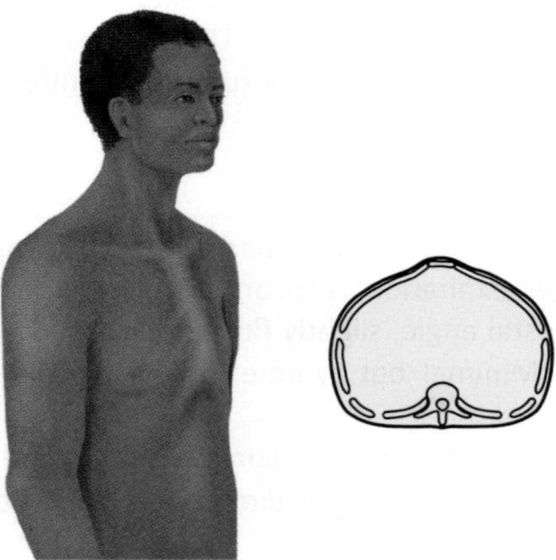

Pectus Carinatum

A forward protrusion of the sternum, with ribs sloping back at either side and vertical depressions along costochondral junctions (pigeon breast). Less common than pectus excavatum, this minor deformity requires no treatment. If severe, surgery may be indicated.

TABLE 18-3 Configurations of the Thorax—cont'd

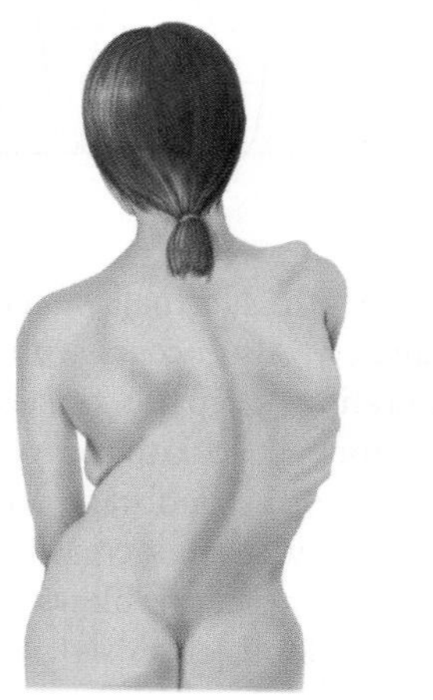
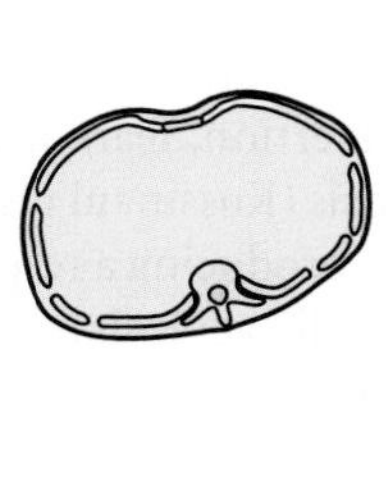

Scoliosis

A lateral S-shaped curvature of the thoracic and lumbar spine, usually with involved vertebrae rotation. Note unequal shoulder and scapular height and unequal hip levels, rib interspaces flared on convex side. More prevalent in adolescent age-groups, especially girls. Mild deformities are asymptomatic. If severe (>45 degrees) deviation is present, scoliosis may reduce lung volume and then person is at risk for impaired cardiopulmonary function. Primary impairment is cosmetic deformity, negatively affecting self-image. Refer early for treatment, often surgery.

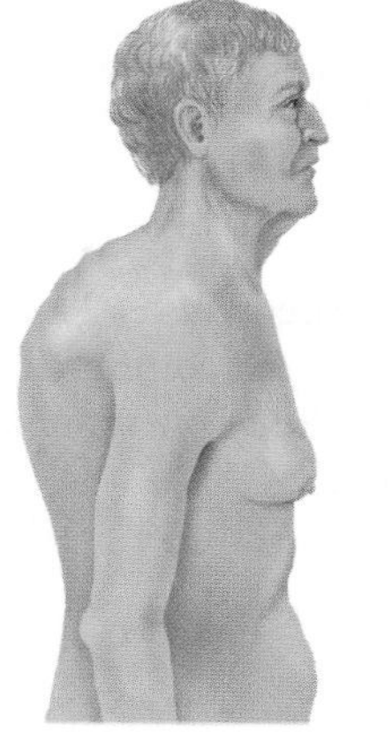
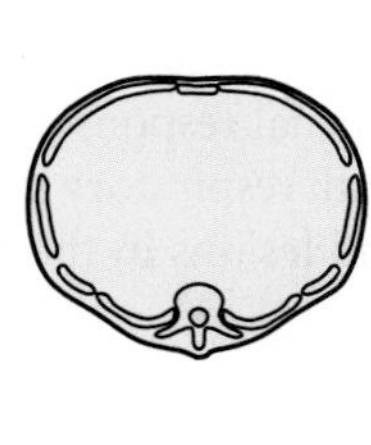

Kyphosis

An exaggerated posterior curvature of the thoracic spine (humpback) that causes significant back pain and limited mobility. Severe deformities impair cardiopulmonary function. If the neck muscles are strong, compensation occurs by hyperextension of head to maintain level of vision.

Kyphosis has been associated with aging, especially the familiar "dowager's hump" of postmenopausal osteoporotic women. However, it is common well before menopause. It is related to physical fitness; women with adequate exercise habits are less likely to have kyphosis.

TABLE 18-4 Respiratory Patterns*

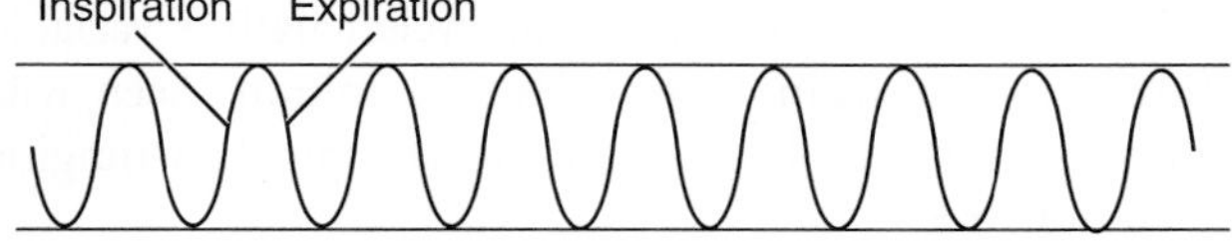

Normal Adult (for Comparison)

Rate—10 to 20 breaths per minute
Depth—500 to 800 mL
Pattern—even
The ratio of pulse to respirations is fairly constant, about 4:1. Both values increase as a normal response to exercise, fear, or fever.
Depth—air moving in and out with each respiration.

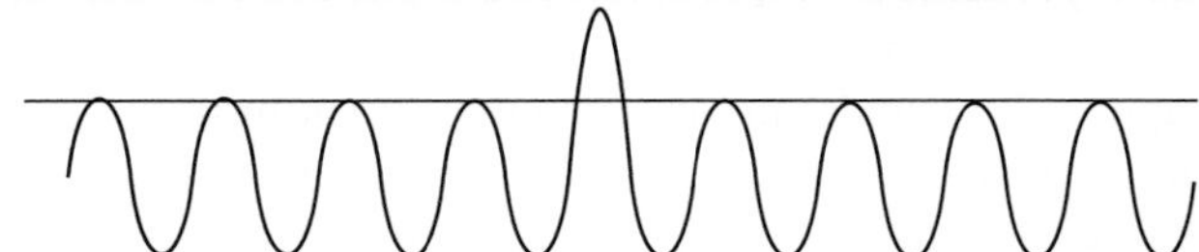

Sigh

Occasional sighs punctuate the normal breathing pattern and are purposeful to expand alveoli. Frequent sighs may indicate emotional dysfunction. Frequent sighs also may lead to hyperventilation and dizziness.

*Assess the (1) rate, (2) depth (tidal volume), and (3) pattern.

Continued

TABLE 18-4 Respiratory Patterns—cont'd

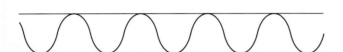

Tachypnea

Rapid, shallow breathing. Increased rate, >24 per minute. This is a normal response to fever, fear, or exercise. Rate also increases with respiratory insufficiency, pneumonia, alkalosis, pleurisy, and lesions in the pons.

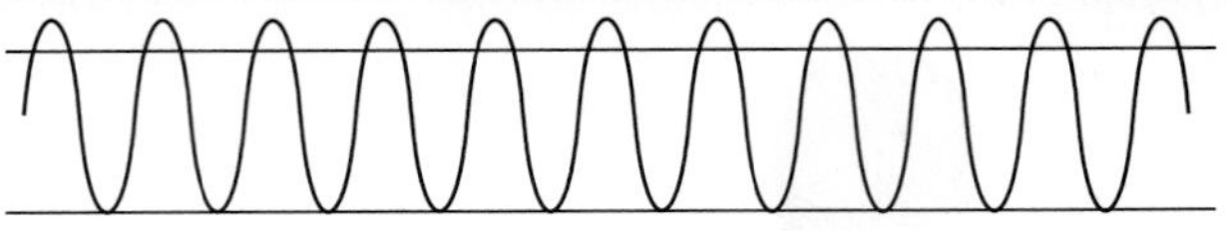

Hyperventilation

Increase in both rate and depth. Normally occurs with extreme exertion, fear, or anxiety. Also occurs with diabetic ketoacidosis (Kussmaul respirations), hepatic coma, salicylate overdose (producing a respiratory alkalosis to compensate for the metabolic acidosis), lesions of the midbrain, and alteration in blood gas concentration (either an increase in CO_2 or a decrease in oxygen). Hyperventilation blows off CO_2, causing a decreased level in the blood (alkalosis).

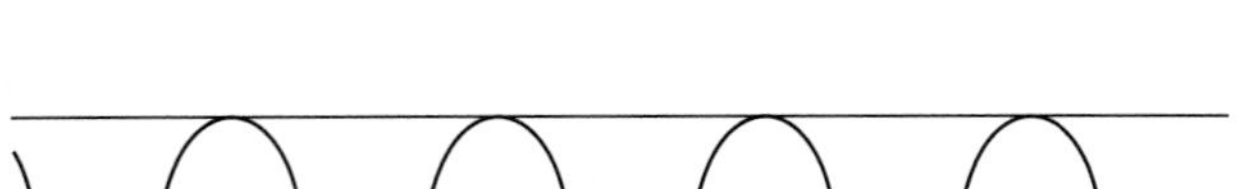

Bradypnea

Slow breathing. A decreased but regular rate (<10 per minute), as in drug-induced depression of the respiratory center in the medulla, increased intracranial pressure, and diabetic coma.

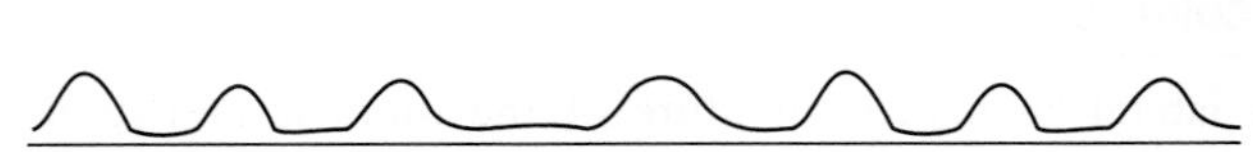

Hypoventilation

An irregular shallow pattern caused by an overdose of narcotics or anesthetics. May also occur with prolonged bedrest or conscious splinting of the chest to avoid respiratory pain.

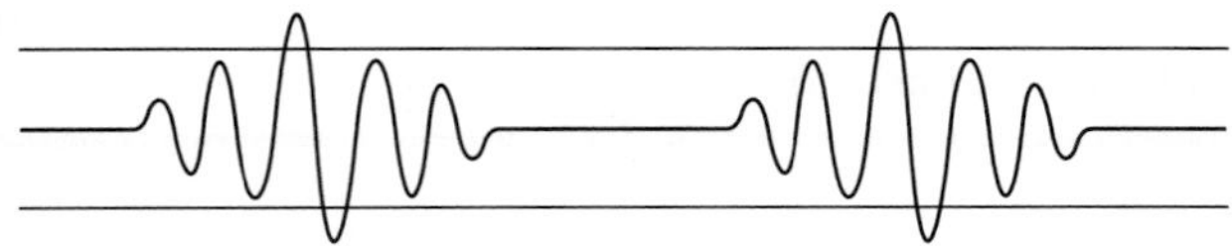

Cheyne-Stokes Respiration

A cycle in which respirations gradually wax and wane in a regular pattern, increasing in rate and depth and then decreasing. The breathing periods last 30 to 45 seconds, with periods of apnea (20 seconds) alternating the cycle. The most common cause is severe heart failure; other causes are renal failure, meningitis, drug overdose, and increased intracranial pressure. Occurs normally in infants and aging persons during sleep.

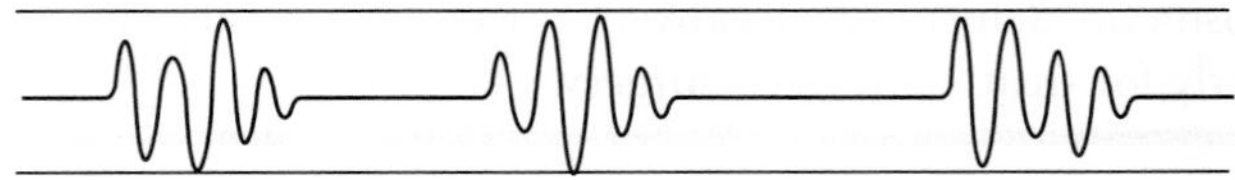

Biot's Respiration

Similar to Cheyne-Stokes respiration, except that the pattern is irregular. A series of normal respirations (three to four) is followed by a period of apnea. The cycle length is variable, lasting anywhere from 10 seconds to 1 minute. Seen with head trauma, brain abscess, heat stroke, spinal meningitis, and encephalitis.

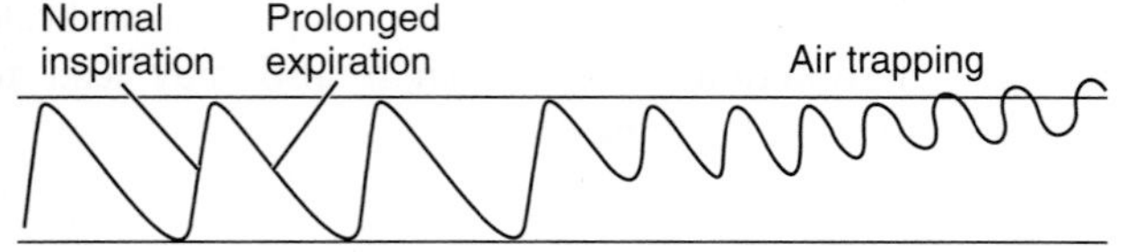

Chronic Obstructive Breathing

Normal inspiration and prolonged expiration to overcome increased airway resistance. In a person with chronic obstructive lung disease, any situation calling for increased heart rate (exercise) may lead to dyspneic episode (air trapping), because then the person does not have enough time for full expiration.

TABLE 18-5 Abnormal Tactile Fremitus

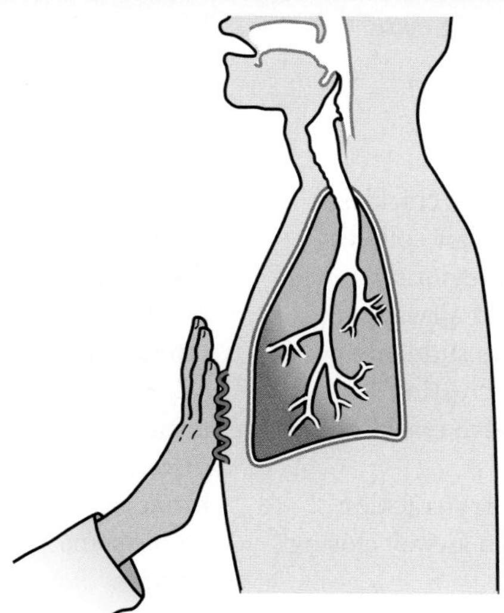

Increased Tactile Fremitus

Occurs with conditions that increase the density of lung tissue, thereby making a better conducting medium for vibrations (e.g., compression or consolidation [pneumonia]). There must be a patent bronchus and consolidation must extend to lung surface for increased fremitus to be apparent.

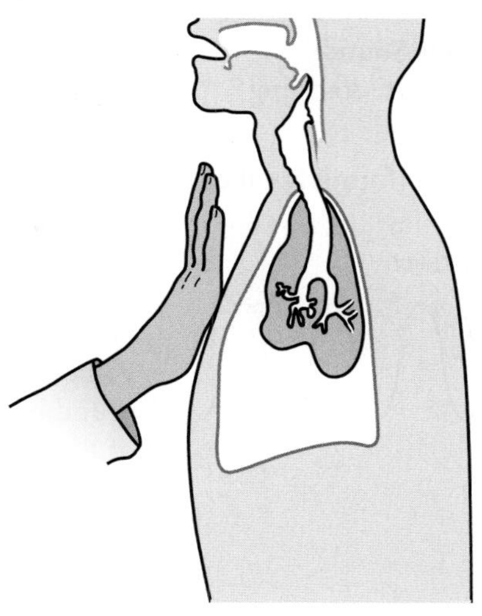

Decreased Tactile Fremitus

Occurs when anything obstructs transmission of vibrations (e.g., an obstructed bronchus, pleural effusion or thickening, pneumothorax, and emphysema). Any barrier that gets in the way of the sound and your palpating hand decreases fremitus.

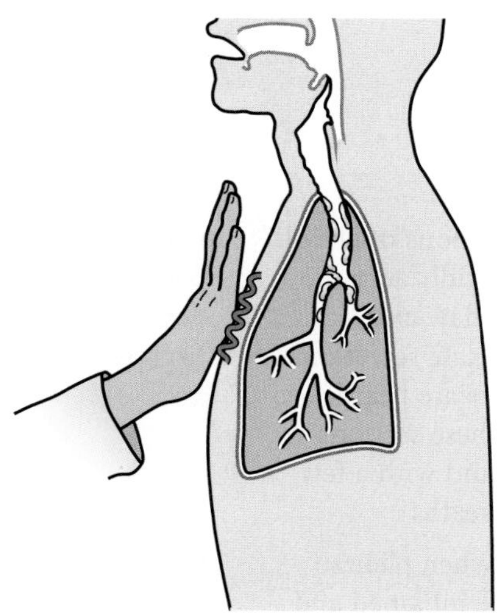

Rhonchal Fremitus

Vibration felt when inhaled air passes through thick secretions in the larger bronchi. This may decrease somewhat by coughing.

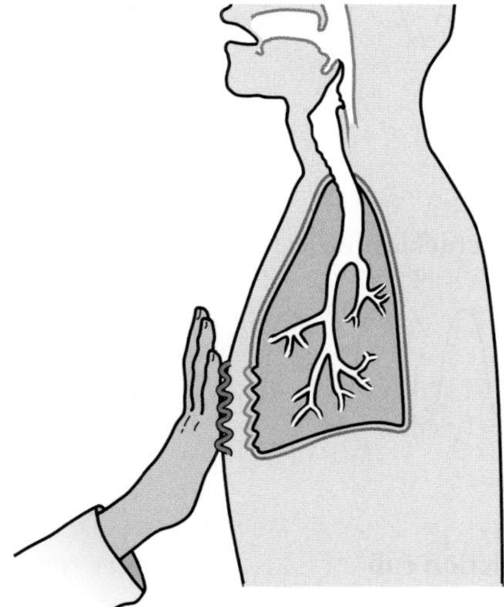

Pleural Friction Fremitus

Produced when inflammation of the parietal or visceral pleura causes a decrease in the normal lubricating fluid. Then the opposing surfaces make a coarse grating sound when rubbed together during breathing. Although this sound is best detected by auscultation, it may sometimes be palpable and feels like two pieces of leather grating together. It is synchronous with respiratory excursion. Also called a *palpable friction rub.*

TABLE 18-6 Adventitious Lung Sounds

Sound	Description	Mechanism	Clinical Example
Discontinuous Sounds These are discrete, crackling sounds.			
Crackles—fine (formerly called *rales*) Expiration Inspiration	Discontinuous, high-pitched, short crackling, popping sounds heard during inspiration that are not cleared by coughing; you can simulate this sound by rolling a strand of hair between your fingers near your ear or by moistening your thumb and index finger and separating them near your ear	Inspiratory crackles: inhaled air collides with previously deflated airways; airways suddenly pop open, creating explosive crackling sound Expiratory crackles: sudden airway closing[24]	*Late inspiratory crackles* occur with restrictive disease: pneumonia, heart failure, and interstitial fibrosis *Early inspiratory crackles* occur with obstructive disease: chronic bronchitis, asthma, and emphysema *Posturally induced crackles* (PICs) are fine crackles that appear with a change from sitting to the supine position or with a change from supine to supine with legs elevated
Crackles—coarse (coarse rales)	Loud, low-pitched, bubbling and gurgling sounds that start in early inspiration and may be present in expiration; may decrease somewhat by suctioning or coughing but will reappear shortly—sounds like opening a Velcro fastener	Inhaled air collides with secretions in the trachea and large bronchi	Pulmonary edema, pneumonia, pulmonary fibrosis, and the terminally ill who have a depressed cough reflex
Atelectatic crackles (atelectatic rales)	Sounds like fine crackles but do not last and are not pathologic; disappear after the first few breaths; heard in axillae and bases (usually dependent) of lungs	When sections of alveoli are not fully aerated, they deflate and accumulate secretions. Crackles are heard when these sections re-expand with a few deep breaths	In aging adults, in bedridden persons, or in persons just aroused from sleep
Pleural friction rub	A very superficial sound that is coarse and low pitched; it has a grating quality as if two pieces of leather are being rubbed together; sounds just like crackles, but *close* to the ear; sounds louder if you push the stethoscope harder onto the chest wall; sound is inspiratory and expiratory	Caused when pleurae become inflamed and lose their normal lubricating fluid; their opposing roughened pleural surfaces rub together during respiration; heard best in anterolateral wall where greatest lung mobility exists	Pleuritis, accompanied by pain with breathing (rub disappears after a few days if pleural fluid accumulates and separates pleurae)

TABLE 18-6 Adventitious Lung Sounds—cont'd

Sound	Description	Mechanism	Clinical Example
Continuous Sounds These are connected, musical sounds.			
Wheeze—high-pitched (sibilant)	High-pitched, musical squeaking sounds that sound polyphonic (multiple notes as in a musical chord); predominate in expiration but may occur in both expiration and inspiration	Air squeezed or compressed through passageways narrowed almost to closure by collapsing, swelling, secretions, or tumors; the passageway walls oscillate in apposition between the closed and barely open positions; the resulting sound is similar to a vibrating reed	Diffuse airway obstruction from acute asthma or chronic emphysema
Wheeze—low-pitched (sonorous rhonchi)	Low-pitched; monophonic single note, musical snoring, moaning sounds; they are heard throughout the cycle, although they are more prominent on expiration; may clear somewhat by coughing	Airflow obstruction as described by the vibrating reed mechanism above; the pitch of the wheeze cannot be correlated to the size of the passageway that generates it	Bronchitis, single bronchus obstruction from airway tumor
Stridor	High-pitched, monophonic, inspiratory, crowing sound, louder in neck than over chest wall	Originating in larynx or trachea, upper airway obstruction from swollen, inflamed tissues or lodged foreign body	Croup and acute epiglottitis in children, and foreign inhalation, obstructed airway may be life-threatening

ABNORMAL FINDINGS
FOR ADVANCED PRACTICE

TABLE 18-7 Voice Sounds

Technique	Normal Finding	Abnormal Finding
Bronchophony Ask the person to repeat "ninety-nine" while you listen with the stethoscope over the chest wall; listen especially if you suspect pathology	Normal voice transmission is soft, muffled, and indistinct; you can hear sound through the stethoscope but cannot distinguish exactly what is being said	Pathology that increases lung density will enhance transmission of voice sounds; you auscultate a clear "ninety-nine" The words are more distinct than normal and sound close to your ear

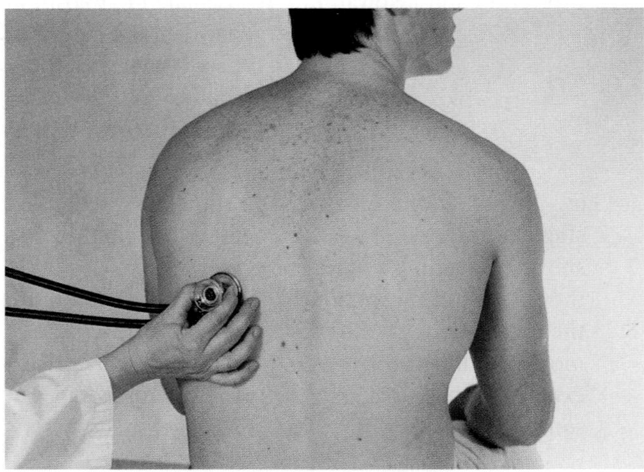

Technique	Normal Finding	Abnormal Finding
Egophony (Greek: "the voice of a goat") Auscultate the chest while the person phonates a long "ee-ee-ee-ee" sound	Normally, you should hear "eeeeeeee" through your stethoscope	Over area of consolidation or compression, the spoken "eeee" sound changes to a bleating long "aaaaa" sound
Whispered Pectoriloquy Ask the person to whisper a phrase like "one-two-three" as you auscultate	The normal response is faint, muffled, and almost inaudible	With only small amounts of consolidation, the whispered voice is transmitted very clearly and distinctly, although still somewhat faint; it sounds as if the person is whispering right into your stethoscope, "one-two-three"

TABLE 18-8 Assessment of Common Respiratory Conditions

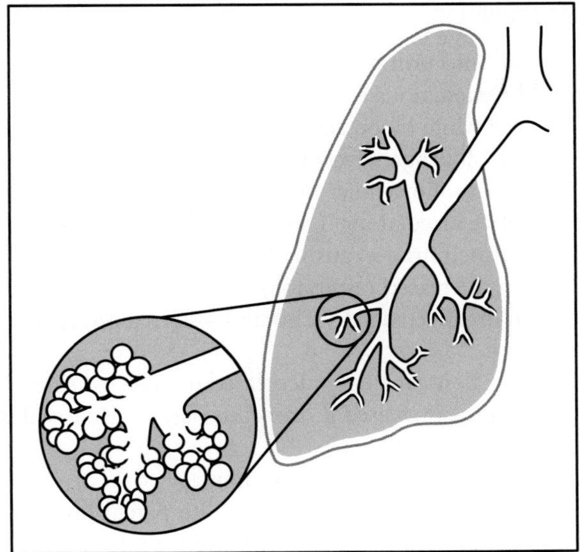

Normal Lung (for comparison)

Inspection Anteroposterior < transverse diameter, relaxed posture, normal musculature; rate 10 to 18 breaths per minute, regular, no cyanosis or pallor.
Palpation Symmetric chest expansion. Tactile fremitus present and equal bilaterally, diminishing toward periphery. No lumps, masses, or tenderness.
Percussion Resonant. Diaphragmatic excursion 3 to 5 cm and equal bilaterally.
Auscultation Vesicular over peripheral fields. Bronchovesicular parasternally (anterior) and between scapulae (posterior). Infant and young child—bronchovesicular throughout.
Adventitious Sounds None.

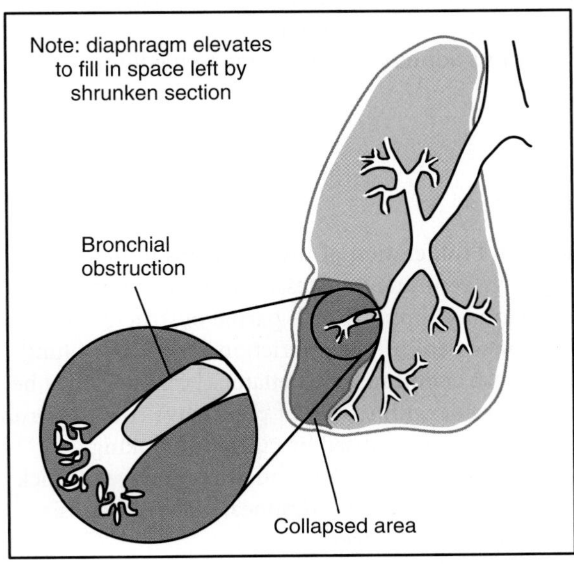

Atelectasis (Collapse)

Condition Collapsed shrunken section of alveoli or an entire lung as a result of (1) airway obstruction (e.g., the bronchus is completely blocked by thick exudate, aspirated foreign body, or tumor), the alveolar air beyond it is gradually absorbed by the pulmonary capillaries, and the alveolar walls cave in; (2) compression on the lung; and (3) lack of surfactant (hyaline membrane disease).
Inspection Cough. Lag on expansion on affected side. Increased respiratory rate and pulse. Possible cyanosis.
Palpation Chest expansion decreased on affected side. Tactile fremitus decreased or absent over area. With large collapse, tracheal shift toward affected side.
Percussion Dull over area (remainder of thorax sometimes may have hyperresonant note).
Auscultation Breath sounds decreased vesicular or absent over area. Voice sounds variable, usually decreased or absent over affected area.
Adventitious Sounds None if bronchus is obstructed. Occasional fine crackles if bronchus is patent.

Continued

TABLE 18-8 **Assessment of Common Respiratory Conditions—cont'd**

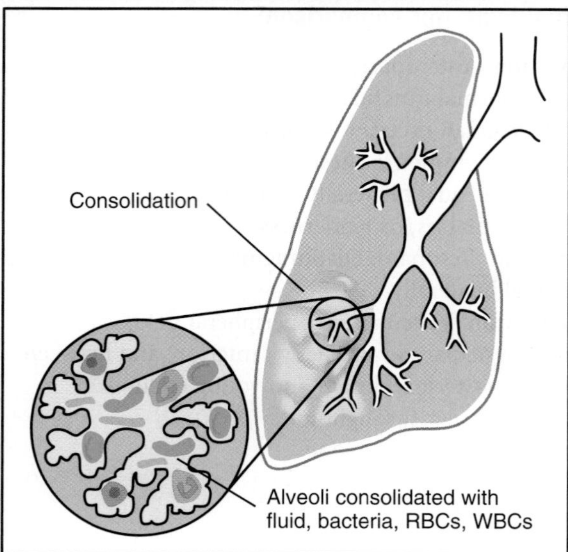

Lobar Pneumonia

Condition Infection in lung parenchyma leaves alveolar membrane edematous and porous, so red blood cells (RBCs) and white blood cells (WBCs) pass from blood to alveoli. Alveoli progressively fill up (become consolidated) with bacteria, solid cellular debris, fluid, and blood cells, which replace alveolar air. This decreases surface area of the respiratory membrane, causing hypoxemia.
Inspection Increased respiratory rate. Guarding and lag on expansion on affected side. Children—sternal retraction, nasal flaring.
Palpation Chest expansion decreased on affected side. Tactile fremitus increased if bronchus patent, decreased if bronchus obstructed.
Percussion Dull over lobar pneumonia.
Auscultation Breath sounds louder with patent bronchus, as if coming directly from larynx. Voice sounds have increased clarity; bronchophony, egophony, whispered pectoriloquy present. Children—diminished breath sounds may occur early in pneumonia.
Adventitious Sounds Crackles, fine to medium.

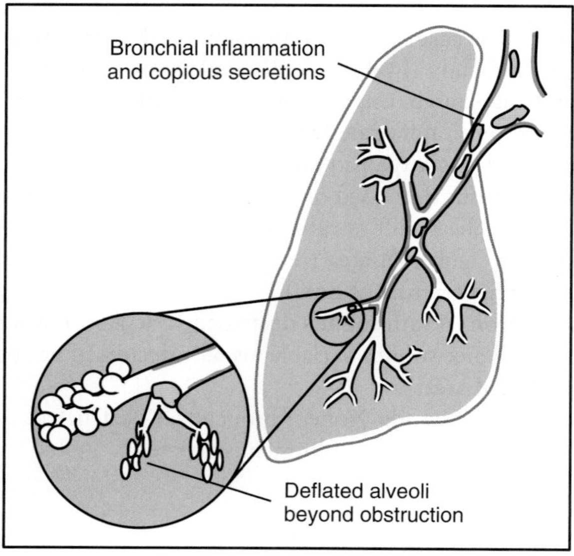

Bronchitis

Condition Proliferation of mucus glands in the passageways, resulting in excessive mucus secretion. Inflammation of bronchi with partial obstruction of bronchi by secretions or constrictions. Sections of lung distal to obstruction may be deflated. Bronchitis may be acute or chronic with recurrent productive cough. Chronic bronchitis is usually caused by cigarette smoking.
Inspection Hacking, rasping cough productive of thick mucoid sputum. Chronic—dyspnea, fatigue, cyanosis, possible clubbing of fingers.
Palpation Tactile fremitus normal.
Percussion Resonant.
Auscultation Normal vesicular. Voice sounds normal. Chronic—prolonged expiration.
Adventitious Sounds Crackles over deflated areas. May have wheeze.

TABLE 18-8 Assessment of Common Respiratory Conditions—cont'd

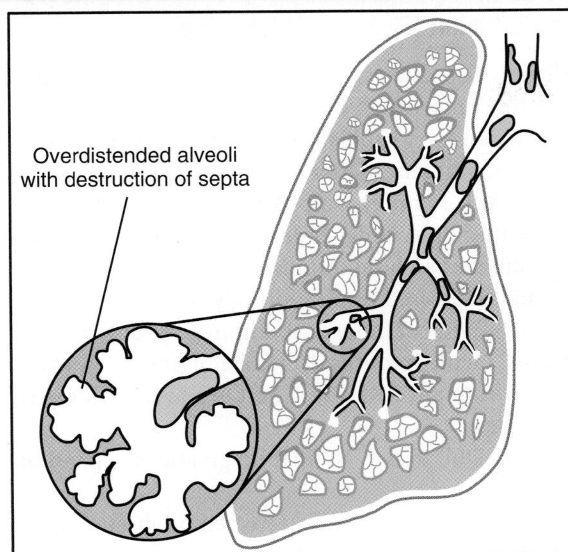

Emphysema

Condition Caused by destruction of pulmonary connective tissue (elastin, collagen); characterized by permanent enlargement of air sacs distal to terminal bronchioles and rupture of interalveolar walls. This increases airway resistance, especially on expiration—producing a hyperinflated lung and an increase in lung volume. Cigarette smoking accounts for 80% to 90% of cases of emphysema.
Inspection Increased anteroposterior diameter. Barrel chest. Use of accessory muscles to aid respiration. Tripod position. Shortness of breath, especially on exertion. Respiratory distress. Tachypnea.
Palpation Decreased tactile fremitus and chest expansion.
Percussion Hyperresonant. Decreased diaphragmatic excursion.
Auscultation Decreased breath sounds. May have prolonged expiration. Muffled heart sounds resulting from overdistention of lungs.
Adventitious Sounds Usually none; occasionally, wheeze.

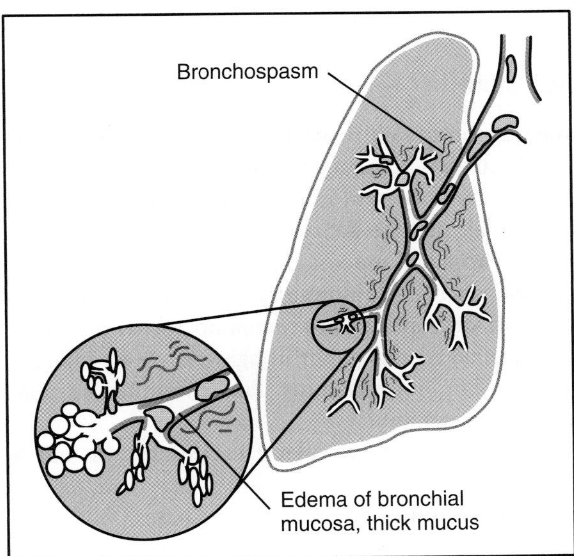

Asthma (Reactive Airway Disease)

Condition An allergic hypersensitivity to certain inhaled allergens (pollen), irritants (tobacco, ozone), microbes, stress, or exercise that produces a complex response characterized by bronchospasm and inflammation, edema in walls of bronchioles, and secretion of highly viscous mucus into airways. These factors greatly increase airway resistance, especially during expiration, and produce the symptoms of wheezing, dyspnea, and chest tightness.
Inspection During severe attack: increased respiratory rate, shortness of breath with audible wheeze, use of accessory neck muscles, cyanosis, apprehension, retraction of intercostal spaces. Expiration labored, prolonged. When chronic, may have barrel chest.
Palpation Tactile fremitus decreased, tachycardia.
Percussion Resonant. May be hyperresonant if chronic.
Auscultation Diminished air movement. Breath sounds decreased, with prolonged expiration. Voice sounds decreased.
Adventitious Sounds Bilateral wheezing on expiration, sometimes inspiratory and expiratory wheezing.

Continued

TABLE 18-8 Assessment of Common Respiratory Conditions—cont'd

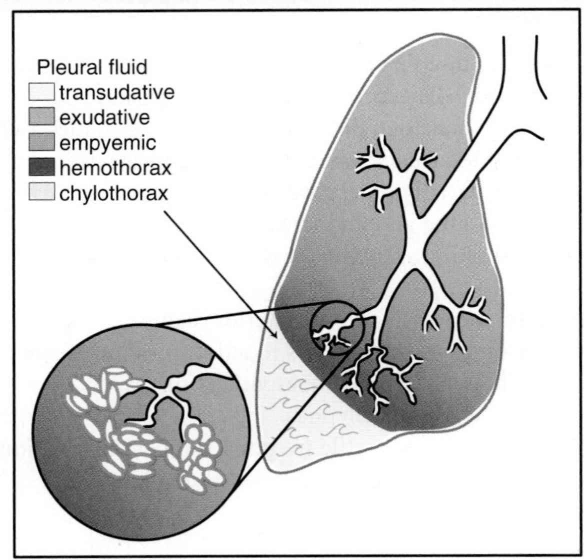

Pleural Effusion (Fluid) or Thickening

Condition Collection of excess fluid in the intrapleural space, with compression of overlying lung tissue. Effusion may contain watery capillary fluid (transudative), protein (exudative), purulent matter (empyemic), blood (hemothorax), or milky lymphatic fluid (chylothorax). Gravity settles fluid in dependent areas of thorax. Presence of fluid subdues all lung sounds.
Inspection Increased respirations, dyspnea; may have dry cough, tachycardia, cyanosis, abdominal distention.
Palpation Tactile fremitus decreased or absent. Tracheal shift away from affected side. Chest expansion decreased on affected side.
Percussion Dull to flat. No diaphragmatic excursion on affected side.
Auscultation Breath sounds decreased or absent. Voice sounds decreased or absent. When remainder of lung is compressed near the effusion, may have bronchial breath sounds over the compression along with bronchophony, egophony, whispered pectoriloquy.
Adventitious Sounds None.

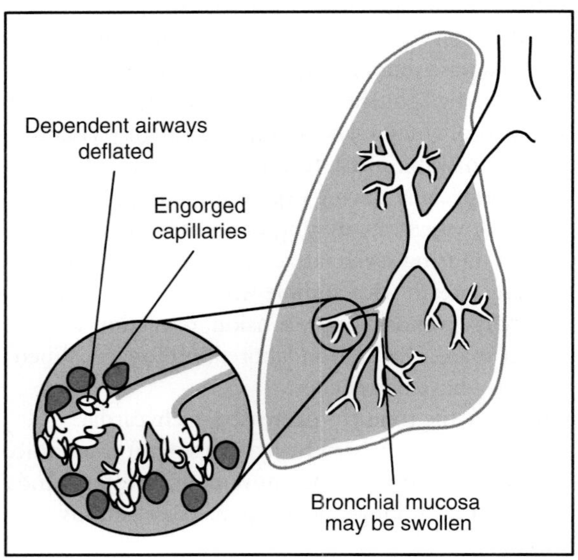

Heart Failure

Condition Pump failure with increasing pressure of cardiac overload causes pulmonary congestion or an increased amount of blood present in pulmonary capillaries. Dependent air sacs are deflated. Pulmonary capillaries engorged. Bronchial mucosa may be swollen.
Inspection Increased respiratory rate, shortness of breath on exertion, orthopnea, paroxysmal nocturnal dyspnea, nocturia, ankle edema, pallor in light-skinned people.
Palpation Skin moist, clammy. Tactile fremitus normal.
Percussion Resonant.
Auscultation Normal vesicular. Heart sounds include S_3 gallop.
Adventitious Sounds Crackles at lung bases.

TABLE 18-8 Assessment of Common Respiratory Conditions—cont'd

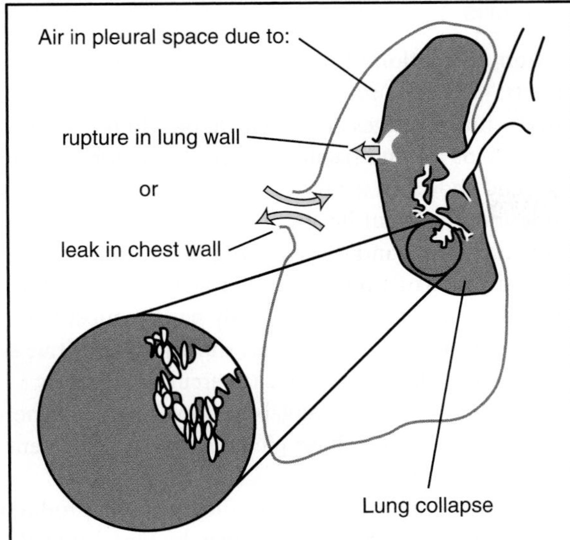

Pneumothorax

Condition Free air in pleural space causes partial or complete lung collapse. Air in pleural space neutralizes the usual negative pressure present; thus lung collapses. Usually unilateral. Pneumothorax can be (1) **spontaneous** (air enters pleural space through rupture in lung wall, (2) **traumatic** (air enters through opening or injury in chest wall), or (3) **tension** (trapped air in pleural space increases, compressing lung and shifting mediastinum to the unaffected side).
Inspection Unequal chest expansion. If large, tachypnea, cyanosis, apprehension, bulging in interspaces.
Palpation Tactile fremitus decreased or absent. Tracheal shift to opposite side (unaffected side). Chest expansion decreased on affected side. Tachycardia, decreased BP.
Percussion Hyperresonant. Decreased diaphragmatic excursion.
Auscultation Breath sounds decreased or absent. Voice sounds decreased or absent.
Adventitious Sounds None.

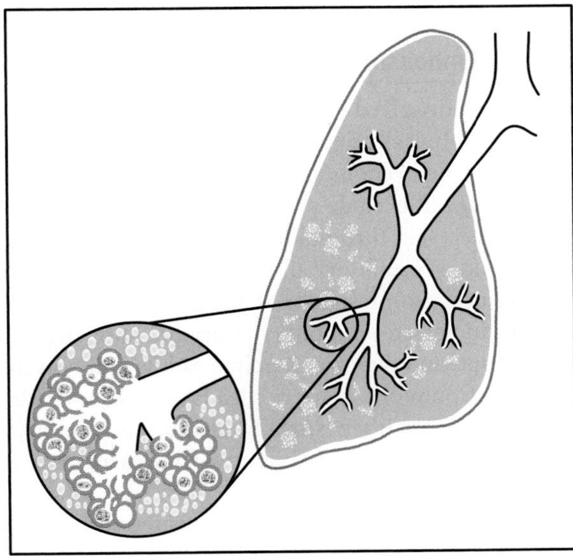

Pneumocystis jiroveci (P. carinii) Pneumonia

Condition This virulent form of pneumonia is a protozoal infection associated with AIDS. The parasite *P. jiroveci (P. carinii)* is common in the United States and harmless to most people, except to the immunocompromised, in whom a diffuse interstitial pneumonitis ensues. Cysts containing the organism and macrophages form in alveolar spaces, alveolar walls thicken, and the disease spreads to bilateral interstitial infiltrates of foamy, protein-rich fluid.
Inspection Anxiety, shortness of breath, dyspnea on exertion, malaise are common; also tachypnea; fever; a dry, nonproductive cough; intercostal retractions in children; cyanosis.
Palpation Decreased chest expansion.
Percussion Dull over areas of diffuse infiltrate.
Auscultation Breath sounds may be diminished.
Adventitious Sounds Crackles may be present but often are absent.

Continued

TABLE 18-8 **Assessment of Common Respiratory Conditions—cont'd**

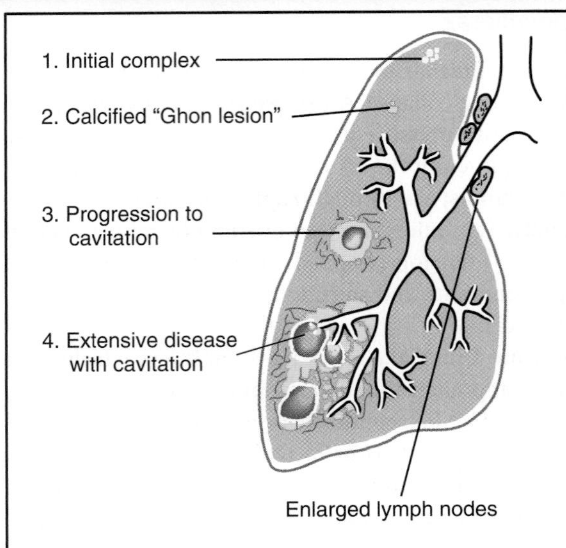

Tuberculosis

Condition Inhalation of tubercle bacilli into the alveolar wall starts: (1) Initial complex is acute inflammatory response—macrophages engulf bacilli but do not kill them. Tubercle forms around bacilli. (2) Scar tissue forms, lesion calcifies and shows on x-ray. (3) Reactivation of previously healed lesion. Dormant bacilli now multiply, producing necrosis, cavitation, and caseous lung tissue (cheeselike). (4) Extensive destruction as lesion erodes into bronchus, forming air-filled cavity. Apex usually has the most damage.
Subjective Initially asymptomatic, showing as positive skin test or on x-ray film. Progressive tuberculosis involves weight loss, anorexia, easy fatigability, low-grade afternoon fevers, night sweats. May have pleural effusion, recurrent lower respiratory infections.
Inspection Cough initially nonproductive, later productive of purulent, yellow-green sputum, may be blood tinged. Dyspnea, orthopnea, fatigue, weakness.
Palpation Skin moist at night from night sweats.
Percussion Resonant initially. Dull over any effusion.
Auscultation Normal or decreased vesicular breath sounds.
Adventitious Sounds Crackles over upper lobes common, persist following full expiration and cough.

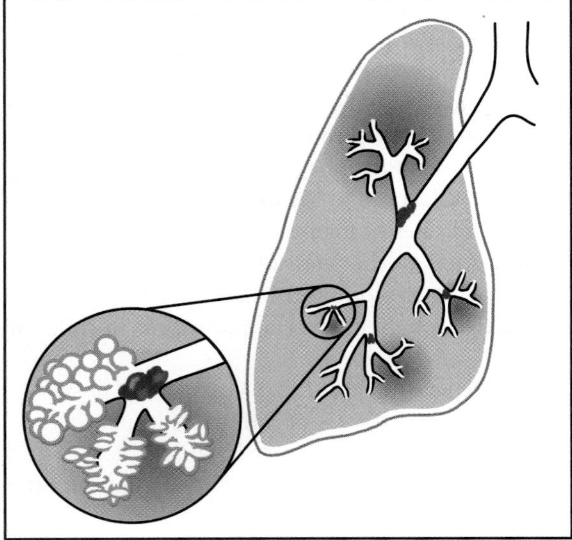

Pulmonary Embolism

Condition Undissolved materials (e.g., thrombus or air bubbles, fat globules) originating in legs or pelvis detach and travel through venous system returning blood to right heart and lodge to occlude pulmonary vessels. Over 95% arise from deep vein thrombi in lower legs as a result of stasis of blood, vessel injury, or hypercoagulability. Pulmonary occlusion results in ischemia of downstream lung tissue, increased pulmonary artery pressure, decreased cardiac output, and hypoxia. Rarely, a saddle embolus in bifurcation of pulmonary arteries leads to sudden death from hypoxia. More often, small to medium pulmonary branches occlude, leading to dyspnea. These may resolve by fibrolytic activity.
Subjective Chest pain, worse on deep inspiration, dyspnea.
Inspection Apprehensive, restless, anxiety, mental status changes, cyanosis, tachypnea, cough, hemoptysis, PaO_2 <80% on pulse oximetry. Arterial blood gases show respiratory alkalosis.
Palpation Diaphoresis, hypotension.
Auscultation Tachycardia, accentuated pulmonic component of S_2 heart sound.
Adventitious Sounds Crackles, wheezes.

TABLE 18-8 **Assessment of Common Respiratory Conditions—cont'd**

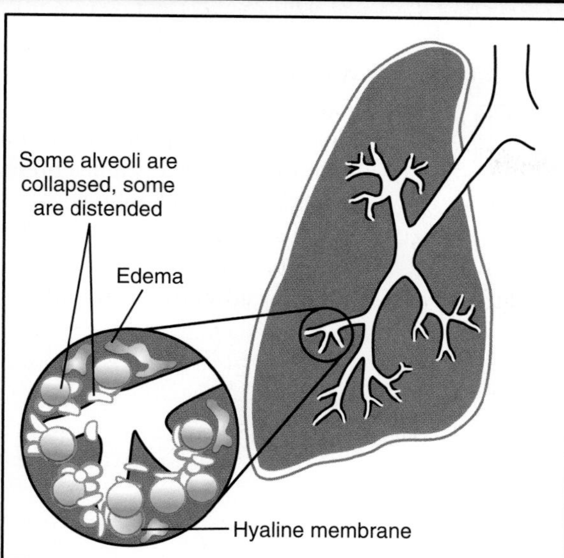

Acute Respiratory Distress Syndrome (ARDS)

Condition An acute pulmonary insult (trauma, gastric acid aspiration, shock, sepsis) damages alveolar capillary membrane, leading to increased permeability of pulmonary capillaries and alveolar epithelium and to pulmonary edema. Gross examination (autopsy) would show dark red, firm, airless tissue, with some alveoli collapsed, and hyaline membranes lining the distended alveoli.
Subjective Acute onset of dyspnea, apprehension.
Inspection Restlessness; disorientation; rapid, shallow breathing; productive cough, thin, frothy sputum; retractions of intercostal spaces and sternum. Decreased PaO_2, blood gases show respiratory alkalosis, x-ray films show diffuse pulmonary infiltrates; a late sign is cyanosis.
Palpation Hypotension.
Auscultation Tachycardia.
Adventitious Sounds Crackles, rhonchi.

BIBLIOGRAPHY

1. Arvas, A., Bas, V., & Gur, E. (2009). The impact of passive smoking on the development of lower respiratory tract infection in infancy. *Turkish Pediatrics Archive, 44*(1), 12-17.
2. Bauldoff, G. S., & Diaz, P. T. (2006). Improving outcomes for COPD patients. *Nurse Practitioner, 31*(8), 27-43.
3. Benninger, C., & McCallister, J. (2010). Asthma in pregnancy: reading between the lines. *Nurse Practitoner, 35*(4), 10-20.
4. Best, D. (2009). Technical report: secondhand and prenatal tobacco smoke exposure. *Pediatrics, 124*(5):e1017-e1044.
5. Centers for Disease Control and Prevention. (2006). *MMWR. Morbidity and Mortality Weekly Report, 55*, 305-308. Retrieved May 10, 2010, from www.cdc.gov/mmwr/preview/mmwrhtml/mm5511a3.htm#top.
6. Centers for Disease Control and Prevention. (2008). *Trends in tuberculosis—United States, 2008. MMWR. Morbidity and Mortality Weekly Report, 58*(10), 249-253.
7. Corbridge, S., & Corbridge, T. C. (2010). Asthma in adolescents and adults. *American Journal of Nursing, 110*(5), 28-40.
8. Crocker, D., Brown, C., Moolenaar, R., et al. (2009). Racial and ethnic disparities in asthma medication usage and health-care utilization: data from the National Asthma Survey. *Chest, 136*(4), 1063-1071.
9. Cunningham, F. G., Leveno, K., Bloom, S., et al. (2010). *Williams obstetrics* (23rd ed.). New York: McGraw-Hill Professional.
10. Du, H., Newton, P. J., Salamonson, Y., et al. (2009). A review of the six-minute walk test: its implication as a self-administered assessment tool. *European Journal of Cardiovascular Nursing, 8*(1), 2-8.
11. Enright, P. L. (2003). The six-minute walk test. *Respiratory Care, 48*, 783-785.
12. Gorman, B. K., & Chu, M. (2009). Racial and ethnic differences in adult prevalence, problems, and medical care. *Ethnicity & Health, 14*(5), 527-552.
13. Gribble, E. A., & Williams, A. (2010). Multi-drug-resistant TB: what NPs need to know. *Nurse Practitioner, 35*(3), 14-23.
14. Haberg, S. E., Bentdal, Y. E., London, S. J., et al. (2010). Prenatal and postnatal parental smoking and acute otitis media in early childhood. *Acta Paediatrica, 99*(1), 99-105.
15. Hart, A. M., Patti, A., Noggle, B., et al. (2008). Acute respiratory infections and antimicrobial resistance. *American Journal of Nursing, 108*(6), 56-66.
16. Kelly, A. (2009). Treatment of primary spontaneous pneumothorax. *Current Opinion in Pulmonary Medicine, 15*, 376-379.
17. Kung, Y. M. (2010). A close-up view of flu. *Nurse Practitioner, 35*(4), 47-52.
18. Langston, S. B., & Appel, S. J. (2010). Smoking cessation: snub out CAD. *The Nurse Practitioner, 35*(4), 43-46.
19. Loudon, R. G. (1987). The lung exam. *Clinics in Chest Medicine, 8*, 265-272.
20. Mendyk, M. K. (2008). Community-associated MRSA. *Nurse Practitioner, 33*(3), 26-32.
21. Olubummo, C. (2008). Asthma epidemic: tighten your treatment options. *The Nurse Practitioner, 33*(8), 12-18.
22. Simon, B. M. (2007). Lung cancer diagnosis in primary care. *Nurse Practitioner, 32*, 43-49.
23. Sleiman, P. M. A., Flory, J., Imielinshi, M., et al. (2010). Variants of DENND1B associated with asthma in children. *New England Journal of Medicine, 362*(1), 36-44.
24. Vyshedskiy, A., Alhashem, R. M., Paciej, R., et al. (2009). Mechanism of inspiratory and expiratory crackles. *Chest, 135*(1), 156-164.

Summary Checklist: Thorax and Lung Examination

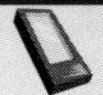 For a PDA-downloadable version, go to http://evolve.elsevier.com/Jarvis/.

1. **Inspection**
   Thoracic cage
   Respirations
   Skin color and condition
   Person's position
   Facial expression
   Level of consciousness
2. **Palpation**
   Confirm symmetric expansion
   Tactile fremitus
   Detect any lumps, masses, tenderness
3. **Percussion**
   Percuss over lung fields
   Estimate diaphragmatic excursion
4. **Auscultation**
   Assess normal breath sounds
   Note any abnormal breath sounds
   If abnormal breath sounds present, perform bronchophony, whispered pectoriloquy, egophony
   Note any adventitious sounds

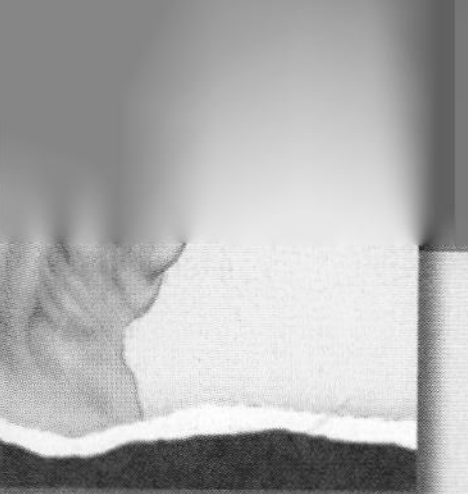

19

Heart and Neck Vessels

evolve WEBSITE

http://evolve.elsevier.com/Jarvis/

- Animations
- Audio—Heart Sounds
- Audio Key Points
- Bedside Assessment Summary Checklist
- Case Study
  Chest Pain
  Shortness of Breath
- Health Promotion Guide
  Heart Disease
- NCLEX Review Questions
- Physical Examination Summary Checklist
- Quick Assessment for Common Conditions
  Congestive Heart Failure (CHF)
  Hyperlipidemia
  Myocardial Infarction
- Video—Assessment
  Neck Vessels and Heart

OUTLINE

Structure and Function, 455

Position and Surface Landmarks
Heart Wall, Chambers, and Valves
Direction of Blood Flow
Cardiac Cycle
Heart Sounds
Conduction
Pumping Ability
The Neck Vessels

Subjective Data, 467

Health History Questions

Objective Data, 470

Preparation
The Neck Vessels
The Precordium

Documentation and Critical Thinking, 484

Abnormal Findings, 486

Abnormal Findings for Advanced Practice, 487

STRUCTURE AND FUNCTION

The cardiovascular system consists of the **heart** (a muscular pump) and the **blood vessels.** The blood vessels are arranged in two continuous loops, the *pulmonary circulation* and the *systemic circulation* (Fig. 19-1). When the heart contracts, it pumps blood simultaneously into both loops.

POSITION AND SURFACE LANDMARKS

The **precordium** is the area on the anterior chest directly overlying the heart and great vessels (Fig. 19-2). The great vessels are the major arteries and veins connected to the heart. The heart and great vessels are located between the lungs in the middle third of the thoracic cage (**mediastinum**). The heart extends from the 2nd to 5th intercostal space and from the right border of the sternum to the left midclavicular line.

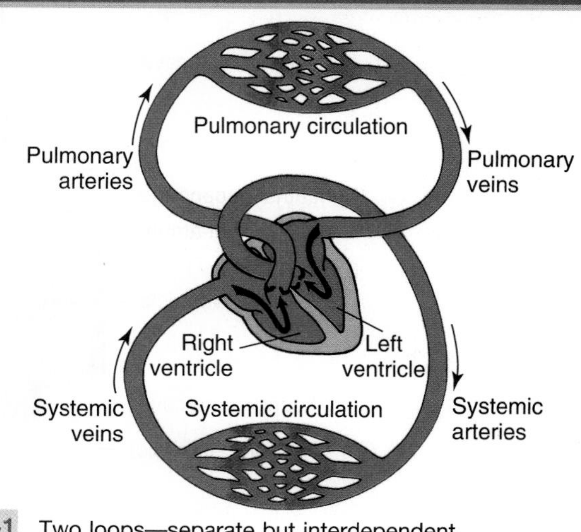

19-1 Two loops—separate but interdependent.

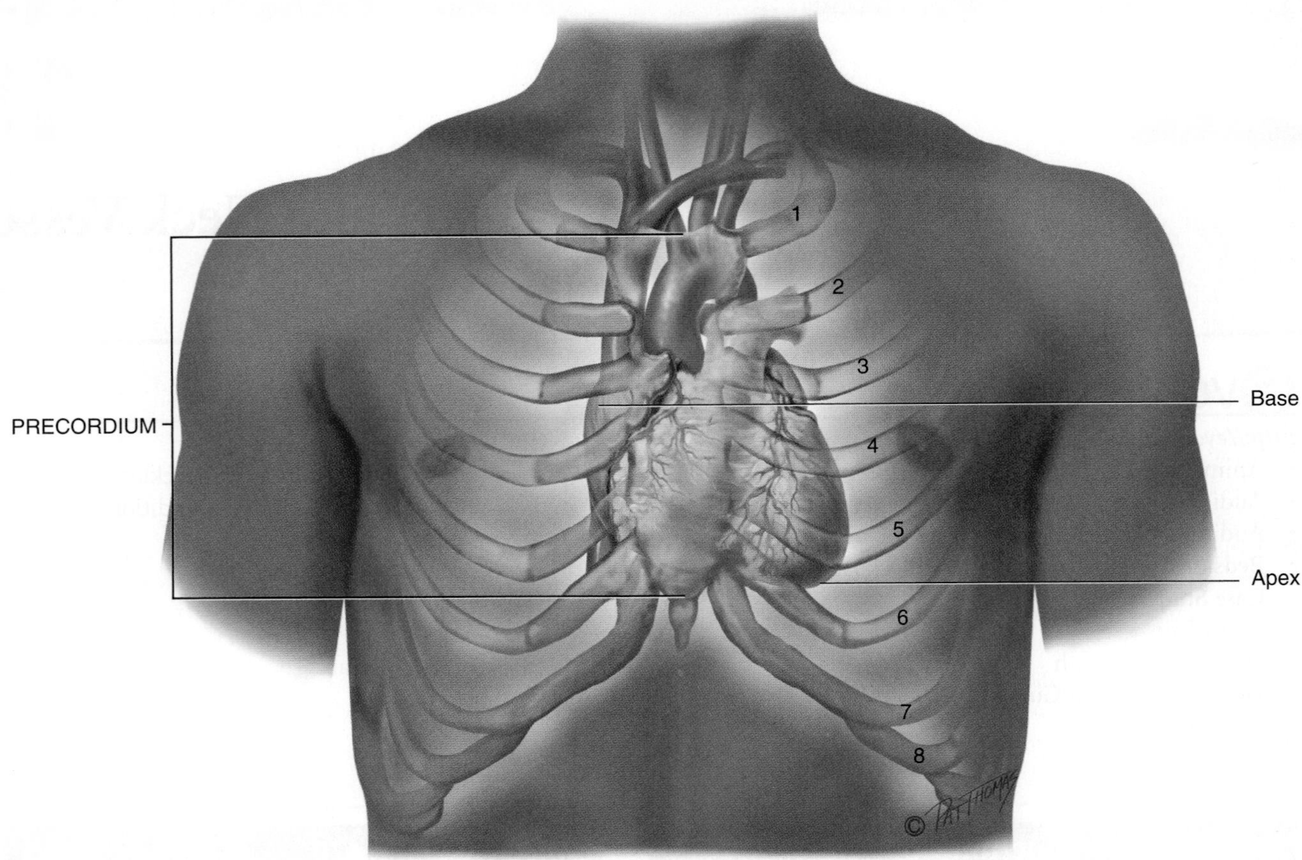

19-2

Think of the heart as an upside-down triangle in the chest. The "top" of the heart is the broader *base,* and the "bottom" is the *apex,* which points down and to the left (Fig. 19-3). During contraction, the apex beats against the chest wall, producing an apical impulse. This is palpable in most people, normally at the fifth intercostal space, 7 to 9 cm from the midsternal line.

Inside the body, the heart is rotated so that its right side is anterior and its left side is mostly posterior. Of the heart's four chambers, the right ventricle forms the greatest area of anterior cardiac surface. The left ventricle lies behind the right ventricle and forms the apex and slender area of the left border. The right atrium lies to the right and above the right ventricle and forms the right border. The left atrium is located

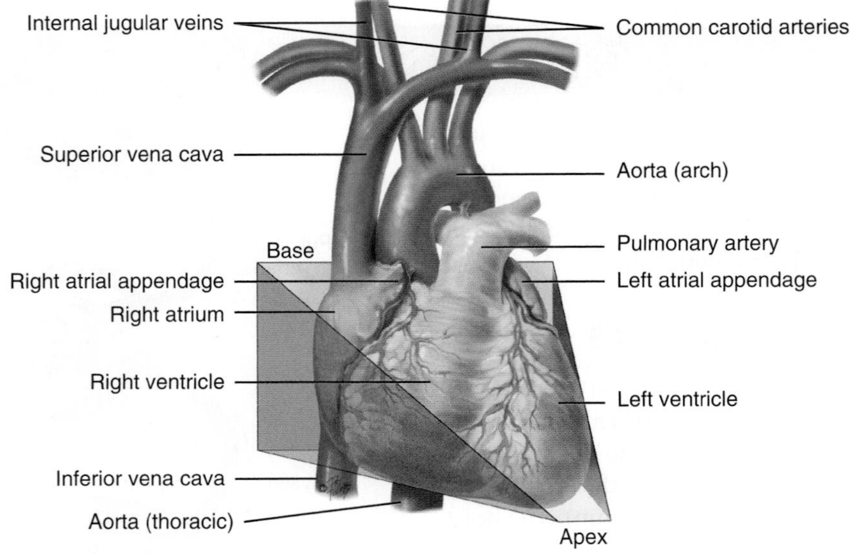

19-3

posteriorly, with only a small portion, the left atrial appendage, showing anteriorly.

The **great vessels** lie bunched above the base of the heart. The **superior** and **inferior vena cava** return unoxygenated venous blood to the right side of the heart. The **pulmonary artery** leaves the right ventricle, bifurcates, and carries the venous blood to the lungs. The **pulmonary veins** return the freshly oxygenated blood to the left side of the heart, and the **aorta** carries it out to the body. The aorta ascends from the left ventricle, arches back at the level of the sternal angle, and descends behind the heart.

HEART WALL, CHAMBERS, AND VALVES

The **heart wall** has numerous layers. The **pericardium** is a tough, fibrous, double-walled sac that surrounds and protects the heart (see its cut edge in Fig. 19-4). It has two layers that contain a few milliliters of serous *pericardial fluid.* This ensures smooth, friction-free movement of the heart muscle. The pericardium is adherent to the great vessels, esophagus, sternum, and pleurae and is anchored to the diaphragm. The **myocardium** is the muscular wall of the heart; it does the pumping. The **endocardium** is the thin layer of endothelial tissue that lines the inner surface of the heart chambers and valves.

The common metaphor is to think of the heart as a pump. But consider that the heart is actually *two* pumps; the right side of the heart pumps blood into the lungs, and the left side of the heart simultaneously pumps blood into the body. The two pumps are separated by an impermeable wall, the septum. Each side has an **atrium** and a **ventricle.** The atrium (Latin for "anteroom") is a thin-walled reservoir for holding blood, and the thick-walled ventricle is the muscular pumping chamber. (It is common to use the following abbreviations to refer to the chambers: *RA,* right atrium; *RV,* right ventricle; *LA,* left atrium; and *LV,* left ventricle.)

The four **chambers** are separated by swinging-door–like structures, called *valves,* whose main purpose is to prevent backflow of blood. The valves are unidirectional; they can open only one way. The valves open and close *passively* in response to pressure gradients in the moving blood.

There are four **valves** in the heart (see Fig. 19-4). The two **atrioventricular** (AV) valves separate the atria and the ventricles. The right AV valve is the **tricuspid,** and the left AV valve is the bicuspid or **mitral** valve (so named because it resembles a bishop's mitred cap). The valves' thin leaflets are anchored by collagenous fibers (**chordae tendineae**) to papillary muscles embedded in the ventricle floor. The AV valves open during the heart's filling phase, or **diastole,** to allow the ventricles to fill with blood. During the pumping phase, or **systole,** the AV valves close to prevent regurgitation of blood back up into the atria. The papillary muscles contract at this time, so that the valve leaflets meet and unite to form a perfect seal without turning themselves inside out.

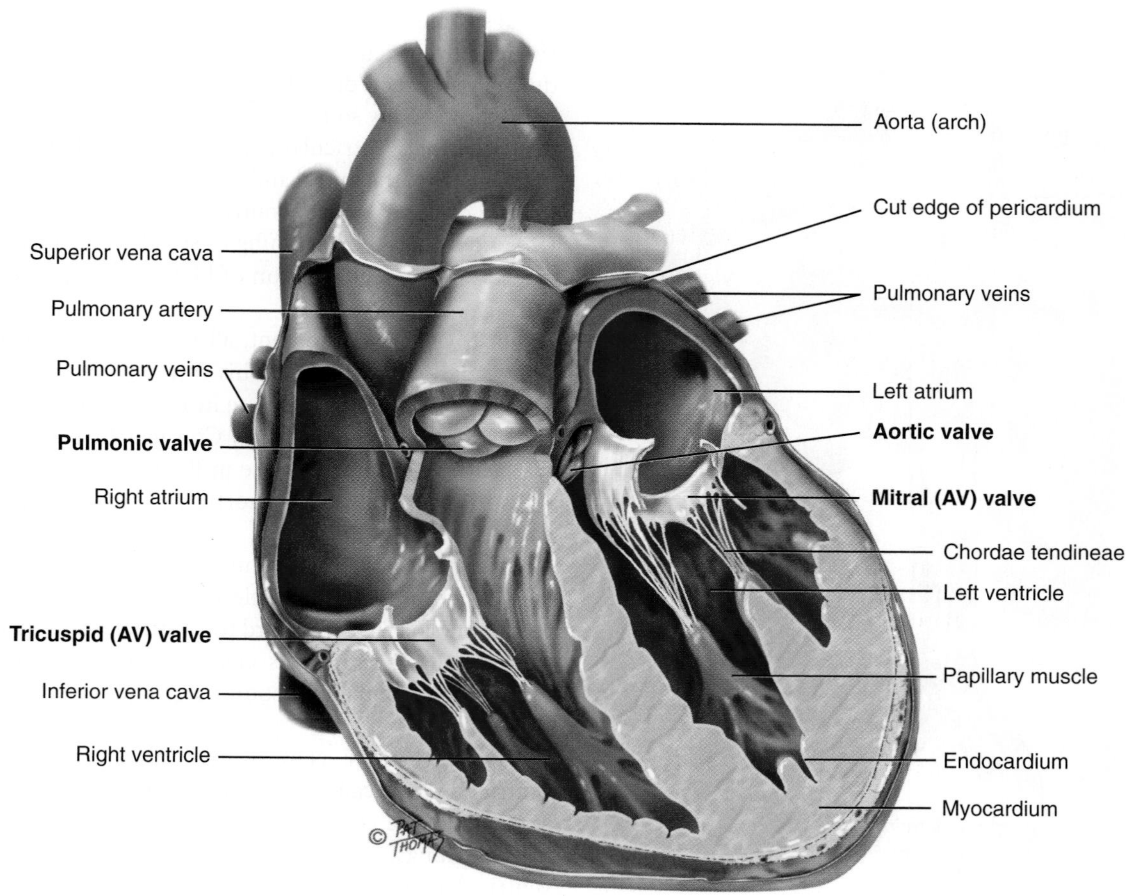

19-4

The **semilunar** (SL) valves are set between the ventricles and the arteries. Each valve has three cusps that look like half moons. The SL valves are the **pulmonic** valve in the right side of the heart and the **aortic** valve in the left side of the heart. They open during pumping, or **systole,** to allow blood to be ejected from the heart.

Note: There are no valves between the vena cava and the right atrium nor between the pulmonary veins and the left atrium. For this reason, abnormally high pressure in the left side of the heart gives a person symptoms of pulmonary congestion, and abnormally high pressure in the right side of the heart shows in the neck veins and abdomen.

DIRECTION OF BLOOD FLOW

Think of an unoxygenated red blood cell being drained downstream into the vena cava. It is swept along with the flow of venous blood and follows the route illustrated in Fig. 19-5.

1. From liver to right atrium (RA) through inferior vena cava
   Superior vena cava drains venous blood from the head and upper extremities
   From RA, venous blood travels through tricuspid valve to right ventricle (RV)
2. From RV, venous blood flows through pulmonic valve to pulmonary artery
   Pulmonary artery delivers unoxygenated blood to lungs

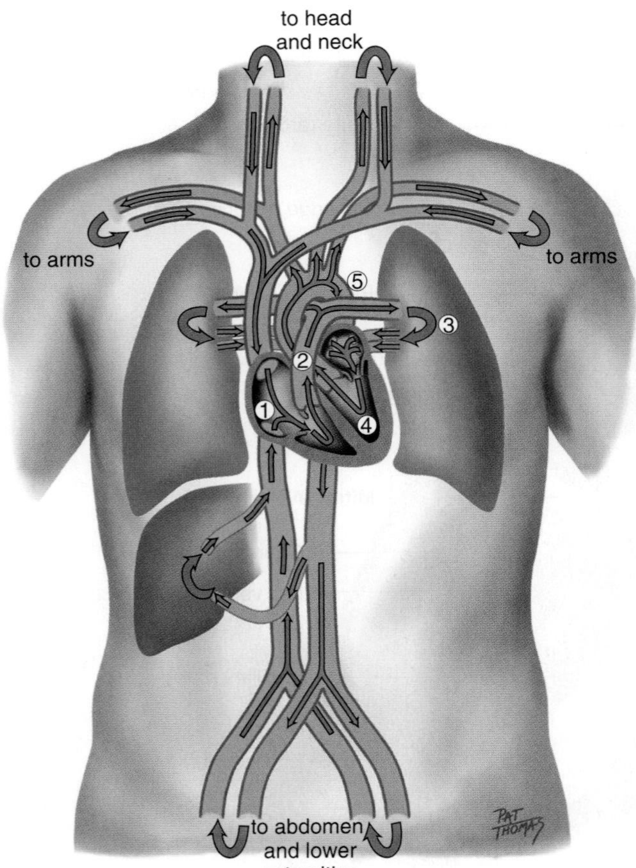

19-5

3. Lungs oxygenate blood
   Pulmonary veins return fresh blood to left atrium (LA)
4. From LA, arterial blood travels through mitral valve to left ventricle (LV)
   LV ejects blood through aortic valve into aorta
5. Aorta delivers oxygenated blood to body

Remember that the circulation is a continuous loop. The blood is kept moving along by continually shifting pressure gradients. The blood flows from an area of higher pressure to one of lower pressure.

CARDIAC CYCLE

The rhythmic movement of blood through the heart is the **cardiac cycle.** It has two phases, **diastole** and **systole.** In **diastole,** the ventricles relax and fill with blood. This takes up two thirds of the cardiac cycle. The heart's contraction is **systole.** During systole, blood is pumped from the ventricles and fills the pulmonary and systemic arteries. This is one third of the cardiac cycle.

Diastole. In diastole, the ventricles are relaxed and the AV valves (i.e., the tricuspid and mitral) are open (Fig. 19-6). (Opening of the normal valve is acoustically silent.) The pressure in the atria is higher than that in the ventricles, so blood pours rapidly into the ventricles. This first passive filling phase is called **early** or **protodiastolic filling.**

Toward the end of diastole, the atria contract and push the last amount of blood (about 25% of stroke volume) into the ventricles. This active filling phase is called **presystole,** or **atrial systole,** or sometimes the "atrial kick." It causes a small rise in left ventricular pressure. (Note that atrial systole occurs during ventricular diastole, a confusing but important point.)

Systole. Now so much blood has been pumped into the ventricles that ventricular pressure is finally higher than that in the atria, so the mitral and tricuspid valves swing shut. The closure of the AV valves contributes to the first heart sound (**S_1**) and signals the beginning of systole. The AV valves close to prevent any regurgitation of blood back up into the atria during contraction.

For a very brief moment, all four valves are closed. The ventricular walls contract. This contraction against a closed system works to build pressure inside the ventricles to a high level **(isometric contraction).** Consider first the left side of the heart. When the pressure in the ventricle finally exceeds pressure in the aorta, the aortic valve opens and blood is ejected rapidly.

After the ventricle's contents are ejected, its pressure falls. When pressure falls below pressure in the aorta, some blood flows backward toward the ventricle, causing the aortic valve to swing shut. This closure of the semilunar valves causes the second heart sound (**S_2**) and signals the end of systole.

Diastole Again. Now all four valves are closed and the ventricles relax (called **isometric** or **isovolumic relaxation**). Meanwhile, the atria have been filling with blood delivered from the lungs. Atrial pressure is now higher than the relaxed ventricular pressure. The mitral valve drifts open, and diastolic filling begins again.

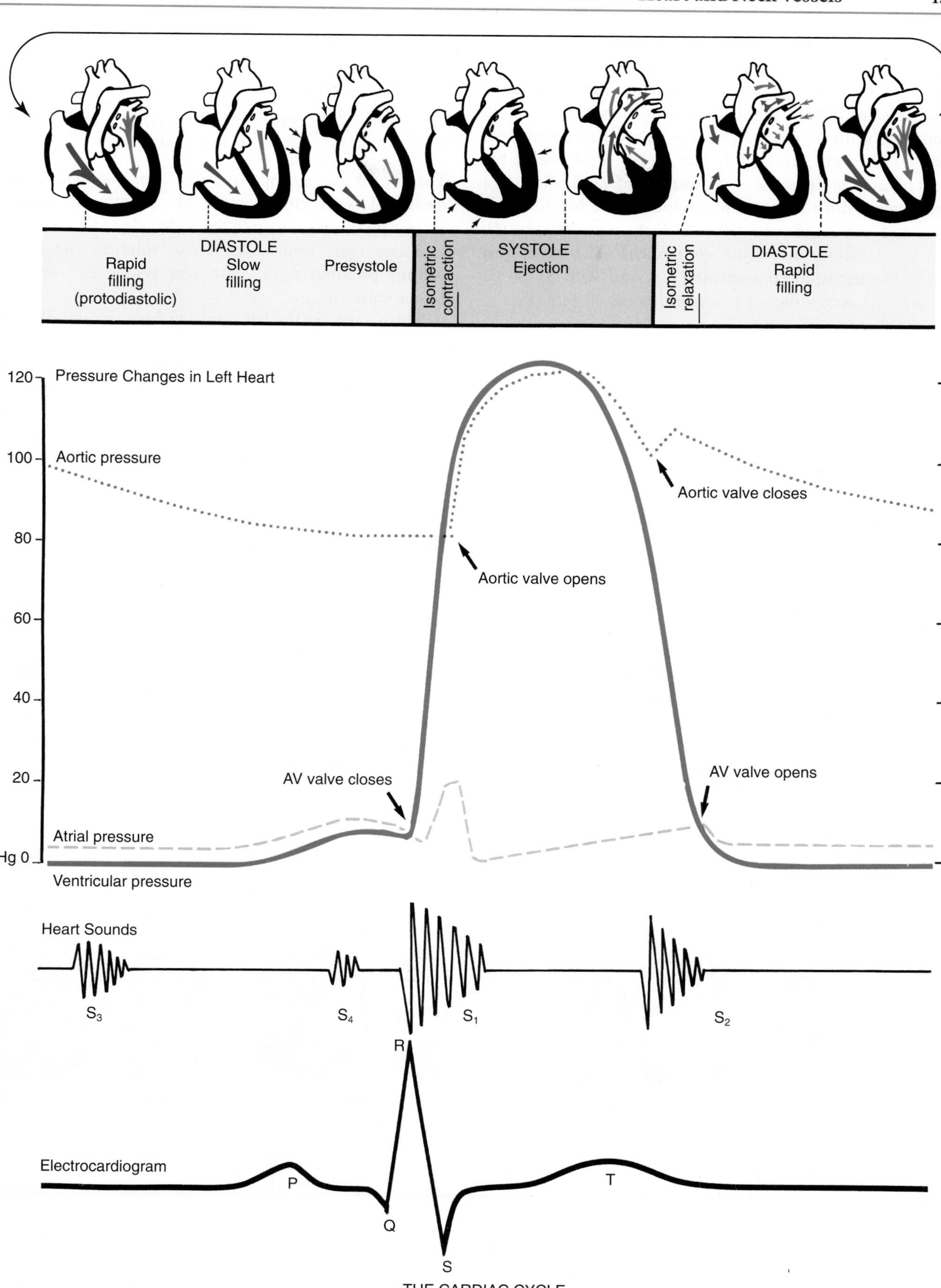

DIASTOLE
Rapid filling (protodiastolic)
Slow filling
Presystole
Isometric contraction
SYSTOLE
Ejection
Isometric relaxation
DIASTOLE
Rapid filling
Pressure Changes in Left Heart
120
100
80
60
40
20
mm Hg 0
Aortic pressure
Aortic valve closes
Aortic valve opens
AV valve closes
AV valve opens
Atrial pressure
Ventricular pressure
Heart Sounds
S_3
S_4
S_1
S_2
Electrocardiogram
P
Q
R
S
T
THE CARDIAC CYCLE

19-6

Events in the Right and Left Sides. The same events are happening at the same time in the right side of the heart, but pressures in the right side of the heart are much lower than those of the left side because less energy is needed to pump blood to its destination, the pulmonary circulation. Also, events occur just slightly later in the right side of the heart because of the route of myocardial depolarization. As a result, two distinct components to each of the heart sounds exist, and sometimes you can hear them separately. In the first heart sound, the mitral component (**M_1**) closes just before the tricuspid component (**T_1**). And with **S_2**, aortic closure (**A_2**) occurs slightly before pulmonic closure (**P_2**).

HEART SOUNDS

Events in the cardiac cycle generate sounds that can be heard through a stethoscope over the chest wall. These include normal heart sounds and, occasionally, extra heart sounds and murmurs (Fig. 19-7).

Normal Heart Sounds

The **first heart sound** (S_1) occurs with closure of the AV valves and thus signals the beginning of systole. The mitral component of the first sound (M_1) slightly precedes the tricuspid component (T_1), but you usually hear these two components fused as one sound. You can hear S_1 over all the precordium, but usually it is loudest at the apex.

The **second heart sound** (S_2) occurs with closure of the semilunar valves and signals the end of systole. The aortic component of the second sound (A_2) slightly precedes the pulmonic component (P_2). Although it is heard over all the precordium, S_2 is loudest at the base.

Effect of Respiration. The volume of right and left ventricular systole is just about equal, but this can be affected by respiration. To learn this, consider the phrase:

Mo**R**e to the **R**ight heart,
Less to the **L**eft

That means that during inspiration, intrathoracic pressure is decreased. This pushes more blood into the vena cava, increasing venous return to the right side of the heart, which increases right ventricular stroke volume. The increased volume prolongs right ventricular systole and delays pulmonic valve closure.

Meanwhile, on the left side, a greater amount of blood is sequestered in the lungs during inspiration. This momentarily decreases the amount returned to the left side of the heart, decreasing left ventricular stroke volume. The decreased volume shortens left ventricular systole and allows the aortic valve to close a bit earlier. When the aortic valve closes significantly earlier than the pulmonic valve, you can hear the two components separately. This is a *split* S_2.

Extra Heart Sounds

Third Heart Sound (S_3). Normally, diastole is a silent event. However, in some conditions, ventricular filling creates vibrations that can be heard over the chest. These vibrations are S_3. S_3 occurs when the ventricles are resistant to filling during the early rapid filling phase (protodiastole). This occurs immediately after S_2, when the AV valves open and atrial blood first pours into the ventricles. (See a complete discussion of S_3 in Table 19-7 on p. 490.)

Fourth Heart Sound (S_4). S_4 occurs at the end of diastole, at presystole, when the ventricle is resistant to filling. The

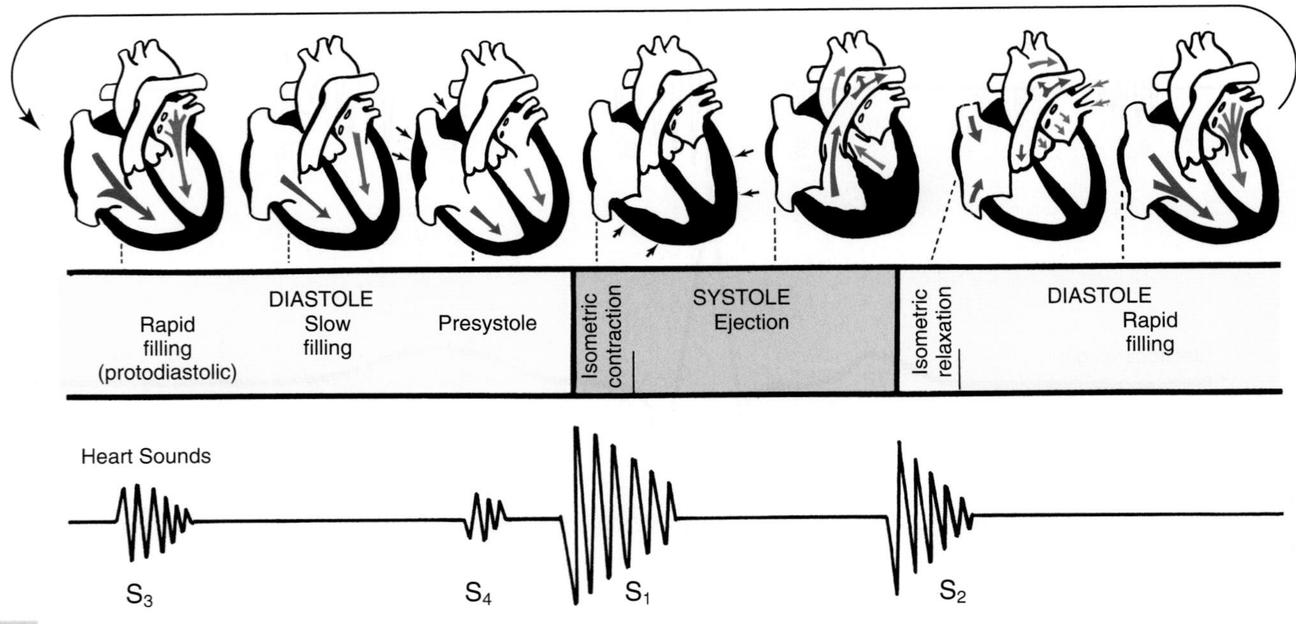

19-7

atria contract and push blood into a noncompliant ventricle. This creates vibrations that are heard as S_4. S_4 occurs just before S_1.

Murmurs

Blood circulating through normal cardiac chambers and valves usually makes no noise. However, some conditions create turbulent blood flow and collision currents. These result in a murmur, much like a pile of stones or a sharp turn in a stream creates a noisy water flow. A murmur is a gentle, blowing, swooshing sound that can be heard on the chest wall. Conditions resulting in a murmur are as follows:

1. Velocity of blood increases (flow murmur) (e.g., in exercise, thyrotoxicosis)
2. Viscosity of blood decreases (e.g., in anemia)
3. Structural defects in the valves (narrowed valve, incompetent valve) or unusual openings occur in the chambers (dilated chamber, wall defect)

Characteristics of Sound

All heart sounds are described by:

1. Frequency (pitch)—heart sounds are described as high pitched or low pitched, although these terms are relative because all are low-frequency sounds, and you need a good stethoscope to hear them
2. Intensity (loudness)—loud or soft
3. Duration—very short for heart sounds; silent periods are longer
4. Timing—systole or diastole

CONDUCTION

Of all organs, the heart has a unique ability—automaticity. The heart can contract by itself, independent of any signals or stimulation from the body. The heart contracts in response to an electrical current conveyed by a conduction system (Fig. 19-8). Specialized cells in the sinoatrial (SA) node near the superior vena cava initiate an electrical impulse. (Because the SA node has an intrinsic rhythm, it is the "pacemaker.") The current flows in an orderly sequence, first across the atria to the AV node low in the atrial septum. There it is delayed slightly so that the atria have time to contract before the ventricles are stimulated. Then the impulse travels to the bundle of His, the right and left bundle branches, and then through the ventricles.

The electrical impulse stimulates the heart to do its work, which is to contract. A small amount of electricity spreads to the body surface, where it can be measured and recorded on the electrocardiograph (ECG). The ECG waves are arbitrarily labeled *PQRST,* which stand for the following elements:

P wave—depolarization of the atria
PR interval—from the beginning of the P wave to the beginning of the QRS complex (the time necessary for atrial depolarization plus time for the impulse to travel through the AV node to the ventricles)
QRS complex—depolarization of the ventricles
T wave—repolarization of the ventricles

Electrical events slightly *precede* the mechanical events in the heart. The ECG juxtaposed on the cardiac cycle is illustrated in Fig. 19-6.

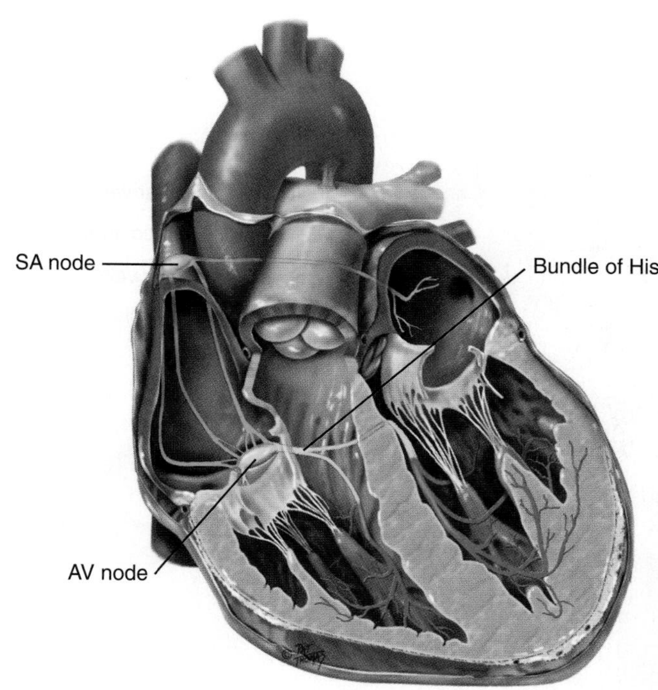

CONDUCTION SYSTEM

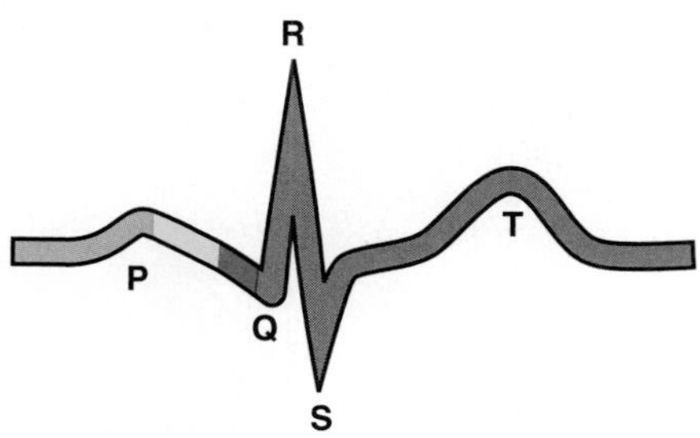

ELECTROCARDIOGRAPH (ECG) WAVE

19-8

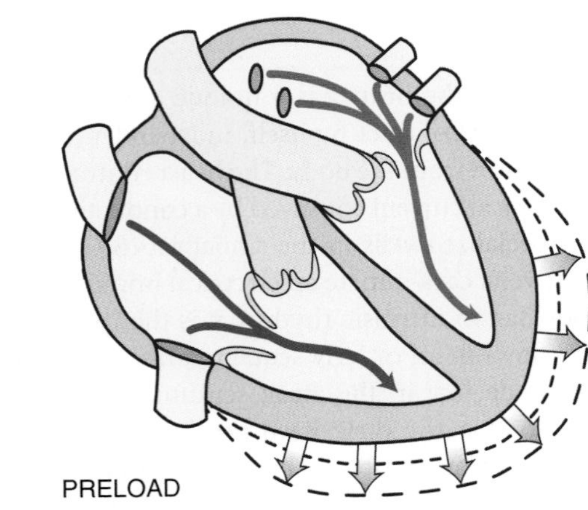

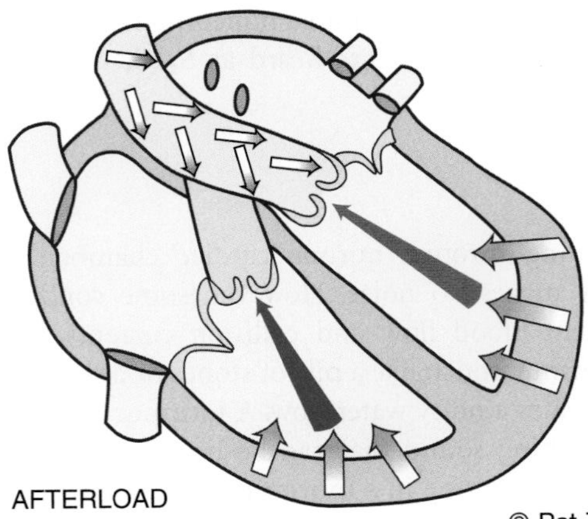

19-9

PUMPING ABILITY

In the resting adult, the heart normally pumps between 4 and 6 L of blood per minute throughout the body. This **cardiac output** equals the volume of blood in each systole (called the *stroke volume*) times the number of beats per minute (rate). This is described as:

$$CO = SV \times R$$

The heart can alter its cardiac output to adapt to the metabolic needs of the body. Preload and afterload affect the heart's ability to increase cardiac output.

Preload is the venous return that builds during diastole. It is the length to which the ventricular muscle is stretched at the end of diastole just before contraction (Fig. 19-9).

When the volume of blood returned to the ventricles is increased (as when exercise stimulates skeletal muscles to contract and force more blood back to the heart), the muscle bundles are stretched beyond their normal resting state to accommodate. The force of this switch is the preload. According to the Frank-Starling law, the greater the stretch, the stronger is the heart's contraction. This increased contractility results in an increased volume of blood ejected (increased stroke volume).

Afterload is the opposing pressure the ventricle must generate to open the aortic valve against the higher aortic pressure. It is the resistance against which the ventricle must pump its blood. Once the ventricle is filled with blood, the ventricular end diastolic pressure is 5 to 10 mm Hg, whereas that in the aorta is 70 to 80 mm Hg. To overcome this difference, the ventricular muscle *tenses* (isovolumic contraction). After the aortic valve opens, rapid ejection occurs.

THE NECK VESSELS

Cardiovascular assessment includes the survey of vascular structures in the neck—the carotid artery and the jugular veins (Fig. 19-10). These vessels reflect the efficiency of cardiac function.

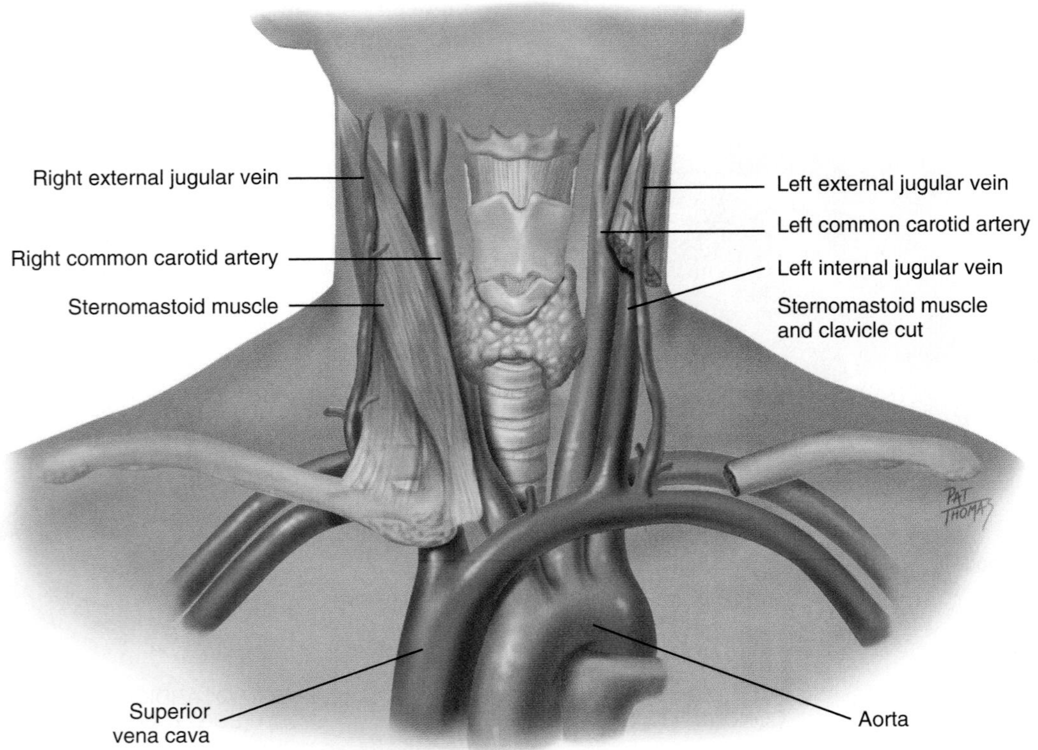

19-10 NECK VESSELS

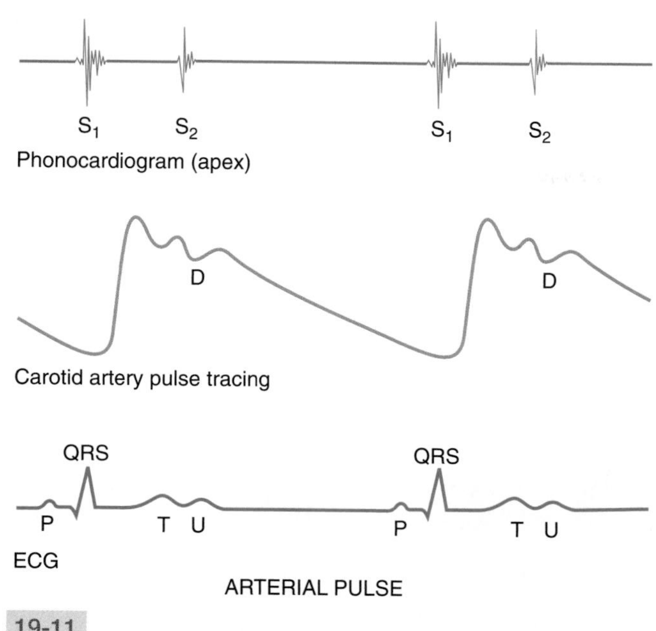

19-11

The Carotid Artery Pulse

Chapter 9 describes the pulse as a pressure wave generated by each systole pumping blood into the aorta. The carotid artery is a central artery—that is, it is close to the heart. Its timing closely coincides with ventricular systole. (Assessment of the peripheral pulses is found in Chapter 20, and blood pressure assessment is found in Chapter 9.)

The **carotid artery** is located in the groove between the trachea and the sternomastoid muscle, medial to and alongside that muscle. Note the characteristics of its waveform (Fig. 19-11): a smooth rapid upstroke, a summit that is rounded and smooth, and a downstroke that is more gradual and that has a dicrotic notch caused by closure of the aortic valve (marked *D* in the figure).

Jugular Venous Pulse and Pressure

The **jugular veins** empty unoxygenated blood directly into the superior vena cava. Because no cardiac valve exists to separate the superior vena cava from the right atrium, the jugular veins give information about activity on the right side of the heart. Specifically, they reflect filling pressure and volume changes. Because volume and pressure increase when the right side of the heart fails to pump efficiently, the jugular veins expose this.

Two jugular veins are present in each side of the neck (see Fig. 19-10). The larger **internal jugular** lies deep and medial to the sternomastoid muscle. It is usually not visible, although its diffuse pulsations may be seen in the sternal notch when the person is supine. The **external jugular** vein is more superficial; it lies lateral to the sternomastoid muscle, above the clavicle.

Although an arterial pulse is caused by a forward propulsion of blood, the jugular pulse is different. The jugular pulse results from a backwash, a waveform moving backward caused by events upstream. The jugular pulse has five components, as shown in Fig 19-12.

The five components of the jugular venous pulse occur because of events in the right side of the heart. The A wave reflects atrial contraction because some blood flows backward to the vena cava during right atrial contraction. The C wave, or ventricular contraction, is backflow from the bulging upward of the tricuspid valve when it closes at the beginning of ventricular systole (not from the neighboring carotid artery pulsation). Next, the X descent shows atrial relaxation when the right ventricle contracts during systole and pulls the bottom of the atria downward. The V wave occurs with passive atrial filling because of the increasing volume in the right atria and increased pressure. Finally, the Y descent reflects passive ventricular filling when the tricuspid valve opens and blood flows from the RA to the RV.

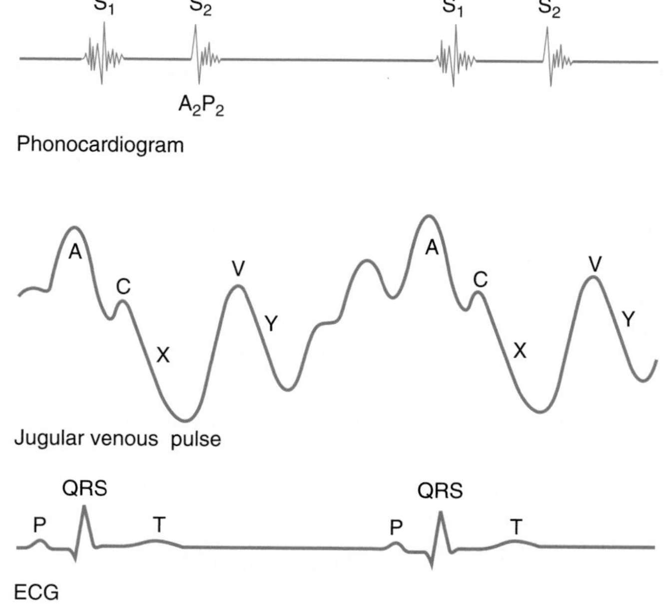

19-12

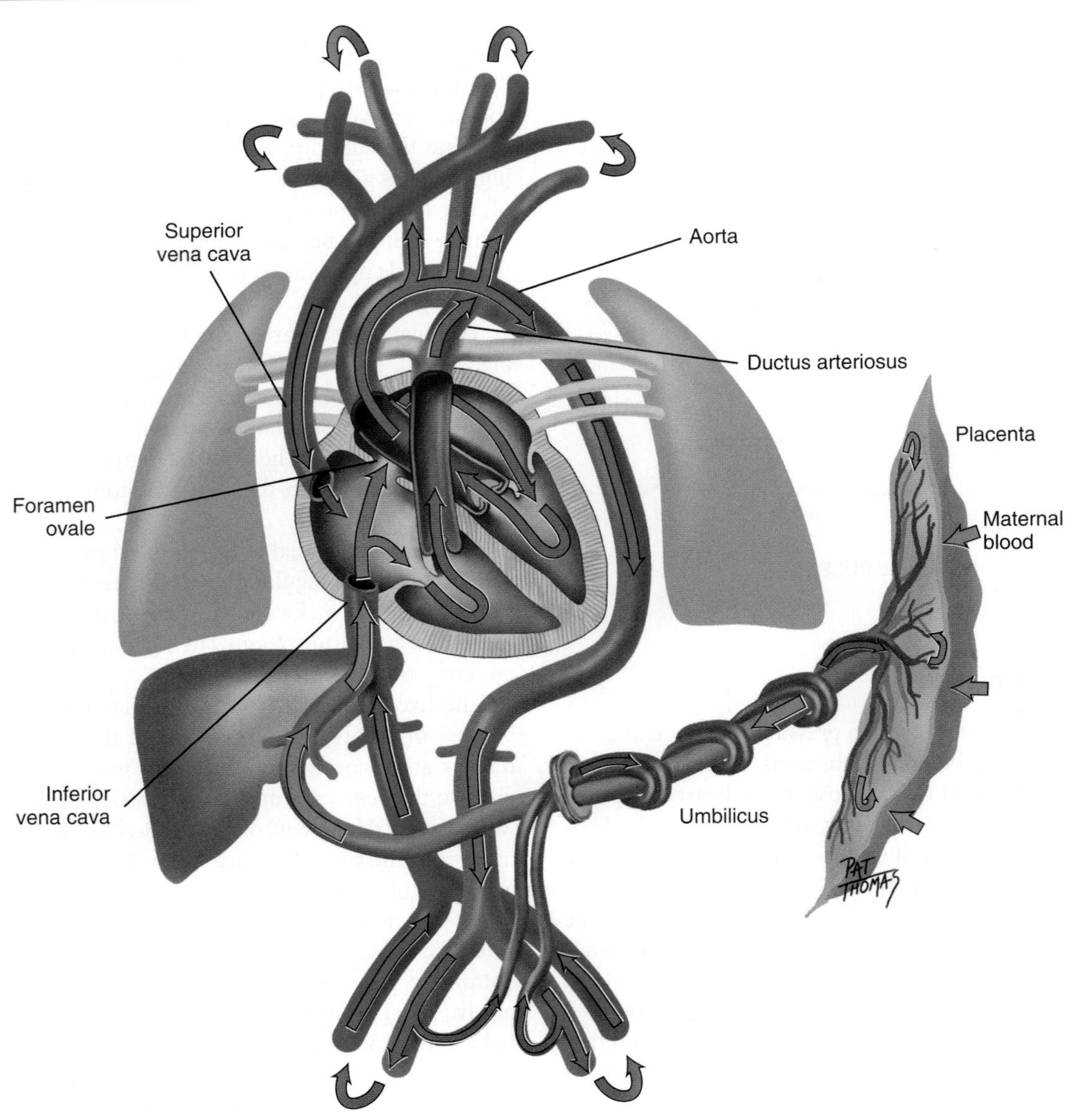

FETAL CIRCULATION

19-13

DEVELOPMENTAL COMPETENCE

Infants and Children

The fetal heart functions early; it begins to beat at the end of 3 weeks' gestation. The lungs are nonfunctional, but the fetal circulation compensates for this (Fig. 19-13). Oxygenation takes place at the placenta, and the arterial blood is returned to the right side of the fetal heart. There is no point in pumping all this freshly oxygenated blood through the lungs, so it is rerouted in two ways. First, about two thirds of it is shunted through an opening in the atrial septum, the **foramen ovale,** into the left side of the heart, where it is pumped out through the aorta. Second, the rest of the oxygenated blood is pumped by the right side of the heart out through the pulmonary artery, but it is detoured through the **ductus arteriosus** to the aorta. Because they are both pumping into the systemic circulation, the right and left ventricles are equal in weight and muscle wall thickness.

Inflation and aeration of the lungs at birth produces circulatory changes. Now the blood is oxygenated through the lungs rather than through the placenta. The foramen ovale closes within the first hour because of the new lower pressure in the right side of the heart than in the left side. The ductus arteriosus closes later, usually within 10 to 15 hours of birth. Now the left ventricle has the greater workload of pumping into the systemic circulation, so that when the baby has reached 1 year of age, the left ventricle's mass increases to reach the adult ratio of 2 : 1, left ventricle to right ventricle.

The heart's position in the chest is more horizontal in the infant than in the adult; thus the apex is higher, located at the fourth left intercostal space (Fig. 19-14). It reaches the adult position when the child reaches age 7 years.

The Pregnant Woman

Blood volume increases by 30% to 40% during pregnancy, with the most rapid expansion occurring during the second

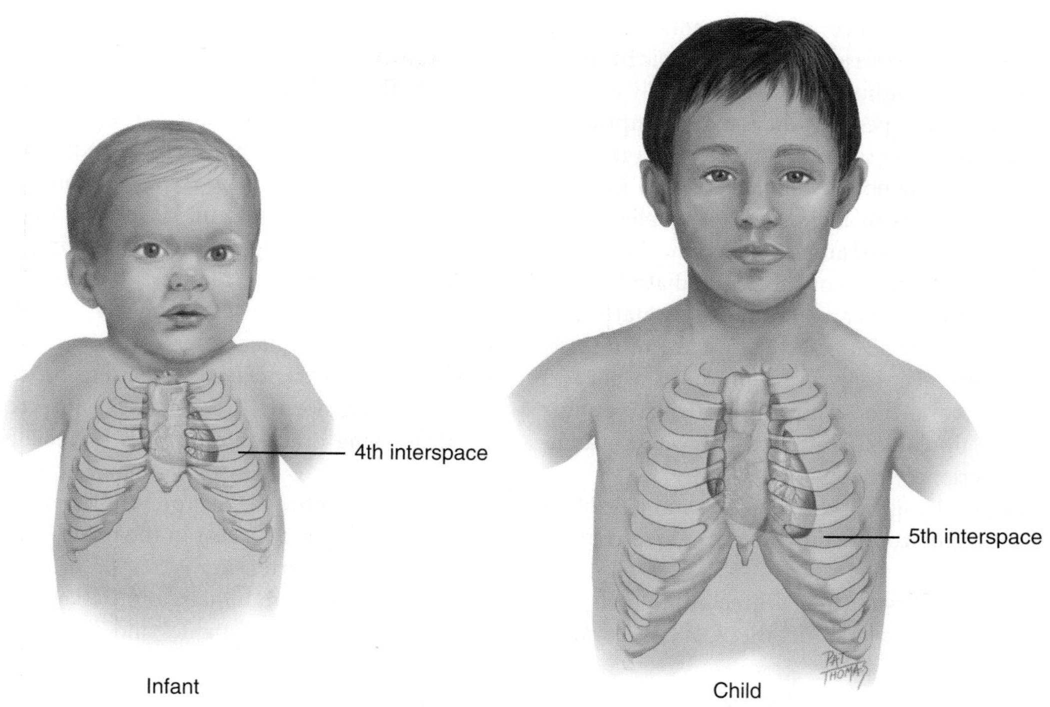

19-14

trimester. This creates an increase in stroke volume and cardiac output and an increased pulse rate of 10 to 15 beats per minute. Despite the increased cardiac output, arterial blood pressure decreases in pregnancy as a result of peripheral vasodilation. The blood pressure drops to its lowest point during the second trimester and then rises after that. The blood pressure varies with the person's position, as described on p. 483.

The Aging Adult

It is difficult to isolate the "aging process" of the cardiovascular system *per se* because it is so closely interrelated with lifestyle, habits, and diseases. We now know that lifestyle is a modifying factor in the development of cardiovascular disease; smoking, diet, alcohol use, exercise patterns, and stress have an influence on coronary artery disease. Lifestyle also affects the aging process; cardiac changes once thought to be due to aging are partially due to the sedentary lifestyle accompanying aging (Fig. 19-15). What is left to be attributed to the aging process alone?

Hemodynamic Changes with Aging

- With aging, there is an increase in systolic blood pressure (BP).[6] This is due to stiffening of the large arteries, which in turn is due to calcification of vessel walls (arteriosclerosis). This stiffening creates an increase in pulse wave velocity because the less compliant arteries cannot store the volume ejected.
- The overall size of the heart does not increase with age, but left ventricular wall thickness increases. This is an adaptive mechanism to accommodate the vascular stiffening mentioned earlier that creates an increased workload on the heart.
- No significant change in diastolic pressure occurs with age. A rising systolic pressure with a relatively constant diastolic pressure increases the pulse pressure (the difference between the two).
- No change in resting heart rate occurs with aging.
- Cardiac output at rest is not changed with aging.
- There is a decreased ability of the heart to augment cardiac output with exercise. This is shown by a decreased maximum heart rate with exercise and diminished sympathetic response. Noncardiac factors also cause a decrease in maximum work performance with aging: decrease in skeletal muscle performance, increase in muscle fatigue, increased sense of dyspnea. Chronic exercise conditioning will modify many of the aging changes in cardiovascular function.[32]

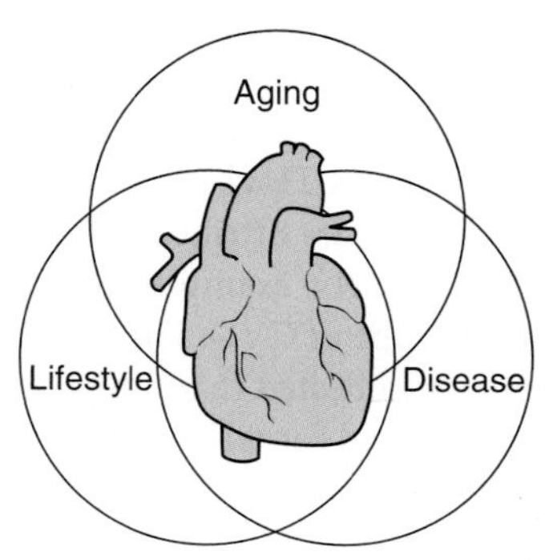

19-15

Dysrhythmias. The presence of supraventricular and ventricular dysrhythmias increases with age. Ectopic beats are common in aging people; although these are usually asymptomatic in healthy older people, they may compromise cardiac output and blood pressure when disease is present.

Tachydysrhythmias may not be tolerated as well in older people. The myocardium is thicker and less compliant, and early diastolic filling is impaired at rest. Thus it may not tolerate a tachycardia as well because of shortened diastole. Also, tachydysrhythmias may further compromise a vital organ whose function has already been affected by aging or disease. For example, a ventricular tachycardia produces a 40% to 70% decrease in cerebral blood flow. Although a younger person may tolerate this, an older person with cerebrovascular disease may experience syncope.[24a]

ECG. Age-related changes in the ECG occur as a result of histologic changes in the conduction system. These changes include:

- Prolonged P-R interval (first-degree AV block) and prolonged Q-T interval, but the QRS interval is unchanged
- Left axis deviation from age-related mild LV hypertrophy and fibrosis in left bundle branch
- Increased incidence of bundle branch block

Although the hemodynamic changes associated with aging alone do not seem severe or portentous, the fact remains that the incidence of cardiovascular disease increases with age. The incidence of coronary artery disease increases sharply with advancing age and accounts for about half of the deaths of older people. Hypertension (systolic >140 mm Hg and/or diastolic >90 mm Hg) and heart failure also increase with age. Certainly, lifestyle habits (smoking, chronic alcohol use, lack of exercise, diet) play a significant role in the acquisition of heart disease. Also, increasing the physical activity of older adults—even at a moderate level—is associated with a reduced risk of death from cardiovascular diseases and respiratory illnesses. Both points underscore the need for health teaching as an important treatment parameter.

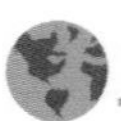

CULTURE AND GENETICS

Prevalence is an estimate of how many people in a stated geographic location have a disease at a given point in time. In the United States, an estimated 81 million people (more than 1 in 3) have one or more forms of cardiovascular heart disease (CVD).[3] The annual rates of first CVD event increase with age. For women, comparable rates occur 10 years later in life than for men, but this gap narrows with advancing age.

Causes of CVD include an interaction of genetic, environmental, and lifestyle factors. However, evidence shows potentially modifiable risk factors attribute to the overwhelming majority of cardiac risk. For example, myocardial infarction (MI) is an important type of CVD. The INTERHEART study covering 52 countries indicated that nine potentially modifiable risk factors accounted for 90% of the population attributable risk for MI in men and 94% in women![47] These nine modifiable risk factors include abnormal lipids, smoking, hypertension, diabetes, abdominal obesity, psychosocial factors, consumption of fruits and vegetables, alcohol use, and regular physical activity.

High Blood Pressure (HBP). Although all adults have some potential CVD risk, some groups (defined by race, ethnicity, gender, socioeconomic status, educational level) carry an excess burden of CVD. **Hypertension** is a systolic blood pressure (SBP) of ≥140 mm Hg or diastolic blood pressure (DBP) of ≥90 mm Hg or currently taking antihypertensive medicine. A higher percentage of men than women have hypertension until age 45 years. From age 45 to 64 years, the percentages are similar; after age 64 years, women have a much higher percentage of hypertension than men have.[3] Also, hypertension is 2 to 3 times more common among women taking oral contraceptives (especially among obese and older women) than in women who do not take them. Among racial groups, the prevalence of hypertension in Blacks is among the highest in the world and it is rising. The prevalence of hypertension is 31.8% for African Americans, 25.3% for American Indians or Alaska natives, 23.3% for whites, and 21% for Hispanics and Asians.[3] Compared with whites, African Americans develop HBP earlier in life and their average BPs are much higher. This results in African Americans having a greater rate of stroke, death due to heart disease, and end-stage kidney disease.

Smoking. In the 40+ years from 1965 to 2004, U.S. smoking rates declined by 50.4% among adults 18 years of age and older.[33] This results in 2008 with 23.1% of men and 18.3% of women being smokers. Nicotine increases the risk of MI and stroke by causing the following: increase in oxygen demand with a concomitant decrease in oxygen supply; an activation of platelets, activation of fibrinogen; and an adverse change in the lipid profile.

Serum Cholesterol. High levels of low-density lipoprotein gradually add to the lipid core of thrombus formation in arteries, which results in MI and stroke. The current cutpoints for cholesterol risk in adults are the following: total cholesterol levels of ≥240 mg/dL are high risk; and levels from 200 to 239 mg/dL are borderline–high risk. The age-adjusted prevalence of total cholesterol levels over 200 mg/dL are as follows: 51.1% of Mexican-American men and 49% of Mexican-American women; 45% of white men and 48.7% of white women; and 40.2% of African American men and 41.8% of African American women.[3]

Obesity. The epidemic of obesity in the United States is well known and is referenced in many chapters of this text. Among Americans ages 20 years and older, the prevalence of overweight or obesity (body mass index [BMI] of ≥25 kg/m^2 for overweight and ≥30.0 for obesity) is as follows: 74.8% of Mexican-American men and 73% of Mexican-American women; 73.7% of African American men and 77.7% of African American women; and 72.4% of white men and 57.5% of white women.

Type 2 Diabetes Mellitus. The risk of CVD is twofold greater among persons with diabetes mellitus (DM) than without DM. The increased prevalence of DM in the United States is being followed by an increasing prevalence of CVD morbidity and mortality.[3] Diabetes causes damage to the large blood vessels that nourish the brain, heart, and extremities; this results in stroke, coronary artery disease, and peripheral vascular disease.

About 13% of African Americans 20 years of age and older have DM. Between 11.8% and 13.1% of Mexican Americans have DM, compared with 6.4% of whites.[3] The most powerful predictor of type 2 DM is obesity, with abdominal (visceral) fat posing a greater risk than lower body obesity poses. Evidence from epidemiologic studies shows a strong genetic factor for DM, but no specific antigen type has yet been identified. In the past, type 2 DM was diagnosed in adults 40 years of age and older, but now we are finding more children with type 2 DM. These children are usually overweight or obese, have a family history of DM, and identify with American Indian, African American, Hispanic, or Asian groups.[3]

SUBJECTIVE DATA

1. Chest pain
2. Dyspnea
3. Orthopnea
4. Cough
5. Fatigue
6. Cyanosis or pallor
7. Edema
8. Nocturia
9. Past cardiac history
10. Family cardiac history
11. Personal habits (cardiac risk factors)

Examiner Asks	Rationale
1. Chest pain. Any **chest pain** or tightness? • Onset: When did it start? How long have you had it *this* time? Had this type of pain before? How often? • Location: Where did the pain start? Does the pain radiate to any other spot? • Character: How would you describe it? Crushing, stabbing, burning, viselike? (Allow the person to offer adjectives before you suggest them.)	Angina, an important cardiac symptom, occurs when the heart's own blood supply cannot keep up with metabolic demand. Chest pain also may have pulmonary, musculoskeletal, or gastrointestinal origin; it is important to differentiate.
(Note if uses clenched fist to describe pain.)	A squeezing "clenched fist" sign is characteristic of angina, but the symptoms below may be anginal equivalents in the absence of chest pain.[37a]
• Pain brought on by: Activity—what type; rest; emotional upset; after eating; during sexual intercourse; with cold weather?	
• Any associated symptoms: Sweating, ashen gray or pale skin, heart skips beat, shortness of breath, nausea or vomiting, racing of heart?	Diaphoresis, cold sweats, pallor, grayness. Palpitations, dyspnea, nausea, tachycardia, fatigue.
• Pain made worse by moving the arms or neck, breathing, lying flat?	Try to differentiate pain of cardiac versus noncardiac origin.
• Pain relieved by rest or nitroglycerin? How many tablets?	
2. Dyspnea. Any shortness of breath? • What type of activity and how much brings on shortness of breath? How much activity brought it on 6 months ago?	**Dyspnea** on exertion (DOE)—quantify exactly (e.g., DOE after walking two level blocks).
• Onset: Does the shortness of breath come on unexpectedly?	Paroxysmal.
• Duration: Constant or does it come and go?	Constant or intermittent.
• Seem to be affected by position: Lying down?	Recumbent.
• Awaken you from sleep at night?	Paroxysmal nocturnal dyspnea (PND) occurs with heart failure. Lying down increases volume of intrathoracic blood, and the weakened heart cannot accommodate the increased load. Typically, the person awakens after 2 hours of sleep with the perception of needing fresh air.
• Does the shortness of breath interfere with activities of daily living?	
3. Orthopnea. How many pillows do you use when sleeping or lying down?	Orthopnea is the need to assume a more upright position to breathe. Note the exact number of pillows used.

Examiner Asks	Rationale
4. **Cough.** Do you have a **cough?** • Duration: How long have you had it? • Frequency: Is it related to time of day? • Type: Dry, hacking, barky, hoarse, or congested? • Do you cough up mucus? Color? Any odor? Blood tinged?	Sputum production, mucoid or purulent. Hemoptysis is often a pulmonary disorder but also occurs with mitral stenosis.
• Associated with: Activity, position (lying down), anxiety, talking? • Does activity make it better or worse (sit, walk, exercise)? • Relieved by rest or medication?	
5. **Fatigue.** Do you seem to tire easily? Able to keep up with your family and co-workers? • Onset: When did fatigue start? Sudden or gradual? Has any *recent* change occurred in energy level? • Fatigue related to time of day: All day, morning, evening?	Fatigue from decreased cardiac output is worse in the evening, whereas fatigue from anxiety or depression occurs all day or is worse in the morning.
6. **Cyanosis or pallor.** Ever noted your facial skin turn blue or ashen?	**Cyanosis** or **pallor** occurs with myocardial infarction or low cardiac output states as a result of decreased tissue perfusion.
7. **Edema.** Any swelling of your feet and legs?	**Edema** is dependent when caused by heart failure.
• Onset: When did you first notice this? • Any recent change? • What time of day does the swelling occur? Do your shoes feel tight at the end of day?	Cardiac edema is worse at evening and better in morning after elevating legs all night.
• How much swelling would you say there is? Are both legs equally swollen?	Cardiac edema is bilateral; unilateral swelling has a local vein cause.
• Does the swelling go away with: Rest, elevation, after a night's sleep? • Any associated symptoms, such as shortness of breath? If so, does the shortness of breath occur before leg swelling or after?	
8. **Nocturia.** Do you awaken at night with an urgent need to urinate? How long has this been occurring? Any recent change?	**Nocturia**—Recumbency at night promotes fluid reabsorption and excretion; this occurs with heart failure in the person who is ambulatory during the day.
9. **Cardiac history.** Any **past history** of: Hypertension, elevated cholesterol or triglycerides, heart murmur, congenital heart disease, rheumatic fever or unexplained joint pains as child or youth, recurrent tonsillitis, anemia? • Ever had heart disease? When was this? Treated by medication or heart surgery? • Last ECG, stress ECG, serum cholesterol measurement, other heart tests?	
10. **Family cardiac history.** Any **family history** of: Hypertension, obesity, diabetes, coronary artery disease (CAD), sudden death at younger age?	
11. **Personal habits (cardiac risk factors).** • Nutrition: Please describe your usual daily diet. (Note if this diet is representative of the basic food groups, the amount of calories, cholesterol,	

Examiner Asks	Rationale
and any additives such as salt.) What is your usual weight? Has there been any recent change? • Smoking: Do you smoke cigarettes or other tobacco? At what age did you start? How many packs per day? For how many years have you smoked this amount? Have you ever tried to quit? If so, how did this go? • Alcohol: How much alcohol do you usually drink each week, or each day? When was your last drink? What was the number of drinks during that episode? Have you ever been told you had a drinking problem? • Exercise: What is your usual amount of exercise each day or week? What type of exercise (state type or sport)? If a sport, what is your usual amount (light, moderate, heavy)? • Drugs: Do you take any antihypertensives, beta-blockers, calcium channel blockers, digoxin, diuretics, aspirin/anticoagulants, over-the-counter or street drugs?	**Risk factors for CAD**—Collect data regarding elevated cholesterol, elevated blood pressure, blood sugar levels above 130 mg/dL or known diabetes mellitus, obesity, cigarette smoking, low activity level, and length of any hormone replacement therapy for postmenopausal women.
Additional History for Infants	
1. How was the mother's health during pregnancy: Any unexplained fever, rubella first trimester, other infection, hypertension, drugs taken?	
2. Have you noted any cyanosis while nursing, crying? Is the baby able to eat, nurse, or finish bottle without tiring?	To screen for heart disease in infant, note fatigue during feeding. Infant with heart failure takes fewer ounces each feeding; becomes dyspneic with sucking; may be diaphoretic, then falls into exhausted sleep; awakens after a short time hungry again.
3. **Growth:** Has this baby grown as expected by growth charts and about the same as siblings or peers?	Poor weight gain.
4. **Activity:** Were this baby's motor milestones achieved as expected? Is the baby able to play without tiring? How many naps does the baby take each day? How long does a nap last?	
Additional History for Children	
1. **Growth:** Has this child grown as expected by growth charts?	Poor weight gain.
2. **Activity:** Is this child able to keep up with siblings or age mates? Is the child willing or reluctant to go out to play? Is the child able to climb stairs, ride a bike, walk a few blocks? Does the child squat to rest during play or to watch television, or assume a knee-chest position while sleeping? Have you noted "blue spells" during exercise?	Fatigue. Record specific limitations. Cyanosis.
3. Has the child had any unexplained joint pains or unexplained fever?	
4. Does the child have frequent headaches, nosebleeds?	
5. Does the child have frequent respiratory infections? How many per year? How are they treated? Have any of these proved to be streptococcal infections?	
6. **Family history:** Does the child have a sibling with heart defect? Is anyone in the child's family known to have chromosomal abnormalities, such as Down syndrome?	

Examiner Asks	Rationale

Additional History for the Pregnant Woman

1. Have you had any high blood pressure during this or earlier pregnancies?
   - What was your usual blood pressure level before pregnancy? How has your blood pressure been monitored during the pregnancy?
   - If high blood pressure, what treatment has been started?
   - Any associated symptoms: Weight gain, protein in urine, swelling in feet, legs, or face?
2. Have you had any faintness or dizziness with this pregnancy?

Additional History for the Aging Adult

1. Do you have any known heart or lung disease: Hypertension, CAD, chronic emphysema, or bronchitis?
   - What efforts to treat this have been started?
   - Usual symptoms changed recently? Does your illness interfere with activities of daily living?
2. Do you take any medications for your illness such as digitalis? Aware of side effects? Have you recently stopped taking your medication? Why?

   Rationale: Noncompliance may be related to side effects or lack of finances.
3. **Environment:** Does your home have any stairs? How often do you need to climb them? Does this have any effect on activities of daily living?

OBJECTIVE DATA

PREPARATION

To evaluate the carotid arteries, the person can be sitting up. To assess the jugular veins and the precordium, the person should be supine with the head and chest slightly elevated.

Stand on the person's right side; this will facilitate your hand placement, viewing of the neck veins, and auscultation of the precordium.

The room must be warm—chilling makes the person uncomfortable, and shivering interferes with heart sounds. Take scrupulous care to ensure *quiet;* heart sounds are very soft, and any ambient room noise masks them.

Ensure the female's privacy by keeping her breasts draped. The female's left breast overrides part of the area you will need to examine. Gently displace the breast upward, or ask the woman to hold it out of the way.

When performing a regional cardiovascular assessment, use this order:

1. Pulse and blood pressure (see Chapter 9)
2. Extremities (see Peripheral Vascular Assessment in Chapter 20)
3. Neck vessels
4. Precordium

The logic of this order is that you will begin observations peripherally and move in toward the heart. For choreography of these steps in the complete physical examination, see Chapter 27.

EQUIPMENT NEEDED

Marking pen
Small centimeter ruler
Stethoscope with diaphragm and bell endpieces
Alcohol wipe (to clean endpiece)

Normal Range of Findings	Abnormal Findings

THE NECK VESSELS

Palpate the Carotid Artery

Located central to the heart, the carotid artery yields important information on cardiac function.

Normal Range of Findings	Abnormal Findings

Palpate each carotid artery medial to the sternomastoid muscle in the neck (Fig. 19-16). Avoid excessive pressure on the carotid sinus area higher in the neck; excessive vagal stimulation here could slow down the heart rate, especially in older adults. Take care to palpate gently. Palpate only one carotid artery at a time to avoid compromising arterial blood to the brain.

Carotid sinus hypersensitivity is the condition in which pressure over the carotid sinus leads to a decreased heart rate, decreased BP, and cerebral ischemia with syncope. This may occur in older adults with hypertension or occlusion of the carotid artery.

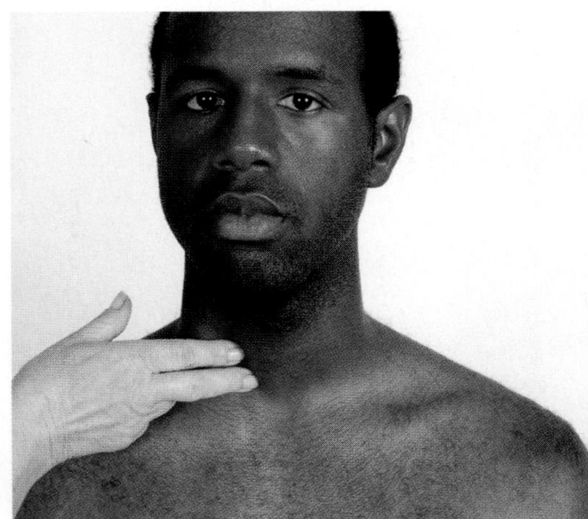

19-16

Feel the contour and amplitude of the pulse. Normally the contour is smooth with a rapid upstroke and slower downstroke, and the normal strength is 2+ or moderate (see Chapter 20). Your findings should be the same bilaterally.

Diminished pulse feels small and weak (decreased stroke volume).

Increased pulse feels full and strong in hyperkinetic states (see Table 20-1, Variations in Pulse Contour, on p. 519).

Auscultate the Carotid Artery

For persons middle-aged or older or who show symptoms or signs of cardiovascular disease, auscultate each carotid artery for the presence of a **bruit** (pronounced bru′-ee) (Fig. 19-17). This is a blowing, swishing sound indicating blood flow turbulence; normally none is present.

A bruit indicates turbulence due to a local vascular cause, such as atherosclerotic narrowing.

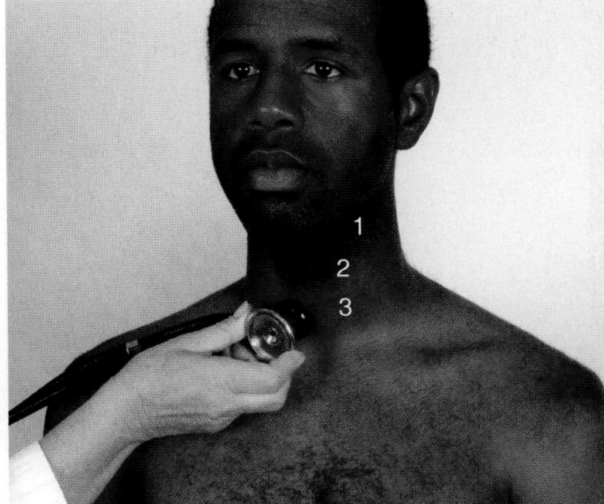

19-17

Keep the neck in a neutral position. Lightly apply the bell of the stethoscope over the carotid artery at three levels: (1) the angle of the jaw, (2) the midcervical area, and (3) the base of the neck (see Fig. 19-17). Avoid compressing the artery because this could create an artificial bruit, and it could compromise circulation if the carotid artery is already narrowed by atherosclerosis. Ask the person to take a breath, exhale, and hold it briefly while you listen so that tracheal breath sounds do not mask or mimic a carotid artery bruit. (Holding the breath on inhalation will also tense the levator scapulae muscles, which makes it hard to hear the carotids.) Sometimes you can hear normal heart sounds transmitted to the neck; do not confuse these with a bruit.

A carotid bruit is audible when the lumen is occluded by ½ to ⅔. Bruit loudness increases as the atherosclerosis worsens until the lumen is occluded by ⅔. After that, bruit loudness decreases. When the lumen is completely occluded, the bruit disappears. Thus absence of a bruit does not ensure absence of a carotid lesion.

Objective Data

Normal Range of Findings

Abnormal Findings

A murmur sounds much the same but is caused by a cardiac disorder. Some aortic valve murmurs (aortic stenosis) radiate to the neck and must be distinguished from a local bruit.

Inspect the Jugular Venous Pulse

From the jugular veins you can assess the **central venous pressure** (CVP) and thus judge the heart's efficiency as a pump. Stand on the person's right side because the veins there have a direct route to the heart. Traditionally we have been taught to use the internal jugular vein pulsations for CVP assessment. However, you may use either the external or the internal jugular veins because measurements in both are similar.[27] You can see the top of the external jugular vein distention overlying the sternomastoid muscle or the pulsation of the internal jugular vein in the sternal notch.

Position the person supine anywhere from a 30- to a 45-degree angle, wherever you can best see the top of the vein or pulsations. In general, the higher the venous pressure is, the higher the position you need. Remove the pillow to avoid flexing the neck; the head should be in the same plane as the trunk. Turn the person's head slightly away from the examined side, and direct a strong light tangentially onto the neck to highlight pulsations and shadows.

Note the external jugular veins overlying the sternomastoid muscle. In some persons, the veins are not visible at all, whereas in others they are full in the supine position. As the person is raised to a sitting position, these external jugulars flatten and disappear, usually at 45 degrees.

Unilateral distention of external jugular veins is due to local cause (kinking or aneurysm).

Full distended external jugular veins above 45 degrees signify increased CVP as with heart failure.

Now look for pulsations of the internal jugular veins in the area of the suprasternal notch or around the origin of the sternomastoid muscle around the clavicle. You must be able to distinguish internal jugular vein pulsation from that of the carotid artery. It is easy to confuse them because they lie close together. Use the guidelines shown in Table 19-1.

TABLE 19-1 Characteristics of Jugular Versus Carotid Pulsations

	Internal Jugular Pulse	Carotid Pulse
1. Location	Lower, more lateral, under or behind the sternomastoid muscle	Higher and medial to this muscle
2. Quality	Undulant and diffuse, two visible waves per cycle	Brisk and localized, one wave per cycle
3. Respiration	Varies with respiration; its level descends during inspiration when intrathoracic pressure is decreased	Does not vary
4. Palpable	No	Yes
5. Pressure	Light pressure at the base of the neck easily obliterates	No change
6. Position of person	Level of pulse drops and disappears as the person is brought to a sitting position	Unaffected

Normal Range of Findings	Abnormal Findings

Estimate the Jugular Venous Pressure

Think of the jugular veins as a CVP manometer attached directly to the right atrium. You can "read" the CVP at the highest level of pulsations (Fig. 19-18). Use the angle of Louis (sternal angle) as an arbitrary reference point, and compare it with the highest level of the distended vein or venous pulsation.

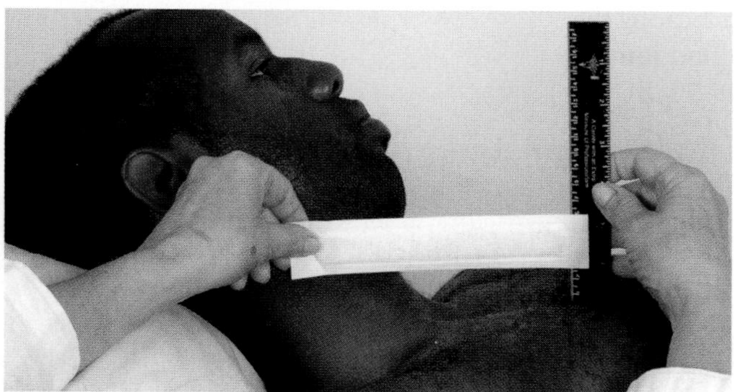

19-18

Hold a vertical ruler on the sternal angle. Align a straight edge on the ruler like a T-square, and adjust the level of the horizontal straight edge to the level of pulsation. Read the level of intersection on the vertical ruler; normal jugular venous pulsation is 2 cm or less above the sternal angle. Also state the person's position, for example, "internal jugular vein pulsations 3 cm above sternal angle when elevated 30 degrees."

Elevated pressure is a level of pulsation that is more than 3 cm above the sternal angle while at 45 degrees. This occurs with heart failure.

If you cannot find the internal jugular veins, use the external jugular veins and note the point where they look collapsed. Be aware that the technique of estimating venous pressure is difficult and is not always a reliable predictor of CVP. Consistency in grading among examiners is difficult to achieve.

If venous pressure is elevated or if you suspect heart failure, perform **hepatojugular reflux** (Fig. 19-19). Position the person comfortably supine, and instruct him or her to breathe quietly through an open mouth. Hold your right hand on the right upper quadrant of the person's abdomen just below the rib cage. Watch the level of jugular pulsation as you push in with your hand. Exert firm sustained pressure for 30 seconds. This displaces venous blood out of the liver sinusoids and adds its volume to the venous system. If the heart is able to pump this additional volume (i.e., if no elevated CVP is present), the jugular veins will rise for a few seconds and then recede back to the previous level.

If heart failure is present, the jugular veins will elevate and stay elevated as long as you push.

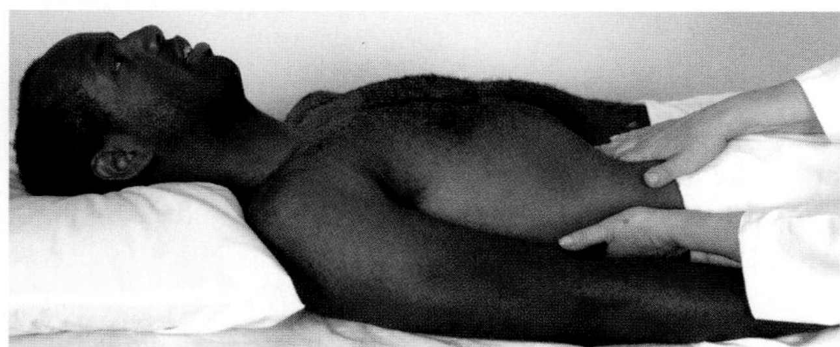

19-19
Hepatojugular reflux.

THE PRECORDIUM

Inspect the Anterior Chest

Arrange tangential lighting to accentuate any flicker of movement.

Pulsations. You may or may not see the **apical impulse,** the pulsation created as the left ventricle rotates against the chest wall during systole. When visible, it occupies the fourth or fifth intercostal space, at or inside the midclavicular line. It is easier to see in children and in those with thinner chest walls.

A **heave** or **lift** is a sustained forceful thrusting of the ventricle during systole. It occurs with ventricular hypertrophy as a result of increased workload. A right ventricular heave is seen at the sternal border; a left ventricular heave is seen at the apex (see Table 19-8, Abnormal Pulsations on the Precordium, p. 492).

Normal Range of Findings	Abnormal Findings

Palpate the Apical Impulse

(This used to be called the *point of maximal impulse,* or *PMI.* Because some abnormal conditions may cause a maximal impulse to be felt elsewhere on the chest, use the term **apical impulse** specifically for the apex beat.)

Localize the apical impulse precisely by using one finger pad (Fig. 19-20, *A*). Asking the person to "exhale and then hold it" aids the examiner in locating the pulsation. You may need to roll the person midway to the left to find it; note that this also displaces the apical impulse farther to the left (Fig. 19-20, *B*).

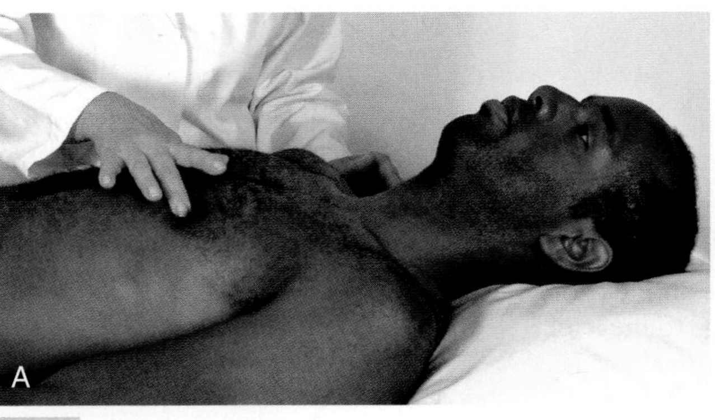

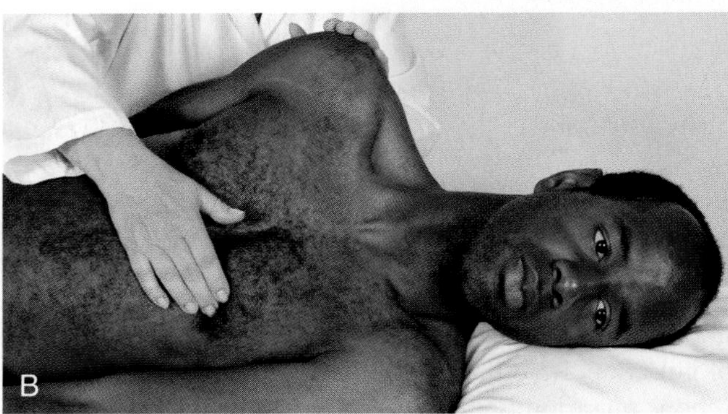

19-20 The apical impulse.

Note:

- *Location*—The apical impulse should occupy only one interspace, the fourth or fifth, and be at or medial to the midclavicular line
- *Size*—Normally 1 × 2 cm
- *Amplitude*—Normally a short, gentle tap
- *Duration*—Short, normally occupies only first half of systole

Cardiac enlargement:

- Left ventricular dilation (volume overload) displaces impulse down and to left and increases size more than one space.
- A **sustained** impulse with increased force and duration but no change in location occurs with left ventricular hypertrophy and no dilation (pressure overload) (see Table 19-8).

The apical impulse is palpable in about half of adults. It is not palpable in obese persons or in persons with thick chest walls. With high cardiac output states (anxiety, fever, hyperthyroidism, anemia), the apical impulse increases in amplitude and duration.

Not palpable with pulmonary emphysema due to overriding lungs.

Palpate Across the Precordium

Using the palmar aspects of your four fingers, gently palpate the apex, the left sternal border, and the base, searching for any other pulsations (Fig. 19-21). Normally none occur. If any are present, note the timing. Use the carotid artery pulsation as a guide, or auscultate as you palpate.

A **thrill** is a palpable vibration. It feels like the throat of a purring cat. The thrill signifies turbulent blood flow and accompanies loud murmurs. Absence of a thrill, however, does not necessarily rule out the presence of a murmur.

Accentuated first and second heart sounds and extra heart sounds also may cause abnormal pulsations.

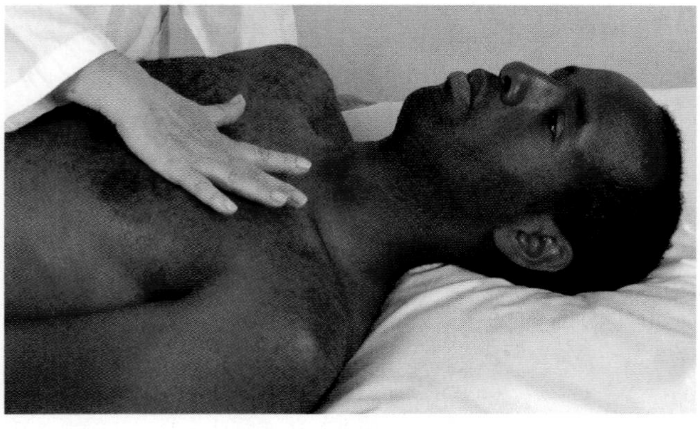

19-21

Normal Range of Findings

Percussion

Percussion is used to outline the heart's borders, but it has been displaced by the chest x-ray or echocardiogram. Evidence shows these are more accurate in detecting heart enlargement. When the right ventricle enlarges, it does so in the anteroposterior diameter, which is better seen on x-ray film. Evidence from numerous comparison studies shows the percussed cardiac border correlates "only moderately" with the true cardiac border.[27] Also, percussion is of limited usefulness with the female breast tissue or in an obese person or a person with a muscular chest wall.

Auscultation

Identify the auscultatory areas where you will listen. These include the four traditional valve "areas" (Fig. 19-22). The valve areas are not over the actual anatomic locations of the valves but are the sites on the chest wall where sounds produced by the valves are best heard. The sound radiates with the direction of blood flow.

Abnormal Findings

Cardiac enlargement is due to increased ventricular volume or wall thickness; it occurs with hypertension, CAD, heart failure, and cardiomyopathy.

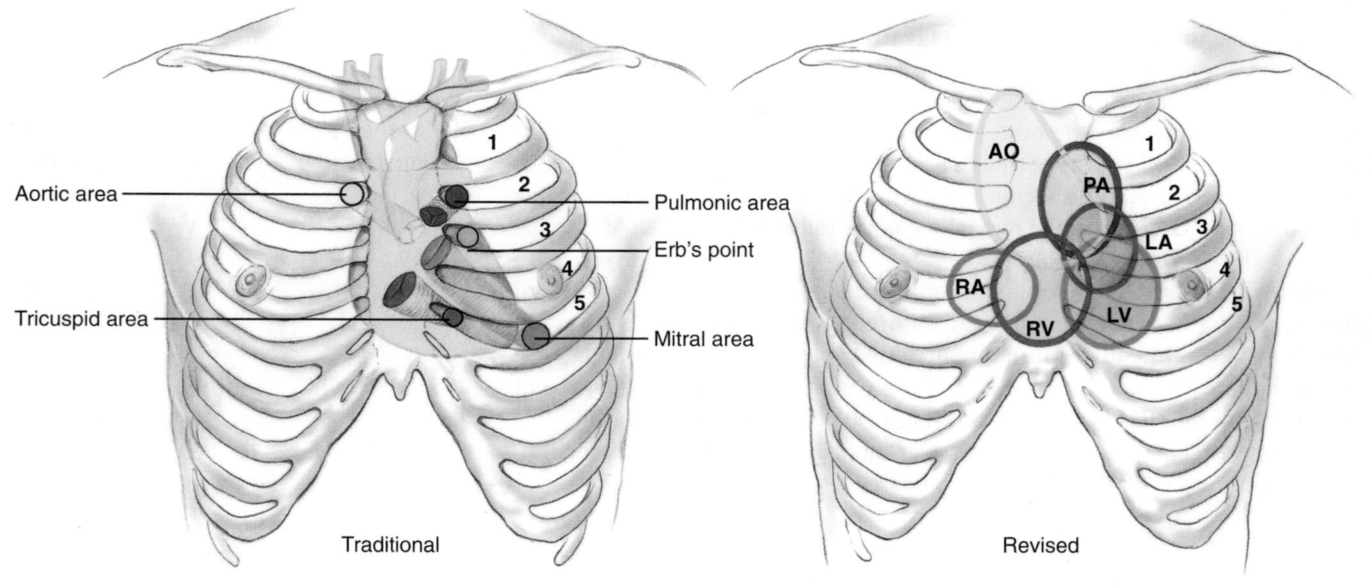

19-22

The valve areas are:

- Second right interspace—aortic valve area
- Second left interspace—pulmonic valve area
- Left lower sternal border—tricuspid valve area
- Fifth interspace at around left midclavicular line—mitral valve area

Do not limit your auscultation to only four locations. Sounds produced by the valves may be heard all over the precordium. (For this reason, many experts even discourage the naming of the valve areas.) Thus learn to inch your stethoscope in a rough Z pattern, from the base of the heart across and down, then over to the apex. Or start at the apex and work your way up. Include the sites shown in Fig. 19-22.

Normal Range of Findings

Recall the characteristics of a good stethoscope (see Chapter 8). Clean the endpieces with an alcohol wipe; you will use both endpieces. Although all heart sounds are low frequency, the diaphragm is for relatively higher pitched sounds and the bell is for relatively lower pitched ones.

Before you begin, alert the person: "I always listen to the heart in a number of places on the chest. Just because I am listening a long time, it does not necessarily mean that something is wrong."

After you place the stethoscope, try closing your eyes briefly to tune out any distractions. Concentrate, and listen selectively to *one sound at a time.* Consider that at least two, and perhaps three or four, sounds may be happening in less than 1 second. You cannot process everything at once. Begin with the diaphragm endpiece and use the following routine: (1) note the rate and rhythm, (2) identify S_1 and S_2, (3) assess S_1 and S_2 separately, (4) listen for extra heart sounds, and (5) listen for murmurs.

Note the Rate and Rhythm. The rate ranges normally from 50 to 90 beats per minute. (Review the full discussion of the pulse in Chapter 9 and the normal rates across age-groups.) The rhythm should be regular, although **sinus arrhythmia** occurs normally in young adults and children. With sinus arrhythmia, the rhythm varies with the person's breathing, increasing at the peak of inspiration and slowing with expiration. Note any other irregular rhythm. If one occurs, check if it has any pattern or if it is totally irregular.

When you notice any irregularity, check for a **pulse deficit** by auscultating the apical beat while simultaneously palpating the radial pulse. Count a serial measurement (one after the other) of apical beat and radial pulse. Normally, every beat you hear at the apex should perfuse to the periphery and be palpable. The two counts should be identical. When different, subtract the radial rate from the apical and record the remainder as the pulse deficit.

Identify S_1 and S_2. This is important because S_1 is the start of systole and thus serves as the reference point for the timing of all other cardiac sounds. Usually, you can identify S_1 instantly because you hear a pair of sounds close together (lub-dup), and S_1 is the first of the pair. This guideline works, except in the cases of the tachydysrhythmias (rates >100 per minute). Then the diastolic filling time is shortened, and the beats are too close together to distinguish. Other guidelines to distinguish S_1 from S_2 are:

- S_1 is louder than S_2 at the apex; S_2 is louder than S_1 at the base.
- S_1 coincides with the carotid artery pulse. Feel the carotid gently as you auscultate at the apex; the sound you hear as you feel each pulse is S_1 (Fig. 19-23).
- S_1 coincides with the R wave (the upstroke of the QRS complex) if the person is on an ECG monitor.

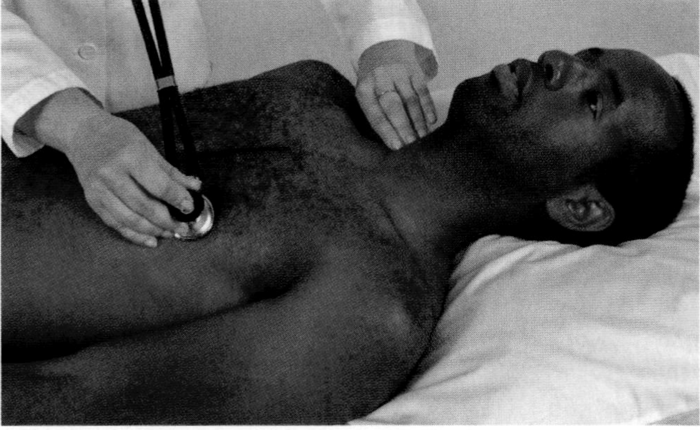

19-23

Abnormal Findings

Premature beat—an isolated beat is early, or a pattern occurs in which every third or fourth beat sounds early.

Irregularly irregular—no pattern to the sounds; beats come rapidly and at random intervals.

A **pulse deficit** signals a weak contraction of the ventricles; it occurs with atrial fibrillation, premature beats, and heart failure.

Normal Range of Findings	Abnormal Findings

Listen to S_1 and S_2 Separately. Note whether each heart sound is normal, accentuated, diminished, or split. Inch your diaphragm across the chest as you do this.

First Heart Sound (S_1). Caused by closure of the AV valves, S_1 signals the beginning of systole. You can hear it over the entire precordium, although it is loudest at the apex (Fig. 19-24). (Sometimes the two sounds are equally loud at the apex, because S_1 is lower pitched than S_2.)

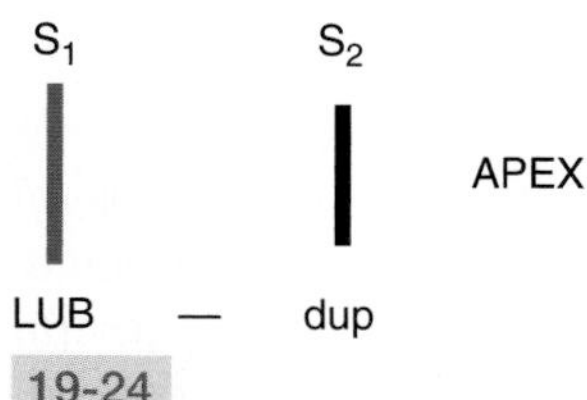

19-24

Causes of accentuated or diminished **S_1** (see Table 19-3, Variations in S_1, on p. 487).

Both heart sounds are diminished with conditions that place an increased amount of tissue between the heart and your stethoscope: emphysema (hyperinflated lungs), obesity, pericardial fluid.

You can hear S_1 with the diaphragm with the person in any position and equally well in inspiration and expiration. A split S_1 is normal, but it occurs rarely. A split S_1 means you are hearing the mitral and tricuspid components separately. It is audible in the tricuspid valve area, the left lower sternal border. The split is very rapid, with the two components only 0.03 second apart.

Second Heart Sound (S_2). The S_2 is associated with closure of the semilunar valves. You can hear it with the diaphragm, over the entire precordium, although S_2 is loudest at the base (Fig. 19-25).

Accentuated or diminished **S_2** (see Table 19-4, Variations in S_2, on p. 488).

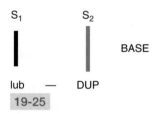

19-25

Splitting of S_2. A split S_2 is a normal phenomenon that occurs toward the end of inspiration in some people. Recall that closure of the aortic and pulmonic valves is nearly synchronous. Because of the effects of respiration on the heart described earlier, inspiration separates the timing of the two valves' closure, and the aortic valve closes 0.06 second before the pulmonic valve. Instead of one DUP, you hear a split sound—T-DUP (Fig. 19-26). During expiration, synchrony returns and the aortic and pulmonic components fuse together. A split S_2 is heard only in the pulmonic valve area, the second left interspace.

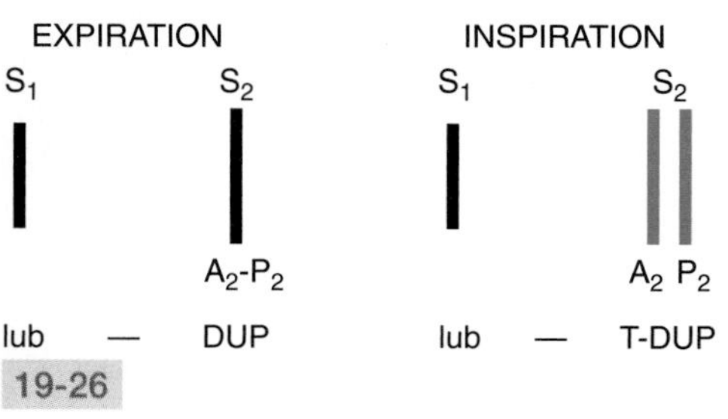

19-26

Objective Data

Normal Range of Findings

When you first hear the split S_2, do *not* be tempted to ask the person to hold his or her breath so that you can concentrate on the sounds. Breath holding will only equalize ejection times in the right and left sides of the heart and cause the split to go away. Instead, concentrate on the split as you watch the person's chest rise up and down with breathing. The split S_2 occurs about every fourth heartbeat, fading in with inhalation and fading out with exhalation.

Focus on Systole, Then on Diastole, and Listen for any Extra Heart Sounds. Listen with the diaphragm, then switch to the bell, covering all auscultatory areas (Fig. 19-27). Usually these are silent periods. When you do detect an extra heart sound, listen carefully to note its timing and characteristics. During systole, the **midsystolic click** (which is associated with mitral valve prolapse) is the most common extra sound (see Table 19-6). The third and fourth heart sounds occur in diastole; either may be normal or abnormal (see Table 19-7).

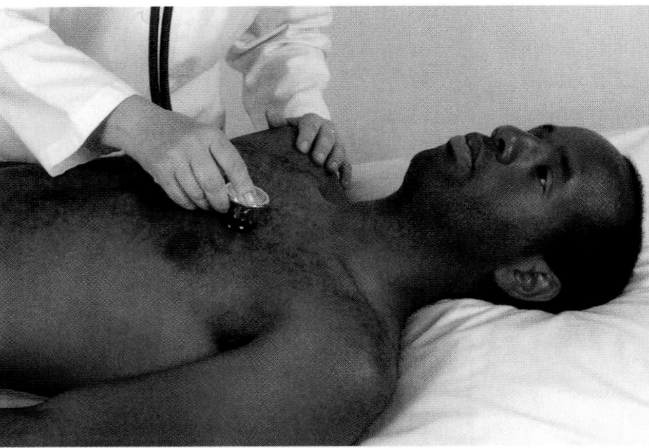

19-27

Listen for Murmurs. A murmur is a blowing, swooshing sound that occurs with turbulent blood flow in the heart or great vessels. Except for the innocent murmurs described, murmurs are abnormal. If you hear a murmur, describe it by indicating these following characteristics:

Timing. It is crucial to define the murmur by its occurrence in systole or diastole. You must be able to identify S_1 and S_2 accurately to do this. Try to further describe the murmur as being in early, mid-, or late systole or diastole; throughout the cardiac event (termed *pansystolic, holosystolic/pandiastolic,* or *holodiastolic*); and whether it obscures or muffles the heart sounds.

Loudness. Describe the intensity in terms of six "grades." For example, record a grade ii murmur as "ii/vi."

Grade i—Barely audible, heard only in a quiet room and then with difficulty
Grade ii—Clearly audible, but faint
Grade iii—Moderately loud, easy to hear
Grade iv—Loud, associated with a thrill palpable on the chest wall
Grade v—Very loud, heard with one corner of the stethoscope lifted off the chest wall
Grade vi—Loudest, still heard with entire stethoscope lifted just off the chest wall

Abnormal Findings

A **fixed split** is unaffected by respiration; the split is always there.

A **paradoxical split** is the opposite of what you would expect; the sounds fuse on inspiration and split on expiration (see Table 19-5, Variations in Split S_2, p. 488).

A pathologic S_3 (ventricular gallop) occurs with heart failure and volume overload; a pathologic S_4 (atrial gallop) occurs with CAD (see Table 19-7, Diastolic Extra Sounds, pp. 490-491, for a full description).

Murmurs may be due to congenital defects and acquired valvular defects. Study Tables 19-9 and 19-10, pp. 492-497, for a complete description.

A systolic murmur may occur with a normal heart or with heart disease; a diastolic murmur always indicates heart disease.

Normal Range of Findings

Pitch. Describe the pitch as high, medium, or low. The pitch depends on the pressure and the rate of blood flow producing the murmur.

Pattern. The intensity may follow a pattern during the cardiac phase, growing louder (crescendo), tapering off (decrescendo), or increasing to a peak and then decreasing (crescendo-decrescendo, or diamond shaped). Because the whole murmur is just milliseconds long, it takes practice to diagnose any pattern.

Quality. Describe the quality as musical, blowing, harsh, or rumbling.

Location. Describe the area of maximum intensity of the murmur (where it is best heard) by noting the valve area or intercostal spaces.

Radiation. The murmur may be transmitted downstream in the direction of blood flow and may be heard in another place on the precordium, the neck, the back, or the axilla.

Posture. Some murmurs disappear or are enhanced by a change in position.

Some murmurs are common in healthy children or adolescents and are termed *innocent* or *functional.* **Innocent** indicates having no valvular or other pathologic cause; **functional** is due to increased blood flow in the heart (e.g., in anemia, fever, pregnancy, hyperthyroidism). The contractile force of the heart is greater in children. This increases blood flow velocity. The increased velocity plus a smaller chest measurement makes an audible murmur.

The innocent murmur is generally soft (grade ii), midsystolic, short, crescendo-decrescendo, and with a vibratory or musical quality ("vooot" sound like fiddle strings). Also, the innocent murmur is heard at the second or third left intercostal space and disappears with sitting, and the young person has no associated signs of cardiac dysfunction.

Although it is important to distinguish innocent murmurs from pathologic ones, it is best to suspect all murmurs as pathologic until they are proved otherwise. Diagnostic tests such as ECG, phonocardiogram, and echocardiogram are needed to establish an accurate diagnosis.

Change Position. After auscultating in the supine position, roll the person toward his or her left side. Listen with the bell at the apex for the presence of any diastolic filling sounds (i.e., the $\mathbf{S_3}$ or $\mathbf{S_4}$) (Fig. 19-28).

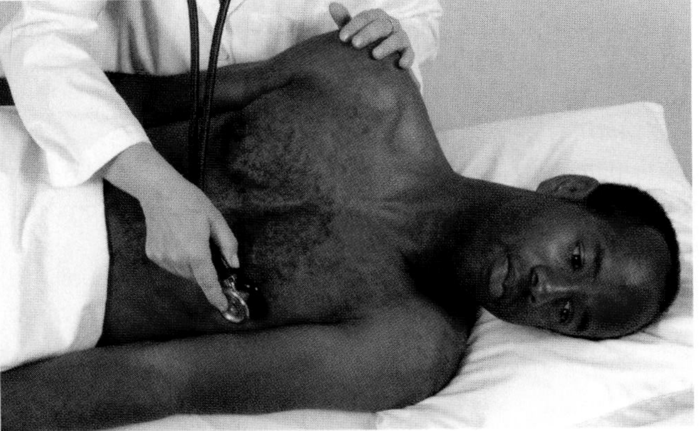

19-28

Abnormal Findings

The murmur of mitral stenosis is rumbling, whereas that of aortic stenosis is harsh (see Table 19-10).

$\mathbf{S_3}$ and $\mathbf{S_4}$, and the murmur of mitral stenosis sometimes may be heard only when on the left side.

Objective Data

Normal Range of Findings	Abnormal Findings

Ask the person to sit up, lean forward slightly, and exhale. Listen with the diaphragm firmly pressed at the base, right, and left sides. Check for the soft, high-pitched, early diastolic murmur of aortic or pulmonic regurgitation (Fig. 19-29).

Murmur of aortic regurgitation sometimes may be heard only when the person is leaning forward in the sitting position.

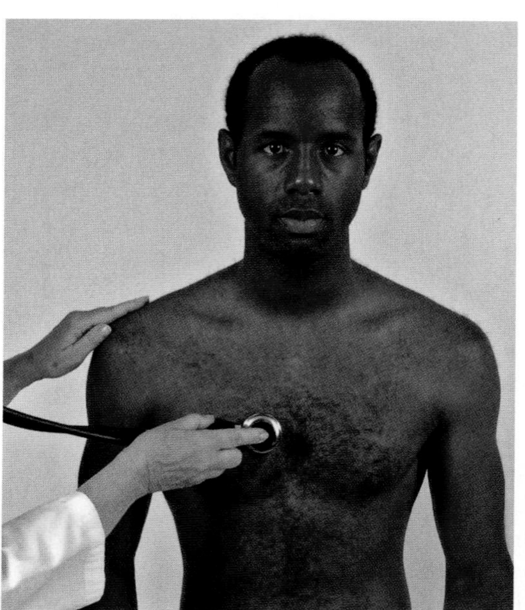

19-29

DEVELOPMENTAL COMPETENCE

Infants

The transition from fetal to pulmonic circulation occurs in the immediate newborn period. Fetal shunts normally close within 10 to 15 hours but may take up to 48 hours. Thus you should assess the cardiovascular system during the first 24 hours and again in 2 to 3 days.

Failure of shunts to close (e.g., patent ductus arteriosus [PDA], atrial septal defect [ASD]); see Table 19-9.

Note any extracardiac signs that may reflect heart status (particularly in the skin), liver size, and respiratory status. The skin color should be pink to pinkish brown, depending on the infant's genetic heritage. If cyanosis occurs, determine its first appearance—at or shortly after birth versus after the neonatal period. Normally, the liver is not enlarged and the respirations are not labored. Also, note the expected parameters of weight gain throughout infancy.

Cyanosis at or just after birth signals oxygen desaturation of congenital heart disease (Table 19-9).

The most important signs of heart failure in an infant are persistent tachycardia, tachypnea, and liver enlargement. Engorged veins, gallop rhythm, and pulsus alternans also are signs. Respiratory crackles (rales) are an important sign in adults but not in infants.

Failure to thrive occurs with cardiac disease.

Palpate the apical impulse to determine the size and position of the heart. Because the infant's heart has a more horizontal placement, expect to palpate the apical impulse at the fourth intercostal space just lateral to the midclavicular line. It may or may not be visible.

The apex is displaced with:

- Cardiac enlargement, shifts to the left
- Pneumothorax, shifts away from the affected side
- Diaphragmatic hernia, shifts usually to right because this hernia occurs more often on the left
- Dextrocardia, a rare anomaly in which the heart is located on right side of chest

Normal Range of Findings

The heart rate is best auscultated because radial pulses are hard to count accurately. Use the small (pediatric size) diaphragm and bell (Fig. 19-30). The heart rate may range from 100 to 180 per minute immediately after birth, then stabilize to an average of 120 to 140 per minute. Infants normally have wide fluctuations with activity, from 170 per minute or more with crying or being active to 70 to 90 per minute with sleeping. Variations are greatest at birth and are even more so with premature babies.

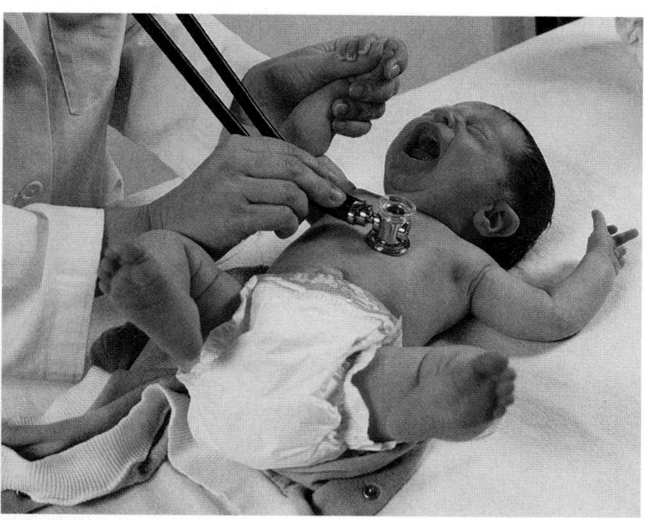

19-30

Expect the heart rhythm to have sinus arrhythmia, the phasic speeding up or slowing down with the respiratory cycle.

Rapid rates make it more challenging to evaluate heart sounds. Expect heart sounds to be louder in infants than in adults because of the infant's thinner chest wall. Also, S_2 has a higher pitch and is sharper than S_1. Splitting of S_2 just after the height of inspiration is common, not at birth, but beginning a few hours after birth.

Murmurs in the immediate newborn period do not necessarily indicate congenital heart disease. Murmurs are relatively common in the first 2 to 3 days because of fetal shunt closure. These murmurs are usually grade i or ii, are systolic, accompany no other signs of cardiac disease, and disappear in 2 to 3 days. The murmur of PDA is a continuous machinery murmur, which disappears by 2 to 3 days. On the other hand, absence of a murmur in the immediate newborn period does not ensure a perfect heart; congenital defects can be present that are not signaled by an early murmur. It is best to listen frequently and to note and describe any murmur according to the characteristics listed on p. 478.

Children

Note any extracardiac or cardiac signs that may indicate heart disease: poor weight gain, developmental delay, persistent tachycardia, tachypnea, dyspnea on exertion, cyanosis, and clubbing. Note that clubbing of fingers and toes usually does not appear until late in the 1st year, even with severe cyanotic defects.

Abnormal Findings

Persistent tachycardia is >200 per minute in newborns, or >150 per minute in infants.

Bradycardia is <90 per minute in newborns or <60 in older infants or children. This causes a serious drop in cardiac output because the small muscle mass of their hearts cannot increase stroke volume significantly.

Investigate any irregularity except sinus arrhythmia.

Fixed split S_2 indicates atrial septal defect (see Table 19-9).

Persistent murmur after 2 to 3 days, holosystolic murmurs or those that last into diastole, and those that are loud—all warrant further evaluation.

Normal Range of Findings

The apical impulse is sometimes visible in children with thin chest walls. Note any obvious bulge or any heave—these are not normal.

Palpate the apical impulse in the fourth intercostal space to the left of the midclavicular line until age 4 years; at the fourth interspace at the midclavicular line from age 4 to 6 years; and in the fifth interspace to the right of the midclavicular line at age 7 years (Fig. 19-31).

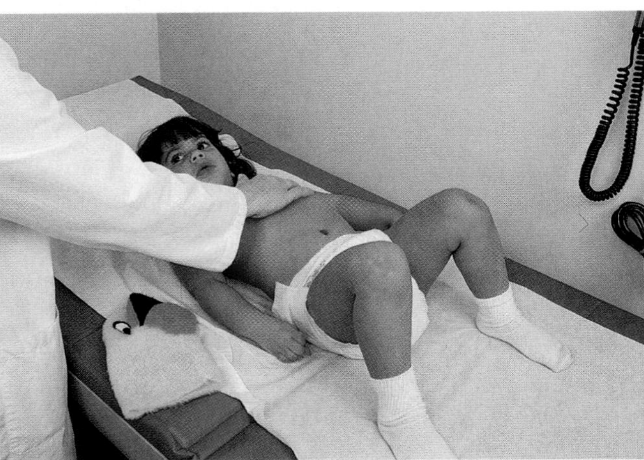

19-31

The average heart rate slows as the child grows older, although it is still variable with rest or activity.

The heart rhythm remains characterized by sinus arrhythmia. Physiologic $\mathbf{S_3}$ is common in children (see Table 19-7). It occurs in early diastole, just after $\mathbf{S_2}$, and is a dull soft sound that is best heard at the apex.

A **venous hum**—due to turbulence of blood flow in the jugular venous system—is common in healthy children and has no pathologic significance. It is a continuous, low-pitched, soft hum that is heard throughout the cycle, although it is loudest in diastole. Listen with the bell over the supraclavicular fossa at the medial third of the clavicle, especially on the right, or over the upper anterior chest.

The venous hum is usually not affected by respiration, may sound louder when the child stands, and is easily obliterated by occluding the jugular veins in the neck with your fingers.

Heart murmurs that are innocent (or functional) in origin are very common through childhood. Some authors say they have a 30% occurrence, and some authors say nearly all children may demonstrate a murmur at some time. Most innocent murmurs have these characteristics: soft, relatively short systolic ejection murmur; medium pitch; vibratory; best heard at the left lower sternal or midsternal border, with no radiation to the apex, base, or back.

For the child whose murmur has been shown to be innocent, it is very important that the parents understand this completely. They need to believe that this murmur is just a "noise" and has no pathologic significance. Otherwise, the parents may become overprotective and limit activity for the child, which may result in the child developing a negative self-concept.

Abnormal Findings

A precordial bulge to the left of the sternum with a hyperdynamic precordium signals cardiac enlargement. The bulge occurs because the cartilaginous rib cage is more compliant.

A substernal heave occurs with right ventricular enlargement; an apical heave occurs with left ventricular hypertrophy.

The apical impulse moves laterally with cardiac enlargement.

Thrill (palpable vibration).

This latter maneuver helps differentiate the venous hum from other cardiac murmurs (e.g., PDA).

Distinguish innocent murmurs from pathologic ones. This may involve referral to another examiner or the performance of diagnostic tests such as the ECG or ultrasonography.

Normal Range of Findings	Abnormal Findings

The Pregnant Woman

The vital signs usually yield an increase in resting pulse rate of 10 to 15 beats per minute and a drop in blood pressure from the normal prepregnancy level. The BP decreases to its lowest point during the second trimester and then slowly rises during the third trimester. The BP varies with position. It is usually lowest in the left lateral recumbent position, a bit higher when supine, and highest when sitting.[10]

Suspect pregnancy-induced hypertension with a sustained rise of 30 mm Hg systolic or 15 mm Hg diastolic under basal conditions.

Inspection of the skin often shows a mild hyperemia in light-skinned women because the increased cutaneous blood flow tries to eliminate the excess heat generated by the increased metabolism. Palpation of the apical impulse is higher and lateral compared with the normal position, because the enlarging uterus elevates the diaphragm and displaces the heart up and to the left and rotates it on its long axis.

Auscultation of the heart sounds shows changes caused by the increased blood volume and workload:

- Heart sounds
  Exaggerated splitting of S_1 and increased loudness of S_1
  A loud, easily heard S_3
- Heart murmurs
  A systolic murmur in 90%, which disappears soon after delivery
  A soft, diastolic murmur heard transiently in 19%
  A continuous murmur from breast vasculature in 10%[10]

The last-mentioned murmur is termed a **mammary souffle** (pronounced soof′ f′l), which occurs near term or when the mother is lactating; it is due to increased blood flow through the internal mammary artery. The murmur is heard in the second, third, or fourth intercostal space; it is continuous, although it is accented in systole. You can obliterate it by pressure with the stethoscope or one finger lateral to the murmur.

Murmurs of aortic valve disease cannot be obliterated.

The ECG has no changes except for a slight left axis deviation due to the change in the heart's position.

The Aging Adult

A gradual rise in systolic blood pressure is common with aging; the diastolic blood pressure stays fairly constant with a resulting widening of pulse pressure. Some older adults experience **orthostatic hypotension,** a sudden drop in blood pressure when rising to sit or stand.

Use caution in palpating and auscultating the carotid artery. Avoid pressure in the carotid sinus area, which could cause a reflex slowing of the heart rate. Also, pressure on the carotid artery could compromise circulation if the artery is already narrowed by atherosclerosis.

When measuring jugular venous pressure, view the right internal jugular vein. The aorta stiffens, dilates, and elongates with aging, which may compress the left neck veins and obscure pulsations on the left side.[15a]

The chest often increases in anteroposterior diameter with aging. This makes it more difficult to palpate the apical impulse and to hear the splitting of S_2. The S_4 often occurs in older people with no known cardiac disease. Systolic murmurs are common, occurring in over 50% of aging people.[15a]

The S_3 is associated with heart failure and is always abnormal over age 35 years (see Table 19-7).

Occasional premature ectopic beats are common and do not necessarily indicate underlying heart disease. When in doubt, obtain an ECG. However, consider that the ECG records for only one isolated minute in time and may need to be supplemented by a test of 24-hour ambulatory heart monitoring.

PROMOTING A HEALTHY LIFESTYLE: WOMEN AND HEART ATTACKS

The Heart Truth

When someone complains of chest pain or pain radiating down the left arm, we think heart attack. After all, these are the symptoms that typically occur, aren't they? Well, yes and no. They are the most "typical" symptoms men have when having a myocardial infarction (MI), but not women. For women, symptoms can be quite different. A woman's "atypical" symptoms may be one of the reasons that more women are dying from heart disease than men these days. According to the Women's Heart Foundation, almost a third of women experience no chest pain at all when having a heart attack. Instead, 71% of women report flu-like symptoms, including extreme fatigue, for up to a month before the attack. Women are more likely to feel a hot or cold burning sensation or a tenderness to touch in their back, shoulders, arms, or jaw—not sharp pain. Women's symptoms often include nausea, vomiting, indigestion, and shortness of breath, which are easy to attribute to something other than the heart. The evidence now shows that women tend to minimize their symptoms or attribute them to something else. This may be due to a lack of awareness.

The Heart Truth® is a national awareness and prevention campaign about heart disease in women sponsored by the *National Heart, Lung, and Blood Institute* (NHLBI). The campaign includes three components: (1) professional education, (2) patient education, and (3) public awareness. At *The Heart Truth®* website, health professionals can access both clinical and patient education resources. Of particular interest are the clinical assessment tools, including a Risk Status, LDL, and Drug-Therapy Guide; a 10-year heart attack calculator; and a body mass index (BMI) calculator, which are either available online or as an applications for a pocket PC. For patients, there is the *Heart Truth E-zine*, the NHBLI quarterly electronic publication that provides new information about heart disease research and heart-healthy recipes. Patients can also download the *The Healthy Heart Handbook for Women*.

The Red Dress® is the centerpiece of *The Heart Truth®* and the primary message of the campaign is *Heart Disease Doesn't Care What You Wear—It's the #1 Killer of Women®*. The idea behind using a red dress as the symbol was to draw attention to the idea that heart disease was not only a man's issue. National *Wear Red Day®* is the first Friday in February. Plan to wear red and raise awareness. You may save a life!

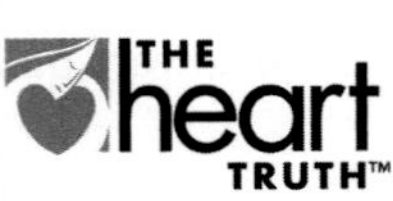

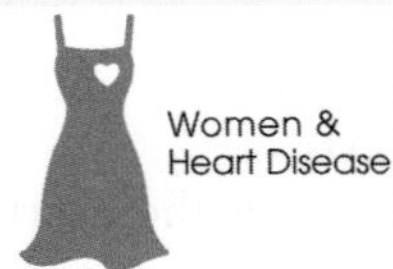

®, ™ The Heart Truth, its logo, The Red Dress, and Heart Disease Doesn't Care What You Wear—It's the #1 Killer of Women are trademarks of NHBLI/ HHS. ®National Wear Red Day is a registered trademark of NHBLI/HHS and AHA.

Resources

American Heart Association. Website: www.americanheart.org.

National Institutes of Health National Heart, Lung, and Blood Institute. Website: www.nhlbi.nih.gov.

The Healthy Heart Handbook for Women. Website: www.nhlbi.nih.gov/health/public/heart/other/hhw/index.htm.

The Heart Truth: Awareness and Prevention. Website: www.womenshealth.gov/hearttruth/.

The Heart Truth E-zine. Website: www.nhlbi.nih.gov/educational/hearttruth/materials/newsletter.htm.

Women's Heart Foundation. Website: www.womensheart.org/.

DOCUMENTATION AND CRITICAL THINKING

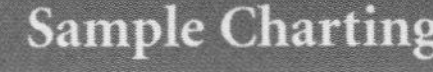

Sample Charting

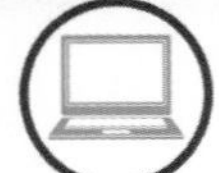

SUBJECTIVE

No chest pain, dyspnea, orthopnea, cough, fatigue, or edema. No history of hypertension, abnormal blood tests, heart murmur, or rheumatic fever in self. Last ECG 2 yrs. PTA, result normal. No stress ECG or other heart tests.

Family history—Father with obesity, smoking, and hypertension, treated $\bar{c}$ diuretic medication. No other family history significant for cardiovascular disease.

Personal habits—Diet balanced in 4 food groups, 2 to 3 c. regular coffee/day; no smoking; alcohol, 1 to 2 beers occasionally on weekend; exercise, runs 2 miles, 3 to 4 ×/week; no prescription or OTC medications or street drugs.

OBJECTIVE

Neck: Carotids 2+ and = bilaterally. Internal jugular vein pulsations present when supine and disappear when elevated to a 45° position.
Precordium: Inspection. No visible pulsations, no heave or lift.
Palpation: Apical impulse in 5th ics at left midclavicular line, no thrill.
Auscultation: Rate 68 beats per minute, rhythm regular, S_1-S_2 are normal, not diminished or accentuated, no S_3, no S_4 or other extra sounds, no murmurs.

ASSESSMENT

Neck vessels healthy by inspection and auscultation
Heart sounds normal

Focused Assessment: Clinical Case Study

Mr. N.V. is a 53-year-old white male woodcutter admitted to the CCU at University Medical Center (UMC) with chest pain.

SUBJECTIVE

1 year PTA—N.V. admitted to UMC with crushing substernal chest pain, radiating to L shoulder, accompanied by nausea, vomiting, diaphoresis.

Diagnosed as MI, hospitalized 7 days, discharged with nitroglycerin prn for anginal pain.

Did not return to work. Activity included walking 1 mile/day, hunting. Had occasional episodes of chest pain with exercise, relieved by rest.

1 day PTA—had increasing frequency of chest pain, about every 2 hours, lasting few minutes, saw pain as warning to go to MD.
Day of admission—severe substernal chest pain ("like someone sitting on my chest") unrelieved by rest. Saw personal MD, while in office had episode of chest pain similar to last year's, accompanied by diaphoresis, no N & V or SOB, relieved by 1 nitroglycerin. Transferred to UMC by paramedics. No further pain since admission 2 hours ago.
Family hx—mother died of MI at age 57.
Personal habits—smokes 1½ pack cigarettes daily × 34 years, no alcohol, diet—trying to limit fat and fried food, still high in added salt.

OBJECTIVE

Extremities: Skin pink, no cyanosis. Upper extrem.—capillary refill sluggish, no clubbing. Lower extrem.—no edema, no hair growth 10 cm below knee bilaterally.
Pulses—

Carotid	Brachial	Radial	Femoral	Popliteal	P.T.	D.P.	
2+	2+	2+	2+	0	0	1+	All = Bilaterally

B/P R arm 104/66 mm Hg
Neck: External jugulars flat. Internal jugular pulsations present when supine and absent when elevated to 45°.
Precordium: Inspection. Apical impulse visible 5th ics, 7 cm left of midsternal line, no heave.
Palpation: Apical impulse palpable in 5th and 6th ics. No thrill.
Auscultation: Apical rate 92 bpm regular, S_1-S_2 are normal, not diminished or accentuated, no S_3 or S_4, grade iii/vi systolic murmur present at left lower sternal border.

ASSESSMENT

Substernal chest pain
Systolic murmur
Ineffective tissue perfusion R/T interruption in flow
Decreased cardiac output R/T reduction in stroke volume

ABNORMAL FINDINGS

TABLE 19-2 Clinical Portrait of Heart Failure

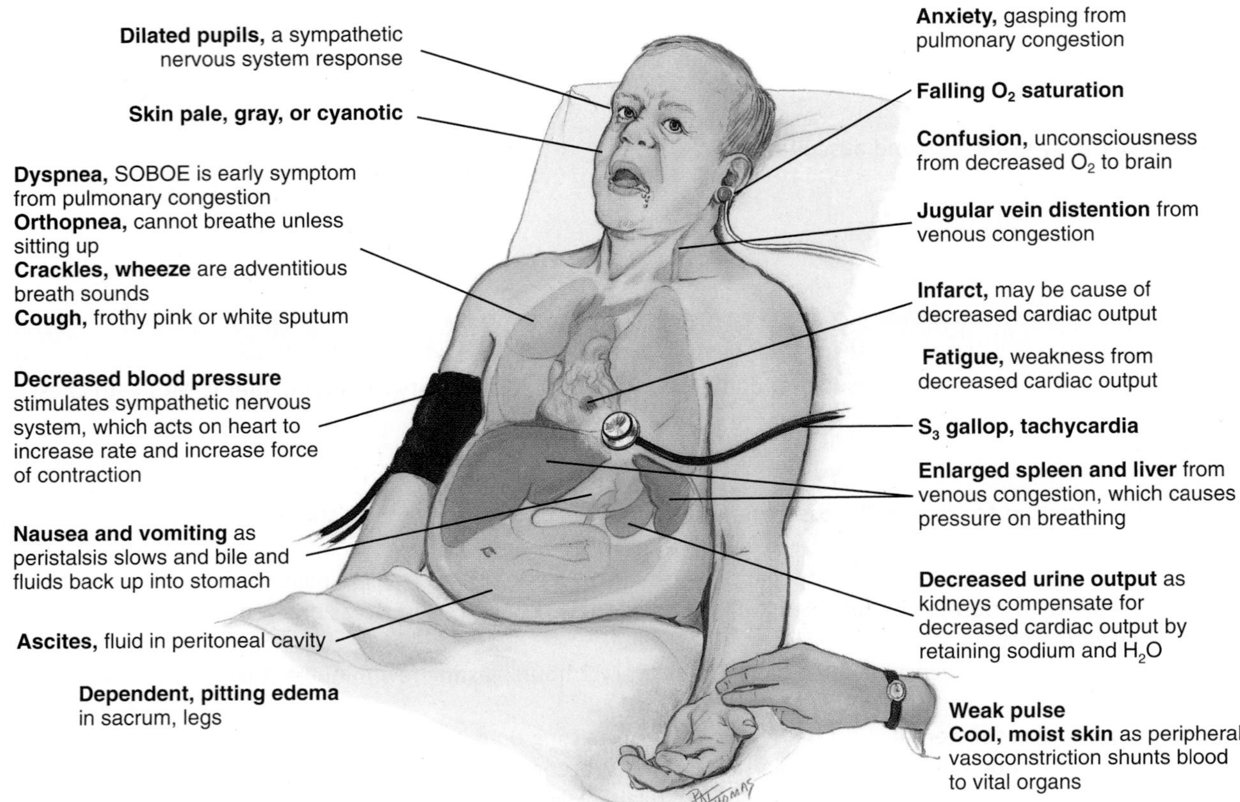
Dilated pupils, a sympathetic nervous system response
Skin pale, gray, or cyanotic
Dyspnea, SOBOE is early symptom from pulmonary congestion
Orthopnea, cannot breathe unless sitting up
Crackles, wheeze are adventitious breath sounds
Cough, frothy pink or white sputum
Decreased blood pressure stimulates sympathetic nervous system, which acts on heart to increase rate and increase force of contraction
Nausea and vomiting as peristalsis slows and bile and fluids back up into stomach
Ascites, fluid in peritoneal cavity
Dependent, pitting edema in sacrum, legs
Anxiety, gasping from pulmonary congestion
Falling O_2 saturation
Confusion, unconsciousness from decreased O_2 to brain
Jugular vein distention from venous congestion
Infarct, may be cause of decreased cardiac output
Fatigue, weakness from decreased cardiac output
S_3 gallop, tachycardia
Enlarged spleen and liver from venous congestion, which causes pressure on breathing
Decreased urine output as kidneys compensate for decreased cardiac output by retaining sodium and H_2O
Weak pulse
Cool, moist skin as peripheral vasoconstriction shunts blood to vital organs

Decreased cardiac output occurs when the heart fails as a pump, and the circulation becomes backed up and congested.
Signs and symptoms of heart failure come from two basic mechanisms: (1) the heart's inability to pump enough blood to meet the metabolic demands of the body; and (2) the kidney's compensatory mechanisms of abnormal retention of sodium and water to compensate for the decreased cardiac output. This increases blood volume and venous return, which causes further congestion.
Onset of heart failure may be: (1) *acute,* as following a myocardial infarction when direct damage to the heart's contracting ability has occurred; or (2) *chronic,* as with hypertension, when the ventricles must pump against chronically increased pressure.

SOBOE, Shortness of breath on exertion.

ABNORMAL FINDINGS
FOR ADVANCED PRACTICE

TABLE 19-3 Variations in S_1

The intensity of $\mathbf{S_1}$ depends on three factors: (1) position of AV valve at the start of systole, (2) structure of the valve leaflets, and (3) how quickly pressure rises in the ventricle.

	Factor	Examples
Loud (Accentuated) S_1 S_1 S_2	1. Position of AV valve at start of systole—wide open and no time to drift together	Hyperkinetic states where blood velocity is increased: exercise, fever, anemia, hyperthyroidism
	2. Change in valve structure—calcification of valve, needs increasing ventricular pressure to close the valve against increased atrial pressure	Mitral stenosis with leaflets still mobile
Faint (Diminished) S_1 S_1 S_2	1. Position of AV valve—delayed conduction from atria to ventricles. Mitral valve drifts shut before ventricular contraction closes it	First-degree heart block (prolonged PR interval)
	2. Change in valve structure—extreme calcification, which limits mobility	Mitral insufficiency
	3. More forceful atrial contraction into noncompliant ventricle; delays or diminishes ventricular contraction	Severe hypertension—systemic or pulmonary
Varying Intensity of S_1 S_1 S_2 S_1 S_2	1. Position of AV valve varies before closing from beat to beat	Atrial fibrillation—irregularly irregular rhythm
	2. Atria and ventricles beat independently	Complete heart block with changing PR interval
Split S_1 S_1 S_2 T M	Mitral and tricuspid components are heard separately	Normal but uncommon

Abnormal Findings

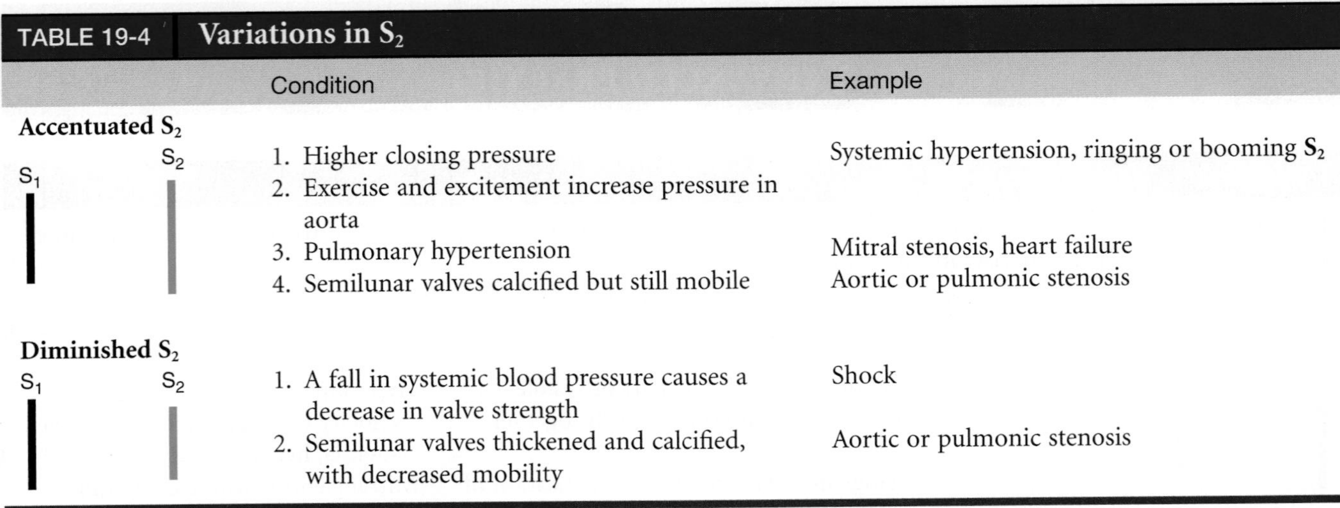

TABLE 19-4 Variations in S_2

	Condition	Example
Accentuated S_2	1. Higher closing pressure	Systemic hypertension, ringing or booming S_2
	2. Exercise and excitement increase pressure in aorta	
	3. Pulmonary hypertension	Mitral stenosis, heart failure
	4. Semilunar valves calcified but still mobile	Aortic or pulmonic stenosis
Diminished S_2	1. A fall in systemic blood pressure causes a decrease in valve strength	Shock
	2. Semilunar valves thickened and calcified, with decreased mobility	Aortic or pulmonic stenosis

TABLE 19-5 Variations in Split S_2

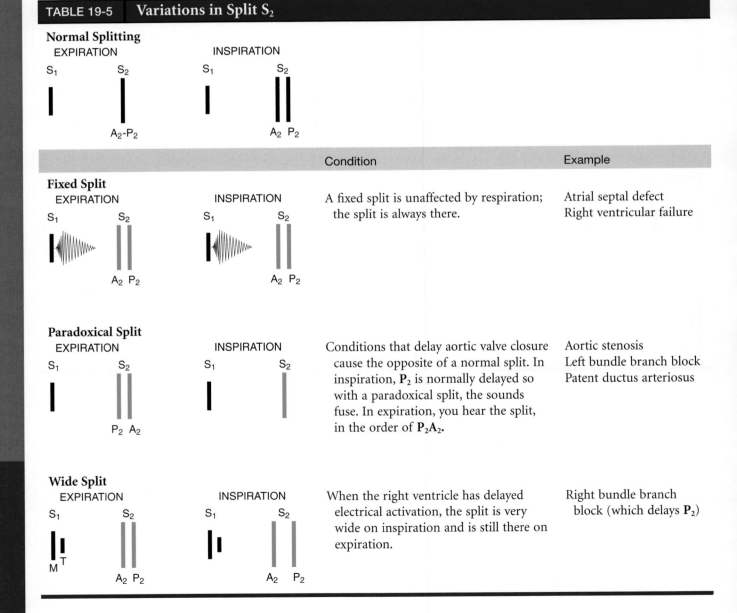

Normal Splitting

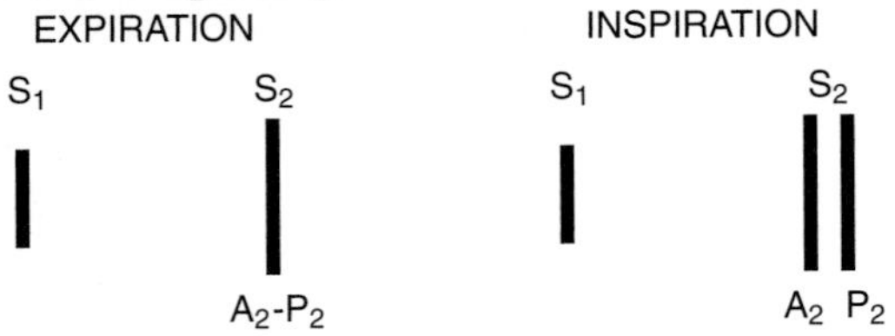

EXPIRATION: S_1 S_2 (A_2-P_2)

INSPIRATION: S_1 S_2 (A_2 P_2)

	Condition	Example
Fixed Split 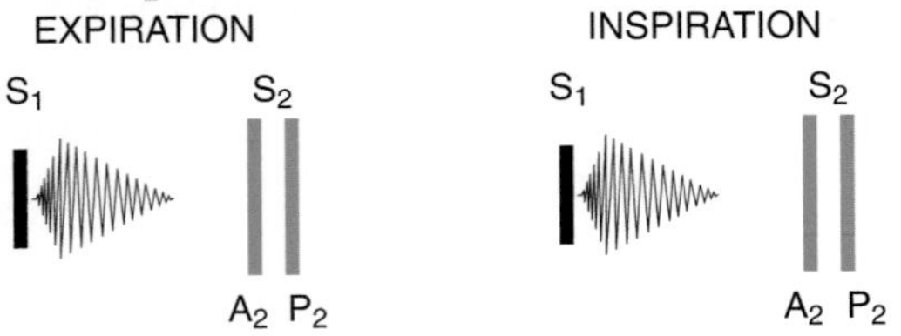 (EXPIRATION: S_1 S_2, A_2 P_2; INSPIRATION: S_1 S_2, A_2 P_2)	A fixed split is unaffected by respiration; the split is always there.	Atrial septal defect Right ventricular failure
Paradoxical Split 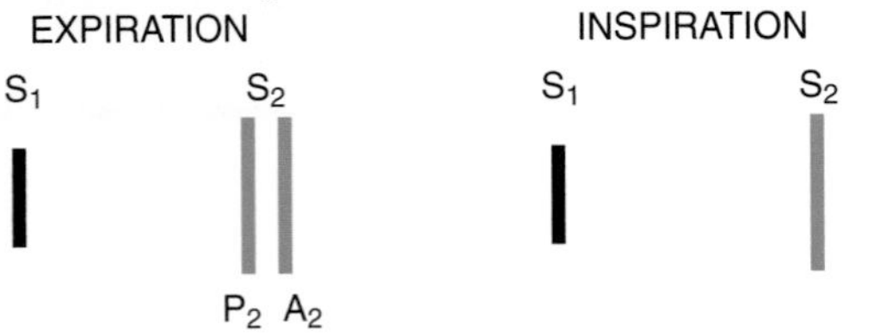 (EXPIRATION: S_1 S_2, P_2 A_2; INSPIRATION: S_1 S_2)	Conditions that delay aortic valve closure cause the opposite of a normal split. In inspiration, P_2 is normally delayed so with a paradoxical split, the sounds fuse. In expiration, you hear the split, in the order of $\mathbf{P_2A_2}$.	Aortic stenosis Left bundle branch block Patent ductus arteriosus
Wide Split 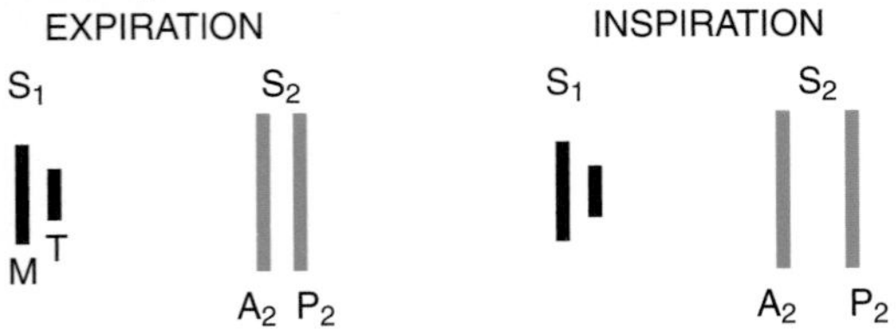 (EXPIRATION: S_1 (M T) S_2, A_2 P_2; INSPIRATION: S_1 S_2, A_2 P_2)	When the right ventricle has delayed electrical activation, the split is very wide on inspiration and is still there on expiration.	Right bundle branch block (which delays $\mathbf{P_2}$)

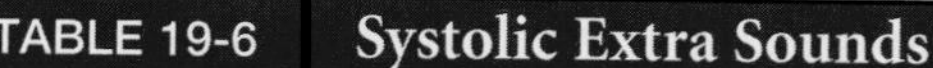

TABLE 19-6 Systolic Extra Sounds

Early systolic:
- Ejection click
- Aortic prosthetic valve sounds

Mid-/late systolic:
- Midsystolic (mitral) click

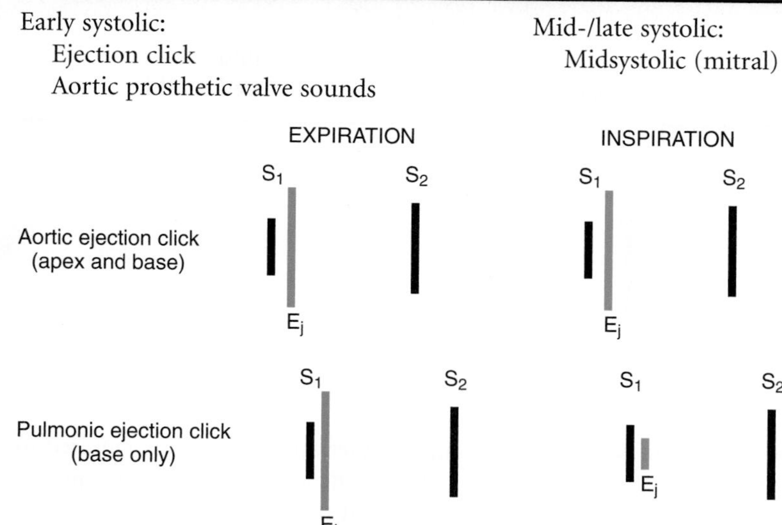

Ejection Click

The ejection click occurs early in systole at the start of ejection because it results from opening of the semilunar valves. Normally, the SL valves open silently, but in the presence of stenosis (e.g., aortic stenosis, pulmonic stenosis), their opening makes a sound. It is short and high pitched, with a click quality, and is heard better with the diaphragm.

The aortic ejection click is heard at the second right interspace and apex and may be loudest at the apex. Its intensity does not change with respiration. The pulmonic ejection click is best heard in the second left interspace and often grows softer with inspiration.

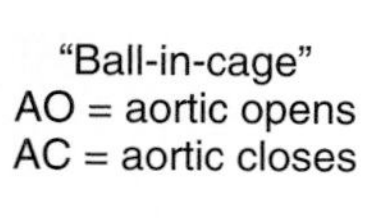

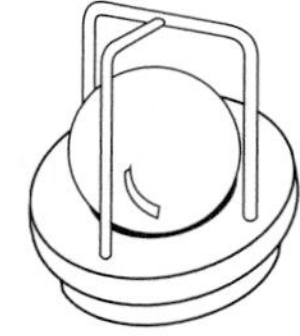

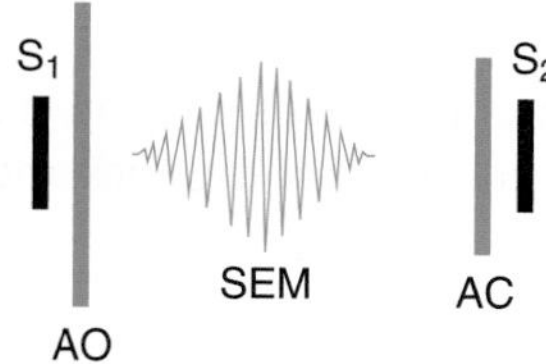

Aortic Prosthetic Valve Sounds

As a sequela of modern technologic intervention for heart problems, some people now have *iatrogenically* induced heart sounds. The opening of a mechanical aortic ball-in-cage prosthesis produces an early systolic sound. This sound is less intense with a tilting disk prosthesis and is absent with a biologic tissue prosthesis (e.g., porcine).

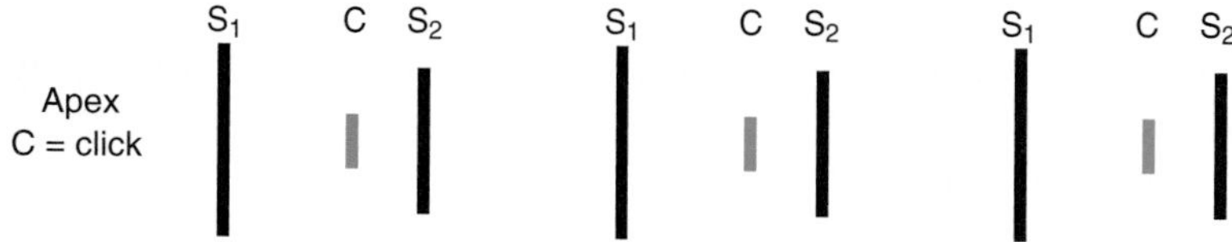

Midsystolic Click

Although it is systolic, this is not an ejection click. It is associated with **mitral valve prolapse,** in which the mitral valve leaflets not only close with contraction but balloon back up into the left atrium. During ballooning, the sudden tensing of the valve leaflets and the chordae tendineae creates the click.

The sound occurs in mid- to late systole and is short and high pitched, with a click quality. It is best heard with the diaphragm, at the apex, but also may be heard at the left lower sternal border. The click usually is followed by a systolic murmur. The click and murmur move with postural change; when the person assumes a squatting position, the click may move closer to **S_2**, and the murmur may sound louder and delayed. The Valsalva maneuver also moves the click closer to **S_2**.

TABLE 19-7 Diastolic Extra Sounds

Early diastole:	Mid-diastole:	Late diastole:
Opening snap	Third heart sound	Fourth heart sound
Mitral prosthetic valve sound	Summation sound ($S_3 + S_4$)	Pacemaker-induced sound

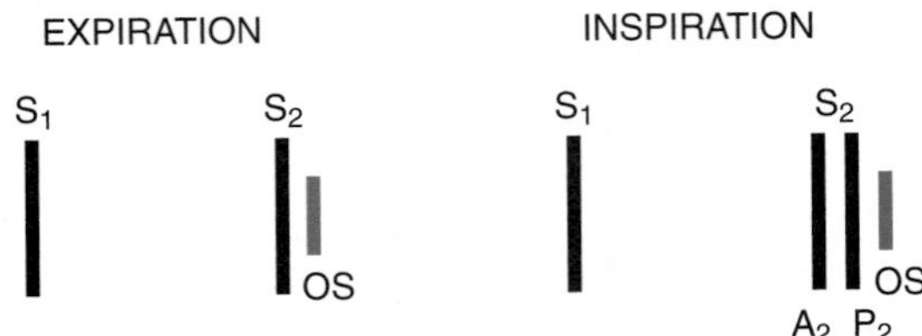

Opening Snap

Normally the opening of the AV valves is silent. In the presence of stenosis, increasingly higher atrial pressure is required to open the valve. The deformed valve opens with a noise: the opening snap. It is sharp and high pitched, with a snapping quality. It sounds after S_2 and is best heard with the diaphragm at the third or fourth left interspace at the sternal border, less well at the apex.

The opening snap usually is not an isolated sound. As a sign of mitral stenosis, the opening snap usually ushers in the low-pitched diastolic rumbling murmur of that condition.

"Ball-in-cage"
MO = mitral prosthesis opens
MC = S_1
S_1 S_2
MC SEM MO

Mitral Prosthetic Valve Sound

An iatrogenic sound, the opening of a ball-in-cage mitral prosthesis gives an early diastolic sound: an opening click just after S_2. It is loud, is heard over the whole precordium, and is loudest at the apex and left lower sternal border.

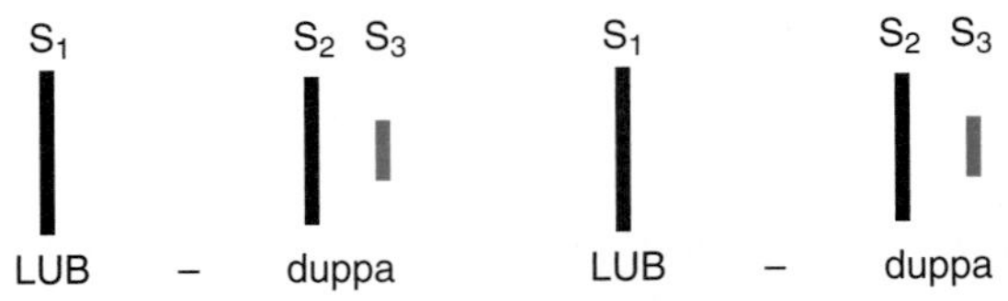

Third Heart Sound

The S_3 is a ventricular filling sound. It occurs in early diastole during the rapid filling phase. Your hearing quickly accommodates to the S_3, so it is best heard when you listen initially. It sounds after S_2 but later than an opening snap would be. It is a dull, soft sound, and it is low pitched, like "distant thunder." It is heard best in a quiet room, at the apex, with the bell held lightly (just enough to form a seal), and with the person in the left lateral position.

The S_3 can be confused with a split S_2. Use these guidelines to distinguish the S_3:

- *Location*—The S_3 is heard at the apex or left lower sternal border; the split S_2 at the base.
- *Respiratory variation*—The S_3 does not vary in timing with respirations; the split S_2 does.
- *Pitch*—The S_3 is lower pitched; the pitch of the split S_2 stays the same.

The S_3 may be normal (physiologic) or abnormal (pathologic). The **physiologic** S_3 is heard frequently in children and young adults; it occasionally may persist after age 40 years, especially in women. The normal S_3 usually disappears when the person sits up.

In adults, the S_3 is usually abnormal. The **pathologic** S_3 is also called a **ventricular gallop** or an S_3 gallop, and it persists when sitting up. The S_3 indicates decreased compliance of the ventricles, as in heart failure. The S_3 may be the earliest sign of heart failure. The S_3 may originate from either the left or the right ventricle; a left-sided S_3 is heard at the apex in the left lateral position, and a right-sided S_3 is heard at the left lower sternal border with the person supine and is louder in inspiration.

The S_3 occurs also with conditions of volume overload, such as mitral regurgitation and aortic or tricuspid regurgitation. The S_3 is also found in high cardiac output states in the absence of heart disease, such as hyperthyroidism, anemia, and pregnancy. When the primary condition is corrected, the gallop disappears.

TABLE 19-7 **Diastolic Extra Sounds—cont'd**

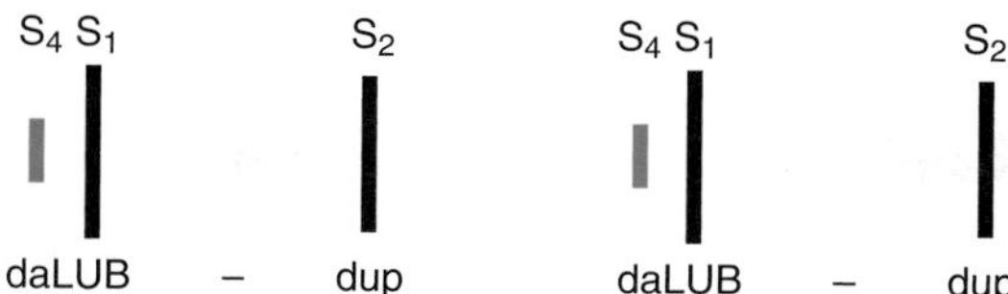

Fourth Heart Sound

The $\mathbf{S_4}$ is a ventricular filling sound. It occurs when the atria contract late in diastole. It is heard immediately before $\mathbf{S_1}$. This is a very soft sound, of very low pitch. You need a good bell, and you must listen for it. It is heard best at the apex, with the person in left lateral position.

A **physiologic** $\mathbf{S_4}$ may occur in adults older than 40 or 50 years with no evidence of cardiovascular disease, especially after exercise.

A **pathologic** $\mathbf{S_4}$ is termed an **atrial gallop** or an $\mathbf{S_4}$ **gallop**. It occurs with decreased compliance of the ventricle (e.g., coronary artery disease, cardiomyopathy) and with systolic overload (afterload), including outflow obstruction to the ventricle (aortic stenosis) and systemic hypertension. A left-sided $\mathbf{S_4}$ occurs with these conditions. It is heard best at the apex, in the left lateral position.

A right-sided $\mathbf{S_4}$ is less common. It is heard at the left lower sternal border and may increase with inspiration. It occurs with pulmonary stenosis or pulmonary hypertension.

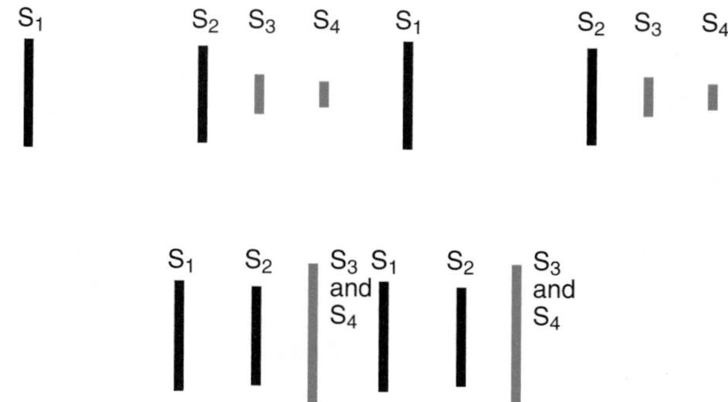

Summation Sound

When both the pathologic $\mathbf{S_3}$ and $\mathbf{S_4}$ are present, a quadruple rhythm is heard. Often, in cases of cardiac stress, one response is tachycardia. During rapid rates, the diastolic filling time shortens and the $\mathbf{S_3}$ and $\mathbf{S_4}$ move closer together. They sound superimposed in mid-diastole, and you hear one loud, prolonged, summated sound, often louder than either $\mathbf{S_1}$ or $\mathbf{S_2}$.

EXTRACARDIAC SOUNDS

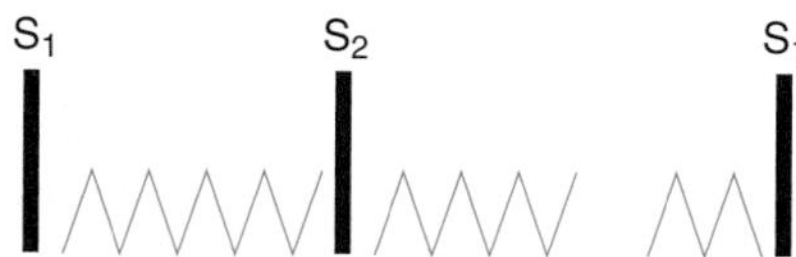

Pericardial Friction Rub

Inflammation of the pericardium gives rise to a friction rub. The sound is high pitched and scratchy, like sandpaper being rubbed. It is best heard with the diaphragm, with the person sitting up and leaning forward, and with the breath held in expiration.

A friction rub can be heard any place on the precordium but usually is best heard at the apex and left lower sternal border, places where the pericardium comes in close contact with the chest wall. Timing may be systolic and diastolic. The friction rub of pericarditis is common during the 1st week after a myocardial infarction and may last only a few hours.

TABLE 19-8 Abnormal Pulsations on the Precordium

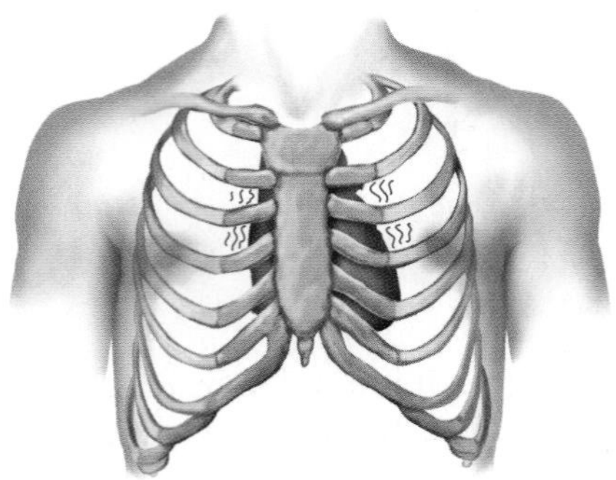

Base

A **thrill** in the second and third right interspaces occurs with severe aortic stenosis and systemic hypertension.

A **thrill** in the second and third left interspaces occurs with pulmonic stenosis and pulmonic hypertension.

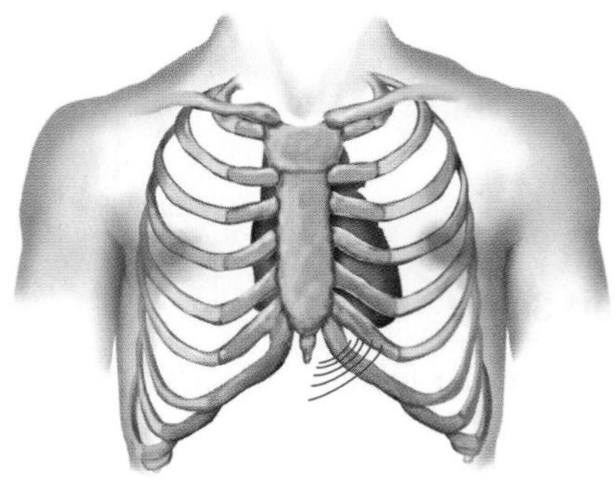

Left Sternal Border

A **lift (heave)** occurs with right ventricular hypertrophy, as found in pulmonic valve disease, pulmonic hypertension, and chronic lung disease. You feel a diffuse lifting impulse during systole at the left lower sternal border. It may be associated with retraction at the apex because the left ventricle is rotated posteriorly by the enlarged right ventricle.

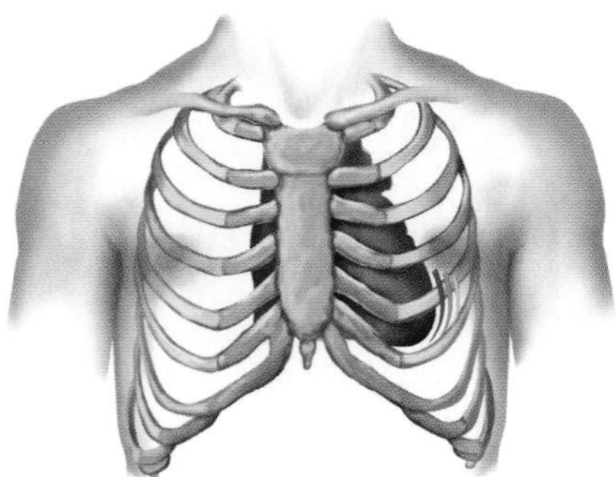

Apex

Cardiac enlargement displaces the apical impulse laterally and over a wider area when left ventricular hypertrophy and dilation are present. This is **volume overload,** as in mitral regurgitation, aortic regurgitation, and left-to-right shunts.

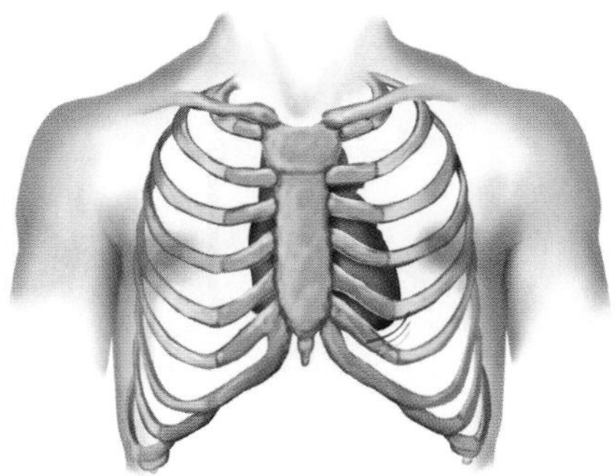

Apex

The apical impulse is increased in force and duration but is not necessarily displaced to the left when left ventricular hypertrophy occurs alone without dilation. This is **pressure overload,** as found in aortic stenosis or systemic hypertension.

Images © Pat Thomas, 2006.

TABLE 19-9 Congenital Heart Defects

	Description	Clinical Data
Patent Ductus Arteriosus (PDA) 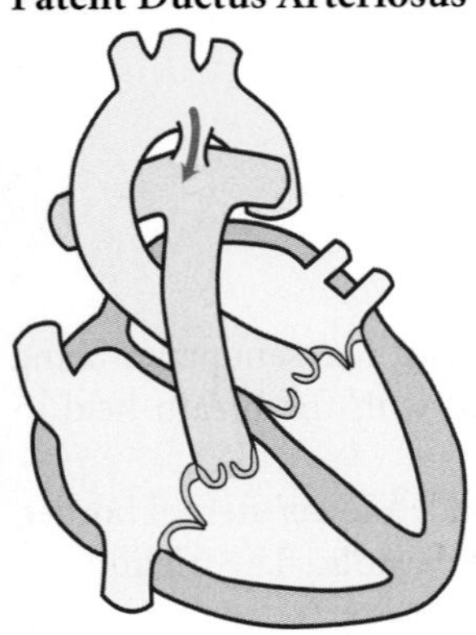	Persistence of the channel joining left pulmonary artery to aorta. This is normal in the fetus and usually closes spontaneously within hours of birth.	S: Usually no symptoms in early childhood; growth and development are normal. O: Blood pressure has wide pulse pressure and bounding peripheral pulses from rapid runoff of blood into low-resistance pulmonary bed during diastole. Thrill often palpable at left upper sternal border. The continuous murmur heard in systole and diastole is called a *machinery murmur.*

TABLE 19-9 Congenital Heart Defects—cont'd

	Description	Clinical Data
Atrial Septal Defect (ASD) 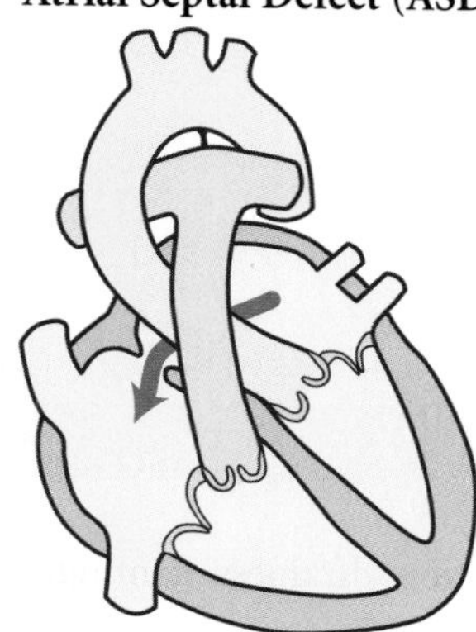	Abnormal opening in the atrial septum, resulting usually in left-to-right shunt and causing large increase in pulmonary blood flow.	S: Defect is remarkably well tolerated. Symptoms in infants are rare; growth and development normal. Children and young adults have mild fatigue and DOE. O: Sternal lift often present. $\mathbf{S_2}$ has fixed split, with $\mathbf{P_2}$ often louder than $\mathbf{A_2}$. Murmur is systolic, ejection, medium pitch, best heard at base in second left interspace. Murmur caused not by shunt itself but by increased blood flow through pulmonic valve.
Ventricular Septal Defect (VSD) 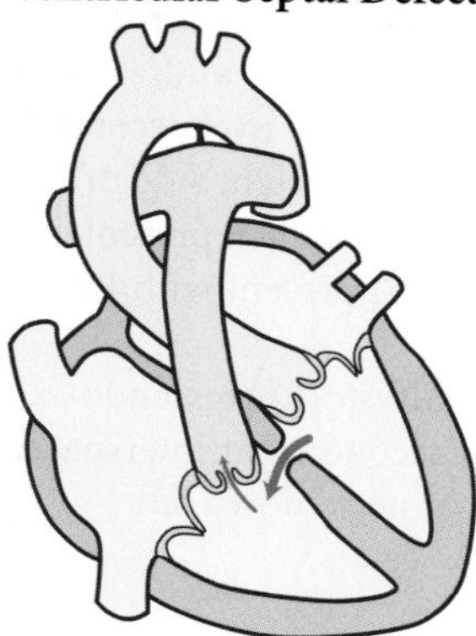	Abnormal opening in septum between the ventricles, usually subaortic area. The size and exact position vary considerably.	S: Small defects are asymptomatic. Infants with large defects have poor growth, slow weight gain; later look pale, thin, delicate. May have feeding problems; DOE; frequent respiratory infections; and when the condition is severe, heart failure. O: Loud, harsh holosystolic murmur, best heard at left lower sternal border, may be accompanied by thrill. Large defects also have soft diastolic murmur at apex (mitral flow murmur) due to increased blood flow through mitral valve.
Tetralogy of Fallot 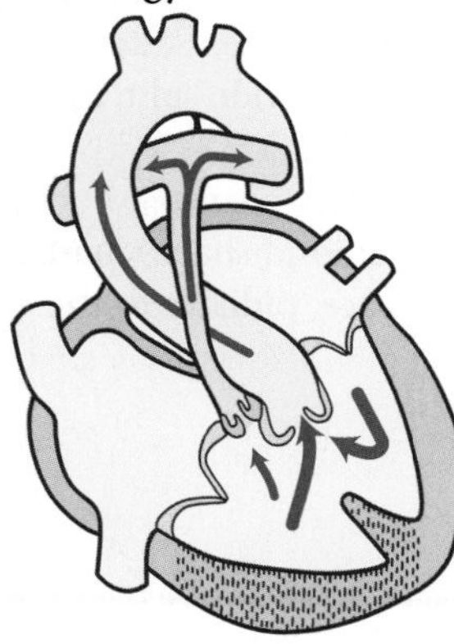	Four components: (1) right ventricular outflow stenosis, (2) VSD, (3) right ventricular hypertrophy, and (4) overriding aorta. *Result:* shunts a lot of venous blood directly into aorta away from pulmonary system, so blood never gets oxygenated.	S: Severe cyanosis, not in first months of life but develops as infant grows and RV outflow (i.e., pulmonic) stenosis gets worse. Cyanosis with crying and exertion at first, then at rest. Uses squatting posture after starts walking. DOE common. Development is slowed. O: Thrill palpable at left lower sternal border. $\mathbf{S_1}$ normal; $\mathbf{S_2}$ has $\mathbf{A_2}$ loud and $\mathbf{P_2}$ diminished or absent. Murmur is systolic, loud, crescendo-decrescendo.
Coarctation of the Aorta 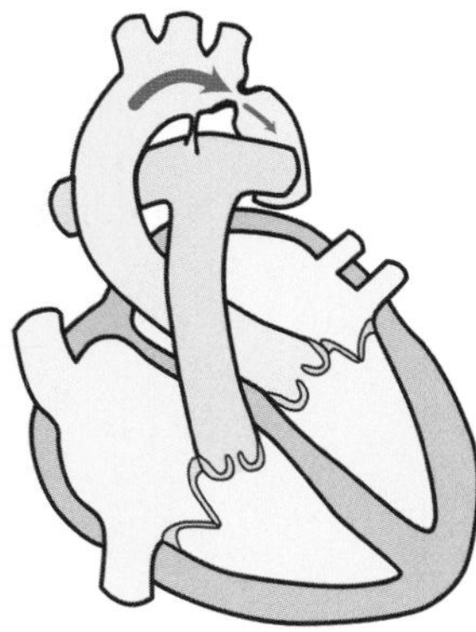	Severe narrowing of descending aorta, usually at the junction of the ductus arteriosus and the aortic arch, just distal to the origin of the left subclavian artery. Results in increased workload on left ventricle. Associated with defects of aortic valve in most cases, as well as associated patent ductus arteriosus; and associated ventricular septal defect.	S: In infants with associated lesions or symptoms, diagnosis occurs in first few months as symptoms of heart failure develop. For asymptomatic children and adolescents, growth and development are normal. Diagnosis usually incidental due to blood pressure findings. Adolescents may complain of vague lower extremity cramping that is worse with exercise. O: Upper extremity hypertension over 20 mm Hg higher than lower extremity measures is a hallmark of coarctation. Another important sign is absent or greatly diminished femoral pulses. A systolic murmur is heard best at the left sternal border, radiating to the back.

S, Subjective data; *O*, objective data.

TABLE 19-10 Murmurs Due to Valvular Defects

Midsystolic Ejection Murmurs

Due to forward flow through semilunar valves

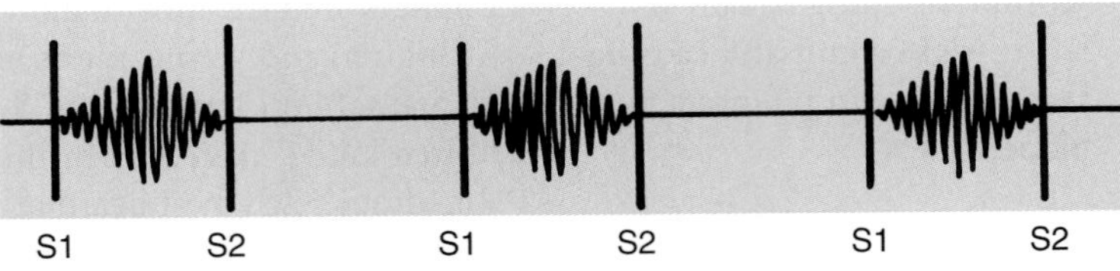

	Description	Clinical Data
Aortic Stenosis 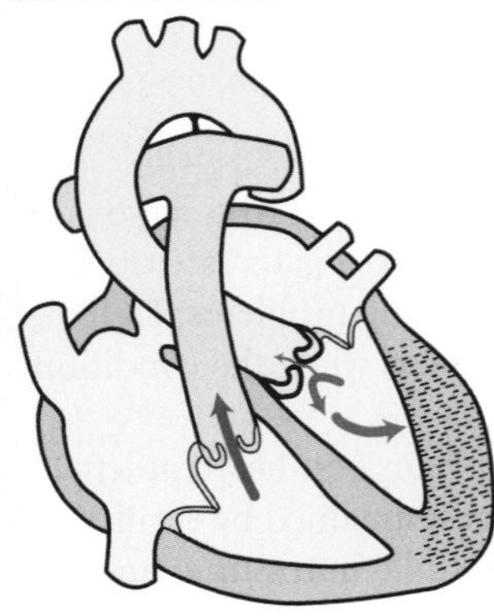	Calcification of aortic valve cusps restricts forward flow of blood during systole; LV hypertrophy develops.	S: Fatigue, DOE, palpitation, dizziness, fainting, anginal pain. O: Pallor, slow diminished radial pulse, low blood pressure, and auscultatory gap are common. Apical impulse sustained and displaced to left. Thrill in systole over second and third right interspaces and right side of neck. $\mathbf{S_1}$ normal, often ejection click present, often paradoxical split $\mathbf{S_2}$, $\mathbf{S_4}$ present with LV hypertrophy. Murmur: Loud, harsh, midsystolic, crescendo-decrescendo, loudest at second right interspace, radiates widely to side of neck, down left sternal border, or apex.
Pulmonic Stenosis 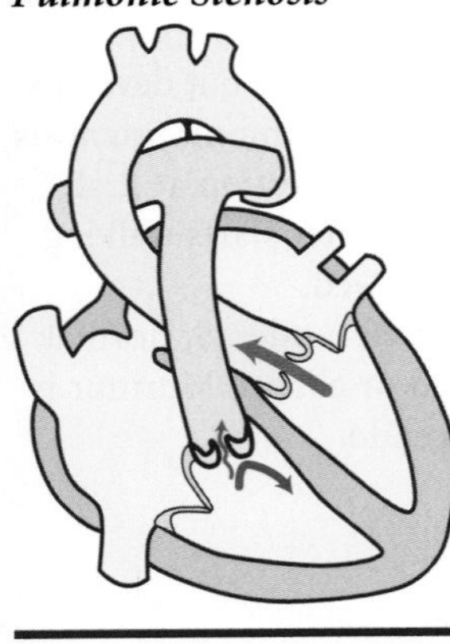	Calcification of pulmonic valve restricts forward flow of blood.	O: Thrill in systole at second and third left interspace, ejection click often present after $\mathbf{S_1}$, diminished $\mathbf{S_2}$ and usually with wide split, $\mathbf{S_4}$ common with RV hypertrophy. Murmur: Systolic, medium pitch, coarse, crescendo-decrescendo (diamond shape), best heard at second left interspace, radiates to the left and neck.

S, Subjective data; *O*, objective data.

TABLE 19-10 Murmurs Due to Valvular Defects—cont'd

Pansystolic Regurgitant Murmurs

Due to backward flow of blood from area of higher pressure to one of lower pressure

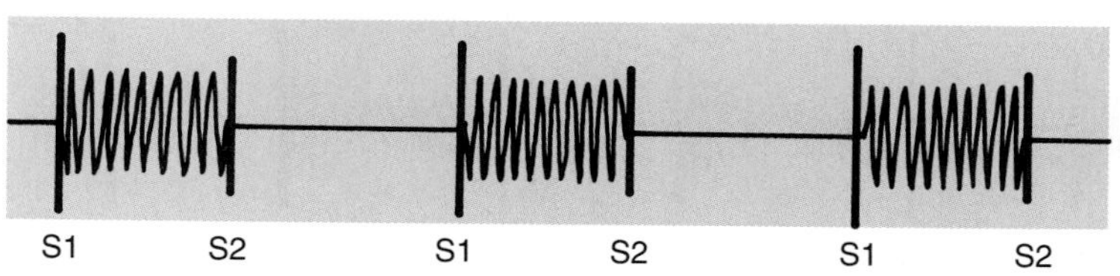

	Description	Clinical Data
Mitral Regurgitation 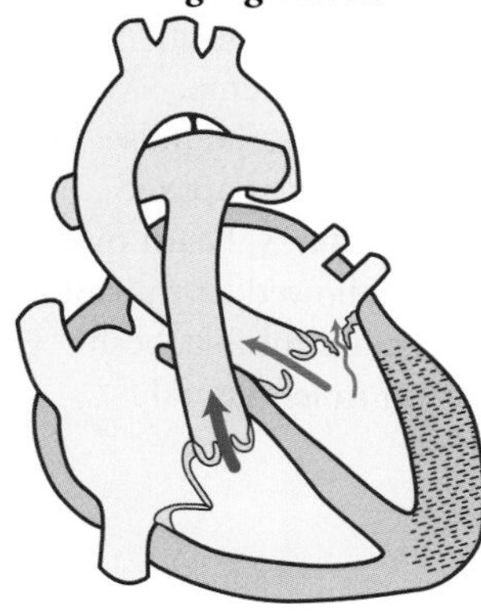	Stream of blood regurgitates back into LA during systole through incompetent mitral valve. In diastole, blood passes back into LV again along with new flow; results in LV dilation and hypertrophy.	S: Fatigue, palpitation, orthopnea, PND. O: Thrill in systole at apex. Lift at apex. Apical impulse displaced down and to left. $\mathbf{S_1}$ diminished, $\mathbf{S_2}$ accentuated, $\mathbf{S_3}$ at apex often present. Murmur: Pansystolic, often loud, blowing, best heard at apex, radiates well to left axilla.
Tricuspid Regurgitation 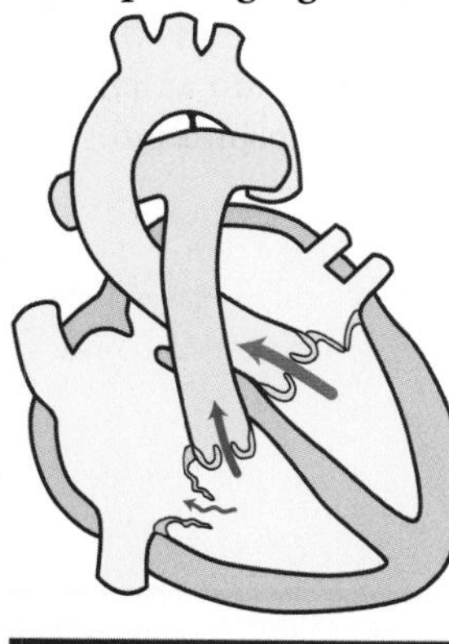	Backflow of blood through incompetent tricuspid valve into RA.	O: Engorged pulsating neck veins, liver enlarged. Lift at sternum if RV hypertrophy present, often thrill at left lower sternal border. Murmur: Soft, blowing, pansystolic, best heard at left lower sternal border, increases with inspiration.

S, Subjective data; *O,* objective data.

Images © Pat Thomas, 2006.

Continued

TABLE 19-10 Murmurs Due to Valvular Defects—cont'd

Diastolic Rumbles of AV Valves

Filling murmurs at low pressures, best heard with bell lightly touching skin

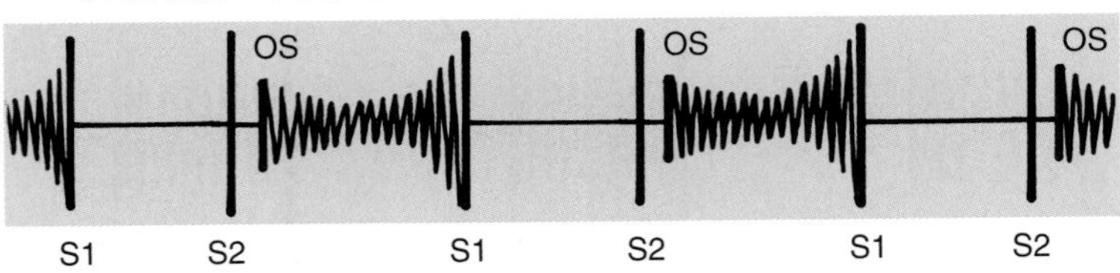

	Description	Clinical Data
Mitral Stenosis 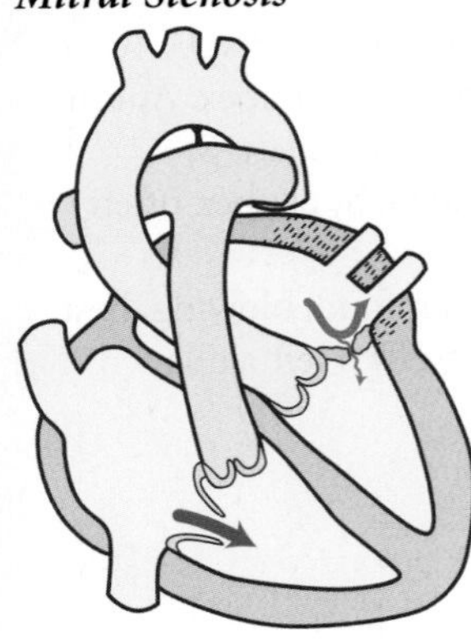	Calcified mitral valve will not open properly, impedes forward flow of blood into LV during diastole. Results in LA enlarged and LA pressure increased.	S: Fatigue, palpitations, DOE, orthopnea, occasional PND or pulmonary edema. O: Diminished, often irregular arterial pulse. Lift at apex, diastolic thrill common at apex. $\mathbf{S_1}$ accentuated; opening snap after $\mathbf{S_2}$ heard over wide area of precordium, followed by murmur. Murmur: Low-pitched diastolic rumble, best heard at apex, with person in left lateral position; does not radiate.
Tricuspid Stenosis 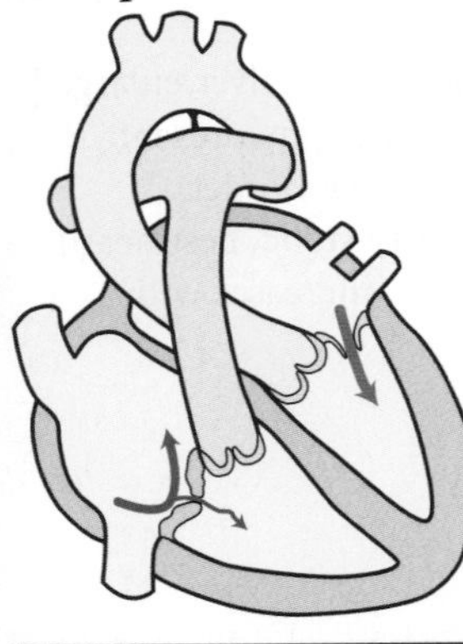	Calcification of tricuspid valve impedes forward flow into RV during diastole.	O: Diminished arterial pulse, jugular venous pulse prominent. Murmur: Diastolic rumble; best heard at left lower sternal border; louder in inspiration.

S, Subjective data; *O*, objective data.

TABLE 19-10 Murmurs Due to Valvular Defects—cont'd

Early Diastolic Murmurs
Due to SL valve incompetence

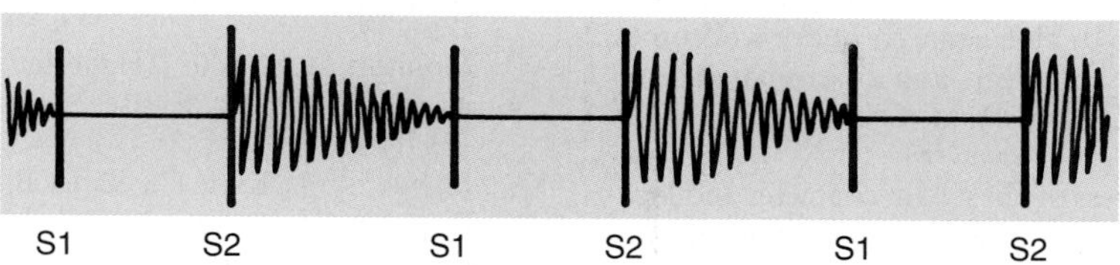

	Description	Clinical Data
Aortic Regurgitation 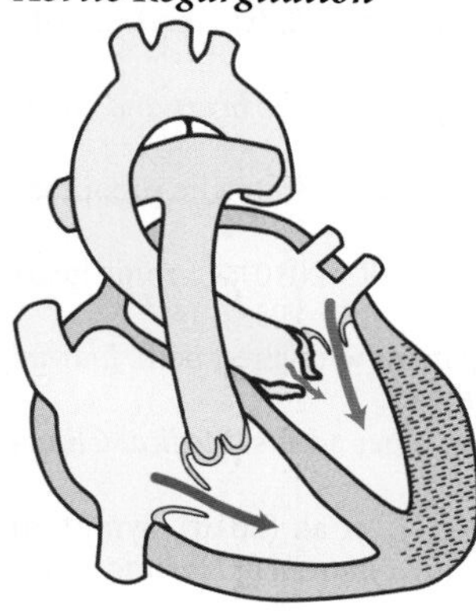	Stream of blood regurgitates back through incompetent aortic valve into LV during diastole. LV dilation and hypertrophy due to increased LV stroke volume. Rapid ejection of large stroke volume into poorly filled aorta, then rapid runoff in diastole as part of blood pushed back into LV.	S: Only minor symptoms for many years, then rapid deterioration: DOE, PND, angina, dizziness. O: Bounding "water-hammer" pulse in carotid, brachial, and femoral arteries. Blood pressure has wide pulse pressure. Pulsations in cervical and suprasternal area, apical impulse displaced to left and down, apical impulse feels brief. Murmur starts almost simultaneously with $\mathbf{S_2}$: soft high pitched, blowing diastolic, decrescendo, best heard at third left interspace at base, as person sits up and leans forward, radiates down.
Pulmonic Regurgitation 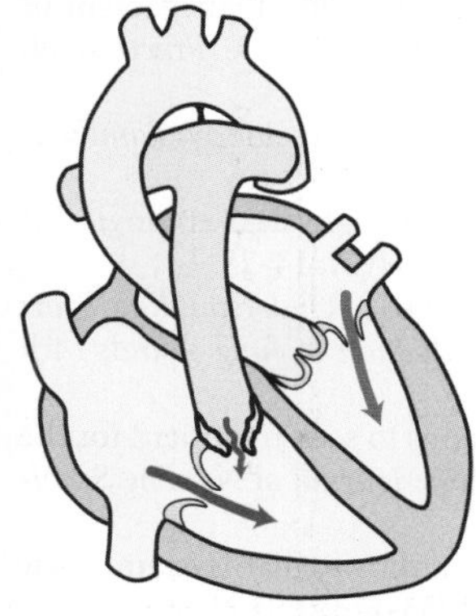	Backflow of blood through incompetent pulmonic valve, from pulmonary artery to RV.	Murmur has same timing and characteristics as that of aortic regurgitation, and is hard to distinguish on physical examination.

S, Subjective data; *O*, objective data.

Abnormal Findings

BIBLIOGRAPHY

1. Acelajado, M. C., & Oparil, S. (2009). Hypertension in the elderly. *Clinics in Geriatric Medicine, 25*(3), 391-412.
2. Allman, E., Berry, D., & Nasir, L. (2009). Depression and coping in heart failure patients. *Journal of Cardiovascular Nursing, 24*(2), 106-117.
3. American Heart Association. (2010). *Heart disease and stroke statistics, 2010.* Retrieved May 2010, from www.americanheart.org/downloadable/heart.
4. Andrews, T. D., Cook, S. S., Baumeister, M., et al. (2010). ARVC: help prevent sudden death. *Nurse Practitioner, 35*(2), 26-33.
5. Armbrister, K. A. (2008). Self-management: improving heart failure outcomes. *Nurse Practitioner, 33*(11), 20-28.
6. Aronow, W. S. (2006). Heart disease and aging. *Medical Clinics of North America, 90*(1), 849-862.
7. Braveman, P. A., Cubbin, C., Egerter, S., et al. (2010). Socioeconomic disparities in health in the United States: what the patterns tell us. *American Journal of Public Health, 100*(Suppl. 1), S186-S196.
8. Brown, D. W., Giles, W. H., & Croft, J. B. (2009). Association of cardiac auscultatory findings with coronary heart disease mortality. *North American Journal of Medical Sciences, 1,* 327-332.
9. Conn, R. D., & O'Keefe, J. H. (2009). Cardiac physical diagnosis in the digital age: an important but increasingly neglected skill (from stethoscopes to microchips). *American Journal of Cardiology, 104*(4), 590-595.
10. Cunningham, F. G., Leveno, K. J., Bloom, S. L., et al. (2010). *Williams obstetrics* (23rd ed.). New York: McGraw-Hill.

11. Dakin, C. L. (2008). New approaches to heart failure in the ED. *American Journal of Nursing, 108*(3), 68-71.
12. Dimeff, R. J. (2009). High school athlete with family history of sudden cardiac death. *Consultant, 49*(2), 79-80.
13. Dracup, K., McKinley, S., Doering, L. V., et al. (2008). Acute coronary syndrome: what do patients know? *Archives of Internal Medicine, 168*(10), 1049-1054.
14. Dressler, D. K. (2009). Death by clot: acute coronary syndromes, ischemic stroke, pulmonary embolism, and disseminated intravascular coagulation. *AACN Advanced Critical Care, 20*(2), 166-176.
15. Eslick, G. D. (2005). Usefulness of chest pain character and location as diagnostic indicators of an acute coronary syndrome. *American Journal of Cardiology, 95*(1), 1228-1231.
15a. Fleg, J. L. (1990). Diagnostic evaluations. In W. B. Abrams & R. Berkow (Eds.), *The Merck manual of geriatrics*. Rahway, NJ: Merck, Sharp, & Dohme.
16. Fleiner, S. (2006). Recognition and stabilization of neonates with congenital heart disease. *Newborn and Infant Nursing Reviews, 6*(3), 137-150.
17. Grossman, V. G. A., & McGowan, B. A. (2008). Postural orthostatic tachycardia syndrome. *American Journal of Nursing, 108*(8), 58-60.
18. Hartas, G., Tsounias, E., & Gupta-Malhotra, M. (2009). Approach to diagnosing congenital cardiac disorders. *Critical Care Nursing Clinics of North America, 21*(1), 27-36.
19. Hayman, L. L., Kamau, M. W., & Stuart-Shor, E. M. (2009). The heart of the matter: reducing CVD risk. *Nurse Practitioner, 34*(5), 31-35.
20. Klein, D. G. (2005). Thoracic aortic aneurysms. *Journal of Cardiovascular Nursing, 20*, 245-250.
21. Kliegman, R. M., Behrman, R. E., Jenson, H. B., et al. (2007). *Nelson textbook of pediatrics* (18th ed.). Philadelphia: Saunders.
22. Klieman, L., Hyde, S., & Berra, K. (2006). Cardiovascular disease risk reduction in older adults. *Journal of Cardiovascular Nursing, 21*, 527-539.
23. Kumar, A., & Cannon, C. P. (2009). Acute coronary syndromes. *Mayo Clinic Proceedings, 84*(10), 917-938.
24. Lembo, N. J., Dell'Italia, L. J., Crawford, M. H., et al. (1988). Bedside diagnosis of systolic murmurs. *New England Journal of Medicine, 318*(24), 1572-1578.
24a. Libby, P., Bonow, R. O., Mann, D. L., et al. (2008). *Braunwald's heart disease: a textbook of cardiovascular medicine* (8th ed.). Philadelphia: Saunders.
25. Lloyd-Jones, D. M., Hong, Y., Labarthe, D., et al. (2010). Defining and setting national goals for cardiovascular health promotion and disease reduction. *Circulation, 121*(1), 586-613.
26. Matthews, K. A., Crawford, S. L., Chae, C. U., et al. (2009). Are changes in cardiovascular disease risk factors in midlife women due to chronological aging or to the menopausal transition? *Journal of the American College of Cardiology, 54*, 2366-2373.
27. McGee, S. (2007). *Evidence based physical diagnosis* (2nd ed.). Philadelphia: Saunders.
28. Moe, G. W., & Tu, J. (2010). Heart failure in the ethnic minorities. *Current Opinion in Cardiology, 2*, 124-130.
29. Mosack, V., & Steinke, E. E. (2009). Trends in sexual concerns after myocardial infarction. *Journal of Cardiovascular Nursing, 24*(2), 162-170.
30. Mosley, W., & Lloyd-Jones, D. M. (2009). Epidemiology of hypertension in the elderly. *Clinics in Geriatric Medicine, 25*(2), 179-189.
31. Moulton, S. A. (2009). Hypertension in African Americans and its related chronic diseases. *Journal of Cultural Diversity, 16*(4), 165-170.
32. Muster, A. J., Kim, H., Kane, B., et al. (2009). Ten-year echo/Doppler determination of the benefits of aerobic exercise after the age of 65 years. *Echocardiography, 27*(1), 5-10.
33. National Center for Health Statistics. (2009). *Health, United States, 2008 with chartbook*. Hyattsville, MD: Author. Retrieved May 20, 2010, from www.cdc.gov/nchs/data/hus/hus08.pdf.
34. Overbaugh, K. J. (2009). Acute coronary syndrome. *American Journal of Nursing, 109*(5), 42-52.
35. Perloff, J. K. (2000). *Physical examination of the heart and circulation* (3rd ed.). Philadelphia: Saunders.
36. Poletti, J. M. (2009). Carotid bruit on an orthopedic preoperative exam. *Nurse Practitioner, 34*(3), 8-11.
37. Ramani, G. V., Uber, P. A., & Mehra, M. R. (2010). Chronic heart failure. *Mayo Clinic Proceedings, 85*(2), 180-195.
37a. Reigle, J. (2005). Evaluating the patient with chest pain. *Journal of Cardiovascular Nursing, 20*, 226-231.
38. Rich, M. W. (2006). Heart failure in older adults. *Medical Clinics of North America, 90*(5), 863-885.
39. Riegel, B., Dickson, V. V., Cameron, J., et al. (2010). Symptom recognition in elders with heart failure. *Journal of Nursing Scholarship, 42*(1), 92-100.
40. Sen, B., McNab, A., & Burdess, C. (2009). Identifying and managing patients with acute coronary conditions. *Emergency Nurse, 17*(7), 18-23.
41. Stewart, D., & Casida, J. (2010). Diagnosis and management of an adult patient with atrial septal defect. *Nurse Practitioner, 35*(2), 8-11.
42. Tanaka, H. (2009). Habitual exercise for the elderly. *Family & Community Health, 32*(Suppl. 1), S57-S65.
43. Thompson, J. (2006). Psychological and physical etiologies of heart palpitations. *Nurse Practitioner, 31*(2), 14-25.
44. Tilkian, A. G., & Conover, M. B. (2001). *Understanding heart sounds and murmurs with an introduction to lung sounds* (4th ed.). Philadelphia: Saunders.
45. Turris, S. A. (2009). Women's decisions to seek treatment for the symptoms of potential cardiac illness. *Journal of Nursing Scholarship, 41*(1), 5-12.
46. Wei, J. Y. (1992). Age and the cardiovascular system. *New England Journal of Medicine, 327*, 1735-1739.
47. Yusuf, S., Hawken, S., Ounpuu, S., et al. (2004). Effect of potentially modifiable risk factors associated with myocardial infarction in 52 countries (the INTERHEART study). *Lancet, 364*, 937-952.

Summary Checklist: Heart and Neck Vessels Exam

For a PDA-downloadable version, go to http://evolve.elsevier.com/Jarvis/.

Neck

1. Carotid pulse—Observe and palpate
2. Observe jugular venous pulse
3. Estimate jugular venous pressure

Precordium

Inspection and palpation

1. Describe location of apical impulse
2. Note any heave (lift) or thrill

Auscultation

1. Identify anatomic areas where you listen
2. Note rate and rhythm of heartbeat
3. Identify S_1 and S_2 and note any variation
4. Listen in systole and diastole for any extra heart sounds
5. Listen in systole and diastole for any murmurs
6. Repeat sequence with bell
7. Listen at the apex with person in left lateral position
8. Listen at the base with person in sitting position

20

Peripheral Vascular System and Lymphatic System

evolve WEBSITE

http://evolve.elsevier.com/Jarvis/

- Animations
- Audio Key Points
- Bedside Assessment Summary Checklist
- Health Promotion Guide
  Foot Care
  High Blood Pressure
- NCLEX Review Questions
- Physical Examination Summary Checklist
- Quick Assessment for Common Conditions
  Deep Vein Thrombosis

OUTLINE

Structure and Function, 499

Arteries
Veins
Venous Flow
Lymphatics

Subjective Data, 505

Health History Questions

Objective Data, 506

Preparation
The Arms
The Legs

Documentation and Critical Thinking, 518

Abnormal Findings, 519

Abnormal Findings for Advanced Practice, 520

STRUCTURE AND FUNCTION

The vascular system consists of the vessels of the body. Vessels are tubes for transporting fluid, such as the blood or lymph. Any disease in the vascular system creates problems with delivery of oxygen and nutrients to the tissues or elimination of carbon dioxide and waste products from cellular metabolism.

ARTERIES

The heart pumps freshly oxygenated blood through the arteries to all body tissues. The pumping heart makes this a high-pressure system. The artery walls are strong, tough, and tense to withstand pressure demands. Arteries contain elastic fibers, which allow their walls to stretch with systole and recoil with diastole. Arteries also contain muscle fibers (vascular smooth muscle, or VSM), which control the amount of blood delivered to the tissues. The VSM contracts or dilates, which changes the diameter of the arteries to control the rate of blood flow.

Each heartbeat creates a pressure wave, which makes the arteries expand and then recoil. It is the recoil that propels blood through like a wave. All arteries have this pressure wave,

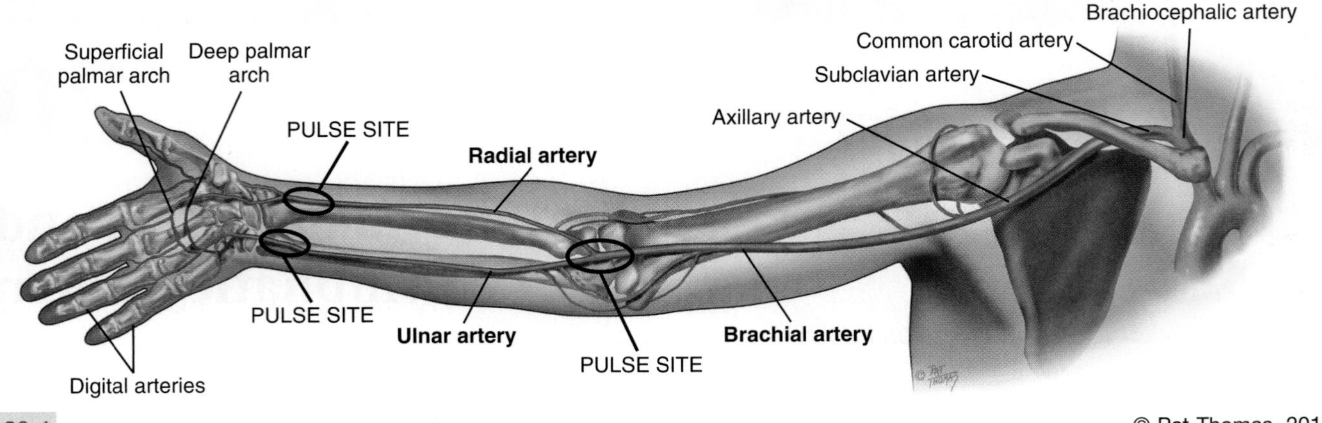

20-1 © Pat Thomas, 2010.

or **pulse,** throughout their length, but you can feel it only at body sites where the artery lies close to the skin and over a bone. The following arteries are accessible to examination.

Temporal Artery. The temporal artery is palpated in front of the ear, as discussed in Chapter 13.

Carotid Artery. The carotid artery is palpated in the groove between the sternomastoid muscle and the trachea and is discussed in Chapter 19.

Arteries in the Arm. The major artery supplying the arm is the **brachial** artery, which runs in the biceps-triceps furrow of the upper arm and surfaces at the antecubital fossa in the elbow medial to the biceps tendon (Fig. 20-1). Immediately below the elbow, the brachial artery bifurcates into the **ulnar** and **radial** arteries. These run distally and form two arches supplying the hand; these are called the *superficial* and *deep palmar arches.* The radial pulse lies just medial to the radius at the wrist; the ulnar artery is in the same relation to the ulna, but it is deeper and often difficult to feel.

Arteries in the Leg. The major artery to the leg is the **femoral** artery, which passes under the inguinal ligament (Fig. 20-2). The femoral artery travels down the thigh. At the lower thigh, it courses posteriorly; then it is termed the **popliteal** artery. Below the knee, the popliteal artery divides. The anterior tibial artery travels down the front of the leg on to the dorsum of the foot, where it becomes the **dorsalis pedis.** In back of the leg, the **posterior tibial** artery travels down behind the medial malleolus and in the foot forms the plantar arteries.

The function of the arteries is to supply oxygen and essential nutrients to the tissues. **Ischemia** is a deficient supply of oxygenated arterial blood to a tissue caused by obstruction of a blood vessel. A complete blockage leads to death of the distal tissue. A partial blockage creates an insufficient supply, and the ischemia may be apparent only at exercise when oxygen needs increase.

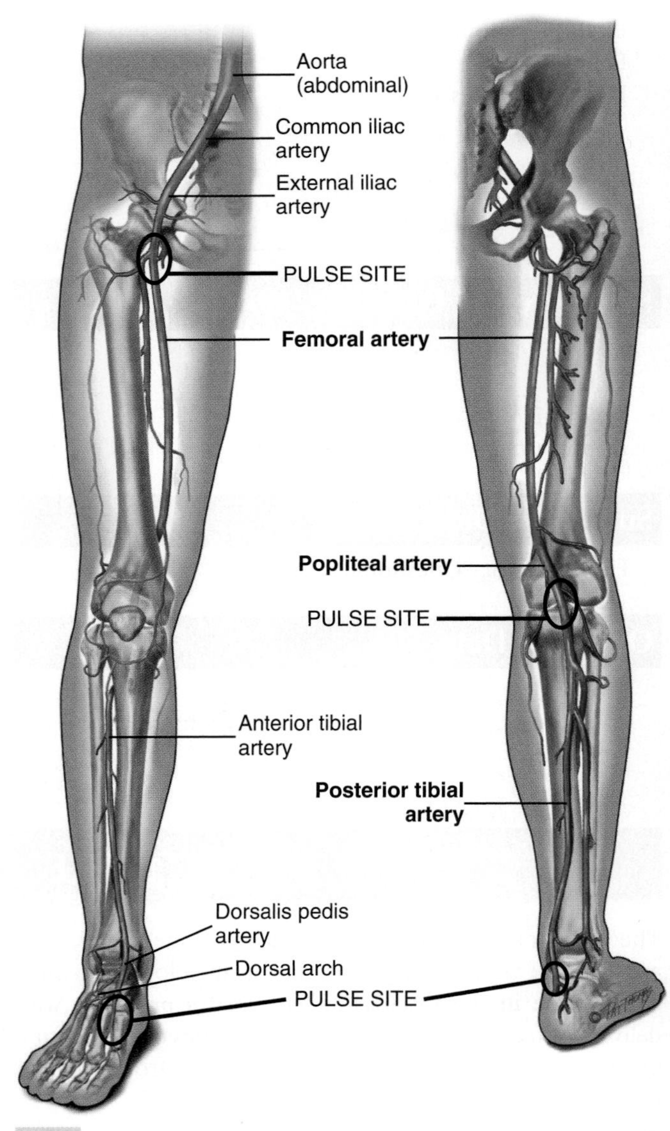

20-2 Arteries in the leg. © Pat Thomas, 2010.

VEINS

The course of veins parallels that of arteries, but the body has more veins and they lie closer to the skin surface. The following veins are accessible to examination.

Jugular Veins. Assessment of the jugular veins is presented in Chapter 19.

Veins in the Arm. Each arm has two sets of veins: superficial and deep. The superficial veins are in the subcutaneous tissue and are responsible for most of the venous return.

Veins in the Leg. The legs have three types of veins (Fig. 20-3):

1. The **deep veins** run alongside the deep arteries and conduct most of the venous return from the legs. These are the **femoral** and **popliteal** veins. As long as these veins remain intact, the superficial veins can be excised without harming the circulation.
2. The **superficial veins** are the **great** and **small saphenous** veins. The great saphenous vein, inside the leg, starts at the medial side of the dorsum of the foot. You can see it ascend in front of the medial malleolus; then it crosses the tibia obliquely and ascends along the medial side of the thigh. The small saphenous vein, outside the leg, starts on the lateral side of the dorsum of the foot, ascends behind the lateral malleolus, up the back of the leg, where it joins the popliteal vein.
3. **Perforators** (not illustrated) are connecting veins that join the two sets. They also have one-way valves that route blood from the superficial into the deep veins.

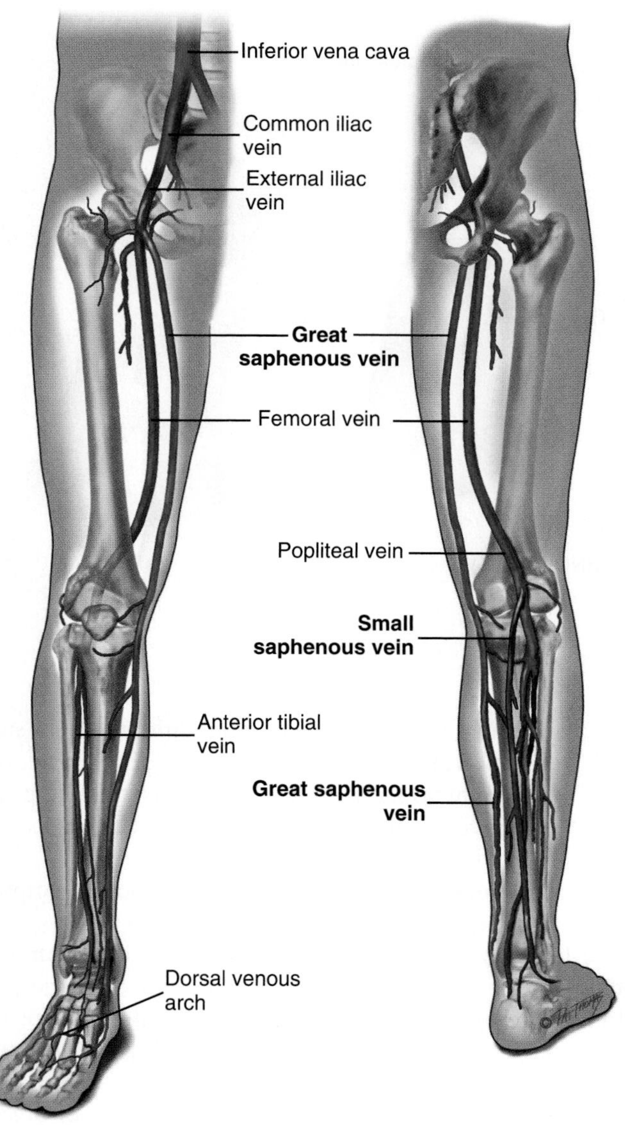

20-3 Veins in the leg. © Pat Thomas, 2010.

VENOUS FLOW

Veins drain the deoxygenated blood and its waste products from the tissues and return it to the heart. Unlike the arteries, veins are a low-pressure system. Because veins do not have a pump to generate their blood flow, the veins need a mechanism to keep blood moving (Fig. 20-4). This is accomplished by (1) the contracting skeletal muscles that milk the blood proximally, back toward the heart; (2) the pressure gradient caused by breathing, in which inspiration makes the thoracic pressure decrease and the abdominal pressure increase; and (3) the intraluminal valves, which ensure unidirectional flow. Each valve is a paired semilunar pocket that opens toward the heart and closes tightly when filled to prevent backflow of blood.

In the legs, this mechanism is called the "calf pump," or "peripheral heart." While walking, the calf muscles alternately contract (systole) and relax (diastole). In the contraction phase, the gastrocnemius and soleus muscles squeeze the veins and direct the blood flow proximally. Because of the valves, venous blood flows just one way—toward the heart.

Besides the presence of intraluminal valves, venous structure differs from arterial structure. Because venous pressure is lower, walls of the veins are thinner than those of the arteries. Veins have a larger diameter and are more distensible; they can expand and hold more blood when blood volume increases. This is a compensatory mechanism to reduce stress on the heart. Because of this ability to stretch, veins are called **capacitance vessels.**

Efficient venous return depends on contracting skeletal muscles, competent valves in the veins, and a patent lumen. Problems with any of these three elements lead to venous stasis. At risk for venous disease are people who undergo prolonged standing, sitting, or bedrest, because they do not benefit from the milking action that walking accomplishes. Hypercoagulable states and vein wall trauma are other factors that increase risk for venous disease. Also, dilated and tortuous (varicose) veins create **incompetent valves,** wherein the lumen is so wide the valve cusps cannot approximate. This condition increases venous pressure, which further dilates the vein. Some people have a genetic predisposition to

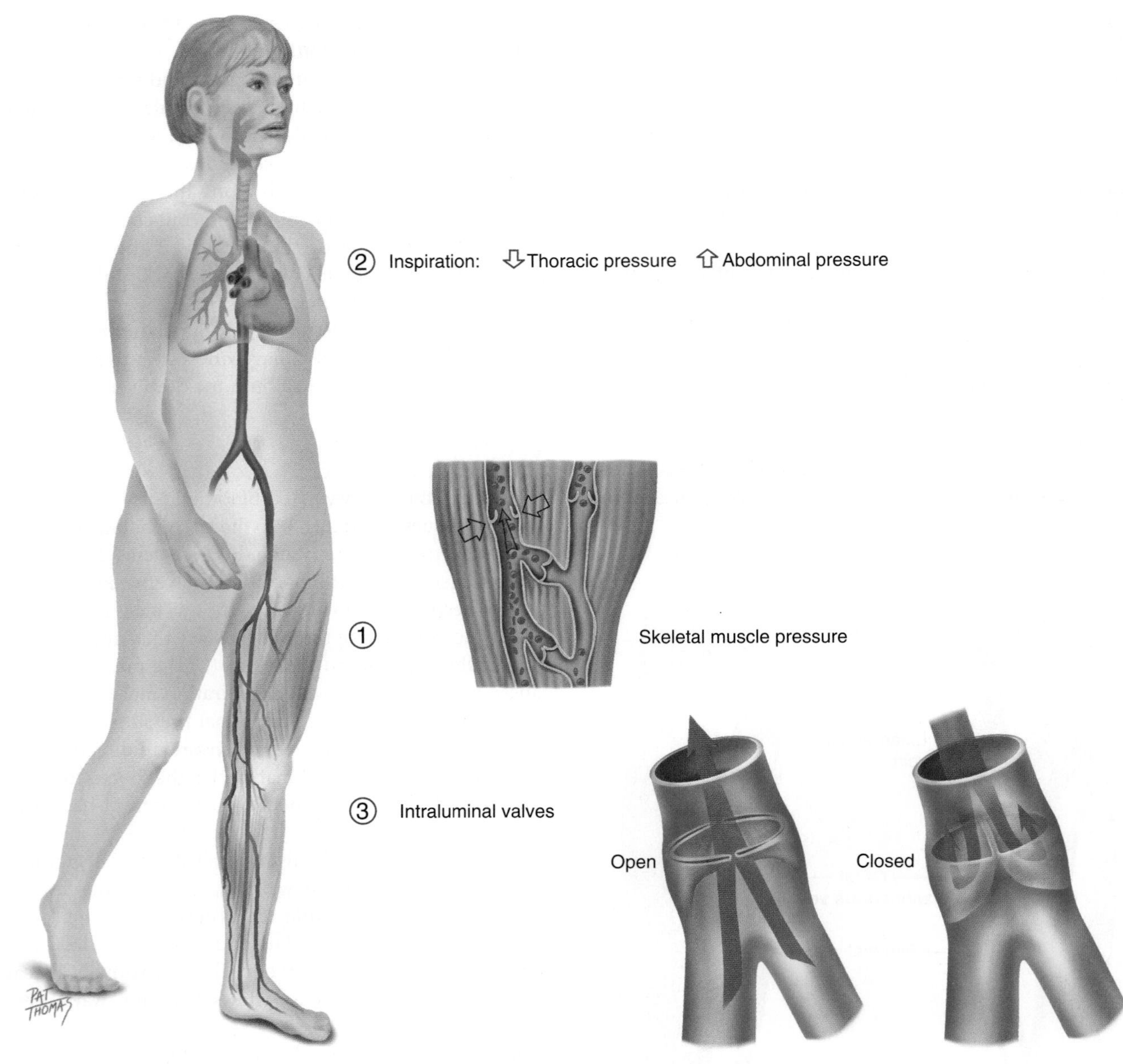

MECHANISMS OF VENOUS FLOW

20-4

varicose veins, but obesity and pregnancy are increased risk factors.

LYMPHATICS

The lymphatics form a completely separate vessel system, which retrieves excess fluid from the tissue spaces and returns it to the bloodstream (Fig. 20-5). During circulation, the blood pressure pushes somewhat more fluid out of the capillaries than the veins can absorb. Without lymphatic drainage, fluid would build up in the interstitial spaces and produce edema.

The vessels converge and drain into two main trunks, which empty into the venous system at the subclavian veins (see Fig. 20-5):

1. The **right lymphatic duct** empties into the right subclavian vein. It drains the right side of the head and neck, right arm, right side of the thorax, right lung and pleura, right side of the heart, and right upper section of the liver.
2. The **thoracic duct** drains the rest of the body. It empties into the left subclavian vein.

The functions of the lymphatic system are (1) to conserve fluid and plasma proteins that leak out of the capillaries, (2) to form a major part of the immune system that defends the body against disease, and (3) to absorb lipids from the intestinal tract.

The immune system is a complicated network of organs and cells that work together to protect the body. The immune system detects and eliminates foreign pathogens, both those that come in from the environment and those arising from inside (abnormal or mutant cells). It accomplishes this by phagocytosis (digestion) of the substances by neutrophils and monocytes/macrophages and by production of specific antibodies or specific immune responses by the lymphocytes.

The lymphatic vessels have a unique structure. Lymphatic capillaries start as microscopic open-ended tubes, which siphon interstitial fluid. The capillaries converge to form vessels. The vessels, like veins, drain into larger ones. The vessels have valves, so flow is one way from the tissue spaces into the bloodstream. The many valves make the vessels look beaded. The flow of lymph is slow compared with that of the blood. Lymph flow is propelled by contracting skeletal muscles, by pressure changes secondary to breathing, and by contraction of the vessel walls themselves.

Lymph nodes are small, oval clumps of lymphatic tissue located at intervals along the vessels. Most nodes are arranged in groups, both deep and superficial, in the body. Nodes filter the fluid before it is returned to the bloodstream and filter out microorganisms that could be harmful to the body. The pathogens are exposed to B and T lymphocytes in the lymph nodes. The lymphocytes mount an antigen-specific response to eliminate the pathogens. With local inflammation, the nodes in that area become swollen and tender.

The superficial groups of nodes are accessible to inspection and palpation and give clues to the status of the lymphatic system:

- **Cervical nodes** drain the head and neck and are described in Chapter 13.
- **Axillary nodes** drain the breast and upper arm. They are described in Chapter 17.
- The **epitrochlear node** is in the antecubital fossa and drains the hand and lower arm.
- The **inguinal nodes** in the groin drain most of the lymph of the lower extremity, the external genitalia, and the anterior abdominal wall.

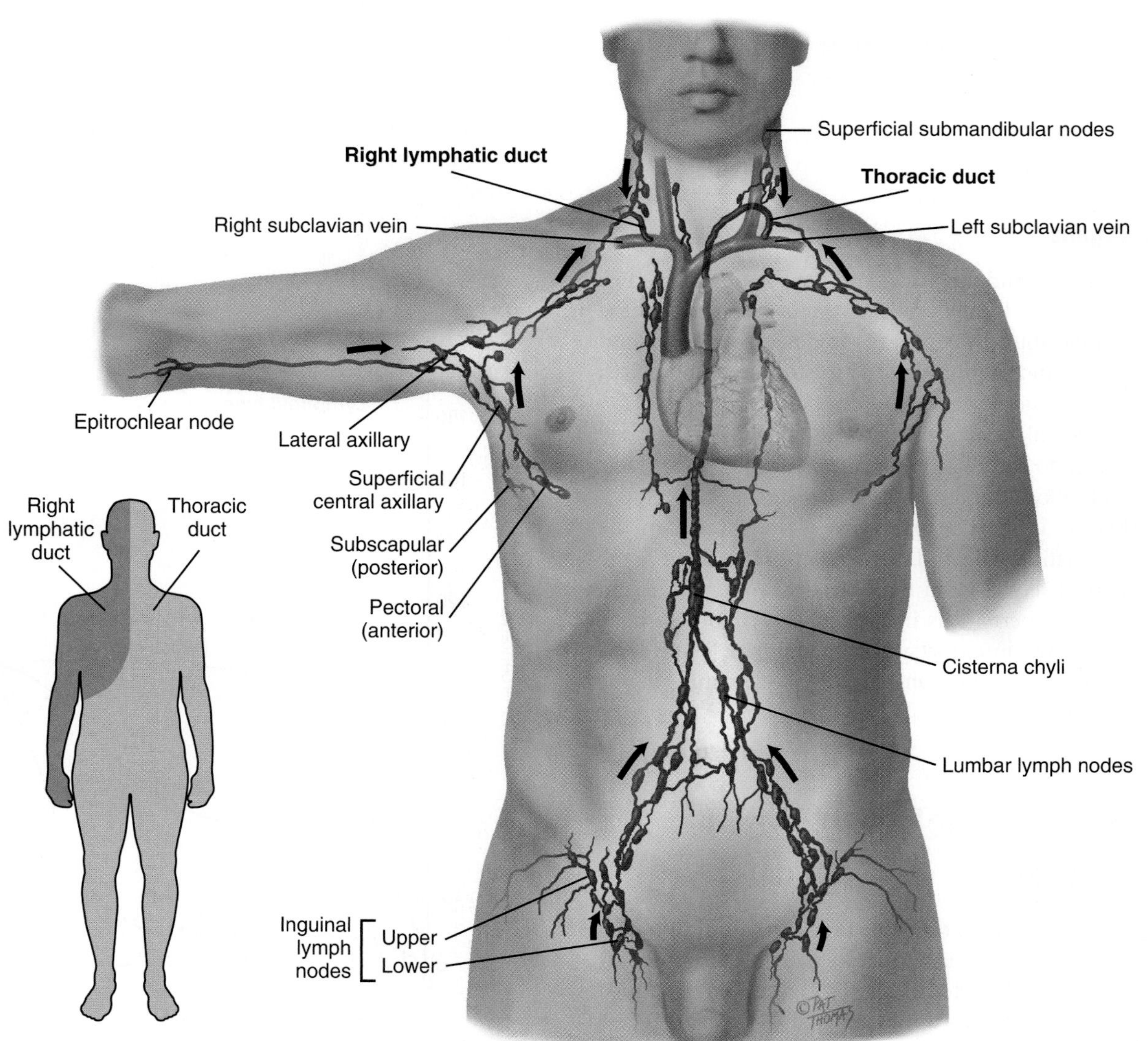

20-5 LYMPHATIC DUCTS AND DRAINAGE PATTERNS © Pat Thomas, 2010.

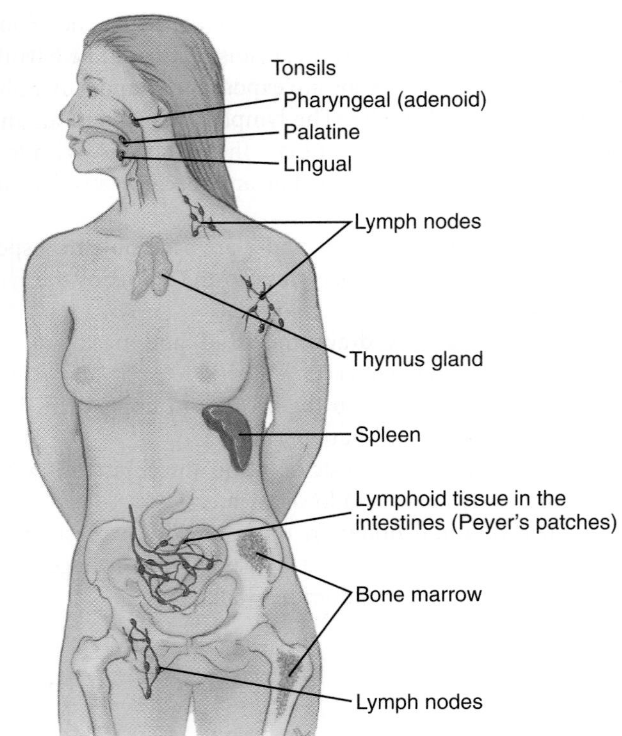

RELATED ORGANS IN IMMUNE SYSTEM
20-6

Related Organs

The spleen, tonsils, and thymus aid the lymphatic system (Fig. 20-6). The **spleen** is located in the left upper quadrant of the abdomen. It has four functions: (1) to destroy old red blood cells; (2) to produce antibodies; (3) to store red blood cells; and (4) to filter microorganisms from the blood.

The **tonsils** (palatine, pharyngeal, and lingual) are located at the entrance to the respiratory and gastrointestinal tracts and respond to local inflammation.

The **thymus** is the flat, pink-gray gland located in the superior mediastinum behind the sternum and in front of the aorta. It is relatively large in the fetus and young child and atrophies after puberty. It is important in developing the T lymphocytes of the immune system in children. The B lymphocytes originate in the bone marrow and mature in the lymphoid tissue.

DEVELOPMENTAL COMPETENCE

Infants and Children

The lymphatic system has the same function in children as in adults. Lymphoid tissue has a unique growth pattern compared with other body systems (Fig. 20-7). It is well developed at birth and grows rapidly until age 10 or 11 years. By age 6 years, the lymphoid tissue reaches adult size; it surpasses adult size by puberty, and then it slowly atrophies. It is possible that the excessive antigen stimulation in children causes the early rapid growth.

Lymph nodes are relatively large in children, and the superficial ones often are palpable even when the child is healthy. With infection, excessive swelling and hyperplasia occur. Enlarged tonsils are familiar signs in respiratory infections. The excessive lymphoid response also may account for the common childhood symptom of abdominal pain with seemingly unrelated problems such as upper respiratory infections. Possibly the inflammation of mesenteric lymph nodes produces the abdominal pain.

The Pregnant Woman

Hormonal changes cause vasodilation and the resulting drop in blood pressure described in Chapter 19. The growing uterus obstructs drainage of the iliac veins and the inferior vena cava. This condition causes low blood flow and increases venous pressure. This, in turn, causes dependent edema, varicosities in the legs and vulva, and hemorrhoids.

The Aging Adult

Peripheral blood vessels grow more rigid with age, resulting in a condition called **arteriosclerosis.** This condition produces the rise in systolic blood pressure discussed in Chapter 9. Do not confuse this process with another one, **atherosclerosis,** or the deposition of fatty plaques on the intima of the arteries.

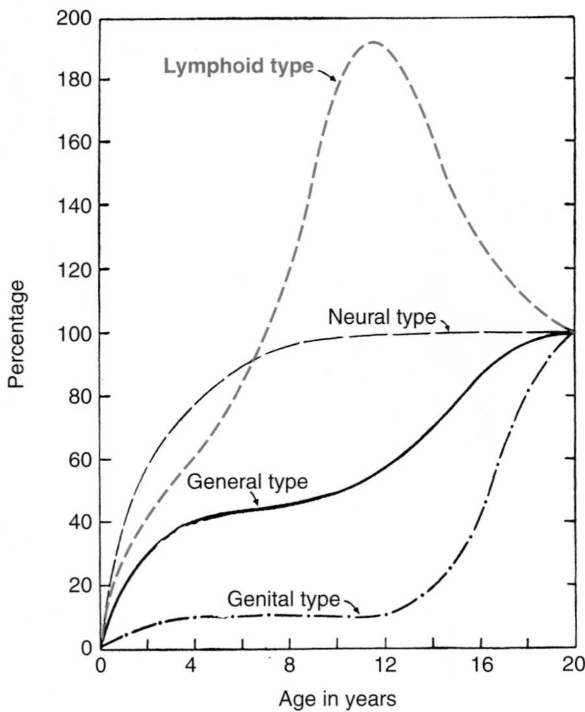

20-7 Comparison of growth rates of three types of tissues in the body.

Aging produces a progressive enlargement of the intramuscular calf veins. Prolonged bedrest, prolonged immobilization, and heart failure increase the risk for deep venous thrombosis and subsequent pulmonary embolism. These conditions are common in aging and also with malignancy and myocardial infarction (MI). Low-dose anticoagulant medication reduces the risk for venous thromboembolism.

Loss of lymphatic tissue leads to fewer numbers of lymph nodes in older people and to a decrease in the size of remaining nodes.

SUBJECTIVE DATA

1. Leg pain or cramps
2. Skin changes on arms or legs
3. Swelling
4. Lymph node enlargement
5. Medications

Examiner Asks	Rationale
1. Leg pain or cramps. Any leg pain (cramps)? Where?	
• Describe the type of pain; is it burning, aching, cramping, stabbing? Did this come on gradually or suddenly?	Peripheral vascular disease (PVD)—see pain profiles in Table 20-3, p. 521.
• Is it aggravated by activity, walking?	
• How many blocks (stairs) does it take to produce this pain?	**Claudication distance** is the number of blocks walked or stairs climbed to produce pain.
• Has this amount changed recently?	Note sudden decrease in claudication distance or pain not relieved by rest.
• Is the pain worse with elevation? Worse with cool temperatures?	
• Does the pain wake you up at night?	Night leg pain is common in aging adults. It may indicate the ischemic rest pain of PVD, severe night muscle cramping (usually the calf), or the restless leg syndrome.
• Any recent change in exercise, a new exercise, increasing exercise?	Pain of musculoskeletal origin rather than vascular.
• What relieves this pain: dangling, walking, rubbing? Is the leg pain associated with any skin changes?	
• Is it associated with any change in sexual function (males)?	Aortoiliac occlusion is associated with impotence (Leriche syndrome).
• Any history of vascular problems, heart problems, diabetes, obesity, pregnancy, smoking, trauma, prolonged standing, or bedrest?	
2. Skin changes on arms or legs. Any **skin changes** on arms or legs? What color: redness, pallor, blueness, brown discolorations?	
• Any change in temperature—excess warmth or coolness?	Coolness is associated with arterial disease.
• Do your leg veins look bulging and crooked? How have you treated these? Do you use support hose?	Varicose veins.
• Any leg sores or ulcers? Where on the leg? Any pain with the leg ulcer?	Leg ulcers occur with chronic arterial and chronic venous disease (see Table 20-4 p. 522).
3. Swelling in the arms or legs. Swelling in one or both legs? When did this swelling start?	**Edema** is bilateral when the cause is generalized (heart failure) or unilateral when it is the result of a local obstruction or inflammation.
• What time of day is the swelling at its worst: morning, or after up most of the day?	
• Does the swelling come and go, or is it constant?	
• What seems to bring it on: trauma, standing all day, sitting?	
• What relieves swelling: elevation, support hose?	
• Is swelling associated with pain, heat, redness, ulceration, hardened skin?	

Examiner Asks	Rationale
4. **Lymph node enlargement.** Any "swollen glands" (lumps, kernels)? Where in body? How long have you had them? • Any recent change? • How do they feel to you: hard, soft? • Are the swollen glands associated with pain, local infection?	Enlarged lymph nodes occur with infection, malignancies, and immunologic diseases.
5. **Medications.** What medications are you taking (e.g., oral contraceptives, hormone replacement)?	

OBJECTIVE DATA

PREPARATION

During a complete physical examination, examine the arms at the very beginning when you are checking the vital signs—the person is sitting. Examine the legs directly after the abdominal examination while the person is still supine. Then stand the person up to evaluate the leg veins.

Examination of the arms and legs includes peripheral vascular characteristics (following here), the skin (see Chapter 12), musculoskeletal findings (see Chapter 22), and neurologic findings (see Chapter 23). A method of integrating these steps is discussed in Chapter 27.

Room temperature should be about 22° C (72° F) and draftless to prevent vasodilation or vasoconstriction.

Use inspection and palpation. Compare your findings with the opposite extremity.

EQUIPMENT NEEDED

Occasionally need:
Paper tape measure
Tourniquet or blood pressure cuff
Stethoscope
Doppler ultrasonic stethoscope

Normal Range of Findings	Abnormal Findings
INSPECT AND PALPATE THE ARMS	
Lift both the person's hands in your hands. Inspect, then turn the person's hands over, noting color of skin and nail beds; temperature, texture, and turgor of skin; and the presence of any lesions, edema, or clubbing. Use the **profile sign** (viewing the finger from the side) to detect early clubbing. The normal nail-bed angle is 160 degrees. (See Chapter 12 for a full discussion of skin color, lesions, and clubbing.)	Flattening of angle and clubbing (diffuse enlargement of terminal phalanges) occur with congenital cyanotic heart disease and cor pulmonale.
With the person's hands near the level of his or her heart, check **capillary refill.** This is an index of peripheral perfusion and cardiac output. Depress and blanch the nail beds; release and note the time for color return. Usually, the vessels refill within a fraction of a second. Consider it normal if the color returns in less than 1 or 2 seconds. Note conditions that can skew your findings: a cool room, decreased body temperature, cigarette smoking, peripheral edema, and anemia.	Refill lasting more than 1 or 2 seconds signifies vasoconstriction or decreased cardiac output (hypovolemia, heart failure, shock). The hands are cold, clammy, and pale.
The two arms should be symmetric in size.	Edema of upper extremities occurs when lymphatic drainage is obstructed, which may occur after breast surgery (see Table 20-2 on p. 520).

Normal Range of Findings

Note the presence of any scars on hands and arms. Many occur normally with usual childhood abrasions or with occupations involving hand tools.

Palpate both radial pulses, noting rate, rhythm, elasticity of vessel wall, and equal force (Fig. 20-8). Grade the force (amplitude) on a 3-point scale:

3+, increased, full, bounding
2+, **normal**
1+, weak
0, absent

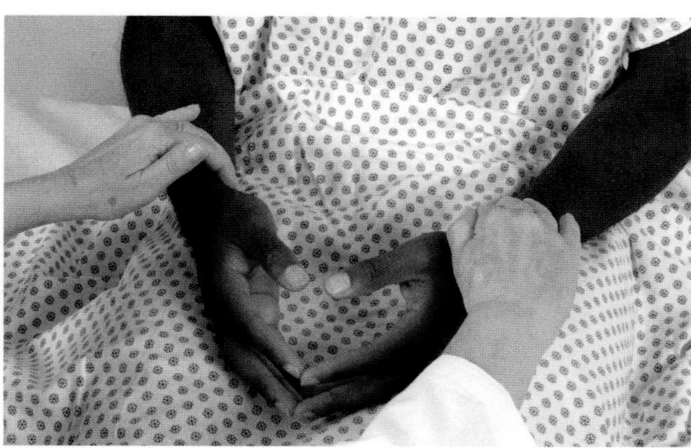

20-8

It usually is not necessary to palpate the ulnar pulses. If indicated, reach your hand under the person's arm and palpate along the medial side of the inner forearm (Fig. 20-9), although the ulnar pulses often are not palpable in the normal person.

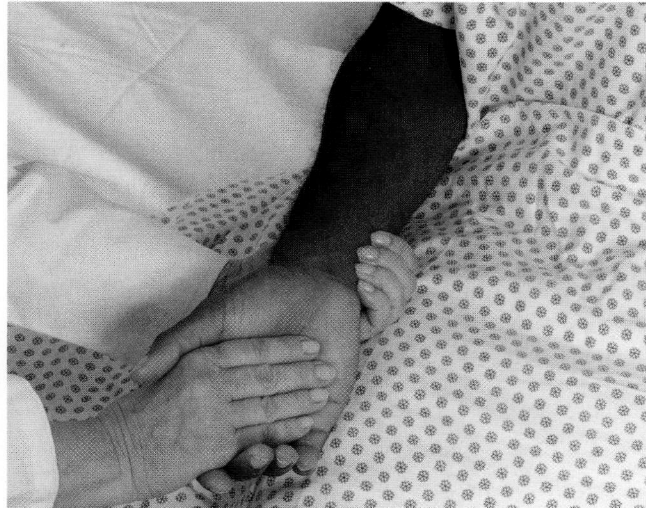

20-9 Palpate ulnar pulse.

Abnormal Findings

Needle tracks in hands, arms, antecubital fossae occur with IV drug use; linear scars in wrists may signify past self-inflicted injury.

Full, bounding pulse (3+) occurs with hyperkinetic states (exercise, anxiety, fever), anemia, and hyperthyroidism.

Weak, "thready" pulse (1+) occurs with shock and peripheral arterial disease. See Table 20-1 on p. 519 for illustrations of these and irregular pulse rhythms.

Normal Range of Findings	Abnormal Findings

Palpate the brachial pulses—their force should be equal bilaterally (Fig. 20-10).

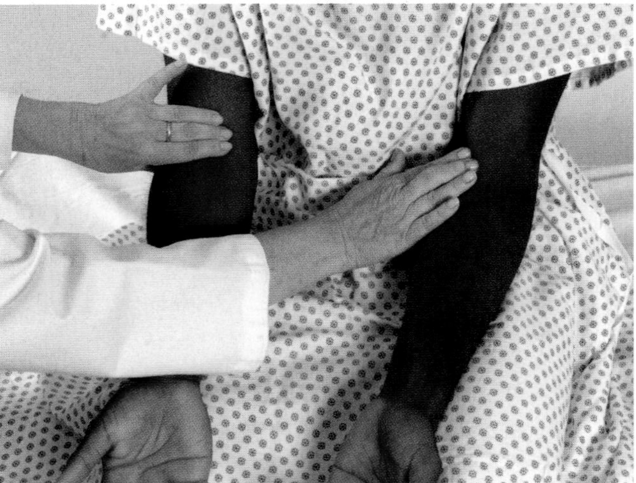

20-10

Check the epitrochlear lymph nodes in the depression above and behind the medial condyle of the humerus. Do this by "shaking hands" with the person and reaching your other hand under the person's elbow to the groove between the biceps and triceps muscles, above the medial epicondyle (Fig. 20-11). These nodes are not palpable normally.

An enlarged epitrochlear node occurs with infection of the hand or forearm.

Epitrochlear nodes occur in conditions of generalized lymphadenopathy: lymphoma, chronic lymphocytic leukemia, sarcoidosis, infections, mononucleosis.

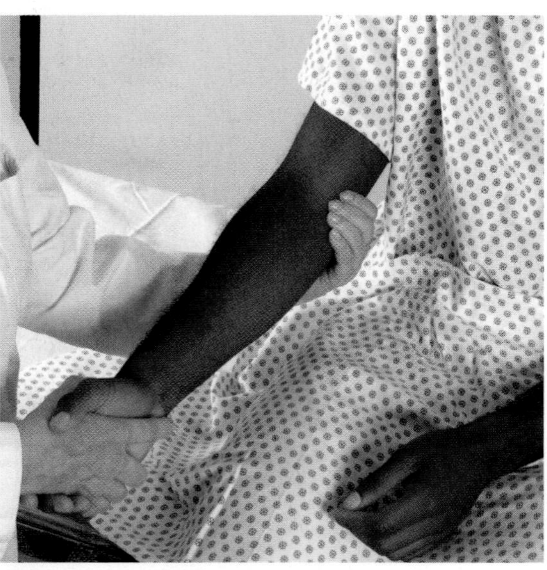

20-11 Search epitrochlear area.

Normal Range of Findings	Abnormal Findings
The **modified Allen test** is used to evaluate the adequacy of collateral circulation before cannulating the radial artery (Fig. 20-12). (A) Firmly occlude both the ulnar and radial arteries of one hand while the person makes a fist several times. This causes the hand to blanch. (B) Ask the person to open the hand without hyperextending it; then release pressure on the ulnar artery while maintaining pressure on the radial artery. Adequate circulation is suggested by a palmar blush, a return to the hand's normal color in approximately 2 to 5 seconds. Although this test is simple and useful, it is relatively crude and subject to error—that is, you must occlude both arteries uniformly with 11 pounds of pressure for the test to be accurate.	(C) Pallor persists or a sluggish return to color suggests occlusion of the collateral arterial flow. Avoid radial artery cannulation until adequate circulation is shown.

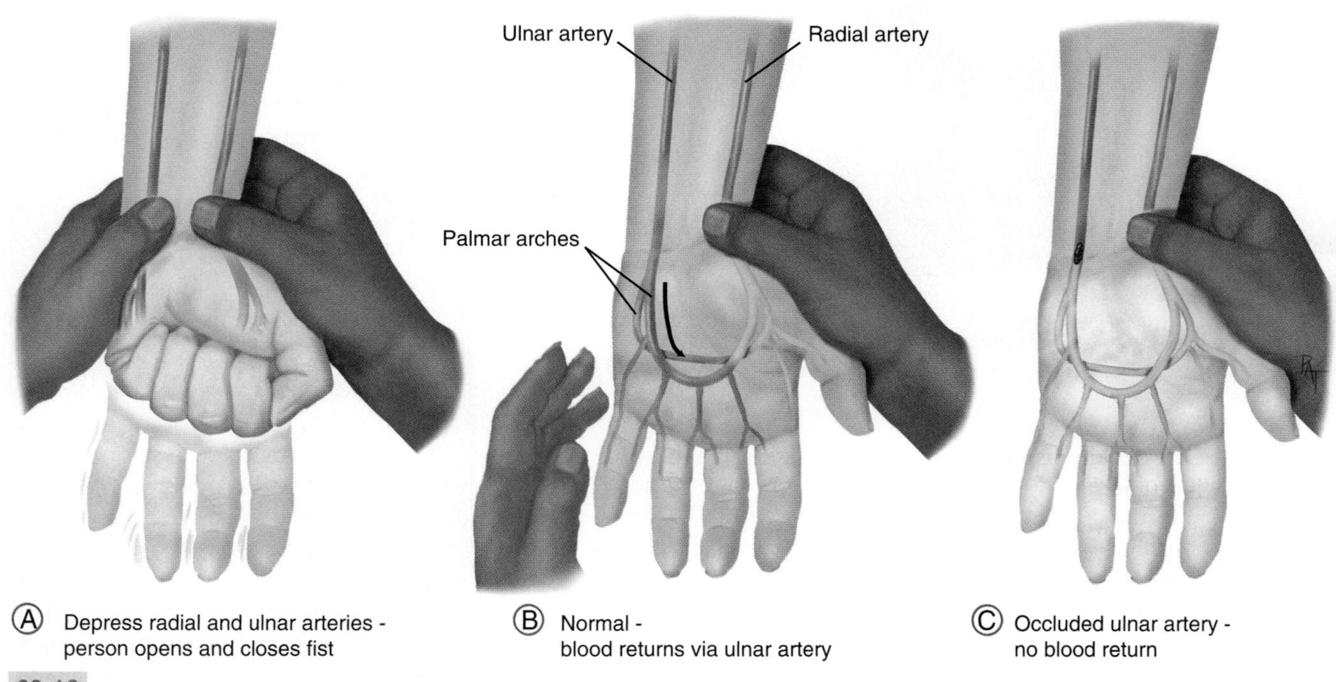

Ⓐ Depress radial and ulnar arteries - person opens and closes fist
Ⓑ Normal - blood returns via ulnar artery
Ⓒ Occluded ulnar artery - no blood return

20-12

Limitations of the modified Allen test are that it is subjective and requires patient cooperation that may not occur in emergency or critical care situations—just the times you need to cannulate the radial artery. The laser Doppler gives a quantifiable measurement of blood flow that is recordable and reproducible.[6] A small, flat probe is taped to the palm at the end of the patient's index finger. A baseline value for blood flow is recorded and then compared for change when the two arteries are occluded.

INSPECT AND PALPATE THE LEGS

Normal Range of Findings	Abnormal Findings
Uncover the legs while keeping the genitalia draped. Inspect both legs together, noting skin color, hair distribution, venous pattern, size (swelling or atrophy), and any skin lesions or ulcers.	Pallor with vasoconstriction; erythema with vasodilation; cyanosis.
Normally, hair covers the legs. Even if leg hair is shaved, you will still note hair on the dorsa of the toes.	Malnutrition: thin, shiny, atrophic skin; thick-ridged nails; loss of hair; ulcers; gangrene. Malnutrition, pallor, and coolness occur with arterial insufficiency.

Objective Data

Normal Range of Findings	Abnormal Findings

The venous pattern normally is flat and barely visible. Note obvious varicosities, although these are best assessed while standing.

Both legs should be symmetric in size without any swelling or atrophy. If the lower legs look asymmetric or if deep venous thrombosis is suspected, measure the calf circumference with a non-stretchable tape measure (Fig. 20-13). Measure at the widest point, taking care to measure the other leg in exactly the same place—the same number of centimeters down from the patella or other landmark. If lymphedema is suspected, measure also at the ankle, distal calf, knee, and thigh. Record your findings in centimeters.

Diffuse bilateral edema occurs with systemic illnesses.

Acute, unilateral, painful swelling and asymmetry of calves of 1 cm or more is abnormal; refer the person to determine whether deep venous thrombosis is present.

Asymmetry of 1 to 3 cm occurs with mild lymphedema; 3 to 5 cm with moderate lymphedema; and more than 5 cm with severe lymphedema (see Table 20-2).

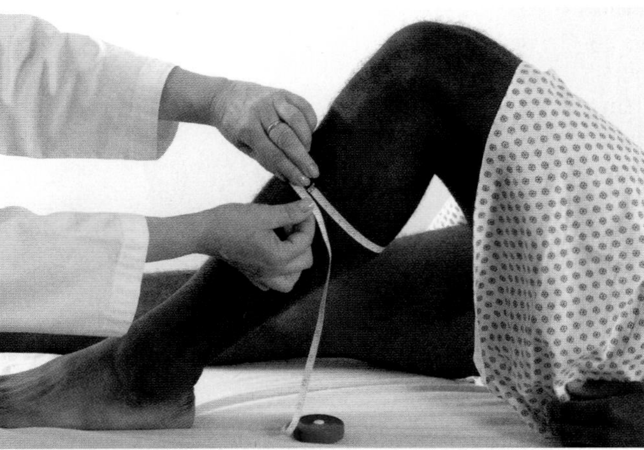

20-13

In the presence of skin discoloration, skin ulcers, or gangrene, note the size and the exact location.

Brown discoloration occurs with chronic venous stasis due to hemosiderin deposits from red blood cell degradation.

Venous ulcers occur usually at medial malleolus because of bacterial invasion of poorly drained tissues (see Table 20-4).

With arterial deficit, ulcers occur on tips of toes, metatarsal heads, and lateral malleoli.

Palpate for temperature along the legs down to the feet, comparing symmetric spots (Fig. 20-14). The skin should be warm and equal bilaterally. Bilateral cool feet may be due to environmental factors such as cool room temperature, apprehension, and cigarette smoking. If any increase in temperature is present higher up the leg, note if it is gradual or abrupt.

A unilateral cool foot or leg or a sudden temperature drop as you move down the leg occurs with arterial deficit.

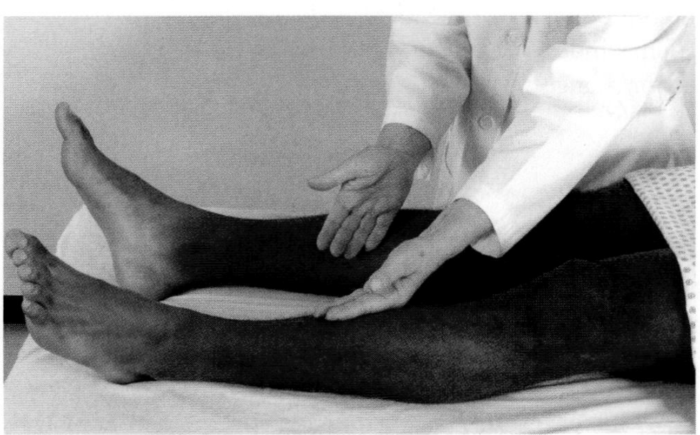

20-14

Normal Range of Findings

Flex the person's knee, and then gently compress the gastrocnemius (calf) muscle anteriorly against the tibia; no tenderness should be present. Or you may sharply dorsiflex the foot toward the tibia. Flexing the knee first exerts pressure on the posterior tibial vein. Normally this does not cause pain.

Palpate the inguinal lymph nodes. It is not unusual to find palpable nodes that are small (1 cm or less), movable, and nontender.

Palpate these peripheral arteries in both legs: femoral, popliteal, dorsalis pedis, and posterior tibial. Grade the force on the 3-point scale. Locate the **femoral arteries** just below the inguinal ligament halfway between the pubis and anterior superior iliac spines (Fig. 20-15). To help expose the femoral area, particularly in obese people, ask the person to bend his or her knees to the side in a froglike position. Press firmly and then slowly release, noting the pulse tap under your fingertips. If this pulse is weak or diminished, auscultate the site for a bruit.

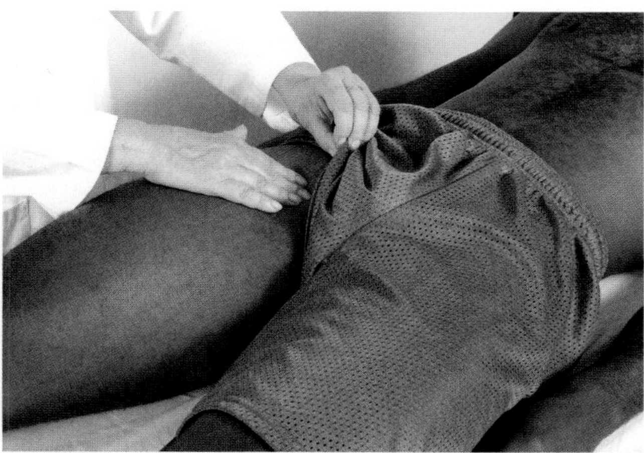

20-15 Femoral pulse.

The **popliteal pulse** is a more diffuse pulse and can be difficult to localize. With the leg extended but relaxed, anchor your thumbs on the knee and curl your fingers around into the popliteal fossa (Fig. 20-16). Press your fingers forward hard to compress the artery against the bone (the lower edge of the femur or the upper edge of the tibia). Often it is just lateral to the medial tendon.

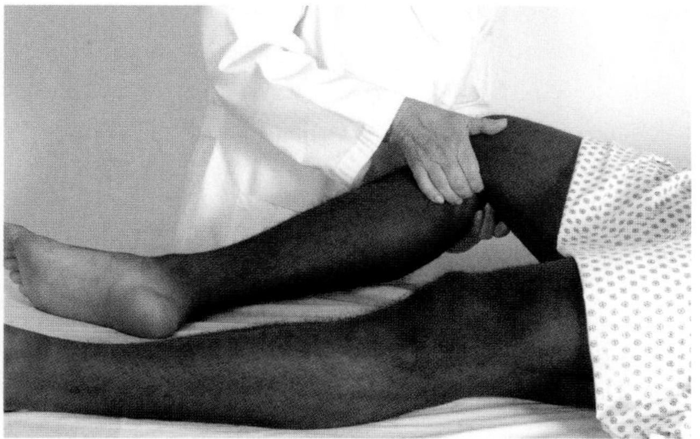

20-16 Popliteal pulse.

Abnormal Findings

Calf pain with these maneuvers is a positive **Homan sign,** which occurs in about 35% of cases of deep vein thrombosis. It is not specific for this condition because it occurs also with superficial phlebitis, Achilles tendinitis, gastrocnemius and plantar muscle injury, and lumbosacral disorders.

Enlarged nodes, tender, or fixed in area.

A bruit occurs with turbulent blood flow, indicating partial occlusion (see Table 20-5).

Normal Range of Findings	Abnormal Findings

If you have difficulty, turn the person prone and lift up the lower leg (Fig. 20-17). Let the leg relax against your arm, and press in deeply with your two thumbs. Often a normal popliteal pulse is impossible to palpate.

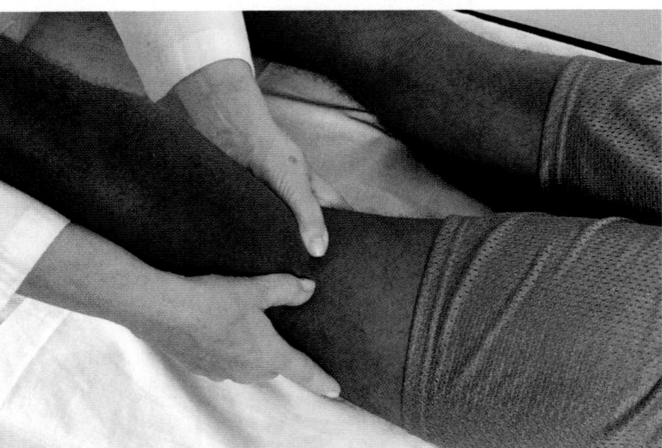

20-17

For the **posterior tibial** pulse, curve your fingers around the medial malleolus (Fig. 20-18). You will feel the tapping right behind it in the groove between the malleolus and the Achilles tendon. If you cannot, try passive dorsiflexion of the foot to make the pulse more accessible.

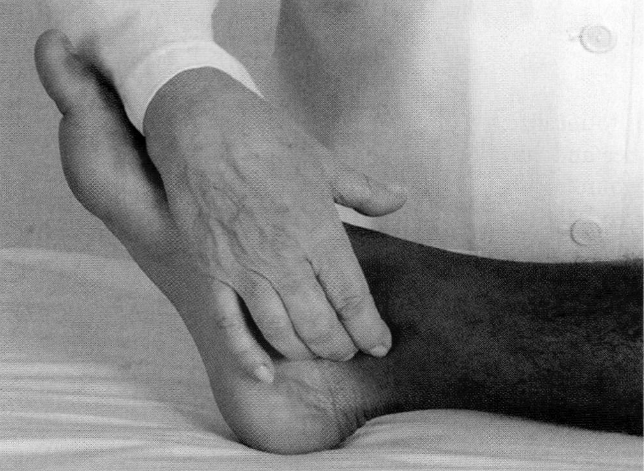

20-18 Posterior tibial pulse.

The **dorsalis pedis** pulse requires a very light touch. Normally it is just lateral to and parallel with the extensor tendon of the big toe (Fig. 20-19). Do not mistake the pulse in your own fingertips for that of the person.

Normal Range of Findings	Abnormal Findings

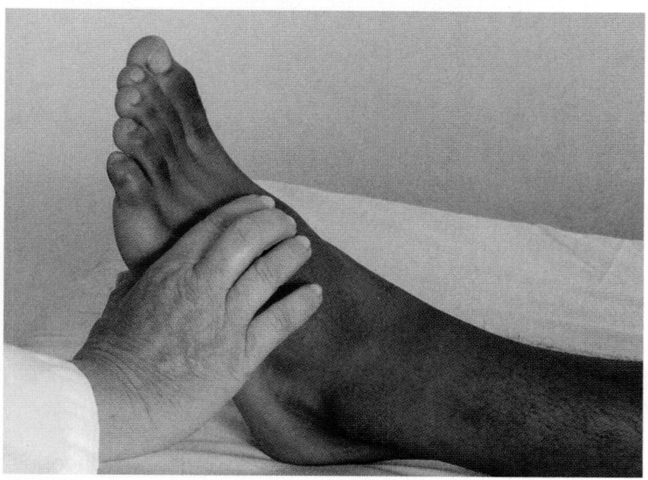

20-19 Dorsalis pedis pulse.

In adults older than 45 years, occasionally either the dorsalis pedis or the posterior tibial pulse may be hard to find, but not both on the same foot.

Check for pretibial edema. Firmly depress the skin over the tibia or the medial malleolus for 5 seconds and release (Fig. 20-20, *A*). Normally, your finger should leave no indentation, although a pit commonly is seen if the person has been standing all day or during pregnancy.

Bilateral, dependent pitting edema occurs with heart failure, diabetic neuropathy, and hepatic cirrhosis (Fig. 20-20, *B*).

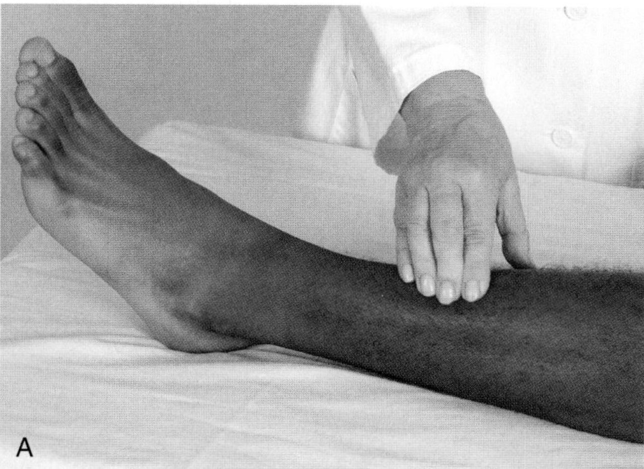

20-20 **A,** Check pretibial edema.

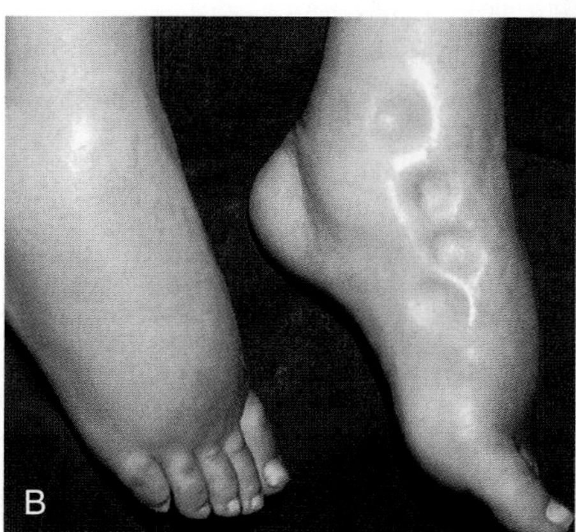

B, Pitting edema.

If pitting edema is present, grade it on the following scale:

1+ Mild pitting, slight indentation, no perceptible swelling of the leg
2+ Moderate pitting, indentation subsides rapidly
3+ Deep pitting, indentation remains for a short time, leg looks swollen
4+ Very deep pitting, indentation lasts a long time, leg is grossly swollen and distorted

Unilateral edema occurs with occlusion of a deep vein. Unilateral or bilateral edema occurs with lymphatic obstruction. With these factors, it is "brawny" or nonpitting and feels hard to the touch.

Normal Range of Findings	Abnormal Findings

This classic method of capturing pit depth and recovery time is commonly used. But it has not been proven to be an objective, reliable, or sensitive measurement for edema. The amount of pressure used is arbitrary, as is the judgment of the depth and rate of pitting. In a recent comparison of 8 different methods of edema assessment, Brodovicz et al[2] found this traditional clinical assessment to be unreliable, with low to average inter-examiner agreement. More reliable methods to quantify edema were the water displacement method (which is time-consuming and cumbersome in clinical practice) and ankle circumference. Ankle circumference was measured using a non-stretchable tape at a point 7 cm proximal to the midpoint of the medial malleolus. Because peripheral edema is a common clinical sign in a great number of conditions, it is important to detect true changes in the most accurate way available. Be aware of the limitations of traditional assessment methods, and check with your own institution to conform with a consistently used scale.

Ask the person to stand so that you can assess the venous system. Note any visible, dilated, and tortuous veins.

Varicosities occur in the saphenous veins (see Table 20-5).

Manual Compression Test

While the person is still standing, test the length of the varicose vein to determine whether its valves are competent (Fig. 20-21). Place one hand on the lower part of the varicose vein, and compress the vein with your other hand about 15 to 20 cm higher. Competent valves will prevent a wave transmission, and your distal (lower) fingers will feel no change.

A palpable wave transmission occurs when the valves are incompetent.

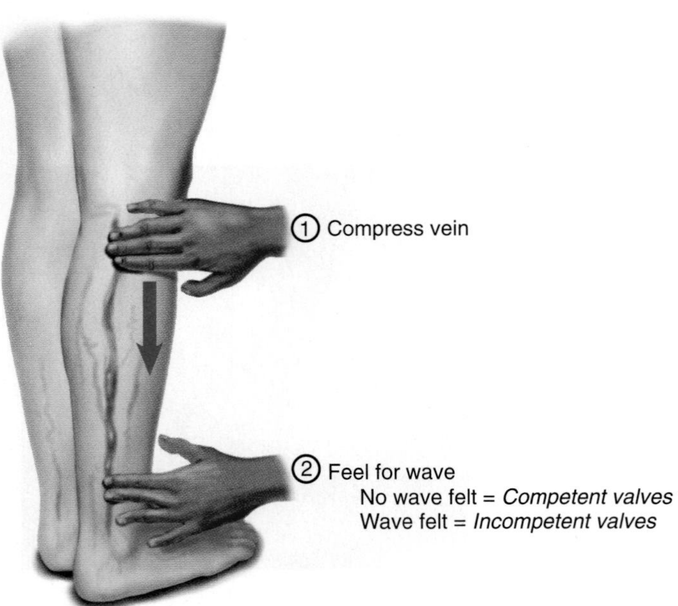

20-21 Manual compression test. ©Pat Thomas, 2006.

Color Changes

If you suspect an arterial deficit, raise the legs about 30 cm (12 inches) off the table and ask the person to wag the feet for about 30 seconds to drain off venous blood (Fig. 20-22). The skin color now reflects only the contribution of arterial blood. A light-skinned person's feet normally will look a little pale but still should be pink. A dark-skinned person's feet are more difficult to evaluate, but the soles should reveal extreme color change.

Normal Range of Findings

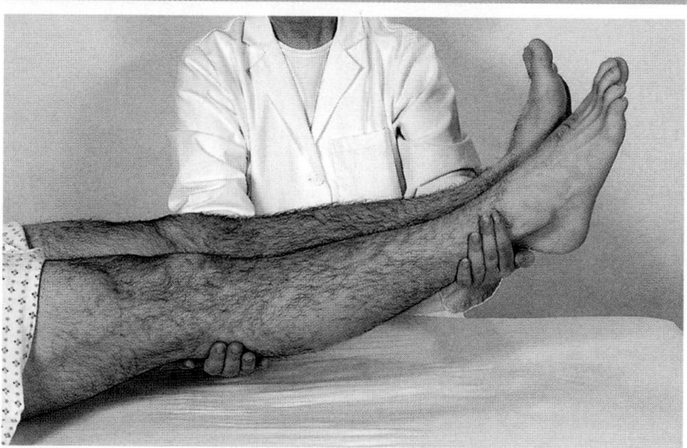
20-22

Now have the person sit up with the legs over the side of the table (Fig. 20-23, *A*). Compare the color of both feet. Note the time it takes for color to return to the feet—the normal time is 10 seconds or less. Note also the time it takes for the superficial veins around the feet to fill—the normal time is about 15 seconds. This test is unreliable if the person has concomitant venous disease with incompetent valves.

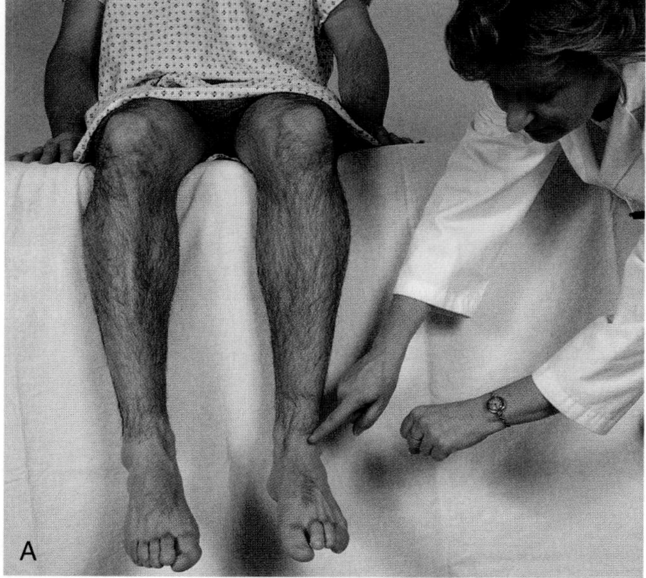

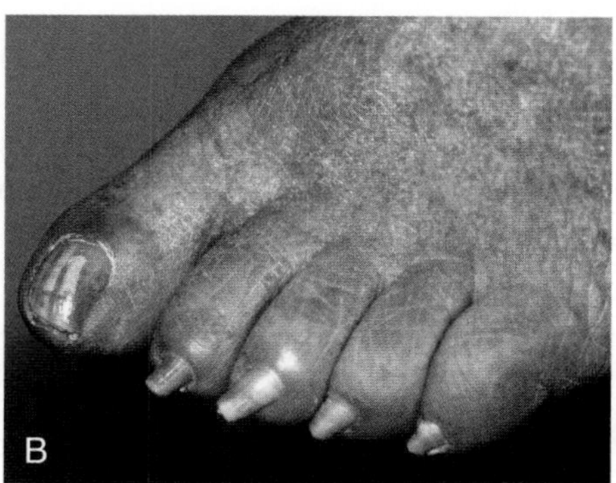

20-23

Test the lower legs for strength (see Chapter 22). Test the lower legs for sensation (see Chapter 23).

Abnormal Findings

Elevational pallor (marked) indicates arterial insufficiency.

Dependent rubor (deep blue-red color) occurs with severe arterial insufficiency (Fig. 20-23, *B*). Chronic hypoxia produces a loss of vasomotor tone and a pooling of blood in the veins.

Delayed venous filling occurs with arterial insufficiency.

Motor loss occurs with severe arterial deficit.

Sensory loss occurs with arterial deficit, especially diabetes.

Normal Range of Findings

The Doppler Ultrasonic Stethoscope

Use this device to detect a weak peripheral pulse, to monitor blood pressure in infants or children, or to measure a low blood pressure or blood pressure in a lower extremity (Fig. 20-24). The Doppler stethoscope magnifies pulsatile sounds from the heart and blood vessels. Position the person supine, with the legs externally rotated so you can reach the medial ankles easily. Place a drop of coupling gel on the end of the handheld transducer. Place the transducer over a pulse site at a 90-degree angle. Apply very light pressure; locate the pulse site by the swishing, whooshing sound.

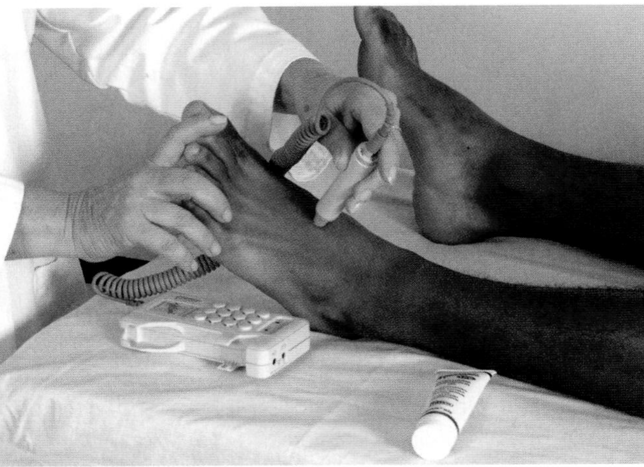

20-24

The Ankle-Brachial Index (ABI)

Use of the Doppler stethoscope is a highly specific, noninvasive, and readily available way to determine the extent of peripheral arterial disease (PAD). The patient is supine. Apply a regular arm blood pressure cuff above the ankle and determine the systolic pressure in either the posterior tibial or dorsalis pedis artery. Then divide that figure by the systolic pressure of the brachial artery.

(Take brachial systolic pressures in both arms and use the higher measurement.) The normal ankle pressure is slightly greater than or equal to the brachial pressure; thus a normal ABI is usually 1.0 to 1.2. For example,

$$\frac{\text{132 ankle systolic pressure}}{\text{124 arm systolic pressure}} = \text{1.06 or 106\%, indicating no flow reduction}$$

In people with diabetes mellitus, the ABI is less reliable because of calcification (which makes their arteries non-compressible) and may give a falsely high ankle pressure. Thus the presence or severity of PAD may be underestimated.[8]

DEVELOPMENTAL COMPETENCE

Infants and Children

Transient acrocyanosis and skin mottling at birth are discussed in Chapter 12. Pulse force should be normal and symmetric. Pulse force also should be the same in the upper and lower extremities.

Abnormal Findings

An ABI of 0.90 or less indicates peripheral arterial disease (PAD):

- 0.90 to 0.70—mild claudication
- 0.70 to 0.40—moderate to severe claudication
- 0.40 to 0.30—severe claudication, usually with rest pain except in the presence of diabetic neuropathy
- <0.30—ischemia, with impending loss of tissue

Weak pulses occur with vasoconstriction of diminished cardiac output.

Full, bounding pulses occur with patent ductus arteriosus as a result of the large left-to-right shunt.

Diminished or absent femoral pulses while upper extremity pulses are normal suggest coarctation of aorta.

Objective Data

Normal Range of Findings	Abnormal Findings
Palpable lymph nodes occur often in healthy infants and children. They are small, firm (shotty), mobile, and nontender. They may be the sequelae of past infection, such as inguinal nodes from a diaper rash or cervical nodes from a respiratory infection. Vaccinations also can produce local lymphadenopathy. Note characteristics of any palpable nodes and whether they are local or generalized.	Enlarged, warm, tender nodes indicate current infection. Look for source of infection.
The Pregnant Woman Expect diffuse bilateral pitting edema in the lower extremities, especially at the end of the day and into the third trimester. Nearly 80% of pregnant women have some peripheral edema.[9] Varicose veins in the legs also are common in the third trimester.	Remain alert for generalized edema plus hypertension, which suggests pre-eclampsia, a dangerous obstetric condition.
The Aging Adult The dorsalis pedis and posterior tibial pulse may become more difficult to find. Trophic changes associated with arterial insufficiency (thin, shiny skin; thick-ridged nails; loss of hair on lower legs) also occur normally with aging.	

Objective Data

PROMOTING A HEALTHY LIFESTYLE: FOOT CARE

Take Care of Your Feet!

According to the National Institutes of Aging (NIA), foot problems are often the first sign of more serious health conditions such as arthritis, diabetes, and nerve or circulatory disorders. Although health care providers advise patients to take care of their feet, they often do not take the time to explain what "good" foot care entails. According to both the NIA and the American Podiatric Medical Association (APMA), "good" foot care entails the following:

- Checking your feet every day.
  - When individuals are unable to see the bottoms of their feet, they need to be instructed to use a mirror or to ask someone to help them.
  - A good time to examine feet is after a shower or bath. Feet should be dried carefully, especially between the toes. Each foot should be examined for red spots or sensitive areas, discoloration of skin or nails, ingrown nails, pain, cuts, swelling, or blisters.
  - Toenails should be kept trimmed, straight across, and filed at the edges with an emery board or nail file.
  - Be careful with nail polish. Although freshly applied nail polish does not increase the number of bacteria, chipped nail polish may support the growth of larger numbers of organisms on nails. This is especially important for individuals who already are at risk for infection. Also, do not use nail polish to cover up discolored nails. Nail polish locks out moisture and keeps the nail bed from being able to "breathe."
- Keeping blood flowing to your feet.
  - Walking is one of the best exercises for overall circulation.
  - When an individual is not able to walk, putting the feet up when sitting or lying down, stretching, wiggling toes, having a gentle foot massage, and warm foot bath are great alternatives.
  - Do not cross legs for long periods.
  - Do not smoke.
- Wearing shoes that fit and are comfortable.
  - The best time to measure feet is toward the end of the day, when feet tend to be the largest.
  - Individuals often have one foot that is larger than the other. It is recommended that shoes are fit to the larger foot.
  - Select shoes that are shaped like one's feet. The ball of the foot should fit comfortably into the widest part of the shoe. Toes should not be crowded.
  - For women, low-heeled shoes are safer and less damaging than high-heeled shoes.
- Keeping skin soft and smooth.
  - A thin coat of skin lotion over the tops and bottoms of one's feet help keep skin soft and smooth. However, this extra moisture should not go between the toes.
  - Use mild soap.
  - Be careful about adding oils to bath water. They can make your feet and the bathtub both very slippery.

Resources

American Orthopedic Foot and Ankle Society. Website: www.aofas.org.

American Podiatric Medical Association. Website: www.apma.org.

Foot Care Pamphlet. Website: www.nia.nih.gov/HealthInformation/Publications/footcare.htm.

National Institute on Aging. Website: www.nia.nih.gov/.

Pedicure Pointers. Website: www.apma.org/Pedicure-Pointers.

DOCUMENTATION AND CRITICAL THINKING

Sample Charting

SUBJECTIVE

No leg pain, no skin changes, no swelling or lymph node enlargement. No history of heart or vascular problems, diabetes, or obesity. Does not smoke. On no medications.

OBJECTIVE

Inspection: Extremities have pink-tan color without redness, cyanosis, or any skin lesions. Extremity size is symmetric without swelling or atrophy.

Palpation: Temperature is warm and = bilaterally. All pulses present, 2+ and = bilaterally. No lymphadenopathy.

ASSESSMENT

Healthy tissue integrity
Effective tissue perfusion

Focused Assessment: Clinical Case Study

James K. is a 43-year-old, married, white, male city sanitation worker, admitted to University Medical Center today for "bypass surgery tomorrow to fix my aorta and these black toes."

SUBJECTIVE

6 years PTA—motorcycle accident with handlebars jammed into groin. Treated and released at local hospital. No apparent injury, although M.D. now thinks accident may have precipitated present stenosis of aorta.

1 year PTA—radiating pain in right calf on walking 1 mile. Pain relieved by stopping walking.

3 months PTA—problems with sex; unable to maintain erection during intercourse.

1 month PTA—leg pain present after walking 2 blocks. Numbness and tingling in right foot and calf. Tips of three toes on right foot look black. Saw M.D. Diagnostic studies showed stenosis of aorta "below vessels that go to my kidneys."

Present—leg pain at rest, constant and severe, worse at night, partially relieved by dangling leg over side of bed.

Past History—no history of heart or vessel disease, hypertension, diabetes, obesity.

Personal habits—smokes cigarettes, 3 packs per day (PPD) × 23 years. Now cut down to 1 PPD.

Walking is part of occupation, although has been driving city truck past 3 months due to leg pain. On no medications.

OBJECTIVE

Inspection: Lower extremity size = bilaterally with no swelling or atrophy. No varicosities. Color L leg pink-tan, R leg pink-tan when supine, but marked pallor to R foot on elevation. Black gangrene at tips of R 2nd, 3rd, 4th toes. Leg hair present but absent on involved toes.

Palpation: R foot cool and temperature gradually warms as proceed palpating up R leg.

Pulses: Femorals, both 1+; popliteals, both 0; posterior tibial, both 0 but present with Doppler; dorsalis pedis 0, but left dorsalis pedis is present with Doppler, and right is not present with Doppler.

ASSESSMENT

Ischemic rest pain R leg
Ineffective tissue perfusion R/T interruption of flow
Impaired tissue integrity R/T altered circulation
Activity intolerance R/T leg pain
Sexual dysfunction R/T effects of disease

ABNORMAL FINDINGS

TABLE 20-1 Variations in Pulse Contour

Description	Associated With
Weak, "Thready" Pulse—1+ Hard to palpate, need to search for it, may fade in and out, easily obliterated by pressure.	Decreased cardiac output, peripheral arterial disease, aortic valve stenosis
Full, Bounding Pulse—3+ Easily palpable, pounds under your fingertips.	Hyperkinetic states (exercise, anxiety, fever), anemia, hyperthyroidism
Water-Hammer (Corrigan) Pulse—3+ Greater than normal force, then collapses suddenly.	Aortic valve regurgitation, patent ductus arteriosus
Pulsus Bigeminus Rhythm is coupled, every other beat comes early, or normal beat followed by premature beat. Force of premature beat is decreased because of shortened cardiac filling time.	Conduction disturbance (e.g., premature ventricular contraction, premature atrial contraction)
Pulsus Alternans Rhythm is regular, but force varies with alternating beats of large and small amplitude.	When heart rate (HR) is normal, pulsus alternans occurs with severe left ventricular failure, which in turn is due to ischemic heart disease, valvular heart disease, chronic hypertension, or cardiomyopathy
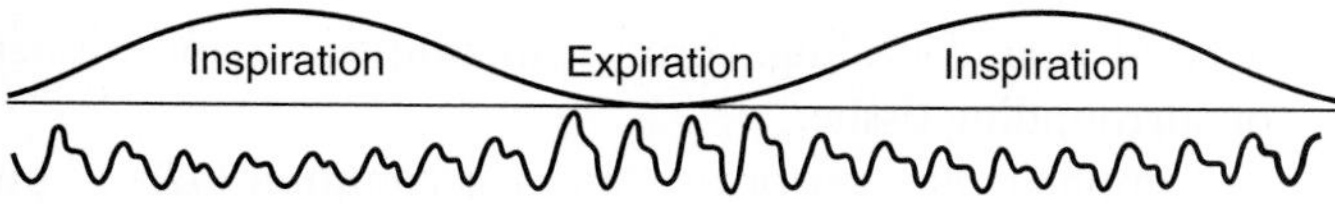 **Pulsus Paradoxus** Beats have weaker amplitude with inspiration, stronger with expiration. Best determined during blood pressure measurement; reading decreases (>10 mm Hg) during inspiration and increases with expiration.	A common finding in cardiac tamponade (pericardial effusion in which high pressure compresses the heart and blocks cardiac output); also in severe bronchospasm of acute asthma
Pulsus Bisferiens Each pulse has two strong systolic peaks, with a dip in between. Best assessed at the carotid artery.	Aortic valve stenosis plus regurgitation

ABNORMAL FINDINGS FOR ADVANCED PRACTICE

TABLE 20-2 Peripheral Vascular Disease in the Arms

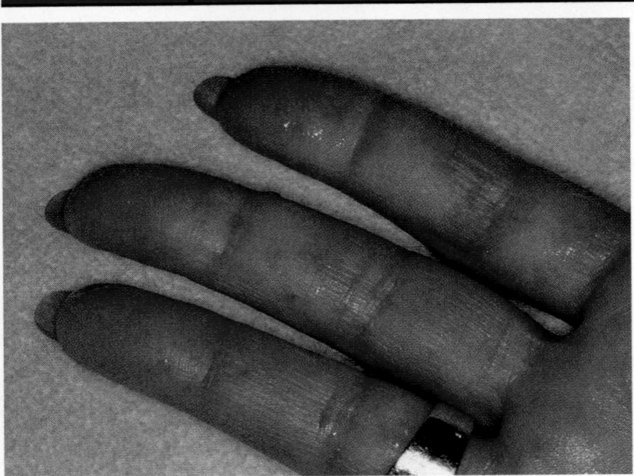

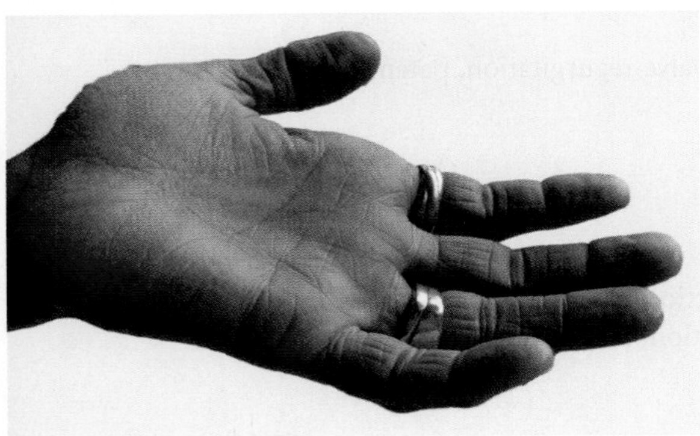

Raynaud's Phenomenon

Episodes of abrupt, progressive tricolor change of the fingers in response to cold, vibration, or stress: (1) white (pallor) in top figure from arteriospasm and resulting deficit in supply; (2) blue (cyanosis) in lower figure from slight relaxation of the spasm that allows a slow trickle of blood through the capillaries and increased oxygen extraction of hemoglobin; (3) finally, red (rubor) in heel of hand due to return of blood into the dilated capillary bed or reactive hyperemia.

May have cold, numbness, or pain along with pallor or cyanosis stage; then burning, throbbing pain, swelling along with rubor. Lasts minutes to hours; occurs bilaterally. Several drugs predispose to the episodes, and smoking can increase the symptoms.

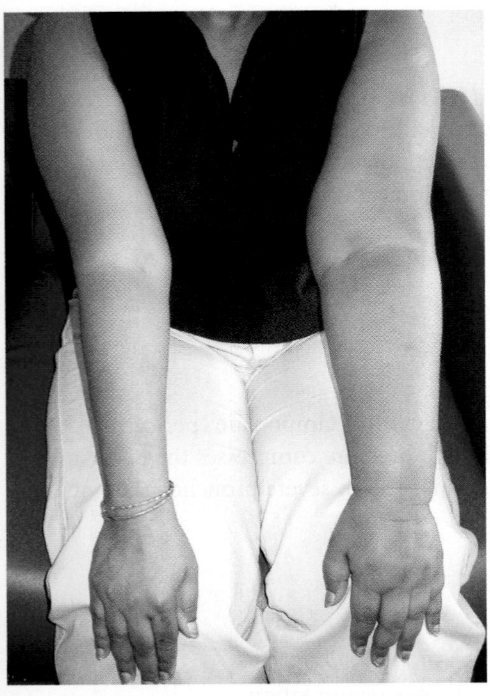

Lymphedema

Lymphedema is high-protein swelling of the limb, most commonly due to breast cancer treatment. Surgical removal of lymph nodes or damage to lymph nodes and vessels with radiation therapy impedes drainage of lymph. Protein-rich lymph builds up in the interstitial spaces, which further raises local colloid oncotic pressure and promotes more fluid leakage. Stagnant lymphatic fluid increases risk for infection, delayed wound healing, chronic inflammation, and fibrosis of surrounding tissue.

Lymphedema after breast cancer is common (42%)[13] but usually mild. Early symptoms include self-reported sensations of a tired, thick, heavy arm, jewelry too tight, swelling, or tingling. Objective data include a unilateral swelling, nonpitting brawny edema, with overlying skin indurated. Early recognition is important because there is evidence to support effective interventions, such as complete decongestive physiotherapy, compression bandaging, and others.[18] Without treatment, lymphedema is chronic and progressive, which is psychologically demoralizing as a threat to body image and constant reminder of the cancer.

TABLE 20-3 **Pain Profiles of Peripheral Vascular Disease**

Symptom Analysis	Chronic **Arterial** Symptoms	Acute **Arterial** Symptoms
Arterial disease causes symptoms and signs of oxygen deficit.		
Location	Deep muscle pain, usually in calf, but may be lower leg or dorsum of foot	Varies, distal to occlusion, may involve entire leg
Character	Intermittent claudication, feels like "cramp," "numbness and tingling," "feeling of cold"	Throbbing
Onset and duration	Chronic pain, onset gradual after exertion	Sudden onset (within 1 hr)
Aggravating factors	Activity (walking, stairs); "Claudication distance" is specific number of blocks, stairs it takes to produce pain Elevation (rest pain indicates severe involvement)	
Relieving factors	Rest (usually within 2 min [e.g., standing]) Dangling (severe involvement)	
Associated symptoms	Cool, pale skin	Six Ps: pain, pallor, pulselessness, paresthesia, poikilothermia (coldness), paralysis (indicates severe)
Those at risk	Older adults, more males than females, inherited predisposition, history of hypertension, smoking, diabetes, hypercholesterolemia, obesity, vascular disease	History of vascular surgery; arterial invasive procedure; abdominal aneurysm (emboli); trauma, including injured arteries; chronic atrial fibrillation

	Chronic **Venous** Symptoms	Acute **Venous** Symptoms
Venous disease causes symptoms and signs of metabolic waste buildup.		
Location	Calf, lower leg	Calf
Character	Aching, tiredness, feeling of fullness	Intense, sharp; deep muscle tender to touch
Onset and duration	Chronic pain, increases at end of day	Sudden onset (within 1 hr)
Aggravating factors	Prolonged standing, sitting	Pain may increase with sharp dorsiflexion of foot
Relieving factors	Elevation, lying, walking	
Associated symptoms	Edema, varicosities, weeping ulcers at ankles	Red, warm, swollen leg
Those at risk	Job with prolonged standing or sitting; obesity; pregnancy; prolonged bedrest; history of heart failure, varicosities, or thrombophlebitis; veins crushed by trauma or surgery	

TABLE 20-4 Leg Ulcers: Arterial, Venous, or Diabetic

Chronic Arterial Insufficiency

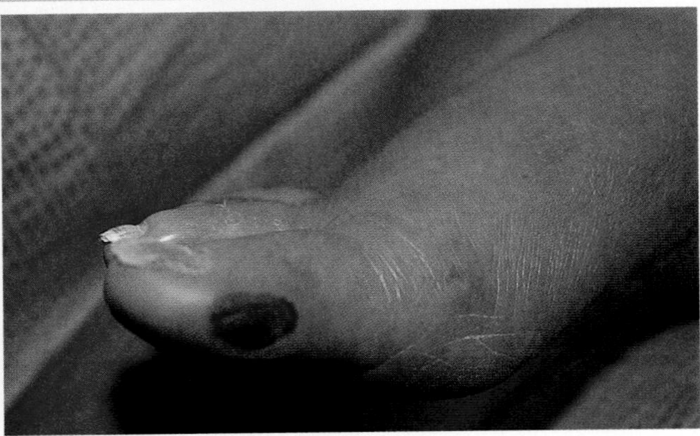

Arterial—Ischemic Ulcer

Buildup of fatty plaques on intima (atherosclerosis) plus hardening and calcification of arterial wall (arteriosclerosis).

S: Deep muscle pain in calf or foot, claudication (pain with walking), pain at rest indicates worsening of condition.
O: Coolness, pallor, elevational pallor, and dependent rubor; diminished pulses; systolic bruits; signs of malnutrition (thin, shiny skin; thick-ridged nails; atrophy of muscles); distal gangrene.

Ulcers occur at toes, metatarsal heads, heels, lateral ankle, and are characterized by pale ischemic base, well-defined edges, and no bleeding.

Chronic Venous Insufficiency

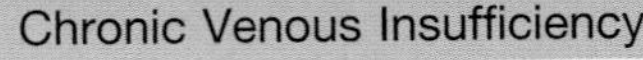

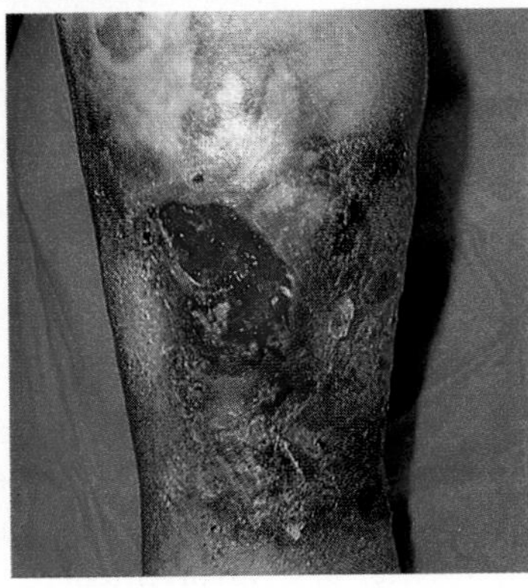

Venous (Stasis) Ulcer

After acute deep vein thrombosis or chronic incompetent valves in deep veins.

S: Aching pain in calf or lower leg, worse at end of the day, worse with prolonged standing or sitting.
O: Firm, brawny edema; coarse, thickened skin; pulses normal; brown pigment discoloration; petechiae; dermatitis. Venous stasis causes increased venous pressure, which then causes red blood cells (RBCs) to leak out of veins and into the skin. The RBCs break down and leave hemosiderin (iron deposits) behind, which are the brown pigment deposits. A weepy, pruritic stasis dermatitis may be present.

Ulcers occur at medial malleolus and are characterized by bleeding, uneven edges.

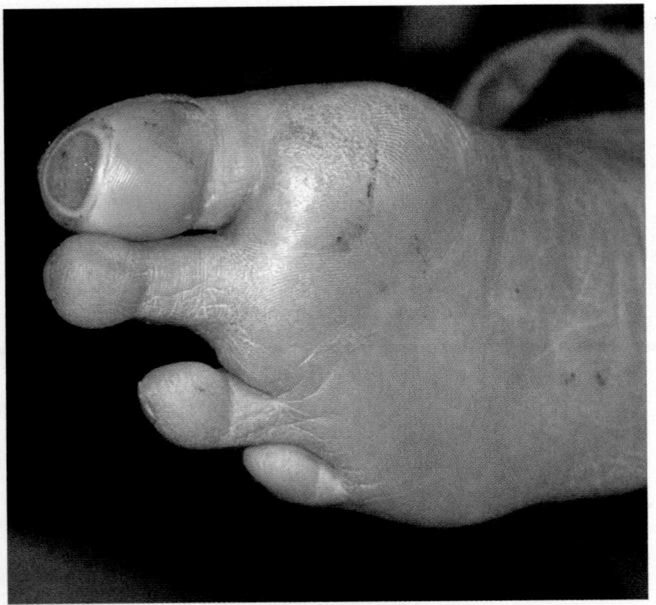

◀ **Diabetes** hastens changes described with ischemic ulcer, with generalized dysfunction in all arterial areas: peripheral, coronary, cerebral, retina, kidney. Peripheral involvement is associated with diabetic neuropathy. Without careful vigilance of pressure points on the feet, ulcer may go unnoticed. Pain and sensation are decreased, and surrounding skin is calloused.

S, Subjective data; *O*, objective data.

TABLE 20-5 Peripheral Vascular Disease in the Legs

Chronic Venous Disease

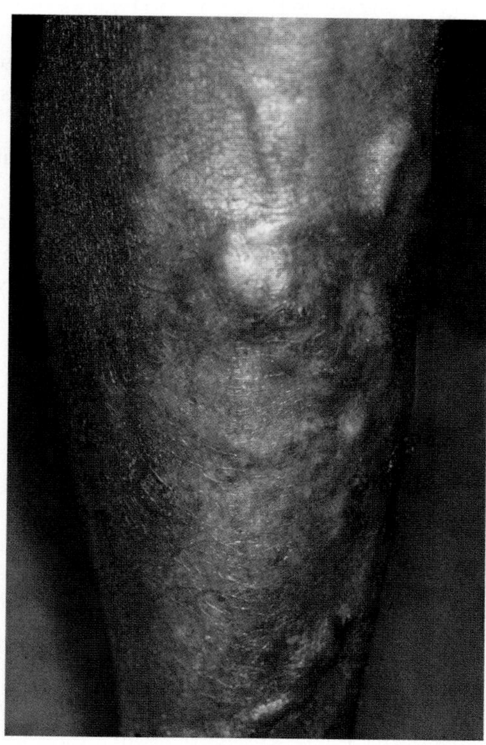

Superficial Varicose Veins

Incompetent valves permit reflux of blood, producing dilated, tortuous veins. Unremitting hydrostatic pressure causes distal valves to be incompetent and causes worsening of the varicosity.

Over age 45 years, occurrence is three times more common in women than in men.

S: Aching, heaviness in calf, easy fatigability, night leg or foot cramps.

O: Dilated, tortuous veins.

Acute Venous Disease

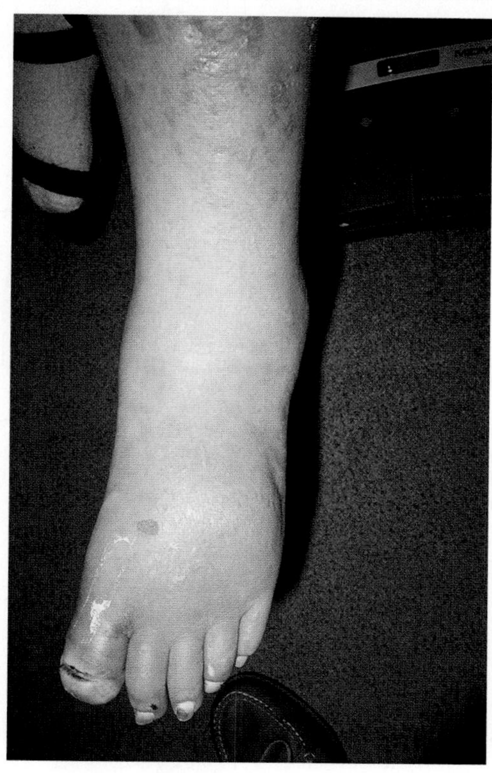

Deep Vein Thrombophlebitis (DVT)

A deep vein is occluded by a thrombus, causing inflammation, blocked venous return, cyanosis, and edema. Virchow's triad is the classic 3 factors that promote thrombogenesis: stasis, hypercoagulability, and endothelial dysfunction.[16] Cause may be prolonged bedrest; history of varicose veins; trauma; infection; cancer; and, in younger women, the use of oral estrogenic contraceptives. Requires emergency referral because of risk for pulmonary embolism. Note that upper-extremity DVT is increasingly common due to frequent use of invasive lines such as central venous catheters.[10]

S: Sudden onset of intense, sharp, deep muscle pain; may increase with sharp dorsiflexion of foot.

O: Increased warmth; swelling (to compare swelling, observe the usual shoe size as in above photo); redness; dependent cyanosis is mild or may be absent; tender to palpation; Homan sign is present only in few cases.

TABLE 20-6 Peripheral Artery Disease

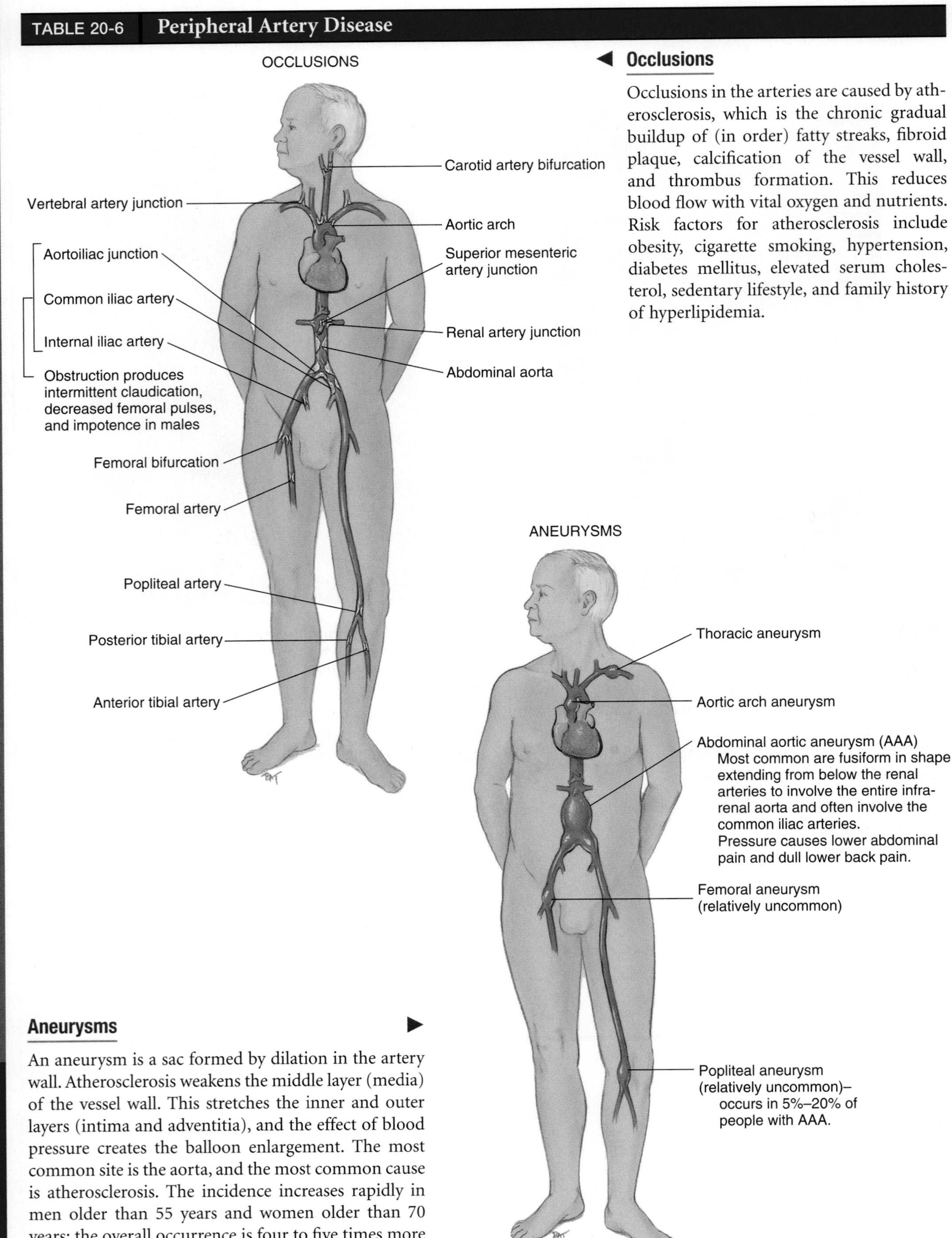

Occlusions

Occlusions in the arteries are caused by atherosclerosis, which is the chronic gradual buildup of (in order) fatty streaks, fibroid plaque, calcification of the vessel wall, and thrombus formation. This reduces blood flow with vital oxygen and nutrients. Risk factors for atherosclerosis include obesity, cigarette smoking, hypertension, diabetes mellitus, elevated serum cholesterol, sedentary lifestyle, and family history of hyperlipidemia.

Aneurysms

An aneurysm is a sac formed by dilation in the artery wall. Atherosclerosis weakens the middle layer (media) of the vessel wall. This stretches the inner and outer layers (intima and adventitia), and the effect of blood pressure creates the balloon enlargement. The most common site is the aorta, and the most common cause is atherosclerosis. The incidence increases rapidly in men older than 55 years and women older than 70 years; the overall occurrence is four to five times more frequent in men.

BIBLIOGRAPHY

1. Aydin, A., Shenbagamurthi, S., & Brem, H. (2009). Lower extremity ulcers: venous, arterial, or diabetic? *Emergency Medicine, 41*(8), 18-24.
2. Brodovicz, K. G., McNaugton, K., Uemura, N., et al. (2009). Reliability and feasibility of methods to quantitatively assess peripheral edema. *Clinical Medicine & Research, 7*(1/2), 21-31.
3. Fahey, V. A. (2004). *Vascular nursing* (4th ed.). Philadelphia: Saunders.
4. Fu, M. R., Ridner, S. H., & Armer, J. (2009). Post–breast cancer lymphedema, Part 1. *American Journal of Nursing, 109*(7), 48-55, 2009.
5. Fu, M. R., Ridner, S. H., & Armer, J. (2009). Post–breast cancer lymphedema, Part 2. *American Journal of Nursing, 109*(8), 34-42.
6. Fuhrman, T. M., & McSweeney, E. (1995). Noninvasive evaluation of the collateral circulation to the hand. *Academic Emergency Medicine, 2*(3), 195-199.
7. Goss, D. E., de Trafford, J., Roberts V. C., et al. (1989). Raised ankle/brachial pressure index in insulin-treated diabetic patients. *Diabetic Medicine, 6*(7), 576-578.
8. Khan, N. A., Rahim, S. A., Anand, S. S., et al. (2006). Does the clinical examination predict lower extremity peripheral arterial disease? *Journal of the American Medical Association, 295,* 536-545.
9. Koo, L. W., Reedy, S., & Smith, J. K. (2010). Patient history key to diagnosing peripheral edema. *Nurse Practitioner, 35*(3), 44-52.
10. Lancaster, S. L., Owens, A., Bryant, A. S., et al. (2010). Upper-extremity deep vein thrombosis. *American Journal of Nursing, 110*(5), 48-52.
11. Meier, A. P., & Cather, J. C. (2010). Blanched fingers. *Proceedings (Baylor University. Medical Center), 23*(1), 73-75.
12. Muir, R. L. (2009). Peripheral arterial disease: pathophysiology, risk factors, diagnosis, treatment, and prevention. *Journal of Vascular Nursing, 27*(2), 26-30.
13. Norman, S. A., Localio, R., Potashnik, S. L., et al. (2009). Lymphedema in breast cancer survivors: incidence, degree, time course, treatment, and symptoms. *Journal of Clinical Oncology, 27*(3), 390-397.
14. Oka, R. K. (2006). Peripheral arterial disease in older adults. *Journal of Cardiovascular Nursing, 21,* 515-520.
15. Ondo, W. G. (2009). Restless legs syndrome. *Neurologic Clinics, 27*(3), 779-799.
16. Osinbowale, O., Ali, L., & Chi, Y. W. (2010). Venous thromboembolism: a clinical review. *Postgraduate Medicine, 122*(2), 54-65.
17. Pearson, T. L. (2010). Ankle brachial index as a prognostic tool for women with coronary artery disease. *Journal of Cardiovascular Nursing, 25*(1), 20-24.
18. Poage, E., Singer, M., Armer, J., et al. (2008). Demystifying lymphedema: development of the lymphedema putting evidence into practice card. *Clinical Journal of Oncology Nursing, 12*(6), 951-964.
19. Scully, M. F., & Lee, A. Y. Y. (2009). The challenge of cancer and thromboembolic disease: current trends and recommendations. *Oncology Exchange, 8*(3), 6-10.
20. Sieggreen, M. (2006). A contemporary approach to peripheral arterial disease. *Nurse Practitioner, 31,* 14-26.

Summary Checklist: Peripheral Vascular Examination

For a PDA-downloadable version, go to http://evolve.elsevier.com/Jarvis/.

1. **Inspect arms for color, size, any lesions.**
2. **Palpate pulses: radial, brachial.**
3. **Check epitrochlear node.**
4. **Inspect legs for color, size, any lesions, trophic skin changes.**
5. **Palpate temperature of feet and legs.**
6. **Palpate inguinal nodes.**
7. **Palpate pulses: femoral, popliteal, posterior tibial, dorsalis pedis.**

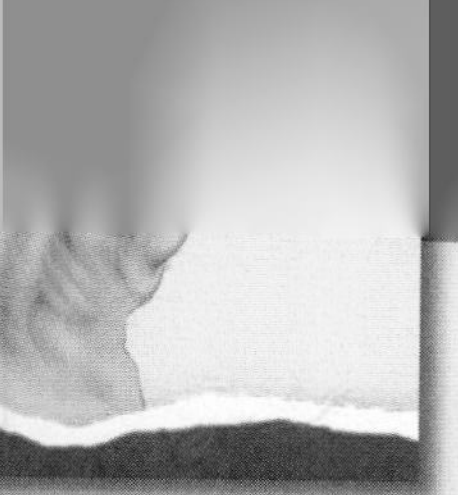

21 Abdomen

evolve WEBSITE

http://evolve.elsevier.com/Jarvis/

- Animations
- Audio—Abdomen Sounds
- Audio Key Points
- Bedside Assessment Summary Checklist
- NCLEX Review Questions
- Physical Examination Summary Checklist
- Quick Assessment for Common Conditions
  Peptic Ulcer Disease
- Video—Assessment
  Abdomen and Inguinal Area

OUTLINE

Structure and Function, 527

Surface Landmarks
Internal Anatomy

Subjective Data , 532

Health History Questions

Objective Data, 536

Preparation
Inspection
Auscultation
Percussion
Palpation

Documentation and Critical Thinking, 555

Abnormal Findings, 557

Abnormal Findings for Advanced Practice, 559

STRUCTURE AND FUNCTION

SURFACE LANDMARKS

The **abdomen** is a large, oval cavity extending from the diaphragm down to the brim of the pelvis. It is bordered in back by the vertebral column and paravertebral muscles and at the sides and front by the lower rib cage and abdominal muscles (Fig. 21-1). Four layers of large, flat muscles form the ventral abdominal wall. These are joined at the midline by a tendinous seam, the **linea alba.** One set, the **rectus abdominis,** forms a strip extending the length of the midline, and its edge is often palpable. The muscles protect and hold the organs in place, and they flex the vertebral column.

INTERNAL ANATOMY

Inside the abdominal cavity, all the internal organs are called the **viscera.** It is important that you know the location of these organs so well that you could draw a map of them on the skin (Fig. 21-2). You must be able to visualize each organ that you listen to or palpate through the abdominal wall.

The **solid viscera** are those that maintain a characteristic shape (liver, pancreas, spleen, adrenal glands, kidneys, ovaries, and uterus). The liver fills most of the right upper quadrant (RUQ) and extends over to the left midclavicular line. The lower edge of the liver and the right kidney normally may be palpable. The ovaries normally are palpable only on bimanual examination during the pelvic examination.

The shape of the **hollow viscera** (stomach, gallbladder, small intestine, colon, and bladder) depends on the contents. They usually are not palpable, although you may feel a colon distended with feces or a bladder distended with urine. The stomach is just below the diaphragm, between the liver and spleen. The gallbladder rests under the posterior surface of the liver, just lateral to the right midclavicular line. Note that

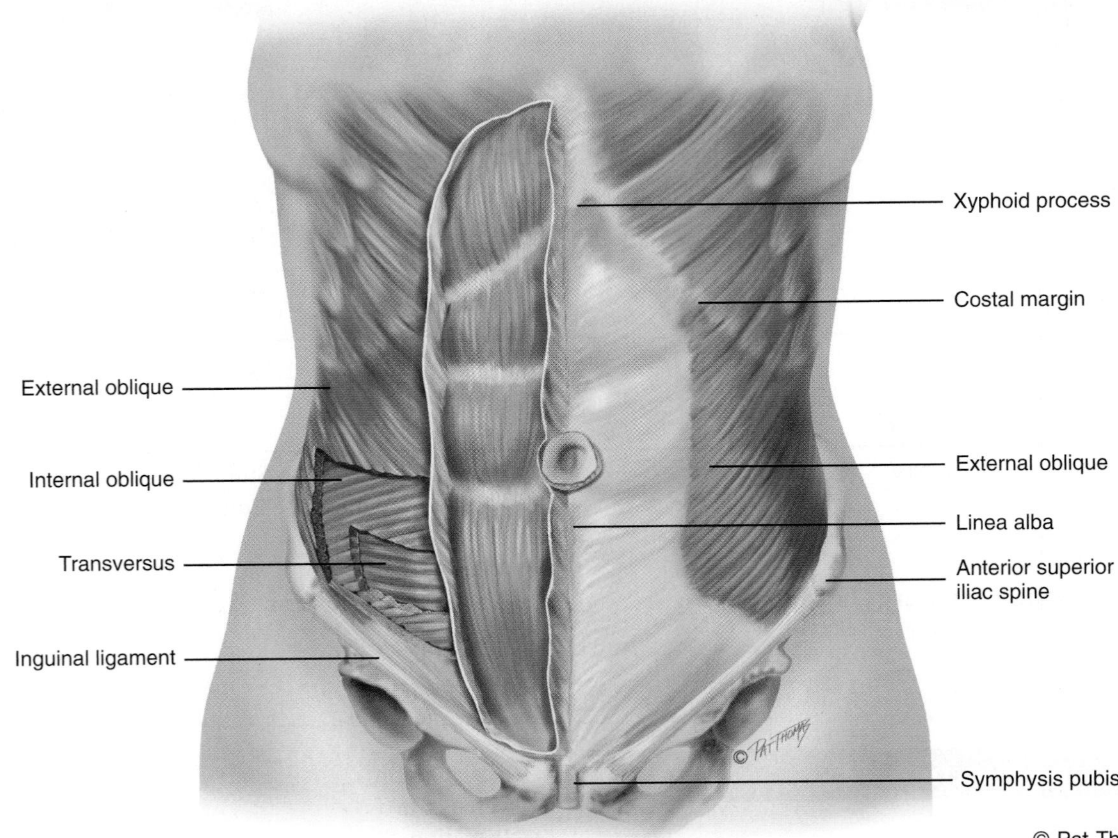
Xyphoid process
Costal margin
External oblique
Internal oblique
External oblique
Linea alba
Transversus
Anterior superior
iliac spine
Inguinal ligament
Symphysis pubis

21-1

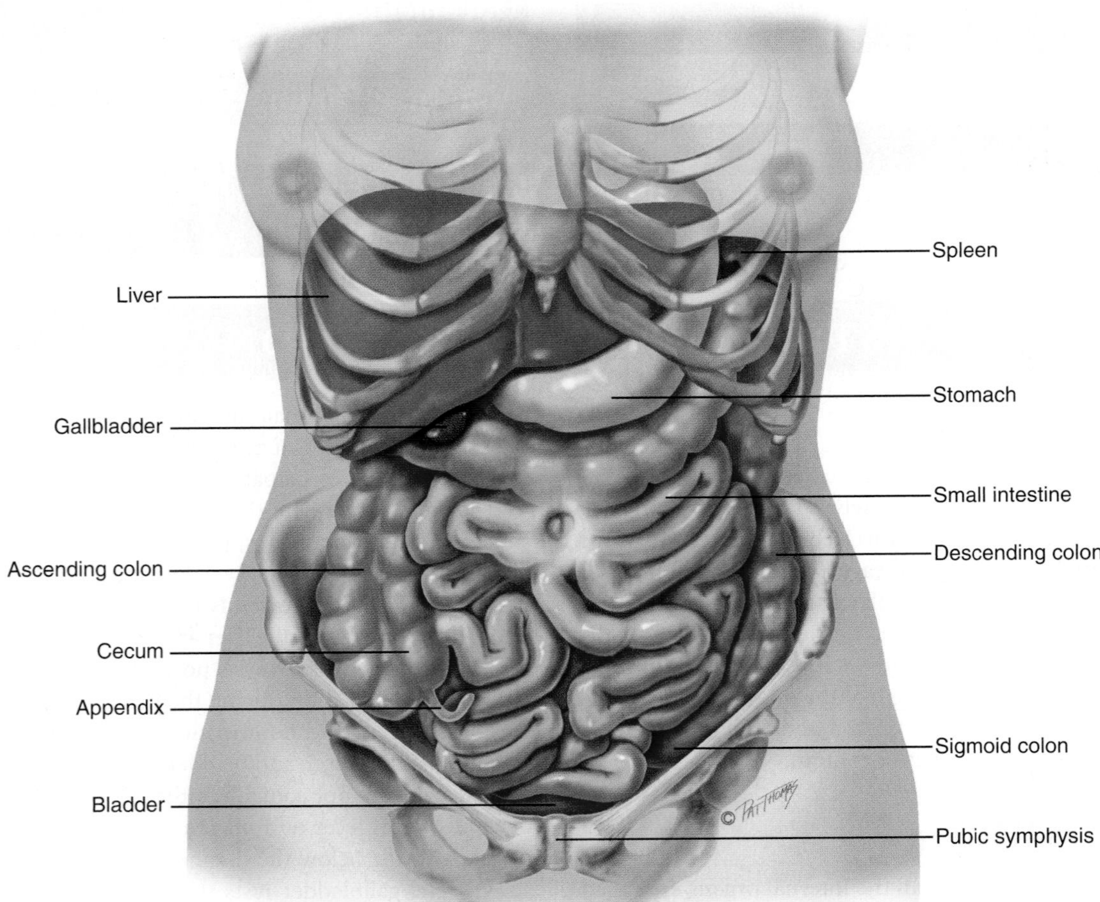
Spleen
Liver
Stomach
Gallbladder
Small intestine
Descending colon
Ascending colon
Cecum
Appendix
Sigmoid colon
Bladder
Pubic symphysis

21-2

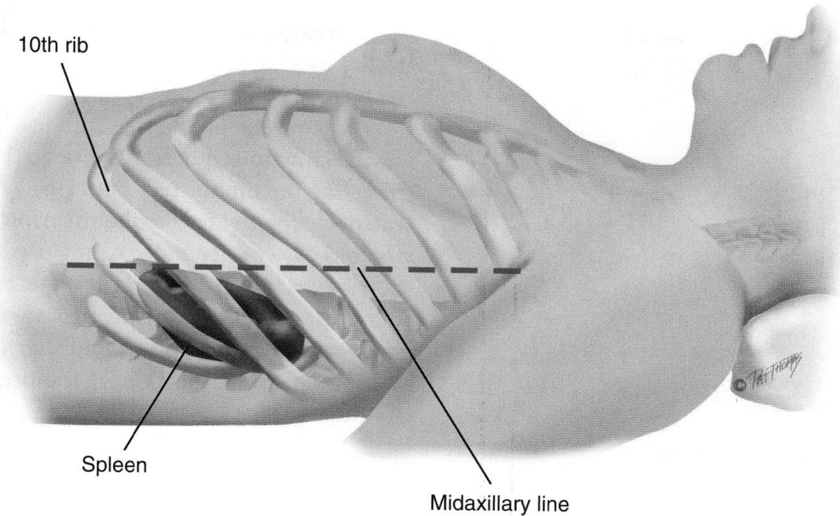

21-3

the small intestine is located in all four quadrants. It extends from the stomach's pyloric valve to the ileocecal valve in the right lower quadrant (RLQ), where it joins the colon.

The **spleen** is a soft mass of lymphatic tissue on the posterolateral wall of the abdominal cavity, immediately under the diaphragm (Fig. 21-3). It lies obliquely with its long axis behind and parallel to the tenth rib, lateral to the midaxillary line. Its width extends from the ninth to the eleventh rib, about 7 cm. It is not palpable normally. If it becomes enlarged, its lower pole moves downward and toward the midline.

The **aorta** is just to the left of midline in the upper part of the abdomen (Fig. 21-4). It descends behind the peritoneum, and at 2 cm below the umbilicus, it bifurcates into the right and left common iliac arteries opposite the fourth lumbar vertebra. You can palpate the aortic pulsations easily in the upper anterior abdominal wall. The right and left iliac arteries

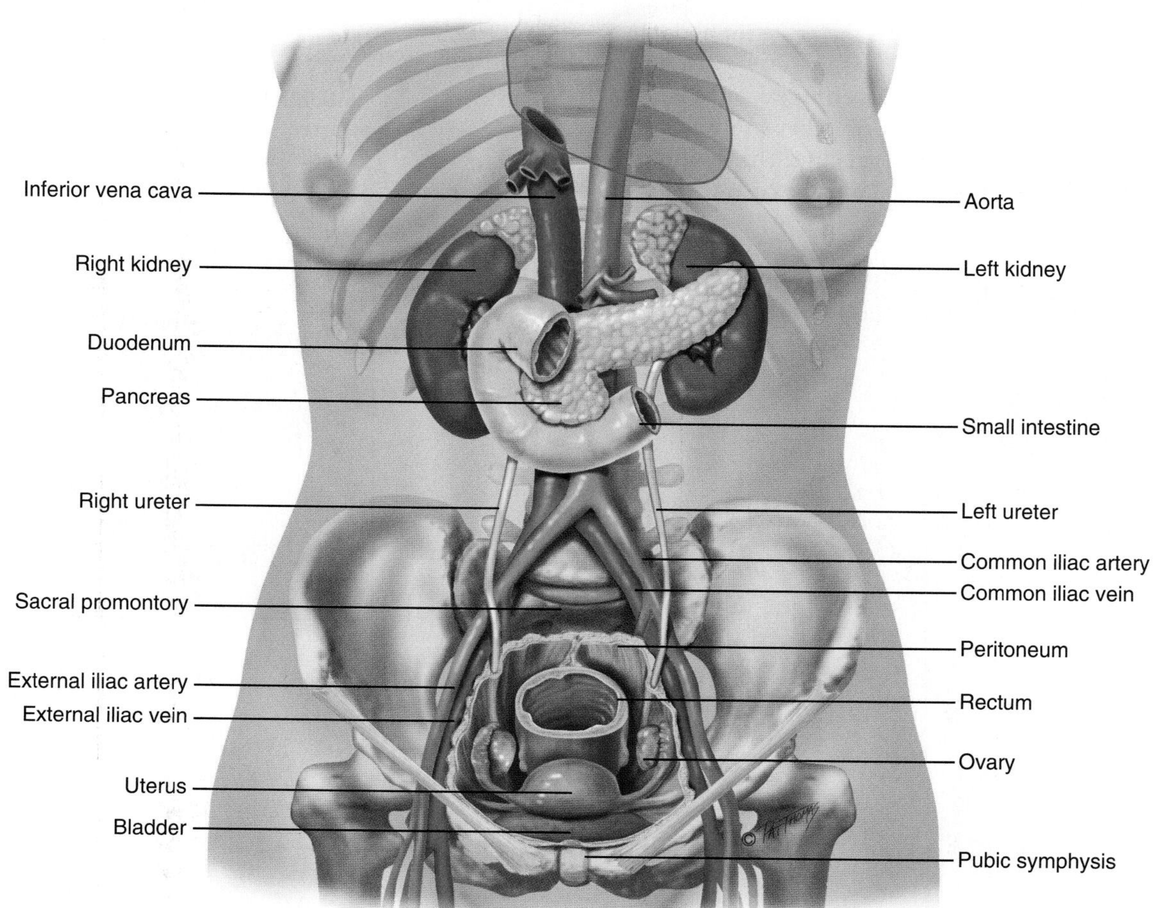

21-4

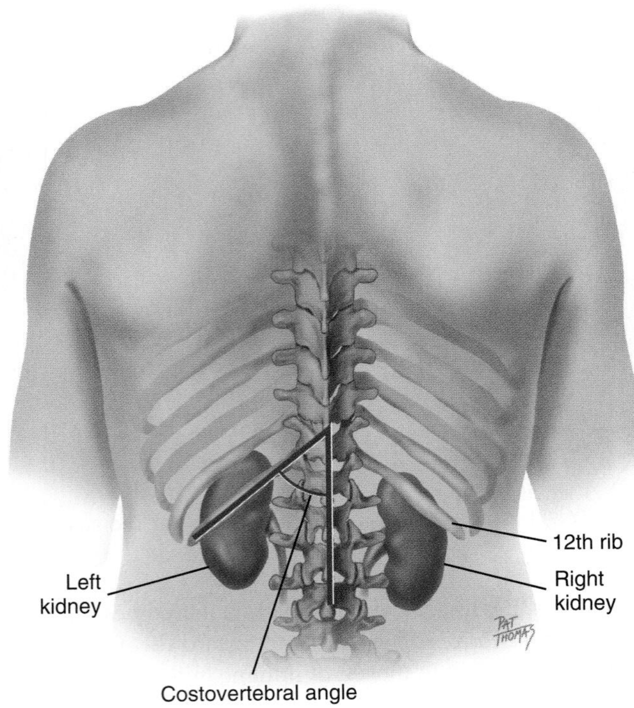

21-5

become the femoral arteries in the groin area. Their pulsations are easily palpated as well, at a point halfway between the anterior superior iliac spine and the symphysis pubis.

The **pancreas** is a soft, lobulated gland located behind the stomach. It stretches obliquely across the posterior abdominal wall to the left upper quadrant.

The bean-shaped **kidneys** are retroperitoneal, or posterior to the abdominal contents (Fig. 21-5). They are well protected by the posterior ribs and musculature. The twelfth rib forms an angle with the vertebral column, the **costovertebral angle.** The left kidney lies here at the eleventh and twelfth ribs. Because of the placement of the liver, the right kidney rests 1 to 2 cm lower than the left kidney and sometimes may be palpable.

For convenience in description, the abdominal wall is divided into **four quadrants** by a vertical and a horizontal line bisecting the umbilicus (Fig. 21-6). (An older, more complicated scheme divided the abdomen into nine regions. Although the old system generally is not used, some regional names persist, such as **epigastric** for the area between the costal margins, **umbilical** for the area around the umbilicus, and **hypogastric** or **suprapubic** for the area above the pubic bone.)

The anatomic location of the organs by quadrants is as follows:

RIGHT UPPER QUADRANT (RUQ)
Liver
Gallbladder
Duodenum
Head of pancreas
Right kidney and adrenal
Hepatic flexure of colon
Part of ascending and transverse colon

LEFT UPPER QUADRANT (LUQ)
Stomach
Spleen
Left lobe of liver
Body of pancreas
Left kidney and adrenal
Splenic flexure of colon
Part of transverse and descending colon

RIGHT LOWER QUADRANT (RLQ)
Cecum
Appendix
Right ovary and tube
Right ureter
Right spermatic cord

LEFT LOWER QUADRANT (LLQ)
Part of descending colon
Sigmoid colon
Left ovary and tube
Left ureter
Left spermatic cord

MIDLINE
Aorta
Uterus (if enlarged)
Bladder (if distended)

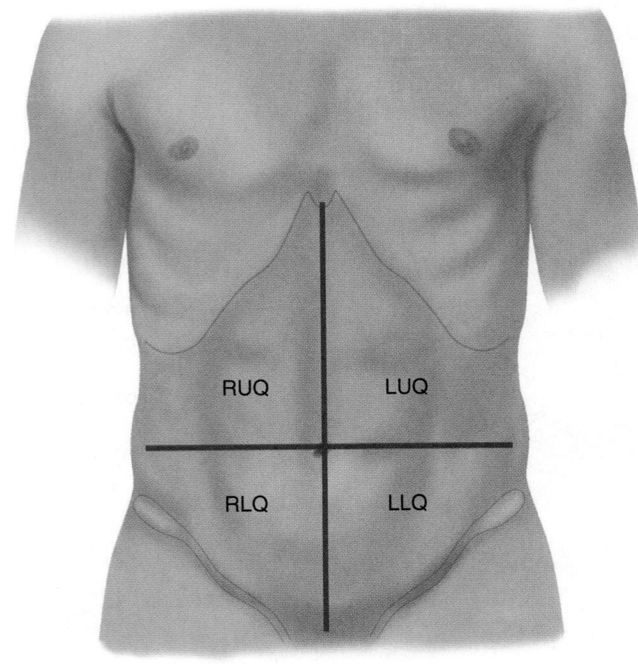

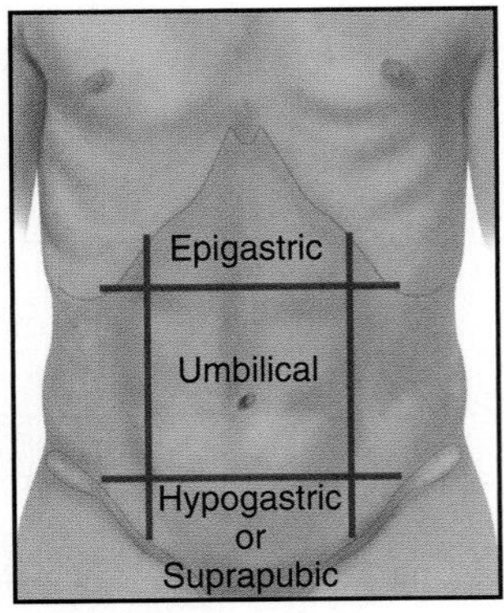

21-6 Four quadrants

DEVELOPMENTAL COMPETENCE

Infants and Children

In the newborn, the umbilical cord shows prominently on the abdomen. It contains two arteries and one vein. The liver takes up proportionately more space in the abdomen at birth than in later life. In healthy term neonates, the lower edge may be palpated 0.5 to 2.5 cm below the right costal margin. Age-related values of expected liver span are listed in the Objective Data section. The urinary bladder is located higher in the abdomen than in the adult. It lies between the symphysis and the umbilicus. Also, during early childhood, the abdominal wall is less muscular, so the organs may be easier to palpate.

The Pregnant Woman

Nausea and vomiting, or "morning sickness," is an early sign of pregnancy for most pregnant women, starting between the first and second missed periods. The cause is unknown but may be due to hormone changes such as the production of human chorionic gonadotropin (hCG). Another symptom is "acid indigestion" or heartburn (pyrosis) caused by esophageal reflux. Gastrointestinal motility decreases, which prolongs gastric emptying time. The decreased motility causes more water to be reabsorbed from the colon, which leads to constipation. The constipation, as well as increased venous pressure in the lower pelvis, may lead to hemorrhoids.

The enlarging uterus displaces the intestines upward and posteriorly. Bowel sounds are diminished. Traditional thinking was that the appendix was displaced upward and to the right. But clinical evidence has contradicted this and have shown that pregnancy does not change the location of the appendix.[19,33] Any appendicitis-related pain during pregnancy would still be felt in the right lower quadrant. Finally, skin changes on the abdomen, such as striae and linea nigra, are discussed later in this chapter on p. 537 and in Chapter 12.

The Aging Adult

Aging alters the appearance of the abdominal wall. During and after middle age, some fat accumulates in the suprapubic area in females as a result of decreased estrogen levels. Males also show some fat deposits in the abdominal area, resulting in the "big belly." This accentuates in adults with a more sedentary lifestyle.

With further aging, adipose tissue is redistributed away from the face and extremities and to the abdomen and hips. The abdominal musculature relaxes.

Changes of aging occur in the gastrointestinal system but do not significantly affect function as long as no disease is present.

- Salivation decreases, causing a dry mouth and a decreased sense of taste (discussed in Chapter 16).
- Esophageal emptying is delayed. If an aging person is fed in the supine position, this increases risk for aspiration.
- Gastric acid secretion decreases with aging. This may cause pernicious anemia (because it interferes with vitamin B_{12} absorption), iron deficiency anemia, and malabsorption of calcium.
- The incidence of gallstones increases with age, occurring in 10% to 20% of middle-aged and older adults, being more common in females.
- Liver size decreases by 25% between the ages of 20 and 70 years, although most liver function remains normal. Drug metabolism by the liver is impaired, in part because by age 65, blood flow through the liver is decreased by 33%.[12] Therefore the liver metabolism that is responsible for the enzymatic oxidation, reduction, and hydrolysis of drugs is substantially decreased with age. Prolonged liver metabolism causes increased side effects (e.g., older people taking benzodiazepines scored lower on functional status measures and had increased risk for hip fracture).[38]
- Aging persons frequently report constipation; most prevalence estimates are between 12% and 19%.[18] Because there is confusion as to what defines constipation, the Rome criteria[28] have been developed as standardized symptom criteria. These symptoms include reduced stool frequency (less than 3 bowel movements per week), as well as other common and troubling associated symptoms (i.e., straining, lumpy or hard stool, feeling of incomplete evacuation, feeling of anorectal blockage, use of manual maneuvers).

Common causes of constipation include decreased physical activity, inadequate intake of water, a low-fiber diet, side effects of medications (opioids, tricyclic antidepressants), irritable bowel syndrome, bowel obstruction, hypothyroidism, and inadequate toilet facilities (i.e., difficulty ambulating to the toilet may cause the person to deliberately retain the stool until it becomes hard and difficult to pass).

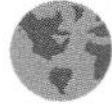

CULTURE AND GENETICS

Lactase is the digestive enzyme necessary for absorption of the carbohydrate *lactose* (milk sugar). In some racial groups, lactase activity is high at birth but declines to low levels by adulthood. These people are **lactose intolerant** and have abdominal pain, bloating, and flatulence when milk products are consumed. Millions of American adults have the potential for lactose-intolerance symptoms, and traditional estimated rates were that 15% of whites, 50% of Mexican Americans, and 80% of African Americans had the condition. Yet a recent study found the prevalence rates in practical life settings is significantly lower than previously estimated rates.[36] When subjects were screened for symptoms following a typical serving of dairy food in the home setting, lactose-intolerance prevalence estimates were 7.72% for whites, 19.5% for African Americans, and 10% for Hispanics.[36] This is clinically significant because dairy foods meet crucial nutritional requirements including calcium, magnesium, and potassium. If people perceive themselves to be lactose intolerant based on racial heritage, the lowered calcium intake may affect bone health. Health care providers should encourage low-fat or fat-free daily foods and monitor any symptoms.

Obesity is the accumulation of excess body fat. Obesity is caused by a complex interaction of genetic predisposition, dietary intake, physical inactivity, and what is now called an "obesogenic" environment[16] (one that encourages large portions of high-fat, energy-dense food). The prevalence of obesity has increased in the United States and globally. Currently, one third of American adults are obese (BMI $\geq$30 kg/m^2), and by 2015, the estimates are that 40% or more U.S. adults will be obese.[44]

Data from the National Health and Nutrition Examination Survey (NHANES) show significant differences among racial/ethnic groups.[37] Among children, Mexican-American boys had a greater prevalence of overweight than had white or Black boys. Mexican-American and Black girls were significantly more likely to be overweight than white girls. No differences were found in overweight rates in men of various racial groups. But in adult women, Mexican Americans and African Americans were significantly more likely to be obese than were whites.

Obesity in adults results in comorbidities of type 2 diabetes and cardiovascular disease. Obese children have an increased risk for asthma, diabetes, liver disease, cardiovascular disease, sleep apnea, and joint problems, and they risk becoming obese adults.[25] Controlling the obesity epidemic will be important in containing health care costs. Do Americans view obesity as a threat in the same way they now view the dangers of smoking? A change in public awareness and public thinking to regard obesity as a "common enemy" has been proposed to garner public support.[25] The areas for needed change are vast and include personal, community, and government strategies. Recommendations include the following[25]:

> *Making healthful food and beverages more widely available; providing access to healthier food by locating stores in underserved areas; and decreasing the availability of less healthful food and beverages. ... discourage consumption of sugar-sweetened beverages; increased support for breastfeeding; linkages between local farms and institutions to increase fruit and vegetable consumption; shifts in agricultural policy; and improved community infrastructure to promote biking, walking, and use of public transit.*

SUBJECTIVE DATA

1. Appetite
2. Dysphagia
3. Food intolerance
4. Abdominal pain
5. Nausea/vomiting
6. Bowel habits
7. Past abdominal history
8. Medications
9. Nutritional assessment

Examiner Asks	Rationale
1. Appetite. • Any change in **appetite?** Is this a loss of appetite? • Any change in weight? How much weight gained or lost? Over what time period? Is the weight loss due to diet?	**Anorexia** is a loss of appetite from gastrointestinal (GI) disease, as a side effect to some medications, with pregnancy, or with psychological disorders.
2. Dysphagia. • Any difficulty swallowing? When did you first notice this?	**Dysphagia** occurs with disorders of the throat or esophagus.
3. Food intolerance. • Are there any foods you cannot eat? What happens if you do eat them: allergic reaction, heartburn, belching, bloating, indigestion? • Do you use antacids? How often?	**Food intolerance** (e.g., lactase deficiency resulting in bloating or excessive gas after taking milk products). **Pyrosis** (heartburn), a burning sensation in esophagus and stomach, from reflux of gastric acid. Eructation (belching).
4. Abdominal pain. • Any **abdominal pain?** Please point to it. • Is the pain in one spot, or does it move around? • How did it start? How long have you had it? • Constant, or does it come and go? Occur before or after meals? Does it peak? When?	Abdominal pain may be *visceral* from an internal organ (dull, general, poorly localized); *parietal* from inflammation of overlying peritoneum (sharp, precisely localized, aggravated by movement); or

Examiner Asks	Rationale
• How would you describe the character: cramping (colic type), burning in pit of stomach, dull, stabbing, aching?	*referred* from a disorder in another site (see Table 21-2 on p. 559). Acute pain requiring urgent diagnosis occurs with appendicitis, cholecystitis, bowel obstruction, or a perforated organ.
• Is the pain relieved by food, or worse after eating?	Chronic pain of gastric ulcers occurs usually on an empty stomach; pain of duodenal ulcers occurs 2 to 3 hours after a meal and is relieved by more food.
• Is the pain associated with menstrual period or irregularities, stress, dietary indiscretion, fatigue, nausea and vomiting, gas, fever, rectal bleeding, frequent urination, vaginal or penile discharge? • What makes the pain worse: food, position, stress, medication, activity? • What have you tried to relieve pain: rest, heating pad, change in position, medication?	
5. Nausea/vomiting.	
• Any **nausea** or **vomiting?** How often? How much comes up? What is the color? Is there an odor?	Nausea/vomiting is common with GI disease, many medications, and with early pregnancy.
• Is it bloody?	Hematemesis occurs with stomach or duodenal ulcers and esophageal varices.
• Is the nausea and vomiting associated with colicky pain, diarrhea, fever, chills?	
• What foods did you eat in the past 24 hours? Where? At home, school, restaurant? Is there anyone else in the family with same symptoms in past 24 hours?	Consider food poisoning.
6. Bowel habits.	
• How often do you have a **bowel movement?** • What is the color? Consistency? • Any diarrhea or constipation? How long? • Any recent change in bowel habits? • Use laxatives? Which ones? How often do you use them?	Assess usual **bowel habits.** Black stools may be tarry due to occult blood (melena) from GI bleeding or nontarry from iron medications. Gray stools occur with hepatitis. Red blood in stools occurs with GI bleeding or localized bleeding around the anus.
7. Past abdominal history.	
• Any **history** of gastrointestinal problems: ulcer, gallbladder disease, hepatitis/jaundice, appendicitis, colitis, hernia? • Ever had any operations in the abdomen? Please describe. • Any problems after surgery? • Any abdominal x-ray studies? How were the results?	
8. Medications.	
• What **medications** are you currently taking? • How about alcohol—how much would you say you drink each day? Each week? When was your last alcoholic drink? • How about cigarettes—do you smoke? How many packs per day? For how long?	Peptic ulcer disease occurs with frequent use of nonsteroidal anti-inflammatory drugs (NSAIDs), alcohol, smoking, and *Helicobacter pylori* infection.

Examiner Asks	Rationale
9. **Nutritional assessment.** • Now I would like to ask you about your diet. Please tell me all the food you ate yesterday, starting with breakfast. • What fresh food markets are located in your neighborhood?	**Nutritional assessment** via 24-hour recall (see Chapter 11 for full discussion). Many inner-city neighborhoods are fresh food "deserts," lacking markets but full of fast-food restaurants.

Additional History for Infants and Children

Examiner Asks	Rationale
1. **Are you breastfeeding or bottle-feeding the baby?** If bottle-feeding, how does baby tolerate the formula?	
2. **What table foods have you introduced?** How does the infant tolerate the food?	Consider a new food as a possible allergen. Adding only one new food at a time to the infant's diet helps identify allergies.
3. **How often does your toddler/child eat?** Does he or she eat regular meals? How do you feel about your child's eating problems? • Please describe all that your child had to eat yesterday, starting with breakfast. What foods does the child eat for snacks?	Irregular eating patterns are common and a source of parental anxiety. As long as the child shows normal growth and development and only nutritious foods are offered, parents may be reassured.
• Does toddler/child ever eat nonfoods: grass, dirt, paint chips?	**Pica:** Although a toddler may attempt nonfoods at some time, he or she should recognize edibles by age 2 years.
4. **Does your child have constipation? How long?** • What is the number of stools/day? Stools/week? • How much water, juice is in the diet? • Does the constipation seem to be associated with toilet training? • What have you tried to treat the constipation?	
5. **Does the child have abdominal pain?** Please describe what you have noticed and when it started.	This symptom is hard to assess with young children. Many conditions of unrelated organ systems are associated with vague abdominal pain (e.g., otitis media). They cannot articulate specific symptoms and often focus on "the tummy." Abdominal pain accompanies inflammation of the bowel, constipation, urinary tract infection, and anxiety.
6. **For the overweight child: How long has weight been a problem?** • At what age did the child first seem overweight? Did any change in diet pattern occur then? • Describe the diet pattern now. • Do any others in family have a similar problem? • How does child feel about his or her own weight?	Reduced physical activity and food marketing practices contribute to current obesity epidemic. Family history of obesity. Assess body image.

Additional History for Adolescents

Examiner Asks	Rationale
1. What do you eat at regular meals? Do you eat breakfast? What do you eat for snacks?	Adolescent takes control of eating and may reject family values (e.g., skipping breakfast, consuming junk foods, soda pop). The only control parents have is to control what food is in the house.
• How many calories do you figure you consume?	You probably cannot change adolescent eating pattern, but you can supply nutritional facts.

Examiner Asks	Rationale
2. What is your exercise pattern?	Boys need an average 4000 cal/day to maintain weight; more calories if exercise is pursued. Girls need 20% fewer calories and the same nutrients as boys. Fast food is high in fat, calories, and salt and has no fiber.
3. If weight is less than body requirements: How much have you lost? By diet, exercise, or how?	Screen any extremely thin teenage girl for **anorexia nervosa,** a serious psychosocial disorder that includes loss of appetite, voluntary starvation, and grave weight loss. This person may augment weight loss by purging (self-induced vomiting) and use of laxatives.
• How do you feel? Tired, hungry? How do you think your body looks?	Denial of these feelings is common. Though thin, this person insists she looks fat, "disgusting." Distorted body image.
• What is your activity pattern?	The anorectic may have healthy activity and exercise but often is hyperactive.
• Is the weight loss associated with any other body change, such as menstrual irregularity?	Amenorrhea is common with anorexia nervosa.
• What do your parents say about your eating? Your friends?	This is a family problem involving control issues. Anyone at risk warrants immediate referral to a physician or psychologist.
Additional History for the Aging Adult	
1. How do you acquire your groceries and prepare your meals?	Assess risk for nutritional deficit: limited access to grocery store, income, or cooking facilities; physical disability (impaired vision, decreased mobility, decreased strength, neurologic deficit).
2. Do you eat alone or share meals with others?	Assess risk for nutritional deficit if living alone; may not bother to prepare all meals; social isolation; depression.
3. Please tell me all that you had to eat yesterday, starting with breakfast.	**NOTE:** 24-hour recall may not be sufficient because daily pattern may vary. Attempt week-long diary of intake. Food pattern may differ during the month if monthly income (e.g., Social Security check) runs out.
• Do you have any trouble swallowing these foods? • What do you do right after eating: walk, take a nap?	
4. How often do your bowels move? • If the person reports constipation: What do you mean by constipation? How much liquid is in your diet? How much bulk or fiber? • Do you take anything for constipation, such as laxatives? Which ones? How often?	
• What medications do you take?	Consider GI side effects (e.g., nausea, upset stomach, anorexia, dry mouth).

OBJECTIVE DATA

PREPARATION

The lighting should include a strong overhead light and a secondary stand light. Expose the abdomen so that it is fully visible. Drape the genitalia and female breasts.

The following measures will enhance abdominal wall relaxation:

- The person should have emptied the bladder, saving a urine specimen if needed.
- Keep the room warm to avoid chilling and tensing of muscles.
- Position the person supine, with the head on a pillow, the knees bent or on pillow, and the arms at the sides or across the chest. (Note: Discourage the person from placing his or her arms over the head because this tenses abdominal musculature.)
- To avoid abdominal tensing, the stethoscope endpiece must be warm, your hands must be warm, and your fingernails must be very short.
- Inquire about any painful areas. Examine such an area last to avoid any muscle guarding.
- Finally, learn to use distraction: Enhance muscle relaxation through breathing exercises; emotive imagery; your low, soothing voice; engaging in conversation or the person relating his or her abdominal history while you palpate.

EQUIPMENT NEEDED

Stethoscope
Small centimeter ruler
Skin-marking pen
Alcohol wipe (to clean endpiece)

Normal Range of Findings

INSPECT THE ABDOMEN

Contour

Stand on the person's right side and look down on the abdomen. Then stoop or sit to gaze across the abdomen. Your head should be slightly higher than the abdomen. Determine the profile from the rib margin to the pubic bone. The contour describes the nutritional state and normally ranges from flat to rounded (Fig. 21-7).

Abnormal Findings

Scaphoid abdomen caves in. Protuberant abdomen, abdominal distention (see Table 21-1, Abdominal Distention, pp. 557-558).

Flat

Scaphoid

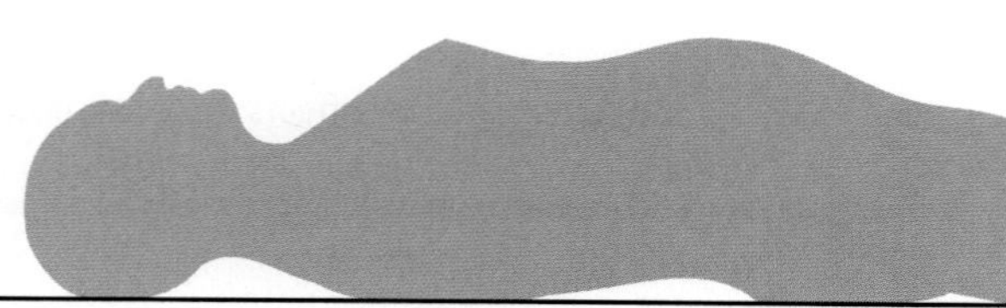

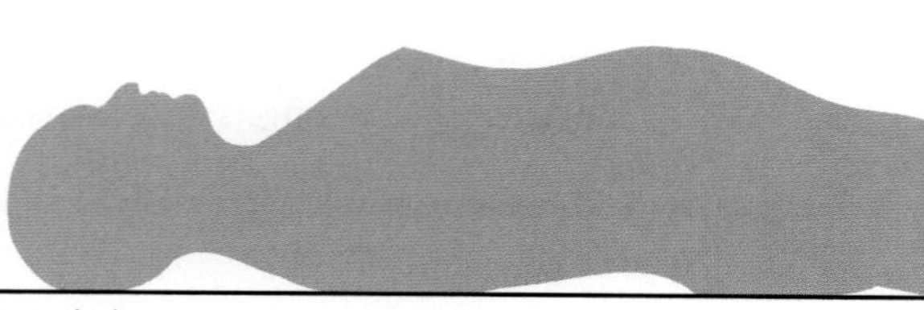

Rounded

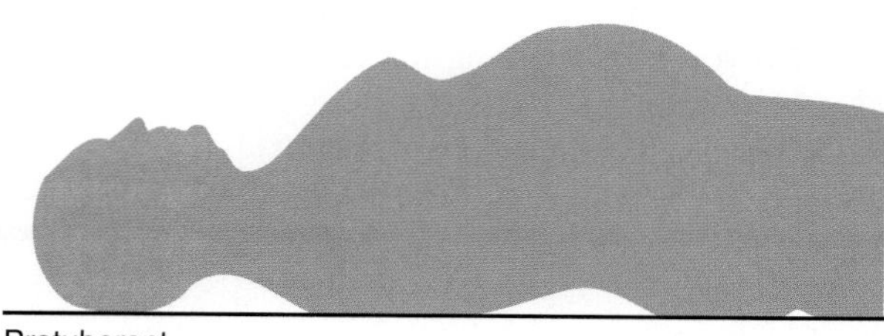

Protuberant

21-7

Normal Range of Findings	Abnormal Findings

Symmetry

Shine a light across the abdomen toward you, or shine it lengthwise across the person. The abdomen should be symmetric bilaterally (Fig. 21-8). Note any localized bulging, visible mass, or asymmetric shape. Even small bulges are highlighted by shadow. Step to the foot of the examination table to recheck symmetry.

Bulges, masses.

Hernia—protrusion of abdominal viscera through abnormal opening in muscle wall (see Table 21-3, Abnormalities on Inspection, p. 560).

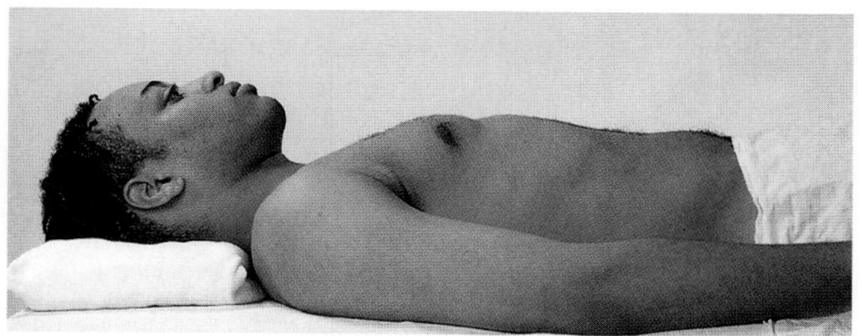

21-8

Ask the person to take a deep breath to further highlight any change. The abdomen should stay smooth and symmetric. Or ask the person to perform a sit-up without pushing up with his or her hands.

Note any localized bulging.

Hernia, enlarged liver or spleen may show.

Umbilicus

Normally it is midline and inverted, with no sign of discoloration, inflammation, or hernia. It becomes everted and pushed upward with pregnancy.

The umbilicus is a common site for piercings in young women. The site should not be red or crusted.

Everted with ascites or underlying mass (see Table 21-1).

Deeply sunken with obesity.

Enlarged, everted with umbilical hernia.

Bluish periumbilical color occurs (though rarely) with intra-abdominal bleeding (Cullen sign).

Skin

The surface is smooth and even, with homogeneous color. This is a good area to judge pigment because it is often protected from sun.

Redness with localized inflammation.

Jaundice (shows best in natural daylight).

Skin glistening and taut with ascites.

One common pigment change is **striae** (lineae albicantes)—silvery white, linear, jagged marks about 1 to 6 cm long (Fig. 21-9). They occur when elastic fibers in the reticular layer of the skin are broken after rapid or prolonged stretching, as in pregnancy or excessive weight gain. Recent striae are pink or blue; then they turn silvery white.

Striae also occur with ascites.

Striae look purple-blue with Cushing syndrome (excess adrenocortical hormone causes the skin to be fragile and easily broken from normal stretching).

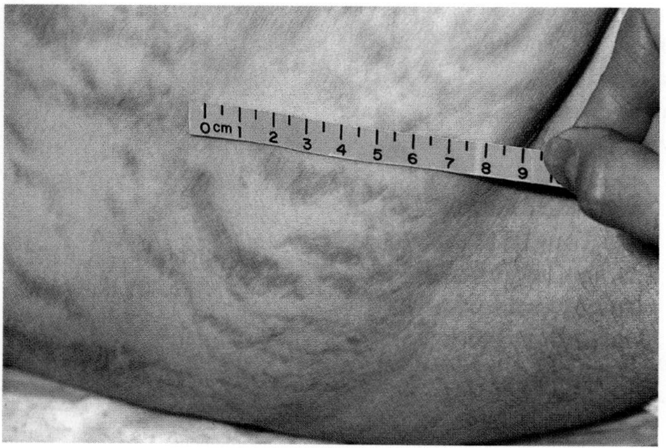

21-9 Striae.

Normal Range of Findings

Pigmented nevi (moles)—circumscribed brown macular or papular areas—are common on the abdomen.

Normally, no lesions are present, although you may note well-healed surgical scars. If a scar is present, draw its location in the person's record, indicating the length in centimeters (Fig. 21-10). (Note: Infrequently, a person may forget a past operation while providing the history. If you note a scar now, ask about it.) A surgical scar alerts you to the possible presence of underlying adhesions and excess fibrous tissue.

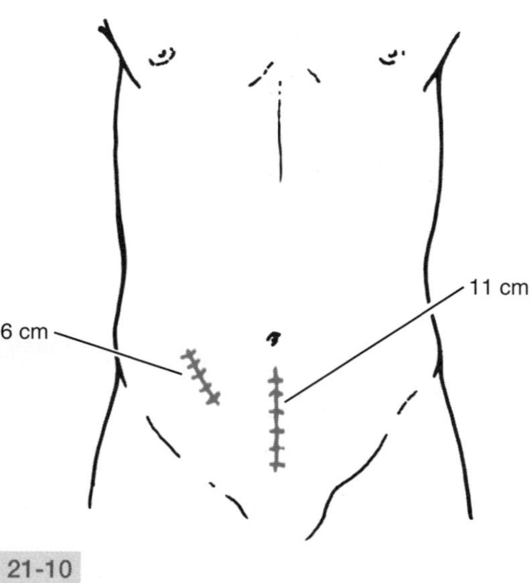

21-10

Veins usually are not seen, but a fine venous network may be visible in thin persons.

Good skin turgor reflects healthy nutrition. Gently pinch up a fold of skin; then release to note the skin's immediate return to original position.

Pulsation or Movement

Normally, you may see the pulsations from the aorta beneath the skin in the epigastric area, particularly in thin persons with good muscle wall relaxation. Respiratory movement also shows in the abdomen, particularly in males. Finally, waves of peristalsis sometimes are visible in very thin persons. They ripple slowly and obliquely across the abdomen.

Hair Distribution

The pattern of pubic hair growth normally has a diamond shape in adult males and an inverted triangle shape in adult females (see Chapters 24 and 26).

Abnormal Findings

Unusual color or change in shape of mole (see Chapter 12).

Petechiae.

Cutaneous angiomas (spider nevi) occur with portal hypertension or liver disease.

Lesions, rashes (see Chapter 12).

Underlying adhesions are inflammatory bands that connect opposite sides of serous surfaces after trauma or surgery.

Prominent, dilated veins occur with portal hypertension, cirrhosis, ascites, or vena caval obstruction. Veins are more visible with malnutrition as a result of thinned adipose tissue.

Poor turgor occurs with dehydration, which often accompanies GI disease.

Marked pulsation of aorta occurs with widened pulse pressure (e.g., hypertension, aortic insufficiency, thyrotoxicosis) and with aortic aneurysm.

Marked visible peristalsis, together with a distended abdomen, indicates intestinal obstruction.

Patterns alter with endocrine or hormone abnormalities, chronic liver disease.

Normal Range of Findings | Abnormal Findings

Demeanor

A comfortable person is relaxed quietly on the examining table and has a benign facial expression and slow, even respirations.

Restlessness and constant turning to find comfort occur with the colicky pain of gastroenteritis or bowel obstruction.

Absolute stillness, resisting any movement, occurs with the pain of peritonitis.

Knees flexed up, facial grimacing, and rapid, uneven respirations also indicate pain.

AUSCULTATE BOWEL SOUNDS AND VASCULAR SOUNDS

Depart from the usual examination sequence and auscultate the abdomen next. This is done because percussion and palpation can increase peristalsis, which would give a false interpretation of bowel sounds. Use the diaphragm endpiece because bowel sounds are relatively high-pitched. Hold the stethoscope lightly against the skin; pushing too hard may stimulate more bowel sounds (Fig. 21-11). Begin in the RLQ at the ileocecal valve area because bowel sounds are normally always present here.

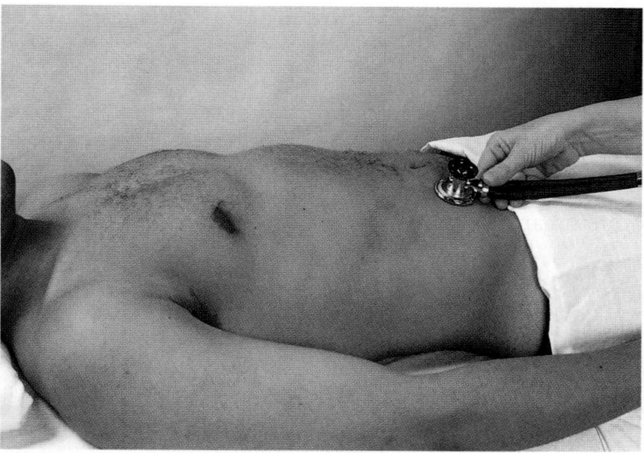

21-11

Bowel Sounds

Note the character and frequency of bowel sounds. Bowel sounds originate from the movement of air and fluid through the small intestine. Depending on the time elapsed since eating, a wide range of normal sounds can occur. Bowel sounds are high-pitched, gurgling, cascading sounds, occurring irregularly anywhere from 5 to 30 times per minute. Do not bother to count them. Judge if they are normal, hypoactive, or hyperactive.

One type of hyperactive bowel sounds is fairly common. This is the hyperperistalsis when you feel your "stomach growling," termed **borborygmus.** A perfectly "silent abdomen" is uncommon; you must listen for 5 minutes by your watch before deciding bowel sounds are completely absent.

Two distinct patterns of abnormal bowel sounds may occur:

1. **Hyperactive sounds** are loud, high-pitched, rushing, tinkling sounds that signal increased motility.
2. **Hypoactive or absent sounds** follow abdominal surgery or with inflammation of the peritoneum (see Table 21-4, Abnormal Bowel Sounds, p. 561).

Objective Data

Normal Range of Findings	Abnormal Findings

Vascular Sounds

As you listen to the abdomen, note the presence of any vascular sounds or **bruits.** Using firmer pressure, check over the aorta, renal arteries, iliac, and femoral arteries, especially in people with hypertension (Fig. 21-12). Usually, no such sound is present. However, a small number of healthy persons (usually younger than 40 years) may have a normal bruit originating from the celiac artery.[30] This is systolic, medium to low in pitch, and heard between the xiphoid process and the umbilicus.

Note location, pitch, and timing of a vascular sound.

A systolic bruit is a pulsatile blowing sound and occurs with stenosis or occlusion of an artery.

Venous hum and peritoneal friction rub are rare (see Table 21-5, Friction Rubs and Vascular Sounds, p. 562).

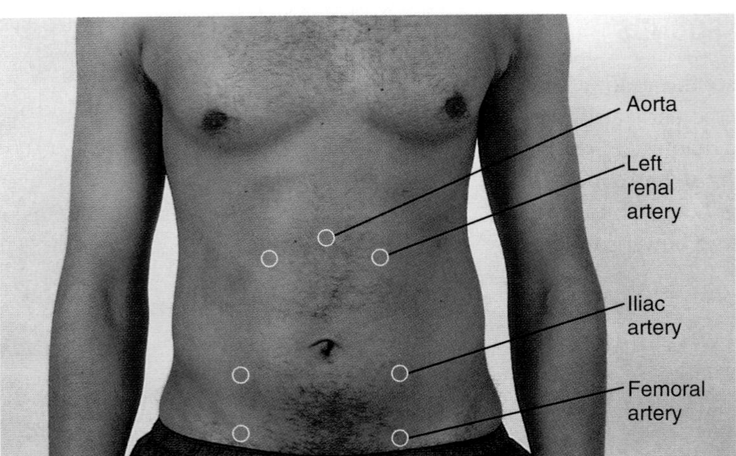

21-12

PERCUSS GENERAL TYMPANY, LIVER SPAN, AND SPLENIC DULLNESS

Percuss to assess the relative density of abdominal contents, to locate organs, and to screen for abnormal fluid or masses.

General Tympany

First, percuss lightly in all four quadrants to determine the prevailing amount of tympany and dullness (Fig. 21-13). Move clockwise. Tympany should predominate because air in the intestines rises to the surface when the person is supine.

Dullness occurs over a distended bladder, adipose tissue, fluid, or a mass.

Hyperresonance is present with gaseous distention.

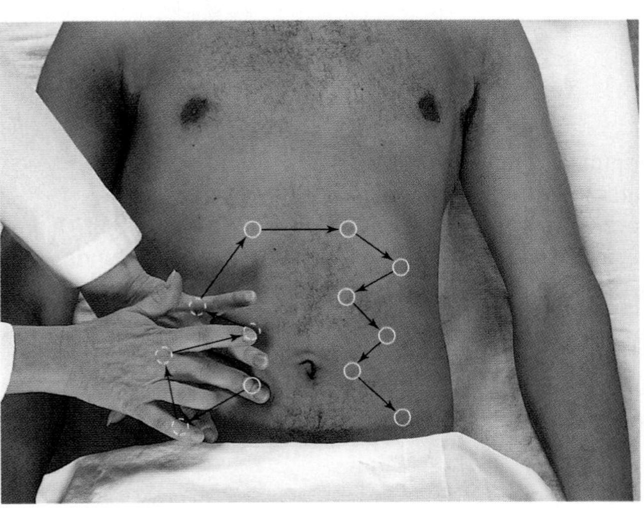

21-13

Normal Range of Findings

Liver Span

Next, percuss to map out the boundaries of certain organs. Measure the height of the liver in the right midclavicular line. (For a consistent placement of the midclavicular line landmark, remember to palpate the acromioclavicular and the sternoclavicular joints and judge the line at a point midway between the two.)

Begin in the area of lung resonance, and percuss down the interspaces until the sound changes to a dull quality (Fig. 21-14). Mark the spot, usually in the fifth intercostal space. Then find abdominal tympany and percuss up in the midclavicular line. Mark where the sound changes from tympany to a dull sound, normally at the right costal margin.

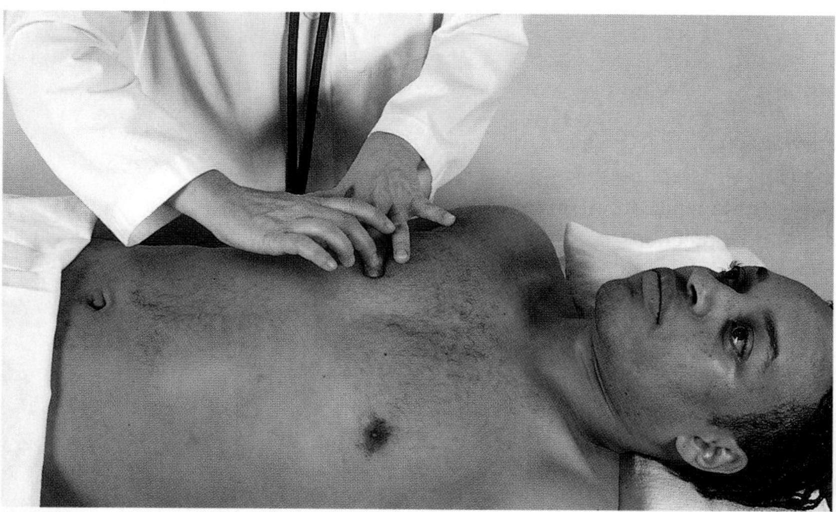

21-14

Measure the distance between the two marks; the normal liver span in the adult ranges from 6 to 12 cm (Fig. 21-15). The height of the liver span correlates with the height of the person; taller people have longer livers. Also males have a larger liver span than females of the same height. Overall, the mean liver span is 10.5 cm for males and 7 cm for females.

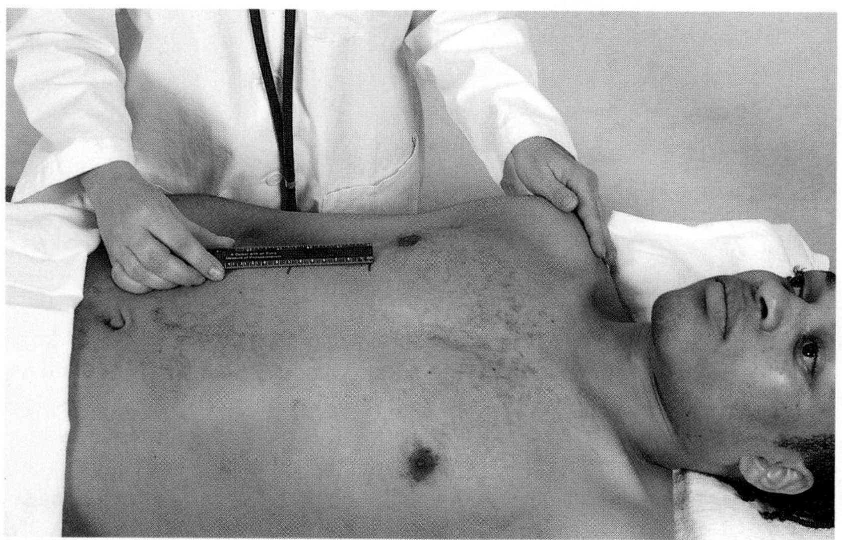

21-15

Abnormal Findings

An enlarged liver span indicates liver enlargement or **hepatomegaly.**

Accurate detection of liver borders is confused by dullness above the fifth intercostal space, which occurs with lung disease (e.g., pleural effusion or consolidation). Accurate detection at the lower border is confused when dullness is pushed up with ascites or pregnancy or with gas distention in the colon, which obscures the lower border.

Normal Range of Findings

One variation occurs in people with chronic emphysema, in which the liver is displaced downward by the hyperinflated lungs. Although you hear a dull percussion note well below the right costal margin, the overall span is still within normal limits.

Clinical estimation of liver span screens for hepatomegaly and monitors changes in liver size. However, this measurement is a gross estimate; the liver span usually is underestimated because of inaccurate detection of the upper border.

Scratch Test. Although traditionally taught, this technique does not work to identify the liver border. It uses a repeated scratching sound from your fingernail along the patient's abdomen; when the sound is magnified in the stethoscope, it was thought to define the lower liver border. However, evidence shows no correlation whatsoever between the liver edge by auscultation of scratches and the actual liver edge by ultrasound.[30,43]

Splenic Dullness

Often the spleen is obscured by stomach contents, but you may locate it by percussing for a dull note from the ninth to eleventh intercostal space just behind the left midaxillary line (Fig. 21-16). The area of splenic dullness normally is not wider than 7 cm in the adult and should not encroach on the normal tympany over the gastric air bubble.

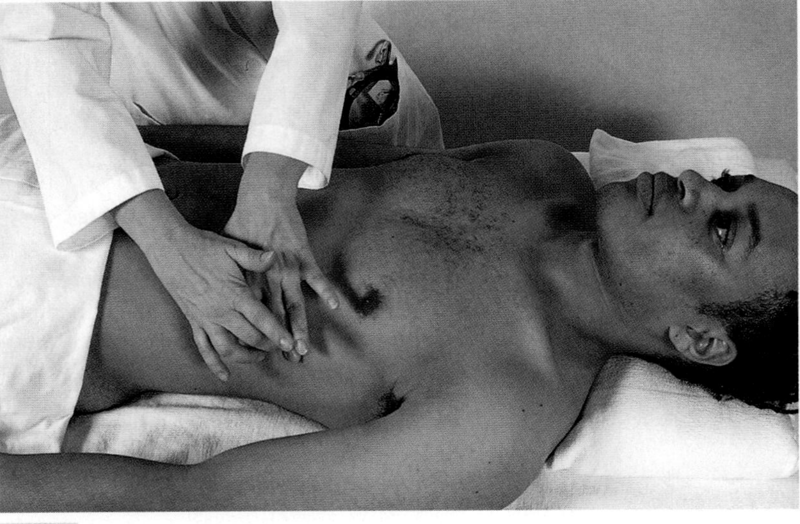

21-16

Now percuss in the lowest interspace in the left *anterior* axillary line. Tympany should result. Ask the person to take a deep breath. Normally, tympany remains through full inspiration.

Abnormal Findings

A dull note forward of the midaxillary line indicates enlargement of the spleen, as occurs with mononucleosis, trauma, and infection.

In this site, the *anterior* axillary line, a change in percussion from tympany to a dull sound with full inspiration is a **positive spleen percussion sign,** indicating splenomegaly. This method will detect mild to moderate splenomegaly before the spleen becomes palpable, as in mononucleosis, malaria, or hepatic cirrhosis.

Normal Range of Findings	Abnormal Findings

Costovertebral Angle Tenderness

Indirect fist percussion causes the tissues to vibrate instead of producing a sound. To assess the kidney, place one hand over the twelfth rib at the costovertebral angle on the back (Fig. 21-17). Thump that hand with the ulnar edge of your other fist. The person normally feels a thud but no pain. (Although this step is explained here with percussion techniques, its usual sequence in a complete examination is with thoracic assessment, when the person is sitting up and you are standing behind.)

Sharp pain occurs with inflammation of the kidney or paranephric area.

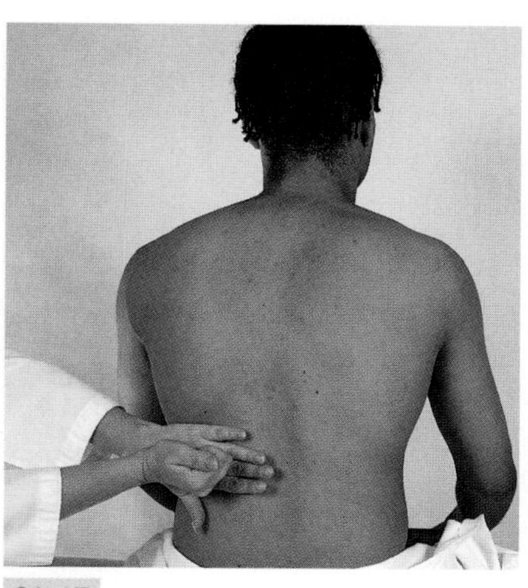

21-17

Special Procedures

At times, you may suspect that a person has ascites (free fluid in the peritoneal cavity) because of a distended abdomen, bulging flanks, and an umbilicus that is protruding and displaced downward. You can differentiate ascites from gaseous distention by performing two percussion tests.

Ascites occurs with heart failure, portal hypertension, cirrhosis, hepatitis, pancreatitis, and cancer.

Fluid Wave. First, test for a **fluid wave** by standing on the person's right side. Place the ulnar edge of another examiner's hand or the patient's own hand firmly on the abdomen in the midline (Fig. 21-18). (This will stop transmission across the skin of the upcoming tap.) Place your left hand on the person's right flank. With your right hand, reach across the abdomen and give the left flank a firm strike.

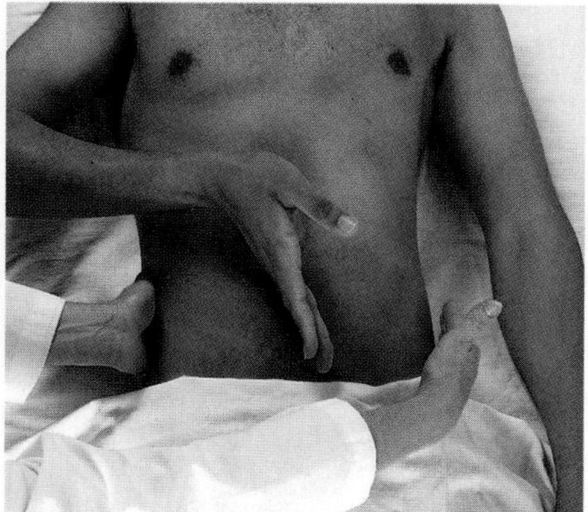

21-18 Fluid wave.

Normal Range of Findings

If ascites is present, the blow will generate a fluid wave through the abdomen and you will feel a distinct tap on your left hand. If the abdomen is distended from gas or adipose tissue, you will feel no change.

Shifting Dullness. The second test for ascites is percussing for **shifting dullness.** In a supine person, ascitic fluid settles by gravity into the flanks, displacing the air-filled bowel upward. You will hear a tympanitic note as you percuss over the top of the abdomen because gas-filled intestines float over the fluid (Fig. 21-19). Then percuss down the side of the abdomen. If fluid is present, the note will change from tympany to dull as you reach its level. Mark this spot.

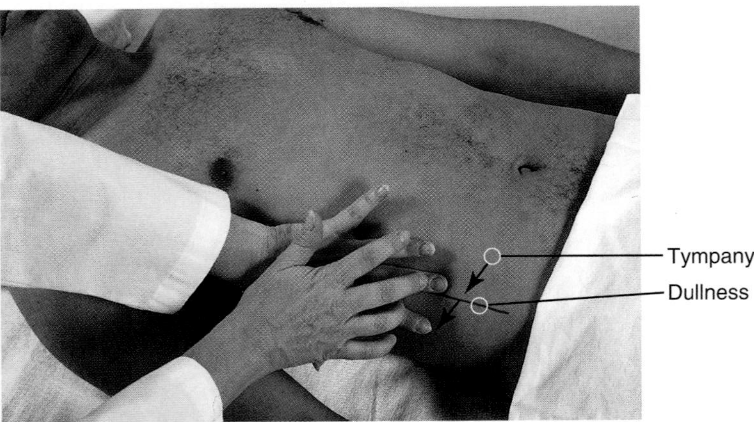

21-19

Now turn the person onto the right side (roll the person toward you) (Fig. 21-20). The fluid will gravitate to the dependent (in this case, right) side, displacing the lighter bowel upward. Begin percussing the upper side of the abdomen and move downward. The sound changes from tympany to a dull sound as you reach the fluid level, but this time the level of dullness is higher, upward toward the umbilicus. This **shifting level of dullness** indicates the presence of fluid.

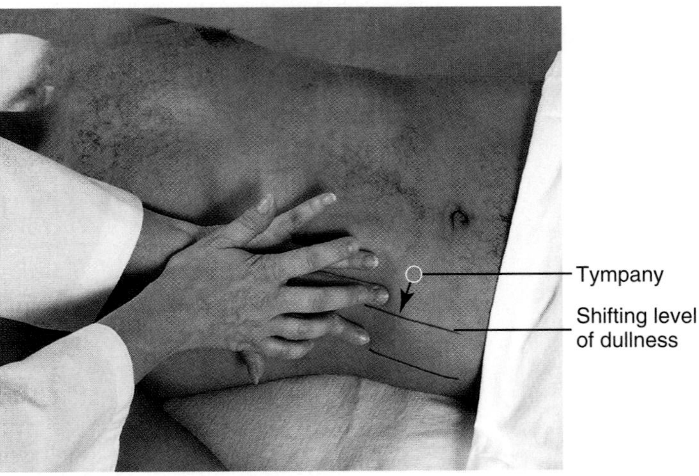

21-20

Abnormal Findings

A positive fluid wave test occurs with large amounts of ascitic fluid.

Shifting dullness is positive with a large volume of ascitic fluid: it will not detect less than 500 mL of fluid.

Normal Range of Findings	Abnormal Findings

Both tests, fluid wave and shifting dullness, are not completely reliable. Ultrasound study is the definitive tool.

PALPATE SURFACE AND DEEP AREAS

Perform palpation to judge the size, location, and consistency of certain organs and to screen for an abnormal mass or tenderness. Review comfort measures on p. 536. Because most people are naturally inclined to protect the abdomen, you need to use additional measures to enhance complete muscle relaxation.

1. Bend the person's knees.
2. Keep your palpating hand low and parallel to the abdomen. Holding the hand high and pointing down would make anyone tense up.
3. Teach the person to breathe slowly (in through the nose, and out through the mouth).
4. Keep your own voice low and soothing. Conversation may relax the person.
5. Try "emotive imagery." For example, you might say, "Now I want you to imagine you are dozing on the beach, with the sun warming your muscles and the sound of the waves lulling you to sleep. Let yourself relax."
6. With a very ticklish person, keep the person's hand under your own with your fingers curled over his or her fingers. Move both hands around as you palpate; people are not ticklish to themselves.
7. Alternatively, perform palpation just after auscultation. Keep the stethoscope in place and curl your fingers around it, palpating as you pretend to auscultate. People do not perceive a stethoscope as a ticklish object. You can slide the stethoscope out when the person is used to being touched.

Light and Deep Palpation

Begin with **light palpation.** With the first four fingers close together, depress the skin about 1 cm (Fig. 21-21). Make a gentle rotary motion, sliding the fingers and skin together. Then lift the fingers (do not drag them) and move clockwise to the next location around the abdomen. The objective here is not to search for organs but to form an overall impression of the skin surface and superficial musculature. Save the examination of any identified tender areas until last. This method avoids pain and the resulting muscle rigidity that would obscure deep palpation later in the examination.

Muscle guarding.
Rigidity.
Large masses.
Tenderness.

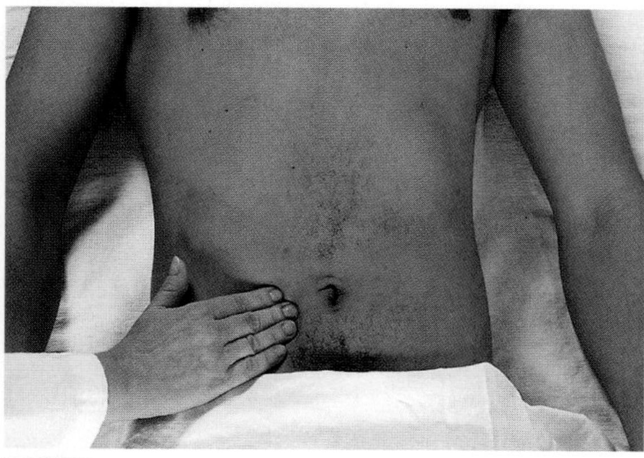
21-21

Normal Range of Findings

As you circle the abdomen, discriminate between voluntary muscle guarding and involuntary rigidity. **Voluntary guarding** occurs when the person is cold, tense, or ticklish. It is bilateral, and you will feel the muscles relax slightly during exhalation. Use the relaxation measures to try to eliminate this type of guarding, or it will interfere with deep palpation. If the rigidity persists, it is probably involuntary.

Now perform **deep palpation** using the same technique described earlier, but push down about 5 to 8 cm (2 to 3 inches) (Fig. 21-22). Moving clockwise, explore the entire abdomen.

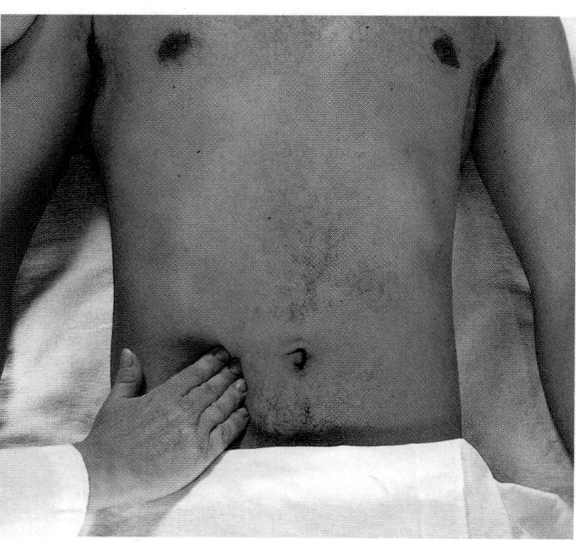

21-22

To overcome the resistance of a very large or obese abdomen, use a bimanual technique. Place your two hands on top of each other (Fig. 21-23). The top hand does the pushing; the bottom hand is relaxed and can concentrate on the sense of palpation. With either technique, note the location, size, consistency, and mobility of any palpable organs and the presence of any abnormal enlargement, tenderness, or masses.

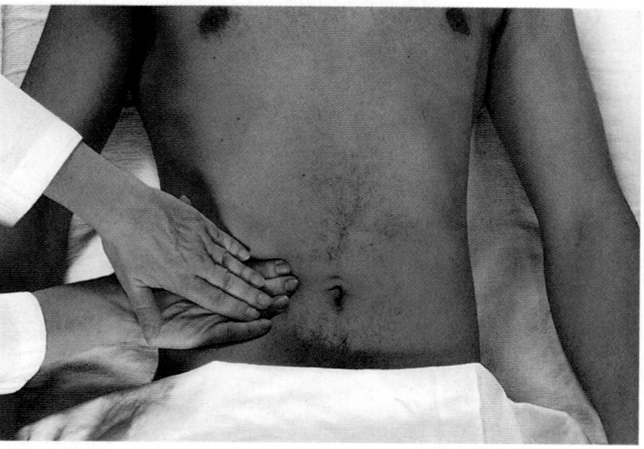

21-23

Abnormal Findings

Involuntary rigidity is a constant, board-like hardness of the muscles. It is a protective mechanism accompanying acute inflammation of the peritoneum. It may be unilateral, and the same area usually becomes painful when the person increases intra-abdominal pressure by attempting a sit-up.

Normal Range of Findings

Making sense of what you are feeling is more difficult than it looks. Inexperienced examiners complain that the abdomen "all feels the same," as if they are pushing their hand into a soft sofa cushion. It helps to memorize the anatomy and visualize what is under each quadrant as you palpate. Also remember that some structures are normally palpable, as illustrated in Fig. 21-24.

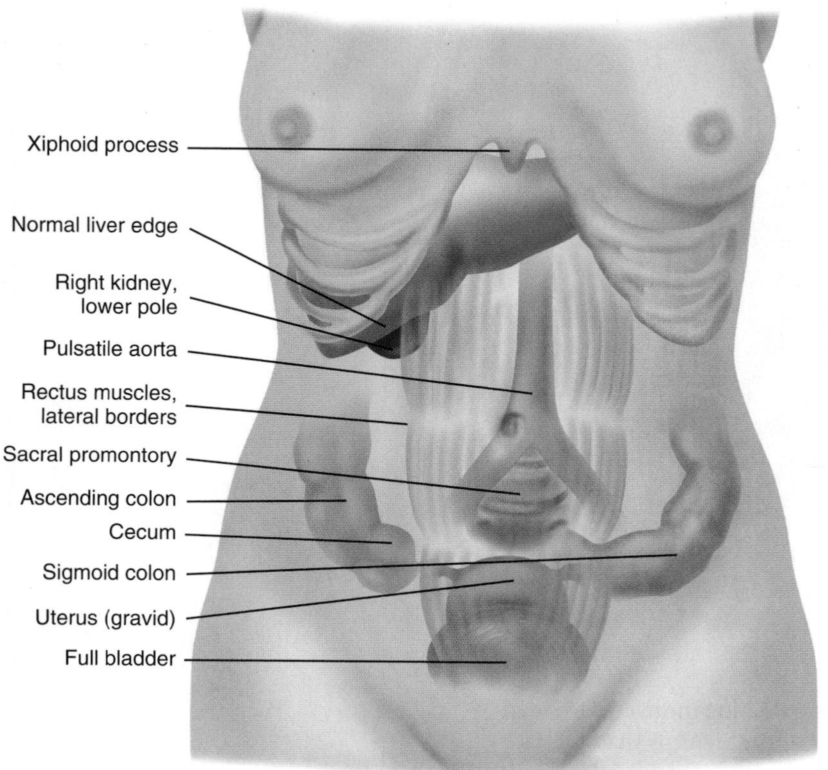

21-24

Mild tenderness normally is present when palpating the sigmoid colon. Any other tenderness should be investigated.

If you identify a mass, first distinguish it from a normally palpable structure or an enlarged organ. Then note the following:

1. Location
2. Size
3. Shape
4. Consistency (soft, firm, hard)
5. Surface (smooth, nodular)
6. Mobility (including movement with respirations)
7. Pulsatility
8. Tenderness

Abnormal Findings

Tenderness occurs with local inflammation, with inflammation of the peritoneum or underlying organ, and with an enlarged organ whose capsule is stretched.

Normal Range of Findings | Abnormal Findings

Liver

Next, palpate for specific organs, beginning with the liver in the RUQ (Fig. 21-25). Place your left hand under the person's back parallel to the eleventh and twelfth ribs and lift up to support the abdominal contents. Place your right hand on the RUQ, with fingers parallel to the midline. Push deeply down and under the right costal margin. Ask the person to breathe slowly. With every exhalation, move your palpating hand up 1 or 2 cm. It is normal to feel the edge of the liver bump your fingertips as the diaphragm pushes it down during inhalation. It feels like a firm, regular ridge. Often, the liver is not palpable and you feel nothing firm.

Except with a depressed diaphragm, a liver palpated more than 1 to 2 cm below the right costal margin is enlarged. Record the number of centimeters it descends and note its consistency (hard, nodular) and tenderness (see Table 21-6, Palpation of Enlarged Organs, on pp. 562-563).

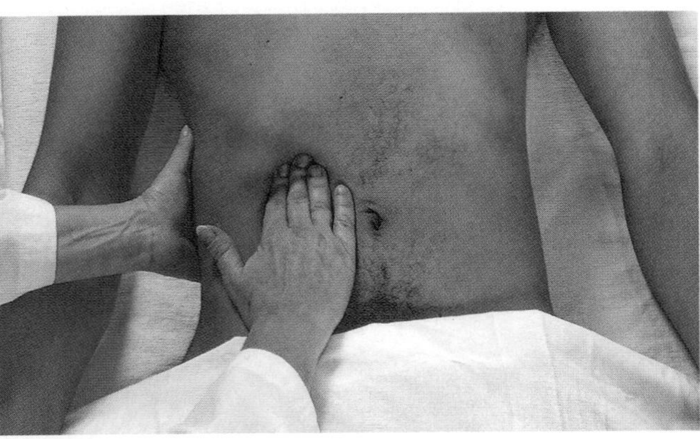

21-25

Hooking Technique. An alternative method of palpating the liver is to stand up at the person's shoulder and swivel your body to the right so that you face the person's feet (Fig. 21-26). Hook your fingers over the costal margin from above. Ask the person to take a deep breath. Try to feel the liver edge bump your fingertips.

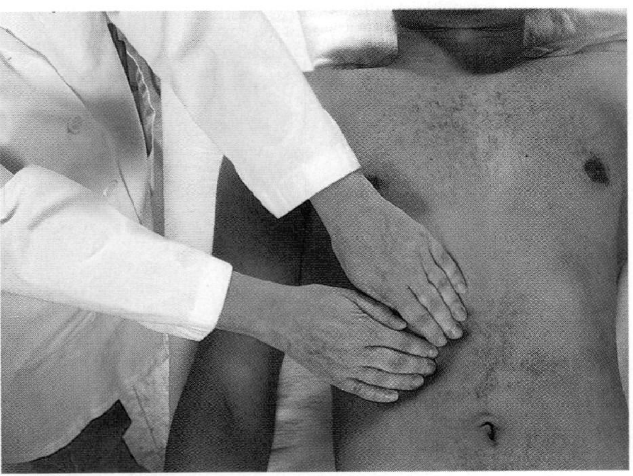

21-26

Normal Range of Findings

Spleen

Normally, the spleen is not palpable and must be enlarged three times its normal size to be felt. To search for it, reach your left hand over the abdomen and behind the left side at the eleventh and twelfth ribs (Fig. 21-27, *A*). Lift up for support. Place your right hand obliquely on the LUQ with the fingers pointing toward the left axilla and just inferior to the rib margin. Push your hand deeply down and under the left costal margin and ask the person to take a deep breath. You should feel nothing firm.

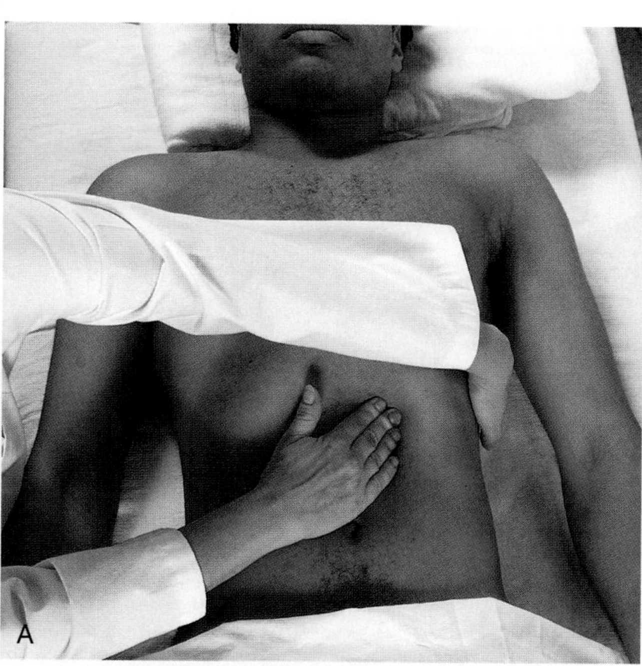

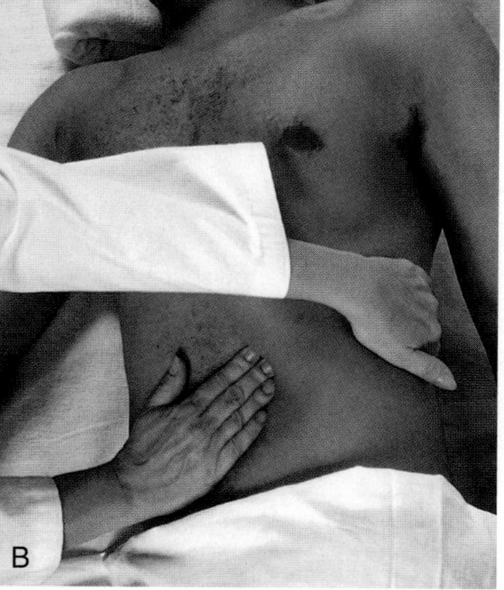

21-27

When enlarged, the spleen slides out and bumps your fingertips. It can grow so large that it extends into the lower quadrants. When this condition is suspected, start low so you will not miss it. An alternative position is to roll the person onto his or her right side to displace the spleen more forward and downward (Fig. 21-27, *B*). Then palpate as described earlier.

Abnormal Findings

The spleen enlarges with mononucleosis, trauma, leukemias, and lymphomas (see Table 21-6). If you feel an enlarged spleen, refer the person but do not continue to palpate it. An enlarged spleen is friable and can rupture easily with overpalpation.

Describe the number of centimeters it extends below the left costal margin.

Normal Range of Findings	Abnormal Findings

Kidneys

Search for the right kidney by placing your hands together in a "duck-bill" position at the person's right flank (Fig. 21-28, *A*). Press your two hands together firmly (you need deeper palpation than that used with the liver or spleen) and ask the person to take a deep breath. In most people, you will feel no change. Occasionally, you may feel the lower pole of the right kidney as a round, smooth mass slide between your fingers. Either condition is normal.

Enlarged kidney.
Kidney mass.

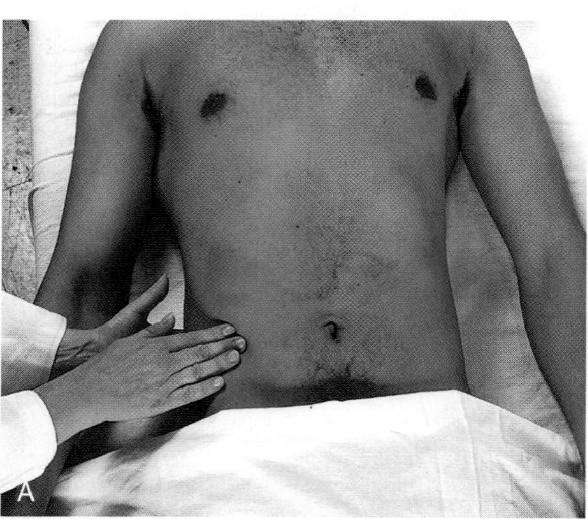
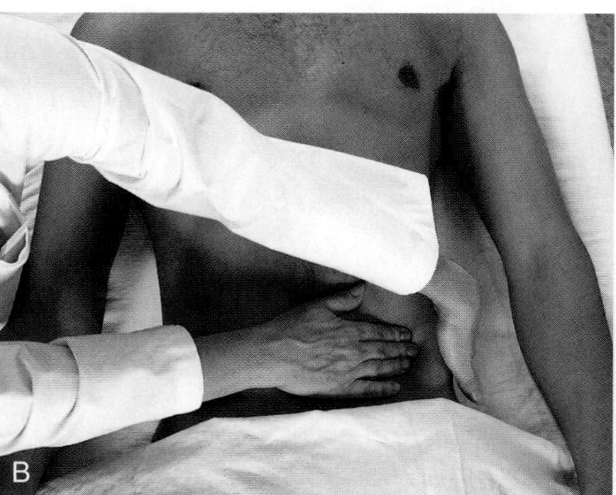
21-28

The left kidney sits 1 cm higher than the right kidney and is not palpable normally. Search for it by reaching your left hand across the abdomen and behind the left flank for support (Fig. 21-28, *B*). Push your right hand deep into the abdomen and ask the person to breathe deeply. You should feel no change with the inhalation.

Aorta

Using your opposing thumb and fingers, palpate the aortic pulsation in the upper abdomen slightly to the left of midline (Fig. 21-29). Normally, it is 2.5 to 4 cm wide in the adult and pulsates in an anterior direction.

Widened with aneurysm (see Tables 21-5 and 21-6).

Prominent lateral pulsation with aortic aneurysm pushes the examiner's two fingers apart.

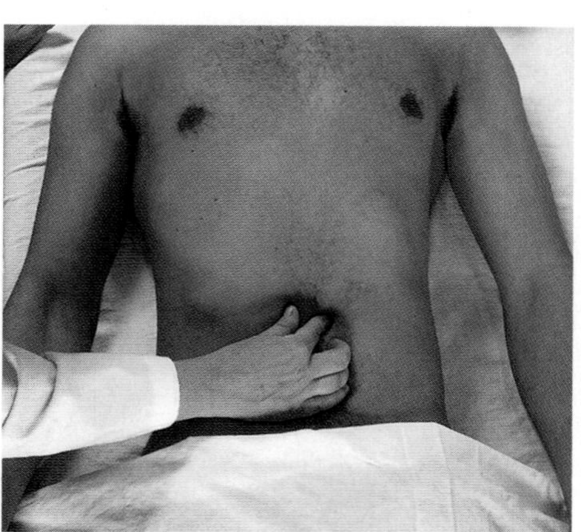
21-29

Normal Range of Findings

Abnormal Findings

Special Procedures for Advanced Practice

Rebound Tenderness (Blumberg Sign). Assess rebound tenderness when the person reports abdominal pain or when you elicit tenderness during palpation. Choose a site away from the painful area. Hold your hand 90 degrees, or perpendicular, to the abdomen. Push down slowly and deeply (Fig. 21-30, *A*); then lift up *quickly* (Fig. 21-30, *B*). This makes structures that are indented by palpation rebound suddenly. A normal, or negative, response is no pain on release of pressure. Perform this test at the end of the examination, because it can cause severe pain and muscle rigidity.

Pain on release of pressure confirms rebound tenderness, which is a reliable sign of peritoneal inflammation. Peritoneal inflammation accompanies appendicitis.

Cough tenderness that is localized to a specific spot also signals peritoneal irritation. Refer the person with suspected appendicitis for computed tomography (CT) scanning.

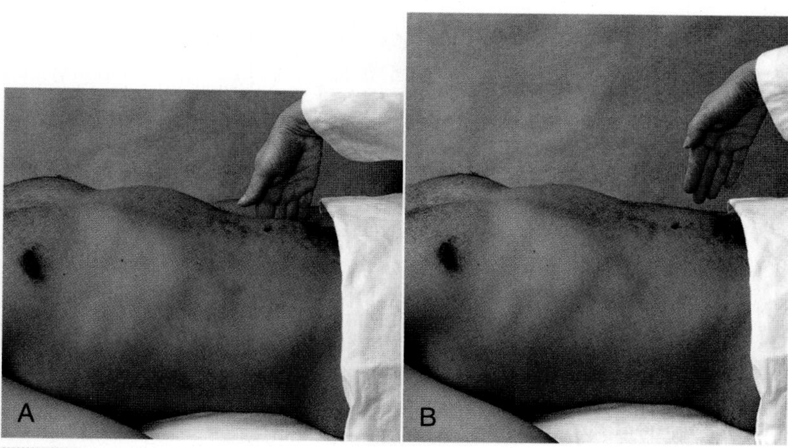

21-30 Rebound tenderness.

Inspiratory Arrest (Murphy Sign). Normally, palpating the liver causes no pain. In a person with inflammation of the gallbladder (cholecystitis), pain occurs. Hold your fingers under the liver border. Ask the person to take a deep breath. A normal response is to complete the deep breath without pain. (Note: This sign is less accurate in patients older than 60 years; evidence shows that 25% of them do not have any abdominal tenderness.[30])

When the test is positive, as the descending liver pushes the inflamed gallbladder onto the examining hand, the person feels sharp pain and abruptly stops inspiration midway.

Iliopsoas Muscle Test. Perform the iliopsoas muscle test when the acute abdominal pain of appendicitis is suspected. With the person supine, lift the right leg straight up, flexing at the hip (Fig. 21-31); then push down over the lower part of the right thigh as the person tries to hold the leg up. When the test is negative, the person feels no change. (Note: Evidence shows that the Obturator Test, another technique that stretches the obturator muscle, does not work to diagnose appendicitis.[30])

When the iliopsoas muscle is inflamed (which occurs with an inflamed or perforated appendix), pain is felt in the right lower quadrant.

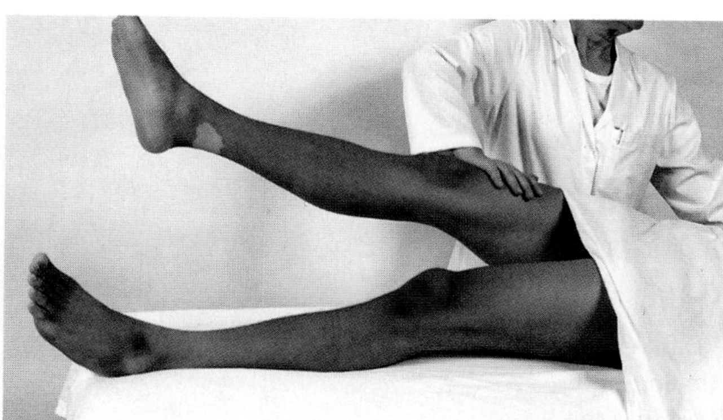

21-31 Iliopsoas muscle test.

Normal Range of Findings	Abnormal Findings

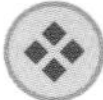

DEVELOPMENTAL COMPETENCE

The Infant

Inspection. The contour of the abdomen is protuberant because of the immature abdominal musculature. The skin contains a fine, superficial venous pattern. This may be visible in lightly pigmented children up to the age of puberty.

Abnormal: Scaphoid shape occurs with dehydration.

Abnormal: Dilated veins.

Inspect the umbilical cord throughout the neonatal period. At birth, it is white and contains two umbilical arteries and one vein surrounded by mucoid connective tissue, called *Wharton's jelly.* The umbilical stump dries within a week, hardens, and falls off by 10 to 14 days. Skin covers the area by 3 to 4 weeks.

Abnormal: The presence of only one artery signals the risk for congenital defects.

Abnormal: Inflammation.

Abnormal: Drainage after cord falls off.

The abdomen should be symmetric, although two bulges are common. You may note an **umbilical hernia.** It appears at 2 to 3 weeks and is especially prominent when the infant cries. The hernia reaches maximum size at 1 month (up to 2.5 cm or 1 inch) and usually disappears by 1 year. Another common variation is **diastasis recti,** a separation of the rectus muscles with a visible bulge along the midline. The condition is more common with Black infants, and it usually disappears by early childhood.

Abnormal: Refer any umbilical hernia larger than 2.5 cm (see Table 21-3); continuing to grow after 1 month; or lasting for more than 2 years in a white child or for more than 7 years in a Black child.

Abnormal: Refer diastasis recti lasting more than 6 years.

The abdomen shows respiratory movement. The only other abdominal movement you should note is occasional peristalsis, which may be visible because of the thin musculature.

Abnormal: Marked peristalsis with pyloric stenosis (see Table 21-4).

Auscultation. Auscultation yields only bowel sounds, the metallic tinkling of peristalsis. No vascular sounds should be heard.

Abnormal: Bruit.

Abnormal: Venous hum.

Percussion. Percussion finds tympany over the stomach (the infant swallows some air with feeding) and dullness over the liver. Percussing the spleen is not done. The abdomen sounds tympanitic, although it is normal to percuss dullness over the bladder. This dullness may extend up to the umbilicus.

Palpation. Aid palpation by flexing the baby's knees with one hand while palpating with the other (Fig. 21-32). Alternatively, you may hold the upper back and flex the neck slightly with one hand. Offer a pacifier to a crying baby.

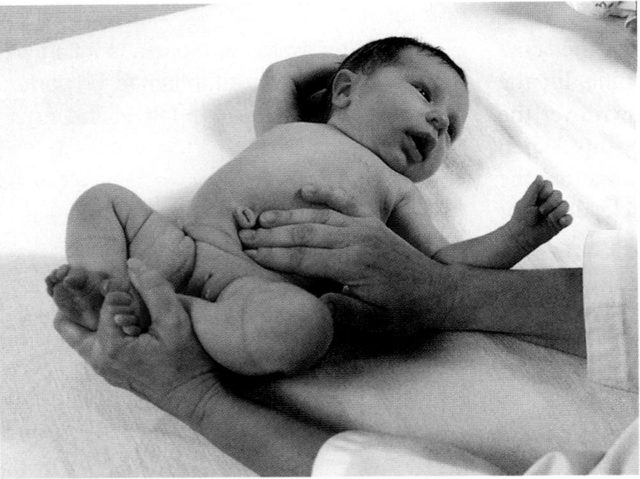

21-32

The liver fills the RUQ. It is normal to feel the liver edge at the right costal margin or 1 to 2 cm below. Normally, you may palpate the spleen tip and both kidneys and the bladder. Also easily palpated are the cecum in the RLQ, and the sigmoid colon, which feels like a sausage in the left inguinal area.

Objective Data

Normal Range of Findings

Make note of the newborn's first stool, a sticky, greenish black meconium stool within 24 hours of birth. By the fourth day, stools of breastfed babies are golden yellow, pasty, and smell like sour milk, whereas those of formula-fed babies are brown-yellow, firmer, and more fecal smelling.

The Child

Younger than 4 years, the abdomen looks protuberant when the child is both supine and standing. After age 4 years, the potbelly remains when standing because of lumbar lordosis but the abdomen looks flat when supine. Normal movement on the abdomen includes respirations, which remain abdominal until 7 years of age.

To palpate the abdomen, position the young child on the parent's lap as you sit knee-to-knee with the parent (Fig. 21-33). Flex the knees up, and elevate the head slightly. The child can "pant like a dog" to further relax abdominal muscles. Hold your entire palm flat on the abdominal surface for a moment before starting palpation. This accustoms the child to being touched. If the child is very ticklish, hold his or her hand under your own as you palpate, or apply the stethoscope and palpate around it.

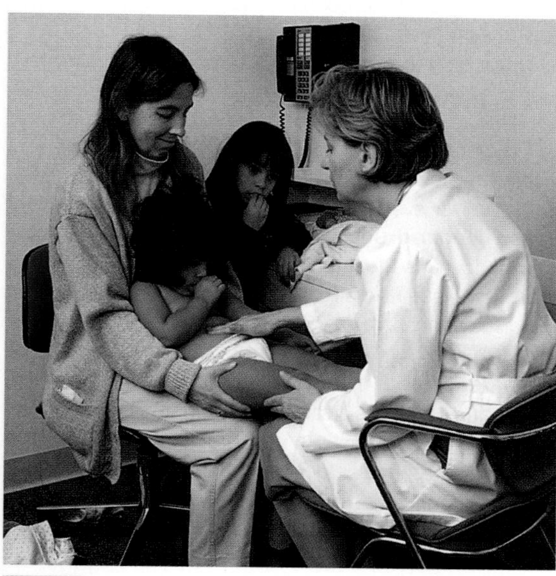

21-33

The liver remains easily palpable 1 to 2 cm below the right costal margin. The edge is soft and sharp and moves easily. On the left, the spleen also is easily palpable with a soft, sharp, movable edge. Usually you can feel 1 to 2 cm of the right kidney and the tip of the left kidney. Percussion of the liver span measures about 3.5 cm at age 2 years, 5 cm at age 6 years, and 6 to 7 cm during adolescence.

In assessing abdominal tenderness, remember that the young child often answers this question affirmatively no matter how the abdomen actually feels. Use objective signs to aid assessment, such as a cry changing in pitch as you palpate, facial grimacing, moving away from you, and guarding.

The school-age child has a slim abdominal shape as he or she loses the potbelly. This slimming trend continues into adolescence. The adolescent easily is embarrassed with exposure of the abdomen, and adequate draping is necessary. The physical findings are the same as those listed for the adult.

Abnormal Findings

A scaphoid abdomen is associated with dehydration or malnutrition.

Younger than 7 years, the absence of abdominal respirations occurs with inflammation of the peritoneum.

Normal Range of Findings	Abnormal Findings
The Aging Adult	
On inspection, you may note increased deposits of subcutaneous fat on the abdomen and hips because it is redistributed away from the extremities. The abdominal musculature is thinner and has less tone than that of the younger adult; thus, in the absence of obesity, you may note peristalsis.	
Because of the thinner, softer abdominal wall, the organs may be easier to palpate (in the absence of obesity). The liver is easier to palpate. Normally, you will feel the liver edge at or just below the costal margin. With distended lungs and a depressed diaphragm, the liver is palpated lower, descending 1 to 2 cm below the costal margin with inhalation. The kidneys are easier to palpate.	Abdominal rigidity with acute abdominal conditions is less common in aging. With an acute abdomen, the aging person often complains of less pain than a younger person would.

PROMOTING A HEALTHY LIFESTYLE

How's Your Liver Doing?

The liver is the largest internal organ in the body. It has an immense capacity to heal and regenerate, but that capacity is not infinite. Signs and symptoms of liver damage and/or disease often are not apparent until the liver has been significantly harmed. The best protection for the liver is prevention!

There are many things an individual can do to protect the liver:

- **Practice safe sex.** Do not have unprotected sex with a male or female.
- **Do not share items that may have bodily fluids on them.** This means needles, razors, nail clippers, cuticle scissors, and toothbrushes. If getting a tattoo, make sure that a new bottle of ink is opened and used for only one individual.
- **Be aware of your environment.** Be careful with aerosol cleaners. Make sure rooms are well ventilated. Wear a mask, hat, or protective clothing when using insecticides, fungicides, paint, or other toxic chemicals. The liver can be damaged by what you breathe or absorb through your skin.
- **Watch your diet and weight.** Obesity can cause a condition called *nonalcoholic fatty liver disease,* which may include cirrhosis.
- **Travel wisely.** Visit a travel medicine clinic before traveling or refer to the CDC *Traveler's Health* website: wwwnc.cdc.gov/travel/default.aspx. The website also informs travelers about health warnings and outbreaks and assists travelers (and their health care providers) in deciding on vaccines, medications, and other measures necessary to prevent illness during international travel. For example, if traveling to an area with an increased rate of hepatitis A, such as South or Central America, Africa, or Asia, get vaccinated, avoid eating any uncooked food and drinking unboiled or unbottled water (that includes ice cubes), and brush your teeth with boiled or bottled water. The CDC website also includes the *Yellow Book*, a valuable reference for those who advise international travelers.
- **Use medications wisely.** Use prescription and over-the-counter medications only when needed. Be sure to take only the recommended doses and strengths. For example, Infant Tylenol, which is a concentrated liquid 3 times stronger than children's strength, should never be substituted for the other.
- **Do not mix medications without consulting a health care provider.** Mixing certain medications can form toxic compounds that can cause liver damage. Be certain that all medications, including over-the-counter and herbal preparations, are reviewed with health care providers.
- **Drink alcohol only in moderation.** Over one drink a day for women or two drinks a day for men over many years may be enough to lead to cirrhosis of the liver. A cirrhotic liver shrinks to a fraction of its former size and ability.
- **Do not mix medications and alcohol.** Acetaminophen can be toxic to the liver even if one drinks in moderation.
- **Do not use illegal drugs.** Cocaine is one of many illegal drugs known to cause liver damage. Further, injection drug users are at increased risk for hepatitis B and hepatitis C infection through the sharing of needles and drug-preparation equipment.
- **Get vaccinated.** Check the CDC website for updated vaccination schedules for travelers, children, and adults. Vaccines are available for both hepatitis A and hepatitis B: www.cdc.gov/vaccines/recs/schedules/default.htm.
- **Be aware of your risk for hepatitis.** The three leading causes of hepatitis are hepatitis A (HAV), hepatitis B (HBV), and hepatitis C (HCV) infection. The *ABCs of Hepatitis* is a 2-page summary chart that identifies persons at risk and reviews routes of transmission, incubation periods, symptoms, screening and vaccination recommendations, and treatment. It is user-friendly and available online at www.aasld.org/patients/Documents/cdchepabc.pdf.

In addition, *Liv and Lucky in Liverland* is a children's workbook (also available as a DVD and VHS in 3-D animation) that features two cartoon characters that teach children (and adults) how important the liver is and how to take care of it. It is available in many different languages and is part of HFI *Foundations for Decision Making*™ training programs developed to inform individuals about life-preserving liver functions and how to modify behaviors and avoid liver-damaging activities.

Resources

Centers for Disease Control and Prevention—Division of Viral Hepatitis. Website: www.cdc.gov/hepatitis/.

Hepatitis Foundation International. Website: www.hepatitisfoundation.org/index.htm.

DOCUMENTATION AND CRITICAL THINKING

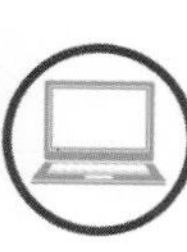

Sample Charting

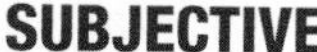

SUBJECTIVE

States appetite is good with no recent change, no dysphagia, no food intolerance, no pain, no nausea/vomiting. Has one formed BM/day. Takes vitamins, no other prescribed or over-the-counter medication. No history of abdominal disease, injury, or surgery. Diet recall of past 24 hours listed at end of history.

OBJECTIVE

Inspection: Abdomen flat, symmetric, with no apparent masses. Skin smooth with no striae, scars, or lesions.
Auscultation: Bowel sounds present, no bruits.
Percussion: Tympany predominates in all four quadrants, liver span is 8 cm in right midclavicular line. Splenic dullness located at tenth intercostal space in left midaxillary line.
Palpation: Abdomen soft, no organomegaly, no masses, no tenderness.

ASSESSMENT

Healthy abdomen, bowel sounds present

Focused Assessment: Clinical Case Study 1

George E. is a 58-year-old unemployed divorced white male with chronic alcoholism who enters the chemical dependency treatment center.

SUBJECTIVE

States past 6 months has been drinking 1 pint whiskey/day. Last alcohol use 1 week PTA, with "5 or 6" drinks that episode. Estranged from family, lives alone. Makes a few meals on hot plate. States never has appetite. Has fatigue and weakness.

OBJECTIVE

Inspection: Appears older than stated age. Oriented, although verbal response time slowed. Weight loss of 12 lb in past 3 mo.
Abdomen protuberant, symmetric, no visible masses. Poor skin turgor. Dilated venous pattern over abdominal wall. Hair sparse in axillary, pubic area.
Auscultation: Bowel sounds present. No vascular sounds.
Percussion: Tympany predominates over abdomen. Liver span is 16 cm in right midclavicular line. No fluid wave. No shifting dullness.
Palpation: Soft. Liver palpable 10 cm below right costal margin, smooth and nontender. No other organomegaly or masses.

ASSESSMENT

Alcohol dependence, severe, with physiologic dependence
Imbalanced nutrition: less than body requirements R/T impaired absorption
Ineffective coping R/T effects of chronic alcoholism
Social isolation

Focused Assessment: Clinical Case Study 2

Edith J. is a 63-year-old retired homemaker with a history of lung cancer with metastasis to the liver.

SUBJECTIVE

Feeling "puffy and bloated" for the past week. States unable to get comfortable. Also short of breath "all the time now." Difficulty sleeping. "I feel like crying all the time now."

OBJECTIVE

Inspection: Weight increase of 8 lb in 1 week. Abdomen is distended with everted umbilicus and bulging flanks. Girth at umbilicus is 85 cm. Prominent dilated venous pattern present over abdomen.

Auscultation: Bowel sounds present, no vascular sounds.

Percussion: When supine, tympany present at dome of abdomen, dullness over flanks. Shifting dullness present. Positive fluid wave present. Liver span is 12 cm in right midclavicular line.

Palpation: Abdominal wall firm, able to feel liver with deep palpation at 6 cm below right costal margin. Liver feels firm, nodular, nontender. 4+ pitting edema in both ankles.

ASSESSMENT

Ascites
Grieving
Ineffective breathing pattern R/T increased intra-abdominal pressure
Pain R/T distended abdomen
Risk for impaired skin integrity R/T ascites, edema, and faulty metabolism
Insomnia

Focused Assessment: Clinical Case Study 3

Dan G. is a 17-year-old Black male high school student who enters the emergency department with abdominal pain for 2 days.

SUBJECTIVE

Two days PTA, Dan noted general abdominal pain in umbilical region. Now pain is sharp and severe, and Dan points to location in right lower quadrant. No BM for 2 days. Nausea and vomiting off and on 1 day.

OBJECTIVE

Inspection: BP 112/70, Temp 38° C, pulse 116, resp 18.

Lying on side with knees drawn up under chin. Resists any movement. Face tight and occasionally grimacing. Cries out with any sudden movement.

Auscultation: No bowel sounds present. No vascular sounds.

Percussion: Tympany. Percussion over RLQ leads to tenderness.

Palpation: Abdominal wall is rigid and boardlike. Extreme tenderness to palpation in RLQ. Rebound tenderness is present in RLQ. Positive iliopsoas muscle test.

ASSESSMENT

Acute abdominal pain in RLQ
Nausea

ABNORMAL FINDINGS

TABLE 21-1 Abdominal Distention

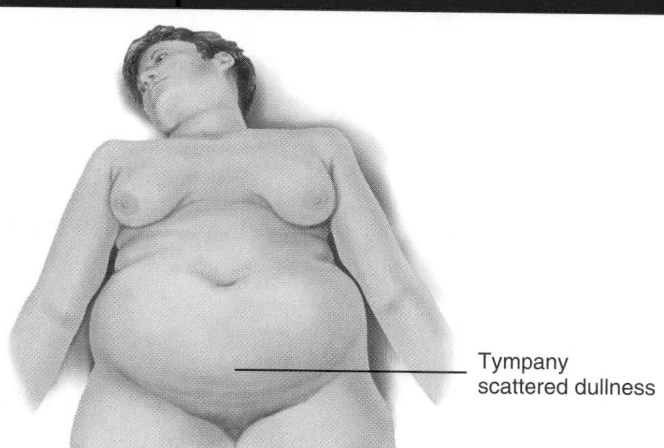

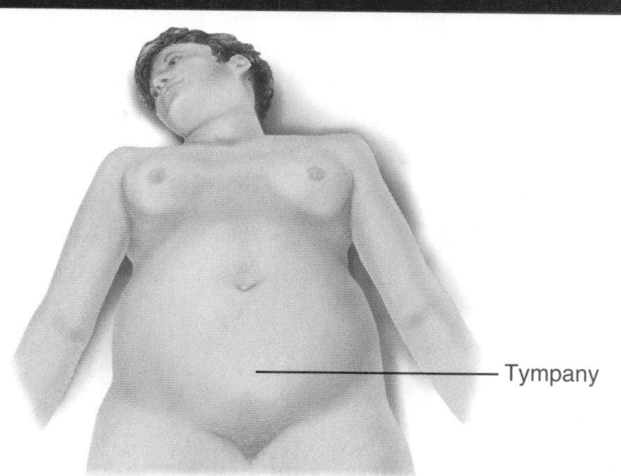

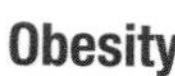

Obesity

Inspection. Uniformly rounded. Umbilicus sunken (it adheres to peritoneum, and layers of fat are superficial to it).
Auscultation. Normal bowel sounds.
Percussion. Tympany. Scattered dullness over adipose tissue.
Palpation. Normal. May be hard to feel through thick abdominal wall.

Air or Gas

Inspection. Single round curve.
Auscultation. Depends on cause of gas, e.g., decreased or absent bowel sounds with ileus; hyperactive with early intestinal obstruction.
Percussion. Tympany over large area.
Palpation. May have muscle spasm of abdominal wall.

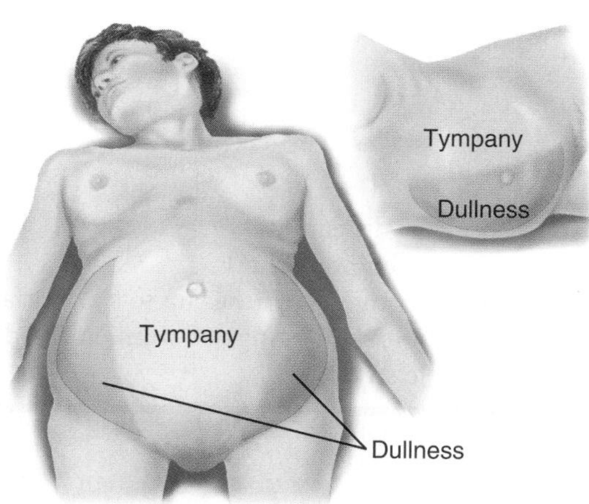

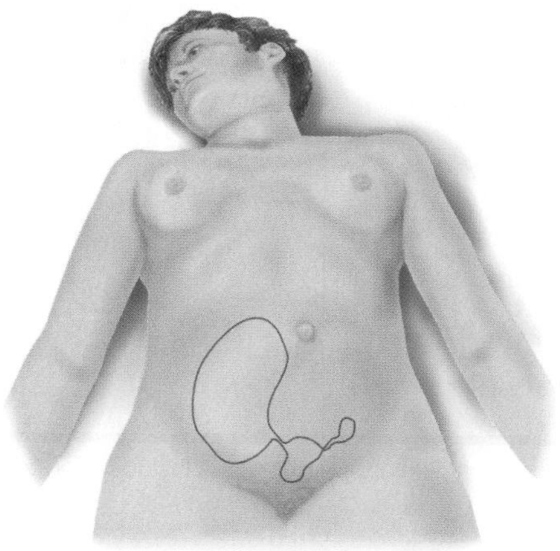

Ascites

Inspection. Single curve. Everted umbilicus. Bulging flanks when supine. Taut, glistening skin; recent weight gain; increase in abdominal girth.
Auscultation. Normal bowel sounds over intestines. Diminished over ascitic fluid.
Percussion. Tympany at top where intestines float. Dull over fluid. Produces fluid wave and shifting dullness.
Palpation. Taut skin and increased intra-abdominal pressure limit palpation.

Ovarian Cyst (Large)

Inspection. Curve in lower half of abdomen, midline. Everted umbilicus.
Auscultation. Normal bowel sounds over upper abdomen where intestines pushed superiorly.
Percussion. Top dull over fluid. Intestines pushed superiorly. Large cyst produces fluid wave and shifting dullness.
Palpation. Transmits aortic pulsation, whereas ascites does not.

Continued

TABLE 21-1 **Abdominal Distention—cont'd**

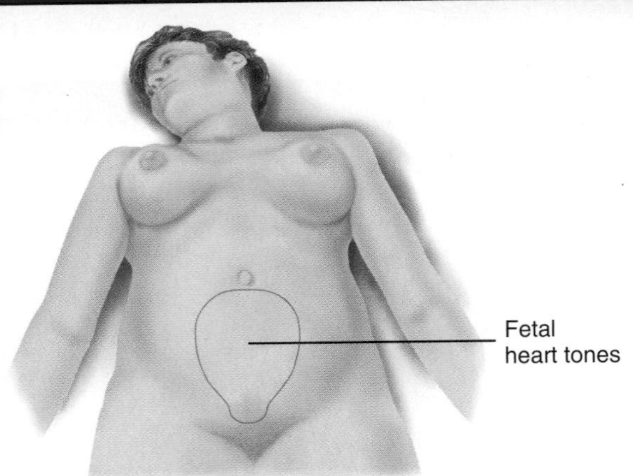

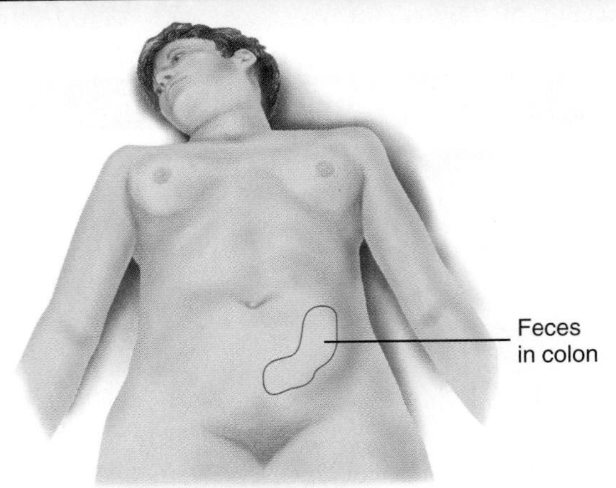

Pregnancy*

Inspection. Single curve. Umbilicus protruding. Breasts engorged.
Auscultation. Fetal heart tones. Bowel sounds diminished.
Percussion. Tympany over intestines. Dull over enlarging uterus.
Palpation. Fetal parts. Fetal movements.

Feces

Inspection. Localized distention.
Auscultation. Normal bowel sounds.
Percussion. Tympany predominates. Scattered dullness over fecal mass.
Palpation. Plastic-like or rope-like mass with feces in intestines.

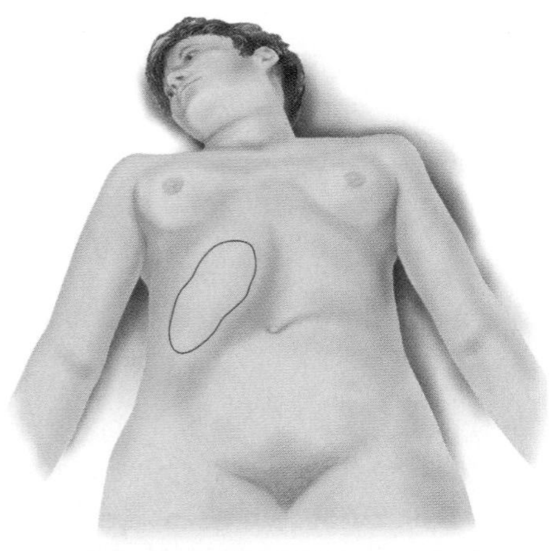

◀ Tumor

Inspection. Localized distention.
Auscultation. Normal bowel sounds.
Percussion. Dull over mass if reaches up to skin surface.
Palpation. Define borders. Distinguish from enlarged organ or normally palpable structure.

*Obviously a normal finding, pregnancy is included for comparison of conditions causing abdominal distention.

ABNORMAL FINDINGS
FOR ADVANCED PRACTICE

TABLE 21-2 Common Sites of Referred Abdominal Pain

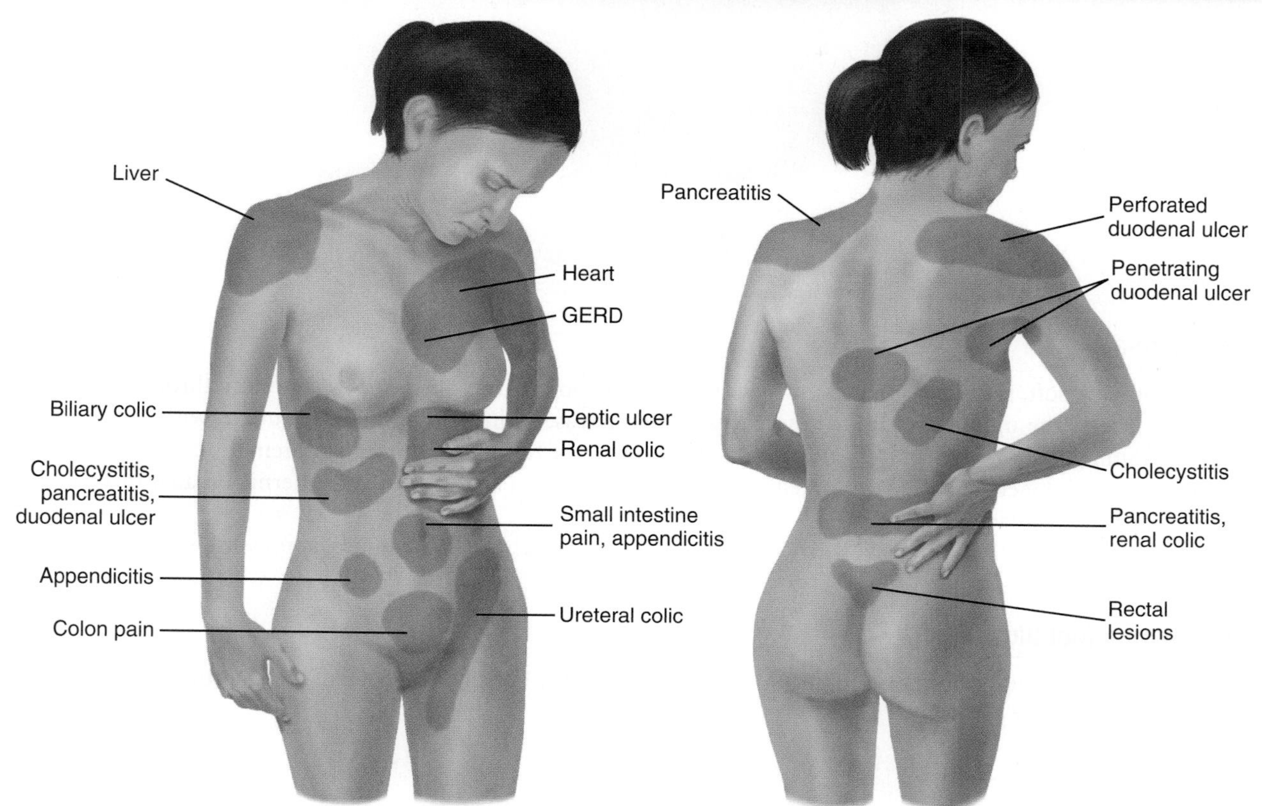

When a person gives a history of abdominal pain, the pain's location may not necessarily be directly over the involved organ. That is because the human brain has no felt image for internal organs. Rather, pain is referred to a site where the organ was located in fetal development. Although the organ migrates during fetal development, its nerves persist in referring sensations from the former location. The following are examples, not a complete list.

Liver. Hepatitis may have mild to moderate, dull pain in right upper quadrant or epigastrium, along with anorexia, nausea, malaise, low-grade fever.
Esophagus. Gastroesophageal reflux disease (GERD) is a complex of symptoms of esophagitis, including burning pain in midepigastrium or behind lower sternum that radiates upward, or "heartburn." Occurs 30 to 60 minutes after eating; aggravated by lying down or bending over.
Gallbladder. Cholecystitis is biliary colic, sudden pain in right upper quadrant that may radiate to right or left scapula, and which builds over time, lasting 2 to 4 hours, after ingestion of fatty foods, alcohol, or caffeine. Associated with nausea and vomiting and with positive Murphy sign or sudden stop in inspiration with RUQ palpation.
Pancreas. Pancreatitis has acute, boring midepigastric pain radiating to the back and sometimes to the left scapula or flank, severe nausea, and vomiting.
Duodenum. Duodenal ulcer typically has dull, aching, gnawing pain, does not radiate, may be relieved by food, and may awaken the person from sleep.
Stomach. Gastric ulcer pain is dull, aching, gnawing epigastric pain, usually brought on by food, radiates to back or substernal area. Pain of perforated ulcer is burning epigastric pain of sudden onset that refers to one or both shoulders.
Appendix. Appendicitis typically starts as dull, diffuse pain in periumbilical region that later shifts to severe, sharp, persistent pain and tenderness localized in RLQ (McBurney point). Pain is aggravated by movement, coughing, deep breathing; associated with anorexia, then nausea and vomiting, fever.
Kidney. Kidney stones prompt a sudden onset of severe, colicky flank or lower abdominal pain.
Small intestine. Gastroenteritis has diffuse, generalized abdominal pain, with nausea, diarrhea.
Colon. Large bowel obstruction has moderate, colicky pain of gradual onset in lower abdomen, bloating. Irritable bowel syndrome (IBS) has sharp or burning, cramping pain over a wide area; does not radiate. Brought on by meals, relieved by bowel movement.

TABLE 21-3 **Abnormalities on Inspection**

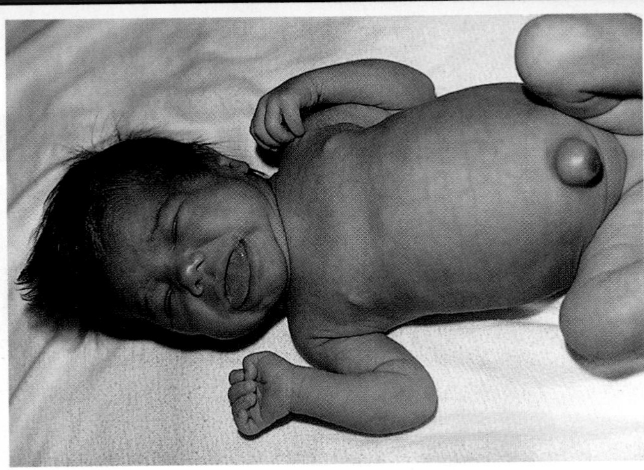

Umbilical Hernia

Umbilical hernia is a soft, skin-covered mass, which is the protrusion of the omentum or intestine through a weakness or incomplete closure in the umbilical ring. It is accentuated by increased intra-abdominal pressure as with crying, coughing, vomiting, or straining, but the bowel rarely incarcerates or strangulates. It is more common in premature infants. Most umbilical hernias resolve spontaneously by 1 year; parents should avoid affixing a belt or coin at the hernia because this will not help closure and may cause contact dermatitis.

In an adult, it occurs with pregnancy, with chronic ascites, or with chronic intrathoracic pressure (e.g., asthma, chronic bronchitis).

Epigastric Hernia (not Illustrated)

A small, fatty nodule at epigastrium in midline, through the linea alba. Usually one can feel it rather than observe it. May be palpable only when standing.

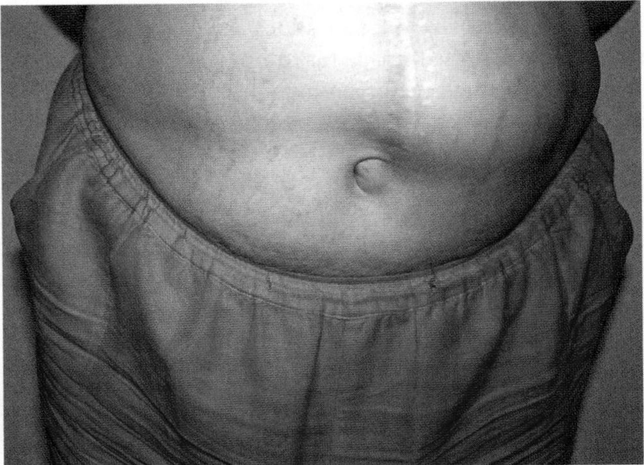

Incisional Hernia

A bulge near an old operative scar that may not show when person is supine but is apparent when the person increases intra-abdominal pressure by a sit-up, by standing, or by the Valsalva maneuver.

Diastasis Recti (not Illustrated)

Diastasis recti, or a midline longitudinal ridge, is a separation of the abdominal rectus muscles. Ridge is revealed when intra-abdominal pressure is increased by raising head while supine. Occurs congenitally and as a result of pregnancy or marked obesity in which prolonged distention or a decrease in muscle tone has occurred. It is not clinically significant.

TABLE 21-4 **Abnormal Bowel Sounds**

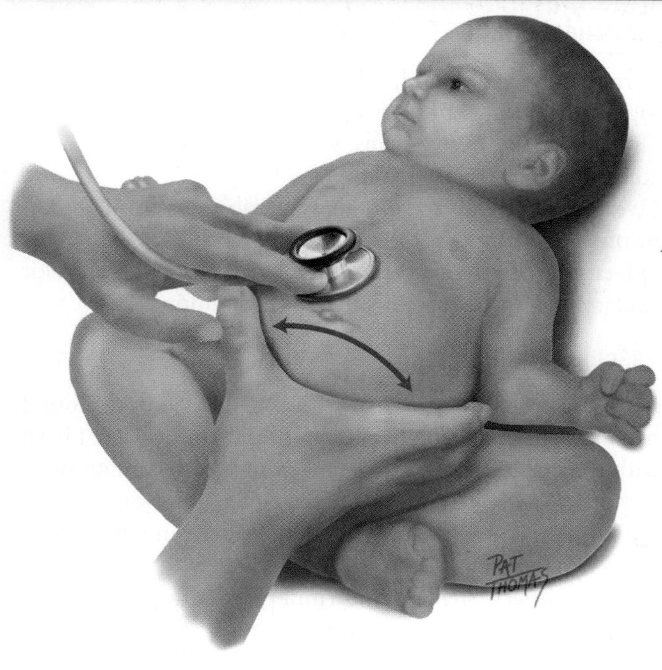

Succussion Splash

Unrelated to peristalsis, this is a very loud splash auscultated over the upper abdomen when the infant is rocked side to side. It indicates increased air and fluid in the stomach, as seen with pyloric obstruction or large hiatus hernia.

Marked peristalsis together with projectile vomiting in the newborn suggests pyloric stenosis, an obstruction of the stomach's pyloric valve. Pyloric stenosis is a congenital defect and appears in the second or third week. After feeding, pronounced peristaltic waves cross from left to right, leading to projectile vomiting. Then one can palpate an olive-sized mass in the RUQ midway between the right costal margin and umbilicus. Refer promptly because of the risk for weight loss.

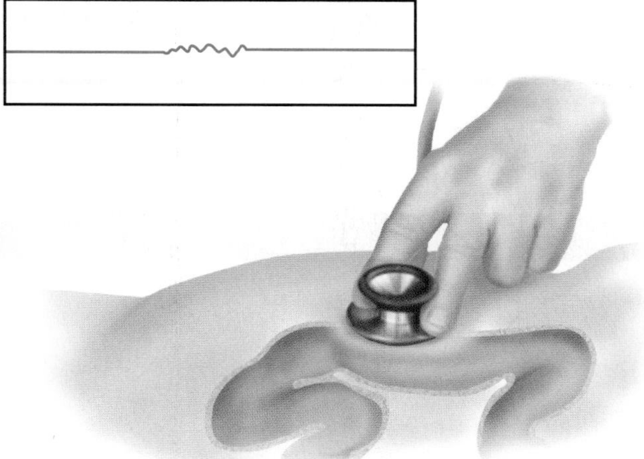

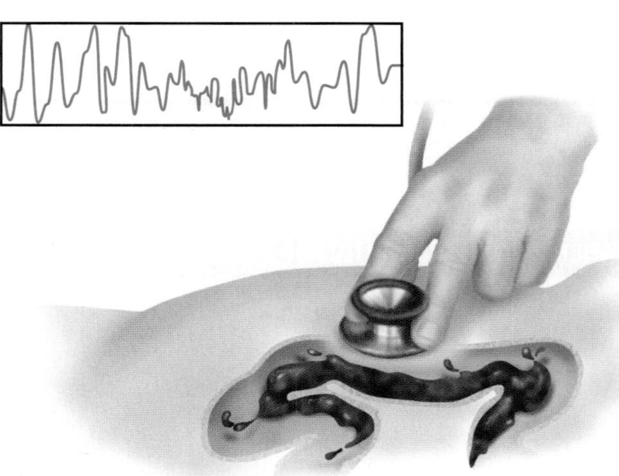

Hypoactive Bowel Sounds

Diminished or absent bowel sounds signal decreased motility as a result of inflammation as seen with peritonitis; from paralytic ileus as following abdominal surgery; or from late bowel obstruction. Occurs also with pneumonia.

Hyperactive Bowel Sounds

Loud, gurgling sounds, "borborygmi," signal increased motility. They occur with early mechanical bowel obstruction (high-pitched), gastroenteritis, brisk diarrhea, laxative use, and subsiding paralytic ileus.

TABLE 21-5 Friction Rubs and Vascular Sounds

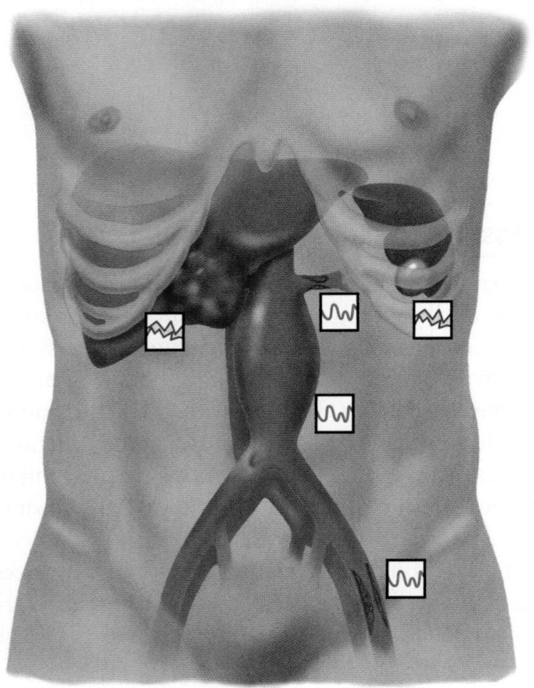

Peritoneal Friction Rub

A rough, grating sound, like two pieces of leather rubbed together, indicates peritoneal inflammation. Occurs rarely. Usually occurs over organs with a large surface area in contact with the peritoneum.

Liver—friction rub over lower right rib cage, from abscess or metastatic tumor.

Spleen—friction rub over lower left rib cage in left anterior axillary line, from abscess, infection, or tumor.

Vascular Sounds

Arterial—a **bruit** indicates turbulent blood flow, as found in constricted, abnormally dilated, or tortuous vessels. Listen with the bell. Occurs with the following three conditions:

Aortic aneurysm—murmur is harsh, systolic, or continuous and accentuated with systole. Note in person with hypertension.

Renal artery stenosis—murmur is midline or toward flank, soft, low to medium pitch.

Partial occlusion of femoral arteries.

Venous hum—occurs rarely. Heard in periumbilical region. Originates from inferior vena cava. Medium pitch, continuous sound, pressure on bell may obliterate it. May have palpable thrill. Occurs with portal hypertension and cirrhotic liver.

TABLE 21-6 Palpation of Enlarged Organs

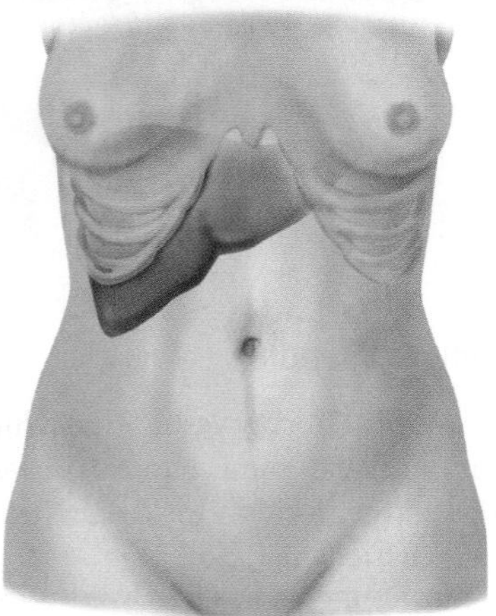

Enlarged Liver

An enlarged, smooth, and nontender liver occurs with fatty infiltration, portal obstruction or cirrhosis, high obstruction of inferior vena cava, and lymphocytic leukemia.

The liver feels enlarged and smooth but is tender to palpation with early heart failure, acute hepatitis, or hepatic abscess.

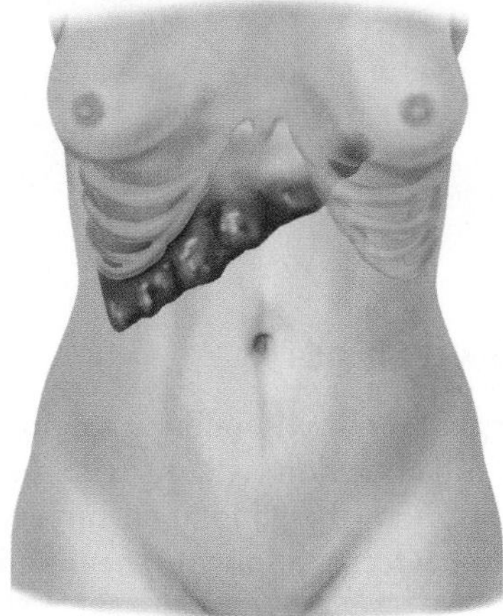

Enlarged Nodular Liver

An enlarged and nodular liver occurs with late portal cirrhosis, metastatic cancer, or tertiary syphilis.

TABLE 21-6 **Palpation of Enlarged Organs—cont'd**

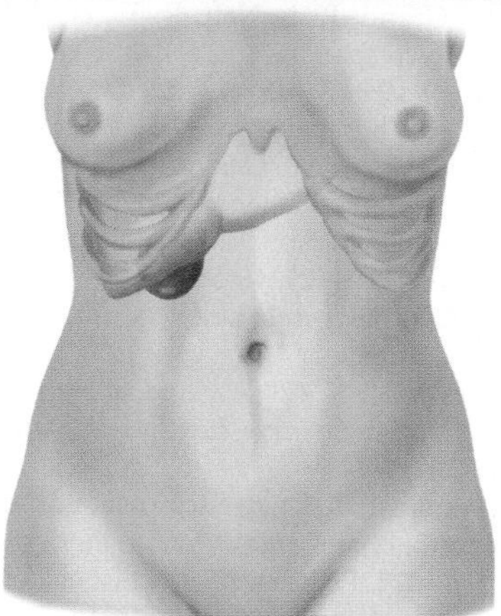

Enlarged Gallbladder

An enlarged, tender gallbladder suggests acute cholecystitis. Feel it behind the liver border as a smooth and firm mass like a sausage, although it may be difficult to palpate because of involuntary rigidity of abdominal muscles. The area is exquisitely painful to fist percussion, and inspiratory arrest (Murphy sign) is present.

An enlarged, nontender gallbladder also feels like a smooth, sausagelike mass. It occurs when the gallbladder is filled with stones, as with common bile duct obstruction.

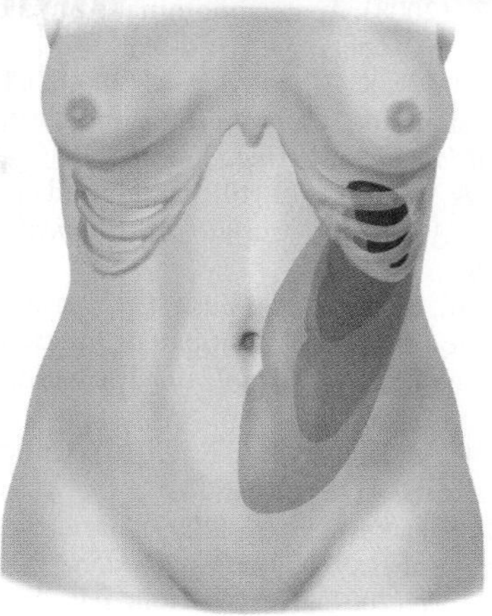

Enlarged Spleen

Because any enlargement superiorly is stopped by the diaphragm, the spleen enlarges down and to the midline. When extreme, it can extend down to the left pelvis. It retains the splenic notch on the medial edge. When splenomegaly occurs with acute infections (mononucleosis), it is moderately enlarged and soft, with rounded edges. When the result of a chronic cause, the enlargement is firm or hard, with sharp edges. An enlarged spleen is usually not tender to palpation; it is tender only if the peritoneum is also inflamed.

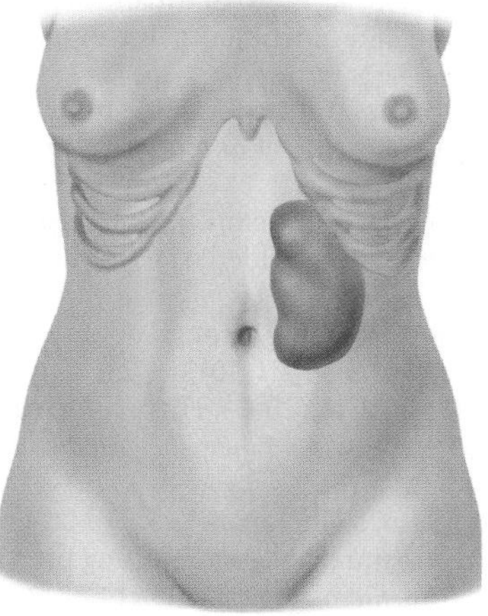

Enlarged Kidney

Enlarged with hydronephrosis, cyst, or neoplasm. May be difficult to distinguish an enlarged kidney from an enlarged spleen because they have a similar shape. Both extend forward and down. However, the spleen may have a sharp edge, whereas the kidney never does. The spleen retains the splenic notch, whereas the kidney has no palpable notch. Percussion over the spleen is dull, whereas over the kidney it is tympanitic because of the overriding bowel.

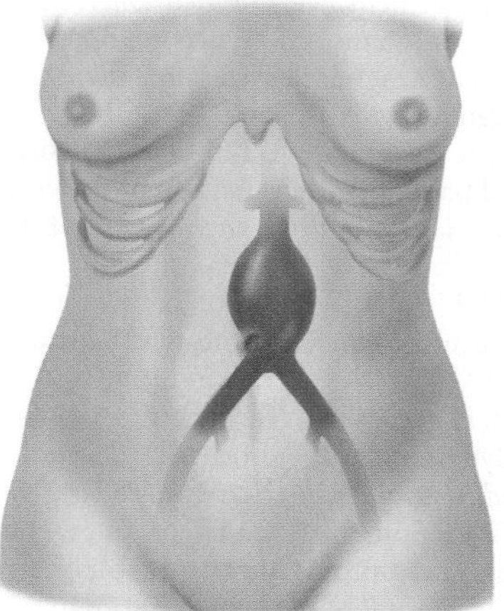

Aortic Aneurysm

Most aortic aneurysms (>95%) are located below the renal arteries and extend to the umbilicus. A focal bulging >5 cm is palpable in about 80% of cases during routine physical examination and feels like a pulsating mass in the upper abdomen just to the left of midline. You will hear a bruit. Femoral pulses are present but decreased.

Additional information on abdominal aneurysm is illustrated in Table 21-5.

BIBLIOGRAPHY

1. Ambinder, M. (2010, May). Beating obesity. *The Atlantic*, 72-83.
2. Amerine, E. (2007). Get optimum outcomes for acute pancreatitis patients. *Nurse Practitioner*, *32*(6), 2007.
3. Anwar, A. (2008). Benzodiazepines: uses, mode of action and prescribing issues. *Nurse Prescribing*, *6*(12), 544-548.
4. Apovian, C. M. (2010). The causes, prevalence, and treatment of obesity revisited in 2009: what have we learned so

far? *American Journal of Clinical Nutrition, 91*(1), 77S-279S.
5. Bartley, M. K. (2008). Acute abdominal pain: a diagnostic challenge. *Nurse Practitioner, 33*(3), 34-39.
6. Becker, A. E., Eddy, K. T., & Perloe, A. (2009). Clarifying criteria for cognitive signs and symptoms for eating disorders in DSM-V. *International Journal of Eating Disorders, 42*(7), 611-619.
7. Biro, F. M., & Wien, M. (2010). Childhood obesity and adult morbidities. *American Journal of Clinical Nutrition, 91*, 1499S-1505S.
8. Bollinger, R. R., Barbas, A. S., Bush, E. L., et al. (2007). Biofilms in the large bowel suggest an apparent function of the human vermiform appendix. *Journal of Theoretical Biology, 249*, 826-831.
9. Brenner, Z. R., & Krenzer, M. E. (2010). Understanding acute pancreatitis. *Nursing, 40*(1), 32-38.
10. Budd, G. M., & Falkenstein, K. (2009). Bariatric surgery: putting the squeeze on obesity. *Nurse Practitioner, 34*(7), 39-46.
11. Fitzgerald, M. A. (2007). Nonalcoholic fatty liver disease. *Nurse Practitioner, 32*(2), 24-25.
12. Frith, J., Jones, D., & Newton, J. L. (2009). Chronic liver disease in an ageing population. *Age and Ageing, 38*(1), 11-18.
13. Gujral, H., & Collantes, R. S. (2009). Understanding viral hepatitis: a guide for primary care. *Nurse Practitioner, 34*(12), 23-32.
14. Halpert, A. D. (2010). Importance of early diagnosis in patients with irritable bowel syndrome. *Postgraduate Medicine, 122*(2), 102-111.
15. Harmon, H. W. (2007). Treatment options for irritable bowel syndrome. *Nurse Practitioner, 32*(7), 39-43.
16. Heber, D. (2010). An integrative view of obesity. *American Journal of Clinical Nutrition, 91*(1), 280S-283S.
17. Heitkemper, M., & Wolff, J. (2007). Challenges in chronic constipation management. *Nurse Practitioner, 32*(4), 36-43.
18. Higgins, P. D., & Johanson, J. F. (2004). Epidemiology of constipation in North America: a systematic review. *American Journal of Gastroenterology, 99*(4), 750-759.
19. Hodjati, H., & Kazerooni, T. (2003). Location of the appendix in the gravid patient: a re-evaluation of the established concept. *International Journal of Gynaecology and Obstetrics, 81*(3), 245-247.
20. Holloway, T. J. (2010). The root of the problem: an irritable bowel or an average American lifestyle? *Gastrointestinal Nursing, 8*(1), 31-37.
21. Howland, R. H. (2009). Effects of aging on pharmacokinetic and pharmacodynamic drug processes. *Journal of Psychosocial Nursing and Mental Health Services, 47*(10), 15-18.
22. Jacobson, B. C., Somers, S. C., Fuchs, C. S., et al. (2006). Body-mass index and symptoms of gastroesophageal reflux in women. *New England Journal of Medicine, 354*, 2340-2348, 2405-2408.
23. Kelso, L. A. (2008). Cirrhosis: caring for patients with end-stage liver failure. *Nurse Practitioner, 33*(7), 24-31.
24. King, J. (2009). Infectious mononucleosis: update and considerations. *Nurse Practitioner, 34*(11), 42-45.
25. Klein, J. D., & Dietz, W. (2010). Childhood obesity: the new tobacco. *Health Affairs, 29*(3), 388-392.
26. Kortgen, A., Recknagel, P., & Bauer, M. (2010). How to assess liver function? *Current Opinion in Critical Care, 16*(2), 126-141.
27. Lawson, E. E., Grand, R. J., Neff, R. K., et al. (1978). Clinical estimation of liver span in infants and children, *Archives of Pediatrics & Adolescent Medicine, 132*, 474-476.
28. Longsterth, G. F., Thompson, W. G., Chey, W. D., et al. (2006). Functional bowel disorders. *Gastroenterology, 130*, 1480-1491.
29. Madsen, D., Sebolt, T., Cullen, L., et al. (2005). Listening to bowel sounds: an evidence-based practice project. *American Journal of Nursing, 105*(12), 40-50.
30. McGee, S. (2007). *Evidence based physical diagnosis* (2nd ed.). Philadelphia: Saunders.
31. Meier, P., & Seitz, H. K. (2008). Age, alcohol metabolism and liver disease. *Current Opinion in Clinical Nutrition and Metabolic Care, 11*(1), 21-26.
32. Miller, S., & Alpert, P. (2006). Assessment and differential diagnosis of abdominal pain. *Nurse Practitioner, 31*, 39-47.
33. Mourad, J., Elliott, J. P., Erickson, L., Lisboa, L. (2000). Appendicitis in pregnancy: new information that contradicts long-held clinical beliefs. *American Journal of Obstetrics and Gynecology, 182*(5), 1027-1029.
34. Murphy, M. A., Colwell, C., Pineda, G., et al. (2010). Abdominal pain: a review of select conditions. *EMS Magazine, 39*(1), 68-74.
35. Nguyen, D. M., & El-Serag, H. B. (2010). The epidemiology of obesity. *Gastroenterology Clinics of North America, 39*(1), 1-7.
36. Nicklas, T. A., Qu H., Hughes, S. O., et al. (2009). Prevalence of self-reported lactose intolerance in a multiethnic sample of adults. *Nutrition Today, 44*(5), 222-229.
37. Ogden, C. L., Carroll, M. D., Curtin, L. R., et al. (2006). Prevalence of overweight and obesity in the United States, 1999-2004. *Journal of the American Medical Association, 295*(13), 1549-1555.
38. Reid, L. D., Johnson, R. E., & Gettman, D. A. (1998). Benzodiazepine exposure and functional status in older people. *Journal of the American Geriatrics Society, 46*, 71-76.
39. Riley, L., & Rubin, M. (2010). A guide to physical examination and history taking of the abdomen. *Gastroenterology Nursing, 33*(2), 167.
40. Schiodt, F. V., Chung, R. T., Schilsky, M. L., et al. (2009). Outcome of acute liver failure in the elderly. *Liver Transplantation, 15*(11), 1481-1487.
41. Sheipe, M. (2006). Breaking through obesity with gastric bypass surgery. *Nurse Practioner, 31*(10), 13-23.
42. Tekwani, K., & Sikka, R. (2009). High-risk chief complaints. III: abdomen and extremities. *Emergency Medicine Clinics of North America, 27*(4), 747-765.
43. Tucker, W. N., Saab, S., Rickman, L. S., & Mathews, W. C. (1997). The scratch test is unreliable for detecting the liver edge. *Journal of Clinical Gastroenterology, 25*, 410-414.
44. Wang, Y., & Beydoun, M. A. (2007). The obesity epidemic in the United States—gender, age, socioeconomic, racial/ethnic, and geographic characteristics: a systematic review and meta-regression analysis. *Epidemiologic Reviews, 29*, 6-28.
45. Zimmerman, P. G. (2008). Is it appendicitis? *American Journal of Nursing, 108*(9), 27-32.

Summary Checklist: Abdomen Examination

 For a PDA-downloadable version, go to http://evolve.elsevier.com/Jarvis/.

1. **Inspection**
   Contour
   Symmetry
   Umbilicus
   Skin
   Pulsation or movement
   Hair distribution
   Demeanor
2. **Auscultation**
   Bowel sounds
   Note any vascular sounds
3. **Percussion**
   Percuss all four quadrants
   Percuss borders of liver, spleen
4. **Palpation**
   Light palpation in all four quadrants
   Deeper palpation in all four quadrants
   Palpate for liver, spleen, kidneys

22

Musculoskeletal System

evolve WEBSITE

http://evolve.elsevier.com/Jarvis/

- Animations
- Audio Key Points
- Bedside Assessment Summary Checklist
- Case Study
  Joint Pain
  Numbness in Hands
- Health Promotion Guide
  Osteoporosis
- NCLEX Review Questions
- Physical Examination Summary Checklist
- Quick Assessment for Common Conditions
  Degenerative Joint Disease (Osteoarthritis)
  Fracture
  Osteoporosis
- Video—Assessment
  Lower Extremities
  Musculoskeletal and Neurologic Systems

OUTLINE

Structure and Function, 565

Components of the Musculoskeletal System

Subjective Data, 574

Health History Questions

Objective Data, 577

Preparation
Order of the Examination
Temporomandibular Joint
Cervical Spine
Upper Extremity
Lower Extremity
Spine

Documentation and Critical Thinking, 607

Abnormal Findings for Advanced Practice, 608

STRUCTURE AND FUNCTION

The musculoskeletal system consists of the body's **bones, joints,** and **muscles.** Humans need this system (1) for *support* to stand erect and (2) for *movement.* The musculoskeletal system also functions (3) to encase and *protect* the inner vital organs (e.g., brain, spinal cord, heart), (4) to *produce* the red blood cells in the bone marrow (hematopoiesis), and (5) as a *reservoir* for *storage* of essential minerals, such as calcium and phosphorus in the bones.

COMPONENTS OF THE MUSCULOSKELETAL SYSTEM

The skeleton is the bony framework of the body. It has 206 bones, which support the body like the posts and beams of a building. **Bone** and cartilage are specialized forms of connective tissue. Bone is hard, rigid, and very dense. Its cells are continually turning over and remodeling. The **joint** (or articulation) is the place of union of two or more bones. Joints are the functional units of the musculoskeletal system because they permit the mobility needed for activities of daily living.

Nonsynovial or Synovial Joints

In **nonsynovial** joints, the bones are united by fibrous tissue or cartilage and are immovable (e.g., the sutures in the skull) or only slightly movable (e.g., the vertebrae). **Synovial** joints are freely movable because they have bones that are separated from each other and are enclosed in a joint cavity (Fig. 22-1).

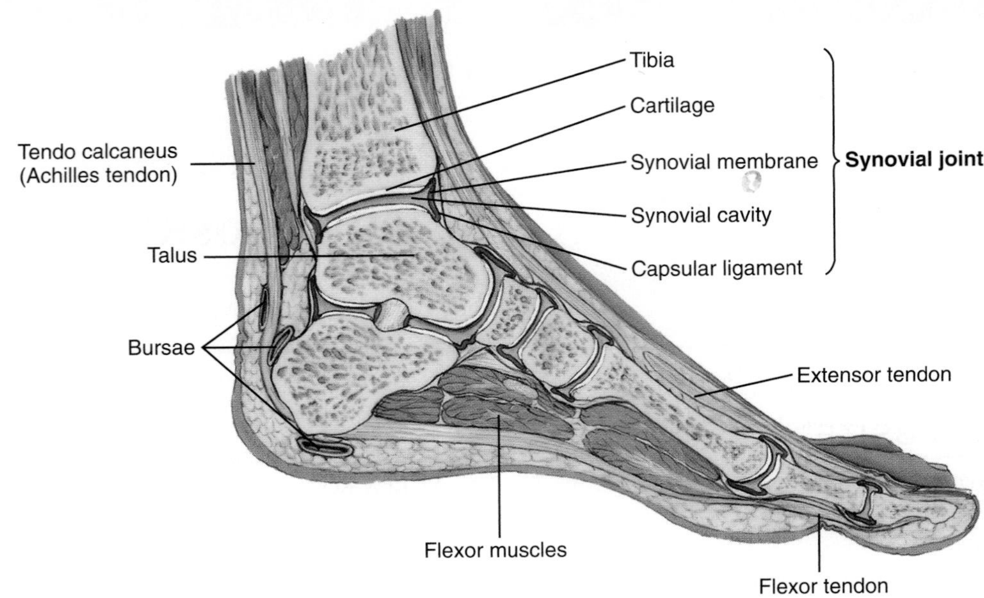

22-1 Synovial joints.

This cavity is filled with a lubricant, or synovial fluid. Just like grease on gears, synovial fluid allows sliding of opposing surfaces, and this sliding permits movement.

In synovial joints, a layer of resilient **cartilage** covers the surface of opposing bones. Cartilage is avascular; it receives nourishment from synovial fluid that circulates during joint movement. It is a very stable connective tissue with a slow cell turnover. It has a tough, firm consistency, yet is flexible. This cartilage cushions the bones and gives a smooth surface to facilitate movement.

The joint is surrounded by a fibrous capsule and is supported by ligaments. **Ligaments** are fibrous bands running directly from one bone to another that strengthen the joint and help prevent movement in undesirable directions. A **bursa** is an enclosed sac filled with viscous synovial fluid, much like a joint. Bursae are located in areas of potential friction (e.g., subacromial bursa of the shoulder, prepatellar bursa of the knee) and help muscles and tendons glide smoothly over bone.

Muscles

Muscles account for 40% to 50% of the body's weight. When they contract, they produce movement. Muscles are of three types: skeletal, smooth, and cardiac. This chapter is concerned with **skeletal,** or voluntary, muscles—those under conscious control.

Each **skeletal muscle** is composed of bundles of muscle fibers, or **fasciculi.** The skeletal muscle is attached to bone by a **tendon**—a strong fibrous cord. Skeletal muscles produce the following movements (Fig. 22-2):

1. Flexion—bending a limb at a joint
2. Extension—straightening a limb at a joint
3. Abduction—moving a limb away from the midline of the body
4. Adduction—moving a limb toward the midline of the body
5. Pronation—turning the forearm so that the palm is down
6. Supination—turning the forearm so that the palm is up
7. Circumduction—moving the arm in a circle around the shoulder
8. Inversion—moving the sole of the foot inward at the ankle
9. Eversion—moving the sole of the foot outward at the ankle
10. Rotation—moving the head around a central axis
11. Protraction—moving a body part forward and parallel to the ground
12. Retraction—moving a body part backward and parallel to the ground
13. Elevation—raising a body part
14. Depression—lowering a body part

Temporomandibular Joint

The temporomandibular joint (TMJ) is the articulation of the mandible and the temporal bone (Fig. 22-3). You can feel it in the depression anterior to the tragus of the ear. The TMJ permits jaw function for speaking and chewing. The joint allows three motions: (1) hinge action to open and close the jaws; (2) gliding action for protrusion and retraction; and (3) gliding for side-to-side movement of the lower jaw.

Flexion
Extension
Abduction
Adduction
Pronation
Supination
Circumduction
Rotation
Eversion
Inversion
Elevation
Depression
Protraction
Retraction

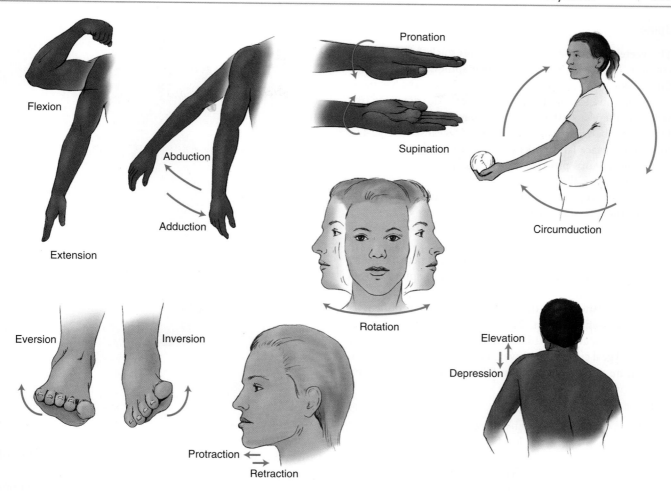

SKELETAL MUSCLE MOVEMENTS

22-2

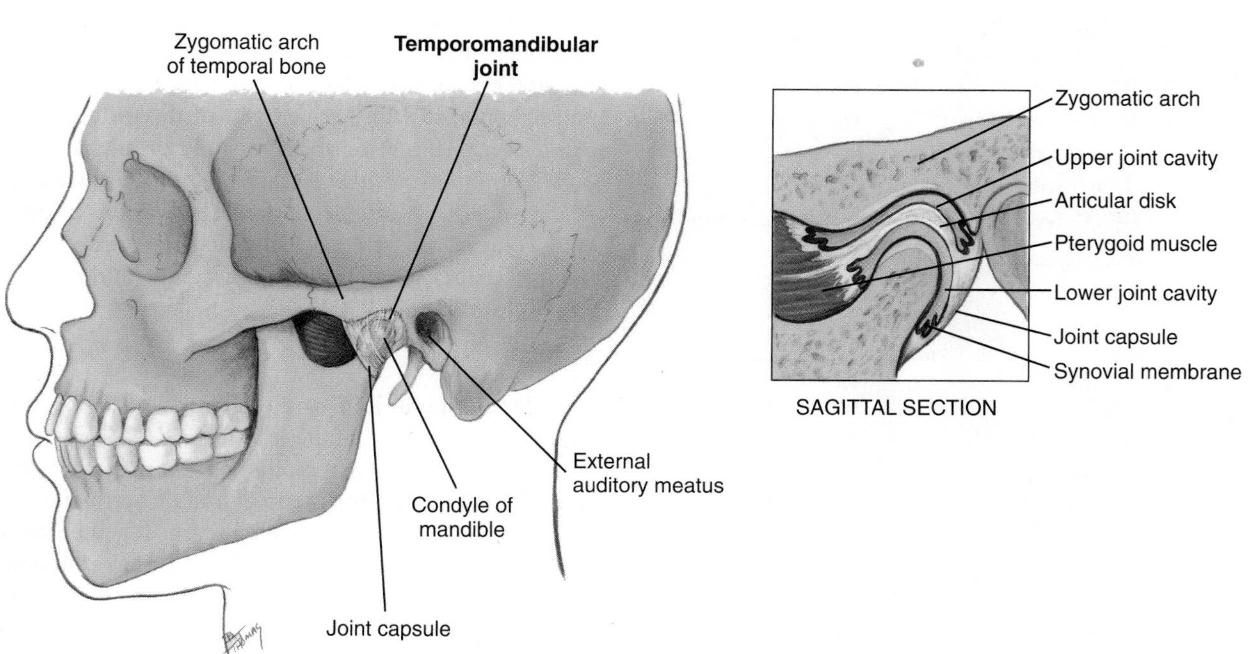

22-3

Spine

The **vertebrae** are 33 connecting bones stacked in a vertical column (Fig. 22-4). You can feel their spinous processes in a furrow down the midline of the back. The furrow has paravertebral muscles mounded on either side down to the sacrum, where it flattens. Humans have 7 cervical, 12 thoracic, 5 lumbar, 5 sacral, and 3 or 4 coccygeal vertebrae. The following surface landmarks will orient you to their levels:

- The spinous processes of C7 and T1 are prominent at the base of the neck.
- The inferior angle of the scapula normally is at the level of the interspace between T7 and T8.
- An imaginary line connecting the highest point on each iliac crest crosses L4.
- An imaginary line joining the two symmetric dimples that overlie the posterior superior iliac spines crosses the sacrum.

A lateral view shows that the vertebral column has four curves (a double-S–shape) (Fig. 22-5). The cervical and lumbar curves are concave (inward or anterior), and the thoracic and sacrococcygeal curves are convex. The balanced or compensatory nature of these curves, together with the resilient intervertebral disks, allows the spine to absorb a great deal of shock.

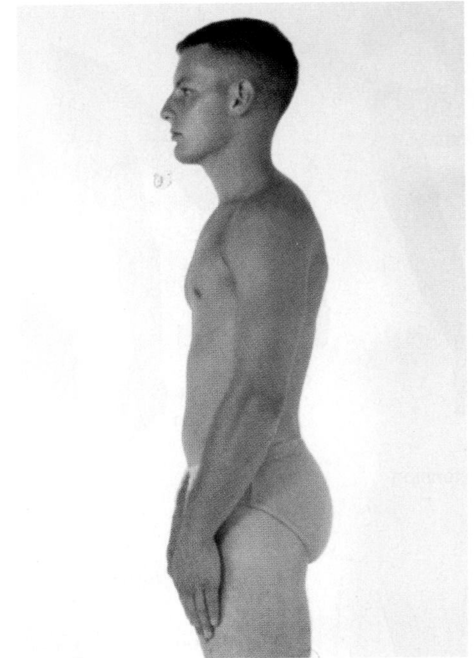

22-5

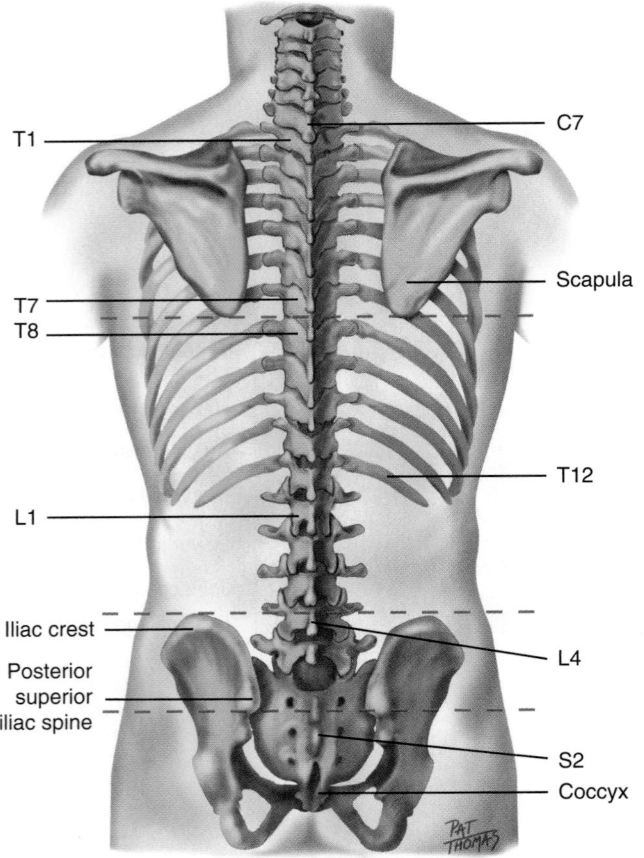

LANDMARKS OF THE SPINE

22-4

The **intervertebral disks** are elastic fibrocartilaginous plates that constitute one fourth of the length of the column (Fig. 22-6). Each disk center has a **nucleus pulposus** made of soft, semifluid, mucoid material that has the consistency of toothpaste in the young adult. The disks cushion the spine like a shock absorber and help it move. As the spine moves, the elasticity of the disks allows compression on one side, with compensatory expansion on the other. Sometimes compression can be too great. The disk then can rupture and the nucleus pulposus can herniate out of the vertebral column, compressing on the spinal nerves and causing pain.

The unique structure of the spine enables both upright posture and flexibility for motion. The motions of the vertebral column are flexion (bending forward), extension (bending back), abduction (to either side), and rotation.

Shoulder

The **glenohumeral joint** is the articulation of the humerus with the glenoid fossa of the scapula (Fig. 22-7). Its ball-and-socket action allows great mobility of the arm on many axes. The joint is enclosed by a group of four powerful muscles and tendons that support and stabilize it. Together these are called the **rotator cuff** of the shoulder. The large **subacromial bursa** helps during abduction of the arm, so that the greater tubercle of the humerus moves easily under the acromion process of the scapula.

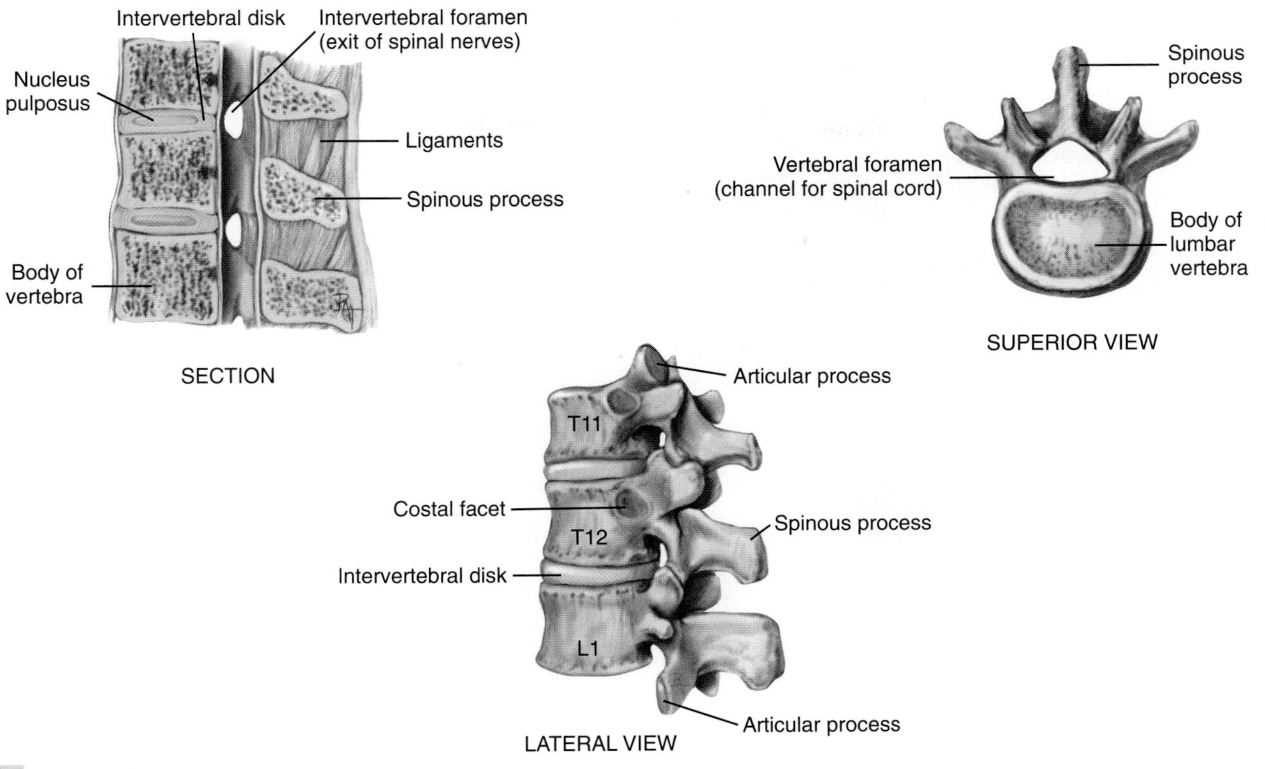
Intervertebral disk
Intervertebral foramen (exit of spinal nerves)
Nucleus pulposus
Ligaments
Spinous process
Body of vertebra
SECTION
Spinous process
Vertebral foramen (channel for spinal cord)
Body of lumbar vertebra
SUPERIOR VIEW
Articular process
T11
Costal facet
T12
Spinous process
Intervertebral disk
L1
Articular process
LATERAL VIEW

22-6 The vertebrae.

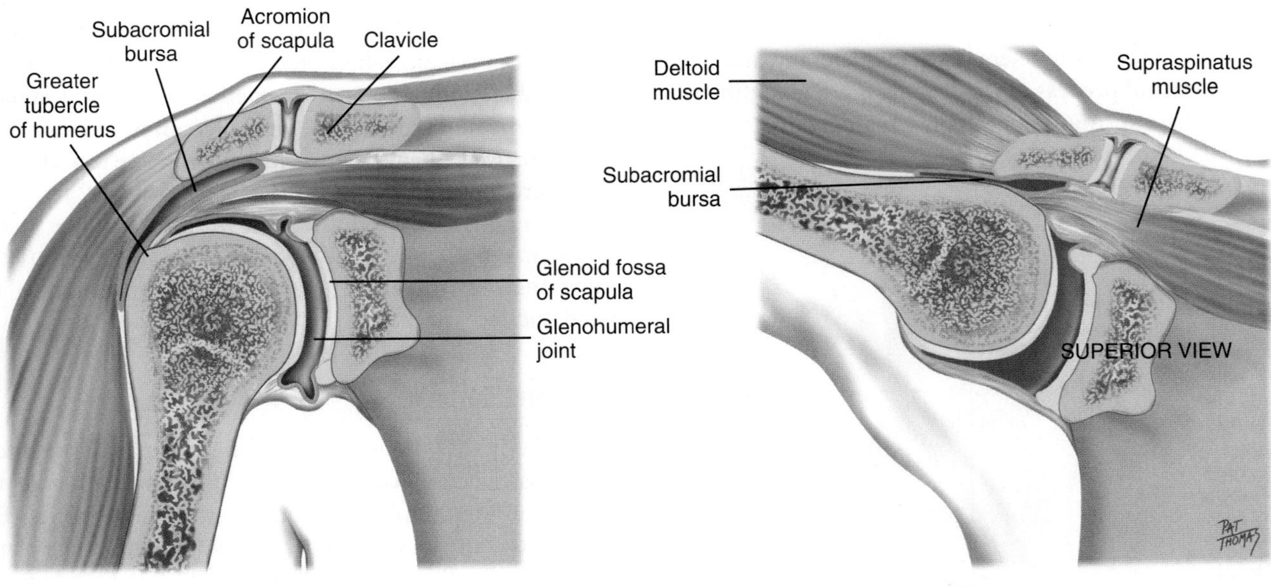
Subacromial bursa
Acromion of scapula
Clavicle
Greater tubercle of humerus
Glenoid fossa of scapula
Glenohumeral joint
SHOULDER JOINT
Deltoid muscle
Supraspinatus muscle
Subacromial bursa
SUPERIOR VIEW
SHOULDER WITH ARM ELEVATED

22-7

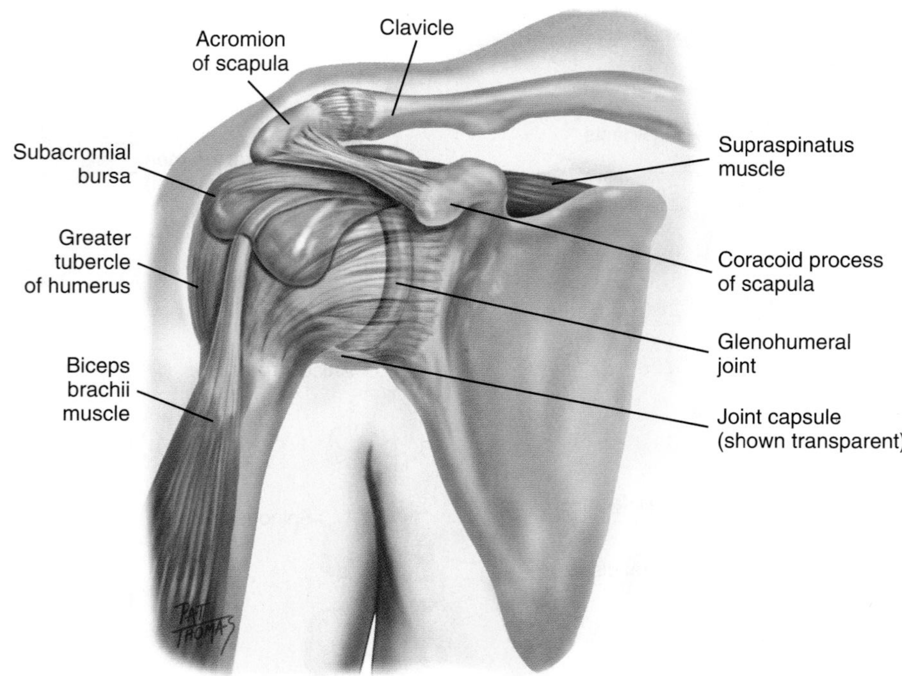

BONY LANDMARKS OF THE SHOULDER – ANTERIOR VIEW

22-8

The bones of the shoulder have palpable landmarks to guide your examination (Fig. 22-8). The scapula and the clavicle connect to form the shoulder girdle. You can feel the bump of the scapula's **acromion process** at the very top of the shoulder. Move your fingers in a small circle outward, down, and around. The next bump is the **greater tubercle** of the humerus a few centimeters down and laterally, and from that the **coracoid process** of the scapula is a few centimeters medially. These surround the deeply situated joint.

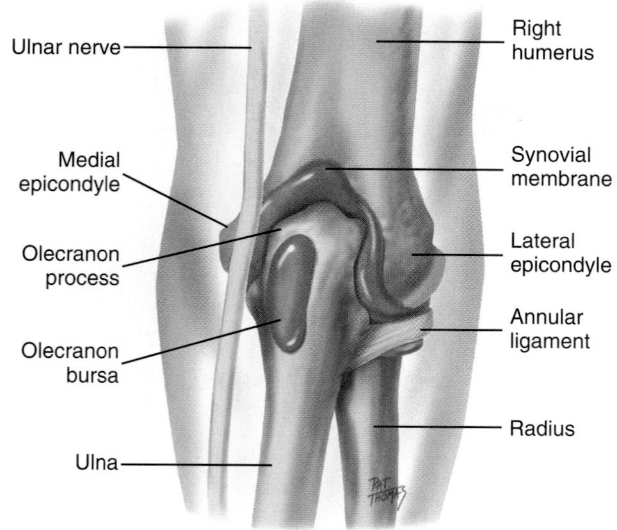

RIGHT ELBOW – POSTERIOR VIEW

22-9

Elbow

The elbow joint contains the three bony articulations of the humerus, radius, and ulna of the forearm (Fig. 22-9). Its hinge action moves the forearm (radius and ulna) on one plane, allowing flexion and extension. The olecranon bursa lies between the olecranon process and the skin.

Palpable landmarks are the **medial** and **lateral epicondyles** of the humerus and the large **olecranon process** of the ulna in between them. The sensitive ulnar nerve runs between the olecranon process and the medial epicondyle.

The radius and ulna articulate with each other at two radioulnar joints, one at the elbow and one at the wrist. These move together to permit pronation and supination of the hand and forearm.

Wrist and Carpals

Of the body's 206 bones, over half are in the hands and feet. The wrist, or **radiocarpal joint,** is the articulation of the radius (on the thumb side) and a row of carpal bones (Fig. 22-10). Its condyloid action permits movement in two planes at right angles: flexion and extension, and side-to-side deviation. You can feel the groove of this joint on the dorsum of the wrist.

The **midcarpal** joint is the articulation between the two parallel rows of carpal bones. It allows flexion, extension, and some rotation. The **metacarpophalangeal** and the **interphalangeal** joints permit finger flexion and extension. The flexor tendons of the wrist and hand are enclosed in synovial sheaths.

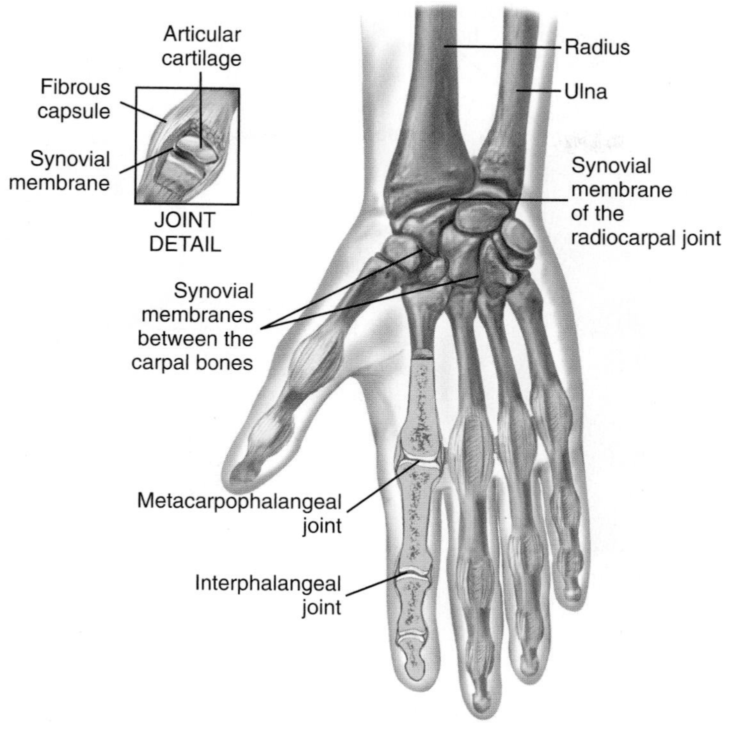

22-10 BONES OF THE HAND – PALMAR VIEW

Hip

The hip joint is the articulation between the acetabulum and the head of the femur (Fig. 22-11). As in the shoulder, ball-and-socket action permits a wide range of motion (ROM) on many axes. The hip has somewhat less ROM than the shoulder, but it has more stability as befits its weight-bearing function. Hip stability is due to powerful muscles that spread over the joint, a strong fibrous articular capsule, and the very deep insertion of the head of the femur. Three bursae facilitate movement.

Palpation of these bony landmarks will guide your examination. You can feel the entire iliac crest, from the **anterior superior iliac spine** to the posterior. The **ischial tuberosity** lies under the gluteus maximus muscle and is palpable when the hip is flexed. The **greater trochanter** of the femur is normally the width of the person's palm below the iliac crest and

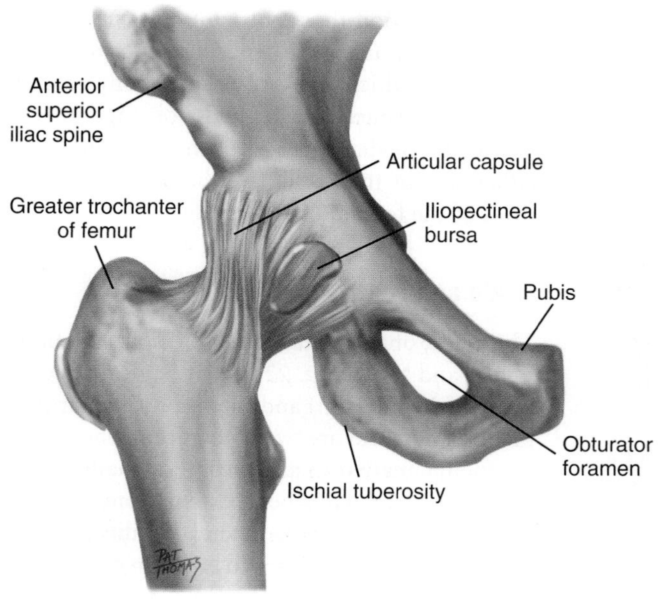

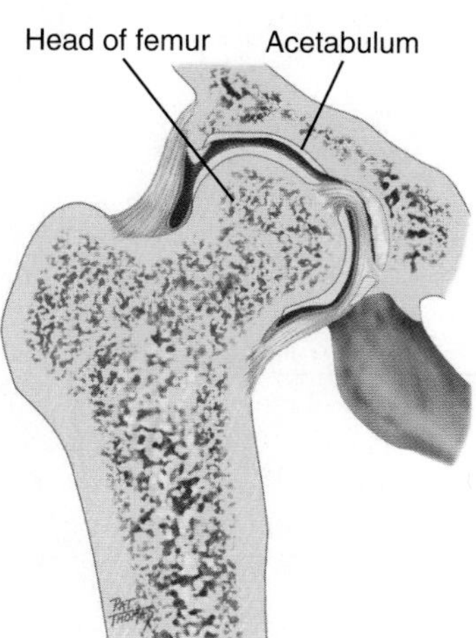

22-11 HIP JOINT

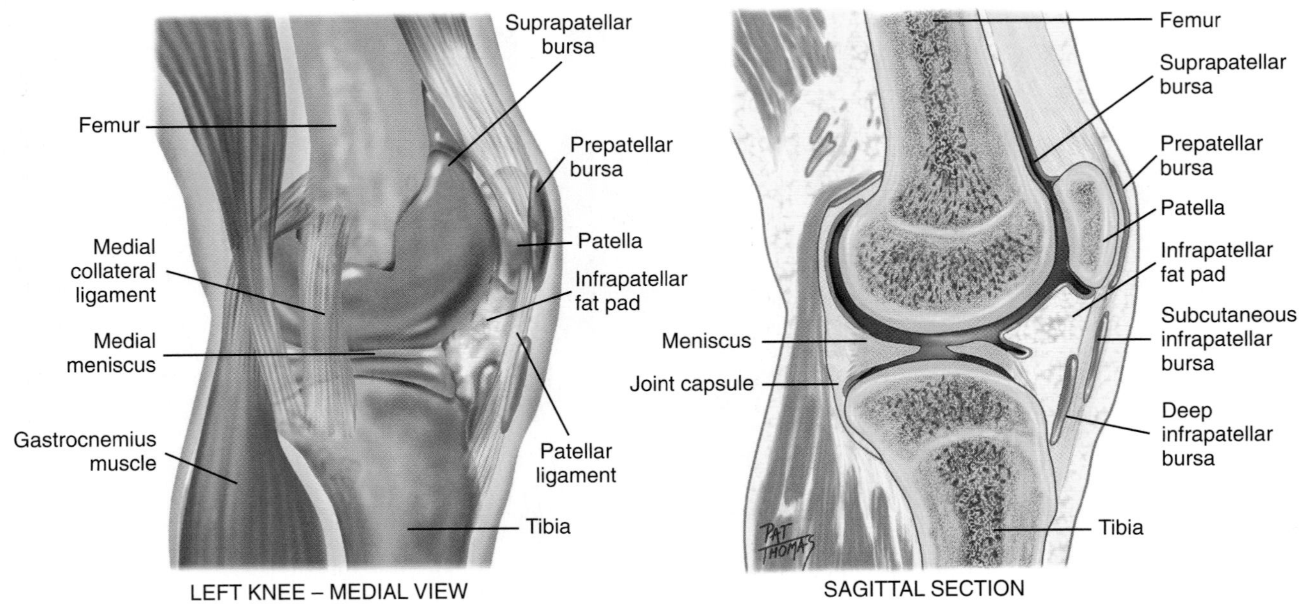

22-12

halfway between the anterior superior iliac spine and the ischial tuberosity. Feel it when the person is standing, in a flat depression on the upper lateral side of the thigh.

Knee

The knee joint is the articulation of three bones—the femur, the tibia, and the patella (kneecap)—in one common articular cavity (Fig. 22-12). It is the largest joint in the body and is complex. It is a hinge joint, permitting flexion and extension of the lower leg on a single plane.

The knee's synovial membrane is the largest in the body. It forms a sac at the superior border of the patella, called the **suprapatellar pouch,** which extends up as much as 6 cm behind the quadriceps muscle. Two wedge-shaped cartilages, called the **medial** and **lateral menisci,** cushion the tibia and femur. The joint is stabilized by two sets of ligaments. The **cruciate ligaments** (not shown) crisscross within the knee; they give anterior and posterior stability and help control rotation. The **collateral ligaments** connect the joint at both sides; they give medial and lateral stability and prevent dislocation. Numerous bursae prevent friction. One, the **prepatellar bursa,** lies between the patella and the skin. The **infrapatellar fat pad** is a small, triangular fat pad below the patella behind the patellar ligament.

Landmarks of the knee joint start with the large **quadriceps** muscle, which you can feel on your anterior and lateral thigh (Fig. 22-13). The muscle's four heads merge into a common tendon that continues down to enclose the round bony patella. Then the tendon inserts down on the **tibial tuberosity,** which you can feel as a bony prominence in the midline. Move to the sides and a bit superiorly and note the lateral and medial condyles of the tibia. Superior to these on either side of the patella are the medial and lateral epicondyles of the femur.

Quadriceps muscle
Lateral epicondyle of femur
Patella
Patellar ligament
Lateral collateral ligament
Medial condyle of tibia
Lateral meniscus
Lateral condyle of tibia
Anterior cruciate ligament (joint opened to show detail)
Fibula
Tibial tuberosity

LANDMARKS OF THE RIGHT KNEE JOINT

22-13

Ankle and Foot

The ankle, or **tibiotalar joint,** is the articulation of the tibia, fibula, and talus (Fig. 22-14). It is a hinge joint, limited to flexion (dorsiflexion) and extension (plantar flexion) on one plane. Landmarks are two bony prominences on either side—the **medial malleolus** and the **lateral malleolus.** Strong, tight medial and lateral ligaments extend from each malleolus onto the foot. These help the lateral stability of the ankle joint, although they may be torn in eversion or inversion sprains of the ankle.

Joints distal to the ankle give additional mobility to the foot. The subtalar joint permits inversion and eversion of the

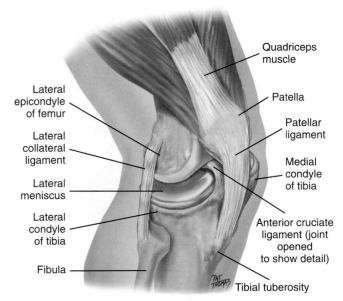

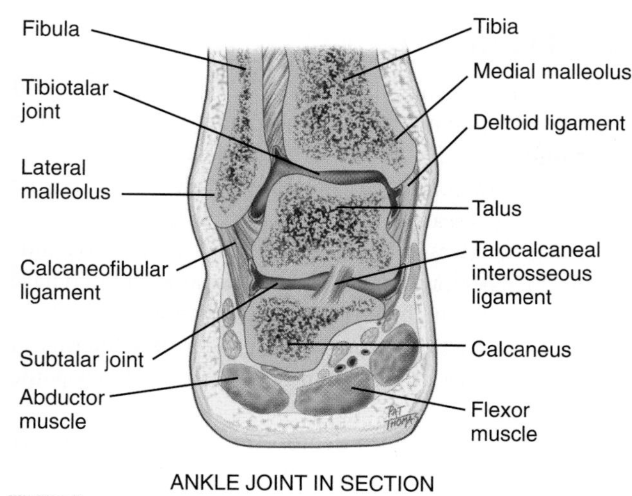

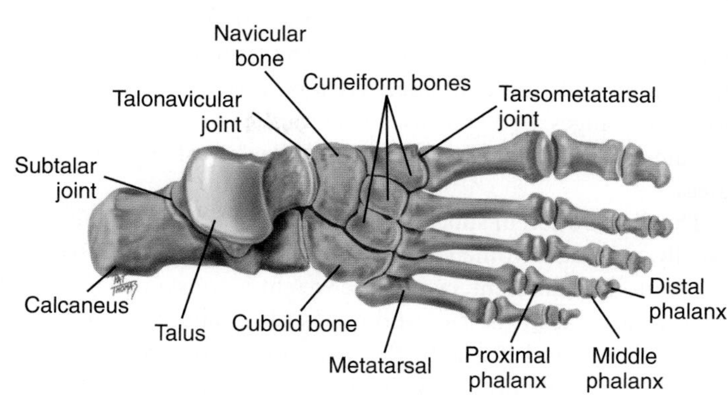

22-14

foot. The foot has a longitudinal arch, with weight-bearing distributed between the parts that touch the ground—the heads of the metatarsals and the calcaneus (heel).

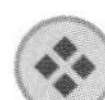

DEVELOPMENTAL COMPETENCE

Infants and Children

By 3 months' gestation, the fetus has formed a "scale model" of the skeleton that is made up of cartilage. During succeeding months in utero, the cartilage ossifies into true bone and starts to grow. Bone growth continues after birth—rapidly during infancy and then steadily during childhood—until adolescence, when both boys and girls undergo a rapid growth spurt.

Long bones grow in two dimensions. They increase in width or diameter by deposition of new bony tissue around the shafts. Lengthening occurs at the **epiphyses,** or growth plates. These specialized growth centers are transverse disks located at the ends of long bone. Any trauma or infection at this location puts the growing child at risk for bone deformity. This longitudinal growth continues until closure of the epiphyses; the last closure occurs at about age 20 years.

Skeletal contour changes are apparent at the vertebral column. At birth, the spine has a single C-shaped curve. At 3 to 4 months, raising the baby's head from prone position develops the anterior curve in the cervical neck region. From 1 year to 18 months, standing erect develops the anterior curve in the lumbar region.

Although the skeleton contributes to linear growth, muscles and fat are significant for weight increase. Individual muscle fibers grow throughout childhood, but growth is marked during the adolescent growth spurt. Then muscles respond to increased secretion of growth hormone, to adrenal androgens, and in boys, to further stimulation by testosterone. Muscles vary in size and strength in different people. This is due to genetic programming, nutrition, and exercise. All through life, muscles increase with use and atrophy with disuse.

The Pregnant Woman

Increased levels of circulating hormones (estrogen, relaxin from the corpus luteum, and corticosteroids) cause increased mobility in the joints. Increased mobility in the sacroiliac, sacrococcygeal, and symphysis pubis joints in the pelvis contributes to the noticeable changes in maternal posture. The most characteristic change is progressive **lordosis,** which compensates for the enlarging fetus; otherwise, the center of balance would shift forward. Lordosis compensates by shifting the weight farther back on the lower extremities. This shift in balance in turn creates strain on the low back muscles, which, in some women, is felt as low back pain during late pregnancy.

Anterior flexion of the neck and slumping of the shoulder girdle are other postural changes that compensate for the lordosis. These upper back changes may put pressure on the ulnar and median nerves during the third trimester. Nerve pressure creates aching, numbness, and weakness in the upper extremities in some women.

The Aging Adult

Bone **remodeling** is a cyclic process of bone resorption and deposition. The balance favors deposition until skeletal maturity at 25 to 35 years when bones mass reaches its peak.[17] After age 40, loss of bone matrix (resorption) occurs more rapidly than new bone formation. The net effect is a gradual loss of bone density, or **osteoporosis.** Although some degree of osteoporosis is nearly universal, women have more than men because for 5 years after menopause, the lack of estrogen leads to accelerated bone loss.

Postural changes are evident with aging, and decreased height is the most noticeable. Long bones do not shorten with age. Decreased height is due to shortening of the vertebral column. This is caused by loss of water content and thinning of the intervertebral disks and by a decrease in the height of individual vertebrae from osteoporosis.

Both men and women can expect a progressive decrease in height beginning at age 40 years in males and age 43 years in females, although this is not significant until age 60 years.[6] A greater decrease occurs in the 70s and 80s as a result of osteoporotic collapse of the vertebrae. The result is a shortening of the trunk and comparatively long extremities. Other postural changes are kyphosis, a backward head tilt to compensate for the kyphosis, and a slight flexion of hips and knees.

The distribution of subcutaneous fat changes through life. Usually, men and women gain weight in their 40s and 50s. The contour is different, even if the weight is constant. They begin to lose fat in the face and deposit it in abdomen and hips. In the 80s and 90s, fat further decreases in the periphery, which is especially noticeable in the forearms and apparent over the abdomen and hips.

Loss of subcutaneous fat leaves bony prominences more marked (e.g., tips of vertebrae, ribs, iliac crests) and body hollows deeper (e.g., cheeks, axillae). An absolute loss in muscle mass occurs; some muscles decrease in size, and some atrophy, producing weakness. The contour of muscles becomes more prominent, and muscle bundles and tendons feel more distinct.

Lifestyle affects musculoskeletal changes; a sedentary lifestyle hastens musculoskeletal changes of aging. However, physical exercise increases skeletal mass and helps prevent or delay osteoporosis. Physical activity delays or prevents bone loss in postmenopausal women in a dose-dependent manner.[19] Fast walking is the best prevention for osteoporosis; the faster the pace, the higher the preventive effect on the risk for hip fracture. The other positive effects of physical activity are improving muscle strength to prevent falls, balance and posture control, decrease in back pain, increase in quality of life, and prevention of cardiovascular disease, cancer, and depression.[19]

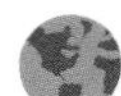

CULTURE AND GENETICS

There are racial/ethnic differences in bone strength and mineral density that may explain the incidence in hip fracture in older adults. African-American adults have a decreased risk for fracture when compared with white adults, and Hispanic women have a decreased risk for fractures than white women have.[2] The differences in fracture rates may be traced to childhood, in which African-American and Hispanic children have shown significantly higher bone strength than white children. This is due to structural properties—greater bone density at specific bone sites in African-American and Hispanic children.[26]

Similar results have been demonstrated in adults: greater bone mass and bone mineral density (BMD) among African-American men than among their white counterparts.[22] Younger Hispanic men had similar bone strength as African Americans, but older Hispanic men had more rapid loss of BMD and strength. The increased bone strength helps explain fracture risk.

Women have been studied regarding age at attaining peak bone mineral density. In the spine, women of all races gained BMD up to 30 to 33 years of age.[3] But at the femoral neck in the hip joint, BMD peaked earlier among white women (≤16 years) than among African Americans (21 years) and Hispanics (20 years). An earlier peak BMD and a more rapid decline following is a trend that may explain the increased fracture risk for white women later in life. These data plus physical activity data discussed earlier suggest that weight-bearing physical activity (e.g., fast walking) is imperative during the reproductive and middle adult years to slow the process of decline in BMD.

SUBJECTIVE DATA

1. Joints
   Pain
   Stiffness
   Swelling, heat, redness
   Limitation of movement
2. Muscles
   Pain (cramps)
   Weakness
3. Bones
   Pain
   Deformity
   Trauma (fractures, sprains, dislocations)
4. Functional assessment (activities of daily living [ADLs])
5. Self-care behaviors

Examiner Asks	Rationale
1. **Joints.**	
• Any problems with your joints? Any **pain?**	**Joint pain** and loss of function are the most common musculoskeletal concerns that prompt a person to seek care.
• Location: Which joints? On one side or both sides?	Rheumatoid arthritis (RA) involves symmetric joints; other musculoskeletal illnesses involve isolated or unilateral joints.
• Quality: What does the pain feel like: aching, stiff, sharp or dull, shooting? Severity: How strong is the pain?	Exquisitely tender with acute inflammation.
• Onset: When did this pain start?	

Examiner Asks	Rationale
• Timing: What time of day does the pain occur? How long does it last? How often does it occur?	RA pain is worse in morning when arising; osteoarthritis is worse later in the day; tendinitis is worse in morning, improves during the day.
• Is the pain aggravated by movement, rest, position, weather? Is the pain relieved by rest, medications, application of heat or ice?	Movement increases most joint pain except in RA, in which movement decreases pain.
• Is the pain associated with chills, fever, recent sore throat, trauma, repetitive activity?	Joint pain 10 to 14 days after an untreated strep throat suggests rheumatic fever. Joint injury occurs from trauma, repetitive motion.
• Any **stiffness** in your joints?	RA stiffness occurs in morning and after rest periods.
• Any **swelling, heat, redness** in the joints?	Suggests acute inflammation.
• Any **limitation of movement** in any joint? Which joint? • Which activities give you problems? (See Functional Assessment below and on p. 605.)	Decreased ROM may be due to joint injury to cartilage or capsule or to muscle contracture.
2. Muscles.	
• Any problems in the muscles, such as any **pain** or **cramping?** Which muscles?	**Myalgia** is usually felt as cramping or aching.
• If in calf muscles: Is the pain with walking? Does it go away with rest?	Suggests intermittent claudication (see Chapter 20).
• Are your muscle aches associated with fever, chills, the "flu"?	Viral illness often includes myalgia.
• Any **weakness** in muscles? • Location: Where is the weakness? How long have you noticed weakness?	Weakness may involve musculoskeletal or neurologic systems (see Chapter 23).
• Do the muscles look smaller there?	Atrophy.
3. Bones.	
• Any **bone pain?** Is the pain affected by movement? • Any **deformity** of any bone or joint? Is the deformity due to injury or trauma? Does the deformity affect ROM? • Any **accidents** or **trauma** ever affected the bones or joints: fractures; joint strain, sprain, dislocation? Which ones? • When did this occur? What treatment was given? Any problems or limitations now as a result? • Any back pain? In which part of your back? Is pain felt anywhere else, like shooting down leg? • Any numbness and tingling? Any limping?	Fracture causes sharp pain that increases with movement. Other bone pain usually feels "dull" and "deep" and is unrelated to movement.
4. Functional assessment (ADL). Do your joint (muscle, bone) problems create any limits on your usual activities of daily living (ADLs)? Which ones? (Note: Ask about each category; if the person answers "yes," ask specifically about each activity in category.)	**Functional assessment** screens the safety of independent living, the need for home health services, and quality of life (see Chapter 30).
• Bathing—getting in and out of the tub, turning faucets? • Toileting—urinating, moving bowels, able to get self on/off toilet, wipe self? • Dressing—doing buttons, zipper, fasten opening behind neck, pulling dress or sweater over head, pulling up pants, tying shoes, getting shoes that fit? • Grooming—shaving, brushing teeth, brushing or fixing hair, applying makeup? • Eating—preparing meals, pouring liquids, cutting up foods, bringing food to mouth, drinking?	Assess any self-care deficit.
• Mobility—walking, walking up or down stairs, getting in/out of bed, getting out of house?	Impaired physical mobility.
• Communicating—talking, using phone, writing?	Impaired verbal communication.

Examiner Asks	Rationale
5. **Self-care behaviors.** Any occupational hazards that could affect the muscles and joints? Does your work involve heavy lifting? Or any repetitive motion or chronic stress to joints? Any efforts to alleviate these?	Assess risk for back pain or carpal tunnel syndrome.
• Tell me about your exercise program. Describe the type of exercise, frequency, the warm-up program. • Any pain during exercise? How do you treat it? • Have you had any recent weight gain? Please describe your usual daily diet. (Note the person's usual caloric intake, all four food groups, daily amount of protein, calcium.) • Are you taking any medications for musculoskeletal system: aspirin, anti-inflammatory, muscle relaxant, pain reliever?	Self-care behaviors.
• If person has chronic disability or crippling illness: How has your illness affected: Your interaction with family Your interaction with friends The way you view yourself	Assess for: • Self-esteem disturbance • Loss of independence • Body image disturbance • Role performance disturbance • Social isolation

Additional History for Infants and Children

Examiner Asks	Rationale
1. Were you told about any trauma to infant during labor and delivery? Did the baby come head first? Was there a need for forceps?	Traumatic delivery increases risk for fractures, (e.g., humerus, clavicle).
2. Did the baby need resuscitation?	Period of anoxia may result in hypotonia of muscles.
3. Were the baby's motor milestones achieved at about the same time as siblings or age-mates?	
4. Has your child ever broken any bones? Any dislocations? How were these treated?	
5. Have you ever noticed any bone deformity? Spinal curvature? Unusual shape of toes or feet? At what age? Have you ever sought treatment for any of these?	

Additional History for Adolescents

Examiner Asks	Rationale
1. Involved in any sports at school or after school? How frequently (times per week)?	Assess safety of sport for child. Note if child's height and weight are adequate for the particular sport (e.g., football).
2. Do you use any special equipment? Does any training program exist for your sport?	Use of safety equipment and presence of adult supervision decrease risk for sports injuries.
3. What is the nature of your daily warm-up?	Lack of adequate warm-up increases risk for sports injury.
4. What do you do if you get hurt?	Students may not report injury or pain for fear of limiting participation in sport.
5. How does your sport fit in with other school demands and other activities?	

Additional History for the Aging Adult

Use the functional assessment history questions in Chapter 4 (pp. 49 to 70) to elicit any loss of function, self-care deficit, or safety risk that may occur as a process of aging or musculoskeletal illness. (Review the complete functional assessment in Chapter 30.)

Examiner Asks	Rationale
1. Any change in weakness over the past months or years?	
2. Any increase in falls or stumbling over the past months or years?	
3. Do you use any mobility aids to help you get around: cane, walker?	

OBJECTIVE DATA

PREPARATION

The purpose of the musculoskeletal examination is to assess function for ADLs and to screen for any abnormalities. You already will have considerable data regarding ADLs through the history. Note additional ADLs data as the person goes through the motions necessary for an examination: gait; posture; how the person sits in a chair, raises from chair, takes off jacket, manipulates small object such as a pen, raises from supine.

A **screening** musculoskeletal examination suffices for most people:

- Inspection and palpation of joints integrated with each body region
- Observation of ROM as person proceeds through motions described earlier
- Age-specific screening measures, such as Ortolani sign for infants or scoliosis screening for adolescents

A **complete** musculoskeletal examination, as described in this chapter, is appropriate for persons with articular disease, a history of musculoskeletal symptoms, or any problems with ADLs.

Make the person comfortable before and throughout the examination. Drape for full visualization of the body part you are examining without needlessly exposing the person.

Take an orderly approach—head to toe, proximal to distal (from the midline outward).

Support each joint at rest. Muscles must be soft and relaxed to assess the joints under them accurately. Take care when examining any inflamed area where rough manipulation could cause pain and muscle spasm. To avoid this, use firm support, gentle movement, and gentle return to a relaxed state.

Compare corresponding paired joints. Expect symmetry of structure and function and normal parameters for that joint.

EQUIPMENT NEEDED

Tape measure
Skin marking pen

Normal Range of Findings	Abnormal Findings
ORDER OF THE EXAMINATION	
Inspection	
Note the **size** and **contour** of the joint. Inspect the skin and tissues over the joints for **color, swelling,** and any **masses** or **deformity.** Presence of swelling is significant and signals joint irritation.	Swelling may be excess joint fluid (effusion), thickening of the synovial lining, inflammation of surrounding soft tissue (bursae, tendons), or bony enlargement. Deformities include **dislocation** (complete loss of contact between the two bones in a joint); **subluxation** (two bones in a joint stay in contact but their alignment is off); **contracture** (shortening of a muscle leading to limited ROM of joint), or **ankylosis** (stiffness or fixation of a joint).

Normal Range of Findings | **Abnormal Findings**

Palpation

Palpate each joint, including its skin for temperature, its muscles, bony articulations, and area of joint capsule. Notice any heat, tenderness, swelling, or masses. Joints normally are not tender to palpation. If any tenderness does occur, try to localize it to specific anatomic structures (e.g., skin, muscles, bursae, ligaments, tendons, fat pads, or joint capsule).

Warmth and tenderness signal inflammation.

The synovial membrane normally is not palpable. When thickened, it feels "doughy" or "boggy." A small amount of fluid is present in the normal joint, but it is not palpable.

Palpable fluid is abnormal. Because fluid is contained in an enclosed sac, if you push on one side of the sac, the fluid will shift and cause a visible bulging on another side.

Range of Motion (ROM)

Ask for **active (voluntary) ROM** while stabilizing the body area proximal to that being moved. Familiarize yourself with the type of each joint and its normal ROM so that you can recognize limitations. If you see a limitation, gently attempt **passive motion** with the person's muscles relaxed and with you moving the body part. Anchor the joint with one hand while your other hand slowly moves it to its limit. The normal ranges of active and passive motion should be the same.

Limitation in ROM is the most sensitive sign of joint disease.[15a] The amount of limitation may alert you to the cause of disease. Articular disease (inside the joint capsule [e.g., arthritis]) produces swelling and tenderness around the whole joint, and it limits all planes of ROM in both active and passive motion. Extra-articular disease (injury to a specific tendon, ligament, nerve) produces swelling and tenderness to that one spot in the joint and affects only certain planes of ROM, especially during active (voluntary) motion.

Joint motion normally causes no tenderness, pain, or crepitation. Do not confuse crepitation with the normal discrete "crack" heard as a tendon or ligament slips over bone during motion, such as when you do a knee bend.

Crepitation is an audible and palpable crunching or grating that accompanies movement. It occurs when the articular surfaces in the joints are roughened, as with rheumatoid arthritis (see Table 22-1, Abnormalities Affecting Multiple Joints, p. 608).

Muscle Testing

Test the strength of the prime mover muscle groups for each joint. Repeat the motions you elicited for active ROM. Now ask the person to flex and hold as you apply opposing force. Muscle strength should be equal bilaterally and should fully resist your opposing force. (Note: Muscle status and joint status are interdependent and should be interpreted together. Chapter 23 discusses the examination of muscles for size and development, tone, and presence of tenderness.)

A wide variability of strength exists among people. You may wish to use a grading system from no voluntary movement to full strength, as shown.

GRADE	DESCRIPTION	% NORMAL	ASSESSMENT
5	Full ROM against gravity, full resistance	100	Normal
4	Full ROM against gravity, some resistance	75	Good
3	Full ROM with gravity	50	Fair
2	Full ROM with gravity eliminated (passive motion)	25	Poor
1	Slight contraction	10	Trace
0	No contraction	0	Zero

Normal Range of Findings

TEMPOROMANDIBULAR JOINT

With the person seated, **inspect** the area just anterior to the ear. Place the tips of your first two fingers in front of each ear and ask the person to open and close the mouth. Drop your fingers into the depressed area over the joint, and note smooth motion of the mandible. An audible and palpable snap or click occurs in many healthy people as the mouth opens (Fig. 22-15). Then ask the person to:

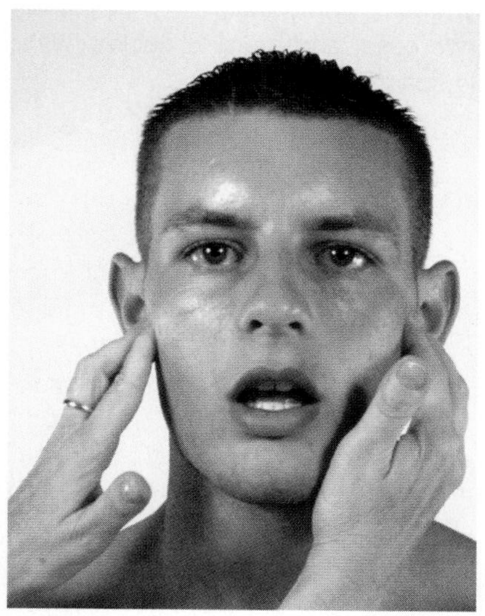

22-15

Instructions to Person	Motion and Expected Range
• Open mouth maximally.	Vertical motion. You can measure the space between the upper and lower incisors. Normal is 3 to 6 cm, or three fingers inserted sideways.
• Partially open mouth, protrude lower jaw, and move it side to side.	Lateral motion. Normal extent is 1 to 2 cm (Fig. 22-16).
• Stick out lower jaw.	Protrude without deviation.

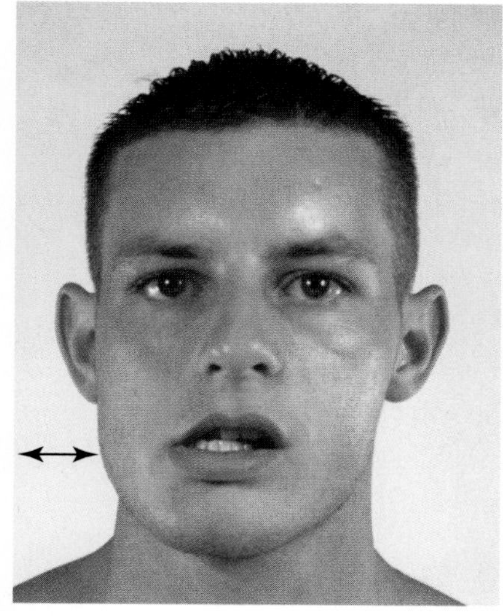

22-16

Abnormal Findings

Swelling looks like a round bulge over the joint, although it must be moderate or marked to be visible.

Crepitus and pain occur with temporomandibular joint dysfunction.

Lateral motion may be lost earlier and more significantly than vertical.

Normal Range of Findings | **Abnormal Findings**

Palpate the contracted temporalis and masseter muscles as the person clenches the teeth. Compare right and left sides for size, firmness, and strength. Ask the person to move the jaw forward and laterally against your resistance and to open mouth against your resistance. This also tests the integrity of cranial nerve V (trigeminal).

CERVICAL SPINE

Inspect the alignment of head and neck. The spine should be straight and the head erect. **Palpate** the spinous processes and the sternomastoid, trapezius, and paravertebral muscles. They should feel firm, with no muscle spasm or tenderness.

Ask the person to follow these motions (Fig. 22-17)*:

Abnormal Findings: Head tilted to one side. Asymmetry of muscles. Tenderness and hard muscles with muscle spasm.

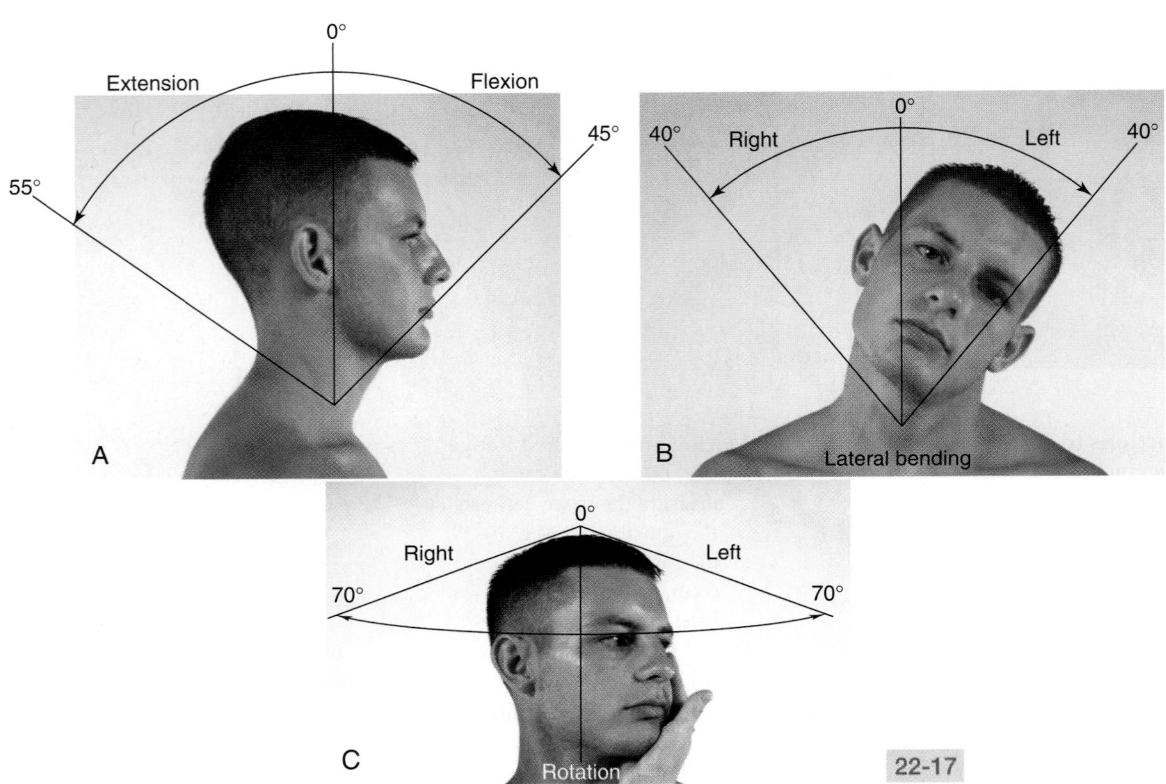

22-17

Instructions to Person	Motion and Expected Range	Abnormal Findings
• Touch chin to chest.	Flexion of 45 degrees (Fig. 22-17, *A*).	Limited ROM.
• Lift the chin toward the ceiling.	Hyperextension of 55 degrees.	
• Touch each ear toward the corresponding shoulder. Do not lift up the shoulder.	Lateral bending of 40 degrees (Fig. 22-17, *B*).	Pain with movement.
• Turn the chin toward each shoulder.	Rotation of 70 degrees (Fig. 22-17, *C*).	

Repeat the motions while applying opposing force. The person normally can maintain flexion against your full resistance. This also tests the integrity of cranial nerve XI (spinal).

Abnormal Findings: The person cannot hold flexion.

*Do not attempt if you suspect neck trauma.

Objective Data

Normal Range of Findings	Abnormal Findings

UPPER EXTREMITY

Shoulder

Inspect and compare both shoulders posteriorly and anteriorly. Check the size and contour of the joint, and compare shoulders for equality of bony landmarks. Normally, no redness, muscular atrophy, deformity, or swelling is present. Check the anterior aspect of the joint capsule and the subacromial bursa for abnormal swelling.

Redness.

Inequality of bony landmarks.

Atrophy, shows as lack of fullness.

Dislocated shoulder loses the normal rounded shape and looks flattened laterally.

Swelling from excess fluid is best seen anteriorly. Considerable fluid must be present to cause a visible distention because the capsule normally is so loose (see Table 22-2, Abnormalities of the Shoulder, p. 609).

Swelling of subacromial bursa is localized under deltoid muscle and may be accentuated when the person tries to abduct the arm.

If the person reports any shoulder pain, ask that he or she point to the spot with the hand of the unaffected side. Be aware that shoulder pain may be from local causes or it may be referred pain from a hiatal hernia or a cardiac or pleural condition, which could be potentially serious. Pain from a local cause is reproducible during the examination by palpation or motion.

While standing in front of the person, **palpate** both shoulders, noting any muscular spasm or atrophy, swelling, heat, or tenderness. Start at the clavicle and methodically explore the acromioclavicular joint, scapula, greater tubercle of the humerus, area of the subacromial bursa, the biceps groove, and the anterior aspect of the glenohumeral joint. Palpate the pyramid-shaped axilla; no adenopathy or masses should be present.

Swelling.

Hard muscles with muscle spasm.

Tenderness or pain.

Test ROM by asking the person to perform four motions (Fig. 22-18). Cup one hand over the shoulder during ROM to note any crepitation; normally none is present.

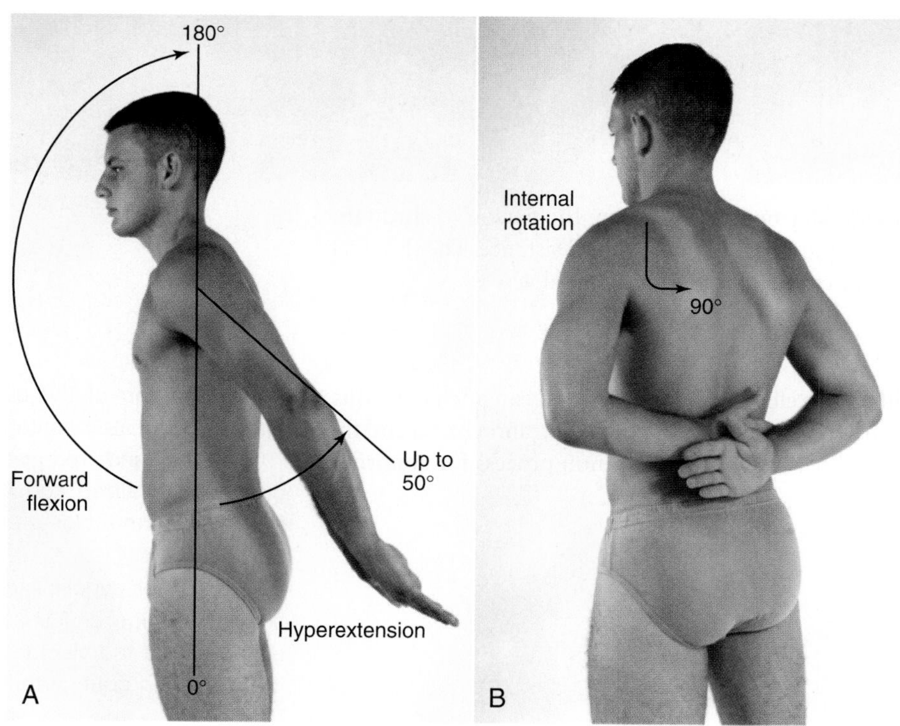

22-18

Objective Data

Normal Range of Findings		Abnormal Findings
Instructions to Person	**Motion and Expected Range**	
• With arms at sides and elbows extended, move both arms forward and up in wide vertical arcs and then move them back.	Forward flexion of 180 degrees. Hyperextension up to 50 degrees (Fig. 22-18, *A*).	Limited ROM. Asymmetry. Pain with motion.
• Rotate arms internally behind back, place back of hands as high as possible toward the scapulae.	Internal rotation of 90 degrees (Fig. 22-18, *B*).	Crepitus with motion. Rotator cuff lesions may cause limited ROM, pain, and muscle spasm during abduction, whereas forward flexion stays fairly normal.
• With arms at sides and elbows extended, raise both arms in wide arcs in the coronal plane. Touch palms together above head.	Abduction of 180 degrees. Adduction of 50 degrees (Fig. 22-18, *C*).	
• Touch both hands behind the head with elbows flexed and rotated posteriorly.	External rotation of 90 degrees (Fig. 22-18, *D*).	

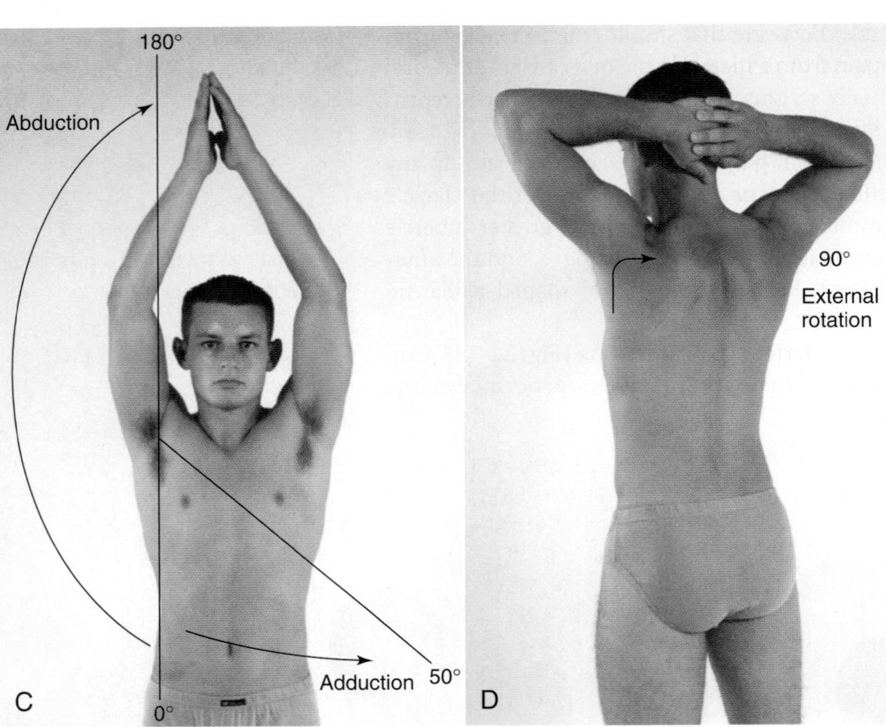

22-18 *Cont'd*

Test the strength of the shoulder muscles by asking the person to shrug the shoulders, flex forward and up, and abduct against your resistance. The shoulder shrug also tests the integrity of cranial nerve XI, the spinal accessory.

Elbow

Inspect the size and contour of the elbow in both flexed and extended positions. Look for any deformity, redness, or swelling. Check the olecranon bursa and the normally present hollows on either side of the olecranon process for abnormal swelling.

Subluxation of the elbow shows the forearm dislocated posteriorly.

Swelling and redness of olecranon bursa are localized and easy to observe because of the close proximity of the bursa to skin.

Effusion or synovial thickening shows first as a bulge or fullness in groove on either side of the olecranon process, and it occurs with gouty arthritis.

Normal Range of Findings

Palpate with the elbow flexed about 70 degrees and as relaxed as possible (Fig. 22-19). Use your left hand to support the person's left forearm, and palpate the extensor surface of the elbow—the olecranon process and the medial and lateral epicondyles of humerus—with your right thumb and fingers.

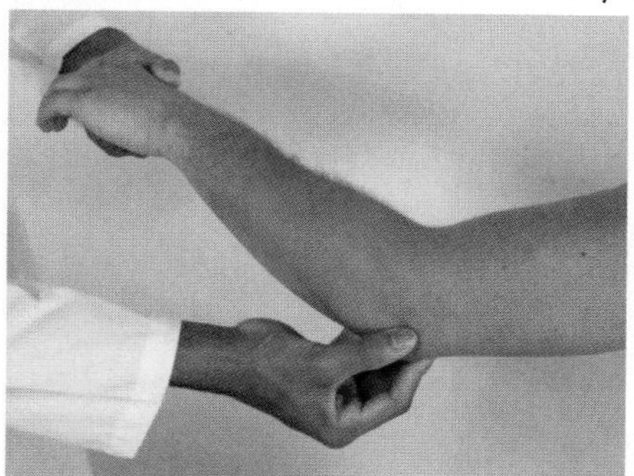

22-19

With your thumb in the lateral groove and your index and middle fingers in the medial groove, palpate either side of the olecranon process using varying pressure. Normally, present tissues and fat pads feel fairly solid. Check for any synovial thickening, swelling, nodules, or tenderness.

Palpate the area of the olecranon bursa for heat, swelling, tenderness, consistency, or nodules.

Test ROM by asking the person to:

Instructions to Person	Motion and Expected Range
• Bend and straighten the elbow (Fig. 22-20).	Flexion of 150 to 160 degrees; extension at 0. Some healthy people lack 5 to 10 degrees of full extension, and others have 5 to 10 degrees of hyperextension.
• Movement of 90 degrees in pronation and supination (Fig. 22-21).	Hold the hand midway; then touch front and back sides of hand to table.

Abnormal Findings

Epicondyles, head of radius, and tendons are common sites of inflammation and local tenderness, or "tennis elbow."

Soft, boggy, or fluctuant swelling in both grooves occurs with synovial thickening or effusion.

Local heat or redness (signs of inflammation) can extend beyond synovial membrane.

Subcutaneous nodules are raised, firm, and nontender, and overlying skin moves freely. Common sites are in the olecranon bursa and along extensor surface of the ulna. These nodules occur with RA (see Table 22-3, Abnormalities of the Elbow, p. 610).

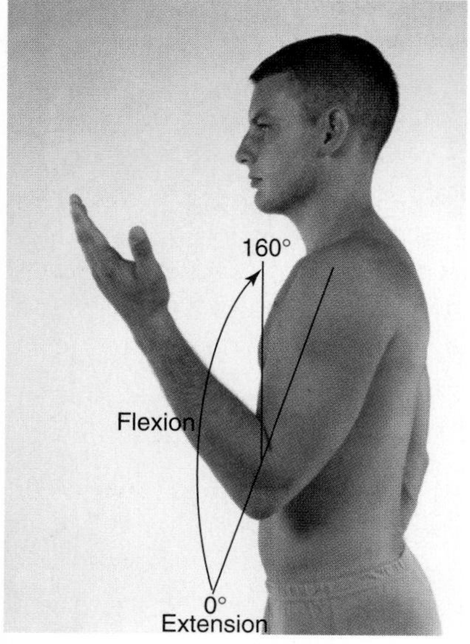

22-20

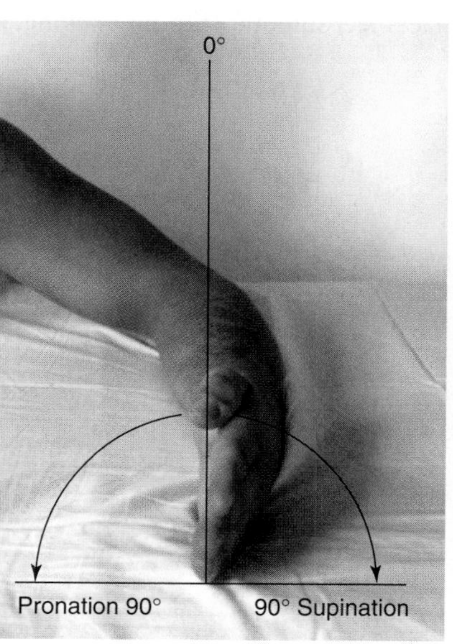

22-21

Objective Data

Normal Range of Findings	Abnormal Findings

While testing **muscle strength,** stabilize the person's arm with one hand (Fig. 22-22). Have the person flex the elbow against your resistance applied just proximal to the wrist. Then ask the person to extend the elbow against your resistance.

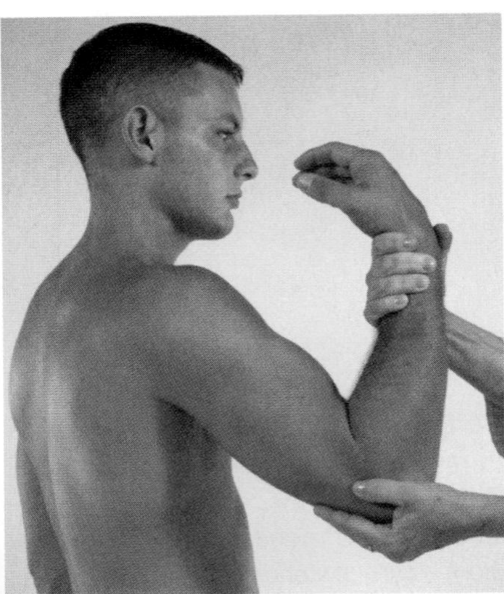

22-22

Wrist and Hand

Inspect the hands and wrists on the dorsal and palmar sides, noting position, contour, and shape. The normal functional position of the hand shows the wrist in slight extension. This way, the fingers can flex efficiently and the thumb can oppose them for grip and manipulation. The fingers lie straight in the same axis as the forearm. Normally, no swelling or redness, deformity, or nodules are present.

The skin looks smooth with knuckle wrinkles present and no swelling or lesions. Muscles are full, with the palm showing a rounded mound proximal to the thumb (the **thenar eminence**) and a smaller rounded mound proximal to the little finger.

Subluxation (partial dislocation) of wrist.

Ulnar deviation; fingers list to ulnar side.

Ankylosis; wrist in extreme flexion.

Dupuytren contracture; flexion contracture of finger(s).

Swan-neck or boutonnière deformity in fingers.

Atrophy of the thenar eminence (see Table 22-4, Abnormalities of the Wrist and Hand, p. 611).

Palpate each joint in the wrist and hands. Facing the person, support the hand with your fingers under it and palpate the wrist firmly with both your thumbs on its dorsum (Fig. 22-23). Make sure the person's wrist is relaxed and in straight alignment. Move your palpating thumbs side to side to identify the normal depressed areas that overlie the joint space. Use gentle but firm pressure. Normally, the joint surfaces feel smooth, with no swelling, bogginess, nodules, or tenderness.

Ganglion cyst in wrist (see Table 22-4).

Synovial swelling on dorsum.

Generalized swelling.

Tenderness.

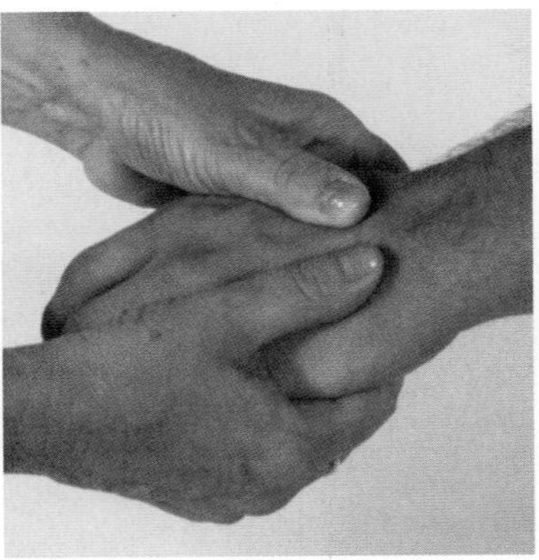

22-23

Normal Range of Findings	Abnormal Findings

Palpate the metacarpophalangeal joints with your thumbs, just distal to and on either side of the knuckle (Fig. 22-24).

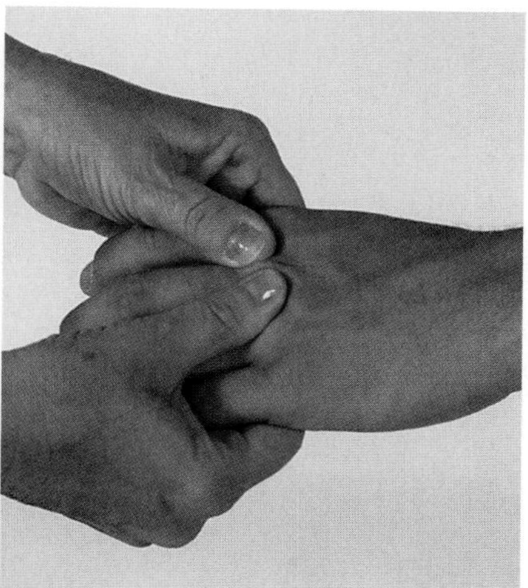

22-24

Use your thumb and index finger in a pinching motion to palpate the sides of the interphalangeal joints (Fig. 22-25). Normally, no synovial thickening, tenderness, warmth, or nodules are present.

Heberden and Bouchard nodules are hard and nontender and occur with osteoarthritis (see Table 22-4).

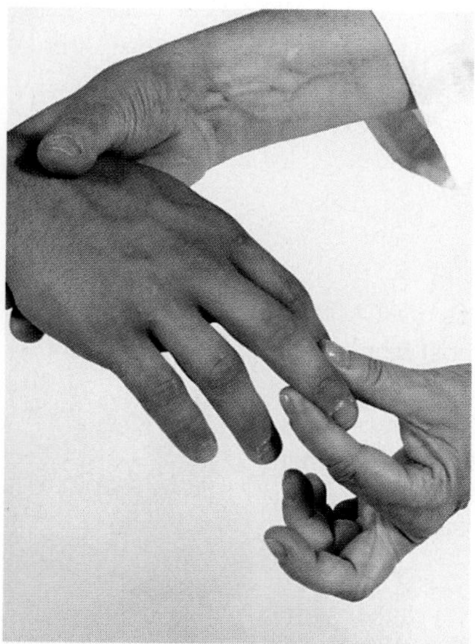

22-25

Normal Range of Findings

Test ROM (Fig. 22-26) by asking the person to:

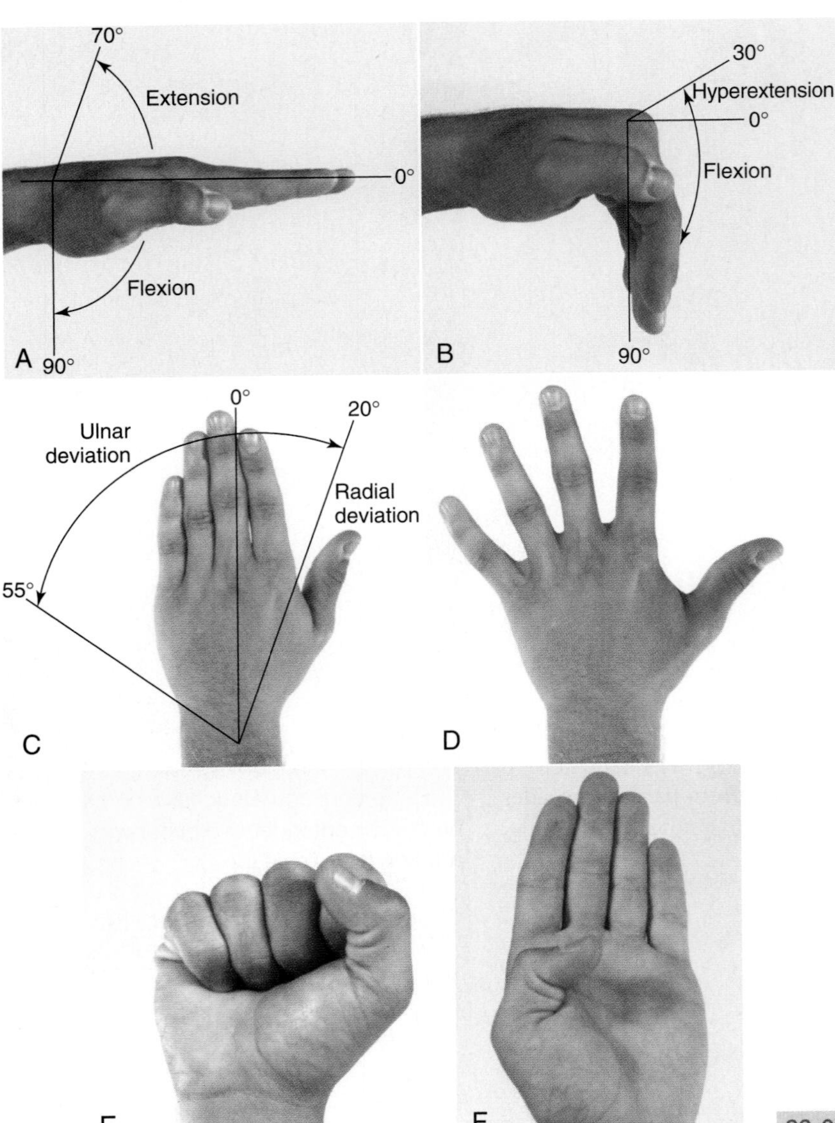

Instructions to Person	Motion and Expected Range
• Bend the hand up at the wrist.	Hyperextension of 70 degrees (Fig. 22-26, *A*).
• Bend hand down at the wrist.	Palmar flexion of 90 degrees.
• Bend the fingers up and down at metacarpophalangeal joints.	Flexion of 90 degrees. Hyperextension of 30 degrees (Fig. 22-26, *B*).
• With palms flat on table, turn them outward and in.	Ulnar deviation of 50 to 60 degrees, and radial deviation of 20 degrees (Fig. 22-26, *C*).
• Spread fingers apart; make a fist.	Abduction of 20 degrees; fist tight. The responses should be equal bilaterally (Fig. 22-26, *D, E*).
• Touch the thumb to each finger and to the base of little finger.	The person is able to perform, and the responses are equal bilaterally (Fig. 22-26, *F*).

Abnormal Findings

Loss of ROM here is the most common and most significant functional loss of the wrist.

Limited motion.

Pain on movement.

Normal Range of Findings

For **muscle testing,** position the person's forearm supinated (palm up) and resting on a table (Fig. 22-27). Stabilize by holding your hand at the person's midforearm. Ask the person to flex the wrist against your resistance at the palm.

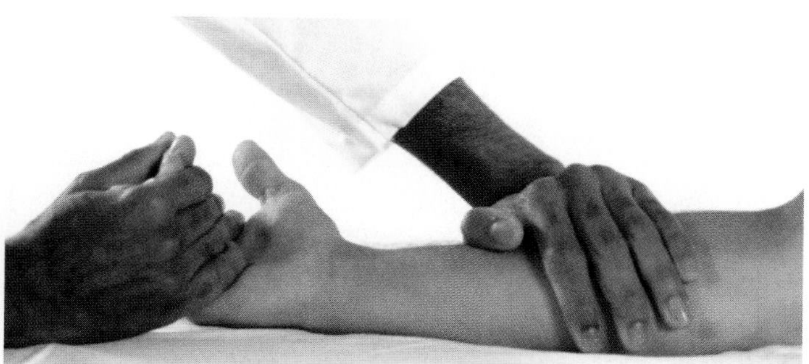

22-27

Phalen Test. Ask the person to hold both hands back to back while flexing the wrists 90 degrees. Acute flexion of the wrist for 60 seconds produces no symptoms in the normal hand (Fig. 22-28).

Tinel Sign. Direct percussion of the location of the median nerve at the wrist produces no symptoms in the normal hand (Fig. 22-29).

Abnormal Findings

Phalen test reproduces numbness and burning in a person with carpal tunnel syndrome (see Table 22-4).

In carpal tunnel syndrome, percussion of the median nerve produces burning and tingling along its distribution, which is a positive Tinel sign.

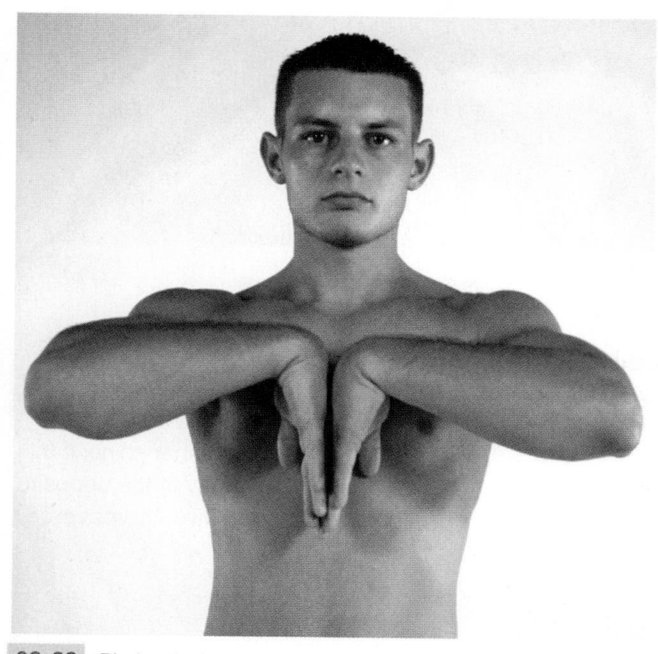

22-28 Phalen test.

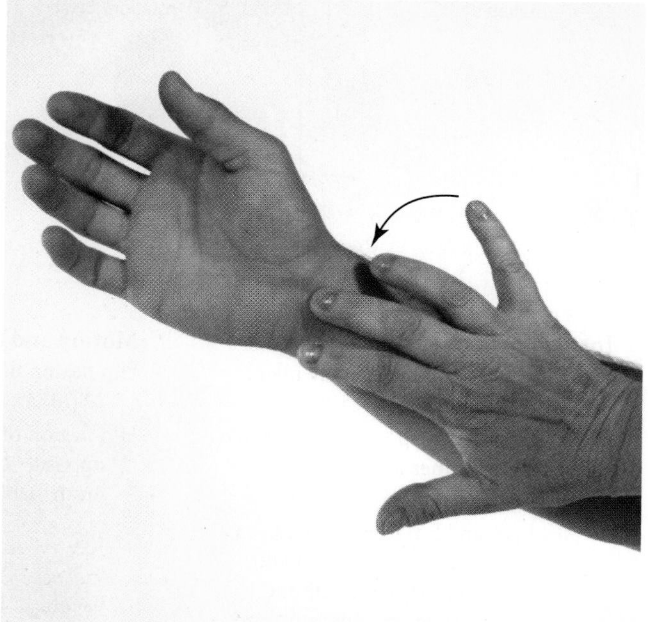

22-29 Tinel sign.

Normal Range of Findings

LOWER EXTREMITY

Hip

Wait to **inspect** the hip joint together with the spine a bit later in the examination as the person stands. At that time, note symmetric levels of iliac crests, gluteal folds, and equally sized buttocks. A smooth, even gait reflects equal leg lengths and functional hip motion.

Help the person into a supine position and **palpate** the hip joints. The joints should feel stable and symmetric, with no tenderness or crepitus.

Assess ROM (Fig. 22-30) by asking the person to:

Abnormal Findings

Pain with palpation.
Crepitation.

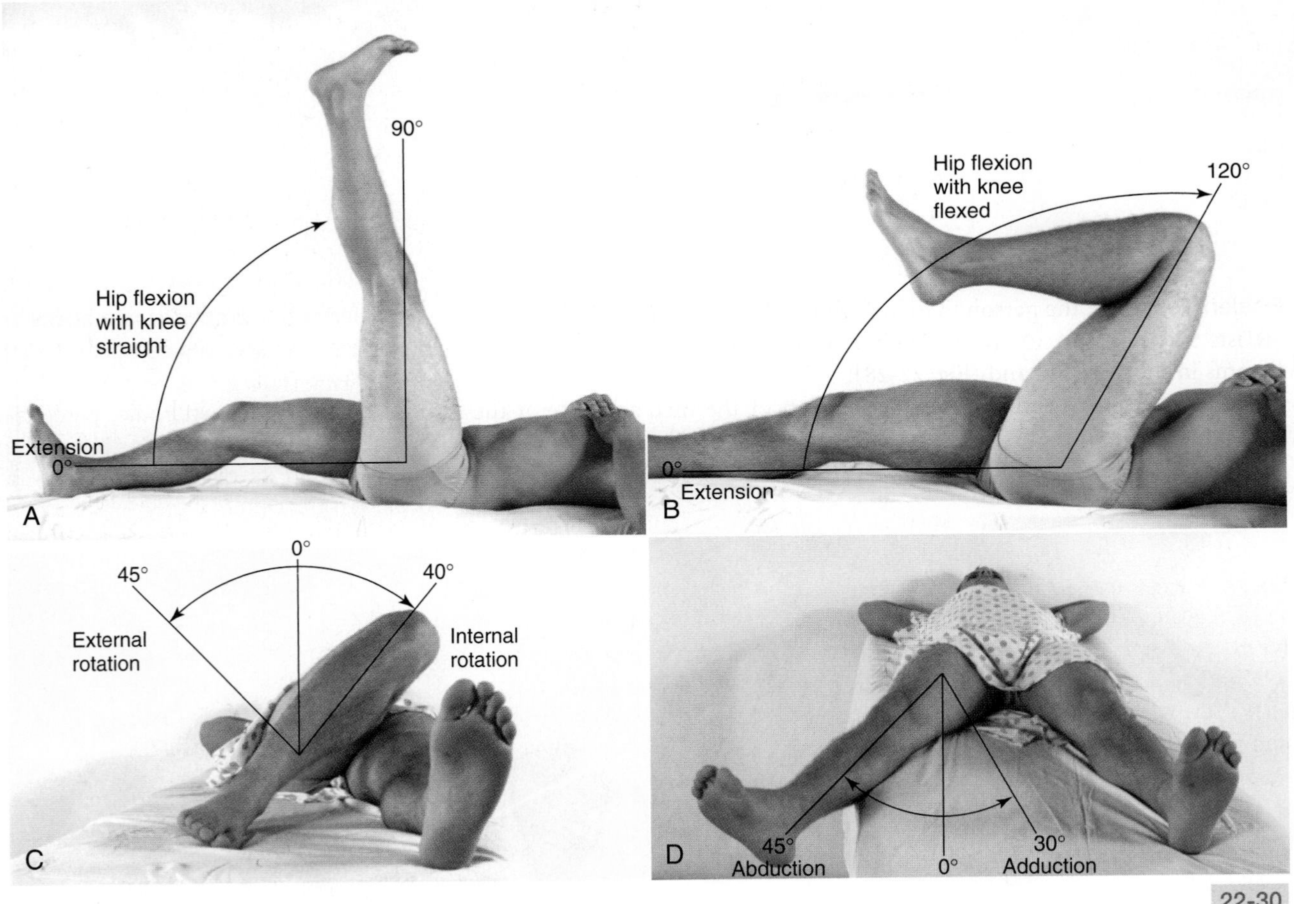

22-30

Instructions to Person

- Raise each leg with knee extended.
- Bend each knee up to the chest while keeping the other leg straight.
- Flex knee and hip to 90 degrees. Stabilize by holding the thigh with one hand and the ankle with the other hand. Swing the foot outward. Swing the foot inward. (Foot and thigh move in opposite directions.)

Motion and Expected Range

Hip flexion of 90 degrees (Fig. 22-30, *A*).

Hip flexion of 120 degrees. The opposite thigh should remain on the table (Fig. 22-30, *B*).

Internal rotation of 40 degrees. External rotation of 45 degrees (Fig. 22-30, *C*).

Abnormal Findings

Limited motion.
Pain with motion.
Flexion flattens the lumbar spine; if this reveals a flexion deformity in the opposite hip, it represents a positive *Thomas test.*

Limited internal rotation of hip is an early and reliable sign of hip disease.

Normal Range of Findings

- Swing leg laterally, then medially, with knee straight. Stabilize pelvis by pushing down on the opposite anterior superior iliac spine.
- When standing (later in examination), swing straight leg back behind body. Stabilize pelvis to eliminate exaggerated lumbar lordosis. The most efficient way is to ask person to bend over the table and to support the trunk on the table. Or the person can lie prone on the table.

Abduction of 40 to 45 degrees. Adduction of 20 to 30 degrees (Fig. 22-30, *D*).

Hyperextension of 15 degrees when stabilized.

Abnormal Findings

Limitation of abduction of the hip while supine is the most common motion dysfunction found in hip disease.

Knee

The person should remain supine with legs extended, although some examiners prefer the knees to be flexed and dangling for **inspection.** The skin normally looks smooth, with even coloring and no lesions.

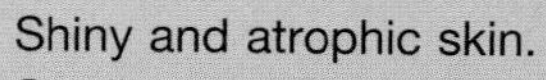

Shiny and atrophic skin.

Swelling or inflammation (see Table 22-5, Abnormalities of the Knee, p. 613).

Lesions (e.g., psoriasis).

Inspect lower leg alignment. The lower leg should extend in the same axis as the thigh.

Angulation deformity:

- Genu varum (bowlegs) (see p. 601)
- Genu valgum (knock knees)
- Flexion contracture

Inspect the knee's shape and contour. Normally, distinct concavities, or hollows, are present on either side of the patella. Check them for any sign of fullness or swelling. Note other locations, such as the prepatellar bursa and the suprapatellar pouch, for any abnormal swelling.

Hollows disappear; then they may bulge with synovial thickening or effusion.

Check the quadriceps muscle in the anterior thigh for any atrophy. Because it is the prime mover of knee extension, this muscle is important for joint stability during weight-bearing.

Atrophy occurs with disuse or chronic disorders. First, it appears in the medial part of the muscle, although it is difficult to note because the vastus medialis is relatively small.

Enhance **palpation** with the knee in the supine position with complete relaxation of the quadriceps muscle. Start high on the anterior thigh, about 10 cm above the patella. Palpate with your left thumb and fingers in a grasping fashion (Fig. 22-31). Proceed down toward the knee, exploring the region of the suprapatellar pouch. Note the consistency of the tissues. The muscles and soft tissues should feel solid, and the joint should feel smooth, with no warmth, tenderness, thickening, or nodularity.

Feels fluctuant or boggy with synovitis of suprapatellar pouch.

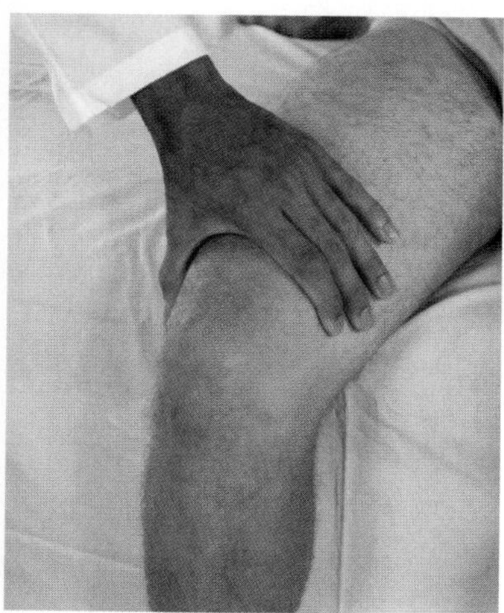

22-31

Normal Range of Findings

When swelling occurs, you need to distinguish whether it is due to soft tissue swelling or increased fluid in the joint. The tests for the bulge sign and ballottement of the patella aid this assessment.

Bulge Sign. For swelling in the suprapatellar pouch, the bulge sign confirms the presence of small amounts of fluid as you try to move the fluid from one side of the joint to the other. Firmly stroke up on the medial aspect of the knee two or three times to displace any fluid (Fig. 22-32, *A*). Tap the lateral aspect (Fig. 22-32, *B*). Watch the medial side in the hollow for a distinct bulge from a fluid wave. Normally, none is present.

Abnormal Findings

The bulge sign occurs with very small amounts of effusion, 4 to 8 mL, from fluid flowing across the joint (Fig. 22-33, *C*).

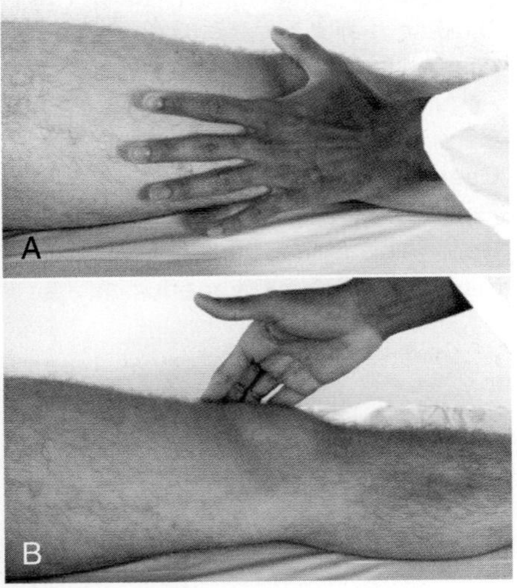

22-32 B, Bulge sign.

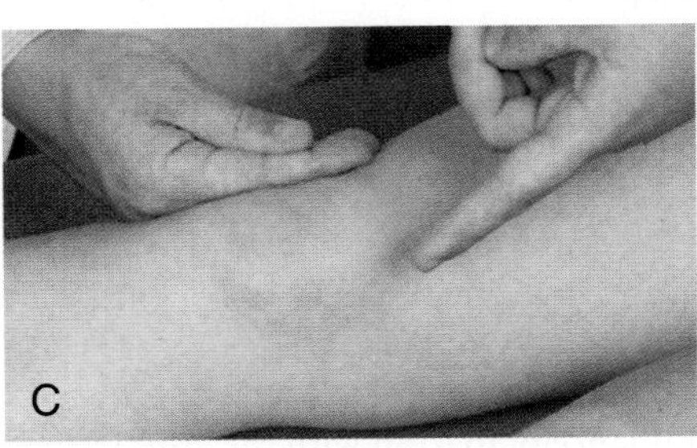

C, Note bulge sign.

Ballottement of the Patella. This test is reliable when larger amounts of fluid are present. Use your left hand to compress the suprapatellar pouch to move any fluid into the knee joint. With your right hand, push the patella sharply against the femur. If no fluid is present, the patella is already snug against the femur (Fig. 22-33, *A*).

If fluid has collected, your tap on the patella moves it through the fluid and you will hear a tap as the patella bumps up on the femoral condyles (Fig. 22-33, *B*).

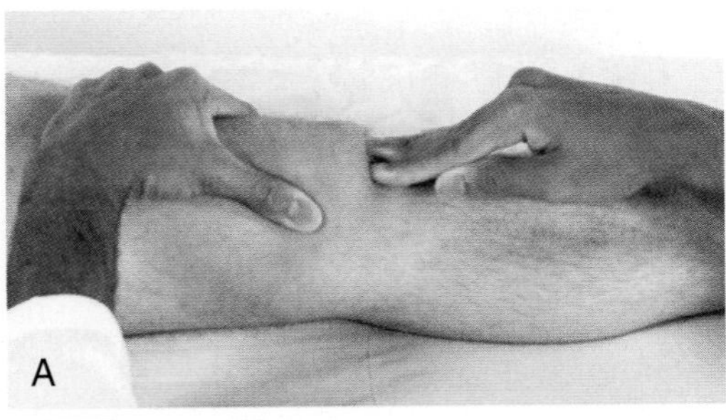

22-33 Ballottement.

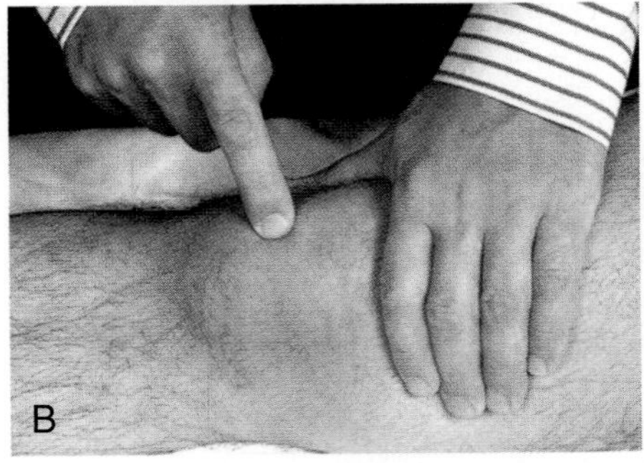

Normal Range of Findings

Continue palpation and explore the tibiofemoral joint (Fig. 22-34). Note smooth joint margins and absence of pain. Palpate the infrapatellar fat pad and the patella. Check for crepitus by holding your hand on the patella as the knee is flexed and extended. Some crepitus in an otherwise asymptomatic knee is not uncommon.

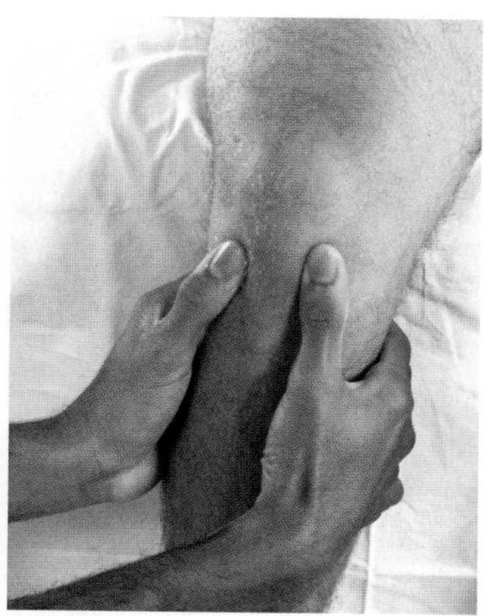

22-34

Check ROM (Fig. 22-35) by asking the person to:

Instructions to Person	Motion and Expected Range
• Bend each knee.	Flexion of 130 to 150 degrees.
• Extend each knee.	A straight line of 0 degrees in some persons; a hyperextension of 15 degrees in others.
• Check knee ROM during ambulation.	

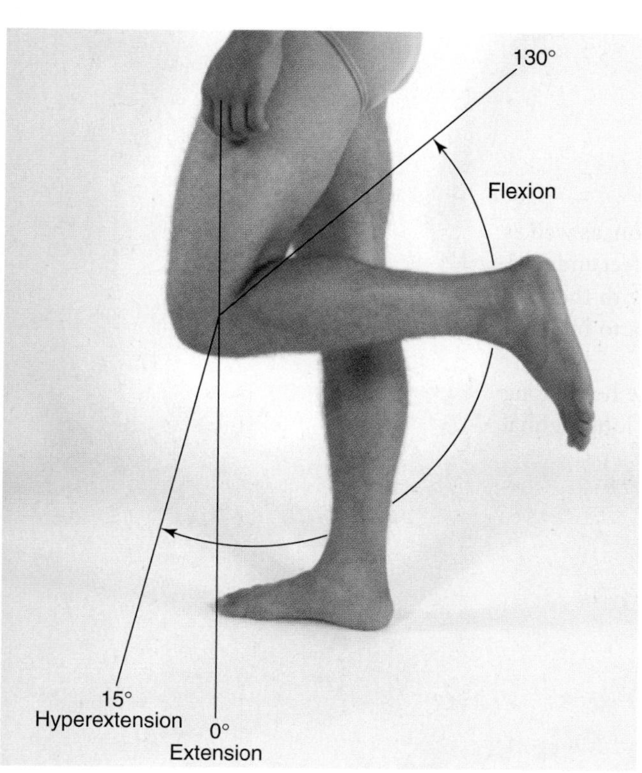

22-35

Abnormal Findings

Irregular bony margins occur with osteoarthritis.

Pain at joint line.

Pronounced crepitus is significant, and it occurs with degenerative diseases of the knee.

Limited ROM.

Contracture.

Pain with motion.

Limp.

Sudden locking—the person is unable to extend the knee fully. This usually occurs with a painful and audible "pop" or "click." Sudden buckling, or "giving way," occurs with ligament injury, which causes weakness and instability.

Normal Range of Findings

Check **muscle strength** by asking the person to maintain knee flexion while you oppose by trying to pull the leg forward. Muscle extension is demonstrated by the person's success in rising from a seated position in a low chair or by rising from a squat without using the hands for support.

Special Test for Meniscal Tears

McMurray Test. Perform this test when the person has reported a history of trauma followed by locking, giving way, or local pain in the knee. Position the person supine as you stand on the affected side. Hold the heel, and flex the knee and hip. Place your other hand on the knee with fingers on the medial side. Rotate the leg in and out to loosen the joint. Externally rotate the leg, and push a valgus (inward) stress on the knee. Then slowly extend the knee. Normally, the leg extends smoothly with no pain (Fig. 22-36).

Abnormal Findings

If you hear or feel a "click," McMurray test is positive for a torn meniscus.

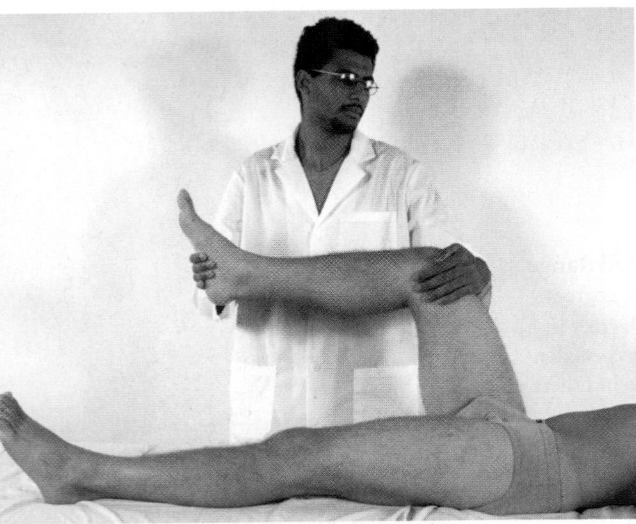

22-36 McMurray test.

Ankle and Foot

Inspect while the person is in a sitting, non–weight-bearing position, as well as when standing and walking. Compare both feet, noting position of feet and toes, contour of joints, and skin characteristics. The foot should align with the long axis of the lower leg; an imaginary line would fall from midpatella to between the first and second toes.

Weight-bearing should fall on the middle of the foot, from the heel, along the midfoot, to between the second and third toes. Most feet have a longitudinal arch, although that can vary normally from "flat feet" to a high instep.

Normal Range of Findings

The toes point straight forward and lie flat. The ankles (malleoli) are smooth bony prominences. Normally, the skin is smooth, with even coloring and no lesions. Note the locations of any calluses or bursal reactions because they reveal areas of abnormal friction. Examining well-worn shoes helps assess areas of wear and accommodation.

Support the ankle by grasping the heel with your fingers while palpating with your thumbs (Fig. 22-38). Explore the joint spaces. They should feel smooth and depressed, with no fullness, swelling, or tenderness.

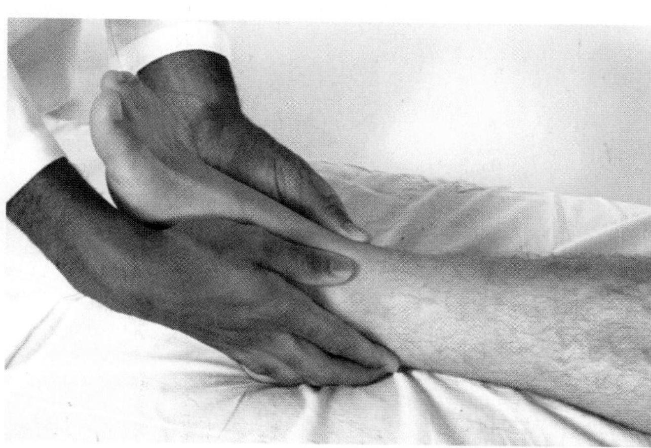

22-38

Palpate the metatarsophalangeal joints between your thumb on the dorsum and your fingers on the plantar surface (Fig. 22-39).

Using a pinching motion of your thumb and forefinger, palpate the interphalangeal joints on the medial and lateral sides of the toes.

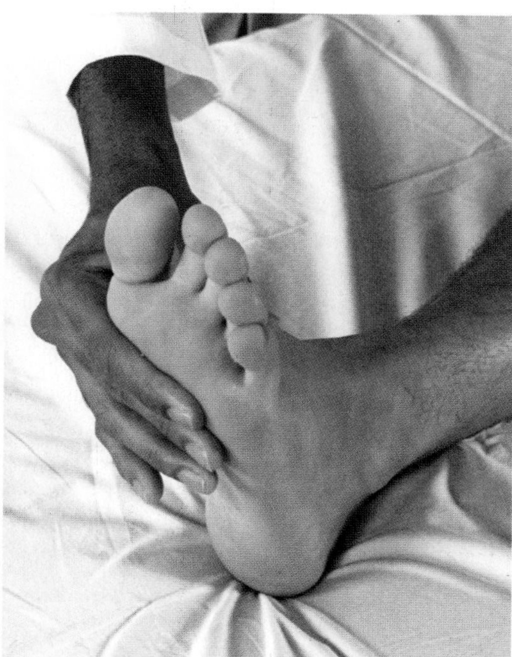

22-39

Abnormal Findings

In **hallux valgus**, the distal part of the great toe is directed *away* from the body midline (Fig. 22-37).

Hammertoes.

Swelling or inflammation.

Calluses. Ulcers (see Table 22-6, Abnormalities of the Ankle and Foot, p. 616).

Swelling or inflammation.

Tenderness.

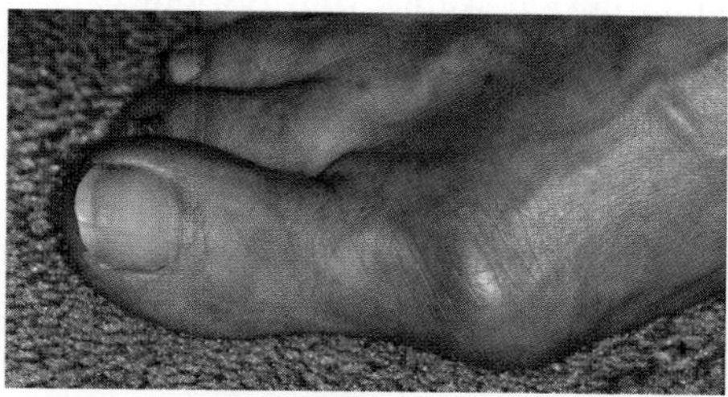

22-37 Hallux valgus with bunion.

Swelling or inflammation.

Tenderness.

Normal Range of Findings	Abnormal Findings

Test ROM (Fig. 22-40) by asking the person to:

Instructions to Person	Motion and Expected Range
• Point toes toward the floor.	Plantar flexion of 45 degrees.
• Point toes toward the nose.	Dorsiflexion of 20 degrees (Fig. 22-40, *A*).
• Turn soles of feet out, then in. (Stabilize the ankle with one hand, hold heel with the other to test the subtalar joint.)	Eversion of 20 degrees. Inversion of 30 degrees (Fig. 22-40, *B*).
• Flex and straighten toes.	

Limited ROM.
Pain with motion.

Assess **muscle strength** by asking the person to maintain dorsiflexion and plantar flexion against your resistance.

Unable to hold flexion.

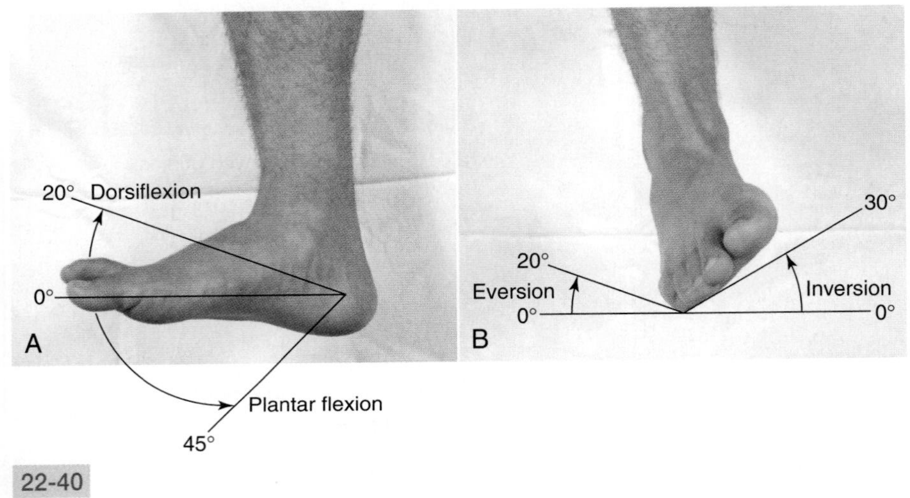

22-40

SPINE

The person should be standing, draped in a gown open at the back. Place yourself far enough back so that you can see the entire back. **Inspect** and note whether the spine is straight (1) by following an imaginary vertical line from the head through the spinous processes and down through the gluteal cleft and (2) by noting equal horizontal positions for the shoulders, scapulae, iliac crests, and gluteal folds and equal spaces between the arm and lateral thorax on the two sides (Fig. 22-41, *A*). The person's knees and feet should be aligned with the trunk and should be pointing forward.

A difference in shoulder elevation and in level of scapulae and iliac crests occurs with scoliosis (see Table 22-7, Abnormalities of the Spine, p. 617).

Normal Range of Findings

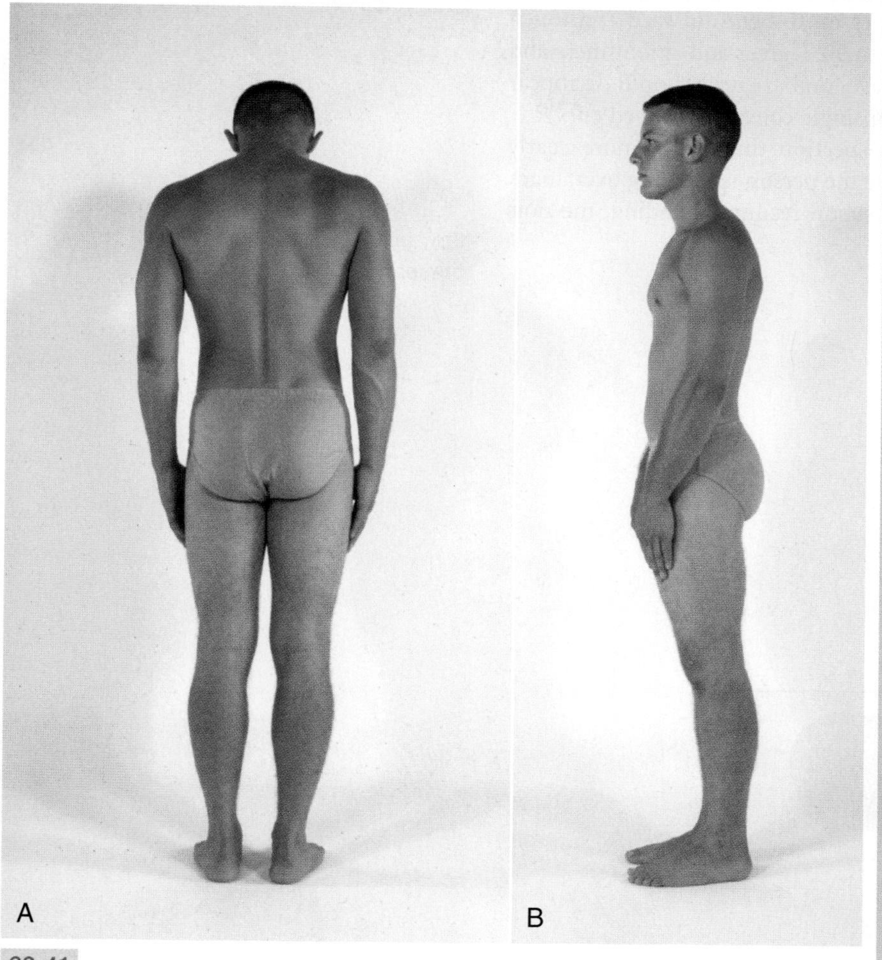

22-41

From the side, note the normal convex thoracic curve and concave lumbar curve (Fig. 22-41, *B*). An enhanced thoracic curve, or kyphosis, is common in aging people. A pronounced lumbar curve, or lordosis, is common in obese people.

Palpate the spinous processes. Normally, they are straight and not tender. Palpate the paravertebral muscles; they should feel firm with no tenderness or spasm.

Abnormal Findings

Lateral tilting and forward bending occur with a herniated nucleus pulposus (see Table 22-7).

Spinal curvature.

Tenderness. Spasm of paravertebral muscles.

Chronic axial skeletal pain occurs with Fibromyalgia Syndrome (see Table 22-9, p. 619).

Normal Range of Findings	Abnormal Findings
Check **ROM** of the spine by asking the person to bend forward and touch the toes (Fig. 22-42). Look for flexion of 75 to 90 degrees and smoothness and symmetry of movement. Note that the concave lumbar curve should disappear with this motion and the back should have a single convex C-shaped curve.	
If you suspect a spinal curvature during inspection, this may be more clearly seen when the person touches the toes. While the person is bending over, mark a dot on each spinous process. When the person resumes standing, the dots should form a straight vertical line.	If the dots form a slight S-shape when the person stands, a spinal curve is present.

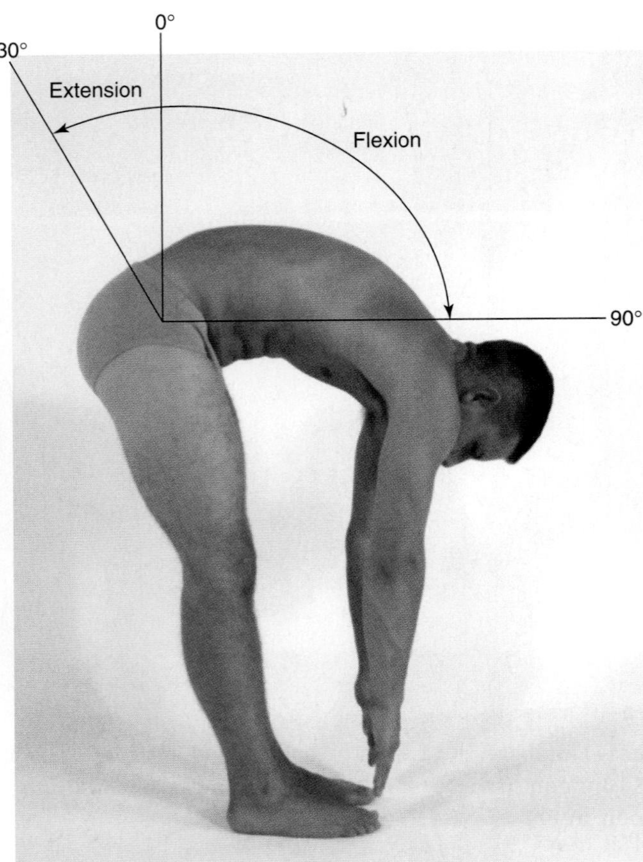

22-42

Stabilize the pelvis with your hands. Check ROM (Fig. 22-43) by asking the person to:

Instructions to Person	Motion and Expected Range	Abnormal Findings
• Bend sideways.	Lateral bending of 35 degrees (Fig. 22-43, *A*).	Limited ROM.
• Bend backward.	Hyperextension of 30 degrees.	Pain with motion.
• Twist shoulders to one side, then the other.	Rotation of 30 degrees, bilaterally (Fig. 22-43, *B*).	

Normal Range of Findings | **Abnormal Findings**

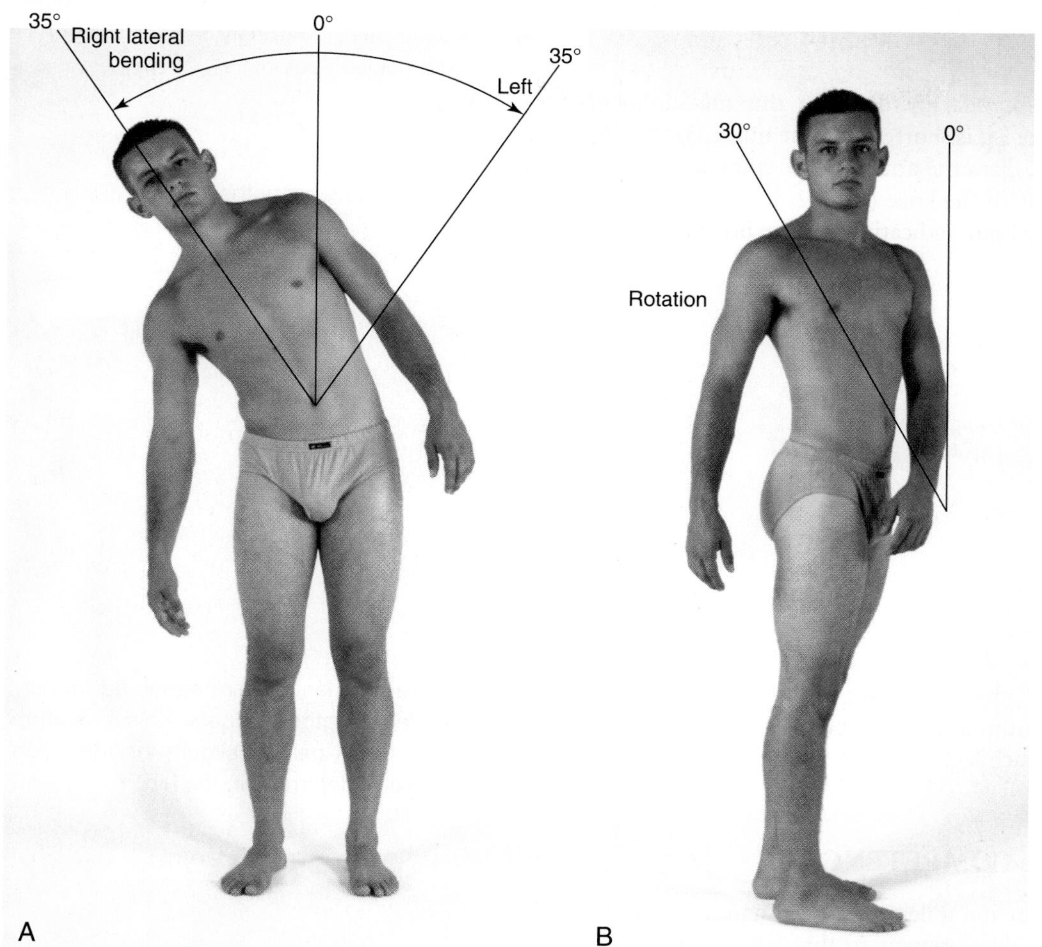

22-43

These maneuvers reveal only gross restriction. Movement is still possible even if some spinal fusion has occurred.

Finally, ask the person to walk on his or her toes for a few steps; then return walking on the heels.

Straight Leg Raising or Lasègue Test. These maneuvers reproduce back and leg pain and help confirm the presence of a herniated nucleus pulposus. Straight leg raising while keeping the knee extended normally produces no pain. Raise the affected leg just short of the point where it produces pain. Then dorsiflex the foot (Fig. 22-44).

Lasègue test is positive if it reproduces sciatic pain. If lifting the affected leg reproduces sciatic pain, it confirms the presence of a herniated nucleus pulposus.

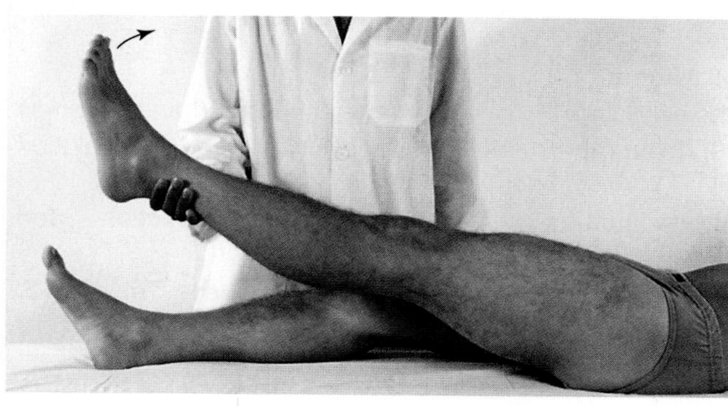

22-44

Normal Range of Findings	Abnormal Findings

Raise the unaffected leg while leaving the other leg flat. Inquire about the involved side.

If lifting the unaffected leg reproduces sciatic pain, it strongly suggests a herniated nucleus pulposus.

Measure Leg Length Discrepancy. Perform this measurement if you need to determine whether one leg is shorter than the other. For *true leg length,* measure between *fixed* points, from the anterior iliac spine to the medial malleolus, crossing the medial side of the knee (Fig. 22-45). Normally, these measurements are equal or within 1 cm, indicating no true bone discrepancy.

Unequal leg lengths.

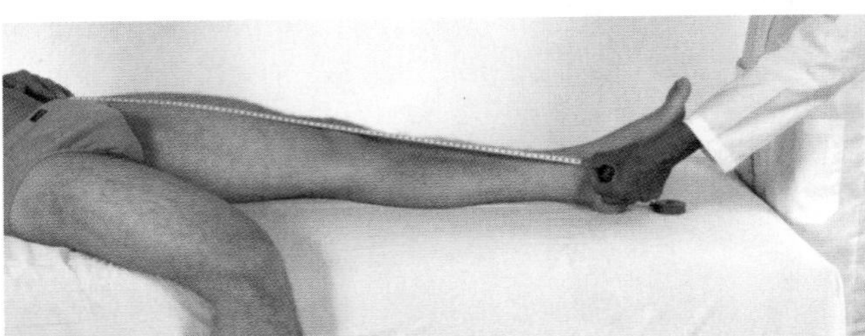

22-45

Sometimes the true leg length is equal but the legs still look unequal. For *apparent leg length,* measure from a nonfixed point (the umbilicus) to a fixed point (medial malleolus) on each leg.

True leg lengths are equal, but apparent leg lengths unequal—this condition occurs with pelvic obliquity or adduction or flexion deformity in the hip.

DEVELOPMENTAL COMPETENCE

Be familiar with the developmental milestones. Keep handy a concise chart of the usual sequence of motor development so that you can refer to expected findings for the age of each child you are examining. Use the Denver II test to screen the fine and gross motor skills for the child's age.

Because some overlap exists between the musculoskeletal and neurologic examinations, the assessments of muscle tone, resting posture, and motor activity are discussed in Chapter 23.

Infants

Examine the infant fully undressed and lying on the back. Take care to place the newborn on a warming table to maintain body temperature.

Feet and Legs. Start with the feet and work your way up the extremities. Note any *positional deformities,* a residual of fetal positioning. Often the newborn's feet are not held straight but, instead, in a varus (apart) or valgus (together) position. It is important to distinguish whether this position is flexible (and thus usually self-correctable) or fixed. Scratch the outside of the bottom of the foot. If the deformity is self-correctable, the foot assumes a normal right angle to the lower leg. Or immobilize the heel with one hand and gently push the forefoot to the neutral position with the other hand. If you can move it to neutral position, it is flexible.

A true deformity is fixed and assumes a right angle only with forced manipulation or not at all.

Note the relationship of the forefoot to the hindfoot. Commonly, the hindfoot is in alignment with the lower leg and just the forefoot angles inward. This forefoot adduction is *metatarsus adductus.* It is usually present at birth and usually resolves spontaneously by age 3 years.

Metatarsus varus—adduction and inversion of forefoot.

Talipes equinovarus (see Table 22-8, Common Congenital or Pediatric Abnormalities, p. 618).

Normal Range of Findings

Check for *tibial torsion,* a twisting of the tibia. Place both feet flat on the table, and push to flex up the knees. With the patella and the tibial tubercle in a straight line, place your fingers on the malleoli. In an infant, note that a line connecting the four malleoli is parallel to the table.

Tibial torsion may originate from intrauterine positioning and then may be exacerbated at a later age by continuous sitting in a reverse tailor position, the "TV squat." This is sitting with the buttocks on the floor and the lower legs splayed back and out on either side.

Hips. Check the hips for *congenital dislocation.* The most reliable method is **Ortolani maneuver,** which should be done at every professional visit until the infant is 1 year old. With the infant supine, flex the knees holding your thumbs on the inner mid-thighs and your fingers outside on the hips touching the greater trochanters. Adduct the legs until your thumbs touch (Fig. 22-46, *A*). Then gently lift and *abduct,* moving the knees apart and down so their lateral aspects touch the table (Fig. 22-46, *B*). This normally feels smooth and has no sound.

Abnormal Findings

More than 20 degrees of deviation; or if lateral malleolus is anterior to medial malleolus, it indicates tibial torsion.

With a dislocated hip, the head of the femur is not cupped in the acetabulum but rests posterior to it.

Hip instability feels like a clunk as the head of the femur pops back into place. This is a *positive Ortolani sign* and warrants referral.

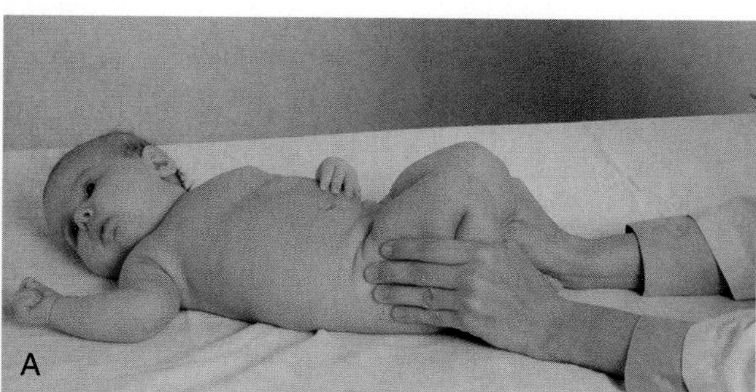
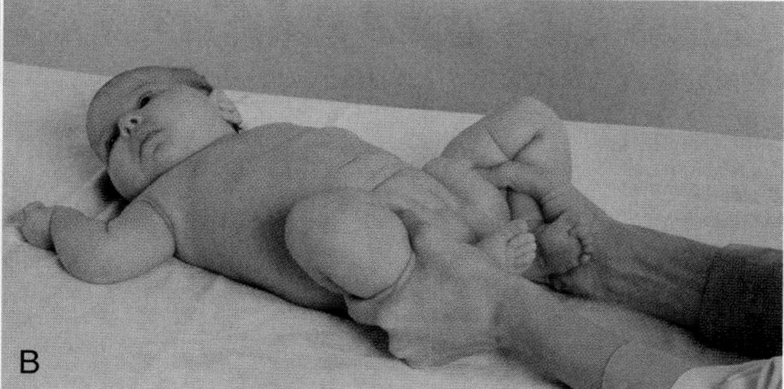

22-46 Ortolani maneuver.

The **Allis test** also is used to check for hip dislocation by comparing leg lengths (Fig. 22-47). Place the baby's feet flat on the table and flex the knees up. Scan the tops of the knees; normally, they are at the same elevation.

Finding one knee significantly lower than the other is a positive indication of Allis' sign and suggests hip dislocation.

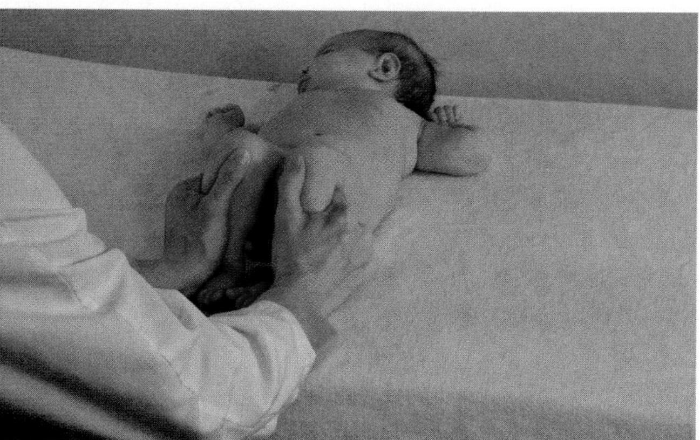

22-47 Allis test.

Objective Data

Normal Range of Findings	Abnormal Findings
Note the gluteal folds. Normally, they are equal on both sides. However, some asymmetry may occur in healthy children.	Unequal gluteal folds may accompany hip dislocation after 2 to 3 months of age.
Hands and Arms. Inspect the hands, noting shape, number, and position of fingers and palmar creases.	Polydactyly is the presence of extra fingers or toes. Syndactyly is webbing between adjacent fingers or toes (see Table 22-4). A simian crease is a single palmar crease that occurs with Down syndrome, accompanied by short broad fingers, incurving of little fingers, and low-set thumbs.
Palpate the length of the clavicles because the clavicle is the bone most frequently fractured during birth. The clavicles should feel smooth, regular, and without crepitus. Also note equal ROM of arms during Moro's reflex.	Fractured clavicle: Note irregularity at the fracture site, crepitus, and angulation. The site has rapid callus formation with a palpable lump within a few weeks. Observe limited arm ROM and unilateral response to Moro's reflex.
Back. Lift up the infant and examine the back. Note the normal single C-curve of the newborn's spine (Fig. 22-48). By 2 months of age, the infant can lift the head while prone. This builds the concave cervical spinal curve and indicates normal forearm strength. Inspect the length of the spine for any tuft of hair, dimple in midline, cyst, or mass. Normally, none are present.	A tuft of hair over a dimple in the midline may indicate spina bifida. A small dimple in the midline—anywhere from the head to the coccyx—suggests dermoid sinus. Mass, such as meningocele.

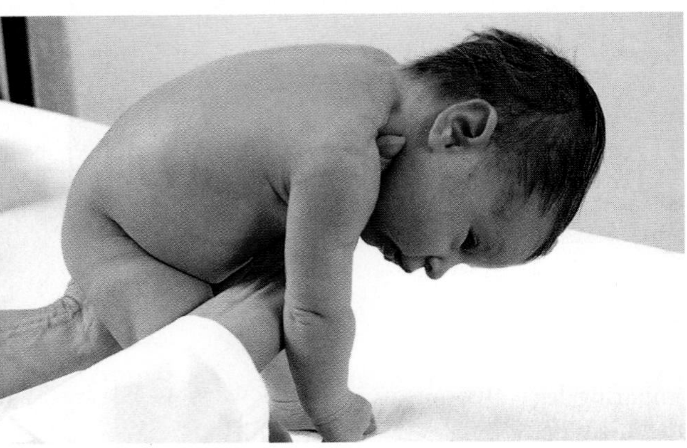

22-48

Normal Range of Findings	Abnormal Findings
Observe ROM through spontaneous movement of extremities.	
Test muscle strength by lifting up the infant with your hands under the axillae (Fig. 22-49). A baby with normal muscle strength wedges securely between your hands.	A baby who starts to "slip" between your hands shows weakness of the shoulder muscles.

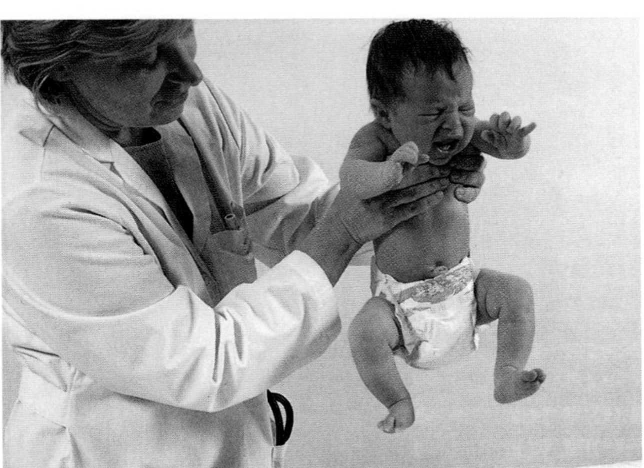

22-49

Normal Range of Findings | Abnormal Findings

Preschool-Age and School-Age Children

Once the infant learns to crawl and then to walk, the waking hours show perpetual motion. This is convenient for your musculoskeletal assessment; you can observe the muscles and joints during spontaneous play before a table-top examination. Most young children enjoy showing off their physical accomplishments. For specific motions, coax the toddler: "Show me how you can walk to Mom," "Climb the step stool." Ask the preschooler to hop on one foot or to jump.

Back. While the child is standing, note the posture. From behind, you should note a "plumb line" from the back of the head, along the spine, to the middle of the sacrum. Shoulders are level within 1 cm, and scapulae are symmetric. From the side, lordosis is common throughout childhood, appearing more pronounced in children with a protuberant abdomen.

Lordosis is marked with muscular dystrophy and rickets.

Legs and Feet. Anteriorly, note the leg position. A "bowlegged" stance *(genu varum)* is a lateral bowing of the legs (Fig. 22-50, *A*). It is present when you measure a persistent space of more than 2.5 cm between the knees when the medial malleoli are together. Genu varum is normal for 1 year after the child begins walking. The child may walk with a waddling gait. This resolves with growth; no treatment is indicated.

Severe bowing or unilateral bowing also occurs with rickets.

"Knock knees" *(genu valgum)* are present when there is more than 2.5 cm between the medial malleoli when the knees are together (Fig. 22-50, *B*). It occurs normally between 2 and 3½ years of age. Also, treatment is not indicated. (Note: To remember the two conditions, remember to link the r's and g's: genu va**r**um—knees apa**r**t; genu val**g**um—knees to**g**ether.)

Genu valgum also occurs with rickets, poliomyelitis, and syphilis.

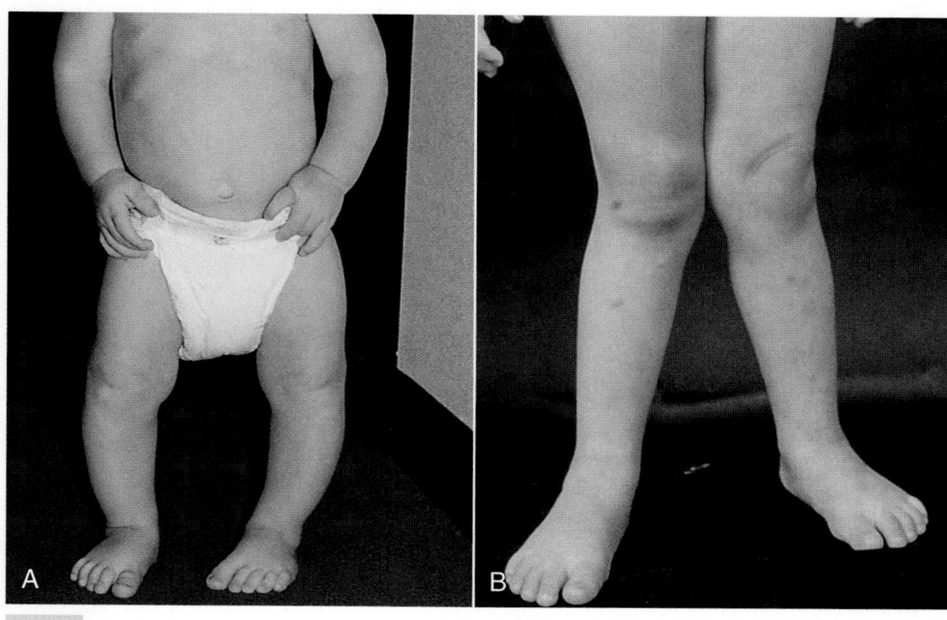

22-50 **A,** Genu varum. **B,** Genu valgum.

Often, parents tell you they are concerned about the child's foot development. The most common questions are about "flatfeet" and "pigeon toes." Flatfoot *(pes planus)* is pronation, or turning in, of the medial side of the foot. The young child may look flatfooted because the normal longitudinal arch is concealed by a fat pad until age 3 years. When standing begins, the child takes a broad-based stance, which causes pronation. Thus pronation is common between 12 and 30 months. You can see it best from behind the child, where the medial side of the foot drops down and in.

Pronation beyond 30 months.

Normal Range of Findings

Pigeon toes, or toeing in, are demonstrated when the child tends to walk on the lateral side of the foot, and the longitudinal arch looks higher than normal. It often starts as a forefoot adduction, which usually corrects spontaneously by age 3 years, as long as the foot is flexible.

Check the child's gait while walking away from and returning to you. Let the child wear socks, because a cold tile floor will distort the usual gait. From 1 to 2 years of age, expect a broad-based gait, with arms out for balance. Weight-bearing falls on the inside of the foot. From 3 years of age, the base narrows and the arms are closer to the sides. Inspect the shoes for spots of greatest wear to aid your judgment of the gait. Normally, the shoes wear more on the outside of the heel and the inside of the toe.

Check the **Trendelenburg sign** to screen progressive subluxation of the hip. Watching from behind, ask the child to stand on one leg, then the other (Fig. 22-51, *A*). Watch the buttocks and iliac crests; they should stay level when weight is shifted. Remember that you are testing the side that is bearing weight.

Abnormal Findings

Toeing in from forefoot adduction that is fixed, or lasts beyond age 3 years.

Toeing in from tibial torsion.

Limp, usually caused by trauma, fatigue, or hip disease.

Abnormal gait patterns (see Chapter 23).

The *positive Trendelenburg* sign occurs with severe subluxation of one hip. When the child stands on the good leg, the pelvis looks level. When the child stands on the affected leg, the pelvis drops toward the "good" side and the opposite buttock falls. The hip abductors on the standing side are too weak to hold the pelvis level (Fig. 22-51, *B*).

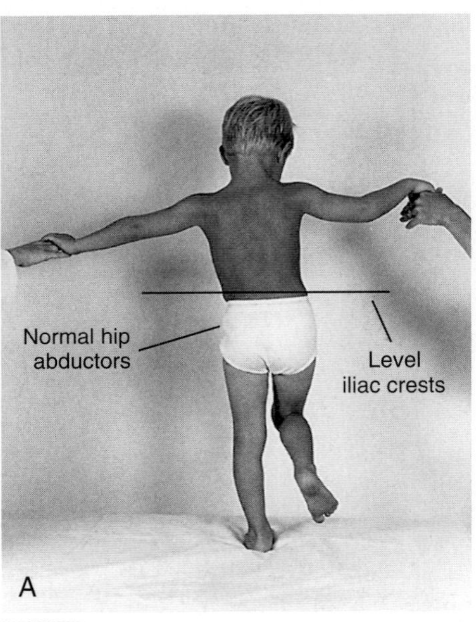

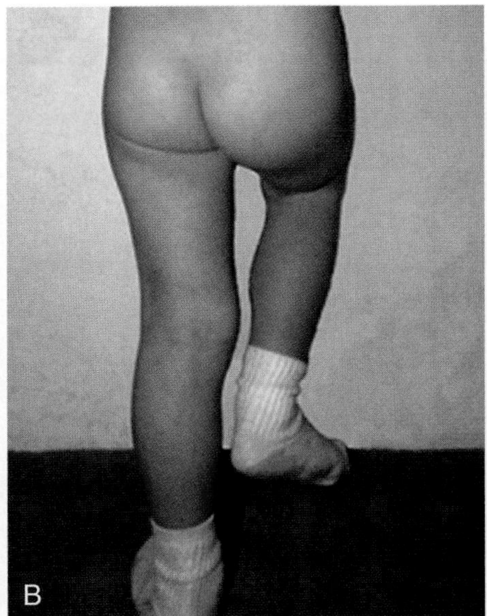

22-51

The child may sit for the remainder of the examination. Start with the feet and hands of the child from 2 to 6 years of age because the child is happy to show these off, and proceed through the examination described earlier.

Particularly, check the arm for full ROM and presence of pain. Look for subluxation of the elbow (head of the radius). This occurs most often between 2 and 4 years of age as a result of forceful removal of clothing or dangling while adults suspend the child by the hands.

Palpate the bones, joints, and muscles of the extremities as described in the adult examination.

Inability to supinate the hand while the arm is flexed, together with pain in elbow, indicates subluxation of the head of the radius.

Pain or tenderness in extremities is usually caused by trauma or infection.

Normal Range of Findings

Abnormal Findings

Fractures are usually due to trauma and are exhibited as an inability to use the area, a deformity, or an excess motion in the involved bone with pain and crepitation.

Enlargement of the tibial tubercles with tenderness suggests Osgood-Schlatter disease (see Table 22-5).

Adolescents

Proceed with the musculoskeletal examination you provide for the adult, except pay special note to spinal posture. Kyphosis is common during adolescence because of chronic poor posture. Be aware of the risk for sports-related injuries with the adolescent, because sports participation and competition often peak with this age-group.

The U.S. Preventive Services Task Force[24] does not support the routine screening of asymptomatic adolescents for idiopathic scoliosis. They found that most cases detected through screening did not progress to clinically significant scoliosis. Also, the harms of unnecessary follow-up visits and psychological adverse effects of brace wear did not offset any potential benefits of screening. However, when idiopathic scoliosis is discovered incidentally or when the teen or parent expresses concern, clinicians should be prepared to evaluate.

Screen for scoliosis with the *forward bend test* (Fig. 22-52). Seat yourself behind the standing child, and ask the child to stand with the feet shoulder-width apart and bend forward slowly to touch the toes. Expect a straight vertical spine while standing and also while bending forward. Posterior ribs should be symmetric, with equal elevation of shoulders, scapulae, and iliac crests. You may wish to mark each spinous process with a felt marker. The lineup of ink dots highlights even a subtle curve.

Scoliosis is most apparent during the preadolescent growth spurt. Asymmetry suggests scoliosis—ribs hump up on one side as child bends forward, and with unequal landmark elevation (see Table 22-7).

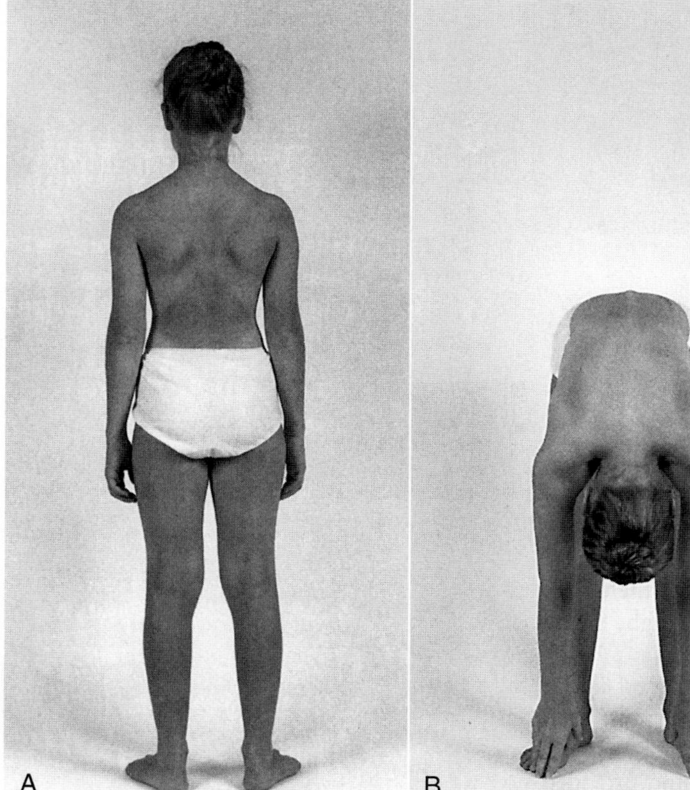

22-52

Normal Range of Findings

The Pregnant Woman

Proceed through the examination described in the adult section. Expected postural changes in pregnancy include progressive lordosis and, toward the third trimester, anterior cervical flexion, kyphosis, and slumped shoulders (Fig. 22-53, *A*). When the pregnancy is at term, the protuberant abdomen and the relaxed mobility in the joints create the characteristic "waddling" gait (Fig. 22-53, *B*).

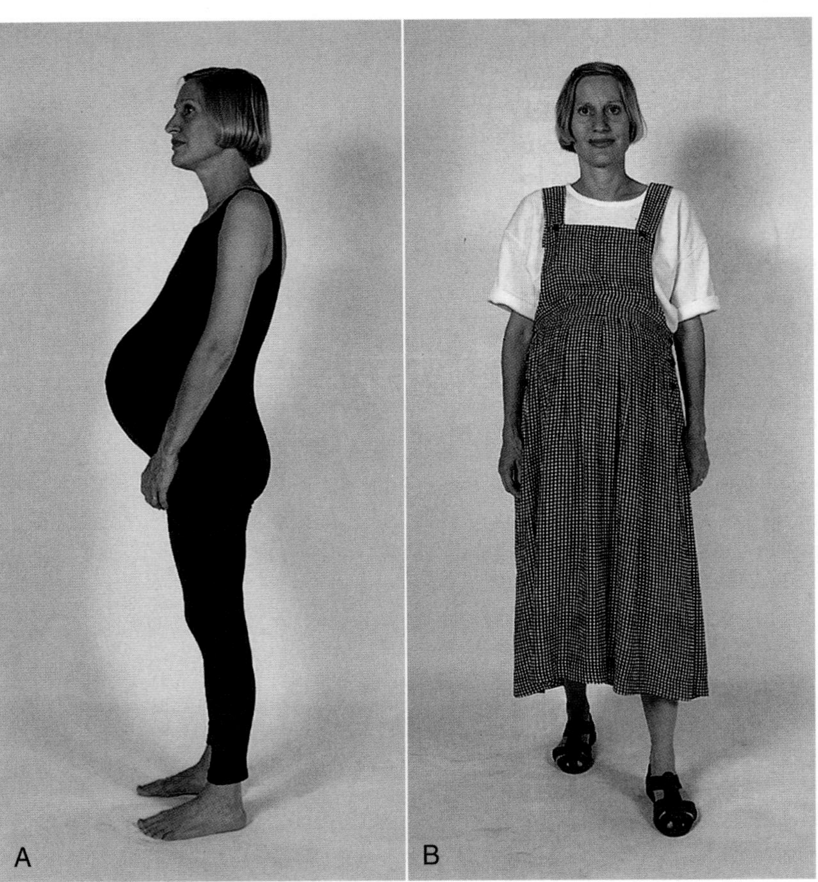

22-53

The Aging Adult

Postural changes include a decrease in height, more apparent in the eighth and ninth decades (Fig. 22-54). "Lengthening of the arm-trunk axis" describes this shortening of the trunk with comparatively long extremities. Kyphosis is common, with a backward head tilt to compensate. This creates the outline of a figure 3 when you view this older adult from the left side. Slight flexion of hips and knees is also common.

Contour changes include a decrease of fat in the body periphery and fat deposition over the abdomen and hips. The bony prominences become more marked.

For most older adults, ROM testing proceeds as described earlier. ROM and muscle strength are much the same as with the younger adult, provided no musculoskeletal illnesses or arthritic changes are present.

Abnormal Findings

Normal Range of Findings	Abnormal Findings

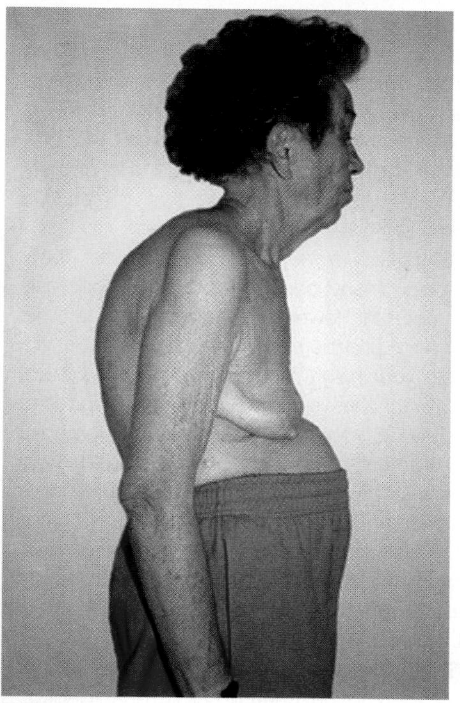

22-54

Functional Assessment. For those with advanced aging changes, arthritic changes, or musculoskeletal disability, perform a **functional assessment for ADLs.** This applies the ROM and muscle strength assessments to the accomplishment of specific activities. You need to determine adequate and safe performance of functions essential for independent home life. See Chapter 30 for further assessments.

Instructions to Person	Common Adaptation for Aging Changes
1. Walk (with shoes on).	Shuffling pattern; swaying; arms out to help balance; broader base of support; person may watch feet.
2. Climb up stairs.	Person holds hand rail; may haul body up with it; may lead with favored (stronger) leg.
3. Walk down stairs.	Holds hand rail, sometimes with both hands. If the person is weak, he or she may descend sideways, lowering the weaker leg first. If the person is unsteady, he or she may watch feet.
4. Pick up object from floor.	Person often bends at waist instead of bending knees; holds furniture to support while bending and straightening.
5. Rise up from sitting in chair.	Person uses arms to push off chair arms, upper trunk leans forward before body straightens, feet planted wide in broad base of support.
6. Rise up from lying in bed.	May roll to one side, push with arms to lift up torso, grab bedside table to increase leverage.

PROMOTING A HEALTHY LIFESTYLE: PREVENTING OSTEOPOROSIS

Don't Overlook Osteoporosis!

Your bones are living tissues that are continually growing and changing. Every day, old bone tissue dissolves and is replaced with new, stronger bone tissue. New bone appears at a faster rate than the old bone disappears. But as we age, the opposite begins to occur. When this happens, bones can become "spongy," weak, and more likely to break with even the slightest twist or bump. This condition is called *osteoporosis.* The bones of the wrist, hip, and spine are most often affected. Prevention of osteoporosis is important because, although there is available treatment for osteoporosis, there is no cure. The National Institutes of Health (NIH) has developed an interactive bone health checkup—*Check Up On Your Bones*—to identify the most common red flags and risk factors, based on the U.S. Surgeon General's Report on Osteoporosis and Bone Health. In addition, the National Osteoporosis Foundation (NOF) shares five steps to prevent osteoporosis. No one step by itself is enough to prevent osteoporosis, but doing all five may.

Five Steps to Bone Health and Osteoporosis Prevention*

1. **DIET.** The bottom line is you need the daily recommended amounts of calcium and vitamin D.
   a. **Drink milk.** Low-fat and skim milk, nonfat yogurt, and reduced-fat cheese are healthy sources of calcium. Fortified milk products also contain vitamin D, which is needed to absorb calcium.
   b. **Go fish.** Canned salmon and sardines that are packed with their bones are also rich in calcium. Further, oily fish such as mackerel is rich in vitamin D.
   c. **Eat greens with gusto.** Leafy green vegetables have a lot of calcium. Fill up on broccoli, kale, Swiss chard, turnip greens, and bok choy. In addition to the calcium, you will also get the benefits of potassium and vitamin K, which help block calcium loss from bones.
   d. **Try soy.** Soy contains calcium and plant estrogens. Try substituting soy flour for regular flour in recipes, nibbling on soybean "nuts," or drinking soy milk.
   e. **Limit caffeine.** Caffeine causes the body to excrete calcium more readily. Caffeine is in coffee, tea, hot chocolate, and many sodas.
   f. **Eat onions.** Although onions are not known to have any nutritive value, they appear to reduce the bone breakdown process that can lead to osteoporosis.
2. **EXERCISE.** The key here is weight-bearing. Your bones and muscles must work against gravity for a bone-building effect. A regular program of weight-bearing exercise for at least 30 minutes three times a week is recommended as the minimum. Try walking, low-impact aerobics, dancing, or stationary cycling. The bonus: by improving your posture, balance, and flexibility, it also reduces your risk for falls. Don't forget sunshine either. Sunshine helps the body produce vitamin D. About 15 minutes of sunshine a day is all that is needed to maintain a good vitamin D supply.
3. **LIFESTYLE.** Avoid smoking and excessive alcohol, and seek help for depression. Smokers have twice the risk for spinal and hip fractures. Further, fractures heal slower in smokers and are more apt to heal improperly. Too much alcohol prevents your body from absorbing calcium. And don't let depression linger. Seek help. Research has shown that women with clinical depression have lower bone densities.
4. **MEDICAL OPTIONS.** Talk to your health care provider about bone health. Although many people consider osteoporosis prevention to be important, fewer than half discuss the topic with their health care providers or undergo bone density screening. Ask that your height be measured on an annual basis. A loss of 1 to 2 inches is an early sign of undiagnosed vertebral fractures and osteoporosis. Seek treatment for those conditions that can threaten bone density, including thyroid disease, certain intestinal and kidney diseases, and some cancers. Also, remember that other medications may contribute to bone loss. These medications include corticosteroids, anticoagulants, thyroid supplements, and certain anticonvulsants. **Bone-density tests** are the only way to predict your fracture risk and diagnose osteoporosis.
5. **SUPPLEMENTS.** When appropriate, take supplemental calcium. Most people do not get enough calcium in their diets, and supplements may help make up the difference. Make sure the supplement contains vitamin D, which helps your body absorb the calcium. For women, your daily requirements vary by age:
   19 to 50 years: 1000 mg calcium; 200 IU vitamin D
   51 to 70 years: 1200 mg calcium; 400 IU vitamin D
   Older than 70 years: 1200 mg calcium; 600 IU vitamin D

Resources

Best Bones Forever. Website: www.bestbonesforever.gov/parents/.
Check Up On Your Bones. Website: www.niams.nih.gov/Health_Info/Bone/Optool/index.asp.
Grocery List. Website: www.bestbonesforever.gov/parents/foods/shopping.cfm.
National Institutes of Health: Osteoporosis and related bone diseases—National Resource Center. Website: www.niams.nih.gov/Health_Info/Bone/.
National Osteoporosis Foundation. Website: www.nof.org/.
U.S. Surgeon General's Report on Osteoporosis and Bone Health. Website: www.surgeongeneral.gov/library/bonehealth/.

Another useful resource for patients is NIH's bilingual novella entitled "Isabel's Story." The story is about a 50-year-old woman who breaks her wrist and discovers through bone densitometry that she has osteoporosis. It is available to download from www.niams.nih.gov/Health_Info/Bone/osteoporosis/Isabel_story.asp.

And, remember, it is never too early to raise awareness about bone health, especially in young girls. NOF has teamed up with the *Best Bones Forever!*™ campaign, which focuses on girls ages 9 to 14. They even provide a printable *Grocery List* that identifies foods high in calcium and vitamin D, as well as a *Calcium Calculator.*

*Source: Bone Health and Osteoporosis: A Report of the Surgeon General, 2004.

DOCUMENTATION AND CRITICAL THINKING

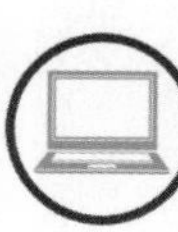

Sample Charting

SUBJECTIVE

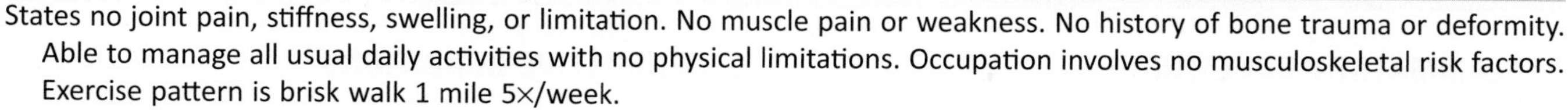

States no joint pain, stiffness, swelling, or limitation. No muscle pain or weakness. No history of bone trauma or deformity. Able to manage all usual daily activities with no physical limitations. Occupation involves no musculoskeletal risk factors. Exercise pattern is brisk walk 1 mile 5×/week.

OBJECTIVE

Joints and muscles symmetric; no swelling, masses, deformity; normal spinal curvature. No tenderness to palpation of joints; no heat, swelling, or masses. Full ROM; movement smooth, no crepitus, no tenderness. Muscle strength—able to maintain flexion against resistance and without tenderness.

ASSESSMENT

Muscles and joints—healthy and functional

Focused Assessment: Clinical Case Study

M.T. is a 45-year-old white female salesperson with a diagnosis of rheumatoid arthritis 3 years PTA, who seeks care now for "swelling and burning pain in my hands" for 1 day.

SUBJECTIVE

M.T. was diagnosed as having rheumatoid arthritis at age 41 years by staff at this agency. Since that time, her "flare-ups" seem to come every 6 to 8 months. Acute episodes involve hand joints and are treated with aspirin, which gives relief. Typically experiences morning stiffness, lasting ½ to 1 hour. Joints feel warm, swollen, tender. Has had weight loss of 15 pounds over past 4 years and feels fatigued much of the time. States should rest more, but "I can't take the time." Daily exercises have been prescribed but doesn't do them regularly. Takes aspirin for acute flare-ups, feels better in a few days, decreases dose by herself.

OBJECTIVE

Body joints within normal limits with exception of joints of wrist and hands. Radiocarpal, metacarpophalangeal, and proximal interphalangeal joints are red, swollen, tender to palpation. Spindle-shaped swelling of proximal interphalangeal joints of third digit right hand and second digit left hand; ulnar deviation of metacarpophalangeal joints.

ASSESSMENT

Acute pain R/T inflammation
Impaired physical mobility R/T inflammation
Deficient knowledge about aspirin treatment R/T lack of exposure
Noncompliance with exercise program R/T lack of perceived benefits of treatment
Noncompliance with advised rest periods R/T lack of perceived benefits of treatment

ABNORMAL FINDINGS FOR ADVANCED PRACTICE

TABLE 22-1 Abnormalities Affecting Multiple Joints

INFLAMMATORY CONDITIONS

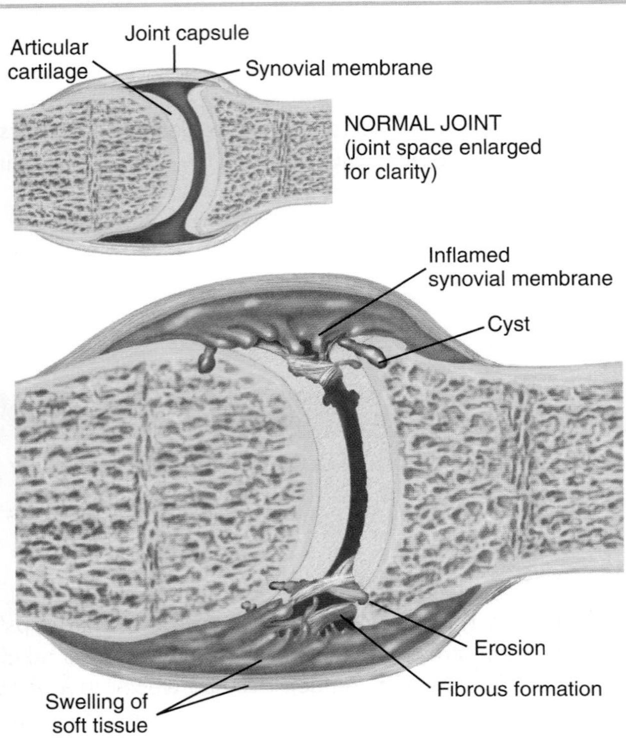

Rheumatoid Arthritis (RA)

This is a chronic, systemic inflammatory disease of joints and surrounding connective tissue. Inflammation of synovial membrane leads to thickening; then to fibrosis, which limits motion; and finally to bony ankylosis. The disorder is symmetric and bilateral and is characterized by heat, redness, swelling, and painful motion of the affected joints. RA is associated with fatigue, weakness, anorexia, weight loss, low-grade fever, and lymphadenopathy. Associated signs are described in the following tables, especially Table 22-4.

Ankylosing Spondylitis (not illustrated)

Chronic, progressive inflammation of spine, sacroiliac, and larger joints of the extremities, leading to bony ankylosis and deformity. A form of RA, this affects primarily men by a 10:1 ratio, in late adolescence or early adulthood. Spasm of paraspinal muscles pulls spine into forward flexion, obliterating cervical and lumbar curves. Thoracic curve exaggerated into single kyphotic rounding. Also includes flexion deformities of hips and knees.

DEGENERATIVE CONDITIONS

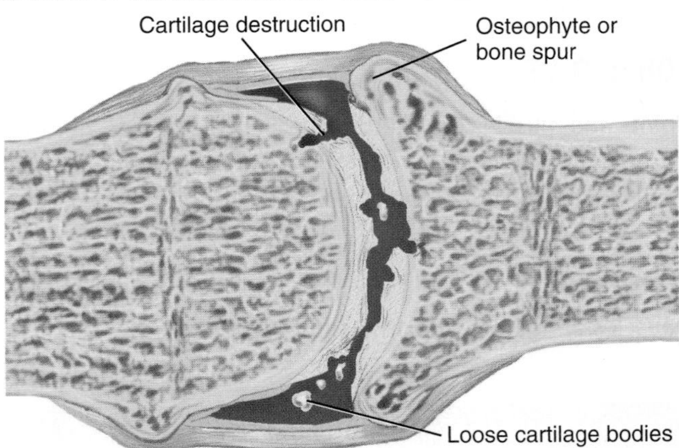

Osteoarthritis (Degenerative Joint Disease)

Noninflammatory, localized, progressive disorder involving deterioration of articular cartilages and subchondral bone and formation of new bone (osteophytes) at joint surfaces. Aging increases incidence; nearly all adults older than 60 years have some radiographic signs of osteoarthritis. Asymmetric joint involvement commonly affects hands, knees, hips, and lumbar and cervical segments of the spine. Affected joints have stiffness, swelling with hard, bony protuberances, pain with motion, and limitation of motion (see Table 22-4).

Osteoporosis

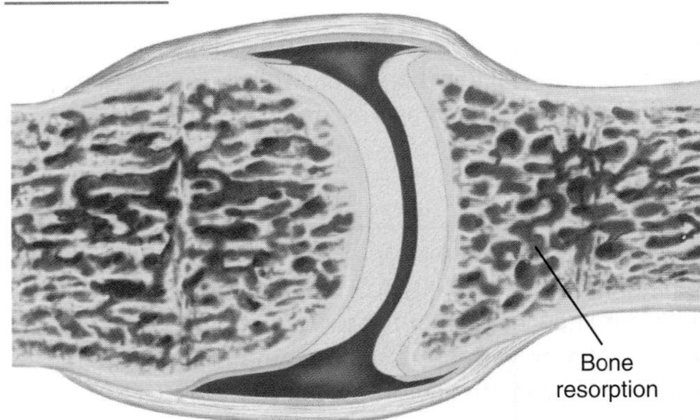

Decrease in skeletal bone mass occurring when rate of bone resorption is greater than that of bone formation. The weakened bone state increases risk for stress fractures, especially at wrist, hip, and vertebrae. Occurs primarily in postmenopausal white women. Osteoporosis risk also is associated with smaller height and weight, younger age at menopause, lack of physical activity, and lack of estrogen in women.

TABLE 22-2 Abnormalities of the Shoulder

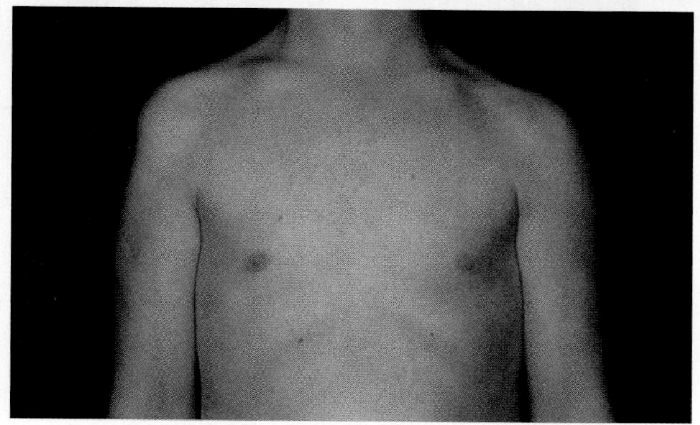

Atrophy

Loss of muscle mass is exhibited as a lack of fullness surrounding the deltoid muscle. In this case, atrophy is due to axillary nerve palsy. Atrophy also occurs from disuse, muscle tissue damage, or motor nerve damage.

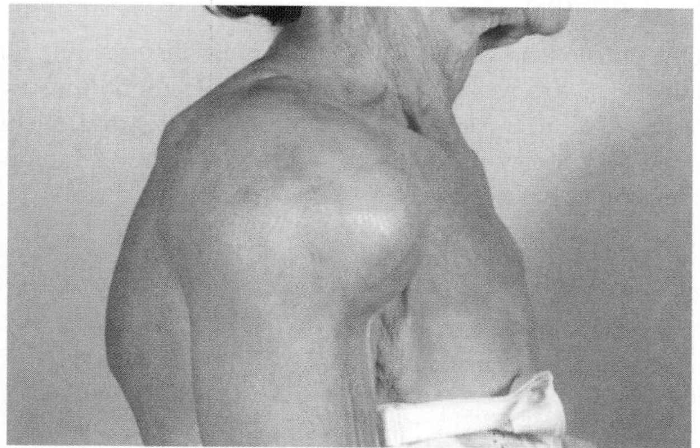

Joint Effusion

Swelling from excess fluid in the joint capsule, here from rheumatoid arthritis. Best observed anteriorly. Fluctuant to palpation. Considerable fluid must be present to cause a visible distention because the capsule normally is so loose.

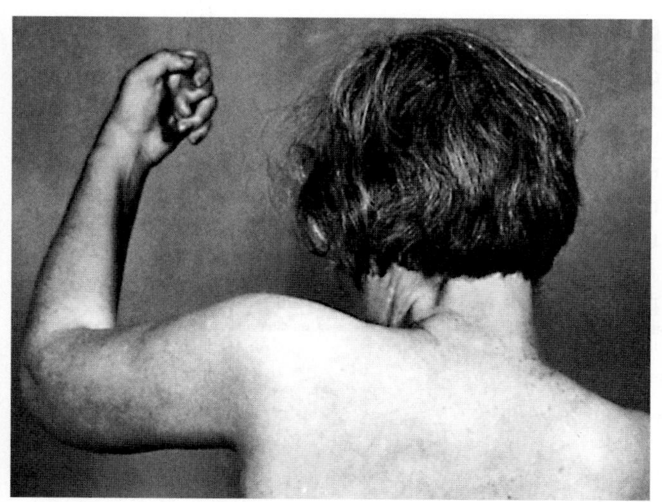

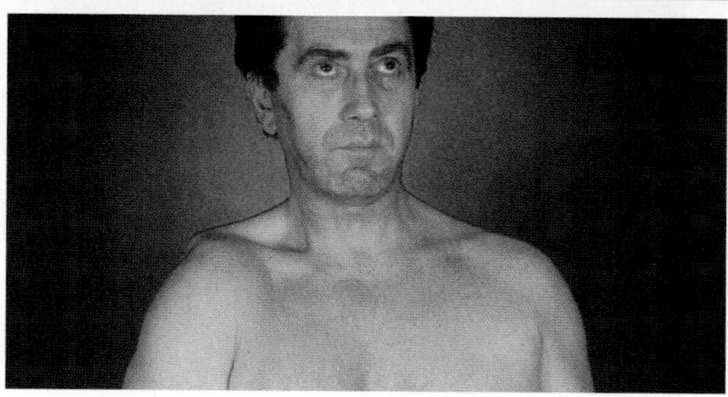

Dislocated Shoulder

Anterior dislocation (95%) is exhibited when hunching the shoulder forward and the tip of the clavicle dislocates. It occurs with trauma involving abduction, extension, and rotation (e.g., falling on an outstretched arm or diving into a pool).

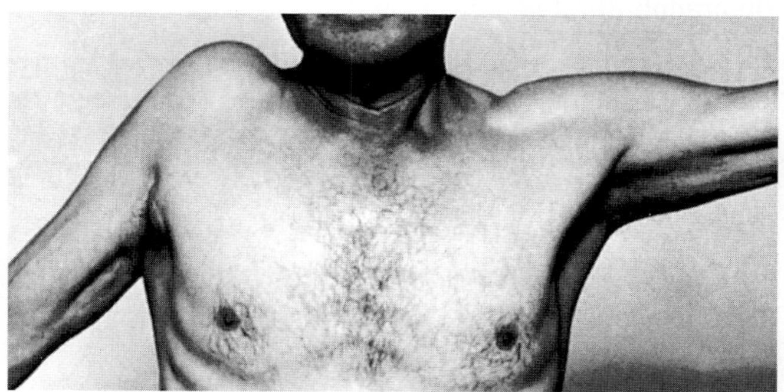

Tear of Rotator Cuff

Characteristic "hunched" position and limited abduction of arm. Occurs from traumatic adduction while arm is held in abduction, or from fall on shoulder, throwing, or heavy lifting. Positive drop arm test: if the arm is passively abducted at the shoulder, the person is unable to sustain the position and the arm falls to the side.

◀ Frozen Shoulder—Adhesive Capsulitis

Fibrous tissues form in the joint capsule, causing stiffness, progressive limitation of motion, and pain. Motion limited in abduction and external rotation; unable to reach overhead. It may lead to atrophy of shoulder girdle muscles. Gradual onset; unknown cause. It is associated with prolonged bedrest or shoulder immobility. May resolve spontaneously.

Subacromial Bursitis (not illustrated)

Inflammation and swelling of subacromial bursa over the shoulder cause limited ROM and pain with motion. Localized swelling under deltoid muscle may increase by partial passive abduction of the arm. Caused by direct trauma, strain during sports, local or systemic inflammatory process, or repetitive motion with injury.

TABLE 22-3 Abnormalities of the Elbow

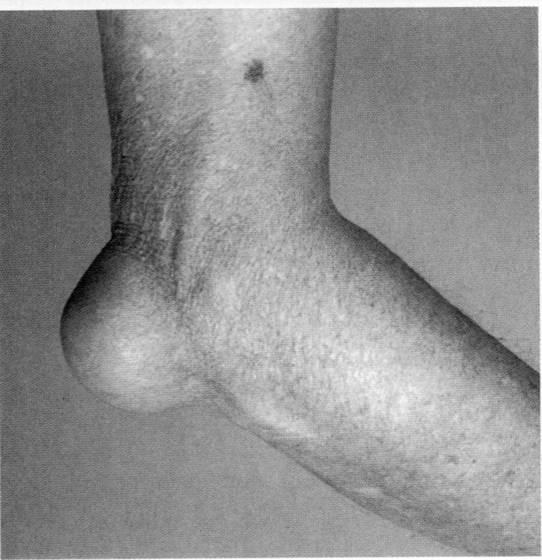

Olecranon Bursitis

Large, soft knob, or "goose egg," and redness from inflammation of olecranon bursa. Localized and easy to see because bursa lies just under skin.

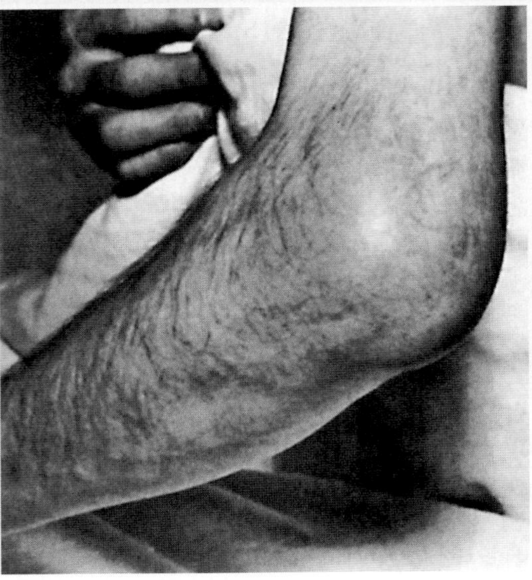

Gouty Arthritis

Joint effusion or synovial thickening, seen first as bulge or fullness in grooves on either side of olecranon process. Redness and heat can extend beyond area of synovial membrane. Soft, boggy, or fluctuant fullness to palpation. Limited extension of elbow.

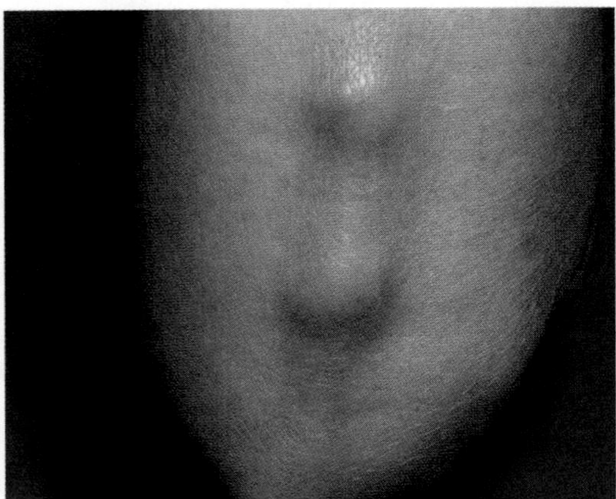

Subcutaneous Nodules

Raised, firm, nontender nodules that occur with rheumatoid arthritis. Common sites are in the olecranon bursa and along extensor surface of arm. The skin slides freely over the nodules.

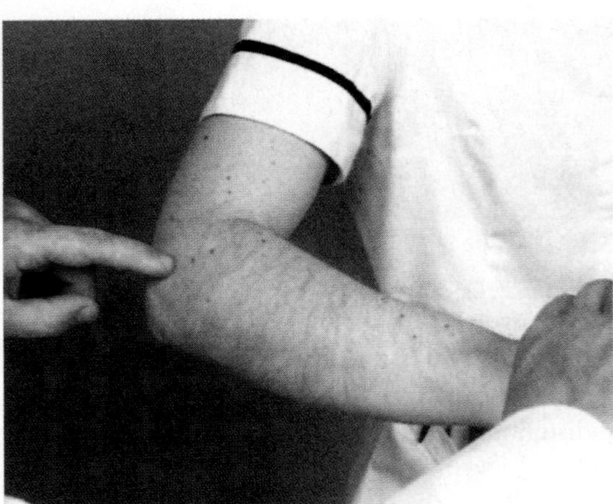

Epicondylitis—Tennis Elbow

Chronic disabling pain at lateral epicondyle of humerus, radiates down extensor surface of forearm. Pain can be located with one finger. Resisting extension of the hand will increase the pain. Occurs with activities combining excessive pronation and supination of forearm with an extended wrist (e.g., racquet sports or using a screwdriver).

Medial epicondylitis is rarer and is due to activity of forced palmar flexion of wrist against resistance.

TABLE 22-4 Abnormalities of the Wrist and Hand

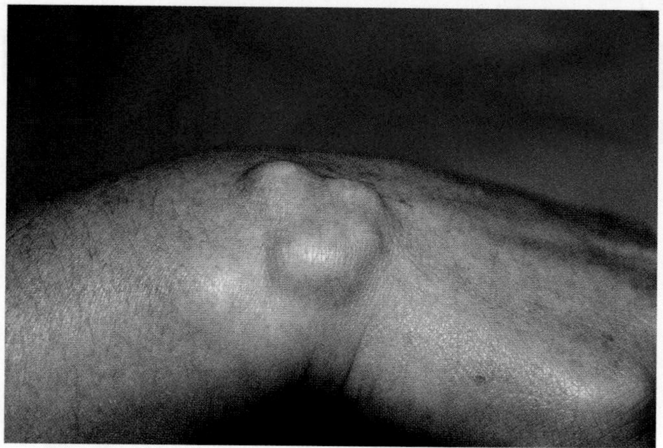

Ganglion Cyst

Round, cystic, nontender nodule overlying a tendon sheath or joint capsule, usually on dorsum of wrist. Flexion makes it more prominent. A common benign tumor; it does not become malignant.

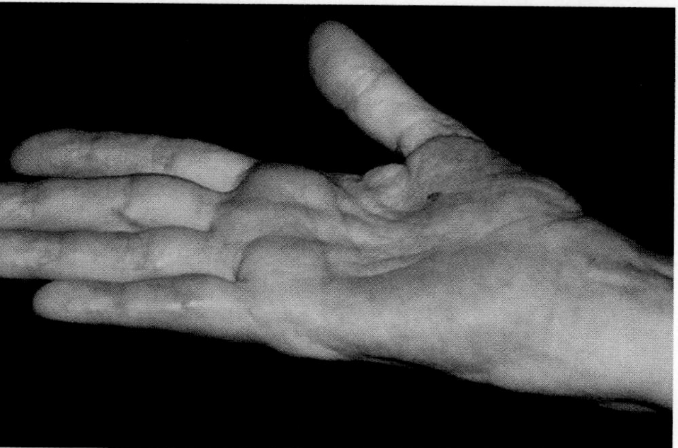

Carpal Tunnel Syndrome with Atrophy of Thenar Eminence

Atrophy occurs from interference with motor function from compression of the median nerve inside the carpal tunnel. Caused by chronic repetitive motion; occurs between 30 and 60 years of age and is five times more common in women than in men. Symptoms of carpal tunnel syndrome include pain, burning and numbness, positive findings on Phalen test, positive indication of Tinel sign, and often atrophy of thenar muscles.

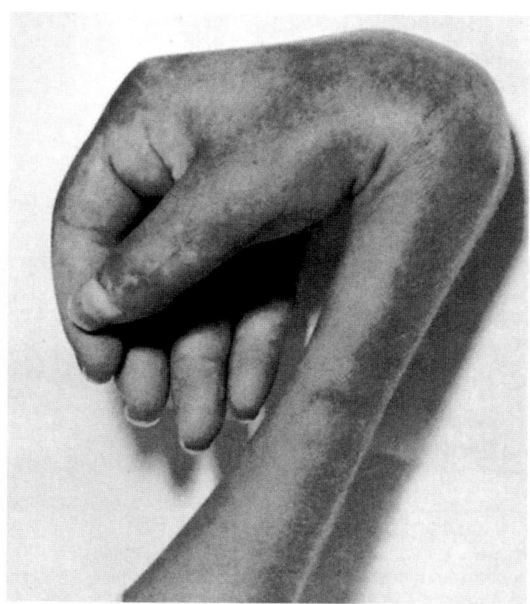

Ankylosis

Wrist in extreme flexion, due to severe rheumatoid arthritis. This is a functionally useless hand because when the wrist is palmar flexed, a good deal of power is lost from the fingers and the thumb cannot oppose the fingers.

Colles Fracture (not illustrated)

Nonarticular fracture of distal radius, with or without fracture of ulna at styloid process. Usually from a fall on an outstretched hand; occurs more often in older women. Wrist looks puffy with "silver fork" deformity, a characteristic hump when viewed from the side.

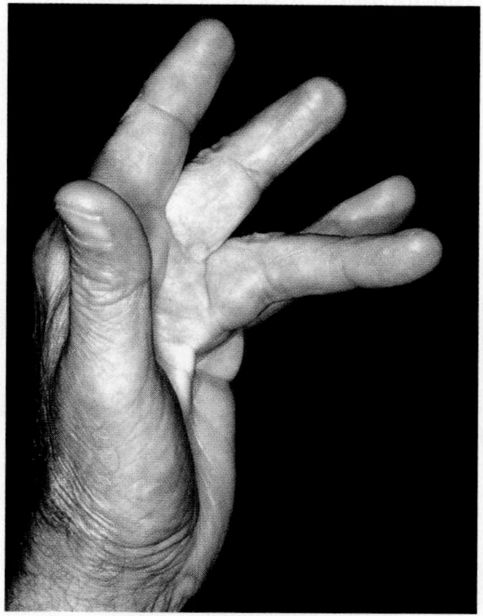

Dupuytren Contracture

Chronic hyperplasia of the palmar fascia causes flexion contractures of the digits, first in the 4th digit, then the 5th digit, and then the 3rd digit. Note the bands that extend from the midpalm to the digits and the puckering of palmar skin. The condition occurs commonly in men older than 40 years and is usually bilateral. It occurs with diabetes, epilepsy, and alcoholic liver disease and as an inherited trait. The contracture is painless but impairs hand function.

Continued

TABLE 22-4 Abnormalities of the Wrist and Hand—cont'd

CONDITIONS CAUSED BY CHRONIC RHEUMATOID ARTHRITIS

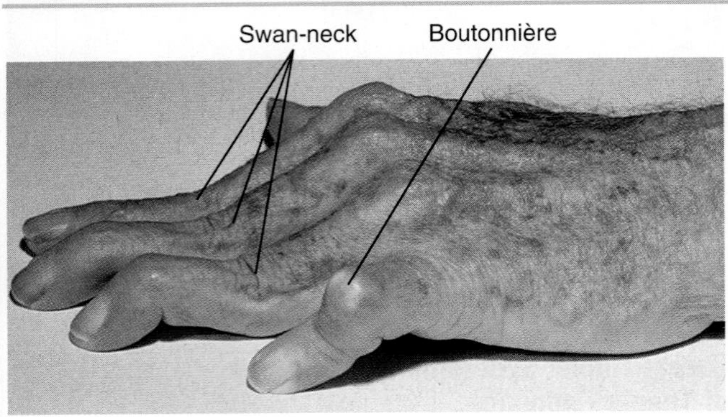

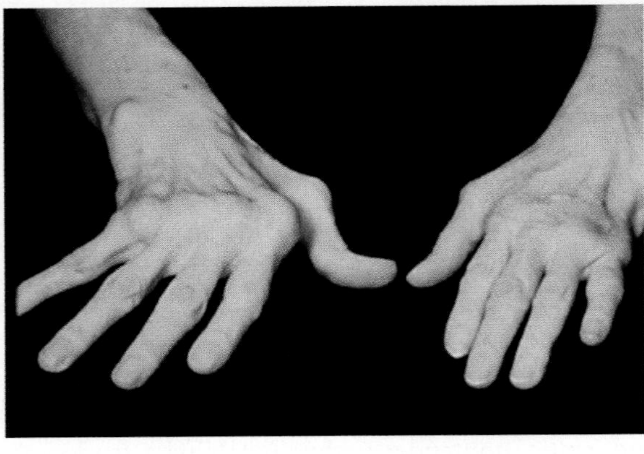

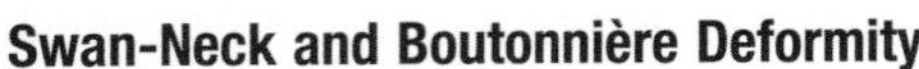

Swan-Neck and Boutonnière Deformity

Flexion contracture resembles curve of a **swan's neck.** Note flexion contracture of metacarpophalangeal joint, then hyperextension of the proximal interphalangeal joint, and flexion of the distal interphalangeal joint. It occurs with chronic rheumatoid arthritis and is often accompanied by ulnar drift of the fingers.

In **boutonnière deformity,** the knuckle looks as if it is being pushed through a buttonhole. It is a relatively common deformity and includes flexion of proximal interphalangeal joint with compensatory hyperextension of distal interphalangeal joint.

Reprinted from the Clinical Slide Collection on the Rheumatic Diseases, © 1991, 1995, 1997. Used by permission of the American College of Rheumatology.

Ulnar Deviation or Drift

Fingers drift to the ulnar side because of stretching of the articular capsule and muscle imbalance. Also note subluxation and swelling in the joints and muscle atrophy on the dorsa of the hands. This is caused by chronic rheumatoid arthritis.

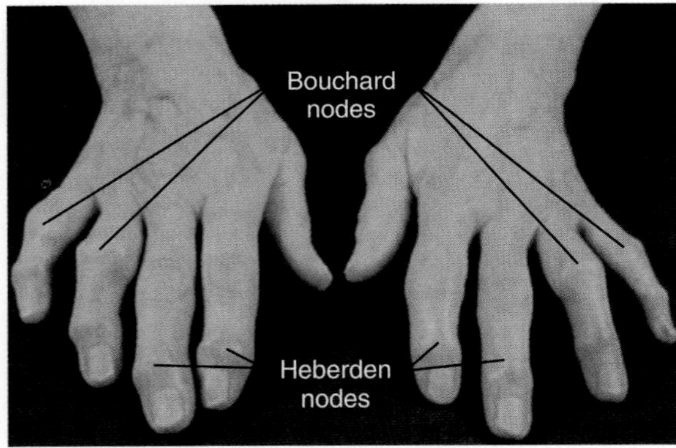

Degenerative Joint Disease, or Osteoarthritis

Osteoarthritis is characterized by hard, nontender nodules, 2 to 3 mm or more. These osteophytes (bony overgrowths) of the distal interphalangeal joints are called *Heberden nodes,* and those of the proximal interphalangeal joints are called *Bouchard nodes.*

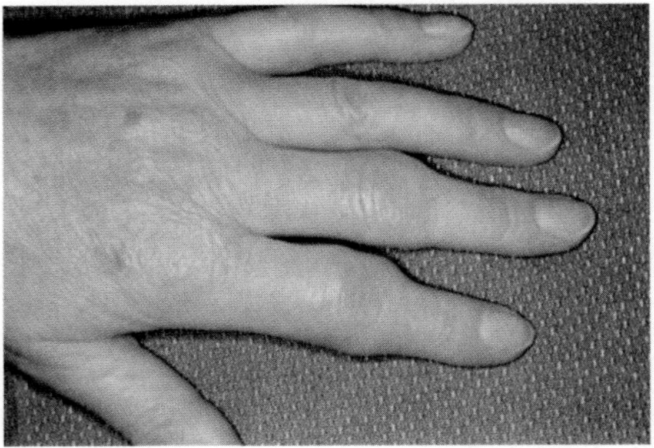

Acute Rheumatoid Arthritis

Painful swelling and stiffness of joints, with fusiform or spindle-shaped swelling of the soft tissue of proximal interphalangeal joints. Fusiform swelling is usually symmetric, the hands are warm, and the veins are engorged. The inflamed joints have a limited range of motion.

TABLE 22-4 Abnormalities of the Wrist and Hand—cont'd

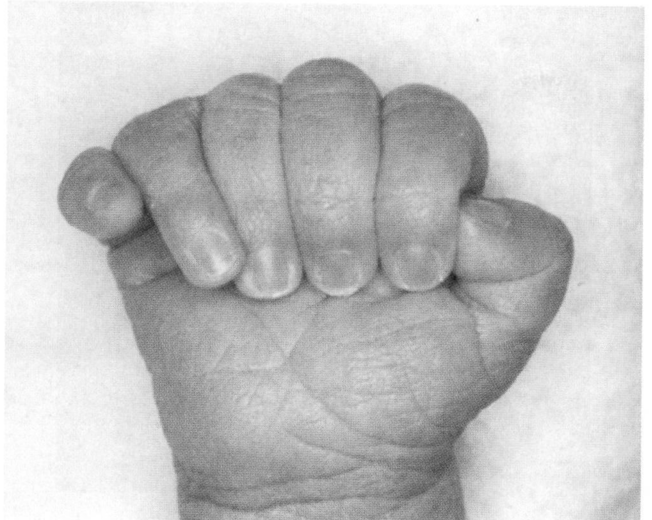

Polydactyly

Extra digits are a congenital deformity, usually occurring at the fifth finger or the thumb. Surgical removal is considered for cosmetic appearance. The 6th finger shown here was not removed because it had full ROM and sensation and a normal appearance.

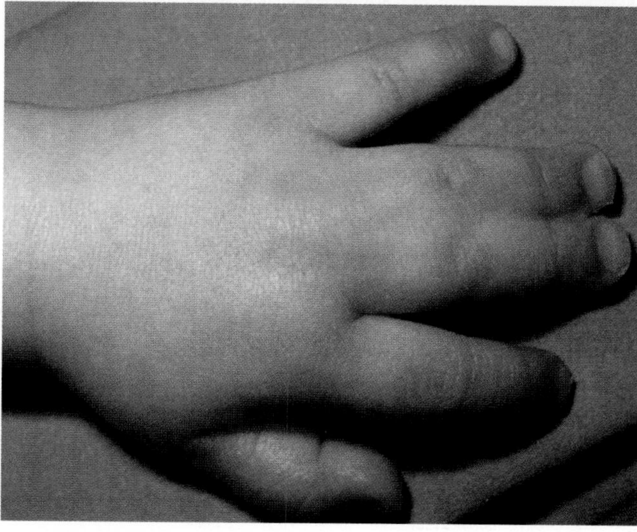

Syndactyly

Webbed fingers are a congenital deformity, usually requiring surgical separation. The metacarpals and phalanges of the webbed fingers are different lengths, and the joints do not line up. To leave the fingers fused would thus limit their flexion and extension.

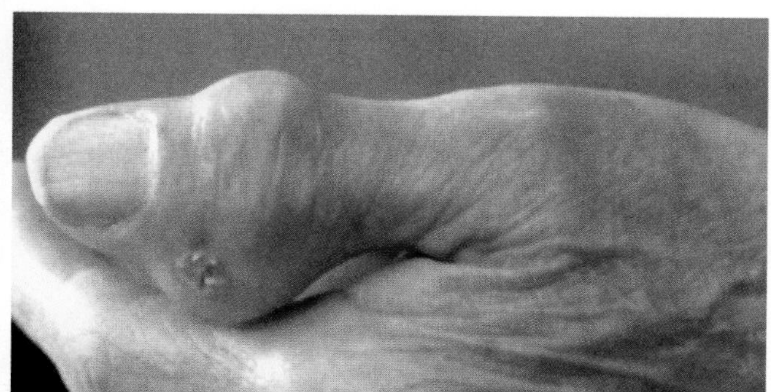

◀ Gout in Thumb

See explanation in Table 22-6.

TABLE 22-5 Abnormalities of the Knee

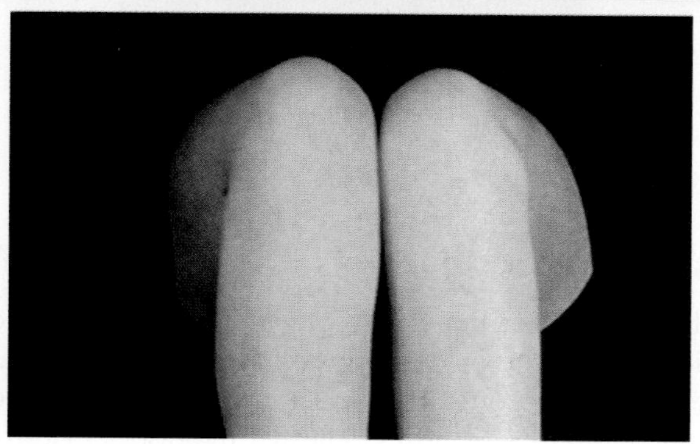

Swelling of Menisci

Localized soft swelling from cyst in lateral meniscus shows at the midpoint of the anterolateral joint line. Semiflexion of the knee makes swelling more prominent.

Continued

TABLE 22-5 Abnormalities of the Knee—cont'd

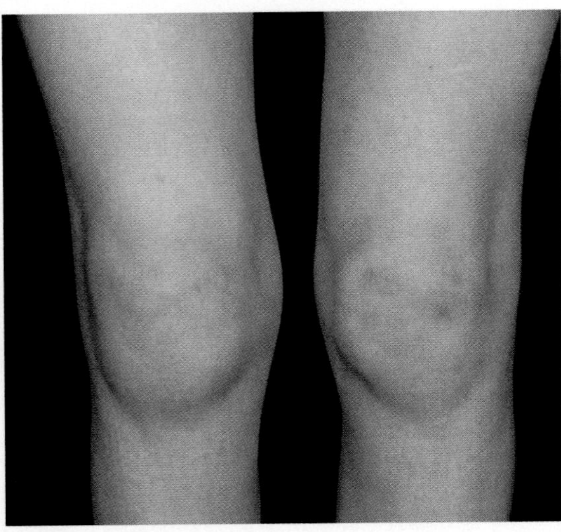

Mild Synovitis

Loss of normal hollows on either side of the patella, which are replaced by mild distention. Occurs with synovial thickening or effusion (excess fluid). Also note mild distention of the suprapatellar pouch.

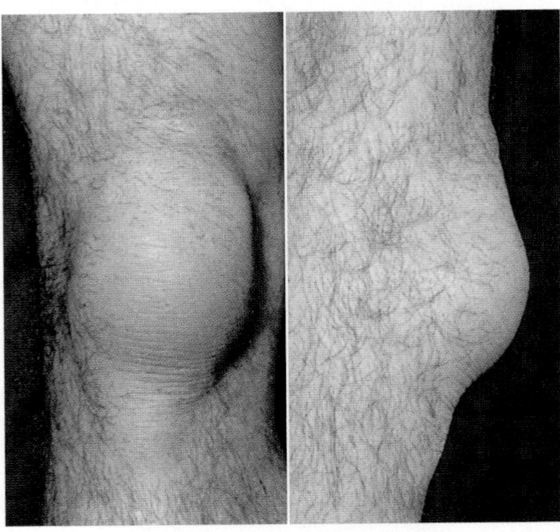

Prepatellar Bursitis

Localized swelling on anterior knee between patella and skin. A tender, fluctuant mass indicates swelling; in some cases, infection spreads to surrounding soft tissue. The condition is limited to the bursa, and the knee joint itself is not involved. Overlying skin may be red, shiny, atrophic, or coarse and thickened.

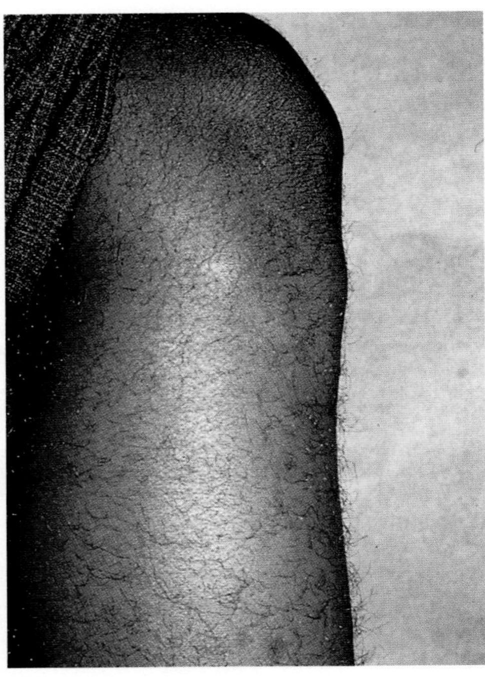

Osgood-Schlatter Disease

Painful swelling of the tibial tubercle just below the knee, probably from repeated stress on the patellar tendon. Occurs most in puberty during rapid growth and most often in males. Pain increases with kicking, running, bike riding, stair climbing, or kneeling. The condition is usually self-limited, and symptoms resolve with rest.

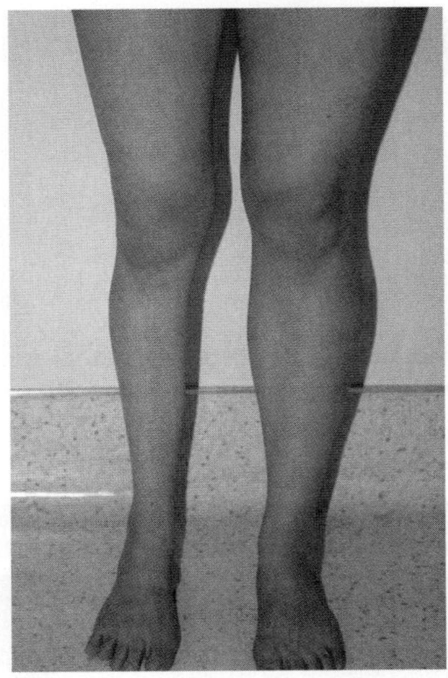

Post Polio Muscle Atrophy

Right leg and foot muscle atrophy as a result of childhood polio. Poliomyelitis epidemics peaked in the United States in the 1940s and 1950s. The development of the oral polio vaccine (1962) has almost eradicated the disease. However, thousands of polio survivors have this muscle atrophy.

TABLE 22-6 **Abnormalities of the Ankle and Foot**

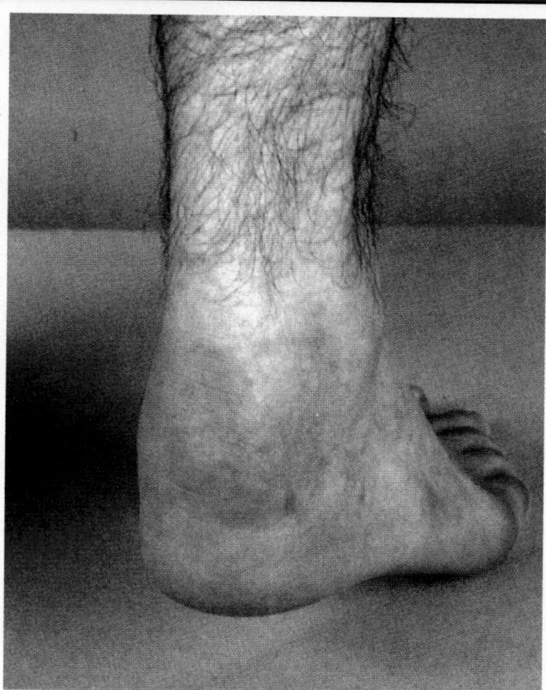

Achilles Tenosynovitis

Inflammation of a tendon sheath near the ankle (here, the Achilles tendon) produces a superficial linear swelling and a localized tenderness along the route of the sheath. Movement of the involved tendon usually causes pain.

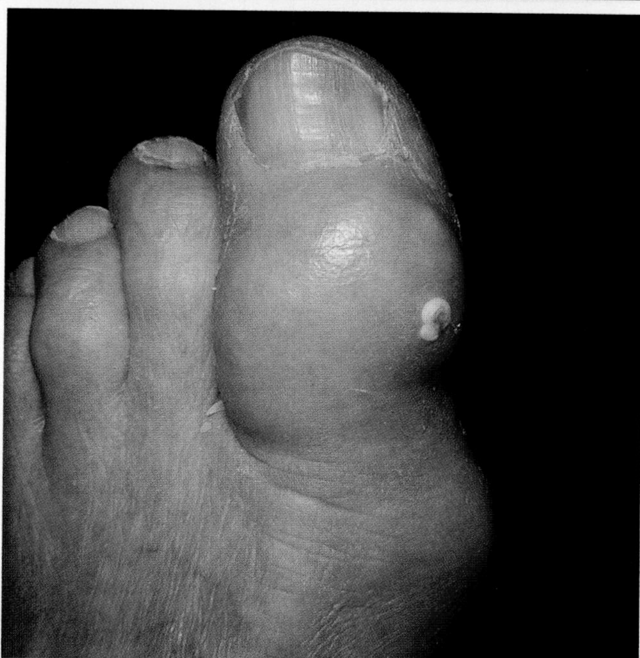

Tophi with Chronic Gout

Hard, painless nodule (tophi) over metatarsophalangeal joint of first toe. Tophi are collections of sodium urate crystals due to chronic gout in and around the joint that cause extreme swelling and joint deformity. They sometimes burst with a chalky discharge.

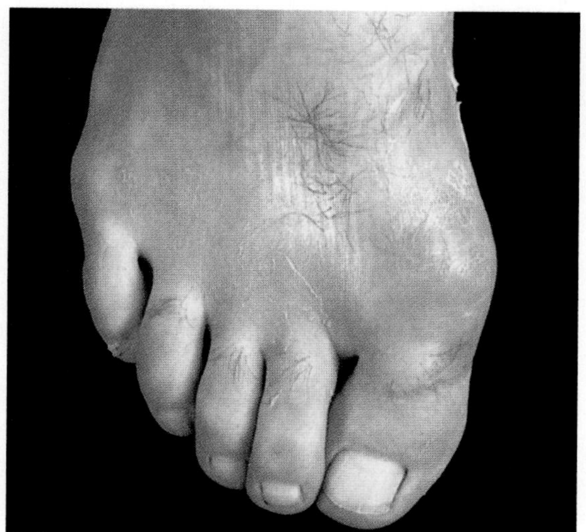

◀ Acute Gout

Acute episode of gout usually involves first the metatarsophalangeal joint. Clinical findings consist of redness, swelling, heat, and extreme tenderness. Gout is a metabolic disorder of disturbed purine metabolism, associated with elevated serum uric acid. It occurs primarily in men older than 40 years.

Continued

TABLE 22-6 Abnormalities of the Ankle and Foot—cont'd

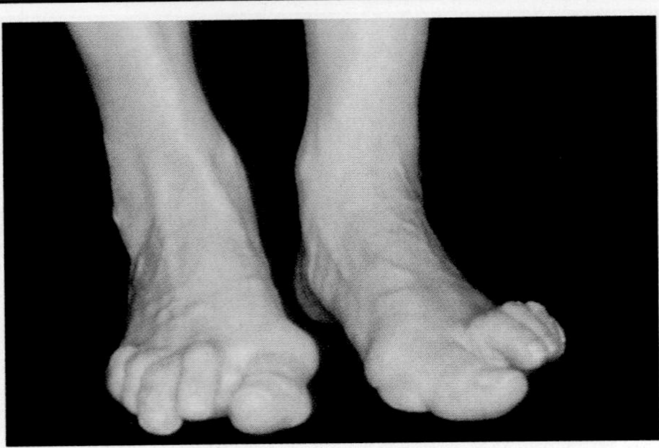

Hallux Valgus with Bunion and Hammertoes

Hallux valgus is a common deformity from rheumatoid arthritis. It is a lateral or outward deviation of the great toe with medial prominence of the head of the first metatarsal. The **bunion** is the inflamed bursa that forms at the pressure point. The great toe loses power to push off while walking; this stresses the second and third metatarsal heads, and they develop calluses and pain. Chronic sequelae include corns, calluses, hammertoes, and joint subluxation.

Note the **hammertoe** deformities in the 2nd, 3rd, 4th, and 5th toes. Often associated with hallux valgus, hammertoe includes hyperextension of the metatarsophalangeal joint and flexion of the proximal interphalangeal joint.

Corns (thickening of soft tissue) develop on the dorsum over the bony prominence from prolonged pressure from shoes.

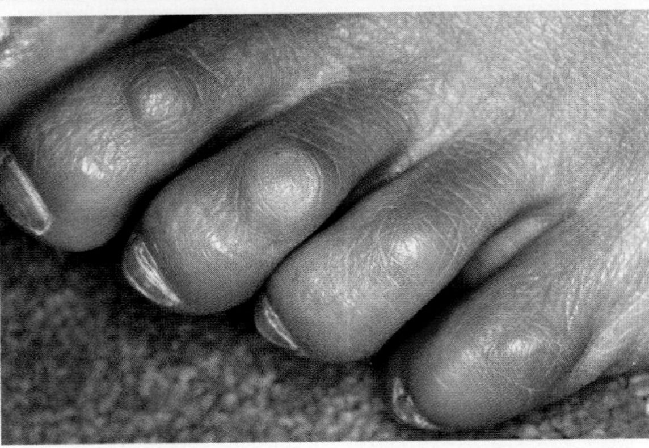

Callus

Hypertrophy of the epithelium develops because of prolonged pressure, commonly on the plantar surface of the first metatarsal head in the hallux valgus deformity or as shown here over the bony prominences of the joints in hammertoes. The condition is not painful.

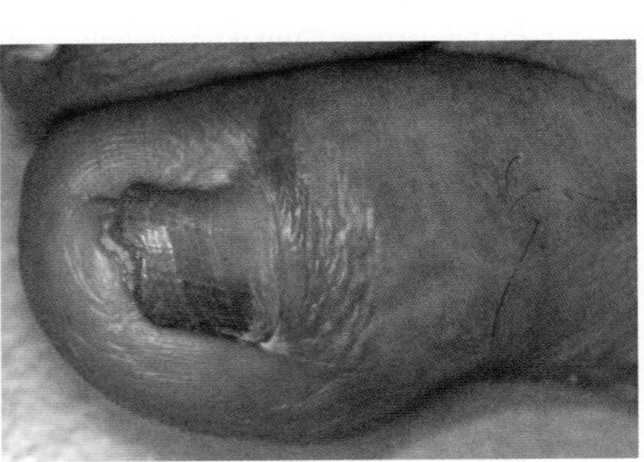

Ingrown Toenail

A misnomer; the nail does not grow in, but the soft tissue grows over the nail and obliterates the groove. It occurs almost always on the great toe on the medial or lateral side. It is due to trimming the nail too short or toe-crowding in tight shoes. The area becomes infected when the nail grows and its corner penetrates the soft tissue.

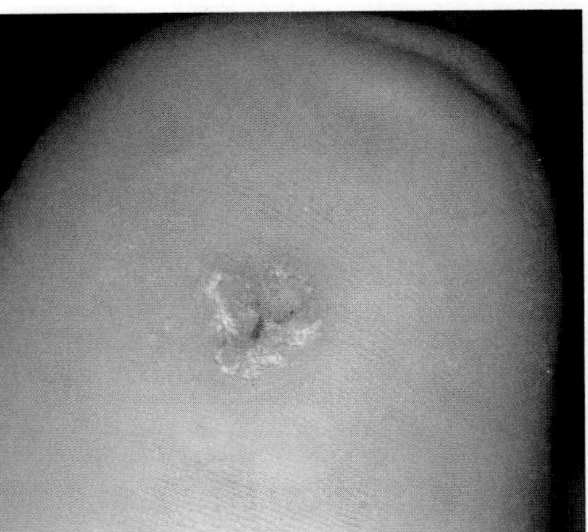

Plantar Wart

Vascular papillomatous growth is probably due to a virus and occurs on the sole of the foot, commonly at the ball. The condition is extremely painful.

TABLE 22-7 Abnormalities of the Spine

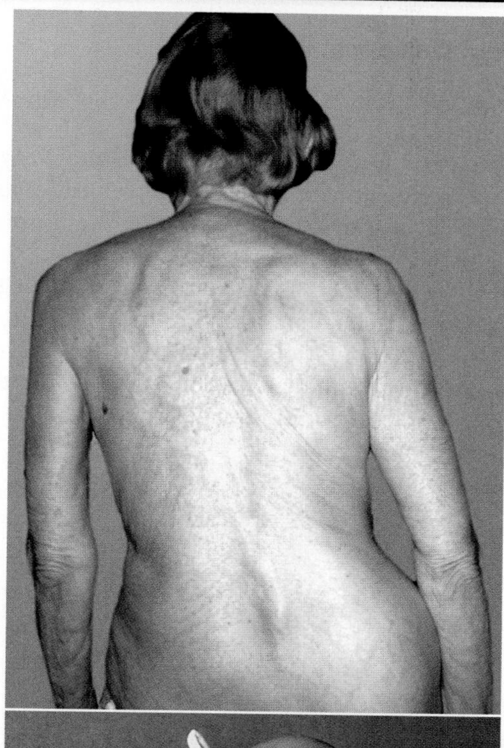

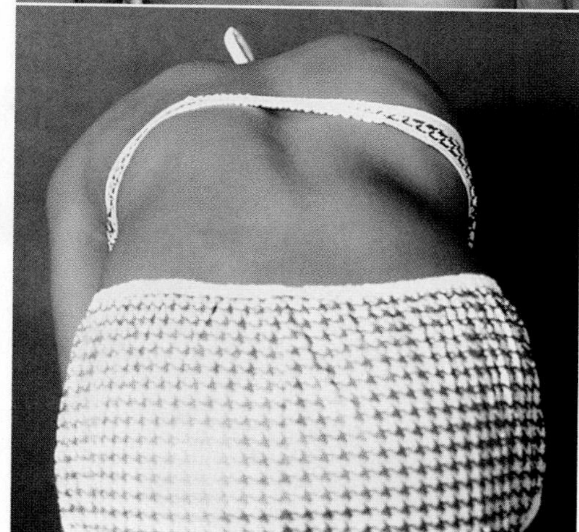

◀ Scoliosis

Lateral curvature of thoracic and lumbar segments of the spine, usually with some rotation of involved vertebral bodies.

Functional scoliosis is flexible; it is apparent with standing and disappears with forward bending. It may be compensatory for other abnormalities such as leg length discrepancy.

Structural scoliosis is fixed; the curvature shows both on standing and on bending forward. Note rib hump with forward flexion. When the person is standing, note unequal shoulder elevation, unequal scapulae, obvious curvature, and unequal hip level. At greatest risk are females 10 years of age through adolescence, during the peak of the growth spurt.

Herniated Nucleus Pulposus ▶

The nucleus pulposus (at the center of the intervertebral disk) ruptures into the spinal canal and puts pressure on the local spinal nerve root. Usually occurs from stress, such as lifting, twisting, continuous flexion with lifting, or fall on buttocks. Occurs mostly in men 20 to 45 years of age. Lumbar herniations occur mainly in interspaces L4 to L5 and L5 to S1. Note: Sciatic pain, numbness, and paresthesia of involved dermatome; listing away from affected side; decreased mobility; low back tenderness; and decreased motor and sensory function in leg. Straight leg raising tests reproduce sciatic pain.

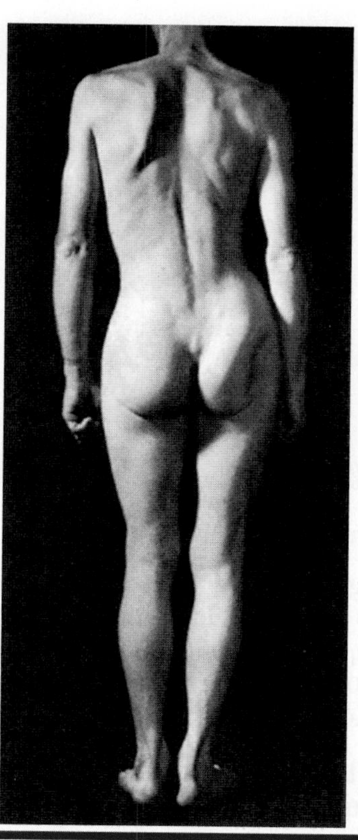

TABLE 22-8 Common Congenital or Pediatric Abnormalities

◀ Congenital Dislocated Hip

Head of the femur is displaced out of the cup-shaped acetabulum.

The degree of the condition varies; subluxation may occur as stretched ligaments allow partial displacement of femoral head, and acetabular dysplasia may develop because of excessive laxity of hip joint capsule.

Occurrence is 1:500 to 1:1000 births; common in girls by 7:1 ratio. Signs include limited abduction of flexed thigh, positive indications of Ortolani and Barlow signs, asymmetric skin creases or gluteal folds, limb length discrepancy, and positive indication of Trendelenburg sign in older children.

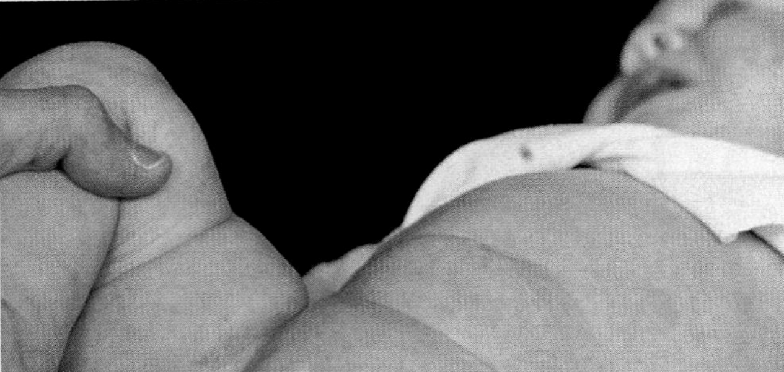

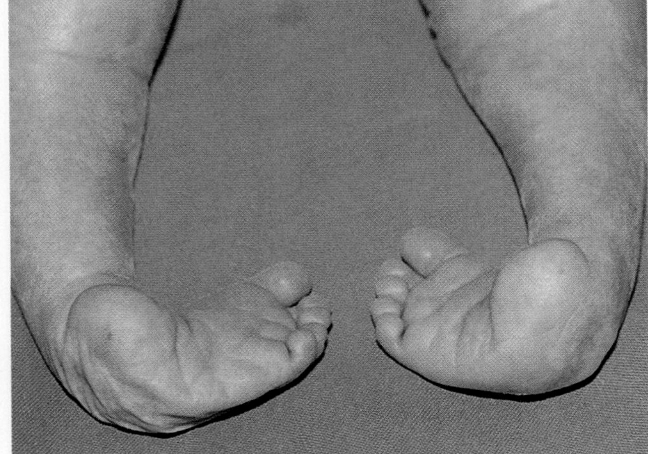

Talipes Equinovarus (Clubfoot)

Congenital, rigid, and fixed malposition of foot, including (1) inversion, (2) forefoot adduction, and (3) foot pointing downward (equinus). A common birth defect, with an incidence of 1:1000 to 3:1000 live births. Males are affected twice as frequently as females.

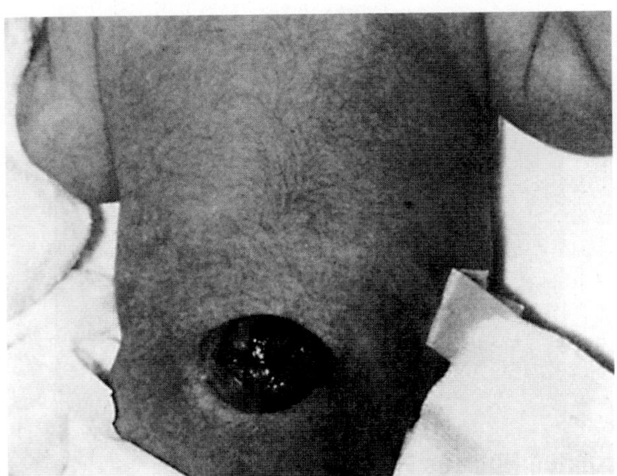

Spina Bifida

Incomplete closure of posterior part of vertebrae results in a neural tube defect. Seriousness varies from skin defect along the spine to protrusion of the sac containing meninges, spinal fluid, or malformed spinal cord. The most serious type is myelomeningocele (shown here), in which the meninges and neural tissue protrude. In these cases, the child is usually paralyzed below the level of the lesion.

Coxa Plana (Legg-Calvé-Perthes Syndrome) (not illustrated)

Avascular necrosis of the femoral head, occurring primarily in males between 3 and 12 years of age, with peak at age 6 years. In initial inflammatory stage, interruption of blood supply to femoral epiphysis occurs, halting growth. Revascularization and healing occur later, but significant residual deformity and dysfunction may be present.

TABLE 22-9 Fibromyalgia Syndrome

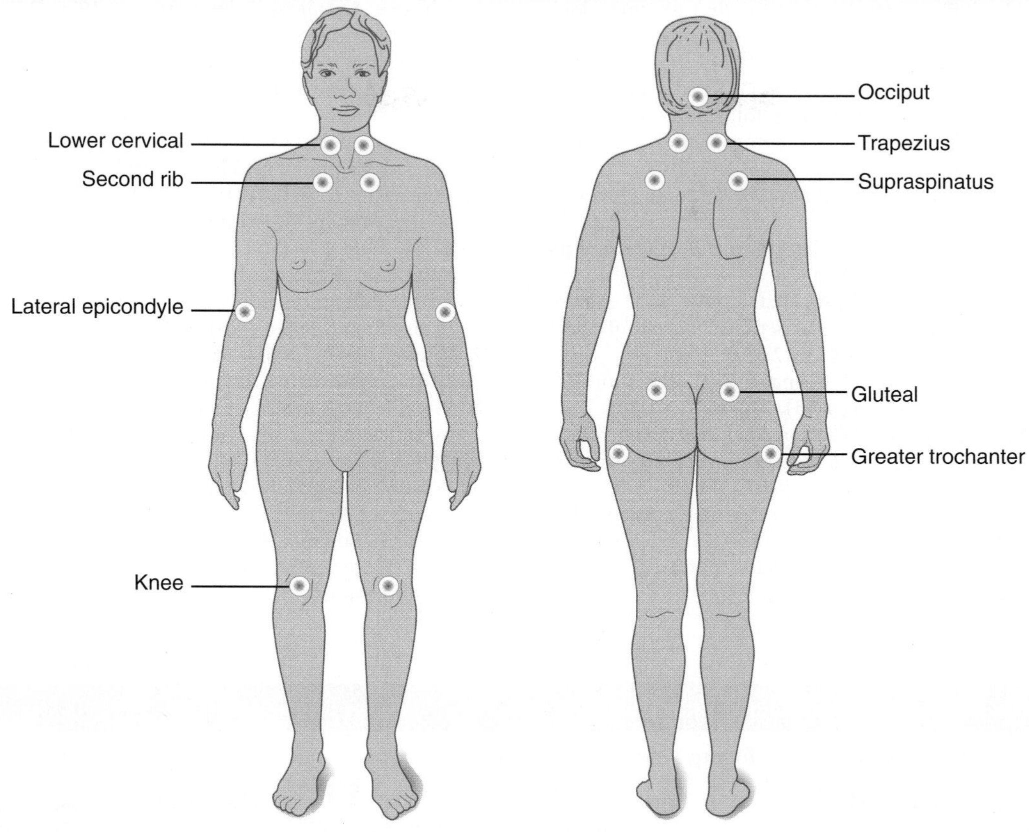

Chronic disorder of unknown cause characterized by widespread musculoskeletal pain lasting 3 months or longer, associated with fatigue, insomnia, and psychosocial distress. Most patients (90%) are adult women. There are two major diagnostic criteria[30]: (1) pain on both sides of the body, above and below the waist, and axial skeletal pain (cervical, thoracic, lumbar spine, or anterior chest); and (2) point tenderness on digital palpation in 11 of 18 specified sites shown above. The examiner presses the thumb of the dominant hand with a force of 4 kg (same as needed to blanch or whiten the nail bed). Burden of illness is high with one third to one fourth of patients receiving disability compensation.

BIBLIOGRAPHY

1. Alexander, I. M. (2009). Pharmacotherapeutic management of osteoporosis and osteopenia. *Nurse Practitioner, 34*(6), 30-42.
2. Barrett-Connor, E., Siris, E. S., Wehren, L.E., et al. (2005). Osteoporosis and fracture risk in women of different ethnic groups. *Journal of Bone and Mineral Research, 20*, 185-194.
3. Berenson, A. B., Rahman, M., & Wilkinson, G. (2009). Racial difference in the correlates of bone mineral content/density and age at peak among reproductive-aged women. *Osteoporosis International, 20*(8), 1439-1449.
4. Broy, S. B., & Myers, A. K. (2010). Identifying and managing osteoporosis: an update. *Journal of Musculoskeletal Medicine, 27*(1), 11-19.
5. Bunout, D., Barrera, G., Pia, M., et al. (2007). Height reduction, determined using knee height measurement as a risk factor or predictive sign for osteoporosis in elderly women. *Nutrition, 23*(11-12), 794-797.
6. Cline, M. G., Meredith, K. E., Boyer, J. T., et al. (1989). Decline of height with age in adults in a general population sample: estimating maximum height and distinguishing birth cohort effects from actual loss of stature with aging. *Human Biology, 61*, 415-425.
7. Cruz, A. I., & Smith, B. G. (2010). Scoliosis in children and adolescence: an update. *Contemporary Pediatrics, 27*(1), 42-52.
8. Dadabhoy, D., McCarberg, B., & Hassett, A. L. (February 2010). Managing fibromyalgia in primary care. *Primary Psychiatry, 17*(2), 2-16.
9. D'Arcy, Y. (2009). Is low back pain getting on your nerves? *Nurse Practitioner, 34*(5), 10-20.
10. Davidson, J., Randall, G. K., & Getz, M. A. (2009). Self-reported height, calculated height, and derived body mass index in assessment of older adults. *Journal of Nutrition for the Elderly, 28*(4), 359-371.
11. Hart, L. (2005). Primary care for patients with neurofibromatosis 1, *Nurse Practitioner, 30*, 38-43.
12. Jacobson, A. F., Myerscough, R. P., DeLambo, K., et al. (2008). Patients' perspectives on total knee replacement: a qualitative study sheds light on pre- and postoperative experiences. *American Journal of Nursing, 108*(5), 54-64.

13. Lee, S. G. (2008). Little arms, big league injuries. *American Journal of Nursing, 33*(4), 24-32.
14. Lewiecki, E. M. (2009). Current and emerging pharmacologic therapies for the management of postmenopausal osteoporosis. *Journal of Women's Health, 18*(10), 1615-1624.
15. Looker, A. C., Melton, III, L. J., Harris, T., et al. (2009). Age, gender, and race/ethnic differences in total body and subregional bone density. *Osteoporosis International, 20*(7), 1141-1149.
15a. McGee, S. (2007). *Evidence-based physical diagnosis* (2nd ed.). St. Louis: Saunders.
16. Olson, A. F. (2007). Osteoporosis detection: is BMD testing the future? *Nurse Practitioner, 32*(6), 20-28.
17. Pigozzi, E., Rizzo, M., Giombini, A., et al. (2009). Bone mineral density and sport: effect of physical activity. *Journal of Sports Medicine and Physical Fitness, 49*(2), 177-183.
18. Scanlon, A., & Maffei, J. (2009). Carpal tunnel syndrome. *The Journal of Neuroscience Nursing, 41*(3), 140-147.
19. Schmitt, N. M., Schmitt, J., & Doren, M. (2009). The role of physical activity in the prevention of osteoporosis in postmenopausal women: an update. *Maturitas, 63*(1), 34-38.
20. Seed, S. M., Dunican, K. C., & Lynch, A. M. (2009). Osteoarthritis: a review of treatment options. *Geriatrics, 64*(10), 20-29.
21. Svara, J. (2009). Weekend warriors: men's sports-related knee injuries. *Nurse Practitioner, 34*(7), 13-24.
22. Travison, T. G., Beck, T. J., Esche, G. R., et al. (2008). Age trends in proximal femur geometry in men: variation by race and ethnicity. *Osteoporosis International, 19*(3), 277-287.
23. U.S. Preventive Services Task Force. (2003). Screening for osteoporosis in postmenopausal women: recommendations and rationale. *American Journal of Nursing, 103*, 73-81.
24. U.S. Preventive Services Task Force. (2005). Screening for idiopathic scoliosis for adolescents: recommendation statement. *American Family Physician, 71*, 1975-1976.
25. Vondracek, S. F. (2010). Managing osteoporosis in postmenopausal women. *American Journal of Health-System Pharmacy, 67*(7), S9-S19.
26. Wetzsteon, R. J., Hughes, J. M., Kaufman, B. C., et al. (2009). Ethnic differences in bone geometry and strength are apparent in childhood. *Bone, 44*(5), 970-975.
27. Whyte, M. P. (2006). Paget's disease of bone. *New England Journal of Medicine, 335*(6), 593-599.
28. Wick, J. M., Konze, J., Alexander, K., et al. (2009). Infantile and juvenile scoliosis: the crooked path to diagnosis and treatment. *AORN Journal, 90*(3), 347-380.
29. Wilson, C. (2005). Rotator cuff versus cervical spine: making the diagnosis. *Nurse Practitioner, 30*, 45-50.
30. Wolfe, F., Smythe, H. A., Yunus, M. B., et al. (1990). The American College of Rheumatology 1990 criteria for the classification of fibromyalgia. *Arthritis and Rheumatism, 33*, 160-172.

Summary Checklist: Musculoskeletal Examination

 For a PDA-downloadable version, go to http://evolve.elsevier.com/Jarvis/.

For each joint to be examined:

1. **Inspection**
   Size and contour of joint
   Skin color and characteristics
2. **Palpation of joint area**
   Skin
   Muscles
   Bony articulations
   Joint capsule
3. **ROM**
   Active
   Passive (if limitation in active ROM is present)
   Measure with goniometer (if abnormality in ROM is present)
4. **Muscle testing**

23

Neurologic System

evolve WEBSITE

http://evolve.elsevier.com/Jarvis/

- Animations
- Audio Key Points
- Bedside Assessment Summary Checklist
- Case Study
  Seizures
- Health Promotion Guide
  Stroke
- NCLEX Review Questions
- Physical Examination Summary Checklist
- Quick Assessment for Common Conditions
  Brain Attack (Stroke, Cerebrovascular Accident)
- Video—Assessment
  Lower Extremities and Neuromuscular Function
  Musculoskeletal and Neurologic Systems

OUTLINE

Structure and Function, 621

The Central Nervous System (CNS)
The Peripheral Nervous System

Subjective Data, 630

Health History Questions

Objective Data, 632

Preparation
Cranial Nerves
The Motor System
The Sensory System
Reflexes
Neurologic Recheck

Documentation and Critical Thinking, 665

Abnormal Findings, 667

Abnormal Findings for Advanced Practice, 672

STRUCTURE AND FUNCTION

The nervous system can be divided into two parts—central and peripheral. The **central nervous system** (CNS) includes the brain and spinal cord. The **peripheral nervous system** includes all the nerve fibers *outside* the brain and spinal cord: the 12 pairs of cranial nerves, the 31 pairs of spinal nerves, and all their branches. The peripheral nervous system carries sensory (**af**ferent) messages *to* the CNS from sensory receptors, motor (**ef**ferent) messages *from* the CNS out to muscles and glands, as well as autonomic messages that govern the internal organs and blood vessels.

THE CENTRAL NERVOUS SYSTEM (CNS)

Cerebral Cortex. The cerebral cortex is the cerebrum's outer layer of nerve cell bodies, which looks like "gray matter" because it lacks myelin. Myelin is the white insulation on the axon that increases the conduction velocity of nerve impulses.

The cerebral cortex is the center for human's highest functions, governing thought, memory, reasoning, sensation, and voluntary movement (Fig. 23-1). Each half of the cerebrum

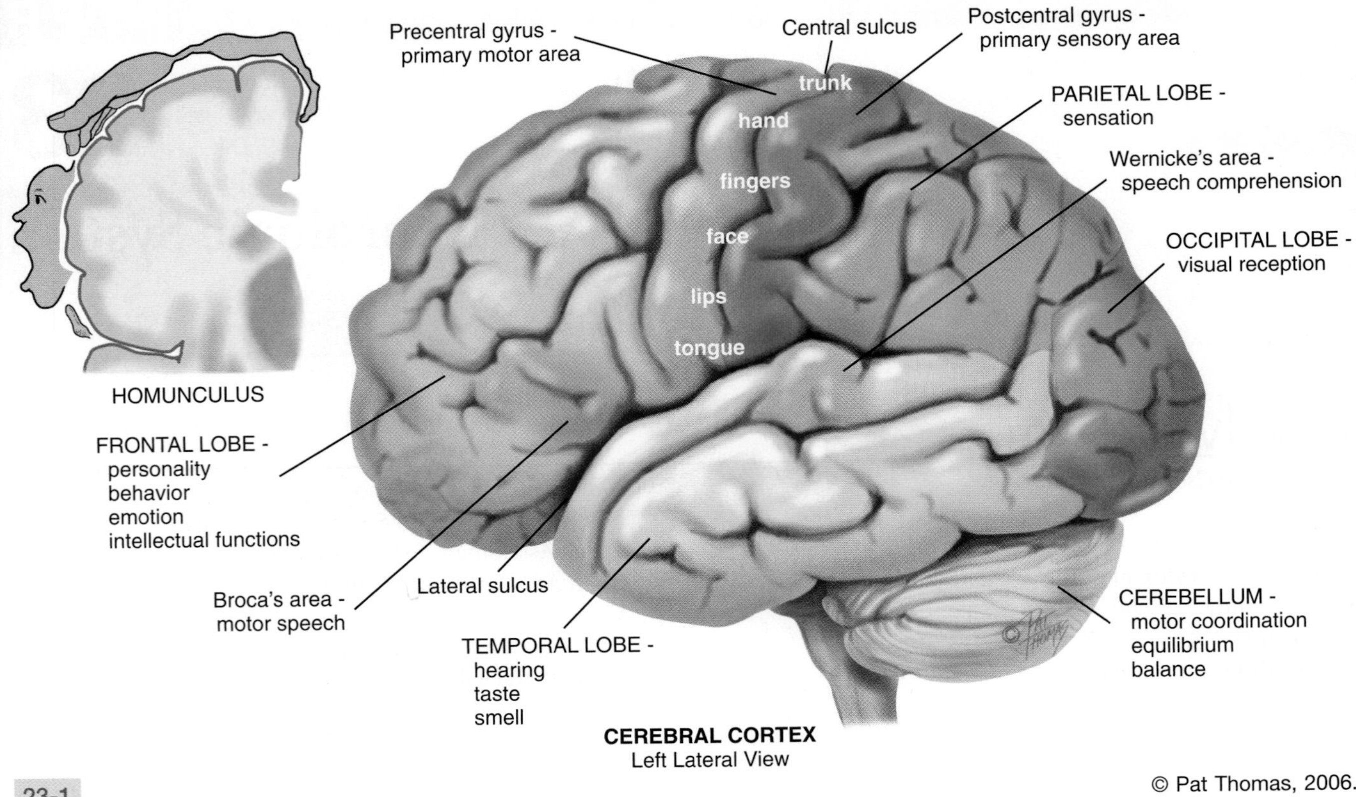

23-1

is a **hemisphere;** the left hemisphere is dominant in most (95%) people, including those who are left-handed.

Each hemisphere is divided into four **lobes:** frontal, parietal, temporal, and occipital. The lobes have certain areas that mediate specific functions.

- The **frontal** lobe has areas concerned with personality, behavior, emotions, and intellectual function.
- The precentral gyrus of the frontal lobe initiates voluntary movement.
- The **parietal** lobe's postcentral gyrus is the primary center for sensation.
- The **occipital** lobe is the primary visual receptor center.
- The **temporal** lobe behind the ear has the primary auditory reception center with functions of hearing, taste, and smell.
- **Wernicke's area** in the temporal lobe is associated with language comprehension. When damaged in the person's dominant hemisphere, *receptive aphasia* results. The person hears sound, but it has no meaning, like hearing a foreign language.
- **Broca's area** in the frontal lobe mediates motor speech. When injured in the dominant hemisphere, *expressive aphasia* results; the person cannot talk. The person can understand language and knows what he or she wants to say, but can produce only a garbled sound.

Damage to any of these specific cortical areas produces a corresponding loss of function: motor weakness, paralysis, loss of sensation, or impaired ability to understand and process language. Damage occurs when the highly specialized neurologic cells are deprived of their blood supply, such as when a cerebral artery becomes occluded or when vascular bleeding or vasospasm occurs.

Basal Ganglia. The basal ganglia are large bands of gray matter buried deep within the two cerebral hemispheres that form the subcortical associated motor system (the extrapyramidal system) (Fig. 23-2). They help to initiate and coordinate movement and control automatic associated movements of the body (e.g., the arm swing alternating with the legs during walking).

Thalamus. The thalamus is the main relay station where the sensory pathways of the spinal cord, cerebellum, and brainstem form **synapses** (sites of contact between two neurons) on their way to the cerebral cortex.

Hypothalamus. The hypothalamus is a major respiratory center with basic vital functions: temperature, appetite, sex drive, heart rate, and blood pressure (BP) control; sleep center; anterior and posterior pituitary gland regulator; and coordinator of autonomic nervous system activity and stress response.

Cerebellum. The cerebellum is a coiled structure located under the occipital lobe that is concerned with motor coordination of voluntary movements, equilibrium (i.e., the postural balance of the body), and muscle tone. It does not initiate movement but coordinates and smoothes it (e.g., the complex and quick coordination of many different muscles

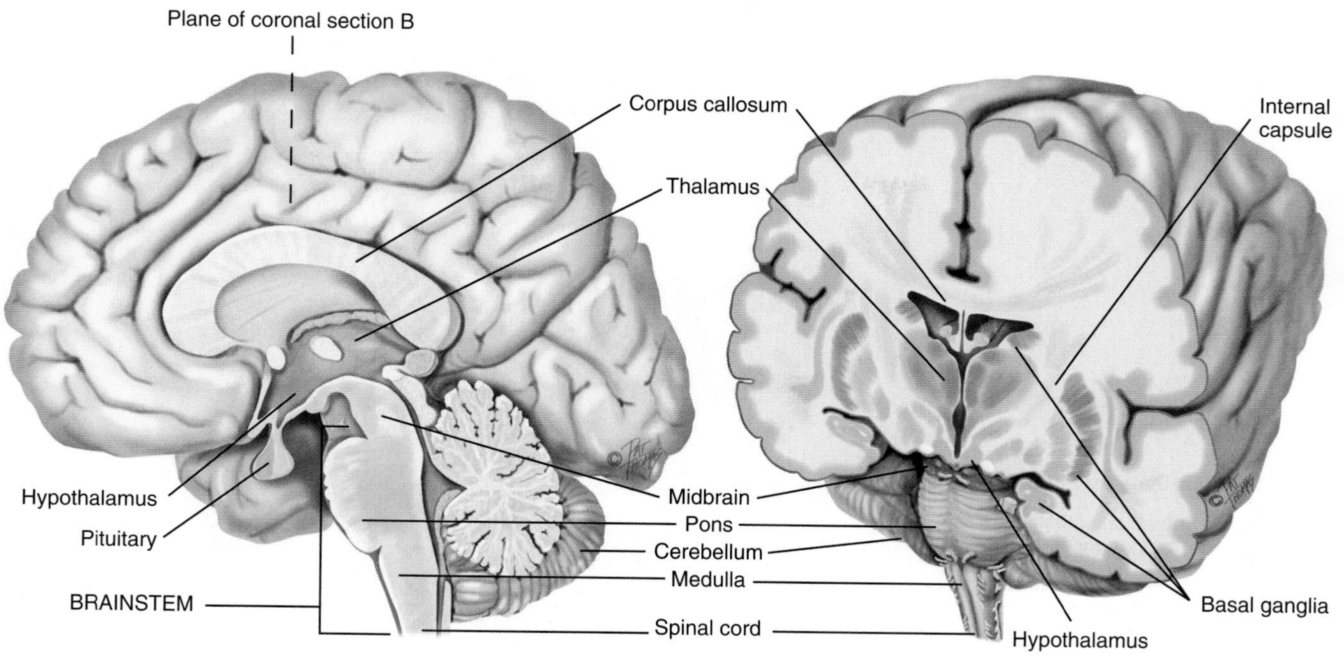

23-2 COMPONENTS OF THE CENTRAL NERVOUS SYSTEM

needed in playing the piano, swimming, or juggling). It is like the "automatic pilot" on an airplane in that it adjusts and corrects the voluntary movements but operates entirely below the conscious level.

Brainstem. The brainstem is the central core of the brain consisting of mostly nerve fibers. Cranial nerves III through XII originate from nuclei in the brainstem. It has three areas:

1. **Midbrain**—the most anterior part of the brainstem that still has the basic tubular structure of the spinal cord. It merges into the thalamus and hypothalamus. It contains many motor neurons and tracts.
2. **Pons**—the enlarged area containing ascending sensory and descending motor tracts. It has two respiratory centers (pneumotaxic and apneustic) that coordinate with the main respiratory center in the medulla.
3. **Medulla**—the continuation of the spinal cord in the brain that contains all ascending and descending fiber tracts. It has vital autonomic centers (respiration, heart, gastrointestinal function), as well as nuclei for cranial nerves VIII through XII. Pyramidal decussation (crossing of the motor fibers) occurs here (see p. 625).

Spinal Cord. The spinal cord is the long, cylindric structure of nervous tissue about as big around as the little finger. It occupies the upper two thirds of the vertebral canal from the medulla to lumbar vertebrae L1-L2. Its white matter is bundles of myelinated axons that form the main highway for ascending and descending fiber tracts that connect the brain to the spinal nerves. It mediates reflexes of posture control, urination, and pain response. Its nerve cell bodies, or gray matter, are arranged in a butterfly shape with anterior and posterior "horns."

The vertebral canal continues down beyond the spinal cord for several inches. The lumbar cistern is inside this space and is the favored spot to withdraw samples of cerebrospinal fluid (CSF).

Pathways of the CNS

Crossed representation is a notable feature of the nerve tracts; the *left* cerebral cortex receives sensory information from and controls motor function to the *right* side of the body, whereas *the right* cerebral cortex likewise interacts with the *left* side of the body. Knowledge of where the fibers cross the midline will help you interpret clinical findings.

Sensory Pathways

Millions of sensory receptors are embroidered into the skin, mucous membranes, muscles, tendons, and viscera. They monitor conscious sensation, internal organ functions, body position, and reflexes. Sensation travels in the afferent fibers in the peripheral nerve, then through the posterior (dorsal) root, and then into the spinal cord. There, it may take one of two routes—the spinothalamic tract or the posterior (dorsal) columns (Fig. 23-3).

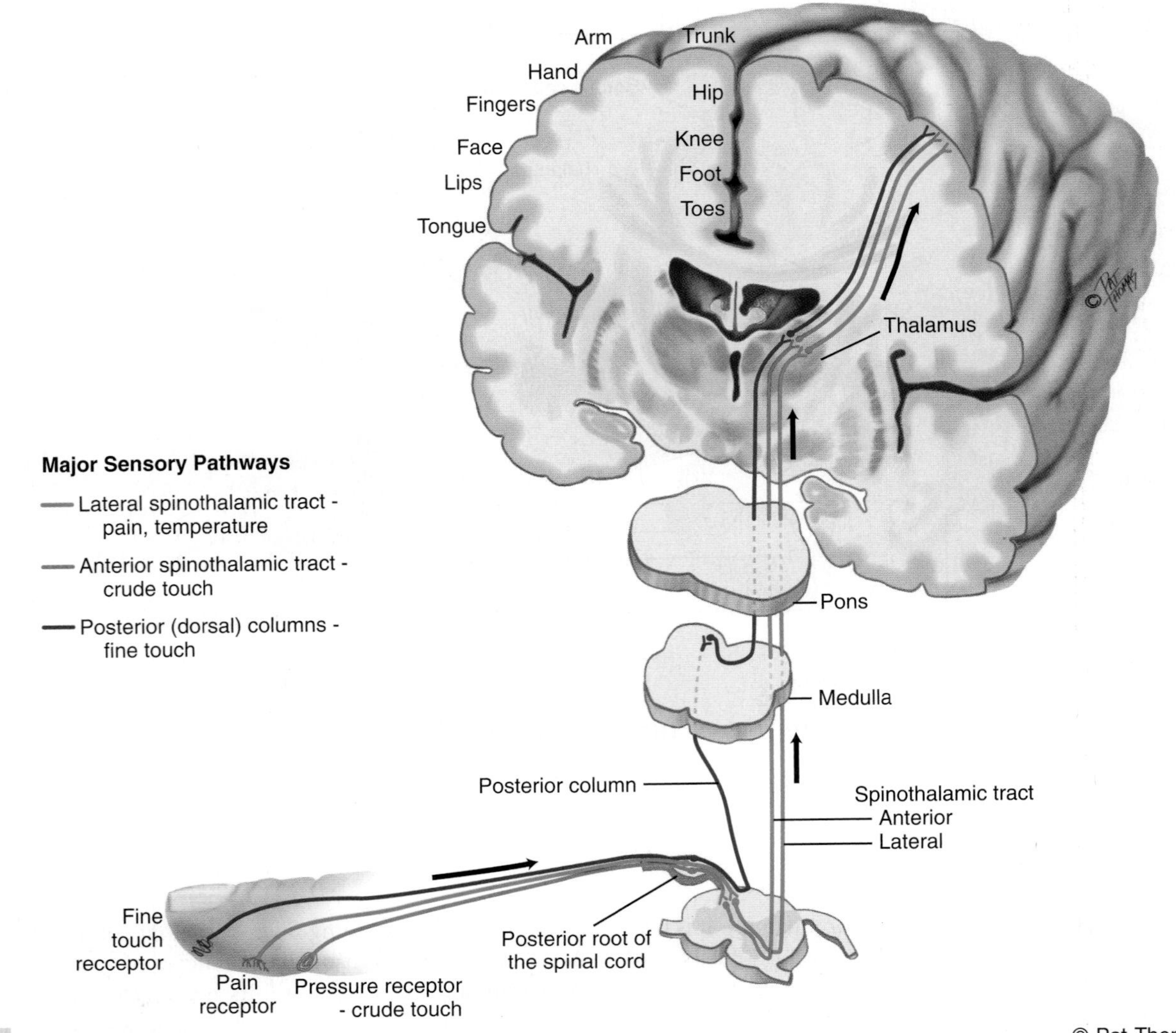

23-3 Sensory pathways.

Spinothalamic Tract. The spinothalamic tract contains sensory fibers that transmit the sensations of pain, temperature, and crude or light touch (i.e., not precisely localized). The fibers enter the dorsal root of the spinal cord and synapse with a second sensory neuron. The second-order neuron fibers cross to the opposite side and ascend up the spinothalamic tract to the thalamus. Fibers carrying pain and temperature sensations ascend the *lateral* spinothalamic tract, whereas those of crude touch form the *anterior* spinothalamic tract. At the thalamus, the fibers synapse with a third sensory neuron, which carries the message to the sensory cortex for full interpretation.

Posterior (Dorsal) Columns. These fibers conduct the sensations of position, vibration, and finely localized touch.

- **Position** (proprioception)—Without looking, you know where your body parts are in space and in relation to each other
- **Vibration—**Feeling vibrating objects
- **Finely localized touch** (stereognosis)—Without looking, you can identify familiar objects by touch

These fibers enter the dorsal root and proceed immediately up the same side of the spinal cord to the brainstem. At the medulla, they synapse with a second sensory neuron and then cross. They travel to the **thalamus,** synapse again, and proceed to the sensory cortex, which localizes the sensation and makes full discrimination.

The sensory cortex is arranged in a specific pattern forming a corresponding "map" of the body (see the homunculus in Fig. 23-1). Pain in the right hand is perceived at its specific spot on the left cortex map. Some organs are absent from the brain map, such as the heart, liver, or spleen. You know you have one but you have no "felt image" of it. Pain originating in these organs is referred, because no felt image exists in which to have pain. Pain is felt "by proxy" by another body part that does have a felt image. For example, pain in the heart is referred to the chest, shoulder, and left arm, which were its neighbors in fetal development. Pain originating in the spleen is felt on the top of the left shoulder.

Motor Pathways

Corticospinal or Pyramidal Tract (Fig. 23-4). The area has been named "pyramidal" because it originates in pyramidal-shaped cells in the motor cortex. Motor nerve fibers originate in the motor cortex and travel to the brainstem, where they cross to the opposite or contralateral side *(pyramidal decussation)* and then pass down in the lateral column of the spinal cord. At each cord level, they synapse with a lower motor neuron contained in the anterior horn of the spinal cord. Ten percent of corticospinal fibers do *not* cross, and these descend in the anterior column of the spinal cord. Corticospinal fibers mediate voluntary movement, particularly very skilled, discrete, purposeful movements, such as writing.

The corticospinal tract is a newer, "higher," motor system that permits humans to have very skilled and purposeful movements. The tract's origin in the motor cortex is arranged in a specific pattern called *somatotopic organization.* It is another body map, this one of a person, or *homunculus,* hanging "upside down" (see Fig. 23-1). Body parts are not equally represented on the map, and the homunculus looks distorted. To use political terms, it is more like an electoral map than a geographic map. That is, body parts whose movements are relatively more important to humans (e.g., the hand) occupy proportionally more space on the brain map.

Extrapyramidal Tracts. The extrapyramidal tracts include all the motor nerve fibers originating in the motor cortex, basal ganglia, brainstem, and spinal cord that are *outside* the pyramidal tract. This is a phylogenetically older, "lower," more primitive motor system. These subcortical motor fibers maintain muscle tone and control body movements, especially gross automatic movements, such as walking.

Cerebellar System. This complex motor system coordinates movement, maintains equilibrium, and helps maintain posture. The cerebellum receives information about the position of muscles and joints, the body's equilibrium, and what kind of motor messages are being sent from the cortex to the muscles. The information is integrated, and the cerebellum uses feedback pathways to exert its control back on the cortex or down to lower motor neurons in the spinal cord. This entire process occurs on a subconscious level.

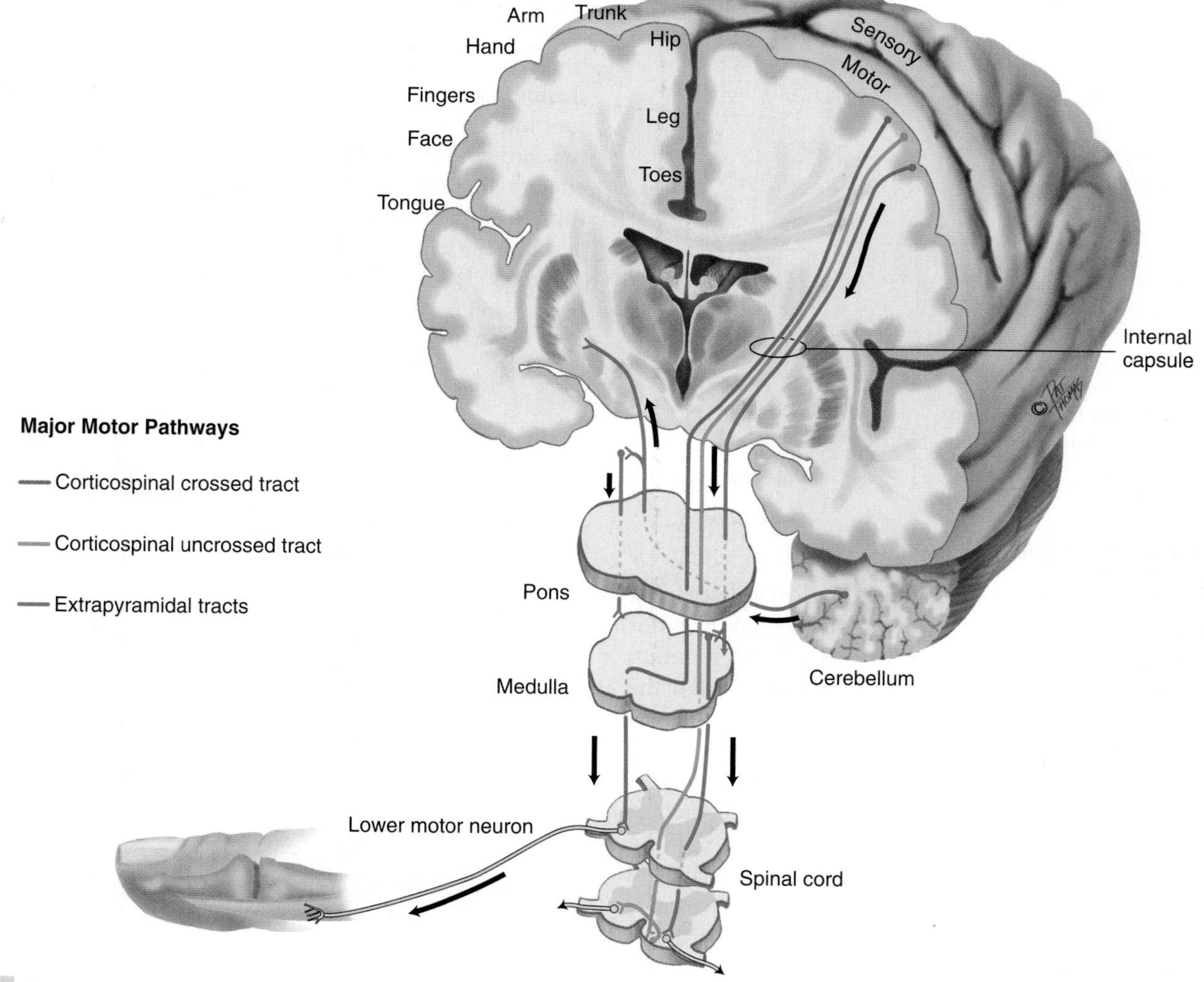

23-4 Motor pathways.

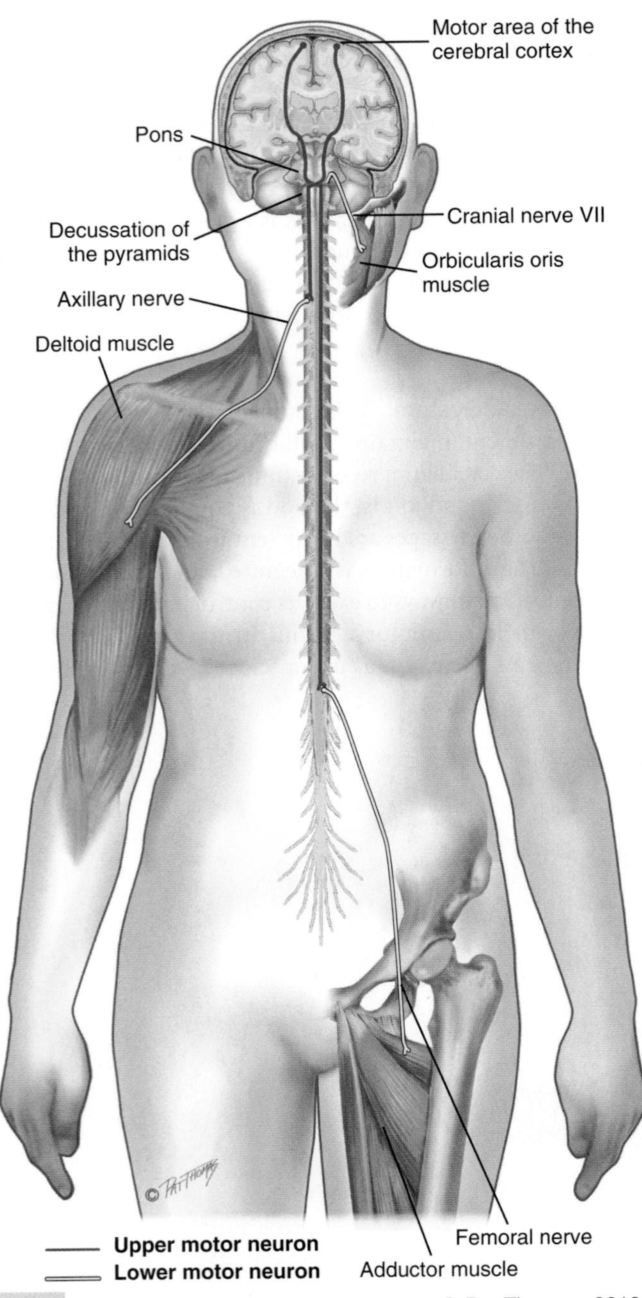

23-5

Upper and Lower Motor Neurons

Upper motor neurons are a complex of all the descending motor fibers that can influence or modify the lower motor neurons. Upper motor neurons are located completely within the CNS. The neurons convey impulses from motor areas of the cerebral cortex to the lower motor neurons in the anterior horn cells of the spinal cord (Fig. 23-5). Examples of upper motor neurons are corticospinal, corticobulbar, and extrapyramidal tracts. Examples of upper motor neuron diseases are cerebrovascular accident, cerebral palsy, and multiple sclerosis.

Lower motor neurons are located mostly in the peripheral nervous system. The cell body of the lower motor neuron is located in the anterior gray column of the spinal cord, but the nerve fiber extends from here to the muscle. The lower motor neuron is the "final common pathway," because it funnels many neural signals here and it provides the final direct contact with the muscles. Any movement must be translated into action by lower motor neuron fibers. Examples of lower motor neurons are cranial nerves and spinal nerves of the peripheral nervous system. Examples of lower motor neuron diseases are spinal cord lesions, poliomyelitis, and amyotrophic lateral sclerosis.

THE PERIPHERAL NERVOUS SYSTEM

A **nerve** is a bundle of fibers *outside* the CNS. The peripheral nerves carry input to the CNS via their sensory afferent fibers and deliver output from the CNS via the efferent fibers.

Reflex Arc

Reflexes are basic defense mechanisms of the nervous system. They are involuntary, operating below the level of conscious control and permitting a quick reaction to potentially painful or damaging situations. Reflexes also help the body maintain balance and appropriate muscle tone. There are four types of reflexes: (1) **Deep tendon reflexes** (myotatic), e.g., patellar [or knee jerk]; (2) **Superficial,** e.g., corneal reflex, abdominal reflex; (3) **Visceral** (organic), e.g., pupillary response to light and accommodation; (4) **Pathologic** (abnormal), e.g., Babinski (or extensor plantar) reflex.

The fibers that mediate the reflex are carried by a specific spinal nerve. In the simplest reflex, tapping the tendon stretches the muscle spindles in the muscle, which activates the sensory afferent nerve. The sensory afferent fibers carry the message from the receptor and travel through the dorsal root into the spinal cord (Fig. 23-6). They synapse directly in the cord with the motor neuron in the anterior horn. Motor efferent fibers leave via the ventral root and travel to the muscle, stimulating a sudden contraction.

The deep tendon (myotatic, or stretch) reflex has five components: (1) an intact sensory nerve (afferent); (2) a functional synapse in the cord; (3) an intact motor nerve fiber

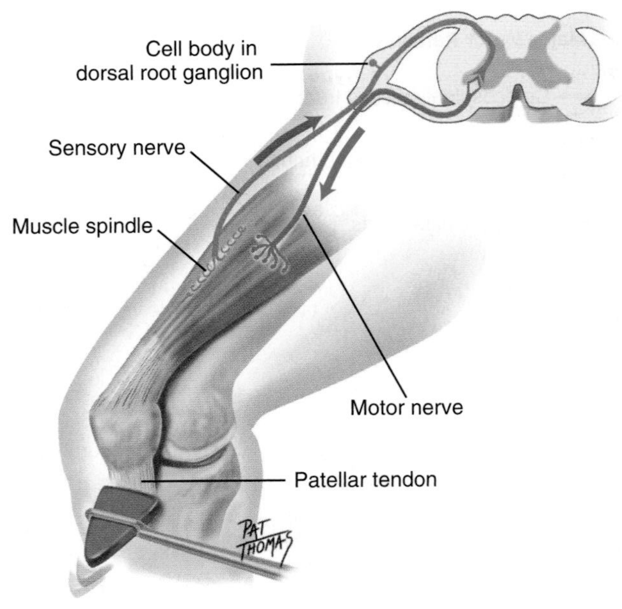

23-6

(efferent); (4) the neuromuscular junction; and (5) a competent muscle.

Cranial Nerves

Cranial nerves enter and exit the brain rather than the spinal cord (Fig. 23-7). Cranial nerves I and II extend from the cerebrum; cranial nerves III through XII extend from the lower diencephalon and brainstem. The 12 pairs of cranial nerves supply primarily the head and neck, except the vagus nerve (Lat. *vagus,* or wanderer, as in "vagabond"), which travels to the heart, respiratory muscles, stomach, and gallbladder.

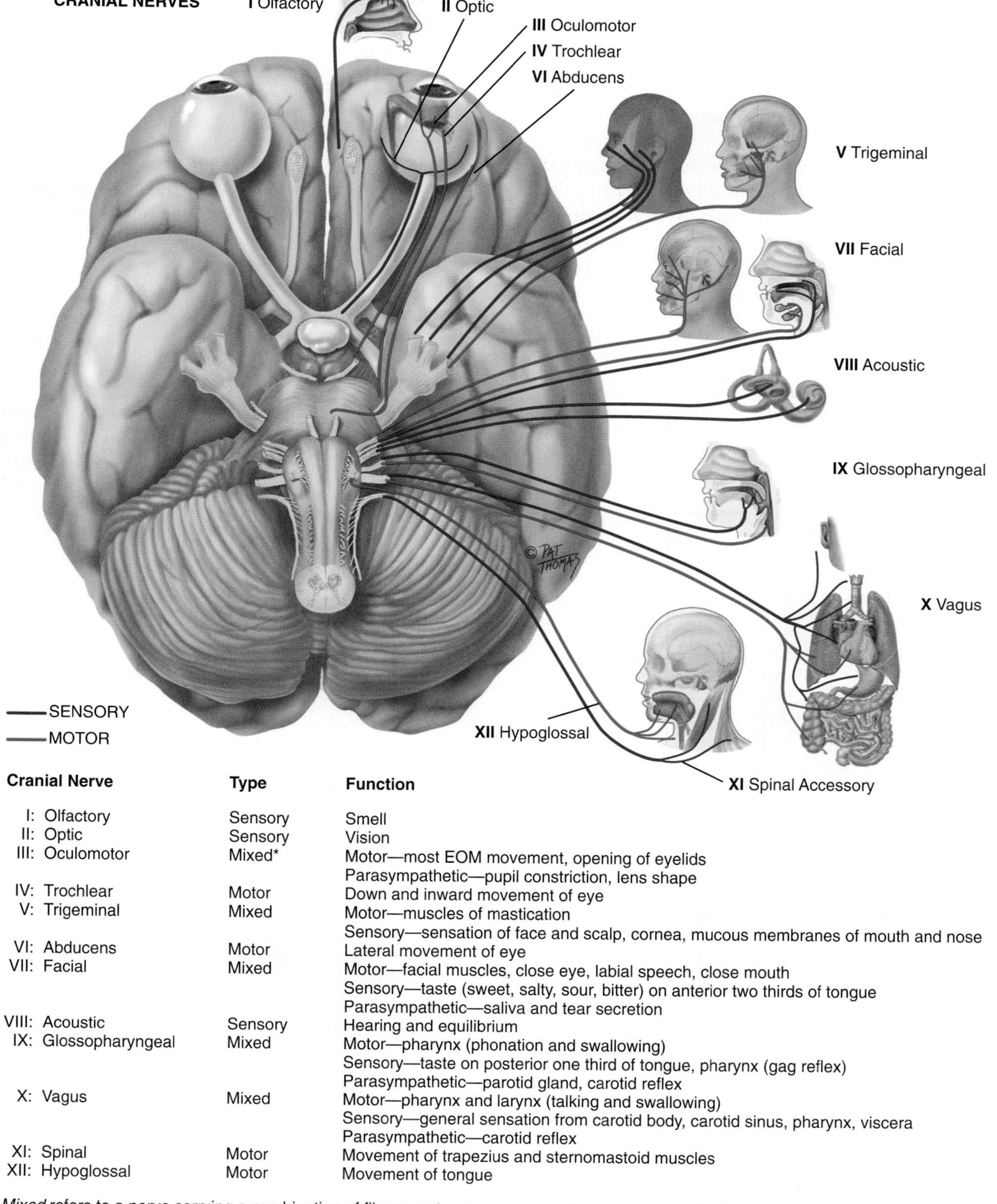

Cranial Nerve	Type	Function
I: Olfactory	Sensory	Smell
II: Optic	Sensory	Vision
III: Oculomotor	Mixed*	Motor—most EOM movement, opening of eyelids Parasympathetic—pupil constriction, lens shape
IV: Trochlear	Motor	Down and inward movement of eye
V: Trigeminal	Mixed	Motor—muscles of mastication Sensory—sensation of face and scalp, cornea, mucous membranes of mouth and nose
VI: Abducens	Motor	Lateral movement of eye
VII: Facial	Mixed	Motor—facial muscles, close eye, labial speech, close mouth Sensory—taste (sweet, salty, sour, bitter) on anterior two thirds of tongue Parasympathetic—saliva and tear secretion
VIII: Acoustic	Sensory	Hearing and equilibrium
IX: Glossopharyngeal	Mixed	Motor—pharynx (phonation and swallowing) Sensory—taste on posterior one third of tongue, pharynx (gag reflex) Parasympathetic—parotid gland, carotid reflex
X: Vagus	Mixed	Motor—pharynx and larynx (talking and swallowing) Sensory—general sensation from carotid body, carotid sinus, pharynx, viscera Parasympathetic—carotid reflex
XI: Spinal	Motor	Movement of trapezius and sternomastoid muscles
XII: Hypoglossal	Motor	Movement of tongue

**Mixed* refers to a nerve carrying a combination of fibers: motor + sensory; motor + parasympathetic; or motor + sensory + parasympathetic.

23-7

Spinal Nerves

The 31 pairs of **spinal nerves** arise from the length of the spinal cord and supply the rest of the body. They are named for the region of the spine from which they exit: 8 cervical, 12 thoracic, 5 lumbar, 5 sacral, and 1 coccygeal. They are "mixed" nerves because they contain both sensory and motor fibers. The nerves enter and exit the cord through roots—sensory afferent fibers through the posterior or dorsal roots, and motor efferent fibers through the anterior or ventral roots.

The nerves exit the spinal cord in an orderly ladder. Each nerve innervates a particular segment of the body. **Dermal segmentation** is the cutaneous distribution of the various spinal nerves.

A **dermatome** is a circumscribed skin area that is supplied mainly from one spinal cord segment through a particular spinal nerve (Fig. 23-8). The dermatomes overlap, which is a form of biologic insurance. That is, if one nerve is severed, most of the sensations can be transmitted by the one above and the one below. Do not attempt to memorize all dermatome segments; just focus on the following as useful landmarks:

- The **thumb, middle finger,** and **fifth finger** are each in the dermatomes of **C6, C7,** and **C8.**
- The **axilla** is at the level of **T1.**
- The **nipple** is at the level of **T4.**
- The **umbilicus** is at the level of **T10.**
- The **groin** is in the region of **L1.**
- The **knee** is at the level of **L4.**

Autonomic Nervous System

The peripheral nervous system is composed of cranial nerves and spinal nerves. These nerves carry fibers that can be divided functionally into two parts—somatic and autonomic. The somatic fibers innervate the skeletal (voluntary) muscles;

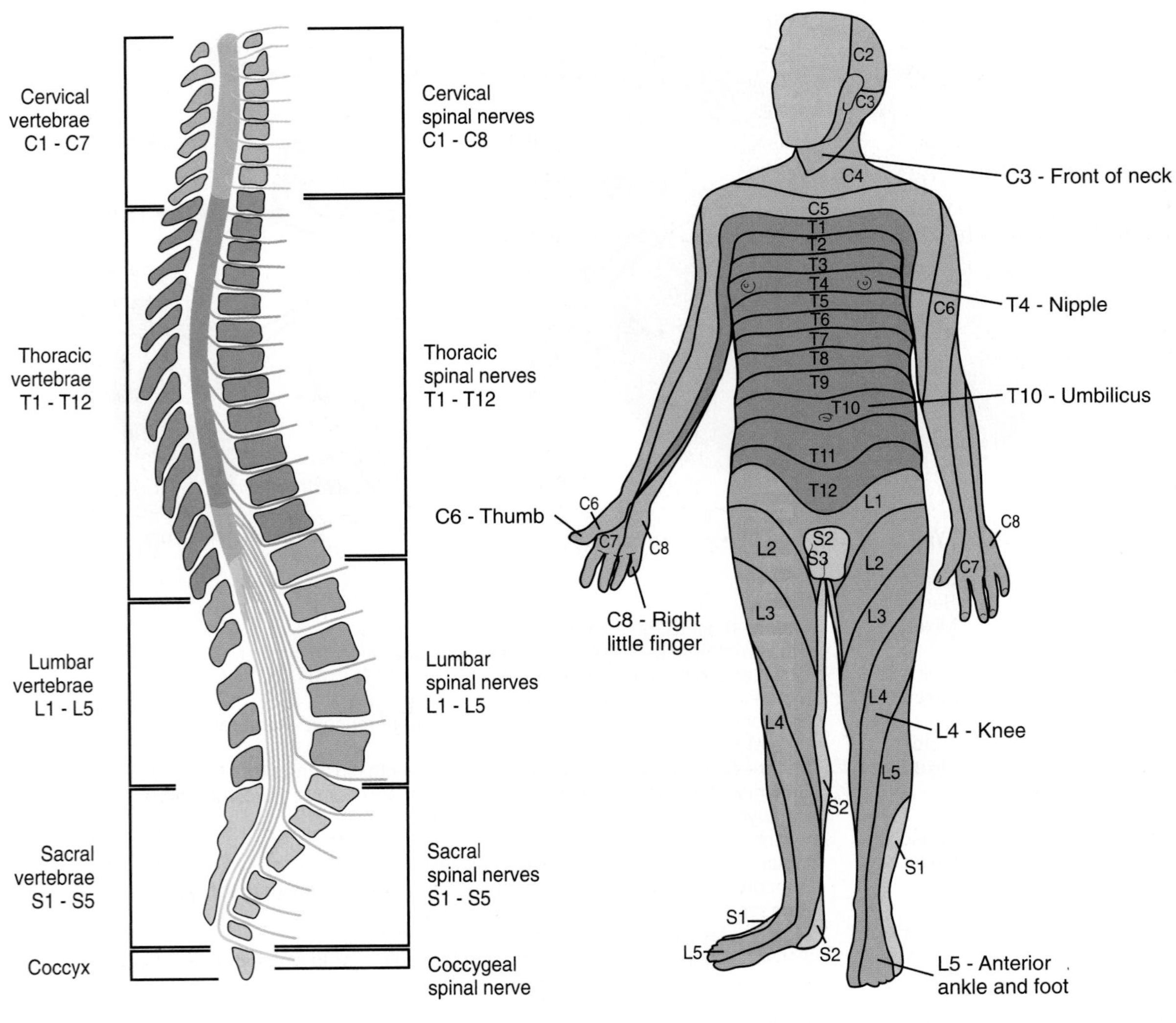

23-8

the autonomic fibers innervate smooth (involuntary) muscles, cardiac muscle, and glands. The autonomic system mediates unconscious activity. Although a description of the autonomic system is beyond the scope of this book, its overall function is to maintain homeostasis of the body.

DEVELOPMENTAL COMPETENCE

Infants

The neurologic system is not completely developed at birth. Motor activity in the newborn is under the control of the spinal cord and medulla. Very little cortical control exists, and the neurons are not yet myelinated. Movements are directed primarily by primitive reflexes. As the cerebral cortex develops during the first year, it inhibits these reflexes and they disappear at predictable times. Persistence of the primitive reflexes is an indication of CNS dysfunction.

The infant's sensory and motor development proceed along with the gradual acquisition of myelin, because myelin is needed to conduct most impulses. The process of myelinization follows a cephalocaudal and proximodistal order (head, neck, trunk, and extremities). This is just the order in which we observe the infant gaining motor control (lifts head, lifts head and shoulders, rolls over, moves whole arm, uses hands, walks). As the milestones are achieved, each is more complex and coordinated. Milestones occur in an orderly sequence, although the exact age of occurrence may vary.

Sensation also is rudimentary at birth. The newborn needs a strong stimulus and then responds by crying and with whole body movements. As myelinization develops, the infant is able to localize the stimulus more precisely and to make a more accurate motor response.

The Aging Adult

The aging process causes a general atrophy with a steady loss of neuron structure in the brain and spinal cord. This causes a decrease in weight and volume with a thinning of the cerebral cortex, reduced subcortical brain structures, and expansion of the ventricles.[9] Neuron loss leads many people older than 65 years to show signs that, in the younger adult, would be considered abnormal, such as general loss of muscle bulk; loss of muscle tone in the face, in the neck, and around the spine; decreased muscle strength; impaired fine coordination and agility; loss of vibratory sense at the ankle; decreased or absent Achilles reflex; loss of position sense at the big toe; pupillary miosis; irregular pupil shape; and decreased pupillary reflexes.

The velocity of nerve conduction decreases between 5% and 10% with aging, making the reaction time slower in some older persons. An increased delay at the synapse also occurs, so the impulse takes longer to travel. As a result, touch and pain sensation, taste, and smell may be diminished.

The motor system may show a general slowing down of movement. Muscle strength and agility decrease. A generalized decrease occurs in muscle bulk, which is most apparent in the dorsal hand muscles. Muscle tremors may occur in the hands, head, and jaw, along with possible repetitive facial grimacing (dyskinesias).

Aging has a progressive decrease in cerebral blood flow and oxygen consumption. In some people, this causes dizziness and a loss of balance with position change. These people need to be taught to get up slowly. Otherwise they have an increased risk for falls and resulting injuries. In addition, older people may forget they fell, which makes it hard to diagnose the cause of the injury.

When they are in good health, aging people walk about as well as they did during their middle and younger years, except more slowly and more deliberately. Some survey the ground for obstacles or uneven terrain. Some show a hesitation and a slightly wayward path.

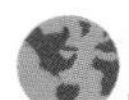

CULTURE AND GENETICS

Stroke is the third most common cause of death in the United States.[19] The overall prevalence of stroke in adults older than 20 years is 2.9%. There is racial/ethnic disparity here because 6% of American Indian/Alaska Natives have had a stroke, 4% of African Americans, 2.6% of Hispanics, 2.3% of whites, and only 1.6% of Asian/Pacific Islanders. Further, African Americans, American Indian/Alaska Natives (AI/AN), Asian/Pacific Islanders, and Hispanics die from stroke at younger ages than do whites.[19]

There is geographic disparity; many states with high stroke mortality are concentrated in the U.S. southeast region, called the "stroke belt." This may occur because of the high proportion of people who live in this region who have two or more of the major modifiable risk factors for stroke (high BP, high cholesterol, diabetes, current smoking, physical inactivity, or obesity). And why would this occur? Perhaps it is a combination of factors: cultural norms for diet and exercise, poverty, lack of economic opportunity, social isolation, lack of access to health care and preventive services.[3]

The disparity in prevalence among racial groups also is attributed to the disproportion in these groups of having risk factors for stroke. The AI/AN men have a higher prevalence of hypertension and high cholesterol than any other racial/ethnic group, and AI/AN women have the highest rate of obesity, current smoking, and diabetes.[4] African Americans also have high rates of stroke, and their risk factors are the following: higher prevalence of hypertension and diabetes than whites, and less likely to have BP controlled or diabetes treated than whites.[19] Because we know these risk factors lead to stroke, it is important to develop community policy to control such things as access to healthful foods, reduced tobacco exposure, opportunities for physical activity, and access to health care and health education.[5]

SUBJECTIVE DATA

1. Headache
2. Head injury
3. Dizziness/vertigo
4. Seizures
5. Tremors
6. Weakness
7. Incoordination
8. Numbness or tingling
9. Difficulty swallowing
10. Difficulty speaking
11. Significant past history
12. Environmental/occupational hazards

Examiner Asks / Rationale

1. **Headache.** Any unusually frequent or severe headaches?
   - When did this start? How often does it occur?
   - Where in your head do you feel the headaches? Do the headaches seem to be associated with anything? (Headache history is discussed in Chapter 13.)

A patient who says "This is the worst headache of my life" needs emergency referral to screen cerebrovascular cause.

2. **Head injury.** Ever had any **head injury?** Please describe.
   - What part of your head was hit?
   - Did you have a loss of consciousness? For how long?

3. **Dizziness/vertigo.** Ever feel light-headed, a swimming sensation, like feeling faint?
   - When have you noticed this? How often does it occur? Does it occur with activity, change in position?
   - Do you ever feel a sensation called **vertigo,** a rotational spinning sensation? (Note: Distinguish vertigo from dizziness.) Do you feel as if the room spins (objective vertigo)? Or do you feel that you are spinning (subjective vertigo)? Did this come on suddenly or gradually?

Syncope is a sudden loss of strength, a temporary loss of consciousness (a faint) due to lack of cerebral blood flow (e.g., low BP).

True **vertigo** is rotational spinning caused by neurologic disease in the vestibular apparatus in the ear or in the vestibular nuclei in the brainstem.

4. **Seizures.** Ever had any convulsions? When did they start? How often do they occur?
   - Course and duration—When a seizure starts, do you have any warning sign? What type of sign?
   - Motor activity—Where in your body do the seizures begin? Do the seizures travel through your body? On one side or both? Does your muscle tone seem tense or limp?
   - Any associated signs—Color change in face or lips, loss of consciousness, for how long, automatisms (eyelid fluttering, eye rolling, lip smacking), incontinence?
   - Postictal phase—After the seizure, are you told you spend time sleeping or have any confusion, weakness, headache, or muscle ache?
   - Precipitating factors—Does anything seem to bring on the seizures: activity, discontinuing medication, fatigue, stress?
   - Are you on any medication?
   - Coping strategies—How have the seizures affected daily life, occupation?

Seizures occur with epilepsy, a paroxysmal disease characterized by altered or loss of consciousness, involuntary muscle movements, and sensory disturbances.

Aura is a subjective sensation that precedes a seizure; it could be auditory, visual, or motor.

5. **Tremors.** Any shakes or **tremors** in the hands or face? When did these start?
   - Do they seem to grow worse with anxiety, intention, or rest?
   - Are they relieved with rest, activity, alcohol? Do they affect daily activities?

Tremor is an involuntary shaking, vibrating, or trembling (see Table 23-5, Abnormalities in Muscle Movement, p. 670).

6. **Weakness.** Any **weakness** or problem moving any body part? Is this generalized or local? Does weakness occur with any particular movement? (For

Paresis is a partial or incomplete paralysis.

Examiner Asks	Rationale
example, with proximal or large muscle weakness, it is hard to get up out of a chair or reach for an object; with distal or small muscle weakness, it is hard to open a jar, write, use scissors, or walk without tripping.)	*Paralysis* is a loss of motor function due to a lesion in the neurologic or muscular system or loss of sensory innervation.
7. Incoordination. Any problem with **coordination?** Any problem with balance when walking? Do you list to one side? Any falling? Which way? Do your legs seem to give way? Any clumsy movement?	*Dysmetria* is the inability to control the distance, power, and speed of a muscular action.
8. Numbness or tingling. Any **numbness or tingling** in any body part? Does it feel like pins and needles? When did this start? Where do you feel it? Does it occur with activity?	*Paresthesia* is an abnormal sensation (e.g., burning, tingling).
9. Difficulty swallowing. Any problem **swallowing?** Occur with solids or liquids? Have you experienced excessive saliva, drooling?	
10. Difficulty speaking. Any problem **speaking:** with forming words or with saying what you intended to say? When did you first notice this? How long did it last?	*Dysarthria* is difficulty forming words; *dysphasia* is difficulty with language comprehension or expression (see Table 5-4, p. 84).
11. Significant past history. **Past history** of: stroke (cerebrovascular accident), spinal cord injury, meningitis or encephalitis, congenital defect, or alcoholism?	
12. Environmental/occupational hazards. Are you exposed to any environmental/occupational hazards: insecticides, organic solvents, lead? • Are you taking any medications now? • How much alcohol do you drink? Each week? Each day? • How about other mood-altering drugs: marijuana, cocaine, barbiturates, tranquilizers?	Review anticonvulsants; anti-tremor, anti-vertigo, pain medication.

Additional History for Infants and Children

Examiner Asks	Rationale
1. Did you (the mother) have any health problems during the pregnancy: any infections or illnesses, medications taken, toxemia, hypertension, alcohol or drug use, diabetes?	Prenatal history may affect infant's neurologic development.
2. Please tell me about this baby's birth. Was the baby at term or premature? Birth weight? • Any birth trauma? Did the baby breathe immediately? • Were you told the baby's Apgar scores? • Any congenital defects?	
3. Reflexes—What have you noticed about the baby's behavior? Do the baby's sucking and swallowing seem coordinated? When you touch the cheek, does the baby turn his or her head toward touch? Does the baby startle with a loud noise or shake of crib? Does the baby grasp your finger?	
4. Does the child seem to have any problem with balance? Have you noted any unexplained falling, clumsy or unsteady gait, progressive muscular weakness, problem with going up or down stairs, problem with getting up from lying position?	If occurs, may not be noticed until starts to walk in late infancy. Screens for muscular dystrophy.
5. Has this child had any seizures? Please describe. Did the seizure occur with a high fever? Did any loss of consciousness occur—how long? How many seizures occurred with this same illness (if occurred with high fever)?	Seizures may occur with high fever in infants and toddlers. Or, seizures may be sign of neurologic disease.

Subjective Data

Examiner Asks	Rationale
6. Did this child's motor or developmental milestones seem to come at about the right age? Does this child seem to be growing and maturing normally to you? How does this child's development compare with siblings or with age-mates?	
7. Do you know if your child has had any environmental exposure to lead?	Chronically elevated lead levels may cause a developmental delay or a loss of a newly acquired skill or be asymptomatic.
8. Have you been told about any learning problems in school: problems with attention span, cannot concentrate, hyperactive?	
9. Any family history of seizure disorder, cerebral palsy, muscular dystrophy?	

Additional History for the Aging Adult

Examiner Asks	Rationale
1. Any problem with dizziness? Does this occur when you first sit or stand up, when you move your head, when you get up and walk just after eating? Does this occur with any of your medications?	Diminished cerebral blood flow and diminished vestibular response may produce staggering with position change, which increases risk for falls.
• (For men) Do you ever get up at night and then feel faint while standing to urinate?	Micturition syncope.
• How does dizziness affect your daily activities? Are you able to drive safely and to maneuver within your house safely?	
• What safety modifications have you applied at home?	
2. Have you noticed any decrease in memory, change in mental function? Have you felt any confusion? Did this seem to come on suddenly or gradually?	Memory loss and cognitive decline are early indicators of Alzheimer disease and can be mistaken for normal cognitive decline of aging[19] (see Table 23-2, 10 Warning Signs of Alzheimer Disease, p. 667).
3. Have you ever noticed any tremor? Is this in your hands or face? Is this worse with anxiety, activity, rest? Does the tremor seem to be relieved with alcohol, activity, rest? Does the tremor interfere with daily or social activities?	Senile tremor is relieved by alcohol, but this is not a recommended treatment. Assess if the person is abusing alcohol in effort to relieve tremor.
4. Have you ever had any sudden vision change, fleeting blindness? Did this occur along with weakness? Did you have any loss of consciousness?	Screen symptoms of stroke.

Objective Data

OBJECTIVE DATA

PREPARATION

Perform a **screening neurologic examination** (items identified in following sections) on seemingly well persons who have no significant subjective findings from the history.

Perform a **complete neurologic examination** on persons who have neurologic concerns (e.g., headache, weakness, loss of coordination) or who have shown signs of neurologic dysfunction.

Perform a **neurologic recheck** examination on persons who have neurologic deficits and require periodic assessments (e.g., hospitalized persons or those in extended care), using the examination sequence beginning on p. 660.

Integrate the steps of the neurologic examination with the examination of each particular part of the body, as much as you are able. For example, test cranial nerves while assessing the head and neck (recall Chapters 13 through

EQUIPMENT NEEDED

Penlight
Tongue blade
Cotton swab
Cotton ball
Tuning fork (128 Hz or 256 Hz)
Percussion hammer
(Possibly) familiar aromatic substances (e.g., peppermint, coffee, vanilla)

16) and superficial abdominal reflexes while assessing the abdomen. When recording your findings, however, consider all neurologic data as a functional unit, and record them all together.

Use the following sequence for the complete neurologic examination:

1. Mental status (see Chapter 5)
2. Cranial nerves
3. Motor system
4. Sensory system
5. Reflexes

Position the person sitting up with the head at your eye level.

Normal Range of Findings	Abnormal Findings

TEST CRANIAL NERVES

Cranial Nerve I—Olfactory Nerve

Do not test routinely. Test the sense of smell in those who report loss of smell, those with head trauma, and those with abnormal mental status, and when the presence of an intracranial lesion is suspected. First, assess patency by occluding one nostril at a time and asking the person to sniff. Then, with the person's eyes closed, occlude one nostril and present an aromatic substance. Use familiar, conveniently obtainable, and non-noxious smells, such as coffee, toothpaste, orange, vanilla, soap, or peppermint. Alcohol wipes smell familiar and are easy to find but are irritating.

Normally, a person can identify an odor on each side of the nose. Smell normally is decreased bilaterally with aging. Any asymmetry in the sense of smell is important.

One cannot test smell when air passages are occluded with upper respiratory infection or with sinusitis.

Anosmia—decrease or loss of smell occurs bilaterally with tobacco smoking, allergic rhinitis, and cocaine use.

Unilateral loss of smell in the absence of nasal disease is *neurogenic anosmia* (see Table 23-3, Abnormalities in Cranial Nerves, p. 668).

Cranial Nerve II—Optic Nerve

Test visual acuity and test visual fields by confrontation (see Chapter 14).

Using the ophthalmoscope, examine the ocular fundus to determine the color, size, and shape of the optic disc (see Chapter 14).

Visual field loss (see Table 14-5, p. 316).

Papilledema with increased intracranial pressure; optic atrophy (see Table 14-9, p. 320).

Cranial Nerves III, IV, and VI—Oculomotor, Trochlear, and Abducens Nerves

Palpebral fissures are usually equal in width or nearly so.

Ptosis (drooping) occurs with myasthenia gravis, dysfunction of cranial nerve III, or Horner syndrome (see Table 14-2).

Check pupils for size, regularity, equality, direct and consensual light reaction, and accommodation (see Chapter 14).

Increasing intracranial pressure causes a sudden, unilateral, dilated and nonreactive pupil.

Assess extraocular movements by the cardinal positions of gaze (see Chapter 14).

Strabismus (deviated gaze) or limited movement (see Table 14-1, p. 311).

Nystagmus is a back-and-forth oscillation of the eyes. End-point nystagmus, a few beats of horizontal nystagmus at extreme lateral gaze, occurs normally. Assess any other nystagmus carefully, noting:

- Presence of nystagmus in one or both eyes.
- *Pendular* movement (oscillations move equally left to right) or *jerk* (a quick phase in one direction, then a slow phase in the other). Classify the jerk nystagmus in the direction of the quick phase.
- Amplitude. Judge whether the degree of movement is fine, medium, or coarse.
- Frequency. Is it constant, or does it fade after a few beats?
- Plane of movement. Horizontal, vertical, rotary, or a combination?

Nystagmus occurs with disease of the vestibular system, cerebellum, or brainstem.

Normal Range of Findings	Abnormal Findings

Cranial Nerve V—Trigeminal Nerve

Motor Function. Assess the muscles of mastication by palpating the temporal and masseter muscles as the person clenches the teeth (Fig. 23-9). Muscles should feel equally strong on both sides. Next, try to separate the jaws by pushing down on the chin; normally you cannot.

Decreased strength on one or both sides.

Asymmetry in jaw movement.

Pain with clenching of teeth.

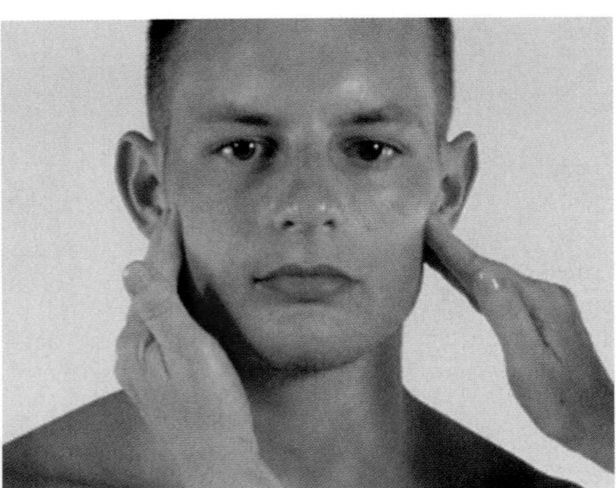

23-9

Sensory Function. With the person's eyes closed, test light touch sensation by touching a cotton wisp to these designated areas on person's face: forehead, cheeks, and chin (Fig. 23-10). Ask the person to say "Now," whenever the touch is felt. This tests all three divisions of the nerve: (1) ophthalmic, (2) maxillary, and (3) mandibular.

Decreased or unequal sensation. With a stroke, sensation of face and body is lost on the opposite side of the lesion.

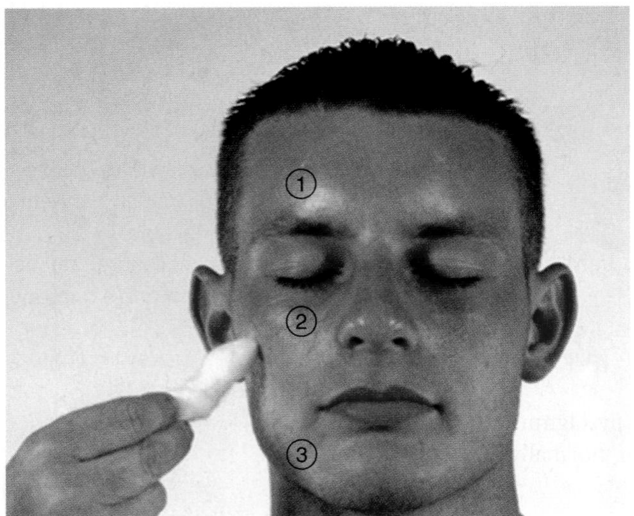

23-10

Corneal Reflex. This test of cranial nerves V and VII was usually omitted unless the person had unilateral sensorineural hearing loss. It involves bringing a wisp of cotton in from the side, lightly touching the cornea, and noting a bilateral blink reflex. However, the corneal reflex may be decreased or absent normally in contact lens wearers and in aging persons. Evidence does not support the usefulness of this test.

The test is limited clinically because an absent blink occurs in only one third of the cases of acoustic neuroma and only then when the tumor has grown quite large.[21a]

Normal Range of Findings

Cranial Nerve VII—Facial Nerve

Motor Function. Note mobility and facial symmetry as the person responds to these requests: smile (Fig. 23-11), frown, close eyes tightly (against your attempt to open them), lift eyebrows, show teeth, and puff cheeks (Fig. 23-12). Then, press the person's puffed cheeks in, and note that the air should escape equally from both sides.

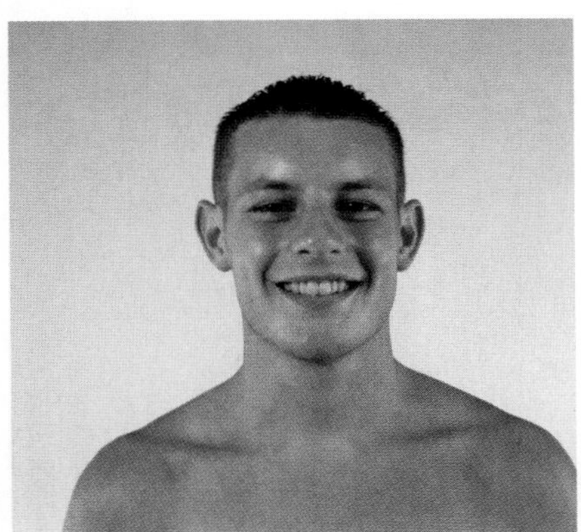

23-11

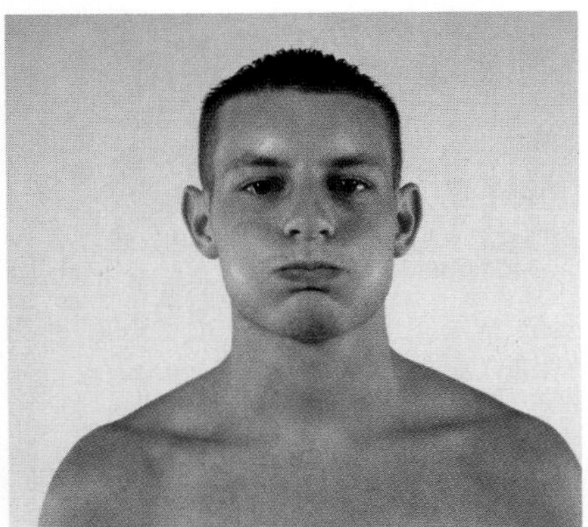

23-12

Sensory Function. Do not test routinely. Test only when you suspect facial nerve injury. When indicated, test sense of taste by applying to the tongue a cotton applicator covered with a solution of sugar, salt, or lemon juice (sour). Ask the person to identify the taste.

Cranial Nerve VIII—Acoustic (Vestibulocochlear) Nerve

Test hearing acuity by the ability to hear normal conversation and by the whispered voice test (see Chapter 15).

Cranial Nerves IX and X—Glossopharyngeal and Vagus Nerves

Motor Function. Depress the tongue with a tongue blade, and note pharyngeal movement as the person says "ahhh" or yawns; the uvula and soft palate should rise in the midline, and the tonsillar pillars should move medially.

Touch the posterior pharyngeal wall with a tongue blade, and note the gag reflex. Also note that the voice sounds smooth and not strained.

Sensory Function. Cranial nerve IX does mediate taste on the posterior one third of the tongue, but technically, this sensation is too difficult to test.

Abnormal Findings

Muscle weakness is shown by flattening of the nasolabial fold, drooping of one side of the face, lower eyelid sagging, and escape of air from only one cheek that is pressed in.

Loss of movement and asymmetry of movement occur with both central nervous system lesions (e.g., brain attack or stroke that affects the lower face on one side) and peripheral nervous system lesions (e.g., Bell's palsy that affects the upper *and* lower face on one side).

Absence or asymmetry of soft palate movement or tonsillar pillar movement. Following a stroke, dysfunction in swallowing may increase risk for aspiration.

Hoarse or brassy voice occurs with vocal cord dysfunction; nasal twang occurs with weakness of soft palate.

Normal Range of Findings	Abnormal Findings

Cranial Nerve XI—Spinal Accessory Nerve

Examine the sternomastoid and trapezius muscles for equal size. Check equal strength by asking the person to rotate the head forcibly against resistance applied to the side of the chin (Fig. 23-13). Then ask the person to shrug the shoulders against resistance (Fig. 23-14). These movements should feel equally strong on both sides.

Atrophy.

Muscle weakness or paralysis occurs with a stroke or following injury to the peripheral nerve (e.g., surgical removal of lymph nodes).

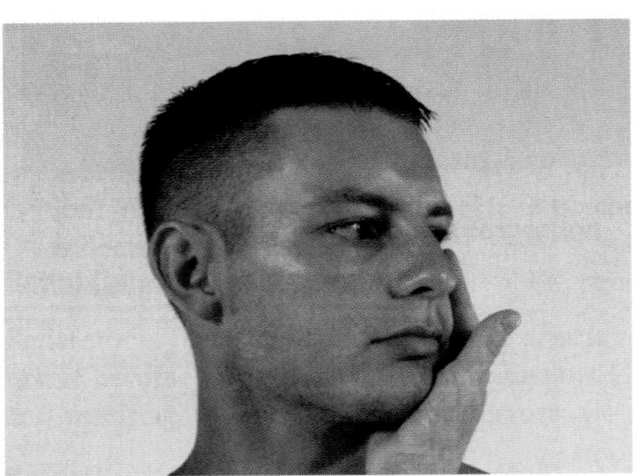

23-13

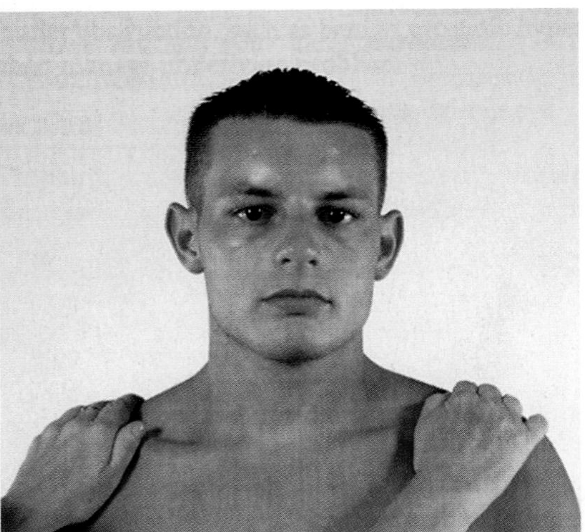

23-14

Cranial Nerve XII—Hypoglossal Nerve

Inspect the tongue. No wasting or tremors should be present. Note the forward thrust in the midline as the person protrudes the tongue. Also ask the person to say "light, tight, dynamite," and note that lingual speech (sounds of letters l, t, d, n) is clear and distinct.

Atrophy. Fasciculations.

Tongue deviates to side with lesions of the hypoglossal nerve (when this occurs, deviation is toward the paralyzed side).

INSPECT AND PALPATE THE MOTOR SYSTEM

Muscles

Size. As you proceed through the examination, inspect all muscle groups for size. Compare the right side with the left. Muscle groups should be within the normal size limits for age and should be symmetric bilaterally. When muscles in the extremities look asymmetric, measure each in centimeters and record the difference. A difference of 1 cm or less is not significant. Note that it is difficult to assess muscle mass in very obese people.

Atrophy—abnormally small muscle with a wasted appearance; occurs with disuse, injury, lower motor neuron disease such as polio, diabetic neuropathy.

Hypertrophy—increased size and strength; occurs with isometric exercise.

Normal Range of Findings	Abnormal Findings
Strength. (See Chapter 22.) Test the power of homologous muscles simultaneously. Test muscle groups of the extremities, neck, and trunk.	Paresis or weakness is diminished strength; paralysis or plegia is absence of strength.
Tone. Tone is the normal degree of tension (contraction) in voluntarily relaxed muscles. It shows as a mild resistance to passive stretch. To test muscle tone, move the extremities through a passive range of motion. First, persuade the person to relax completely, to "go loose like a rag doll." Move each extremity smoothly through a full range of motion. Support the arm at the elbow and the leg at the knee (Fig. 23-15). Normally, you will note a mild, even resistance to movement.	Limited range of motion. Pain with motion. Flaccidity—decreased resistance, hypotonia occur with peripheral weakness. Spasticity and rigidity—types of increased resistance that occur with central weakness (see Table 23-4, Abnormalities in Muscle Tone, p. 669).

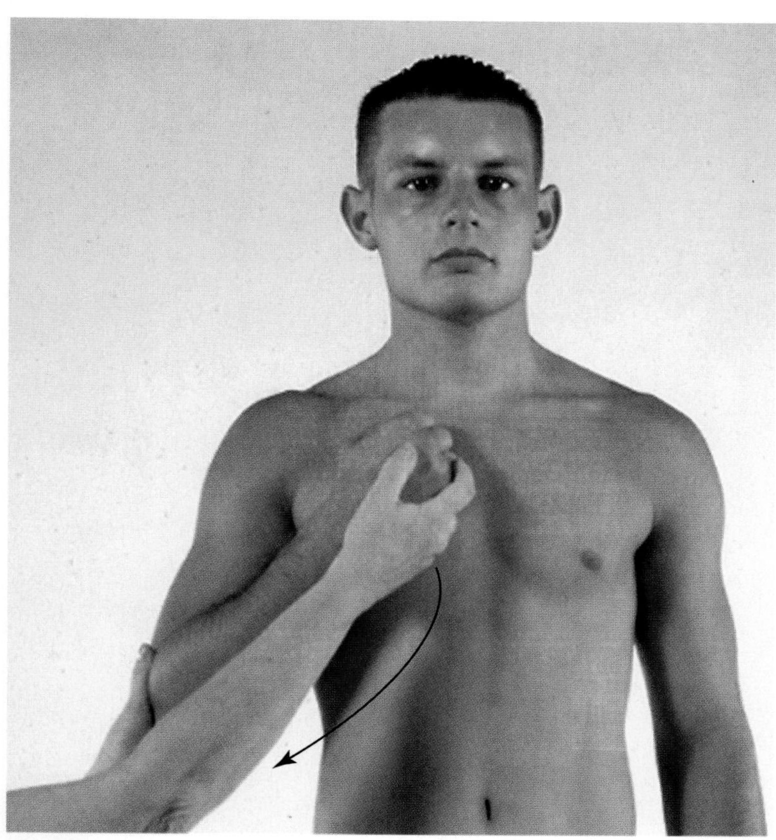

23-15

Normal Range of Findings	Abnormal Findings
Involuntary Movements. Normally, no involuntary movements occur. If they are present, note their location, frequency, rate, and amplitude. Note if the movements can be controlled at will.	Tic, tremor, fasciculation, myoclonus, chorea, and athetosis (see Table 23-5, Abnormalities in Muscle Movement, p. 670).

Cerebellar Function

Balance Tests

Normal Range of Findings	Abnormal Findings
Gait. Observe as the person walks 10 to 20 feet, turns, and returns to the starting point. Normally, the person moves with a sense of freedom. The gait is smooth, rhythmic, and effortless; the opposing arm swing is coordinated; the turns are smooth. The step length is about 15 inches from heel to heel.	Stiff, immobile posture. Staggering or reeling. Wide base of support. Lack of arm swing or rigid arms. Unequal rhythm of steps. Slapping of foot. Scraping of toe of shoe. Ataxia—uncoordinated or unsteady gait (see Table 23-6, Abnormal Gaits, p. 672).

Normal Range of Findings	Abnormal Findings
Ask the person to walk a straight line in a heel-to-toe fashion (tandem walking) (Fig. 23-16). This decreases the base of support and will accentuate any problem with coordination. Normally, the person can walk straight and stay balanced.	Crooked line of walk. Widens base to maintain balance. Staggering, reeling, loss of balance. An ataxia that did not appear with regular gait may appear now. Inability to tandem walk is sensitive for an upper motor neuron lesion, such as multiple sclerosis, and for acute cerebellar dysfunction, such as alcohol intoxication.

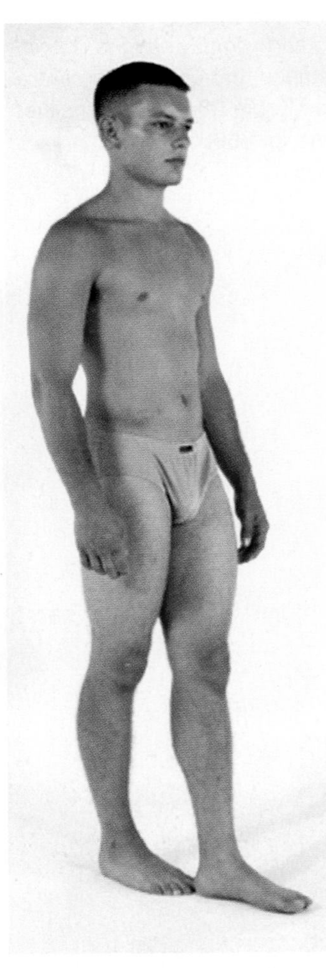

23-16 Tandem walking.

Normal Range of Findings	Abnormal Findings
You may also test for balance by asking the person to walk on his or her toes, then on the heels for a few steps. Normally, plantar flexion and dorsiflexion are strong enough to permit this.	Muscle weakness in the legs prevents this.
The Romberg Test. Ask the person to stand up with feet together and arms at the sides. Once in a stable position, ask the person to close the eyes and to hold the position (Fig. 23-17). Wait about 20 seconds. Normally, a person can maintain posture and balance even with the visual orienting information blocked, although slight swaying may occur. (Stand close to catch the person in case he or she falls.)	Sways, falls, widens base of feet to avoid falling. *Positive* Romberg sign is loss of balance that occurs when closing the eyes. You eliminate the advantage of orientation with the eyes, which had compensated for sensory loss. A positive Romberg sign occurs with cerebellar ataxia (multiple sclerosis, alcohol intoxication), loss of proprioception, and loss of vestibular function.

Normal Range of Findings | **Abnormal Findings**

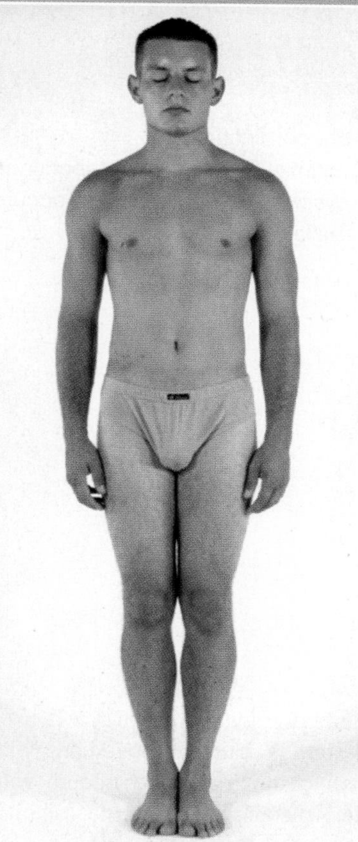

23-17 Romberg test.

Ask the person to perform a shallow knee bend or to hop in place, first on one leg, then the other (Fig. 23-18). This demonstrates normal position sense, muscle strength, and cerebellar function. Note that some individuals cannot hop because of aging or obesity. Alternatively, you can ask them to rise from a chair without using the armrests for support.

Unable to perform knee bend because of weakness in quadriceps muscle or hip extensors.

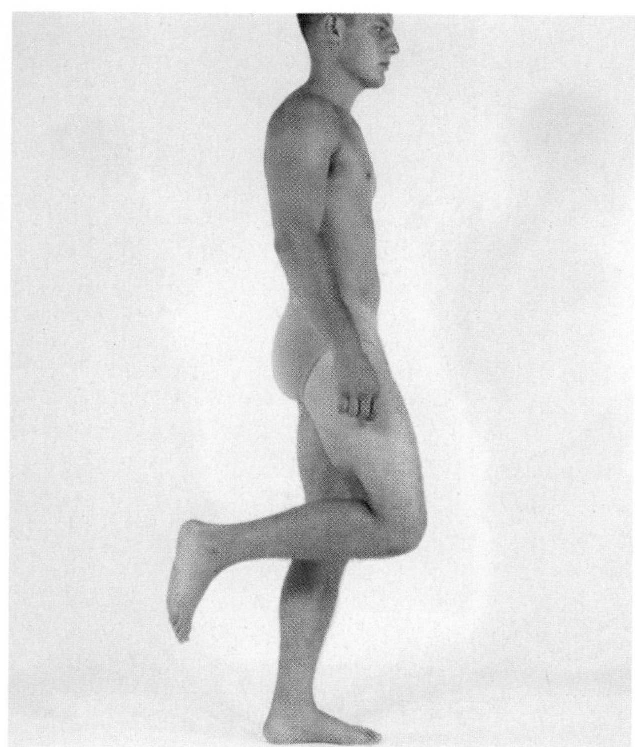

23-18

Normal Range of Findings	Abnormal Findings

Coordination and Skilled Movements

Rapid Alternating Movements (RAM). Ask the person to pat the knees with both hands, lift up, turn hands over, and pat the knees with the backs of the hands (Fig. 23-19). Then ask the person to do this faster. Normally, this is done with equal turning and a quick, rhythmic pace.

Abnormal Findings: Lack of coordination.

Slow, clumsy, and sloppy response is termed *dysdiadochokinesia* and occurs with cerebellar disease.

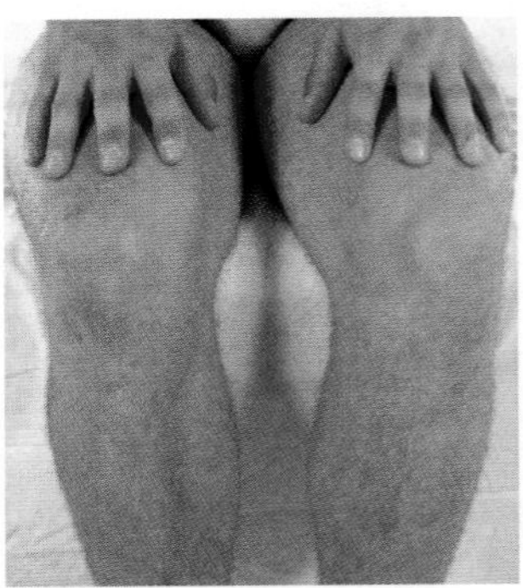

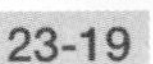

23-19

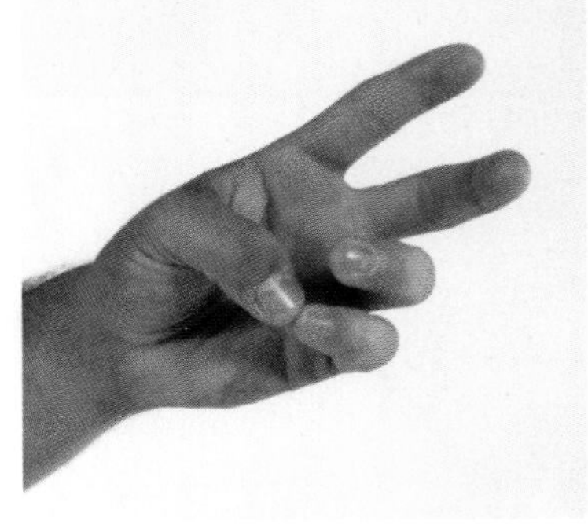

23-20

Alternatively, ask the person to touch the thumb to each finger on the same hand, starting with the index finger, then reverse direction (Fig. 23-20). Normally, this can be done quickly and accurately.

Abnormal Findings: Lack of coordination.

Dysmetria is clumsy movement with overshooting the mark and occurs with cerebellar disorders or acute alcohol intoxication.

Past-pointing is a constant deviation to one side.

Intention tremor when reaching to a visually directed object.

Finger-to-Finger Test. With the person's eyes open, ask that he or she use the index finger to touch your finger, then his or her own nose (Fig. 23-21). After a few times, move your finger to a different spot. The person's movement should be smooth and accurate.

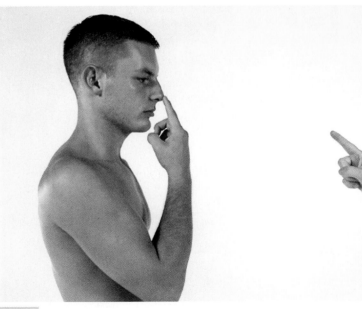

23-21

Normal Range of Findings

Finger-to-Nose Test. Ask the person to close the eyes and to stretch out the arms. Ask the person to touch the tip of his or her nose with each index finger, alternating hands and increasing speed. Normally, this is done with accurate and smooth movement.

Heel-to-Shin Test. Test lower extremity coordination by asking the person, who is in a supine position, to place the heel on the opposite knee and run it down the shin from the knee to the ankle (Fig. 23-22). Normally, the person moves the heel in a straight line down the shin.

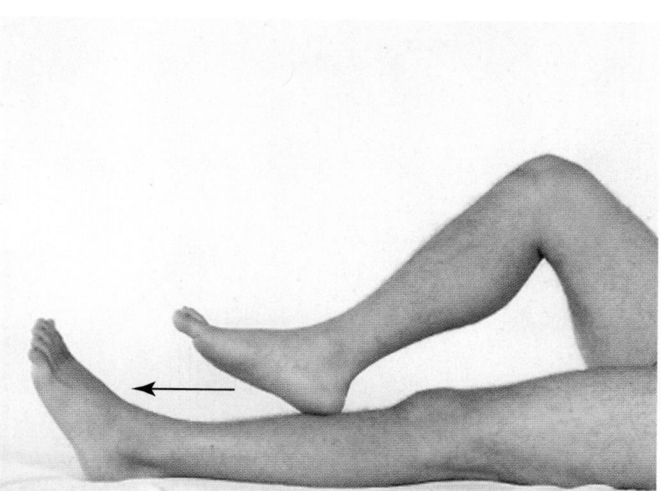

23-22

ASSESS THE SENSORY SYSTEM

Ask the person to identify various sensory stimuli to test the intactness of the peripheral nerve fibers, the sensory tracts, and higher cortical discrimination.

Ensure validity of sensory system testing by making sure the person is alert, cooperative, and comfortable and has an adequate attention span. Otherwise, you may get misleading and invalid results. Testing of the sensory system can be fatiguing. You may need to repeat the examination later or to break it into parts when the person is tired.

You do not need to test the entire skin surface for every sensation. Routine screening procedures include testing superficial pain, light touch, and vibration in a few distal locations and testing stereognosis. This will suffice for all who have not demonstrated any neurologic symptoms or signs. Complete testing of the sensory system is warranted in those with neurologic symptoms (e.g., localized pain, numbness, and tingling) or when you discover abnormalities (e.g., motor deficit). Then, test all sensory modalities and cover most dermatomes of the body.

Compare sensations on symmetric parts of the body. When you find a definite decrease in sensation, map it out by systematic testing in that area. Proceed from the point of decreased sensation toward the sensitive area. By asking the person to tell you where the sensation changes, you can map the exact borders of the deficient area. Draw your results on a diagram.

Avoid asking leading questions such as "Can you feel this pinprick?" This creates an expectation of how the person should feel the sensation, which is called *suggestion.* Instead, use unbiased directions.

The person's eyes should be closed during each of the tests. Take time to explain what will be happening and exactly how you expect the person to respond.

Abnormal Findings

Misses nose. Worsening of coordination when the eyes are closed occurs with cerebellar disease or alcohol intoxication.

Lack of coordination, heel falls off shin, occurs with cerebellar disease.

Note if the topographic pattern of sensory loss is distal (i.e., over the hands and feet in a "glove and stocking" distribution) or if it is over a specific dermatome.

Normal Range of Findings	Abnormal Findings

Spinothalamic Tract

Pain. Pain is tested by the person's ability to perceive a pinprick. Break a tongue blade lengthwise, forming a sharp point at the fractured end and a dull spot at the rounded end. Lightly apply the sharp point or the dull end to the person's body in a random, unpredictable order (Fig. 23-23). Ask the person to say "sharp" or "dull," depending on the sensation felt. (Note that the sharp edge is used to test for pain; the dull edge is used as a general test of the person's responses.)

Hypoalgesia—decreased pain sensation.
Analgesia—absent pain sensation.
Hyperalgesia—increased pain sensation.

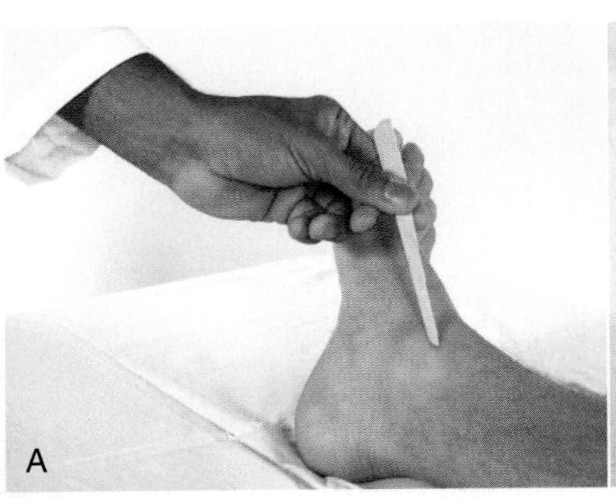
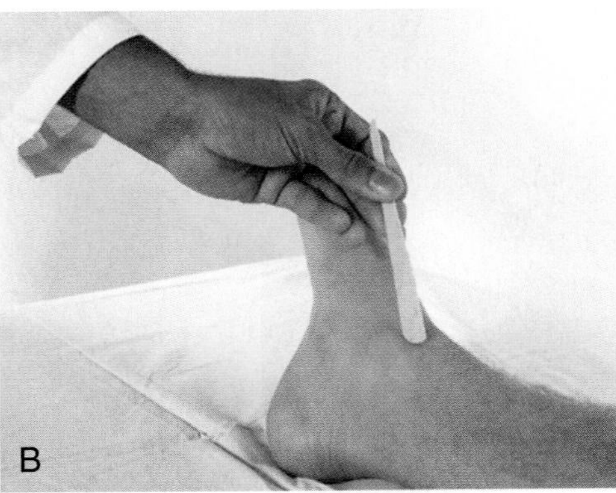

23-23

Let at least 2 seconds elapse between each stimulus to avoid *summation.* With summation, frequent consecutive stimuli are perceived as one strong stimulus. Discard tongue blade to prevent transmitting any possible infection.

Temperature. Test temperature sensation only when pain sensation is abnormal; otherwise, you may omit it because the fiber tracts are much the same. Place the flat side of the tuning fork on the skin; its metal always feels cool. This can alternate with the warmth of your hand.

Light Touch. Apply a wisp of cotton to the skin. Stretch a cotton ball to make a long end, and brush it over the skin in a random order of sites and at irregular intervals (Fig. 23-24). This prevents the person from responding just from repetition. Include the arms, forearms, hands, chest, thighs, and legs. Ask the person to say "now" or "yes" when touch is felt. Compare symmetric points.

Hypoesthesia—decreased touch sensation.
Anesthesia—absent touch sensation.
Hyperesthesia—increased touch sensation.

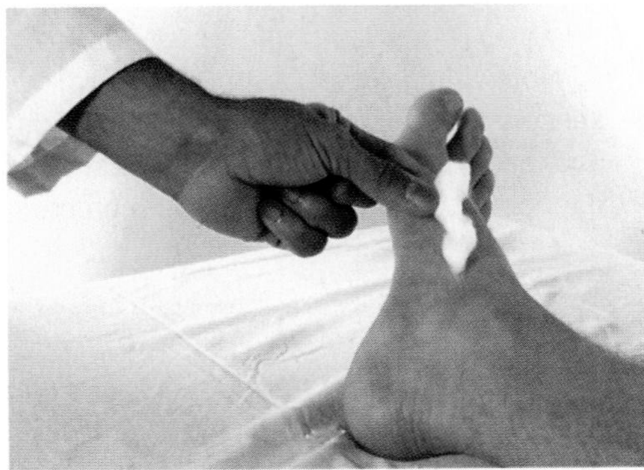

23-24

Normal Range of Findings

Abnormal Findings

Posterior Column Tract

Vibration. Test the person's ability to feel vibrations of a tuning fork over bony prominences. Use a low-pitch tuning fork (128 Hz or 256 Hz) because its vibration has a slower decay. Strike the tuning fork on the heel of your hand, and hold the base on a bony surface of the fingers and great toe (Fig. 23-25). Ask the person to indicate when the vibration starts and stops. If the person feels the normal vibration or buzzing sensation on these distal areas, you may assume proximal spots are normal and proceed no further. If no vibrations are felt, move proximally and test ulnar processes and ankles, patellae, and iliac crests. Compare the right side with the left side. If you find a deficit, note whether it is gradual or abrupt.

Unable to feel vibration. Loss of vibration sense occurs with peripheral neuropathy (e.g., diabetes and alcoholism). Often, this is the first sensation lost.

Peripheral neuropathy is worse at the feet and gradually improves as you move up the leg, as opposed to a specific nerve lesion, which has a clear zone of deficit for its dermatome (see Table 23-9, Patterns of Sensory Loss, p. 675).

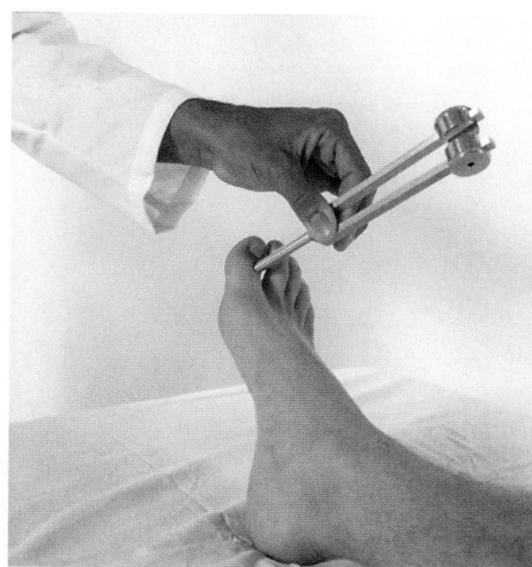

23-25

Position (Kinesthesia). Test the person's ability to perceive passive movements of the extremities. Move a finger or the big toe up and down, and ask the person to tell you which way it is moved (Fig. 23-26). The test is done with the eyes closed, but to be sure it is understood, have the person watch a few trials first. Vary the order of movement up or down. Hold the digit by the sides, since upward or downward pressure on the skin may provide a clue as to how it has been moved. Normally, a person can detect movement of a few millimeters.

Loss of position sense.

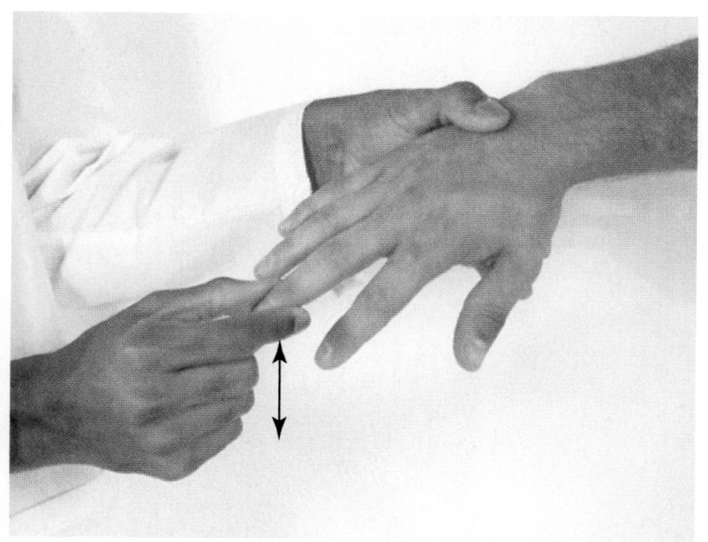

23-26

Objective Data

Normal Range of Findings

Tactile Discrimination (Fine Touch). The following tests also measure the discrimination ability of the sensory cortex. As a prerequisite, the person needs a normal or near-normal sense of touch and position sense.

Stereognosis. Test the person's ability to recognize objects by feeling their forms, sizes, and weights. With the person's eyes closed, place a familiar object (paper clip, key, coin, cotton ball, or pencil) in his or her hand and ask the person to identify it (Fig. 23-27). Normally, a person will explore it with the fingers and correctly name it. Test a different object in each hand; testing the left hand assesses right parietal lobe functioning.

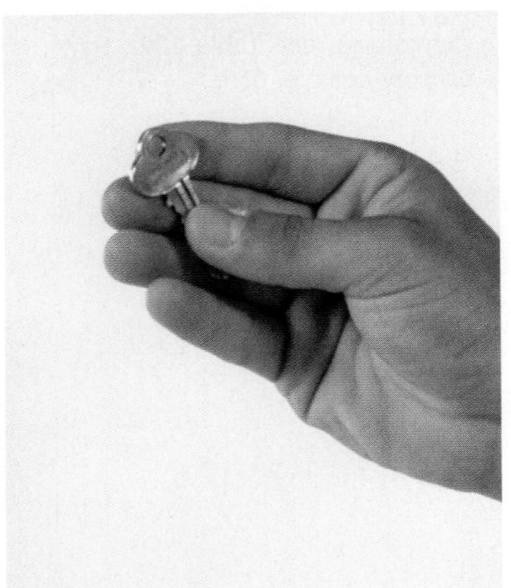

23-27 Stereognosis.

Graphesthesia. Graphesthesia is the ability to "read" a number by having it traced on the skin. With the person's eyes closed, use a blunt instrument to trace a single digit number or a letter on the palm (Fig. 23-28). Ask the person to tell you what it is. Graphesthesia is a good measure of sensory loss if the person cannot make the hand movements needed for stereognosis, as occurs in arthritis.

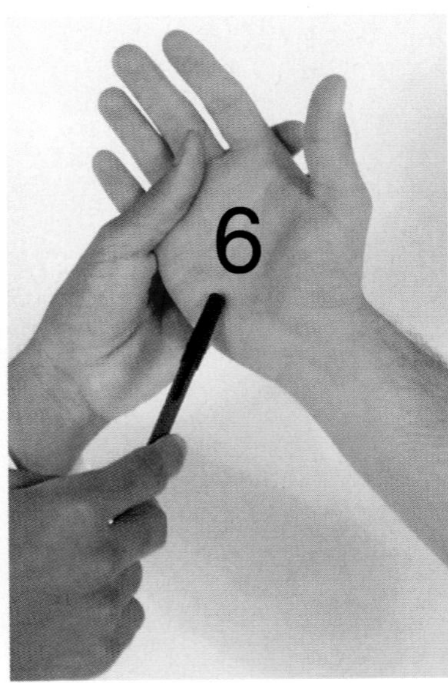

23-28 Graphesthesia.

Abnormal Findings

Problems with tactile discrimination occur with lesions of the sensory cortex or posterior column.

Astereognosis—inability to identify object correctly. Occurs in sensory cortex lesions (e.g., brain attack [stroke]).

Inability to distinguish number occurs with lesions of the sensory cortex.

Normal Range of Findings

Two-Point Discrimination. Test the person's ability to distinguish the separation of two simultaneous pin points on the skin. Apply the two points of an opened paper clip lightly to the skin in ever-closing distances. Note the distance at which the person no longer perceives two separate points. The level of perception varies considerably with the region tested; it is most sensitive in the fingertips (2 to 8 mm) and least sensitive on the upper arms, thighs, and back (40 to 75 mm).

Extinction. Simultaneously touch both sides of the body at the same point. Ask the person to state how many sensations are felt and where they are. Normally, both sensations are felt.

Point Location. Touch the skin, and withdraw the stimulus promptly. Tell the person, "Put your finger where I touched you." You can perform this test simultaneously with light touch sensation.

TEST THE REFLEXES

Stretch, or Deep Tendon Reflexes (DTRs)

Measurement of the stretch reflexes reveals the intactness of the reflex arc at specific spinal levels as well as the normal override on the reflex of the higher cortical levels.

For an adequate response, the limb should be relaxed and the muscle partially stretched. Stimulate the reflex by directing a short, snappy blow of the reflex hammer onto the muscle's insertion tendon. Use a relaxed hold on the hammer.

As with the percussion technique, the action takes place at the wrist. Strike a brief, well-aimed blow, and bounce up promptly; do not let the hammer rest on the tendon. Use the pointed end of the reflex hammer when aiming at a smaller target such as your thumb on the tendon site; use the flat end when the target is wider or to diffuse the impact and prevent pain.

Use just enough force to get a response. Compare right and left sides—the responses should be equal. The reflex response is graded on a 4-point scale:

4+ Very brisk, hyperactive with clonus, indicative of disease
3+ Brisker than average, may indicate disease, probably normal
2+ Average, normal
1+ Diminished, low normal, or occurs only with reinforcement
0 No response

This is a subjective scale and requires some clinical practice. Even then, the scale is not completely reliable because no standard exists to say *how* brisk a reflex should be to warrant a grade of 3+. Also, a wide range of normal exists in reflex responses. Healthy people may have diminished reflexes, or they may have brisk ones. Your best plan is to interpret the DTRs *only* within the context of the rest of the neurologic examination.

Abnormal Findings

An increase in the distance it normally takes to identify two separate points occurs with sensory cortex lesions.

The ability to recognize only one of the stimuli occurs with sensory cortex lesion; the stimulus is extinguished on the side *opposite* the cortex lesion.

With a sensory cortex lesion, the person cannot localize the sensation accurately, even though light touch sensation may be retained.

Clonus is a set of rapid, rhythmic contractions of the same muscle.

Hyperreflexia is the exaggerated reflex seen when the monosynaptic reflex arc is released from the usually inhibiting influence of higher cortical levels. This occurs with upper motor neuron lesions (e.g., a brain attack).

Hyporeflexia, which is the absence of a reflex, is a lower motor neuron problem. It occurs with interruption of sensory afferents or destruction of motor efferents and anterior horn cells (e.g., spinal cord injury).

Normal Range of Findings

Abnormal Findings

Sometimes the reflex response fails to appear. Try further encouragement of relaxation, varying the person's position, or increasing the strength of the blow. **Reinforcement** is another technique to relax the muscles and enhance the response (Fig. 23-29). Ask the person to perform an isometric exercise in a muscle group somewhat away from the one being tested. For example, to enhance a patellar reflex, ask the person to lock the fingers together and "pull as hard as you can." Then strike the tendon. To enhance a biceps response, ask the person to clench the teeth or to grasp the thigh with the opposite hand.

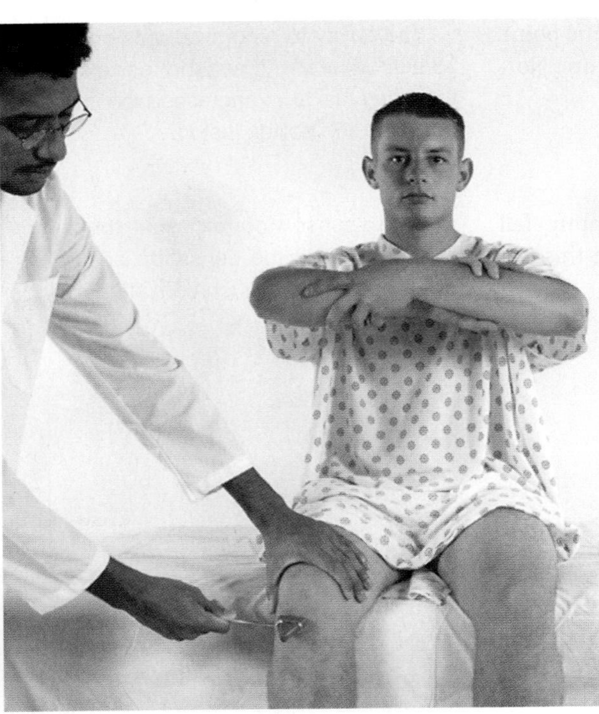

23-29 Reinforcement.

Biceps Reflex (C5 to C6). Support the person's forearm on yours; this position relaxes as well as partially flexes the person's arm. Place your thumb on the biceps tendon and strike a blow on your thumb. You can feel as well as see the normal response, which is contraction of the biceps muscle and flexion of the forearm (Fig. 23-30).

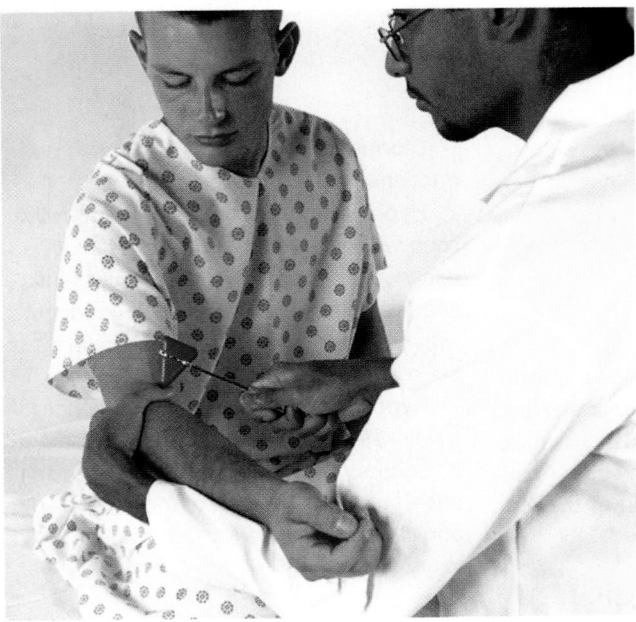

23-30 Biceps reflex.

Normal Range of Findings

Triceps Reflex (C7 to C8). Tell the person to let the arm "just go dead" as you suspend it by holding the upper arm. Strike the triceps tendon directly just above the elbow (Fig. 23-31). The normal response is extension of the forearm. Alternately, hold the person's wrist across the chest to flex the arm at the elbow, and tap the tendon.

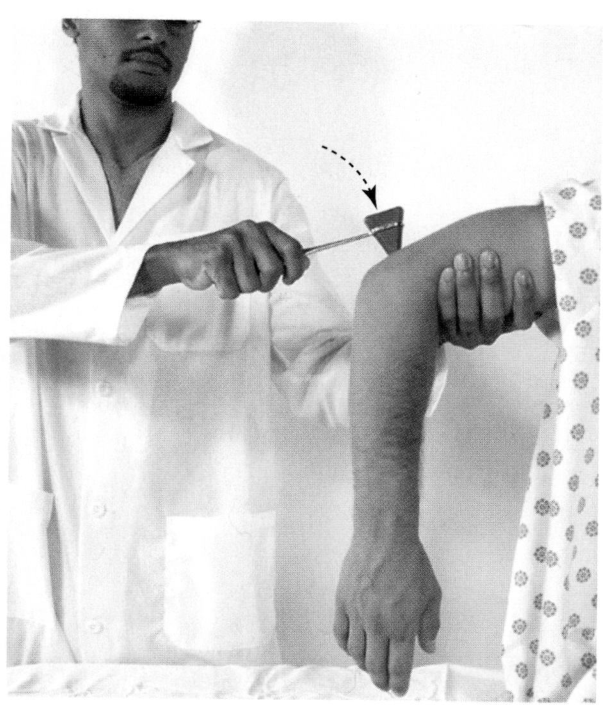

23-31 Triceps reflex.

Brachioradialis Reflex (C5 to C6). Hold the person's thumbs to suspend the forearms in relaxation. Strike the forearm directly, about 2 to 3 cm above the radial styloid process (Fig. 23-32). The normal response is flexion and supination of the forearm.

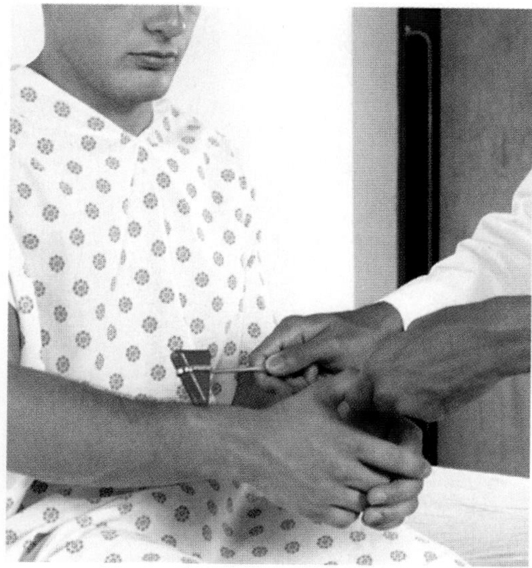

23-32 Brachioradialis reflex.

Abnormal Findings

Normal Range of Findings

Quadriceps Reflex ("Knee Jerk") (L2 to L4). Let the lower legs dangle freely to flex the knee and stretch the tendons. Strike the tendon directly just below the patella (Fig. 23-33). Extension of the lower leg is the expected response. You also will palpate contraction of the quadriceps.

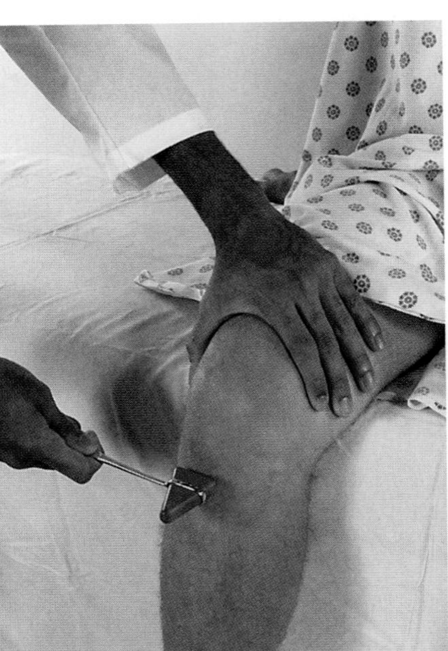

23-33 Quadriceps reflex.

For the person in the supine position, use your own arm as a lever to support the weight of one leg against the other leg (Fig. 23-34). This maneuver also flexes the knee.

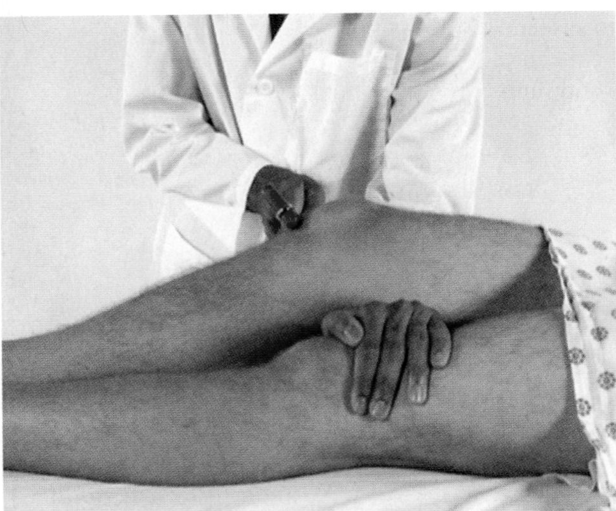

23-34 Supine quadriceps reflex.

Achilles Reflex ("Ankle Jerk") (L5 to S2). Position the person with the knee flexed and the hip externally rotated. Hold the foot in dorsiflexion, and strike the Achilles tendon directly (Fig. 23-35). Feel the normal response as the foot plantar flexes against your hand.

Abnormal Findings

Normal Range of Findings

Abnormal Findings

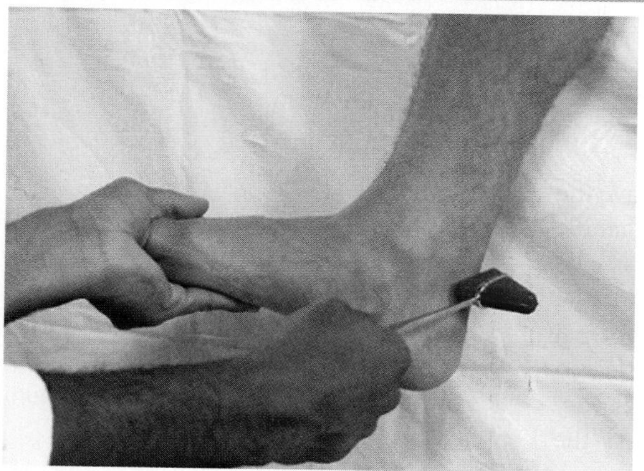
23-35 Achilles reflex.

For the person in the supine position, flex one knee and support that lower leg against the other leg so that it falls "open." Dorsiflex the foot, and tap the tendon (Fig. 23-36).

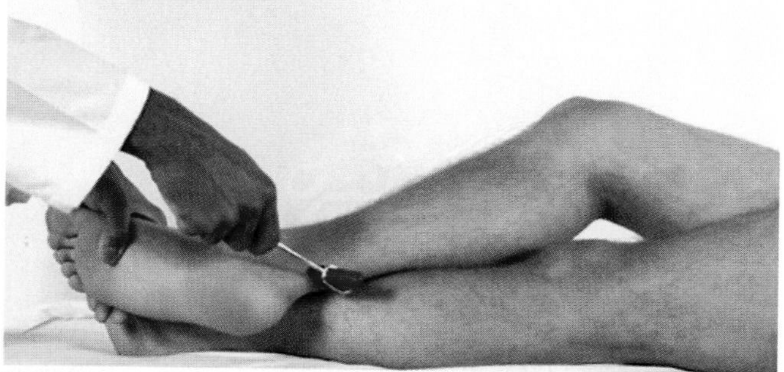
23-36 Supine Achilles reflex.

Clonus. Test for clonus, particularly when the reflexes are hyperactive. Support the lower leg in one hand. With your other hand, move the foot up and down a few times to relax the muscle. Then stretch the muscle by briskly dorsiflexing the foot. Hold the stretch (Fig. 23-37). With a normal response, you feel no further movement. When clonus is present, you will feel and see rapid, rhythmic contractions of the calf muscle and movement of the foot.

Clonus is repeated reflex muscular movements. A hyperactive reflex with sustained clonus (lasting as long as the stretch is held) occurs with upper motor neuron disease.

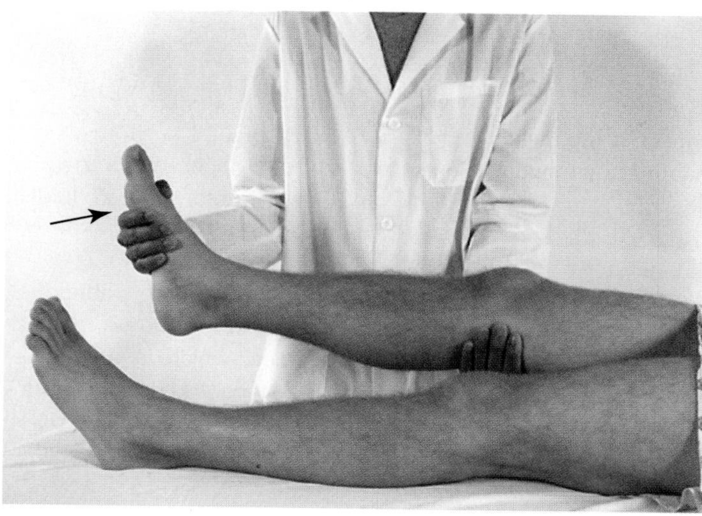
23-37

Normal Range of Findings

Abnormal Findings

Superficial (Cutaneous) Reflexes

Here, the sensory receptors are in the skin rather than in the muscles. The motor response is a localized muscle contraction.

Abdominal Reflexes—Upper (T8 to T10), Lower (T10 to T12). Have the person assume a supine position, with the knees slightly bent. Use the handle end of the reflex hammer, a wood applicator tip, or the end of a split tongue blade to stroke the skin. Move from each corner of the abdomen toward the midline at both the upper and lower abdominal levels (Fig. 23-38). The normal response is ipsilateral contraction of the abdominal muscle with an observed deviation of the umbilicus toward the stroke. When the abdominal wall is very obese, pull the skin to the opposite side and feel it contract toward the stimulus.

Superficial reflexes are absent with diseases of the pyramidal tract (e.g., they are absent on the contralateral side with brain attack).

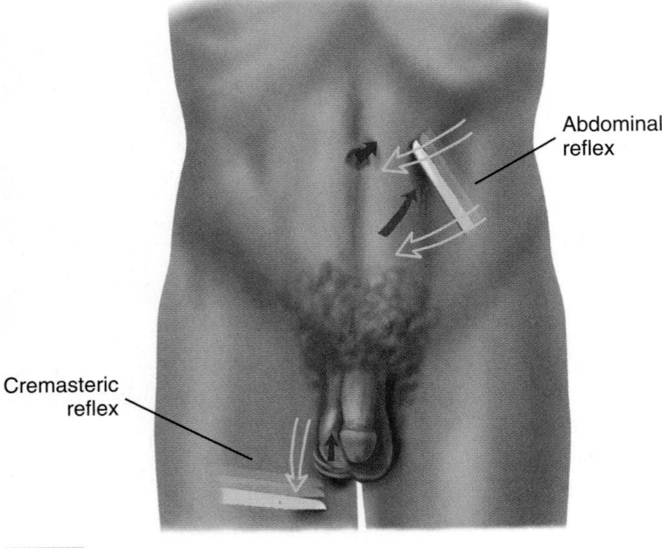

23-38

Cremasteric Reflex (L1 to L2). This is not routinely done. On the male, lightly stroke the inner aspect of the thigh with the reflex hammer or tongue blade (see Fig. 23-38). Note elevation of the ipsilateral testicle.

Absent in both upper motor neuron (UMN) and lower motor neuron (LMN) lesions.

Plantar Reflex (L4 to S2). Position the thigh in slight external rotation. With the reflex hammer, draw a light stroke up the lateral side of the sole of the foot and inward across the ball of the foot, like an upside-down J (Fig. 23-39, *A*). The normal response is plantar flexion of the toes and inversion and flexion of the forefoot.

Except in infancy, the abnormal response is dorsiflexion of the big toe and fanning of all toes, which is a positive Babinski sign, also called "upgoing toes" (Fig. 23-39, *B*). This occurs with UMN disease of the corticospinal (or pyramidal) tract.

Normal Range of Findings | Abnormal Findings

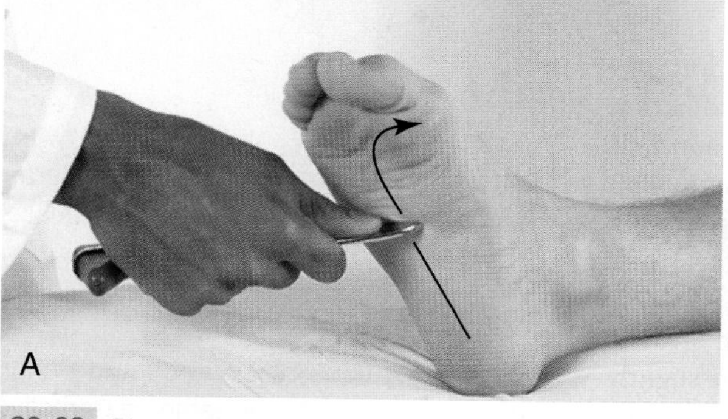

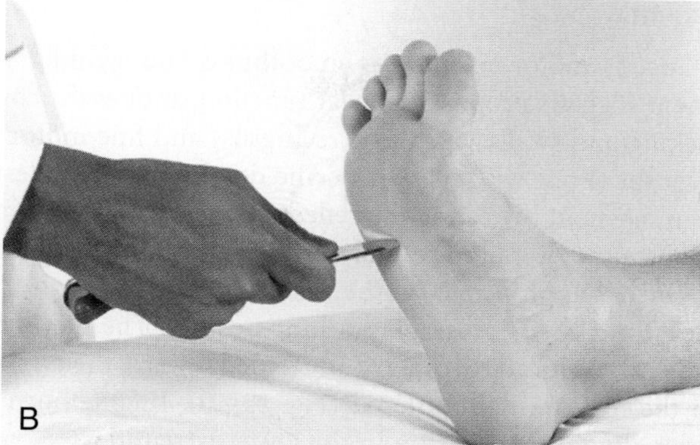

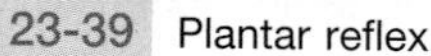
23-39 Plantar reflex.

DEVELOPMENTAL COMPETENCE

Infants (Birth to 12 Months)

The neurologic system shows dramatic growth and development during the first year of life. Assessment includes noting that milestones you normally would expect for each month have indeed been achieved and that the early, more primitive reflexes are eliminated from the baby's repertory when they are supposed to be.

Failure to attain a skill by expected time.

Persistence of reflex behavior beyond the normal time.

At birth, the newborn is very alert, with the eyes open, and demonstrates strong, urgent sucking. The normal cry is loud, lusty, and even angry. The next 2 or 3 days may be spent mostly sleeping as the baby recovers from the birth process. After that, the pattern of sleep and waking activity is highly variable; it depends on the baby's individual body rhythm as well as external stimuli.

A high-pitched, shrill cry or cat-sounding screech occurs with CNS damage.

A weak, groaning cry or expiratory grunt occurs with respiratory distress.

The behavioral assessment should include your observations of the infant's spontaneous waking activity, responses to environmental stimuli, and social interaction with the parents and others.

Lethargy, hyporeactivity, hyperirritability, and parent's report of significant change in behavior all warrant referral.

By 2 months of age, the baby smiles responsively and recognizes the parent's face. Babbling occurs at 4 months, and one or two words (mama, dada) are used nonspecifically after 9 months.

The cranial nerves cannot be tested directly, but you can infer their proper functioning by the maneuvers shown in Table 23-1.

TABLE 23-1 Testing Cranial Nerve Function of Infants

Cranial Nerve	Response
II, III, IV, VI	Optical blink reflex—shine light in open eyes, note rapid closure Size, shape, equality of pupils Regards face or close object Eyes follow movement
V	Rooting reflex, sucking reflex
VII	Facial movements (e.g., wrinkling forehead and nasolabial folds) symmetric when crying or smiling
VIII	Loud noise yields Moro reflex (until 4 mo) Acoustic blink reflex—infant blinks in response to a loud hand clap 30 cm (12 inches) from head (avoid making air current) Eyes follow direction of sound
IX, X	Swallowing, gag reflex Coordinated sucking and swallowing
XII	Pinch nose, infant's mouth will open and tongue rise in midline

Normal Range of Findings

The Motor System

Observe spontaneous motor activity for smoothness and symmetry. Smoothness of movement suggests proper cerebellar function, as does the coordination involved in sucking and swallowing. To screen gross and fine motor coordination, use the Denver II test with its age-specific developmental milestones. You also can assess movement by testing the reflexes listed in the following section. Note their smoothness of response and symmetry. Also, note whether their presence or absence is appropriate for the infant's age.

Assess muscle tone by first observing resting posture. The newborn favors a flexed position; extremities are symmetrically folded inward, the hips are slightly abducted, and the fists are tightly flexed (Fig. 23-40). Infants born by breech delivery, however, do not have flexion in the lower extremities.

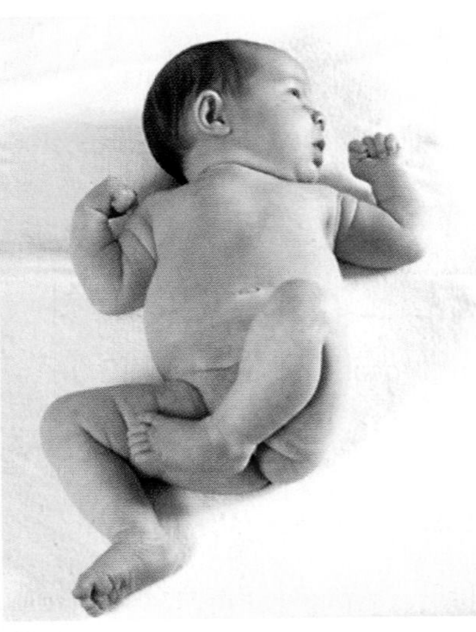

23-40

After 2 months of age, flexion gives way to gradual extension, beginning with the head and continuing in a cephalocaudal direction. Now is the time to check for spasticity; none should be present. Test for spasticity by flexing the infant's knees onto the abdomen and then quickly releasing them. They will unfold but not too quickly. Also, gently push the head forward—the baby should comply.

The fists normally are held in tight flexion for the first 3 months. Then the fists open for part of the time.

A purposeful reach for an object with both hands occurs around 4 months of age, a transfer of an object from hand to hand at 7 months of age, a grasp using fingers and opposing thumb at 9 months of age, and a purposeful release at 10 months of age. Babies are normally ambidextrous for the first 18 months.

Head control is an important milestone in motor development. You can incorporate the following two movements into every infant assessment to check the muscle tone necessary for head control.

First, with the baby supine, pull to a sit holding the wrists and note head control (Fig. 23-41). The newborn will hold the head almost in the same plane as the body, and it will balance briefly when the baby reaches a sitting position and then flop forward. (Even a premature infant shows some head flexion.) At 4 months of age, the head stays in line with the body and does not flop.

Abnormal Findings

Delay in motor activity occurs with brain damage, mental disability, peripheral neuromuscular damage, prolonged illness, and parental neglect

Abnormal postures:

Frog position—hips abducted and almost flat against the table, externally rotated (normal only after breech delivery).

Opisthotonos—head arched back, stiffness of neck, and extension of arms and legs; occurs with meningeal or brainstem irritation and kernicterus (see Table 23-10, Abnormal Postures, p. 676).

Extension of limbs may occur with intracranial hemorrhage.

Any type of continual asymmetry (e.g., asymmetry of upper limbs) occurs with brachial plexus palsy.

Spasticity is an early sign of cerebral palsy. After releasing flexed knees, legs will quickly extend and adduct, even to a "scissoring" motion when spasticity is present. Also, the baby often resists head flexion and extends back against your hand when spasticity is present.

Note persistent one-hand preference in baby younger than 18 months of age, which may indicate a motor deficit on the opposite side.

Because development progresses in a cephalocaudal direction, head lag is an early sign of brain damage.

After 6 months of age, refer any baby with failure to hold head in midline when sitting.

Normal Range of Findings

Abnormal Findings

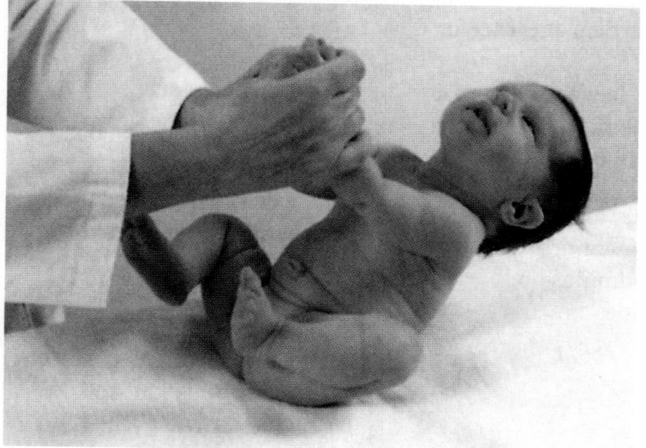

23-41

Second, lift up the baby in a prone position, with one hand supporting the chest (Fig. 23-42). The term newborn holds the head at an angle of 45 degrees or less from horizontal, the back is straight or slightly arched, and the elbows and knees are partly flexed.

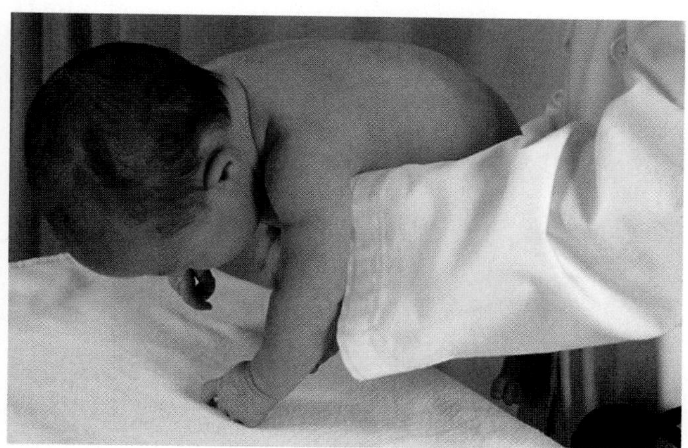

23-42

At 3 months of age, the baby raises the head and arches the back, as in a swan dive. This is the *Landau reflex,* which persists until 1½ years of age (Fig. 23-43).

Head lag, a limp, floppy trunk, and dangling arms and legs.

Absence of the reflex indicates motor weakness, upper motor neuron disease, or mental disability.

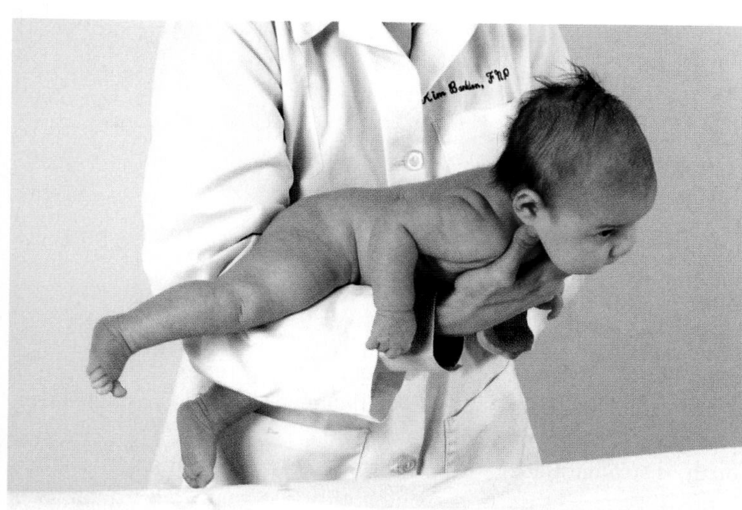

23-43

Normal Range of Findings

Assess muscle strength by noting the strength of sucking and of spontaneous motor activity. Normally, no tremors are present and no continual overshooting of the mark occurs when reaching.

The Sensory System

You will perform very little sensory testing with infants and toddlers. The newborn normally has hypoesthesia and requires a strong stimulus to elicit a response. The baby responds to pain by crying and a general reflex withdrawal of all limbs. By 7 to 9 months of age, the infant can localize the stimulus and shows more specific signs of withdrawal. Other sensory modalities are not tested.

Reflexes

Infantile automatisms are reflexes that have a predictable timetable of appearance and departure. The reflexes most commonly tested are listed in the following section. For the screening examination, you can just check the rooting, grasp, tonic neck, and Moro reflexes.

Rooting Reflex. Brush the infant's cheek near the mouth. Note whether the infant turns the head toward that side and opens the mouth (Fig. 23-44). Appears at birth and disappears at 3 to 4 months.

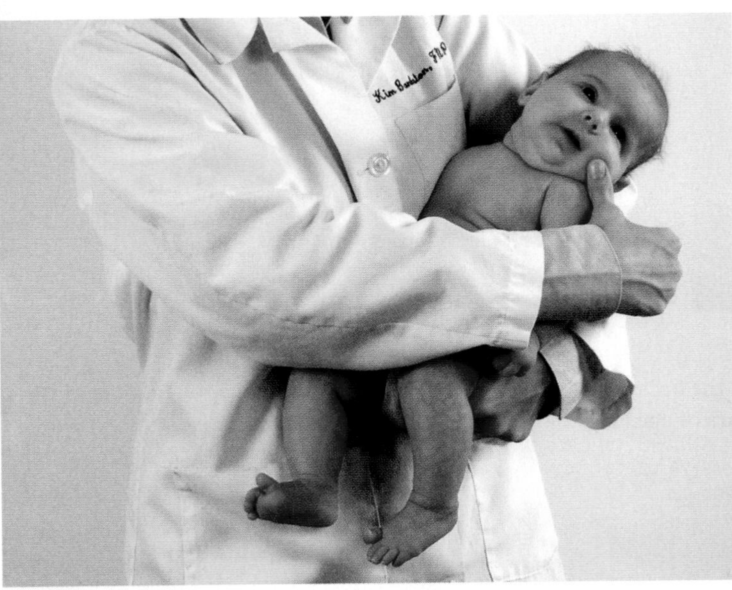

23-44

Sucking Reflex. Touch the lips and offer your gloved little finger to suck. Note strong sucking reflex. The reflex is present at birth and disappears at 10 to 12 months.

Palmar Grasp. Place the baby's head midline to ensure symmetric response. Offer your finger from the baby's ulnar side, away from the thumb. Note tight grasp of all the baby's fingers (Fig. 23-45). Sucking enhances grasp. Often, you can pull baby to a sit from grasp. The reflex is present at birth, is strongest at 1 to 2 months, and disappears at 3 to 4 months.

Abnormal Findings

Unusually rapid withdrawal is *hyperesthesia*, which occurs with spinal cord lesions, CNS infections, increased intracranial pressure, peritonitis.

No withdrawal is decreased sensation, which occurs with decreased consciousness, mental deficiency, spinal cord or peripheral nerve lesions.

The palmar grasp reflex is absent with brain damage and with local muscle or nerve injury.

Persistence of palmar grasp reflex after 4 months of age occurs with frontal lobe lesion.

Normal Range of Findings

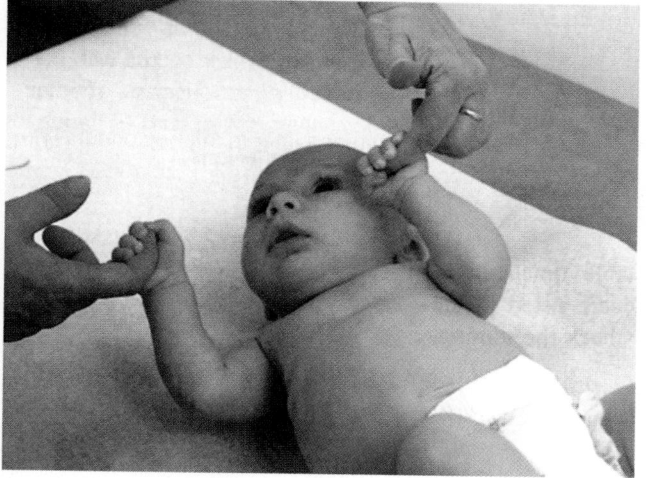

23-45

Plantar Grasp. Touch your thumb at the ball of the baby's foot. Note that the toes curl down tightly (Fig. 23-46). The reflex is present at birth and disappears at 8 to 10 months.

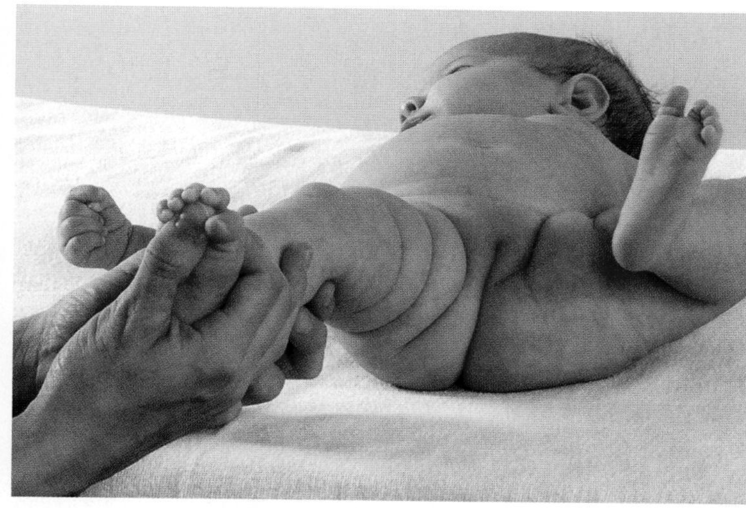

23-46

Babinski Reflex. Stroke your finger up the lateral edge and across the ball of the infant's foot. Note fanning of toes (positive Babinski reflex) (Fig. 23-47). The reflex is present at birth and disappears (changes to the adult response) by 24 months of age (variable).

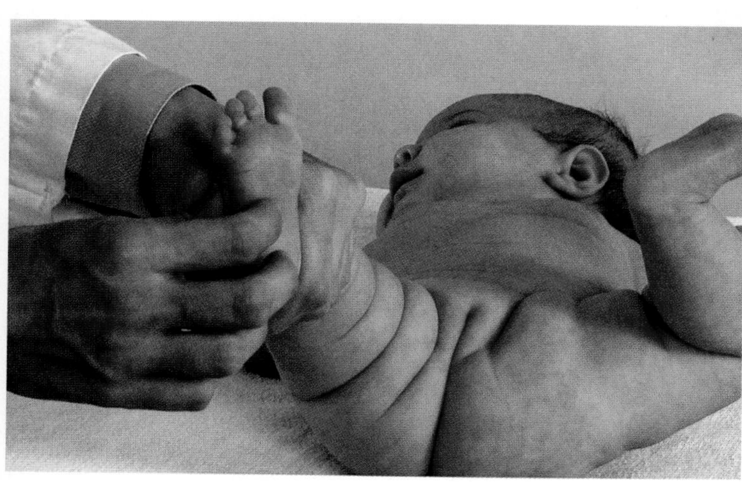

23-47

Abnormal Findings

Positive Babinski reflex after 2 or 2½ years of age occurs with pyramidal tract disease.

Normal Range of Findings

Tonic Neck Reflex. With the baby supine, relaxed, or sleeping, turn the head to one side with the chin over shoulder. Note ipsilateral extension of the arm and leg and flexion of the opposite arm and leg; this is the "fencing" position. If you turn the infant's head to the opposite side, positions will reverse (Fig. 23-48). The reflex appears by 2 to 3 months, decreases at 3 to 4 months, and disappears by 4 to 6 months.

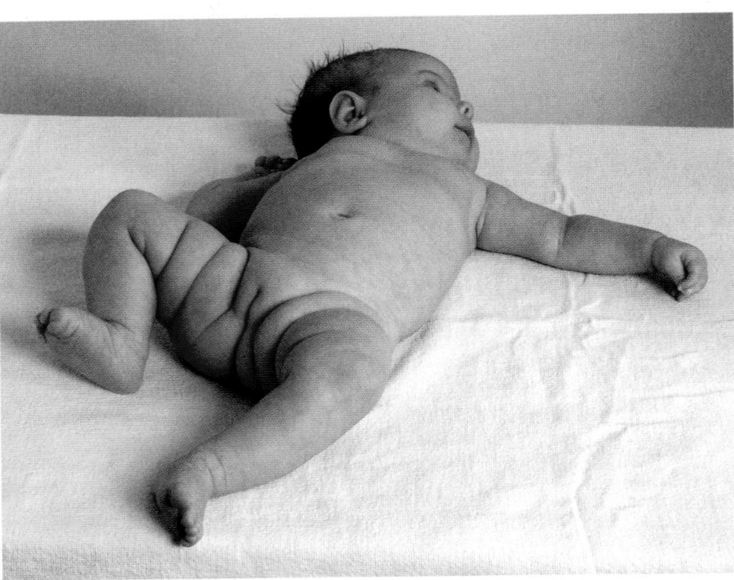

23-48 Tonic neck reflex.

Moro Reflex. Startle the infant by jarring the crib, making a loud noise, or supporting the head and back in a semi-sitting position and quickly lowering the infant to 30 degrees. The baby looks as if he or she is hugging a tree. That is, symmetric abduction and extension of the arms and legs, fanning fingers, and curling of the index finger and thumb to C-position occur. The infant then brings in both arms and legs (Fig. 23-49). The reflex is present at birth and disappears at 1 to 4 months.

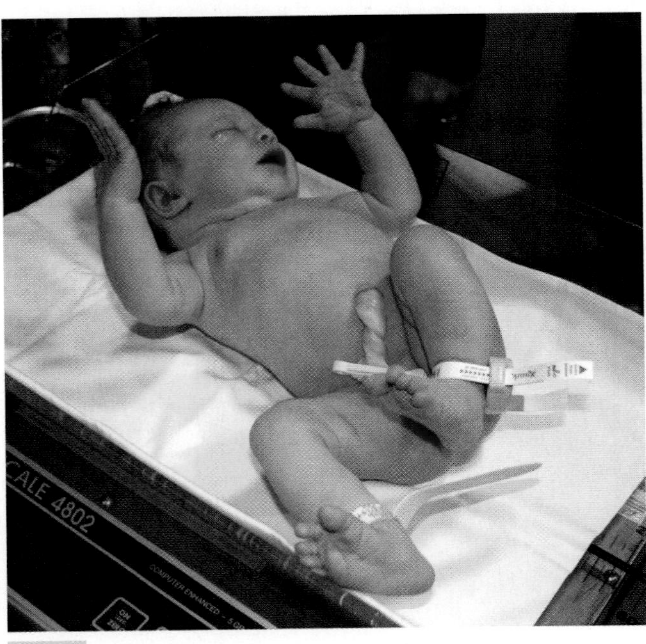

23-49 Moro reflex.

Abnormal Findings

Persistence later in infancy occurs with brain damage.

Absence of the Moro reflex in the newborn or persistence after 5 months of age indicates severe CNS injury.

Absence of movement in just one arm occurs with fracture of the humerus or clavicle and with brachial nerve palsy.

Absence in one leg occurs with a lower spinal cord problem or a dislocated hip.

A hyperactive Moro reflex occurs with tetany or CNS infection.

Normal Range of Findings	Abnormal Findings

Placing Reflex. Hold the infant upright under the arms, close to a table. Let the dorsal "top" of foot touch the underside of table. Note flexing of hip and knee, followed by extension at the hip, to place foot on table (Fig. 23-50). Reflex appears at 4 days after birth.

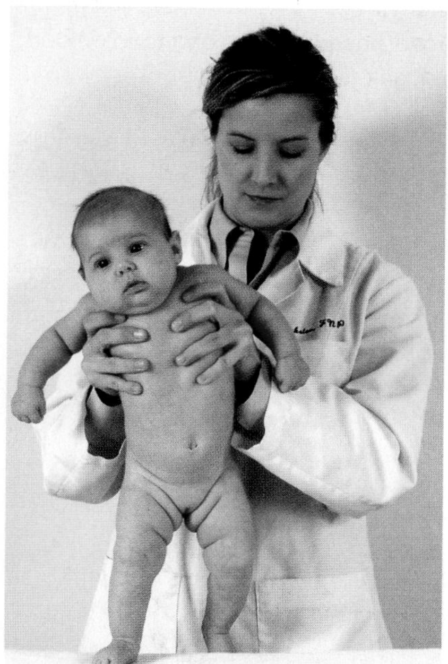

23-50 Placing reflex.

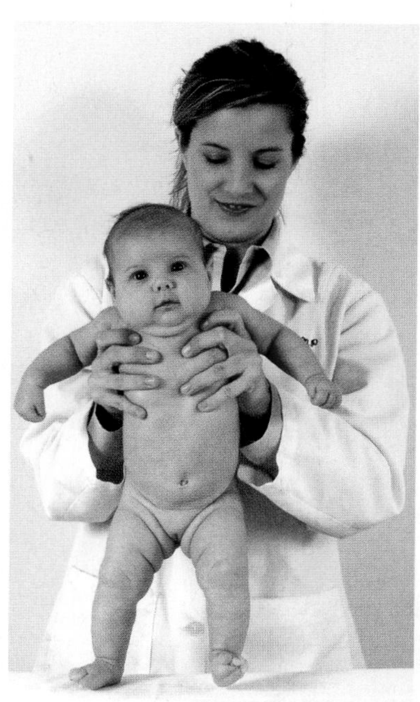

23-51 Stepping reflex.

Stepping Reflex. Hold the infant upright under the arms, with the feet on a flat surface. Note regular alternating steps (Fig. 23-51). The reflex disappears before voluntary walking.

Extensor thrust, or "scissoring"; crossing of lower extremities.

Preschool- and School-Age Children

Use the same sequence of neurologic assessment as with the adult, with the omissions or modifications mentioned in the following section.

Assess the child's general behavior during play activities, reaction to parent, and cooperation with parent and with you. Complete details are described in Chapter 5, Mental Status Assessment.

Smell and taste are almost never tested, but if you need to test the child's sense of smell (cranial nerve I), use a scent familiar to the child such as peanut butter or orange peel. When testing visual fields (cranial nerve II) and cardinal positions of gaze (cranial nerves III, IV, VI), you often need to gently immobilize the head or the child will track with the whole head. Make a game out of asking the child to imitate your funny "faces" (cranial nerve VII); thus the child has fun and you win a friend.

Much of the motor assessment can be derived from watching the child undress and dress and manipulate buttons. This indicates muscle strength, symmetry, joint range of motion, and fine motor skills. Use the Denver II to screen gross and fine motor skills that are appropriate for the child's specific age. Be familiar with developmental milestones for each age.

Muscle hypertrophy or atrophy occurs with muscular dystrophy.

Muscle weakness.

Incoordination.

Normal Range of Findings

Note the child's gait during both walking and running. Allow for the normal wide-based gate of the toddler and the normal knock-kneed walk of the preschooler. Normally, the child can balance on one foot for about 5 seconds by 4 years of age, can balance for 8 to 10 seconds at 5 years of age, and can hop at 4 years. Children enjoy performing these tests (Fig. 23-52).

Abnormal Findings

Causes of motor delay are listed earlier in the infant section.

Staggering, falling.

Weakness climbing up or down stairs occurs with muscular dystrophy.

Broad-based gait beyond toddlerhood, scissor gait (see Table 23-6).

Failure to hop after 5 years of age indicates incoordination of gross motor skill.

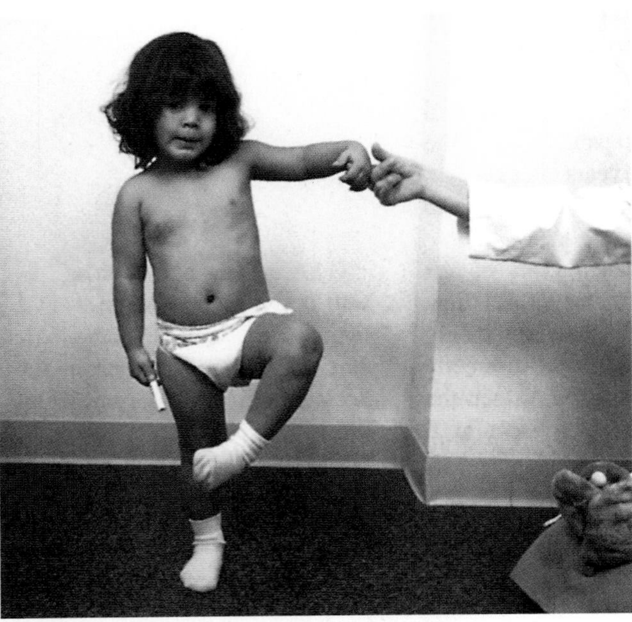

23-52

Observe the child as he or she rises from a supine position on the floor to a sitting position, and then to a stand. Note the muscles of the neck, abdomen, arms, and legs. Normally, the child curls up in the midline to sit up, then pushes off with both hands against the floor to stand (Fig. 23-53, *A*).

Weak pelvic muscles are a sign of muscular dystrophy; from the supine position, the child will roll to one side, bend forward to all four extremities, plant hands on legs, and literally "climb" up himself or herself. This is *Gower's sign* (Fig. 23-53, *B*).

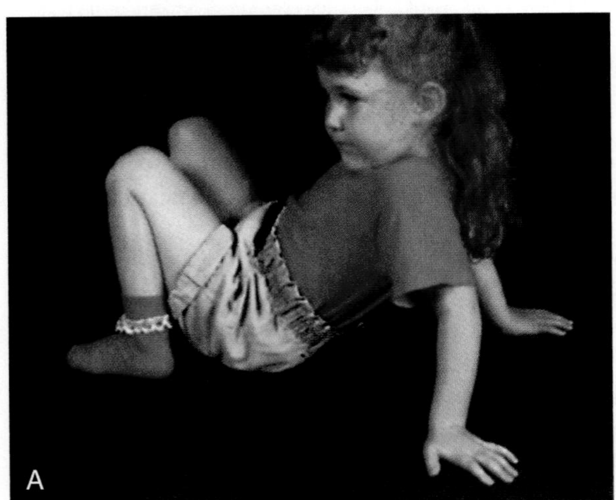

A

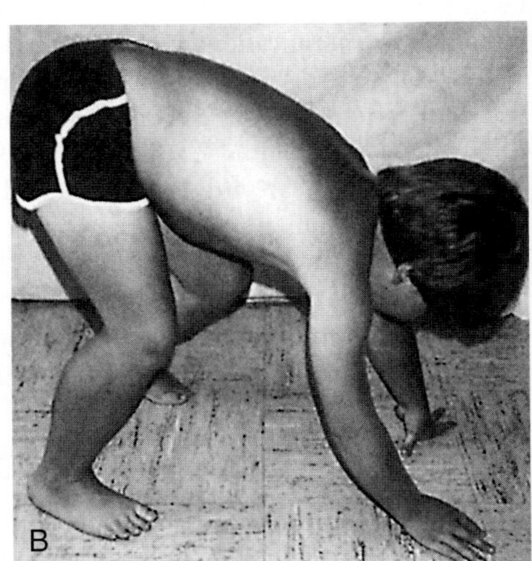

B

23-53

Normal Range of Findings

Assess fine coordination by using the finger-to-nose test if you can be sure the young child understands your directions. Demonstrate the procedure first, then ask the child to do the test with the eyes open and then with the eyes closed. Fine coordination is not fully developed until the child has reached 4 to 6 years of age. Consider it normal if a younger child can bring the finger to within 2 to 5 cm (1 to 2 inches) of the nose.

Testing sensation is very unreliable in toddlers and preschoolers. You may test light touch by asking the child to close the eyes and then to point to the spot where you touch or tickle. Testing of vibration, position, stereognosis, graphesthesia, or two-point discrimination usually is not done on a child younger than 6 years. Also, do not test for perception of superficial pain. In children older than 6 years, you may perform sensory testing as with adults. Use a fractured tongue blade if you need to test superficial pain.

The DTRs usually are not tested in children younger than 5 years due to lack of cooperation in relaxation. When you need to test DTRs in a young child, use your finger to percuss the tendon. Use a reflex hammer only with an older child. Coax the child to relax, or distract and percuss discreetly when the child is not paying attention. The knee jerk is present at birth, then the ankle jerk and brachial reflex appear, and the triceps reflex is present at 6 months.

Abnormal Findings

Failure of the finger-to-nose test with the eyes open indicates gross incoordination; failure of the test with the eyes closed indicates minor incoordination or lack of position sense.

Sensory loss occurs with decreased consciousness, mental deficiency, or spinal cord or peripheral nerve dysfunction.

Hyperactivity of DTRs occurs with upper motor neuron lesion, hypocalcemia, and hyperthyroidism and with muscle spasm associated with early poliomyelitis.

Decreased or absent reflexes occur with a lower motor neuron lesion, muscular dystrophy, and flaccidity or flaccid paralysis.

Clonus may occur with fatigue, but it usually indicates hyperreflexia.

The Aging Adult

Use the same examination as used with the younger adult. Be aware that some aging adults show a slower response to your requests, especially to those calling for coordination of movements. The conditions discussed in the following sections are normal variants due to aging.

Although the cranial nerves mediating taste and smell are not usually tested, they may show some decline in function.

Any decrease in muscle bulk is most apparent in the hand, as seen by guttering between the metacarpals. These dorsal hand muscles often look wasted, even with no apparent arthropathy. The grip strength remains relatively good.

Senile tremors occasionally occur. These benign tremors include an intention tremor of the hands, head nodding (as if saying "yes" or "no"), and tongue protrusion. *Dyskinesias* are the repetitive stereotyped movements in the jaw, lips, or tongue that may accompany senile tremors. No associated rigidity is present.

The gait may be slower and more deliberate than that in the younger person, and it may deviate slightly from a midline path.

The rapid alternating movements (e.g., pronating and supinating the hands on the thigh) may be more difficult to perform by the aging adult.

After 65 years of age, loss of the sensation of vibration at the ankle malleolus is common and is usually accompanied by loss of the ankle jerk. Position sense in the big toe may be lost, although this is less common than vibration loss. Tactile sensation may be impaired. The aging person may need stronger stimuli for light touch and especially for pain.

The DTRs are less brisk. Those in the upper extremities are usually present, but the ankle jerks are commonly lost. Knee jerks may be lost, but this occurs less often. Because aging people find it difficult to relax their limbs, always use reinforcement when eliciting the DTRs.

Hand muscle atrophy is worsened with disuse and degenerative arthropathy.

Distinguish senile tremors from tremors of parkinsonism. The latter includes rigidity and slowness and weakness of voluntary movement.

Absence of a rhythmic reciprocal gait pattern is seen in parkinsonism and hemiparesis (see Table 23-6).

Note any difference in sensation between right and left sides, which may indicate a neurologic deficit.

Normal Range of Findings

The plantar reflex may be absent or difficult to interpret. Often, you will not see a definite normal flexor response. However, you still should consider a definite extensor response to be abnormal.

The superficial abdominal reflexes may be absent, probably because of stretching of the musculature through pregnancy or obesity.

NEUROLOGIC RECHECK

Some hospitalized persons have head trauma or a neurologic deficit due to a systemic disease process. These people must be monitored closely for any improvement or deterioration in neurologic status and for any indication of increasing intracranial pressure. Signs of increasing intracranial pressure signal impending cerebral disaster and death and require early and prompt intervention.

Use an abbreviation of the neurologic examination in the following sequence:

1. Level of consciousness
2. Motor function
3. Pupillary response
4. Vital signs

Level of Consciousness. A *change* in the level of consciousness is the single most important factor in this examination. It is the earliest and most sensitive index of change in neurologic status. Note the ease of *arousal* and the state of awareness, or *orientation*. Assess orientation by asking questions about:

- Person—own name, occupation, names of workers around person, their occupations
- Place—where person is, nature of building, city, state
- Time—day of week, month, year

Vary the questions during repeat assessments so that the person is not merely memorizing answers. Note the quality and the content of the verbal response; articulation, fluency, manner of thinking; and any deficit in language comprehension or production (see Chapter 5).

When the person is intubated and cannot speak, you will have to ask questions that require a nod or shake of the head, for example, "Is this a hospital?" "Are you at home?" "Are we in Texas?"

A person is fully alert when his or her eyes open at your approach or spontaneously; when he or she is oriented to person, place, and time; and when he or she is able to follow verbal commands appropriately.

If the person is not fully alert, increase the amount of stimulus used in this order:

1. Name called
2. Light touch on person's arm
3. Vigorous shake of shoulder
4. Pain applied (pinch nail bed, pinch trapezius muscle, rub your knuckles on the person's sternum)

Record the stimulus used as well as the person's response to it.

Abnormal Findings

A change in consciousness may be subtle. Note any decreasing level of consciousness, disorientation, memory loss, uncooperative behavior, or even complacency in a previously combative person.

Review Table 5-3, Levels of Consciousness, p. 85.

Normal Range of Findings	Abnormal Findings

Motor Function. Check the voluntary movement of each extremity by giving the person specific commands. (This procedure also tests level of consciousness by noting the person's ability to follow commands.)

Ask the person to lift the eyebrows, frown, bare teeth. Note symmetric facial movements and bilateral nasolabial folds (cranial nerve VII).

You can check upper arm strength by checking hand grasps. Ask the person to squeeze your fingers. Offer your two fingers, one on top of the other, so that a strong hand grasp does not hurt your knuckles (Fig. 23-54). Be judicious about asking the person to squeeze your hands; some persons with diffuse brain damage, especially frontal lobe injury, have a grasp that is a reflex only.

A weak grip occurs with UMN and LMN disease and with local hand problems (arthritis, carpal tunnel syndrome).

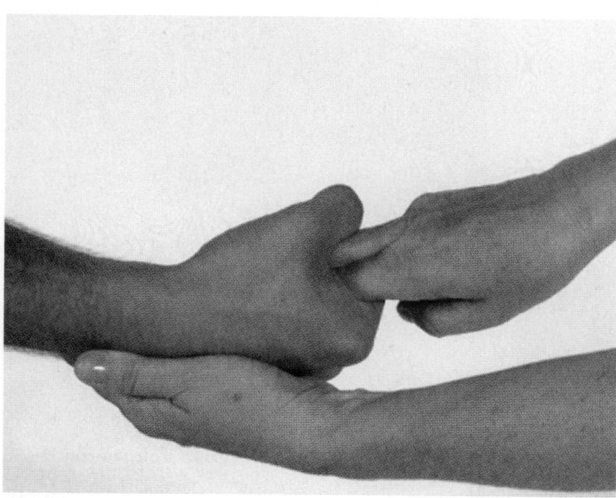

23-54

Alternatively, ask the person to lift each hand or to hold up one finger. You also can check upper extremity strength by palmar drift. Ask the person to extend both arms forward or halfway up, palms up, eyes closed, and hold for 10 to 20 seconds (Fig. 23-55). Normally, the arms stay steady with no downward drift.

Pronator drift is a downward unilateral drift and turning in of the forearm that occurs with mild hemiparesis.

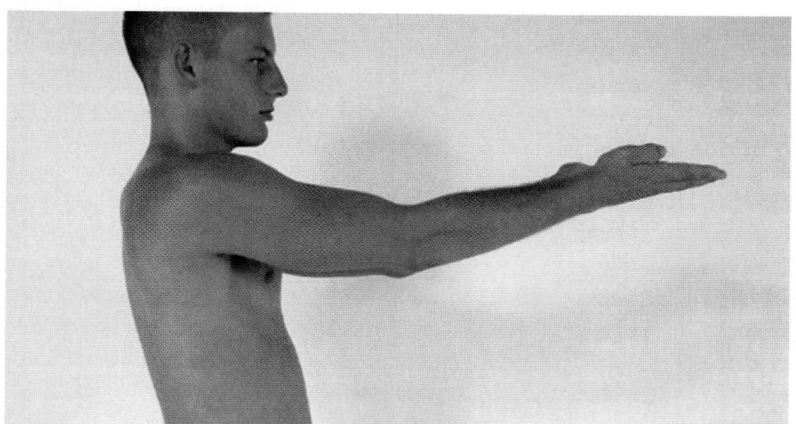

23-55

Objective Data

Normal Range of Findings

Check lower extremities by asking the person to do straight leg raises. Ask the person to lift one leg at a time straight up off the bed (Fig. 23-56). Full strength allows the leg to be lifted 90 degrees. If multiple trauma, pain, or equipment precludes this motion, ask the person to push one foot at a time against your hand's resistance, "like putting your foot on the gas pedal of your car" (Fig. 23-57).

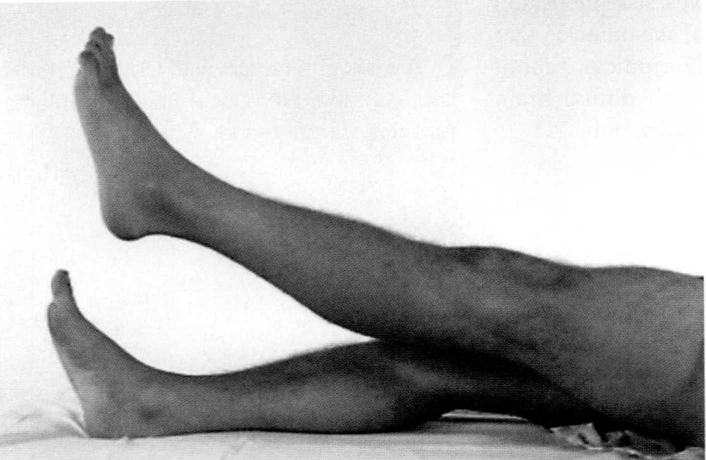

23-56

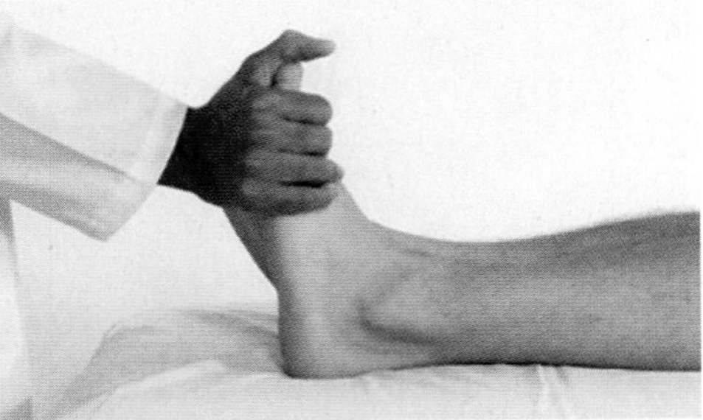

23-57

For the person with decreased level of consciousness, note if movement occurs spontaneously and as a result of noxious stimuli such as pain or suctioning. An attempt to push away your hand after such stimuli is called *localizing* and is characterized as purposeful movement.

Pupillary Response. Note the size, shape, and symmetry of both pupils. Shine a light into each pupil and note the direct and consensual light reflex. Both pupils should constrict briskly. (Allow for the effects of any medication that could affect pupil size and reactivity.) When recording, pupil size is best expressed in millimeters. Tape a millimeter scale onto a tongue blade and hold it next to the person's eyes for the most accurate measurement (Fig. 23-58).

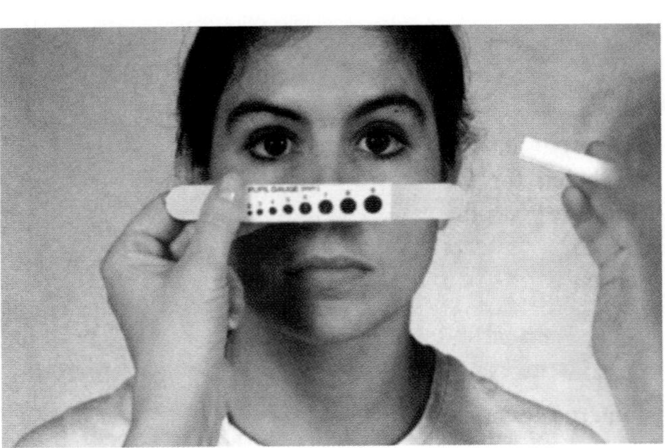

23-58

Abnormal Findings

Any abnormal posturing, decorticate rigidity, or decerebrate rigidity indicates diffuse brain injury (see Table 23-10).

In a brain-injured person, a sudden unilateral dilated and nonreactive pupil is ominous. Cranial nerve III runs parallel to the brainstem. When increasing intracranial pressure pushes the brainstem down (uncal herniation), it puts pressure on cranial nerve III, causing pupil dilation.

Objective Data

Normal Range of Findings

Vital Signs. Measure the temperature, pulse, respiration, and blood pressure as often as the person's condition warrants. Although they are vital to the overall assessment of the critically ill person, pulse and blood pressure are notoriously unreliable parameters of CNS deficit. Any changes are late consequences of rising intracranial pressure.

The Glasgow Coma Scale (GCS). Because the terms describing levels of consciousness are ambiguous, the Glasgow Coma Scale was developed as an accurate and reliable *quantitative* tool (Fig. 23-59). The GCS is a standardized, objective assessment that defines the level of consciousness by giving it a numeric value.

Abnormal Findings

The Cushing reflex shows signs of increasing intracranial pressure: blood pressure—sudden elevation with widening pulse pressure; pulse—decreased rate, slow and bounding.

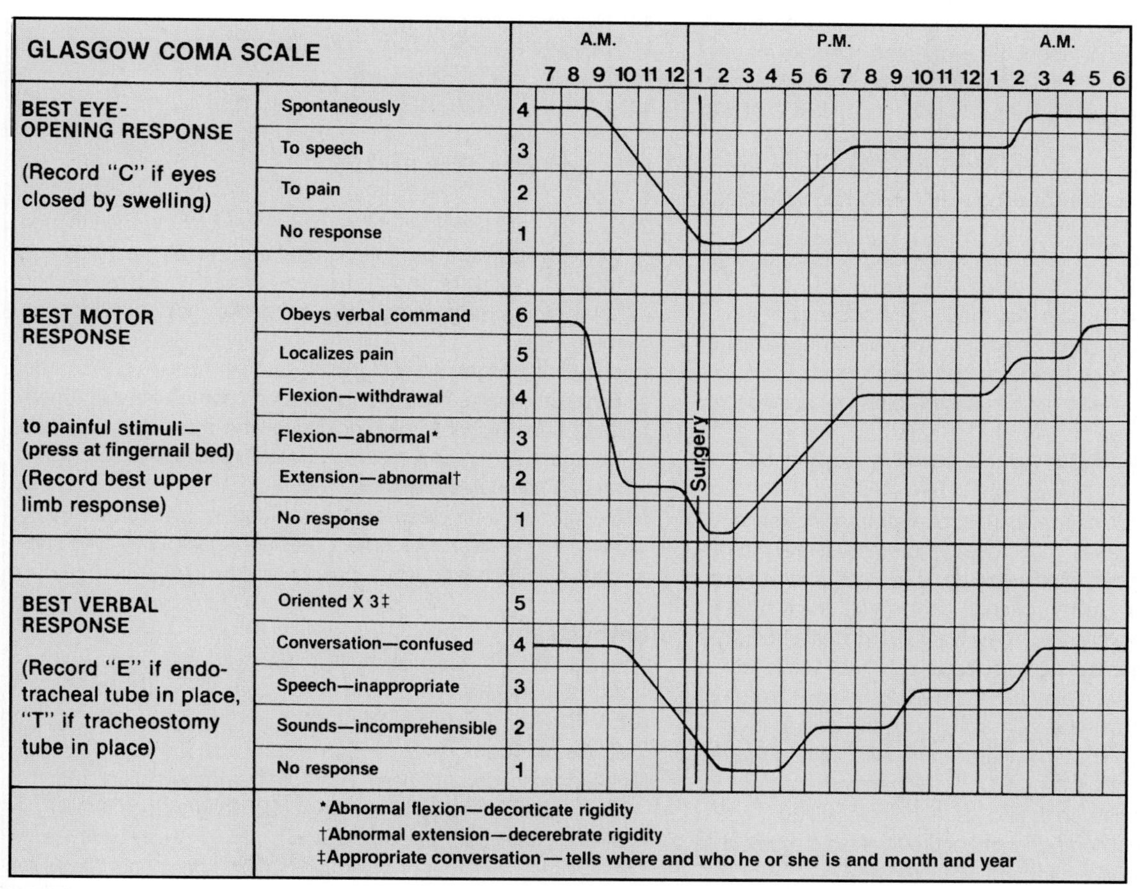

23-59

The scale is divided into three areas: eye opening, verbal response, and motor response. Each area is rated separately, and a number is given for the person's best response. The three numbers are added; the total score reflects the brain's functional level. A fully alert, normal person has a score of 15, whereas a score of 7 or less reflects coma. Serial assessments can be plotted on a graph to illustrate visually whether the person is stable, improving, or deteriorating.

The GCS assesses the functional state of the brain as a whole, not of any particular site in the brain. The scale is easy to learn and master, has good inter-rater reliability, and enhances interprofessional communication by providing a common language.

PROMOTING A HEALTHY LIFESTYLE: STROKE PREVENTION

Symptoms and Non-Modifiable and Well-Documented Modifiable Risk Factors for Stroke

According to the National Institute of Neurological Disorders and Stroke (NINDS), strokes are the leading cause of long-term disability and the third leading cause of death after heart disease and cancer. A stroke, or cerebrovascular accident (CVA), occurs when the blood flow is interrupted to a part of the brain, which is why it is often referred to as a "brain attack." The most common type is an ischemic stroke, occurring when a blood clot blocks a blood vessel in the brain. Less common is a hemorrhagic stroke, which occurs when a blood vessel in the brain ruptures and causes bleeding. The symptoms and aftereffects of a stroke depend on which area of the brain is affected and to what extent. This can make a stroke difficult to diagnose. However, early recognition of symptoms and prompt treatment are essential.

The National Institutes of Health through the NINDS has developed the *Know Stroke. Know the Signs. Act in Time* campaign to help educate the public about the symptoms of stroke and the need to get the individual with symptoms to the hospital quickly. An informational video and community education kit is available at http://stroke.nih.gov/.

Stroke symptoms usually do not hurt, which is why many people ignore them or delay seeking medical attention. Common symptoms of stroke include:

1. Sudden weakness or numbness in the face, arms, or legs, especially when it is on one side of the body
2. Sudden confusion, trouble speaking or understanding
3. Sudden changes in vision, such as blurry vision or partial or complete loss of vision in one or both eyes
4. Sudden trouble walking, dizziness, loss of balance or coordination
5. Sudden severe headache with no reason or explanation

Sometimes people can have a "mini-stroke" or transient ischemic attack (TIA). In these cases, the stroke symptoms last only temporarily and then disappear, often within an hour. Because the symptoms "go away," people too often do not report them or seek medical attention. However, a TIA is a warning sign that should not be ignored. When people experience chest pain, they seek medical attention to rule out a heart attack. Having a TIA should also prompt people to seek medical attention to rule out the possibility of a future "brain attack." The American Stroke Association Professional Education Center offers a CME/CE certified program for health care professionals on the NIH Stroke Scale (NIHSS), which is considered a critical component of acute stroke assessment. It is available as both a computer and a mobile version.

Stroke can strike anyone without any warning. Preventing a stroke is still the best medicine. People need to be aware of their stroke risk and take steps to change the risk factors they can control.

Modifiable Risk Factors

1. History of cardiovascular disease
2. Hypertension
3. Cigarette smoking/smoke
4. Diabetes
5. Atrial fibrillation
6. Other cardiac conditions
7. Dyslipidemia
8. Asymptomatic carotid stenosis
9. Sickle-cell disease
10. Postmenopausal hormone therapy
11. Diet and nutrition
12. Physical inactivity
13. Obesity and fat distribution
14. History of transient ischemic attack (TIA)

Non-modifiable Risk Factors

1. Age
2. Gender—strokes are generally more prevalent in men than in women. However, exceptions are in 35- to 44-year-olds and those 85 years of age and older—groups in which women have slightly greater age-specific stroke incidence than do men
3. Low birth weight
4. Race/Ethnicity—African Americans and some Hispanic Americans have higher stroke incidence and mortality rates than European Americans. Incidence rates are also relatively higher among some Asian groups
5. Genetic factors disorders (e.g., Marfan syndrome, Fabry disease, cerebral autosomal dominant arteriopathy with subcortical infarcts and leukoencephalopathy [CADASIL])

Resources

American Stroke Association. Website: www.strokeassociation.org/STROKEORG/.

Know Stroke. Know the Signs. Act In Time. Website: http://stroke.nih.gov/.

NIHSS downloads. http://learn.heart.org/ihtml/application/student/interface.heart2/nihss.html www.ninds.nih.gov/doctors/NIH_Stroke_Scale.pdf.

The National Institute of Neurological Disorders and Stroke—Stroke Information. www.ninds.nih.gov/disorders/stroke/detail_stroke.htm www.ninds.nih.gov/disorders/stroke/stroke.htm

DOCUMENTATION AND CRITICAL THINKING

Sample Charting

SUBJECTIVE

No unusually frequent or severe headaches, no head injury, dizziness or vertigo, seizures or tremors. No weakness, numbness or tingling, difficulty swallowing or speaking. Has no past history of stroke, spinal cord injury, meningitis, or alcoholism.

OBJECTIVE

Mental Status: Appearance, behavior, and speech appropriate; alert and oriented to person, place, and time; recent and remote memory intact.

Cranial Nerves:

I: Identifies coffee and peppermint.
II: Vision 20/20 left eye, 20/20 right eye; peripheral fields intact by confrontation; fundi normal.
III, IV, VI: EOMs intact, no ptosis or nystagmus; pupils equal, round, react to light and accommodation (PERRLA).
V: Sensation intact and equal bilaterally; jaw strength equal bilaterally.
VII: Facial muscles intact and symmetric.
VIII: Hearing—whispered words heard bilaterally; Weber test—tone is heard midline without lateralization.
IX, X: Swallowing intact, gag reflex present, uvula rises in midline on phonation.
XI: Shoulder shrug, head movement intact and equal bilaterally.
XII: Tongue protrudes midline, no tremors.

Motor: No atrophy, weakness, or tremors. Gait smooth and coordinated, able to tandem walk, negative Romberg. Rapid alternating movements (RAM)—finger-to-nose smoothly intact.

Sensory: Pinprick, light touch, vibration intact. Stereognosis—able to identify key.

Reflexes: Normal abdominal, no Babinski sign, DTRs 2+ and = bilaterally with downgoing toes; see drawing below:

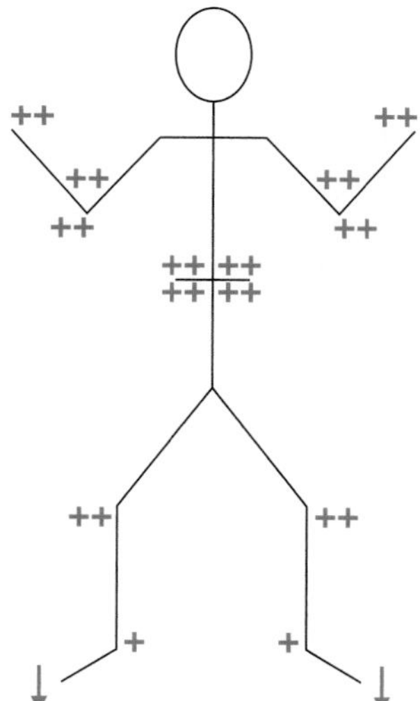

ASSESSMENT

Neurologic system intact, normal function

Focused Assessment: Clinical Case Study

J.T. is a 61-year-old white male carpenter with a large building firm who is admitted to the Rehabilitation Institute with a diagnosis of right hemiplegia and aphasia following a brain attack (CVA) 4 weeks PTA.

SUBJECTIVE

Because of J.T.'s speech dysfunction, history provided by wife.

4 weeks PTA—complaint of severe headache, then sudden onset of collapse and loss of consciousness while at work. Did not strike head as fell. Transported by ambulance to Memorial Hospital where admitting physician said J.T. "probably had a stroke." Right arm and leg were limp, and he remained unconscious. Admitted to critical care unit. Regained consciousness day 3 after admission, unable to move right side, unable to speak clearly or write. Remained in ICU 4 more days until "doctors were sure heart and breathing were steady."

3 weeks PTA—transferred to medical floor where care included physical therapy 2 ×/day and passive ROM 4 ×/day.

Now—some improvement in right motor function. Bowel control achieved with use of commode same time each day (after breakfast). Bladder control improved. Some occasional incontinence, usually when cannot tell people he needs to urinate.

OBJECTIVE

Mental Status: Dressed in jogging suit, sitting in wheelchair, appears alert with appropriate eye contact, listening intently to history. Speech is slow, requires great effort, able to give one-word answers that are appropriate but lack normal tone. Seems to understand all language spoken to him. Follows requests appropriately, within limits of motor weakness.

Cranial Nerves:

II: Acuity normal, fields by confrontation—right homonymous hemianopsia, fundi normal.
III, IV, VI: EOMs intact, no ptosis or nystagmus, PERRLA.
V: Sensation intact to pinprick and light touch. Jaw strength weak on right.
VII: Flat nasolabial fold on right, motor weakness on right lower face. Able to wrinkle forehead bilaterally, but unable to smile or bare teeth on right.
VIII: Hearing intact.
IX, X: Swallowing intact, gag reflex present, uvula rises midline on phonation.
XI: Shoulder shrug, head movement weaker on right.
XII: Tongue protrudes midline, no tremors.

Sensory: Pinprick and light touch present but diminished on right arm and leg. Vibration intact. Position sense impaired on right side. Stereognosis intact.

Motor: Right hand grip weak, right arm drifts, right leg weak, unable to support weight. Spasticity in right arm and leg muscles, limited range of motion on passive motion. Unable to stand up and walk unassisted. Unable to perform finger-to-nose or heel-to-shin on right side, left side smoothly intact.

Reflexes: Hyperactive 4+ with clonus, and upgoing toes in right leg. Abdominal and cremasteric reflexes absent on right.

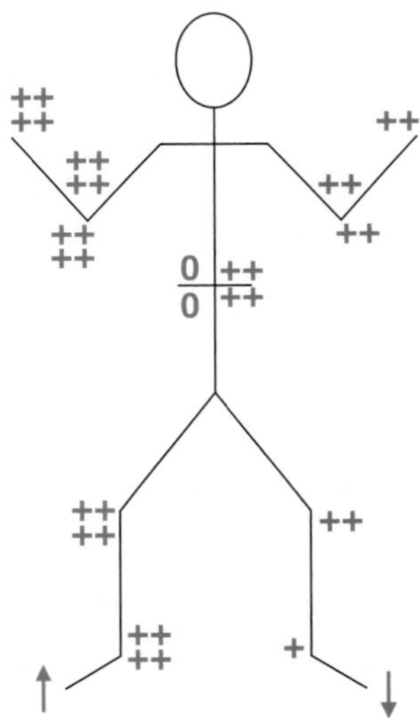

ASSESSMENT

Impaired verbal communication R/T effects of CVA
Impaired physical mobility R/T neuromuscular impairment
Disturbed body image R/T effects of loss of body function
Self-care deficits: feeding, bathing, toileting, dressing/grooming R/T muscular weakness
Disturbed sensory perception (absent right visual fields) R/T neurologic impairment
Risk for injury R/T visual field deficit

ABNORMAL FINDINGS

TABLE 23-2 10 Warning Signs of Alzheimer Disease (Alzheimer's Association, 2006)

		Alzheimer Disease (AD)	Normal Aging
1	MEMORY LOSS	Memory loss: Forgetting recently learned information is one of the most common early signs of dementia. A person begins to forget more often and is unable to recall the information later.	Forgetting names or appointments occasionally
2	LOSING TRACK	Difficulty performing familiar tasks: People with dementia often find it hard to plan or complete everyday tasks. Individuals may lose track of the steps involved in preparing a meal, placing a telephone call, or playing a game.	Occasionally forgetting why you came into a room or what you planned to say
3	FORGETTING WORDS	Problems with language: People with AD often forget simple words or substitute unusual words, making their speech or writing hard to understand. They may be unable to find the toothbrush, for example, and instead ask for "that thing for my mouth."	Sometimes having trouble finding the right word
4	GETTING LOST	Disorientation to time and place: People with AD can become lost in their own neighborhood, forget where they are and how they got there, and not know how to get back home.	Forgetting the day of the week or where you were going
5	POOR JUDGMENT	Poor or decreased judgment: Those with AD may dress inappropriately, wearing several layers on a warm day or little clothing in the cold. They may show poor judgment, like giving away large sums of money to telemarketers.	Making a questionable or debatable decision from time to time
6	ABSTRACT FAILING	Problems with abstract thinking: Someone with AD may have unusual difficulty performing complex mental tasks, such as forgetting what numbers are for and how they should be used.	Finding it challenging to balance a checkbook
7	LOSING THINGS	Misplacing things: A person with AD may put things in unusual places—an iron in the freezer or a wristwatch in the sugar bowl.	Misplacing keys or a wallet temporarily
8	MOOD SWINGS	Changes in mood or behavior: Someone with AD may show rapid mood swings—from calm to tears to anger—for no apparent reason.	Occasionally feeling sad or moody
9	PERSONALITY CHANGE	Changes in personality: The personalities of people with dementia can change dramatically. They may become extremely confused, suspicious, fearful, or dependent on a family member.	People's personalities do change somewhat with age
10	GROWING PASSIVE	Loss of initiative: A person with AD may become very passive, sitting in front of the TV for hours, sleeping more than usual, or not wanting to do usual activities.	Sometimes feeling weary of work or social obligations

Adapted from Leifer, B.P. (2009). Alzheimer's disease: seeing the signs early. *Journal of the Academy of Nurse Practitioners, 21*(11), 588-595.

TABLE 23-3 Abnormalities in Cranial Nerves

Nerve	Test	Abnormal Findings	Possible Causes
I: Olfactory	Identify familiar odors	Anosmia	Upper respiratory infection (temporary); tobacco or cocaine use; fracture of cribriform plate or ethmoid area; frontal lobe lesion; tumor in olfactory bulb or tract
II: Optic	Visual acuity	Defect or absent central vision	Congenital blindness, refractive error, acquired vision loss from numerous diseases (e.g., stroke, diabetes), trauma to globe or orbit (see discussion of cranial nerve III)
	Visual fields	Defect in peripheral vision, hemianopsia	
	Shine light in eye	Absent light reflex	
	Direct inspection	Papilledema	Increased intracranial pressure
		Optic atrophy	Glaucoma
		Retinal lesions	Diabetes
III: Oculomotor	Inspection	Dilated pupil, ptosis, eye turns out and slightly down	Paralysis in cranial nerve III from internal carotid aneurysm, tumor, inflammatory lesions, uncal herniation with increased intracranial pressure
	Extraocular muscle movement	Failure to move eye up, in, down	Ptosis from myasthenia gravis, oculomotor nerve palsy, Horner syndrome
	Shine light in eye	Absent light reflex	Blindness, drug influence, increased intracranial pressure, CNS injury, circulatory arrest, CNS syphilis
IV: Trochlear	Extraocular muscle movement	Failure to turn eye down or out	Fracture of orbit, brainstem tumor
V: Trigeminal	Superficial touch—three divisions	Absent touch and pain, paresthesias	Trauma, tumor, pressure from aneurysm, inflammation, sequelae of alcohol injection for trigeminal neuralgia
	Corneal reflex	No blink	
	Clench teeth	Weakness of masseter or temporalis muscles	Unilateral weakness with cranial nerve V lesion; bilateral weakness with upper or lower motor neuron disorder
VI: Abducens	Extraocular muscle movement to right and left sides	Failure to move laterally, diplopia on lateral gaze	Brainstem tumor or trauma, fracture of orbit
VII: Facial	Wrinkle forehead, close eyes tightly	Absent or asymmetric facial movement	Bell's palsy (lower motor neuron lesion) causes paralysis of entire half of face
	Smile, puff cheeks Identify tastes	Loss of taste	Upper motor neuron lesions (cerebrovascular accident, tumor, inflammatory) cause paralysis of lower half of face, leaving forehead intact Other lower motor neuron causes of paralysis: swelling from ear or meningeal infections

TABLE 23-3 Abnormalities in Cranial Nerves—cont'd

Nerve	Test	Abnormal Findings	Possible Causes
VIII: Acoustic	Hearing acuity	Decrease or loss of hearing	Inflammation, occluded ear canal, otosclerosis, presbycusis, drug toxicity, tumor
IX: Glossopharyngeal	Gag reflex	See cranial nerve X	
X: Vagus	Phonates "ahh"	Uvula deviates to side	Brainstem tumor, neck injury, cranial nerve X lesion
	Gag reflex	No gag reflex	Vocal cord weakness
	Note voice quality	Hoarse or brassy	Soft palate weakness
		Nasal twang	Unilateral cranial nerve X lesion
		Husky	
	Note swallowing	Dysphagia, fluids regurgitate through nose	Bilateral cranial nerve X lesion
XI: Spinal accessory	Turn head, shrug shoulders against resistance	Absent movement of sternomastoid or trapezius muscles	Neck injury, torticollis
XII: Hypoglossal	Protrude tongue	Deviates to side	Lower motor neuron lesion
	Wiggle tongue from side to side	Slowed rate of movement	Bilateral upper motor neuron lesion

TABLE 23-4 Abnormalities in Muscle Tone

Condition	Description	Associated With
Flaccidity	Decreased muscle tone or *hypotonia;* muscle feels limp, soft, and flabby; muscle is weak and easily fatigued; limb feels like a rag doll	Lower motor neuron injury anywhere from the anterior horn cell in the spinal cord to the peripheral nerve (peripheral neuritis, poliomyelitis, Guillain-Barré syndrome); early cerebrovascular accident and spinal cord injury are flaccid at first
Spasticity	Increased tone or *hypertonia;* increased resistance to passive lengthening; then may suddenly give way (clasp-knife phenomenon) like a pocket knife sprung open	Upper motor neuron injury to corticospinal motor tract (e.g., paralysis with stroke develops spasticity days or weeks after incident)
Rigidity	Constant state of resistance (lead-pipe rigidity); resists passive movement in any direction; dystonia	Injury to extrapyramidal motor tracts (e.g., basal ganglia with parkinsonism)
Cogwheel rigidity	Type of rigidity in which the increased tone is released by degrees during passive range of motion so it feels like small, regular jerks	Parkinsonism

TABLE 23-5 Abnormalities in Muscle Movement

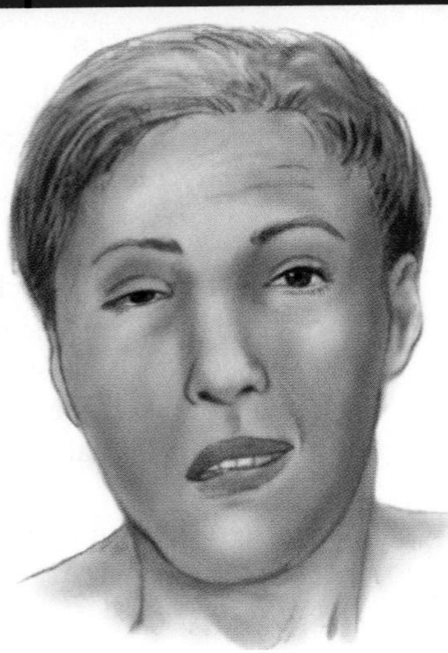

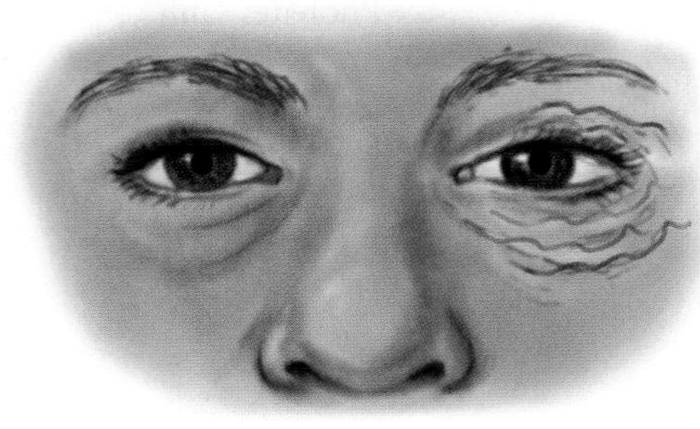

Paralysis

Decreased or loss of motor power due to problem with motor nerve or muscle fibers. Causes: acute—trauma, spinal cord injury, brain attack, poliomyelitis, polyneuritis, Bell's palsy; chronic—muscular dystrophy, diabetic neuropathy, multiple sclerosis; episodic—myasthenia gravis.

Patterns of paralysis: *hemiplegia*—spastic or flaccid paralysis of one side (right or left) of body and extremities; *paraplegia*—symmetric paralysis of both lower extremities; *quadriplegia*—paralysis in all four extremities. *Paresis*—weakness of muscles rather than paralysis.

Fasciculation

Rapid, continuous twitching of resting muscle or part of muscle, without movement of limb, that can be seen by clinicians or felt by patients. Types: fine—occurs with lower motor neuron disease, associated with atrophy and weakness; coarse—occurs with cold exposure or fatigue and is not significant.

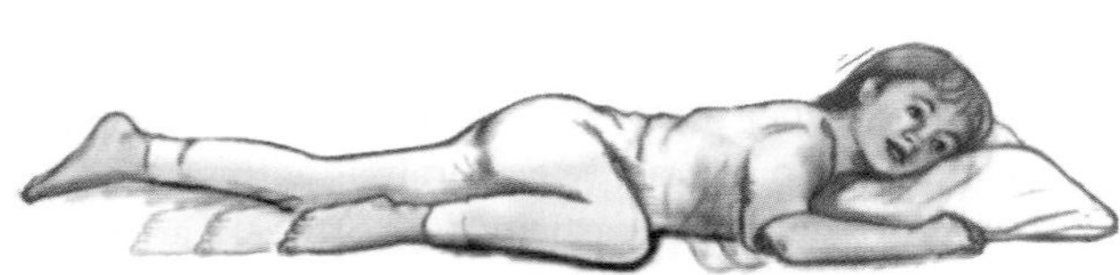

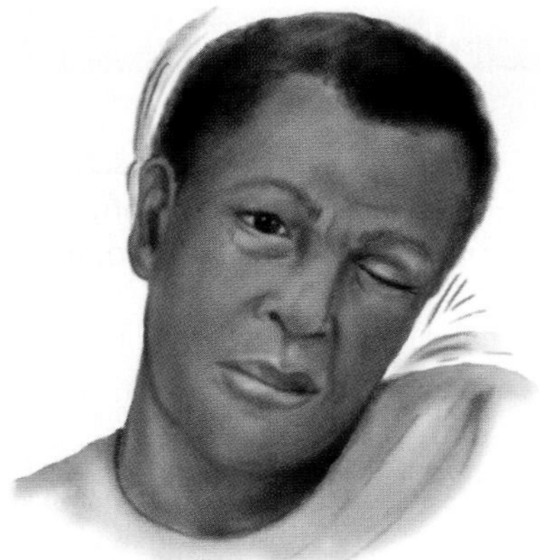

Myoclonus

Rapid, sudden jerk or a short series of jerks at fairly regular intervals. A hiccup is a myoclonus of diaphragm. Single myoclonic arm or leg jerk is normal when the person is falling asleep; myoclonic jerks are severe with grand mal seizures.

Tic

Involuntary, compulsive, repetitive twitching of a muscle group (e.g., wink, grimace, head movement, shoulder shrug); due to a neurologic cause (e.g., tardive dyskinesias, Tourette syndrome) or a psychogenic cause (habit tic).

Seizure Disorder (not illustrated)

A seizure is a time-limited event due to excessive, hypersynchronous discharge of neurons in the brain. This may be due to a clear provocation such as cerebral trauma, structural lesions (tumor, blood clot, infection), hyponatremia, acute alcohol withdrawal, or medication overdose. Also, the condition of epilepsy has unprovoked recurrent seizures due to cerebrovascular disease or in 70% of patients of unknown cause. Generalized seizures involve the entire brain, such as the tonic-clonic or grand mal seizure. This type of seizure has distinct phases: (1) loss of consciousness; (2) tonic phase with muscular rigidity, opening of mouth and eyes, tongue biting, and high-pitched cry; (3) clonic phase with violent muscular contractions, facial grimacing, and increased heart rate; and (4) postictal phase with deep sleeping, disorientation, and confusion.

TABLE 23-5 Abnormalities in Muscle Movement—cont'd

Tremor

Involuntary contraction of opposing muscle groups. Results in rhythmic, back-and-forth movement of one or more joints. May occur at rest or with voluntary movement. All tremors disappear while sleeping. Tremors may be slow (3 to 6 per second) or rapid (10 to 20 per second).

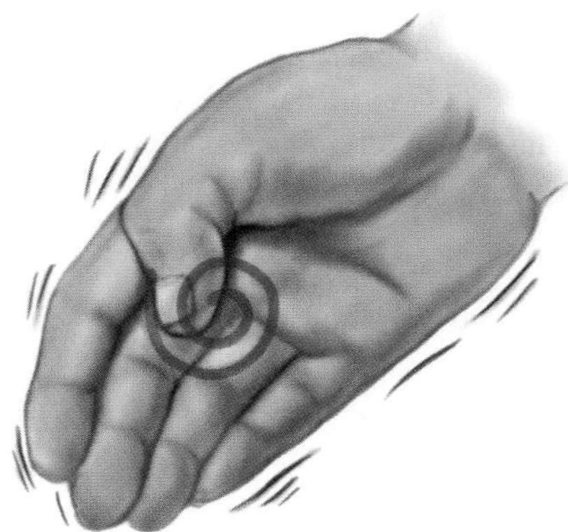

Rest Tremor

This occurs when muscles are quiet and supported against gravity (hand in the lap). Coarse and slow (3 to 6 per second); partly or completely disappears with voluntary movement (e.g., "pill rolling" tremor of parkinsonism, with thumb and opposing fingers).

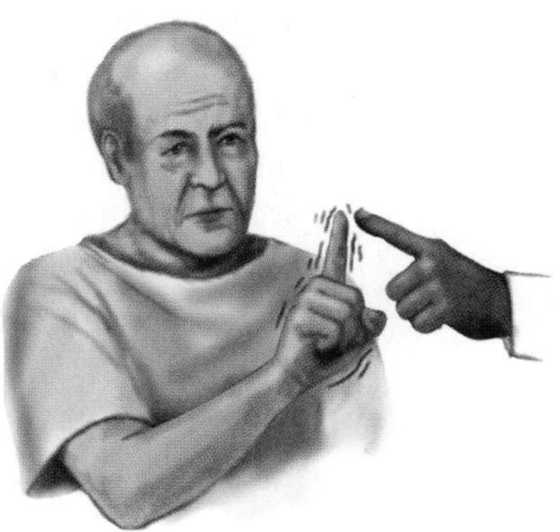

Intention Tremor

Rate varies; worse with voluntary movement as in reaching toward a visually guided target. Occurs with cerebellar disease and multiple sclerosis.

Essential tremor (familial)—a type of intention tremor; most common tremor with older people. Benign (no associated disease) but causes emotional stress in business or social situations. Improves with the administration of sedatives, propranolol, or alcohol, but do discourage alcohol because of the risk for addiction.

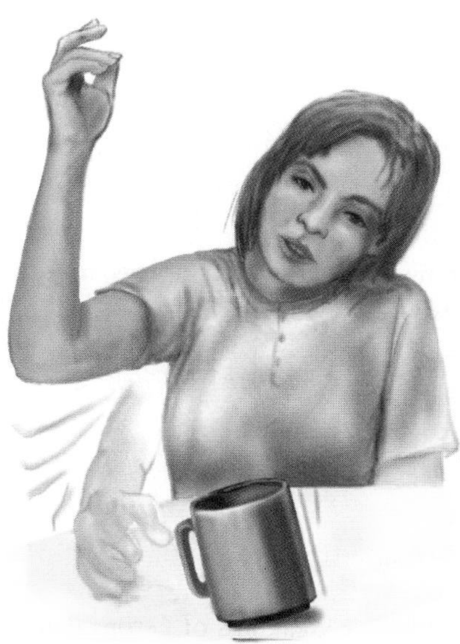

Chorea

Sudden, rapid, jerky, purposeless movement involving limbs, trunk, or face.

Occurs at irregular intervals, not rhythmic or repetitive, more convulsive than a tic. Some are spontaneous, and some are initiated; all are accentuated by voluntary acts. Disappears with sleep. Common with Sydenham's chorea and Huntington's disease.

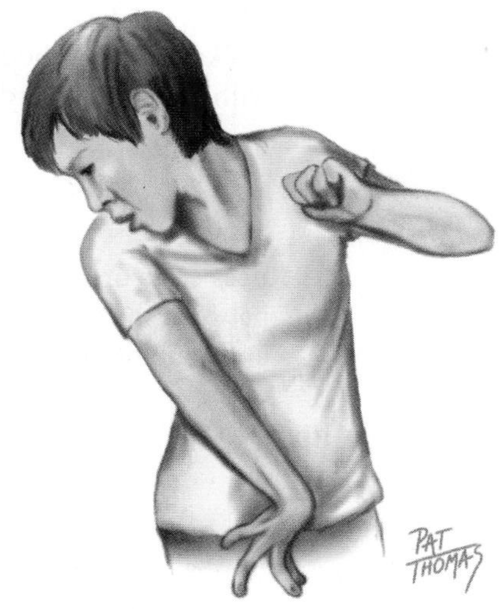

Athetosis

Slow, twisting, writhing, continuous movement, resembling a snake or worm. Involves the distal part of the limb more than the proximal part. Occurs with cerebral palsy. Disappears with sleep. "Athetoid" hand—some fingers are flexed and some are extended.

ABNORMAL FINDINGS
FOR ADVANCED PRACTICE

TABLE 23-6 Abnormal Gaits

Type	Characteristic Appearance	Possible Causes
Spastic Hemiparesis	Arm is immobile against the body, with flexion of the shoulder, elbow, wrist, and fingers and adduction of shoulder, does not swing freely. The leg is stiff and extended and circumducts with each step (drags toe in a semicircle).	Upper motor neuron lesion of the corticospinal tract (e.g., cerebrovascular accident, trauma)
Cerebellar Ataxia	Staggering, wide-based gait; difficulty with turns; uncoordinated movement with positive Romberg sign.	Alcohol or barbiturate effect on cerebellum; cerebellar tumor; multiple sclerosis
Parkinsonian (Festinating)	Posture is stooped; trunk is pitched forward; elbows, hips, and knees are flexed. Steps are short and shuffling. Hesitation to begin walking, and difficult to stop suddenly. The person holds the body rigid. Walks and turns body as one fixed unit. Difficulty with any change in direction.	Parkinsonism
Scissors	Knees cross or are in contact, like holding an orange between the thighs. The person uses short steps, and walking requires effort.	Paraparesis of legs, multiple sclerosis
Steppage or Footdrop	Slapping quality—looks as if walking up stairs and finds no stair there. Lifts knee and foot high and slaps it down hard and flat to compensate for footdrop.	Weakness of peroneal and anterior tibial muscles; due to lower motor neuron lesion at the spinal cord (e.g., poliomyelitis)

TABLE 23-6 Abnormal Gaits—cont'd

Type	Characteristic Appearance	Possible Causes
Waddling	Weak hip muscles—when the person takes a step, the opposite hip drops, which allows compensatory lateral movement of pelvis. Often, the person also has marked lumbar lordosis and a protruding abdomen.	Hip girdle muscle weakness due to muscular dystrophy, dislocation of hips
Short Leg	Leg length discrepancy >2.5 cm (1 inch). Vertical telescoping of affected side, which dips as the person walks. Appearance of gait varies depending on amount of accompanying muscle dysfunction.	Congenital dislocated hip; acquired shortening due to disease, trauma

TABLE 23-7 Characteristics of Upper and Lower Motor Neuron Lesions

	Upper Motor Neuron Lesion	Lower Motor Neuron Lesion
Weakness/paralysis	In muscles corresponding to distribution of damage in pyramidal tract lesion; usually in hand grip, arm extensors, leg flexors	In specific muscles served by damaged spinal segment, ventral root, or peripheral nerve
Location	Descending motor pathways that originate in the motor areas of cerebral cortex and carry impulses to the anterior horn cells of the spinal cord	Nerve cells that originate in the anterior horn of spinal cord or in brainstem and carry impulses by the spinal nerves or cranial nerves to the muscles, the "final common pathway"
Example	Brain attack or cerebrovascular accident	Poliomyelitis, herniated intervertebral disk
Muscle tone	Increased tone; spasticity	Loss of tone, flaccidity
Bulk	May have some atrophy from disuse; otherwise normal	Atrophy (wasting), may be marked
Abnormal movements	None	Fasciculations
Reflexes	Hyperreflexia, ankle clonus; diminished or absent superficial abdominal reflexes; positive Babinski sign	Hyporeflexia or areflexia; no Babinski sign, no pathologic reflexes
Possible nursing diagnoses	Risk for contractures; Impaired Physical Mobility	Impaired Physical Mobility

TABLE 23-8 Patterns of Motor System Dysfunction

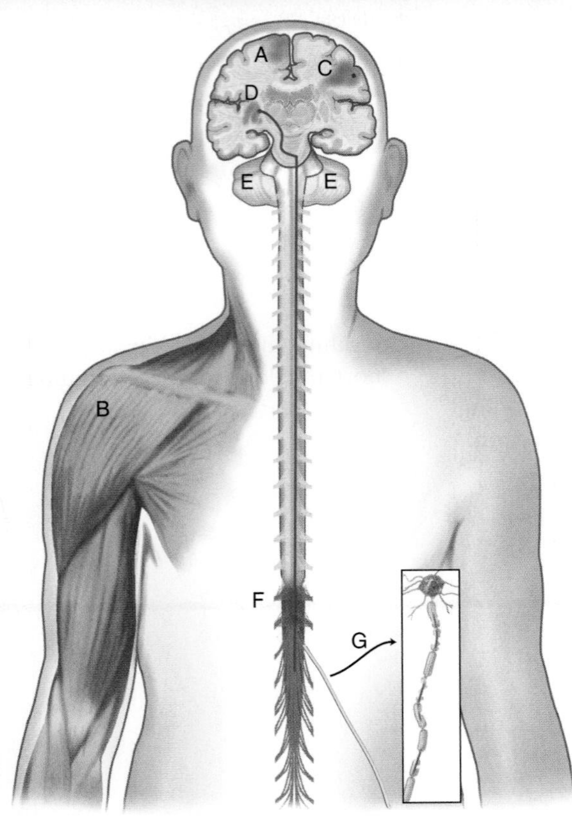

A—Cerebral palsy. Mixed group of paralytic neuromotor disorders of infancy and childhood; due to damage to cerebral cortex caused by a developmental defect, intrauterine meningitis or encephalitis, birth trauma, anoxia, or kernicterus.

B—Muscular dystrophy. Chronic, progressive wasting of skeletal musculature, which produces weakness, contractures and, in severe cases, respiratory dysfunction and death. Onset of symptoms occurs in childhood. Many types exist; the most severe is Duchenne dystrophy, characterized by the waddling gait described in Table 23-6.

C—Hemiplegia. Damage to corticospinal tract (e.g., CVA, or stroke). Upper motor neuron damage occurs above the pyramidal decussation crossover, so motor impairment is on contralateral (opposite) side. Initially flaccid when the lesion is acute; later, the muscles become spastic and abnormal reflexes appear. Characteristic posture: arm—shoulder adducted, elbow flexed, wrist pronated, leg extended; face—weakness only in lower muscles. Hyperreflexia and possible clonus occur on the involved side; loss of corneal, abdominal, and cremasteric reflexes; positive Babinski and Hoffman reflexes.

D—Parkinsonism. Defect of extrapyramidal tracts, in the basal ganglia, with loss of the neurotransmitter *dopamine.* Classic triad of symptoms: tremor, rigidity, bradykinesia. Also slower, monotonous speech and diminutive writing. Body tends to stay immobile; facial expression is flat, staring, expressionless; excessive salivation occurs; reduced eye blinking. Posture is stooped; equilibrium is impaired; loses balance easily; gait is described in Table 23-6. Parkinsonian tremor; cogwheel rigidity on passive range of motion.

E—Cerebellar. A lesion in one hemisphere produces motor abnormalities on the ipsilateral side. Characterized by ataxia, lurching forward of affected side while walking, rapid alternating movements are slow and arrhythmic, finger-to-nose test reveals ataxia and tremor with overshoot or undershoot, and eyes display coarse nystagmus.

F—Paraplegia. Lower motor neuron damage caused by spinal cord injury. A severe injury or complete transection initially produces "spinal shock," which is defined as no movement or reflex activity below the level of the lesion. Gradually, deep tendon reflexes reappear and become increased; flexor spasms of legs occur; and finally, extensor spasms of legs occur; these spasms lead to prevailing extensor tone.

G—Multiple Sclerosis. Chronic, progressive, immune-mediated disease in which axons experience inflammation, demyelination, degeneration and, finally, sclerosis.[6] Structures most frequently involved are the optic nerve, oculomotor nerve, corticospinal tract, posterior column tract, and cerebellum. Thus symptoms are varied but include blurred vision, diplopia, extreme fatigue, weakness, spasticity, numbness and tingling, and loss of balance.

TABLE 23-9 Patterns of Sensory Loss

Type	Characteristics	Possible Causes
Peripheral Neuropathy	Loss of sensation involves all modalities. Loss is most severe distally (feet and hands); response improves as stimulus is moved proximally (glove-and-stocking anesthesia). Anesthesia zone gradually merges into a hypoesthesia zone, and then gradually becomes normal.	Diabetes, chronic alcoholism, nutritional deficiency
Individual Nerves or Roots	Decrease or loss of all sensory modalities. Area of sensory loss corresponds to distribution of the involved nerve.	Trauma, vascular occlusion
Spinal Cord Hemisection (Brown-Séquard Syndrome)	Loss of pain and temperature, contralateral side, starting one to two segments below the level of the lesion. Loss of vibration and position discrimination on the ipsilateral side, below the level of the lesion.	Meningioma, neurofibroma, cervical spondylosis, multiple sclerosis
Complete Transection of the Spinal Cord	Complete loss of *all* sensory modalities below the level of the lesion. Condition is associated with motor paralysis and loss of sphincter control.	Spinal cord trauma, demyelinating disorders, tumor

Continued

TABLE 23-9 Patterns of Sensory Loss—cont'd

Type	Characteristics	Possible Causes
Thalamus	Loss of *all* sensory modalities on the face, arm, and leg on the side contralateral to the lesion.	Vascular occlusion
Cortex	Because pain, vibration, and crude touch are mediated by thalamus, little loss of these sensory functions occurs with a cortex lesion. Loss of discrimination occurs on the contralateral side. Loss of graphesthesia, stereognosis, recognition of shapes and weights, finger finding.	Cerebral cortex, parietal lobe lesion (e.g., CVA, or stroke)

TABLE 23-10 Abnormal Postures

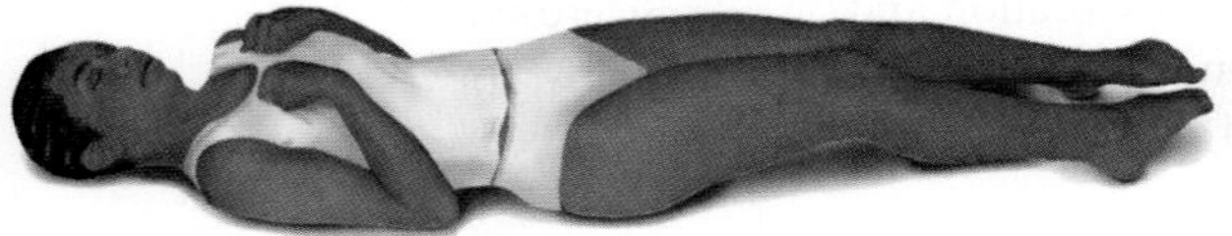

Decorticate Rigidity

Upper extremities—flexion of arm, wrist, and fingers; adduction of arm (i.e., tight against thorax). Lower extremities—extension, internal rotation, plantar flexion. This indicates hemispheric lesion of cerebral cortex.

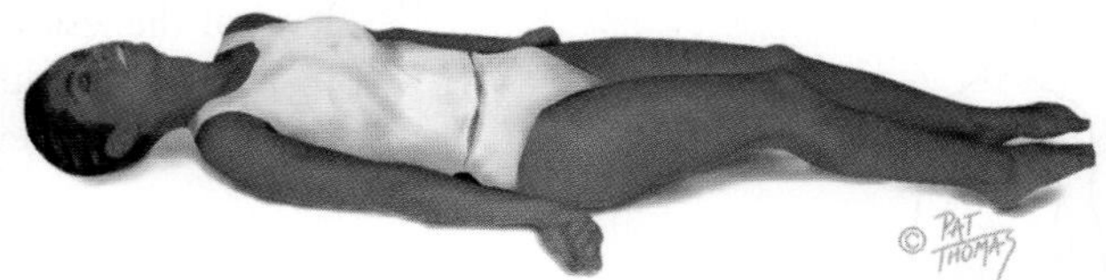

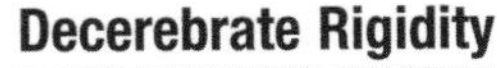

Decerebrate Rigidity

Upper extremities stiffly extended, adducted, internal rotation, palms pronated. Lower extremities stiffly extended, plantar flexion; teeth clenched; hyperextended back. More ominous than decorticate rigidity; indicates lesion in brainstem at midbrain or upper pons.

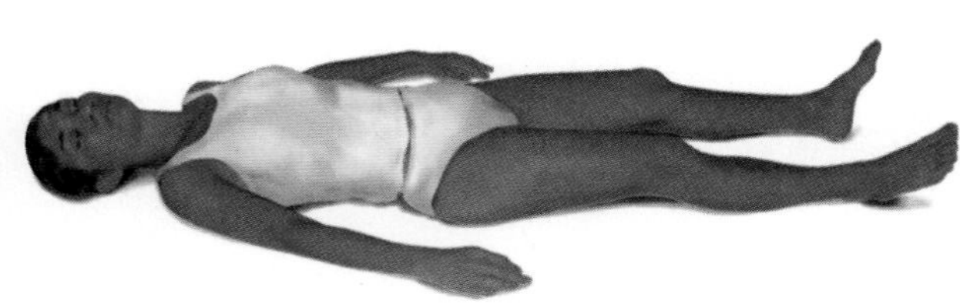

Flaccid Quadriplegia

Complete loss of muscle tone and paralysis of all four extremities, indicating completely nonfunctional brainstem.

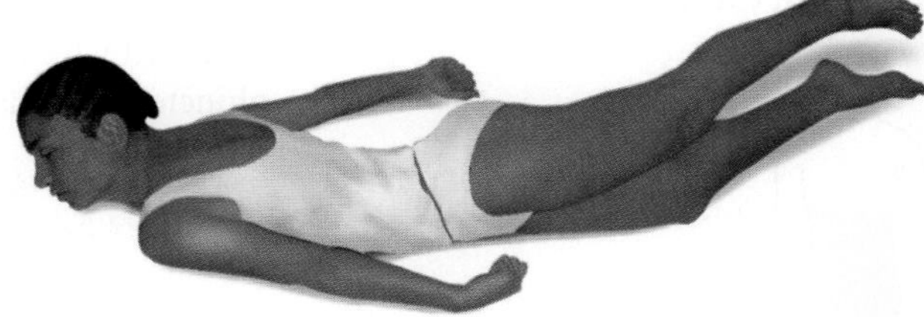

Opisthotonos

Prolonged arching of the back, with head and heels bent backward. This indicates meningeal irritation.

TABLE 23-11 Pathologic Reflexes

Reflex	Method of Testing	Abnormal Response (Reflex is Present)	Indications
Babinski	Stroke lateral aspect and across ball of foot.	Extension of great toe, fanning of toes	Corticospinal (pyramidal) tract disease (e.g., stroke, trauma)
Oppenheim	Using heavy pressure with your thumb and index finger, stroke anterior medial tibial muscle.	Same as above	Same
Gordon	Firmly squeeze calf muscles.	Same as above	Same
Hoffmann	With patient's hand relaxed, wrist dorsiflexed, and fingers slightly flexed, sharply flick nail of distal phalanx of middle or index finger.	Clawing of fingers and thumb	Same
Kernig	In flat-lying supine position, raise leg straight or flex thigh on abdomen, and then extend knee.	Resistance to straightening (because of hamstring spasm), pain down posterior thigh	Meningeal irritation (e.g., meningitis, infections)
Brudzinski	With one hand under the neck and other hand on person's chest, sharply flex chin on chest and watch hips and knees.	Resistance and pain in neck, with flexion of hips and knees	Meningeal irritation (e.g., meningitis, infections)

TABLE 23-12 Frontal Release Signs

Reflex

Snout

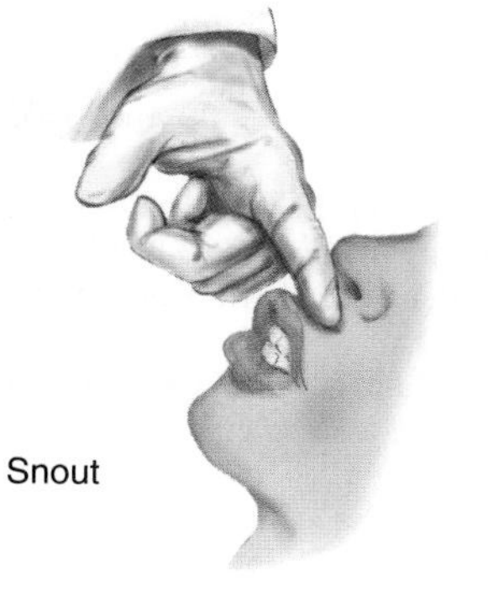

Snout

Method of Testing

Gently percuss oral region

Abnormal Response (Reflex is Present)

Puckers lips

Indications

Frontal lobe disease, cerebral degenerative disease (Alzheimer), amyotrophic sclerosis, corticobulbar lesions

Sucking

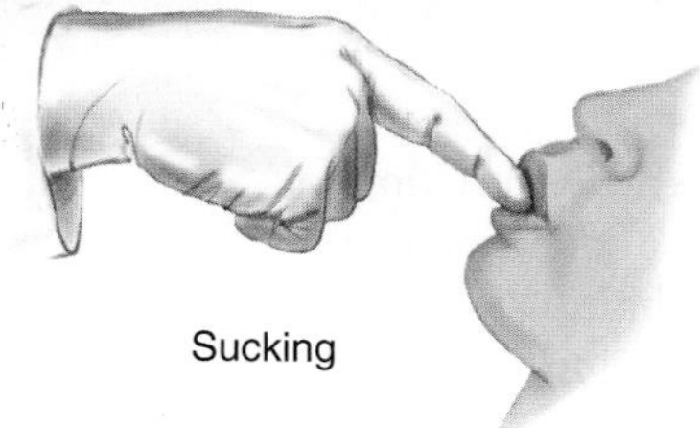

Sucking

Method of Testing

Touch oral region

Abnormal Response (Reflex is Present)

Sucking movement of lips, tongue, jaw, swallowing

Indications

Same as for snout reflex

Grasp

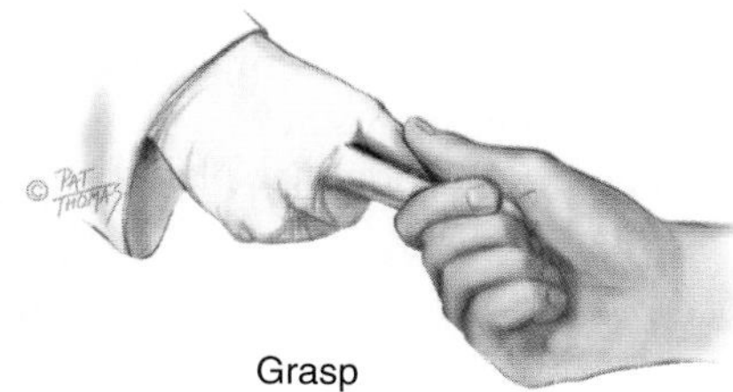

Grasp

Method of Testing

Touch palm with your finger

Abnormal Response (Reflex is Present)

Uncontrolled, forced grasping (grasp is usually last of these signs to appear, so its presence indicates severe disease)

Indications

When unilateral, frontal lobe lesion on contralateral side; when bilateral, diffuse bifrontal lobe disease

BIBLIOGRAPHY

1. Alzheimer's Association. (2010). *10 signs of Alzheimer's*. Retrieved June 9, 2010, from www.alz.org/alzheimers_disease_10_signs_of_alzheimers.asp.
2. Budson, A., & Price, B. (2005). Memory dysfunction. *New England Journal of Medicine, 352*(7), 692-699.
3. Casper, M. L., Barnett, E., Williams, G. I., et al. (2003). *Atlas of stroke mortality: racial, ethnic, and geographic disparities in the United States*. Atlanta: USDHHS. Retrieved June 9, 2010, from www.cdc.gov/dhdsp/library/maps/strokeatlas/index.htm.
4. Centers for Disease Control and Prevention. (2003). Health status of American Indians compared with other racial/ethnic minority populations. *MMWR. Morbidity and Mortality Weekly Report, 52*, 1148-1152.
5. Centers for Disease Control and Prevention. (2007). Prevalence of stroke—United States, 2005. *MMWR. Morbidity and Mortality Weekly Report, 56*(19), 469-474.
6. Courtney, A. M., Treadaway, K., Remington, G., et al. (2009). Multiple sclerosis. *Medical Clinics of North America, 93*(2), 451-476.
7. Criddle, L. M., Bonnono, C., & Fisher, S. K. (2003). Standardizing stroke assessment using the National Institutes of Health stroke scale. *Journal of Emergency Medicine, 29*(6), 541-546.
8. Dahodwala, N., Siderowf, A., Xie, M., et al. (2009). Racial differences in the diagnosis of Parkinson's disease. *Movement Disorders, 24*(8), 1200-1205.
9. Fjell, A. M., Walhovd, K. B., & Fennema-Notestine, C. (2009). One-year brain atrophy evident in healthy aging. *Journal of Neuroscience, 29*(48), 1523-1531.
10. Freedman, M. S., Cohen, B., Dhib-Jalbut, S., et al. (2009). Recognizing and treating suboptimally controlled multiple sclerosis. *Current Medical Research and Opinion, 25*(10), 2459-2470.
11. Freeman, S. H., Kandel, R., & Cruz, L. (2008). Preservation of neuronal number despite age-related cortical brain atrophy in elderly subjects without Alzheimer disease. *Journal of Neuropathology and Experimental Neurology, 67*(12), 1205-1212.
12. Futagi, Y., Toribe, Y., & Suzuki, Y. (2009). Neurological assessment of early infants. *Current Pediatric Reviews, 5*(2), 65-70.
13. Gilden, D. (2004). Clinical practice: Bell's palsy. *New England Journal of Medicine, 351*(13), 1323-1331.
14. Goldstein, L. B., Adams, R. Alberts, M. J., et al. (2006). Primary prevention of ischemic stroke. *Stroke; A Journal of Cerebral Circulation, 37*(6), 1583-1633.
15. Hall, G. R., Gallagher, M., & Dougherty, J. (2009). Integrating roles for successful dementia management. *Nurse Practitioner, 34*(11), 35-41.
16. Hindle, J. V. (2010). Ageing, neurodegeneration and Parkinson's disease. *Age and Ageing, 39*(2), 156-161.
17. Iankova, A. (2006). The Glasgow Coma Scale: clinical application in emergency departments. *Emergency Nurse, 14*(8), 30-35.
18. Leifer, B. P. (2009). Alzheimer's disease: seeing the signs early. *Journal of the Academy of Nurse Practitioners, 21*(11), 588-595.
19. Lloyd-Jones, D., Adams, R. J., Brown, T. M., et al for the AHA. (2010). Heart disease and stroke statistics—2010 update. *Circulation, 121*(7), 948-954.
20. Martin, E. M., Lu, W. C., Helmick, K., et al. (2008). Traumatic brain injuries sustained in Afghanistan and Iraq wars. *American Journal of Nursing, 108*(4), 40-48.
21. McElroy-Cox, C. (2007). Caring for patients with epilepsy. *Nurse Practitioner, 32*(10), 34-41.

21a. McGee, S. (2007). *Evidence-based physical diagnosis*. St. Louis: Saunders.

22. National Center for Health Statistics. (2009). *Health, United States, 2009: in brief*. Centers for Disease Control and Prevention. Retrieved June 12, 2010, from www.cdc.gov/nchs/hus.htm.
23. Palmieri, R. L. (2009). Wrapping your head around cranial nerves. *Nursing, 39*(9), 24-31.
24. Sartorius, D., Le Manach, Y., David, J. S., et al. (2010). Mechanism, Glasgow Coma Scale, age, and arterial pressure (MGAP). *Critical Care Medicine, 38*(3), 831-837.
25. Sauerbeck, L. R. (2006). Primary stroke prevention. *American Journal of Nursing, 106*(11), 40-50.
26. Savva, G. M., Wharton, S. B., Ince, P. G. et al. (2009). Age, neuropathology and dementia. *New England Journal of Medicine, 360*(22), 2302-2309.
27. Schutte, D. L. (2006). Alzheimer disease and genetics: anticipating the questions. *American Journal of Nursing, 106*(12), 40-48.
28. Simmons, S. (2010). Guillain-Barré syndrome: a nursing nightmare that usually ends well. *Nursing, 40*(1), 24-30.
29. Stephens, B. E., Liu, J., Lester, B., et al. (2010). Neurobehavioral assessment predicts motor outcome in preterm infants. *Journal of Pediatrics, 156*(3), 366-371.
30. Struble, L. M. (2010). Tremors: learning to stop the shakes. *Nurse Practitioner, 35*(6), 18-26.
31. Tiemstra, J. D., & Khatkhate, N. (2007). Bell's palsy: diagnosis and management. *American Family Physician, 76*(7), 997-1002.
32. Welsh, M. (2008). Treatment challenges in Parkinson's disease. *Nurse Practitioner, 33*(7), 32-38.
33. Zuercher, M., Ummenhofer, W., & Baltussen, A. (2009). The use of the Glasgow Coma Scale in injury assessment. *Brain Injury, 23*(5), 371-384.

Summary Checklist: Neurologic Examination

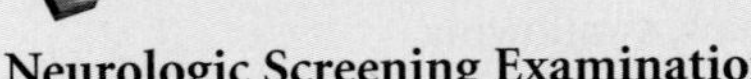
For a PDA-downloadable version, go to http://evolve.elsevier.com/Jarvis/.

Neurologic Screening Examination

1. **Mental status**
2. **Cranial nerves**
   II: Optic
   III, IV, VI: Extraocular muscles
   V: Trigeminal
   VII: Facial mobility
3. **Motor function**
   Gait and balance
   Knee flexion—hop or shallow knee bend
4. **Sensory function**
   Superficial pain and light touch—arms and legs
   Vibration—arms and legs
5. **Reflexes**
   Biceps
   Triceps
   Patellar
   Achilles

Neurologic Complete Examination

1. **Mental status**
2. **Cranial nerves II through XII**
3. **Motor system**
   Muscle size, strength, tone
   Gait and balance
   Rapid alternating movements
4. **Sensory function**
   Superficial pain and light touch
   Vibration
   Position sense
   Stereognosis, graphesthesia, two-point discrimination
5. **Reflexes**
   DTRs: biceps, triceps, brachioradialis, patellar, Achilles
   Superficial: abdominal, plantar

24

Male Genitourinary System

evolve WEBSITE

http://evolve.elsevier.com/Jarvis/

- Animations
- Audio Key Points
- Bedside Assessment Summary Checklist
- Health Promotion Guide
  Sexually Transmitted Infections (STIs)
  Testicular Cancer
- NCLEX Review Questions
- Physical Examination Summary Checklist
- Quick Assessment for Common Conditions
  Renal Calculus (Urolithiasis)
  Urinary Tract Infection
- Video—Assessment
  Male Genitalia and Rectum

OUTLINE

Structure and Function, 679

The Male Genitalia

Subjective Data, 684

Health History Questions

Objective Data, 688

Preparation
The Penis
The Scrotum
Hernia
The Inguinal Lymph Nodes
Self-Care—Testicular Self-Examination (TSE)
Assessing Urinary Function

Documentation and Critical Thinking, 698

Abnormal Findings, 699

Abnormal Findings for Advanced Practice, 701

STRUCTURE AND FUNCTION

THE MALE GENITALIA

The male genital structures include the penis and scrotum externally and the testis, epididymis, and vas deferens internally. Glandular structures accessory to the genital organs (the prostate, seminal vesicles, and bulbourethral glands) are discussed in Chapter 25.

Penis

The **penis** is composed of three cylindric columns of erectile tissue: the two corpora cavernosa on the dorsal side and the corpus spongiosum ventrally (Fig. 24-1). At the distal end of the shaft, the corpus spongiosum expands into a cone of erectile tissue, the **glans.** The shoulder where the glans joins the shaft is the **corona.** The **urethra** is a conduit for both the genital and the urinary systems. It transverses the corpus spongiosum, and its meatus forms a slit at the glans tip. Over the glans, the skin folds in and back on itself forming a hood or flap. This is the **foreskin** or **prepuce.** Often, it is surgically removed shortly after birth by circumcision. The **frenulum** is a fold of the foreskin extending from the urethral meatus ventrally.

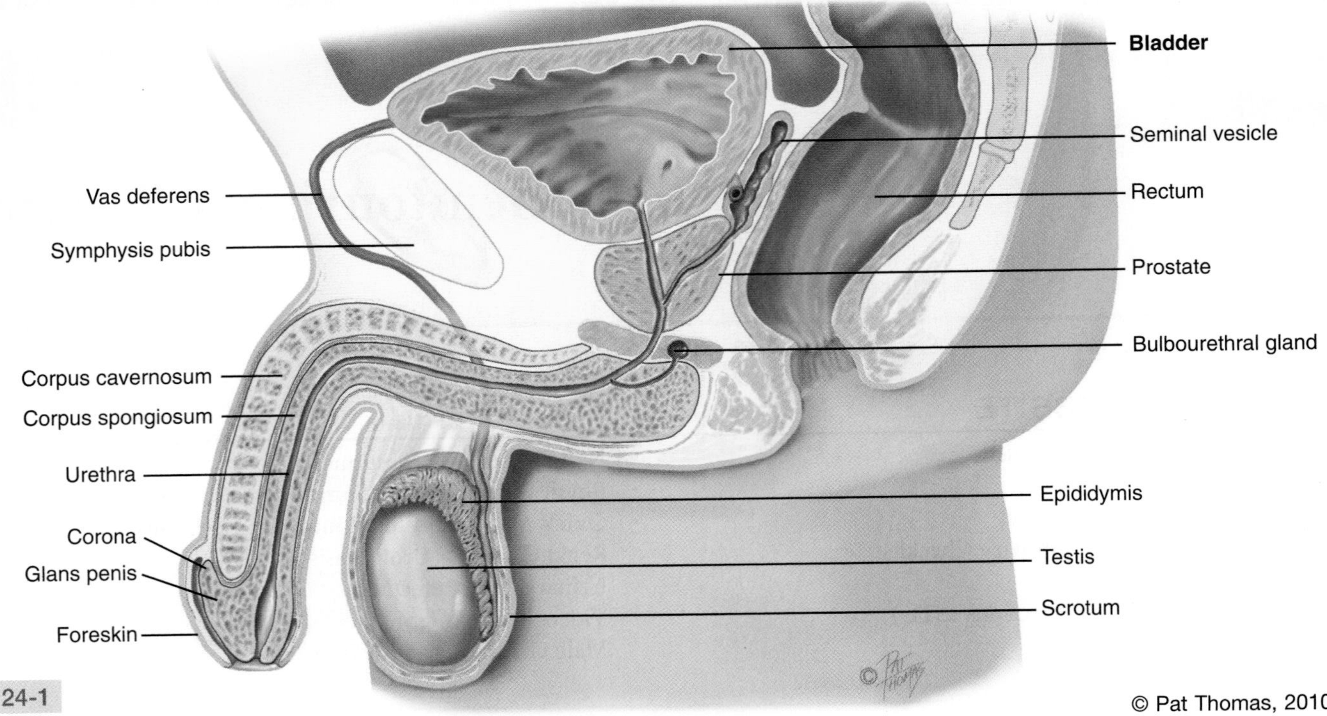

24-1

Scrotum

The **scrotum** is a loose protective sac, which is a continuation of the abdominal wall. After adolescence, the scrotal skin is deeply pigmented and has large sebaceous follicles. The scrotal wall consists of thin skin lying in folds, or **rugae,** and the underlying cremaster muscle. The **cremaster muscle** controls the size of the scrotum by responding to ambient temperature. This is to keep the testes at 3° C below abdominal temperature, the best temperature for producing sperm. When it is cold, the muscle contracts, raising the sac and bringing the testes closer to the body to absorb heat necessary for sperm viability. As a result, the scrotal skin looks corrugated. When it is warmer, the muscle relaxes, the scrotum lowers, and the skin looks smoother.

Inside, a septum separates the sac into two halves. In each scrotal half is a **testis,** which produces sperm. The testis has a solid oval shape, which is compressed laterally and measures 4 to 5 cm long by 3 cm wide in the adult. The testis is suspended vertically by the spermatic cord (Fig. 24-2). The

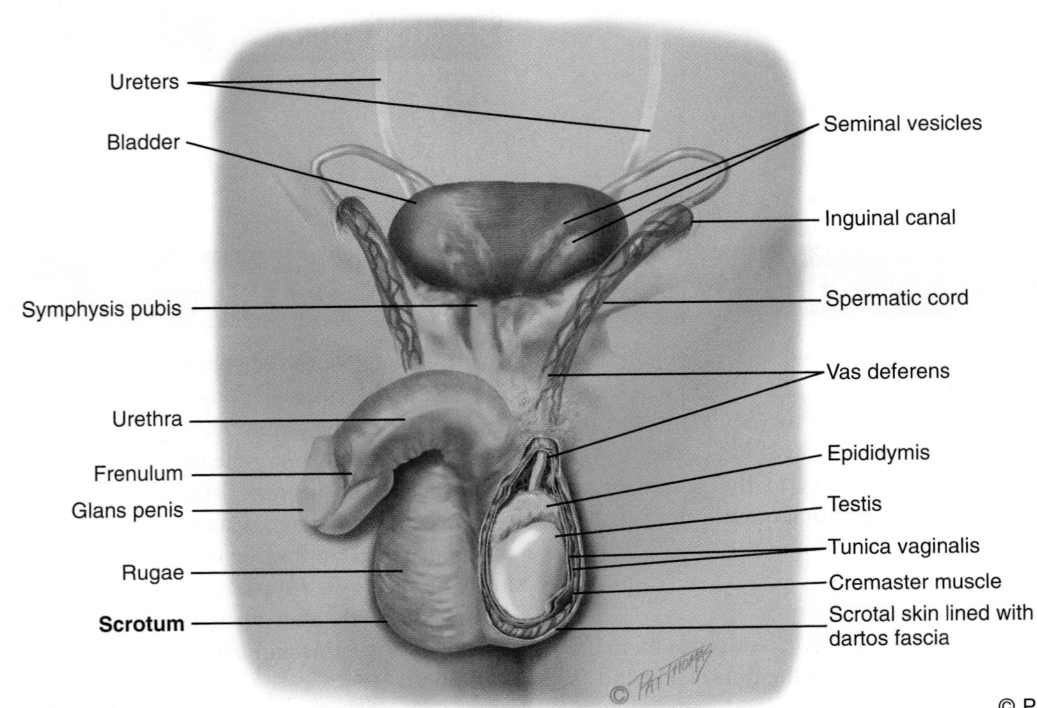

24-2 Male genital structures.

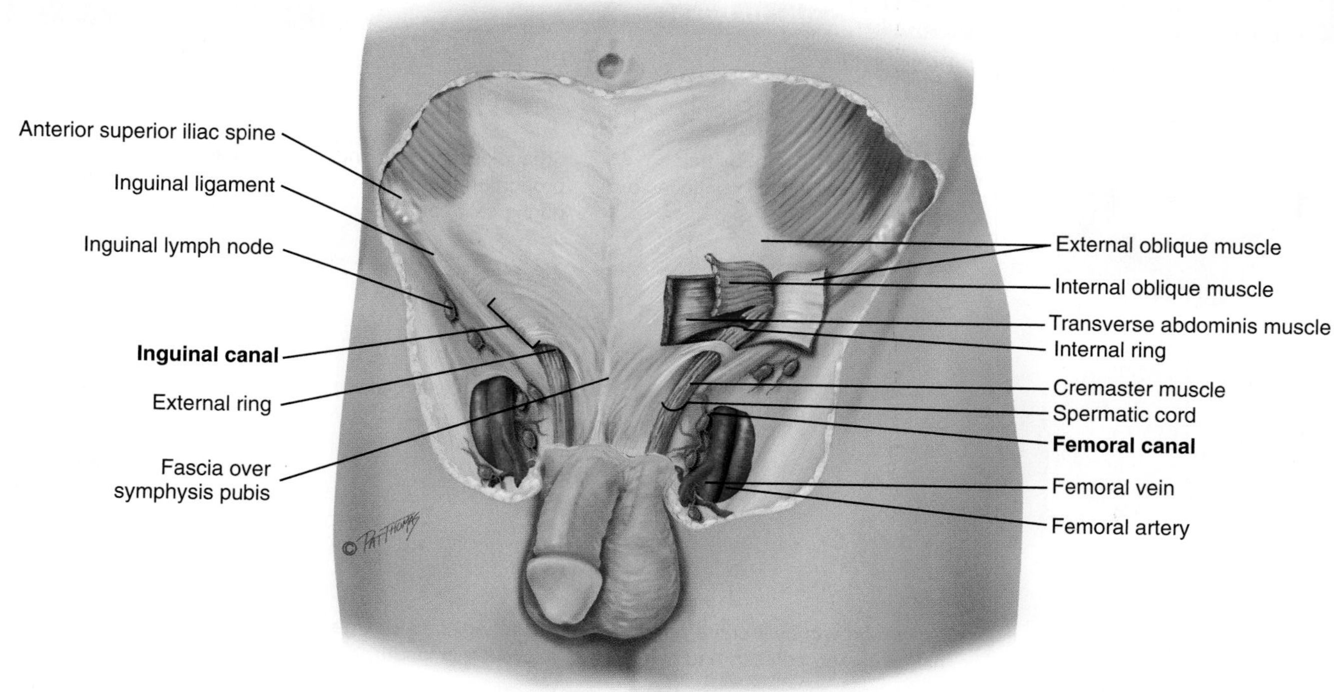

24-3

left testis is lower than the right because the left spermatic cord is longer. Each testis is covered by a double-layered membrane, the tunica vaginalis, which separates it from the scrotal wall. The two layers are lubricated by fluid so that the testis can slide a little within the scrotum; this helps prevent injury.

Sperm are transported along a series of ducts. First, the testis is capped by the **epididymis,** which is a markedly coiled duct system and the main storage site of sperm. It is a comma-shaped structure, curved over the top and the posterior surface of the testis. Occasionally (in 6% to 7% of males), the epididymis is anterior to the testis.

The lower part of the epididymis is continuous with a muscular duct, the **vas deferens.** This duct approximates with other vessels (arteries and veins, lymphatics, nerves) to form the **spermatic cord.** The spermatic cord ascends along the posterior border of the testis and runs through the tunnel of the inguinal canal into the abdomen. Here, the vas deferens continues back and down behind the bladder, where it joins the duct of the seminal vesicle to form the **ejaculatory duct.** This duct empties into the urethra.

The **lymphatics** of the penis and scrotal surface drain into the inguinal lymph nodes, whereas those of the testes drain into the abdomen. Abdominal lymph nodes are not accessible to clinical examination.

Inguinal Area

The **inguinal area,** or groin, is the juncture of the lower abdominal wall and the thigh (Fig. 24-3). Its diagonal borders are the anterior superior iliac spine and the symphysis pubis. Between these landmarks lies the **inguinal ligament** (Poupart ligament). Superior to the ligament lies the **inguinal canal,** a narrow tunnel passing obliquely between layers of abdominal muscle. It is 4 to 6 cm long in the adult. Its openings are an internal ring, located 1 to 2 cm above the midpoint of the inguinal ligament, and an external ring, located just above and lateral to the pubis.

Inferior to the inguinal ligament is the **femoral canal.** It is a potential space located 3 cm medial to and parallel with the femoral artery. You can use the artery as a landmark to find this space.

Knowledge of these anatomic areas in the groin is useful because they are potential sites for a hernia, which is a loop of bowel protruding through a weak spot in the musculature.

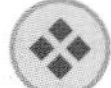

DEVELOPMENTAL COMPETENCE

Infants

Prenatally, the testes develop in the abdominal cavity near the kidneys. During the later months of gestation, the testes migrate, pushing the abdominal wall in front of them and dragging the vas deferens, the blood vessels, and nerves behind. The testes descend along the inguinal canal into the scrotum before birth. At birth, each testis measures 1.5 to 2 cm long and 1 cm wide. Only a slight increase in size occurs during the prepubertal years.

Adolescents

Puberty begins sometime between the ages of 9½ and 13½ years. The first sign is enlargement of the testes. Next, pubic hair appears, and then penis size increases. The stages of

TABLE 24-1 Sexual Maturity Ratings (SMR) in Boys

Developmental Stage	Pubic Hair	Penis	Scrotum
1	No pubic hair; fine body hair on abdomen (vellus hair) continues over pubic area	Preadolescent, size and proportion the same as during childhood	Preadolescent, size and proportion the same as during childhood
2	Few straight, slightly darker hairs at base of penis; hair is long and downy	Little or no enlargement	Testes and scrotum begin to enlarge; scrotal skin reddens and changes in texture
3	Sparse growth over entire pubis; hair is darker, coarser, and curly	Penis begins to enlarge, especially in length	Further enlarged
4	Thick growth over pubic area but not on thighs; hair coarse and curly as in adult	Penis grows in length and diameter, with development of glans	Testes almost fully grown; scrotum darker
5	Growth spread over medial thighs, although not yet up toward umbilicus; after puberty, pubic hair growth continues until the mid-20s, extending up the abdomen toward the umbilicus	Adult size and shape	Adult size and shape

Adapted from Tanner, J.M. (1962). *Growth at adolescence,* Oxford, England: Blackwell Scientific Publications.

development are documented in Tanner's sexual maturity ratings (SMR) (Table 24-1).

The complete change in development from a preadolescent to an adult takes around 3 years, although the normal range is 2 to 5 years (Fig. 24-4). The chart shown in Figure 24-4 is useful in teaching a boy the expected sequence of events and in reassuring him about the wide range of normal ages when these events are experienced.

Data from the NHANES III showed that U.S. boys now have earlier genital maturation and pubic hair growth than traditional Tanner staging.[13] The median age of attaining stage 2 for pubic hair development was 12 years. African-American boys showed pubic hair growth about 9 months earlier than white boys and over 1 year earlier than Mexican-American boys. Toward the end of puberty, or Tanner stage 5, African-American boys were 1 year younger than white or

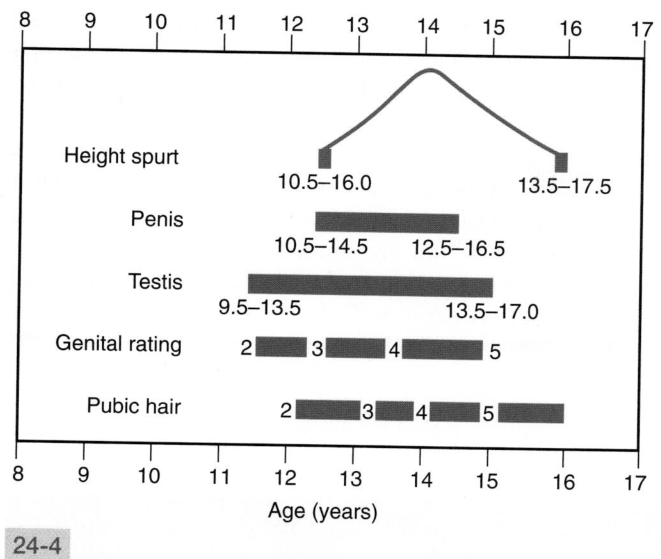

24-4

Mexican-American boys in completing genital development. Although these racial/ethnic differences could not be explained, the study suggested racial differences in the interactions between insulin, glucose, and androgens and racial/ethnic differences in diet, lifestyle, and exposure to environmental factors.

Adults and Aging Adults

The male does not experience a definite end to fertility as the female does. Around age 40 years, the production of sperm begins to decrease, although it continues into the 80s and 90s. After age 55 to 60 years, testosterone production declines very gradually so that resulting physical changes are not evident until later in life.

In the aging male, the amount of pubic hair decreases and the remaining hair turns gray. Penis size decreases. Due to decreased tone of the dartos muscle, the scrotal contents hang lower, the rugae decrease, and the scrotum looks pendulous. The testes decrease in size and are less firm to palpation. Increased connective tissue is present in the tubules, so these become thickened and produce less sperm.

In general, declining testosterone production leaves the older male with a slower and less intense sexual response, and an erection takes longer to develop and is less full or firm. Ejaculation is shorter and less forceful, and the volume of seminal fluid is less than when the man was younger. After ejaculation, rapid detumescence (return to the flaccid state) occurs, especially after 60 years of age. This occurs in a few seconds as compared with minutes or hours in the younger male. The refractory state (when the male is physiologically unable to ejaculate) lasts longer, from 12 to 24 hours as compared with 2 minutes in the younger male.

Sexual Expression in Later Life. Chronologic age by itself should not mean a halt in sexual activity. The just-mentioned physical changes need not interfere with the libido and pleasure from sexual intercourse. The older male is capable of sexual function as long as he is in reasonably good health and has an interested, willing partner. Even chronic illness does not mean a complete end to sexual desire or activity.

The danger is in the male misinterpreting normal age changes as a sexual failure. Once this idea occurs, it may demoralize the man and place undue emphasis on performance rather than on pleasure. In the absence of disease, a withdrawal from sexual activity may be due to loss of spouse; depression; preoccupation with work; marital or family conflict; side effects of medications such as antihypertensives, psychotropics, antidepressants, antispasmodics, sedatives, tranquilizers or narcotics, and estrogens; heavy use of alcohol; lack of privacy (living with adult children or in a nursing home); economic or emotional stress; poor nutrition; or fatigue.

CULTURE AND GENETICS

Circumcision. During pregnancy or the immediate neonatal period, parents will ask you about whether to circumcise the male infant. There are religious and cultural indications for circumcision; other indications include preventing phimosis and inflammation of the glans penis and foreskin, decreasing the incidence of cancer of the penis, and decreasing the incidence of urinary tract infections in infancy.

Circumcision reduces HIV acquisition in men by 53% to 60%, as shown in three randomized trials and numerous observational studies in sub-Saharan Africa,[10,24] and it reduces HIV transmission to uninfected women sexual partners.[27] Further, circumcision significantly reduced the incidence of herpes simplex virus type 2 (HSV-2) and the prevalence of human papillomavirus (HPV).[22] Certain types of HPV cause cervical cancer. The mechanism may be that the presence of the foreskin increases susceptibility to small abrasions, allowing more contact time between pathogens and the mucosa of the partner.[9] The risk for other STIs (*Trichomonas vaginalis*, bacterial vaginosis) is reduced in women with circumcised partners as well.[21]

In the United States, the public health implications of these findings are being debated. Routine neonatal circumcision rates have dropped from a high of 80% after World War II to about 65% of newborns in 1999, in part because the American Academy of Pediatrics does not endorse the procedure. Because of this, Medicaid does not cover routine neonatal circumcision costs in 16 states. This is disadvantageous especially to African-American and Hispanic male infants who are overrepresented in poorer groups whose only medical coverage is Medicaid.

Circumcision carries a very small but possible risk for complications. Most are minor and treatable: pain, bleeding, swelling, or inadequate skin removal. Serious complications are rare and include excess bleeding, wound infection, and urinary retention.[28] Neonates certainly are capable of perceiving pain; therefore parents need to be apprised of pain-relief measures for the circumcision procedure. These include dorsal penile nerve block and a lidocaine-prilocaine cream (EMLA).[29]

Kidney Disease. Chronic kidney disease (CKD) is determined by blood tests, urinalysis, and imaging studies that show decreased kidney function or kidney damage lasting 3 months or longer. This can lead progressively and irreversibly to end-stage renal disease (ESRD), when the person survives only by kidney transplant or dialysis. CKD is a global health problem. It has two main causes, hypertension and diabetes, which comprise 70% or more of patients who progress to ESRD and are having dialysis.

In the United States, the majority of patients with CKD are white; however, racial and ethnic groups are disproportionately affected. When compared with whites, the per million prevalence rates are 47% higher for Hispanics, 230% higher for American Indian/Alaskan Natives, and 420% higher for African Americans.[23] Reasons for these astounding differences are being actively researched. One factor may be long-term underutilization of antihypertensive medications, the renin-angiotensin-aldosterone system (RAAS) inhibitors, by African Americans.[19] Socioeconomic factors also limit access to health care for lower income groups. In the United States, 22% of whites are uninsured or receiving public-funded health care, compared with 55% of Hispanics and 45% of African Americans.[26]

SUBJECTIVE DATA

1. Frequency, urgency, and nocturia
2. Dysuria
3. Hesitancy and straining
4. Urine color
5. Past genitourinary history
6. Penis—pain, lesion, discharge
7. Scrotum, self-care behaviors, lump
8. Sexual activity and contraceptive use
9. Sexually transmitted infection (STI) contact

Examiner Asks	Rationale
1. **Frequency, urgency, and nocturia.** Urinating more often than usual?	**Frequency.** Average adult voids 5-6 ×/day, varying with fluid intake, individual habits. Polyuria—excessive quantity. Oliguria—diminished quantity, <400 mL/24 hours.
• Feel as if you cannot wait to urinate? • Awaken during the night because you need to urinate? How often? Is this a recent change?	**Urgency.** **Nocturia** occurs together with frequency and urgency in urinary tract disorders. Other origins: cardiovascular, habitual, diuretic medication.
2. **Dysuria.** Any pain or burning with urinating?	**Dysuria.** Burning is common with acute cystitis, prostatitis, urethritis.
3. **Hesitancy and straining.** Any trouble starting the urine stream? • Need to strain to start or maintain stream? • Any change in force of stream: narrowing, becoming weaker? • Dribbling, such that you must stand closer to the toilet? • Afterward, do you still feel you need to urinate? • Ever had any urinary tract infections?	**Hesitancy.** Straining. Loss of force and decreased caliber. Terminal dribbling. Sense of residual urine. Recurrent episodes of acute cystitis. These symptoms suggest progressive prostatic obstruction.
4. **Urine color.** Is the usual **urine** clear or discolored, cloudy, foul-smelling, bloody (Fig. 24-5)?	Cloudy in urinary tract infection. Hematuria—a danger sign that warrants further workup.

Examiner Asks | **Rationale**

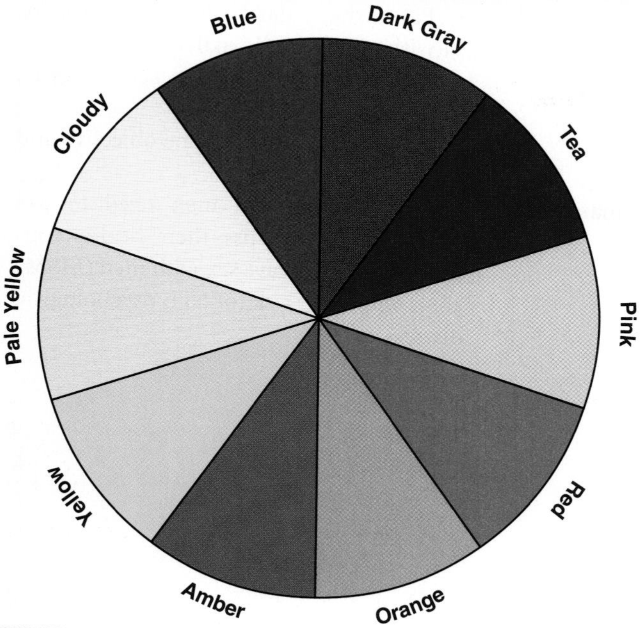

24-5

Some color changes are temporary or harmless. However, for blood in urine or for a color change lasting longer than a day, the person should seek health care. For a complete description, see Table 24-2, Urine Color and Discolorations, p. 699.

5. **Past genitourinary history.** Any difficulty controlling your urine?
   - Accidentally urinate when you sneeze, laugh, cough, or bear down?
   - Any **history** of kidney disease, kidney stones, flank pain, urinary tract infections, prostate trouble?

Urge incontinence—involuntary urine loss from overactive detrusor muscle in bladder. It contracts, causing urgent need to void.

Stress incontinence—involuntary urine loss with physical strain, sneezing, or coughing due to weakness of pelvis floor.

6. **Penis.** Any problem with penis—**pain, lesions?**
   - Any **discharge?** How much? Has that increased or decreased since start?
   - The color? Any odor? Discharge associated with pain or with urination?

Urethral discharge occurs with infection (see Table 24-3, Urinary Problems, p. 700).

7. **Scrotum, self-care behaviors.** Any problem with the scrotum or testicles?
   - Any **lump** or **swelling** on testes?
   - Any change in size of the scrotum? Any history of undescended testicle as infant?
   - Noted any bulge or swelling in the scrotum? For how long? Ever been told you have a hernia? Any dragging, heavy feeling in scrotum?

Concern about any self-discovered mass (spermatocele, hydrocele, varicocele, rarely testicular cancer) alerts you to careful exploration during examination.

Possible hernia.

8. **Sexual activity and contraceptive use.** Are you in a relationship involving sexual intercourse now?
   - Are aspects of sex satisfactory to you and your partner?
   - Are you satisfied with the way you and your partner communicate about sex?
   - Occasionally a man notices a change in ability to have an erection when aroused. Have you noticed any changes?*

Questions about **sexual activity** should be routine in review of body systems for these reasons:

- Communicates that you accept individual's sexual activity and believe it is important.
- Your comfort with discussion prompts person's interest and possibly relief that topic has been introduced.

*At times, phrase your questions so that all is right for the person to acknowledge a problem.

Subjective Data

Examiner Asks	Rationale
• Do you and your partner use a contraceptive? Which method? Is this satisfactory? Any questions about this method?	• Establishes a database for comparisons with any future sexual activities.
• How many sexual partners have you had in the past 6 months?	• Provides opportunity to screen sexual problems. Your questions should be objective and matter-of-fact.
• What is your sexual preference—relationship with a woman, a man, both?	Gay and bisexual men need to feel acceptance to discuss their health concerns. Men who have sex with men (MSM) are at increased risk for STI; psychological distress.
9. STI contact. Any sexual contact with a partner having an STI, such as gonorrhea, herpes, AIDS, chlamydia, venereal warts, syphilis? • When was this contact? Did you get the disease? • How was it treated? Any complications? • Do you use condoms to help prevent STIs? • Any questions or concerns about any of these diseases?	
Additional History for Infants and Children	
1. Does your child have any problem urinating? Urine stream look straight? • Any pain with urinating, crying, or holding the genitals? • Any urinary tract infection?	
2. (If child older than 2 to 2½ years.) Has toilet training started? How is it progressing? • (If child 5 years or older.) Wet the bed at night? Is this a problem for child or for you (parents)? What have you done? How does the child feel about it?	**Nocturnal enuresis**—involuntarily passing urine at night after age 5 to 6 years.
3. Any problem with child's penis or scrotum: sores, swelling, discoloration? • Told if his testes are descended or undescended? • Ever had a hernia or hydrocele? • Swelling in his scrotum during crying or coughing?	
4. (Ask directly to preschooler or young school-age child.) Has anyone ever touched your penis or in between your legs and you did not want them to? Sometimes that happens to children and it's not okay. They should remember that they have not been bad. They should try to tell a big person about it. Can you tell me three different big people you trust who you could talk to?	Screen for sexual abuse. For prevention, teach the child that it is not okay for someone to look at or touch his private parts while telling him it is a secret. Naming three trusted adults will include someone outside the family—important, since most molestation is by a parent.
Additional History for Preadolescents and Adolescents	
Use the following questions regarding sexual growth and development and sexual behavior. First: • Ask questions that seem appropriate for boy's age but be aware that norms vary widely. When you are in doubt, it is better to ask too many questions than to omit something. Children obtain information, often misinformation, from the media, Internet, and peers at surprisingly early ages. You may be sure your information will be more thoughtful and accurate.	

Examiner Asks	Rationale
• Ask direct, matter-of-fact questions. Avoid sounding judgmental. • Start with a *permission statement.* "Often boys your age experience...." This conveys that it is normal and all right to think or feel a certain way. • Try the *ubiquity approach.* "When did you ...?" rather than "Do you ...?" This method is less threatening because it implies that the topic is normal and unexceptional. • Do not be concerned if a boy will not discuss sexuality with you or respond to offers for information. He may not wish to let on that he needs or wants more information. You do well to "open the door." The adolescent may come back at a future time.	
1. Around age 12 to 13 years, but sometimes earlier, boys start to change and grow around the penis and scrotum. What changes have you noticed? Have you ever seen charts and pictures of normal growth patterns for boys? Let us go over these now. Who can you talk to about your body changes and about sex information? How do these talks go? Do you think you get enough information? What about sex education classes at school? How about your parents? Is there a favorite teacher, nurse, doctor, minister, or counselor to whom you can talk?	
2. Boys around age 12 to 13 years (SMR3) have a normal experience of fluid coming out of the penis at night, called nocturnal emissions, or "wet dreams." Have you had this?	An occasional boy confuses this with a sign of STI or feels guilty.
3. Teenage boys have other normal experiences and wonder if they are the only ones who ever had them, like having an erection at embarrassing times, having sexual fantasies, or masturbating. Also, a boy might have a thought about touching another boy's genitals and wonder if this means he might be homosexual. Would you like to talk about any of these things?	A boy may feel guilty about experiencing these things if not informed that they are normal.
4. Often boys your age have questions about sexual activity. What questions do you have? How about things like birth control or STIs such as gonorrhea or herpes? Any questions about these? • Are you dating? Someone steady? Have you had intercourse? Are you using birth control? What kind? • What kind of birth control did you use the *last* time you had intercourse?	Assess level of knowledge. Many boys will not admit they need more knowledge. Avoid the term "having sex." It is ambiguous, and teens can take it to mean anything from foreplay to intercourse. Use behavior-specific words. This particular question often reveals that the teen is not using any method of birth control.
5. Has a nurse or doctor ever taught you how to examine your own testicles to make sure they are healthy?	Assess knowledge of testicular self-examination.
6. Has anyone ever touched your genitals and you did not want them to? Another boy, or an adult, even a relative? Sometimes that happens to teenagers. They should remember it is not their fault. They should tell another adult about it.	
Additional History for the Aging Adult	
1. Any difficulty urinating? Any hesitancy and straining? A weakened force of stream? Any dribbling? Or any incomplete emptying?	Early symptoms of enlarging prostate may be tolerated or ignored. Later symptoms are more dramatic: hematuria, urinary tract infection.

Subjective Data

Examiner Asks	Rationale
2. Do you ever leak water/urine when you don't want to? Do you use pads/tissue to catch urine in your underwear?	Incontinence is any involuntary leaking of urine.
3. Do you need to get up at night to urinate? What medications are you taking? What fluids do you drink in the evening?	Nocturia may be due to diuretic medication, habit, or fluid ingestion 3 hours before bedtime; especially coffee and alcohol have a diuretic effect. Also, fluid retention from mild heart failure or varicose veins produces nocturia because recumbency at night mobilizes fluid.
4. Is it all right to ask you about your sexual function? This is something I ask all the men. For example, it is normal for an erection to develop slowly at this age. This is not a sign of impotence, but a man might wonder if it is. • Any change in your ability to have an erection? • Wanting to have an erection is normal, and it is treatable with medication.	Excluding physical illness, an older man is fully capable of sexual function. But some assume normal changes mean that they are "old men" and withdraw from sexual activity. The older person is not reluctant to discuss sexual activity, and most welcome the opportunity. Depressants to sexual desire and function include antihypertensives, sedatives, tranquilizers, estrogens, and alcohol. Alcohol decreases the sexual response even more dramatically in the older person.

OBJECTIVE DATA

PREPARATION

Position the male standing with undershorts down and appropriate draping. The examiner should be sitting. Alternatively, the male may be supine for the first part of the examination and stand to check for a hernia.

It is normal for a male to feel apprehensive about having his genitalia examined, especially by a female examiner. Younger adolescents usually have more anxiety than older adolescents. But any male may have difficulty dissociating a necessary, matter-of-fact step in the physical examination from the feeling this is an invasion of his privacy. His concerns are similar to those experienced by the female during the examination of the genitalia: modesty, fear of pain, cold hands, negative judgment, or memory of previously uncomfortable examinations. In addition, he may fear comparison with others or fear having an erection during the examination and that this would be misinterpreted by the examiner.

This normal apprehension becomes manifested in different behaviors. Many act resigned and embarrassed and avoid eye contact. An occasional man will laugh and make jokes to cover embarrassment. Also, a man may refuse examination by a female and insist on a male examiner.

Take time to consider these feelings, as well as to explore your own. It is normal for you to feel embarrassed and apprehensive too. You may worry about your age, lack of clinical experience, causing pain, or even that your movements might "cause" an erection. Some examiners feel guilty when this occurs. You need to accept these feelings and work through them so that you can examine the male in a professional way. Discuss these concerns with an experienced examiner. Your demeanor is important. Your unresolved discomfort magnifies any discomfort the man may have.

EQUIPMENT NEEDED

Gloves: wear gloves during every male genitalia examination
Occasionally: glass slide for urethral specimen
Materials for cytology
Flashlight

Your demeanor should be *confident* and relaxed, unhurried yet businesslike. Do not discuss genitourinary history or sexual practices while you are performing the examination. This may be perceived as judgmental. Use a firm, deliberate touch, not a soft, stroking one. If an erection does occur, do *not* stop the examination or leave the room. This only focuses more attention on the erection and increases embarrassment. Reassure the male that this is only a normal physiologic response to touch, just as when the pupil constricts in response to bright light. Proceed with the rest of the examination.

Normal Range of Findings	Abnormal Findings
INSPECT AND PALPATE THE PENIS	
The skin normally looks wrinkled, hairless, and without lesions. The dorsal vein may be apparent (Fig. 24-6).	Inflammation. Lesions: nodules, solitary ulcer (chancre), grouped vesicles or superficial ulcers, wartlike papules (see Table 24-4, Male Genital Lesions, pp. 701-702).

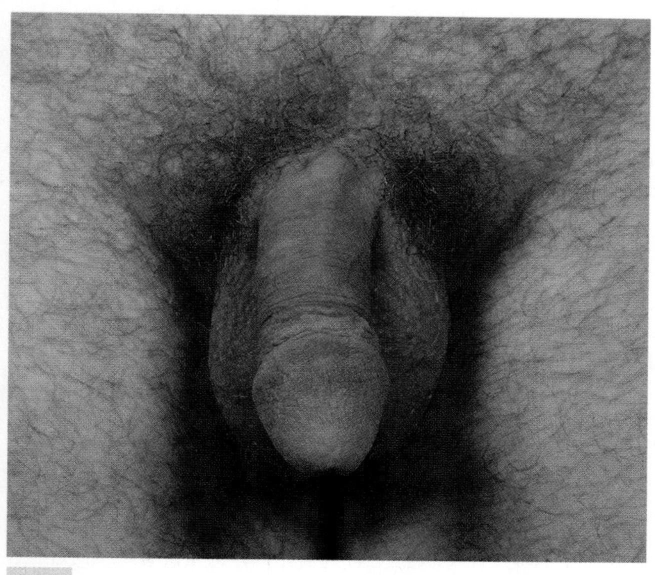

24-6

Normal Range of Findings	Abnormal Findings
The glans looks smooth and without lesions. Ask the uncircumcised male to retract the foreskin, or you retract it. It should move easily. Some cheesy smegma may have collected under the foreskin. After inspection, slide the foreskin back to the original position.	Inflammation. Lesions on glans or corona. **Phimosis**—narrowed opening of prepuce so cannot retract the foreskin. **Paraphimosis**—painful constriction of glans by retracted foreskin.
The urethral meatus is positioned just about centrally.	**Hypospadias**—ventral location of meatus. **Epispadias**—dorsal location of meatus (see Table 24-5, Abnormalities of the Penis, pp. 702-703).
At the base of the penis, pubic hair distribution is consistent with age. Hair is without pest inhabitants.	Pubic lice or nits can be seen with the unaided eye. Excoriated skin usually accompanies.

Objective Data

Normal Range of Findings

Compress the glans anteroposteriorly between your thumb and forefinger (Fig. 24-7). The meatus edge should appear pink, smooth, and without discharge.

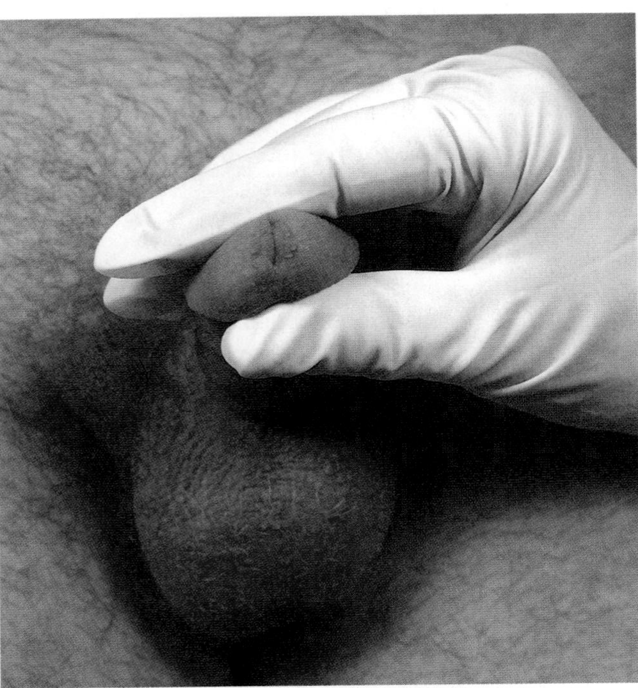

24-7

If you note urethral discharge, collect a smear for microscopic examination and a culture. If no discharge shows but the person gives a history of it, ask him to milk the shaft of the penis. This should produce a drop of discharge.

Palpate the shaft of the penis between your thumb and first two fingers. Normally, the penis feels smooth, semifirm, and nontender.

INSPECT AND PALPATE THE SCROTUM

Inspect the scrotum as the male holds the penis out of the way. Alternatively, you hold the penis out of the way with the back of your hand (Fig. 24-8). Scrotal size varies with ambient room temperature. Asymmetry is normal, with the left scrotal half usually lower than the right.

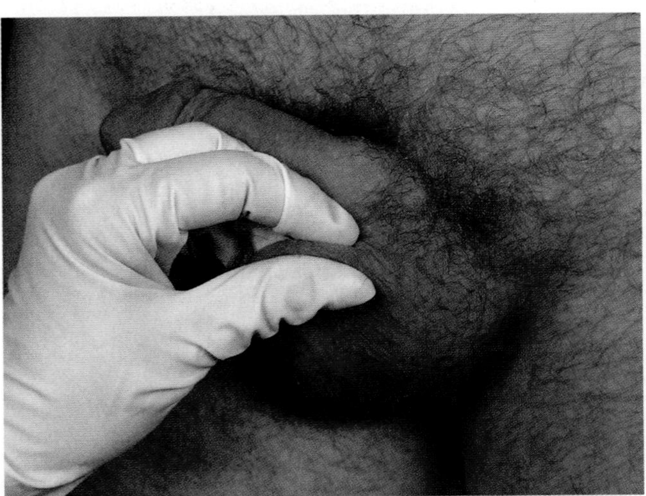

24-8

Abnormal Findings

Stricture—narrowed opening.

Edges that are red, everted, edematous, along with purulent discharge, suggest urethritis (see Table 24-3, p. 700).

Nodule or induration.

Tenderness.

Scrotal swelling (edema) may be taut and pitting. This occurs with heart failure, renal failure, or local inflammation.

Lesions.

Normal Range of Findings

Spread rugae out between your fingers. Lift the sac to inspect the posterior surface. Normally, no scrotal lesions are present, except for the commonly found sebaceous cysts. These are yellowish, 1-cm nodules and are firm, nontender, and often multiple.

Palpate gently each scrotal half between your thumb and first two fingers (Fig. 24-9). The scrotal contents should slide easily. Testes normally feel oval, firm and rubbery, smooth, and equal bilaterally and are freely movable and slightly tender to moderate pressure. Each epididymis normally feels discrete, softer than the testis, smooth, and nontender.

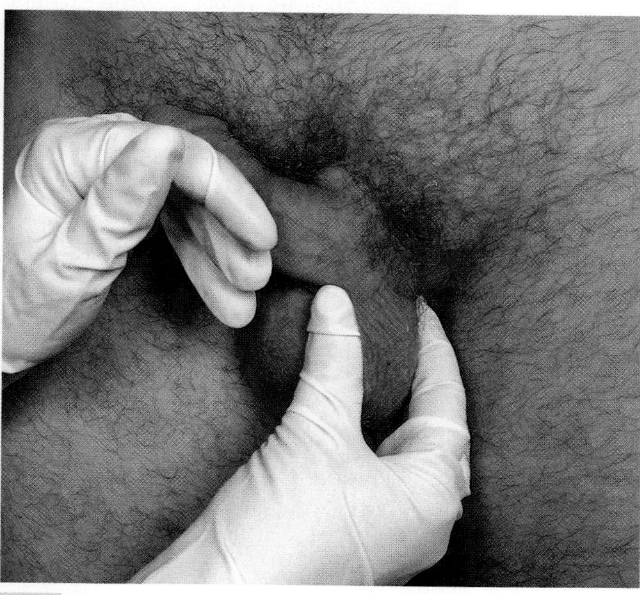

24-9

Palpate each spermatic cord between your thumb and forefinger, along its length from the epididymis up to the external inguinal ring (Fig. 24-10, *A*). You should feel a smooth, nontender cord.

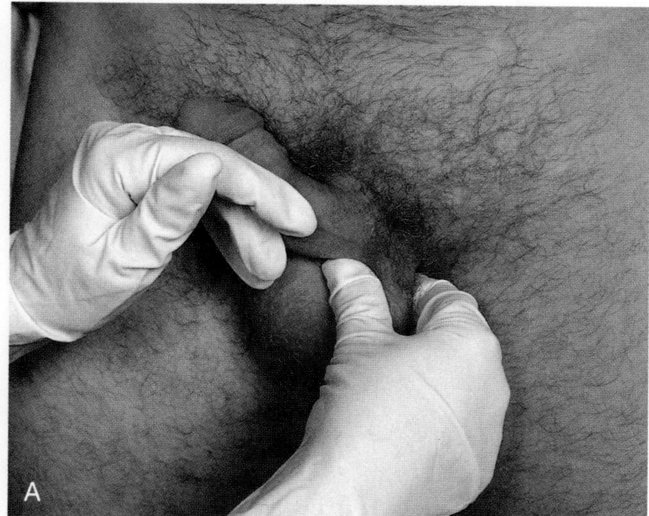

24-10, A

Normally, no other scrotal contents are present. If you do find a mass, note:

- Any tenderness?
- Is the mass distal or proximal to testis?
- Can you place your fingers over it?
- Does it reduce when the person lies down?
- Can you auscultate bowel sounds over it?

Abnormal Findings

Inflammation.

Absent testis—may be a temporary migration or true cryptorchidism (see Table 24-6, Abnormalities in the Scrotum, pp. 704-706).

Atrophied testes—small and soft.

Fixed testes.

Nodules on testes or epididymides.

Marked tenderness.

An indurated, swollen, and tender epididymis indicates epididymitis.

Thickened cord.

Soft, swollen, and tortuous cord—see the discussion of varicocele (Fig. 24-10, *B*).

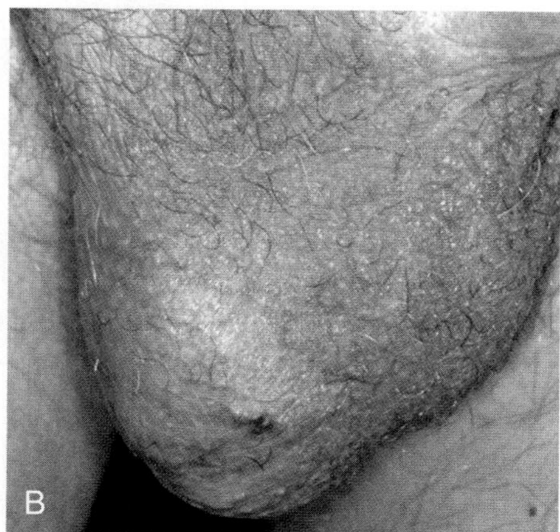

24-10, B Varicocele.

Abnormalities in the scrotum: hernia, tumor, orchitis, epididymitis, hydrocele, spermatocele, varicocele (see Table 24-6).

Objective Data

Normal Range of Findings

Transillumination. Perform this maneuver only if you note a swelling or mass. Darken the room. Shine a strong flashlight from behind the scrotal contents. Normal scrotal contents do not transilluminate.

INSPECT AND PALPATE FOR HERNIA

Inspect the inguinal region for a bulge as the person stands and as he strains down. Normally, none is present.

Palpate the inguinal canal (Fig. 24-11). For the right side, ask the male to shift his weight onto the left (unexamined) leg. Place your right index finger low on the right scrotal half. Palpate up the length of the spermatic cord, invaginating the scrotal skin as you go, to the external inguinal ring. It feels like a triangular slitlike opening, and it may or may not admit your finger. If it will admit your finger, gently insert it into the canal and ask the person to "bear down."* Normally, you feel no change. Repeat the procedure on the left side.

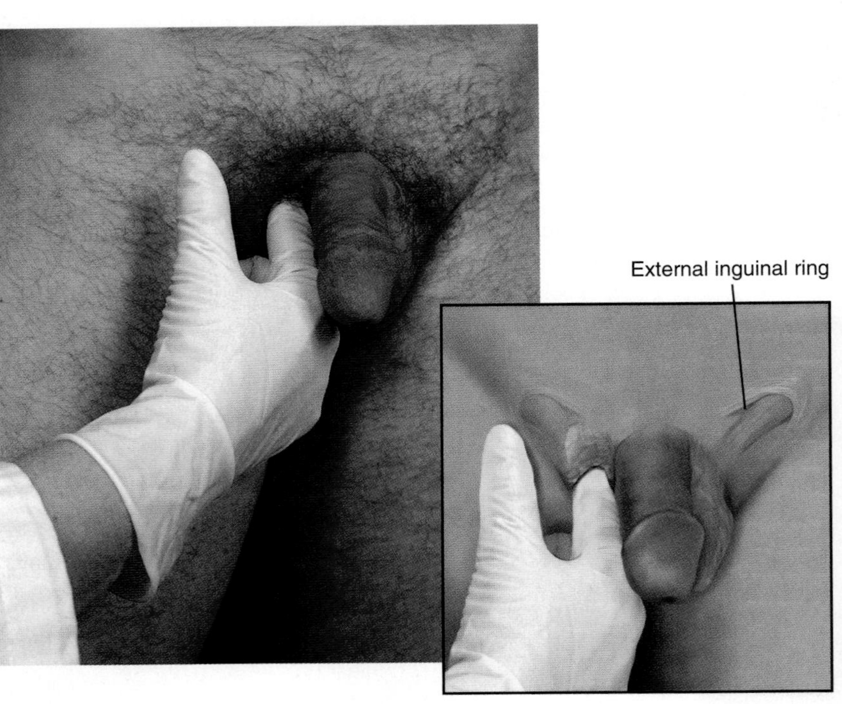

24-11

Palpate the femoral area for a bulge. Normally, you feel none.

*Avoid the old direction, "turn your head and cough." For one thing, a brief cough does not give the steady, increased intra-abdominal pressure you need. For another, the person is likely to cough right in your face.

Abnormal Findings

Serous fluid does transilluminate and shows as a red glow (e.g., hydrocele or spermatocele). Solid tissue and blood do not transilluminate (e.g., hernia, epididymitis, or tumor) (see Table 24-6).

Bulge at external inguinal ring or at femoral canal. (A hernia may be present but easily reduced and may appear only intermittently with an increase in intra-abdominal pressure.)

Palpable herniating mass bumps your fingertip or pushes against the side of your finger (see Table 24-7, Inguinal and Femoral Hernias, p. 707).

Normal Range of Findings

Abnormal Findings

PALPATE INGUINAL LYMPH NODES

Palpate the horizontal chain along the groin inferior to the inguinal ligament and the vertical chain along the upper inner thigh.

It is normal to palpate an isolated node on occasion; it then feels small (<1 cm), soft, discrete, and movable (Fig. 24-12).

Enlarged, hard, matted, fixed nodes.

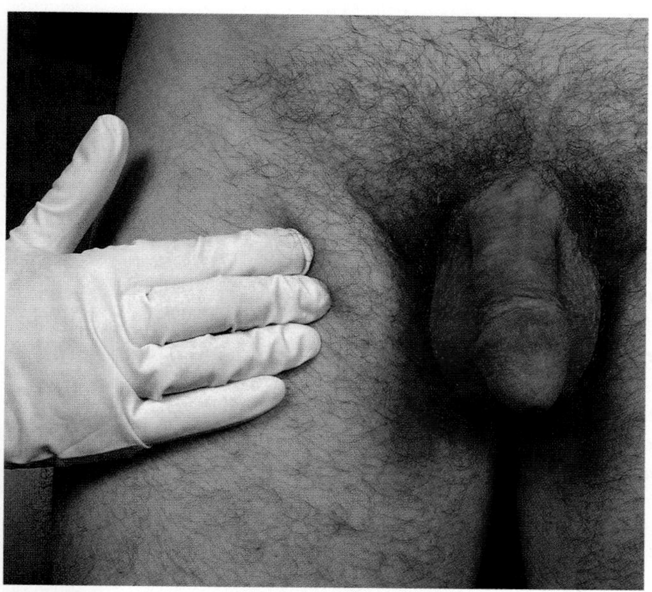

24-12

SELF-CARE—TESTICULAR SELF-EXAMINATION (TSE)

Encourage self-care by teaching every male (from 13 to 14 years old through adulthood) how to examine his own testicles. The overall incidence of testicular cancer is rare, accounting for about 8000 new cases annually. It is rare before age 15 years, peaks during ages 20 to 39 years, and then declines[20] and is associated with a history of cryptorchidism.

Some groups consider teaching TSE controversial because the harms of causing anxiety and unwarranted medical costs[15] exceed the benefits of selective detection of a relatively rare lesion. However, testicular cancer has no early symptoms. When detected early and treated before metastasis, the cure rate is almost 100%. Therefore include the teaching but adjust your message to emphasize familiarity with the young man's own body, rather than only cancer detection, as the goal.

Early detection is enhanced if the male is familiar with his normal consistency. Points to include during health teaching are:

- **T** = timing, once a month
- **S** = shower, warm water relaxes scrotal sac
- **E** = examine, check for changes, report changes immediately

Normal Range of Findings | **Abnormal Findings**

Phrase your teaching something like this (Fig. 24-13):

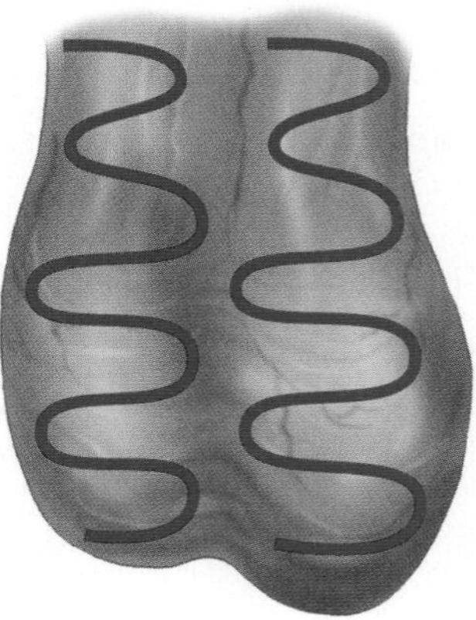

24-13

A good time to examine the testicles is during the shower or bath, when your hands are warm and soapy and the scrotum is warm. Cold hands stimulate a muscle (cremasteric) reflex, retracting the scrotal contents. The procedure is simple. Hold the scrotum in the palm of your hand and gently feel each testicle using your thumb and first two fingers. If it hurts, you are using too much pressure. The testicle is egg-shaped and movable. It feels rubbery with a smooth surface, like a peeled hard-boiled egg. The epididymis is on top and behind the testicle; it feels a bit softer. Abnormal lumps are very rare and usually not worrisome. But, if you ever notice a firm, painless lump, a hard area, or an overall enlarged testicle, call your physician for a further check.

ASSESS URINARY FUNCTION

A urinalysis shows a color of pale yellow to amber due to the presence of urochrome pigments. Normal urine is clear and slightly acidic with a pH range of 4.5 to 8.0. Specific gravity measures the concentration of urine, from very dilute at 1.003 to concentrated at 1.030. There is little or no protein, no glucose, and fewer than 5 red blood cells (RBCs) or white blood cells (WBCs) per high-powered field.

Cloudiness suggests presence of WBCs, bacteria, casts. Certain drugs or foods can change urine color (see Table 24-2). Proteinuria indicates glomerular disease in the nephron. Glycosuria suggests hyperglycemia occurring with diabetes. Increased WBCs occur with urinary tract infection (UTI); increased RBCs occur with UTI, glomerulonephritis, renal calculi, trauma, and cancer.

Serum analysis of kidney function is measured with creatinine, an end-product of muscle metabolism. Normal levels range from 0.7 to 1.5 mg/dL and are fairly constant from day to day. Blood urea nitrogen (BUN) measures urea, an end-product of protein metabolism. It measures 10 to 20 mg/dL and rises with a decrease in fluid volume or an increase in protein intake.

Creatinine measures glomerular filtration rate (GFR). When the GFR decreases by half, the serum creatinine level doubles,[6a] indicating decreased kidney function. The BUN rises with decreased kidney function but is less specific.

Normal Range of Findings	Abnormal Findings

DEVELOPMENTAL COMPETENCE

Infants and Children

For an infant or toddler, perform this procedure right after the abdominal examination. In a preschool-age to young school-age child (3 to 8 years of age), leave underpants on until just before the examination. In an older school-age child or adolescent, offer an extra drape, as with the adult. Reassure child and parents of normal findings.

Inspect the penis and scrotum. Penis size is usually small in infants (2 to 3 cm) (Fig. 24-14) and in young boys until puberty. In the obese boy, the penis looks even smaller because of folds of skin covering the base.

Rarely, a very small penis may be an enlarged clitoris in a genetically female infant.

Redness, swelling, lesions.

Discharge.

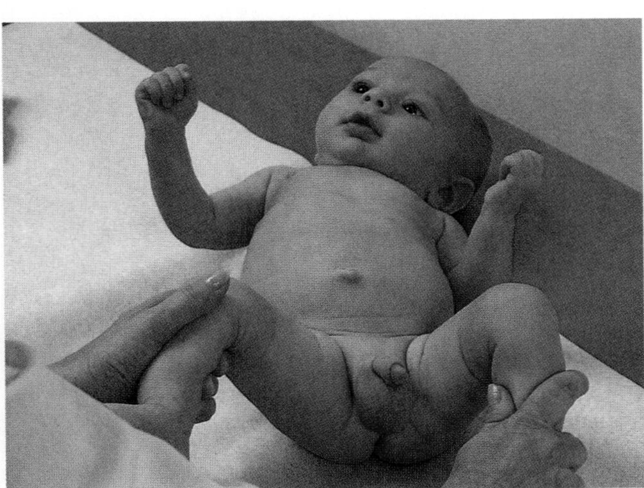

24-14

In the circumcised infant, the glans looks smooth with the meatus centered at the tip. While the child wears diapers, the meatus may become ulcerated from ammonia irritation. This is more common in circumcised infants.

Hypospadias, epispadias (see Table 24-5). Stricture—narrowed opening.

Occasionally, ulceration may produce a stricture, shown by a pinpoint meatus and a narrow stream. This increases the risk for urine obstruction.

If possible, observe the newborn's first voiding to assess strength and direction of stream.

Poor stream is significant, because it may indicate a stricture or neurogenic bladder.

If uncircumcised, the foreskin is normally tight during the first 3 months and should **not** be retracted because of the risk for tearing the membrane attaching the foreskin to the shaft. This leads to scarring and, possibly, to adhesions later in life. In infants older than 3 months, retract the foreskin gently to check the glans and meatus. It should return to its original position easily.

Phimosis—unable to retract the foreskin.

Paraphimosis—the foreskin cannot be slipped forward once it is retracted.

Dirt and smegma collecting under foreskin.

The scrotum looks pink in white infants and dark brown in dark-skinned infants. Rugae are well formed in the full-term infant. Size varies with ambient temperature, but overall, the infant's scrotum looks large in relation to the penis. No bulges, either constant or intermittent, are present.

Normal Range of Findings

Palpate the scrotum and testes. The cremasteric reflex is strong in the infant, pulling the testes up into the inguinal canal and abdomen from exposure to cold, touch, exercise, or emotion. Take care not to elicit the reflex: (1) keep your hands warm and palpate from the external inguinal ring down, and (2) block the inguinal canals with the thumb and forefinger of your other hand to prevent the testes from retracting (Fig. 24-15).

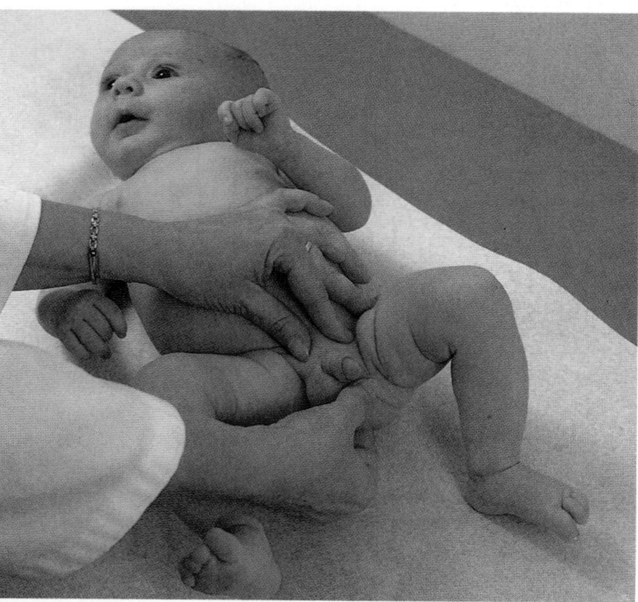

24-15

Normally, the testes are descended and are equal in size bilaterally (1.5 to 2 cm until puberty). It is important to document that you have palpated the testes. Once palpated, they are considered descended, even if they have retracted momentarily at the next visit.

If the scrotal halves feel empty, search for the testes along the inguinal canal and try to milk them down. Ask the toddler or child to squat with the knees flexed up; this pressure may force the testes down. Or, have the young child sit cross-legged to relax the reflex (Fig. 24-16).

Migratory testes (physiologic cryptorchidism) are common because of the strength of the cremasteric reflex and the small mass of the prepubertal testes. Note that the affected side has a normally developed scrotum (with true cryptorchidism, the scrotum is atrophic) and that the testis can be milked down. These testes descend at puberty and are normal.

Palpate the epididymis and spermatic cord as described in the adult section. A common scrotal finding in the boy younger than 2 years is a **hydrocele,** or fluid in the scrotum. It appears as a large scrotum and transilluminates as a faint pink glow. It usually disappears spontaneously.

Abnormal Findings

Cryptorchidism: undescended testes (those that have never descended). Undescended testes are common in premature infants. They occur in 3% to 4% of term infants, although most have descended by 3 months of age. Age at which child should be referred differs among physicians (see Table 24-6).

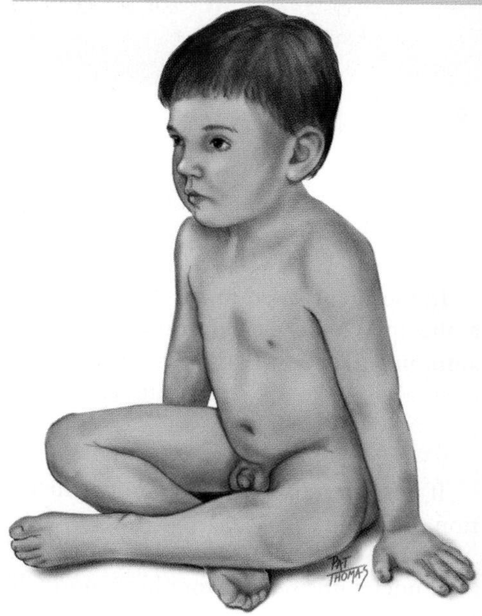

24-16

A hydrocele is a cystic collection of serous fluid in the tunica vaginalis, surrounding the testis. (See Table 24-6.)

Normal Range of Findings	Abnormal Findings

Inspect the inguinal area for a bulge. If you do not see a bulge but the parent gives a positive history of one, try to elicit it by increasing intra-abdominal pressure. Ask the boy to hold his breath and strain down, or have him blow up a balloon.

If a hernia is suspected, palpate the inguinal area. Use your little finger to reach the external inguinal ring.

The Adolescent

The adolescent shows a wide variation in normal development of the genitals. Using the SMR charts, note: (1) enlargement of the testes and scrotum; (2) pubic hair growth; (3) darkening of scrotal color; (4) roughening of scrotal skin; (5) increase in penis length and width; and (6) axillary hair growth.

Be familiar with the normal sequence of growth.

The Aging Adult

In the older male, you may note thinner, graying pubic hair and the decreased size of the penis. The size of the testes may be decreased and may feel less firm. The scrotal sac is pendulous with less rugae. The scrotal skin may become excoriated if the man continually sits on it.

PROMOTING A HEALTHY LIFESTYLE: SCREENING FOR PROSTATE CANCER

Understanding Prostate Changes

The discussion of prostate health and the examination of the prostate gland are unique aspects of male health assessment. Men should be offered the opportunity to discuss changes in their urinary elimination patterns and sexual activity, including ejaculation. These discussions often provide a glimpse of the early signs and symptoms of prostatic changes that may indicate a need for further studies and workup.

The prostate gland goes through two main periods of growth. The first occurs early in puberty, and the second begins after age 25. Although the prostate continues to grow during most of a man's life, the enlargement rarely causes symptoms before age 40. However, more than half of men in their 60s and as many as 90% of men in their 70s will have some symptoms. The gradual enlargement is considered to be a normal part of aging and is often referred to as *benign prostatic hyperplasia (BPH)*. By itself, BPH does not raise an individual's risk for prostate cancer; however, the symptoms of BPH and prostate cancer can be very similar, including hesitant, interrupted, or weak urinary stream; urinary urgency; leaking or dribbling; and increased frequency of urination, especially at night.

Men at increased risk for developing prostate cancer should be offered testing at an earlier age. Two groups that are increased risk for prostate cancer are African-American men and men whose first-degree relatives have had prostate cancer. In African-American men, prostate cancer tends to start younger and grow faster than in men of other racial/ethnicity groups. Men who have a first-degree relative (father, brother, or son) have a 2 to 3 times higher risk for prostate cancer than those without a family history of the disease. The risk for men who have three or more family members with prostate cancer is about 10 times the risk for men without a family history. Also important is the age at diagnosis, because the younger a man's relatives were at diagnosis, the greater his risk is for developing it. So careful history taking is very important. To stay up to date with the latest information about prostate cancer, health care providers and patients should visit the National Cancer Institute (NCI) website.

Prostate cancer is typically detected by testing the blood for *prostate-specific antigen* (PSA) and/or on *digital rectal examination* (DRE). It is recommended that for men without other known risks, a DRE should be offered to men yearly, beginning at age 40, and the PSA yearly, beginning at age 50.

PSA is a substance made by the normal prostate gland. When prostate cancer develops, the PSA level increases. However, benign or non-cancerous enlargement of the prostate (BPH), age, and prostatitis also can cause the PSA to increase. Ejaculation causes a temporary increase in PSA levels, and men need to be instructed to abstain from ejaculation for 2 days before having their PSA level tested. In addition, there are some medications that falsely lower PSA levels, such as finasteride (Proscar) and dutasteride (Avodart). If the PSA is elevated, further laboratory studies and/or a transrectal ultrasound (TRUS) and biopsy may be recommended. A fact sheet about the PSA is available from the National Cancer Institute (NCI).

DRE involves a gloved, lubricated finger being inserted into the rectum. The prostate gland is located just in front of the rectum, making it possible to palpate the surface of the gland manually for bumps or hard areas that may be a developing cancer. Although it is less effective than the PSA blood test in finding prostate cancer, it can sometimes find cancers in men who have normal PSA levels. For this reason, both PSA and DRE are recommended to be done together when screening for prostate cancer.

Resources

National Cancer Institute (NCI). Website: www.cancer.gov/cancertopics/types/prostate.

The Prostate-Specific Antigen (PSA) Test: Questions & Answers. Website: www.cancer.gov/cancertopics/factsheet/Detection/PSA.

Objective Data

DOCUMENTATION AND CRITICAL THINKING

Sample Charting

SUBJECTIVE

Urinates four or five times/day, clear, straw-colored. No nocturia, dysuria, or hesitancy. No pain, lesions, or discharge from penis. Does not do testicular self-examination. No history of genitourinary disease. Sexually active in a monogamous relationship. Sexual life satisfactory to self and partner. Uses birth control via barrier method (partner uses diaphragm). No known STI contact.

OBJECTIVE

No lesions, inflammation, or discharge from penis. Scrotum—testes descended, symmetric, no masses. No inguinal hernia.

ASSESSMENT

Genital structures normal

Focused Assessment: Clinical Case Study

R.C. is a 19-year-old student who 2 days PTA noted acute onset of painful urination, frequency, and urgency. Noted some thick penile discharge.

SUBJECTIVE

States has no side pain, no abdominal pain, no fever, and no genital skin rash. R.C. is concerned he has an STI because of episode of unprotected intercourse with a new partner 6 days PTA. Has no known allergies.

OBJECTIVE

Vital signs 37° C-72-16. No lesions or inflammation around penis or scrotum. Urethral meatus has mild edema with purulent urethral discharge. No pain on palpation of genitalia. Testes symmetric with no masses. No lymphadenopathy.

ASSESSMENT

Urethral discharge
Deficient knowledge about STI prevention R/T lack of information recall

ABNORMAL FINDINGS

TABLE 24-2 Urine Color and Discolorations

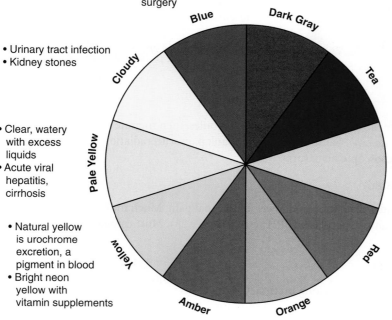

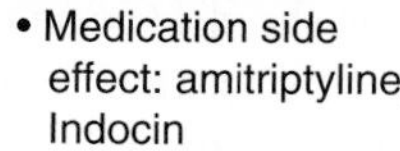

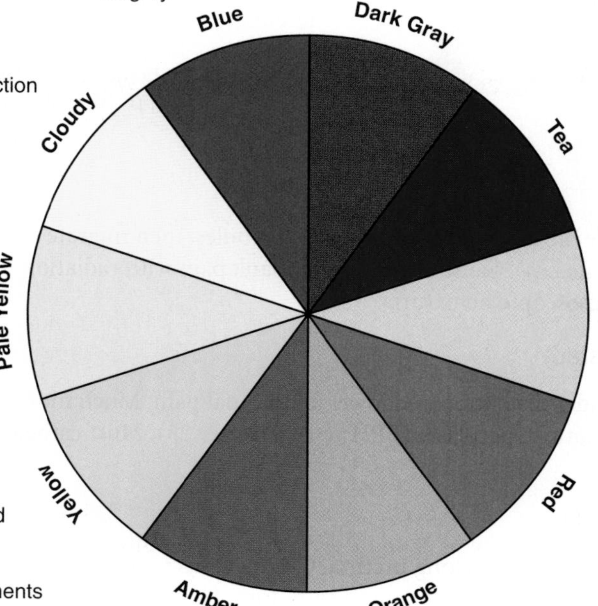

Blue
• Medication side effect: amitriptyline, Indocin
• Foods: asparagus
• Dye after prostate surgery
Dark Gray
• Urine contains melanin, melanuria
Tea
• Liver disease, especially with pale stools, jaundice
• Myoglobinuria
• Some medications or food dyes
• Blood in urine
Pink
• With menses
• Some foods: beets, berries, food dyes
• Some laxatives
• Kidney stones
• Urinary tract infection
Red
• Blood in urine
• Nephritis, cystitis
• Cancer
• Following prostate surgery
Orange
• Medication side effect: rifampin for meningitis, Pyridium, warfarin (Coumadin)
• Some foods, food dyes, laxatives
• Dehydration
• Jaundice (bilirubinemia)
Amber
• Gold or concentrated with dehydration
• Some laxatives
• Food or supplements with B-complex vitamins
Yellow
• Natural yellow is urochrome excretion, a pigment in blood
• Bright neon yellow with vitamin supplements
Pale Yellow
• Clear, watery with excess liquids
• Acute viral hepatitis, cirrhosis
Cloudy
• Urinary tract infection
• Kidney stones

TABLE 24-3 Urinary Problems

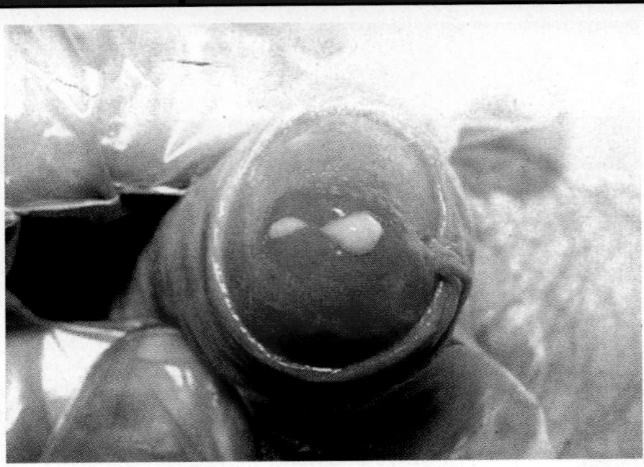

Urethritis (Urethral Discharge and Dysuria)

Infection of urethra causes painful burning urination or pruritus. Meatus edges are reddened, everted, and swollen with purulent discharge. Urine is cloudy with discharge and mucus shreds. Cause determined by culture: (1) gonococcal urethritis has thick, profuse, yellow or gray-brown discharge; (2) nonspecific urethritis (NSU) may have similar discharge but often has scanty, mucoid discharge. Of these, about 50% are caused by chlamydia infection. This is important to differentiate because antibiotic treatment is different.

Reprinted from Edmond, R. (1995). *Colour atlas of infectious diseases* (3rd ed., p. 161). St. Louis: Mosby.

Renal Calculi (not illustrated)

Renal stones (crystals of calcium oxalate or uric acid) form in kidney tubules; then migrate and become urgent when pass into ureter, become lodged, and obstruct urine flow. Cause abrupt severe flank pain with radiation to the groin or abdomen, nausea and vomiting, restlessness, gross or microscopic hematuria.

Acute Urinary Retention (not illustrated)

Abrupt inability to pass urine with bladder distention and lower abdominal pain. Much more common in men due to bladder outlet obstruction, such as benign prostatic hyperplasia (BPH) (see Chapter 25). Must catheterize to relieve acute discomfort; then manage underlying problem.

Urethral Stricture (not illustrated)

Pinpoint, constricted opening at meatus or inside along urethra. Occurs congenitally or secondary to urethral injury. Gradual decrease in force and caliber of urine stream is most common symptom. Shaft feels indurated along ventral aspect at the site of the stricture.

ABNORMAL FINDINGS FOR ADVANCED PRACTICE

TABLE 24-4 Male Genital Lesions

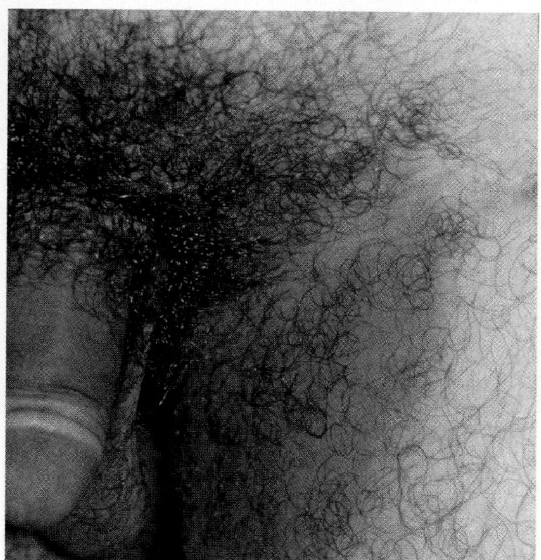

Tinea Cruris

A fungal infection in the crural fold, not extending to scrotum, occurring in postpubertal males ("jock itch") after sweating or wearing layers of occlusive clothing. It forms a red-brown half-moon shape with well-defined borders.

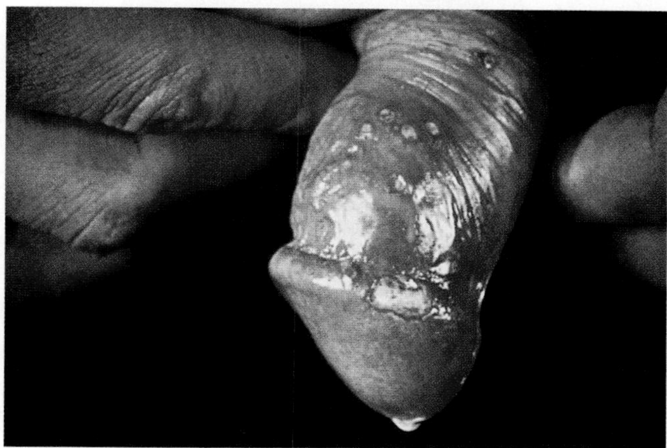

Genital Herpes—HSV-2 Infection

Clusters of small vesicles with surrounding erythema, which are often painful, erupt on the glans or foreskin. These rupture to form superficial ulcers. A sexually transmitted infection (STI), the initial infection lasts 7 to 10 days. The virus remains dormant indefinitely; recurrent infections last 3 to 10 days with milder symptoms.

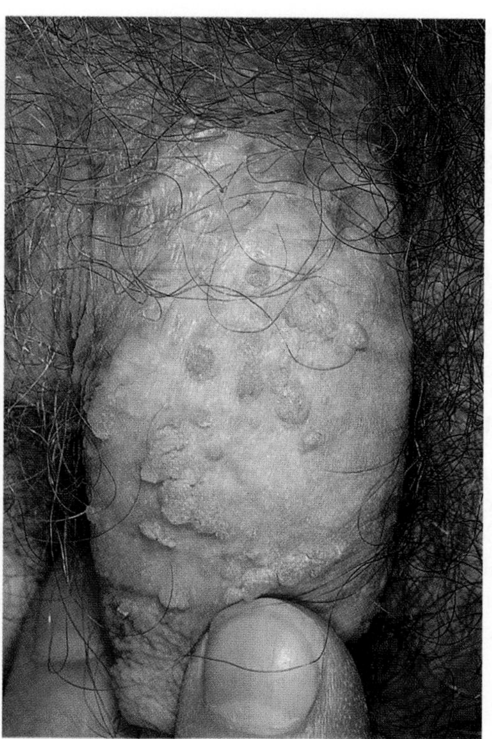

◀ Genital Warts

Soft, pointed, moist, fleshy, painless papules may be single or multiple in a cauliflower-like patch. Color may be gray, pale yellow, or pink in white males, and black or translucent gray-black in Black males. They occur on shaft of penis, behind corona, or around the anus where they may grow into large, grapelike clusters.

These are caused by the human papillomavirus (HPV) and are one of the most common STIs. The HPV infection is correlated with early onset of sexual activity, infrequent use of contraception, and multiple sexual partners.

Continued

TABLE 24-4 Male Genital Lesions—cont'd

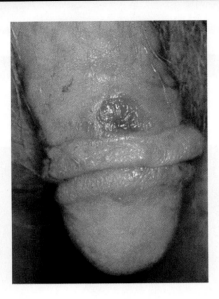

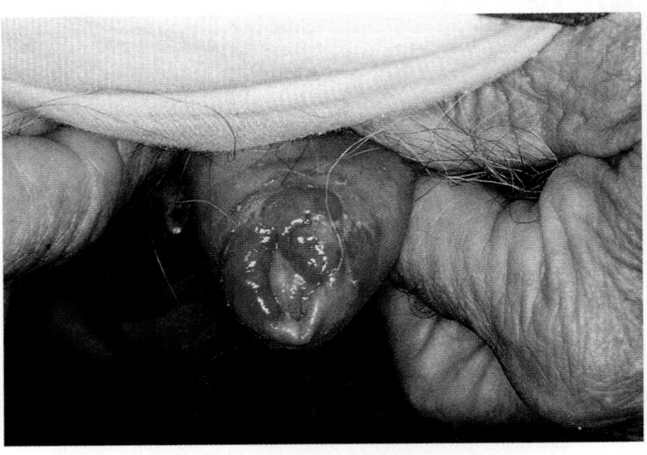

Syphilitic Chancre

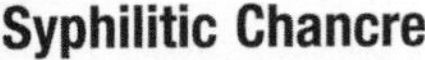

Begins within 2 to 4 weeks of infection, as a small, solitary, silvery papule that erodes to a red, round or oval, superficial ulcer with a yellowish serous discharge. Palpation reveals a nontender indurated base that can be lifted like a button between the thumb and the finger. Lymph nodes enlarge early but are nontender. This is an STI easily treated with penicillin G, but untreated leads to cardiac and neurologic problems, blindness. Almost eradicated in the United States in 1957; epidemics recur cyclically every 7 to 10 years.[17]

Reprinted from Edmond, R. (1995). *Colour atlas of infectious diseases* (3rd ed., p. 173). St. Louis: Mosby.

Carcinoma

Begins as red, raised, warty growth or as an ulcer, with watery discharge. As it grows, may necrose and slough. Usually painless. Almost always on glans or inner lip of foreskin and following chronic inflammation. Enlarged lymph nodes are common.

TABLE 24-5 Abnormalities of the Penis

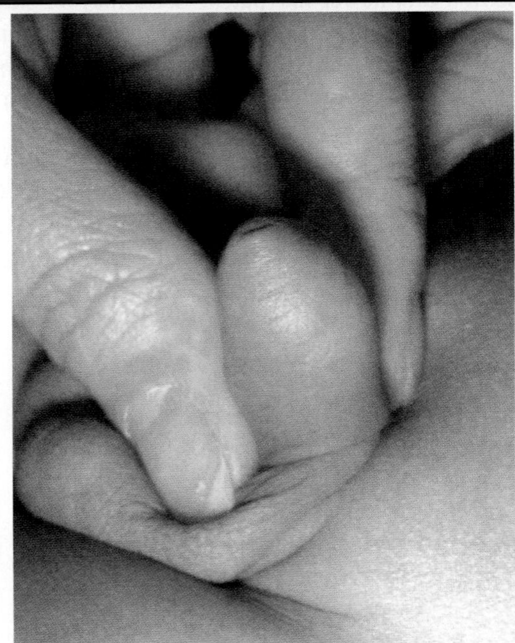

◀ Phimosis

Nonretractable foreskin forming a pointy tip with a tiny orifice. Foreskin is advanced and so tight it is impossible to retract over glans. May be congenital or acquired from adhesions secondary to infection. Poor hygiene leads to retained dirt and smegma, which increases risk for inflammation, calculus formation, obstructive uropathy.

Paraphimosis (not illustrated)

Foreskin is retracted and fixed. Once retracted behind glans, a tight or inflamed foreskin cannot return to its original position. Constriction impedes circulation, so glans swells. A medical emergency; the constricting band prevents venous and lymphatic return from the glans and compromises arterial circulation.

TABLE 24-5 Abnormalities of the Penis—cont'd

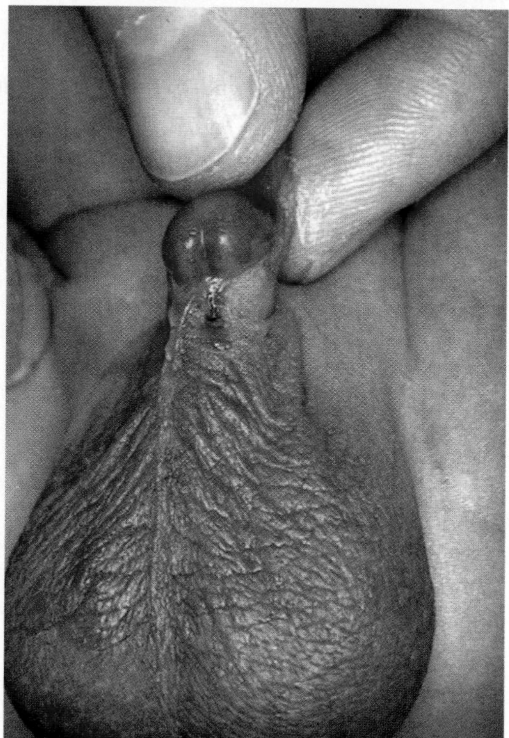

Hypospadias

Urethral meatus opens on the ventral (under) side of glans, shaft, or at the penoscrotal junction. A groove extends from the meatus to the normal location at the tip. This is a congenital defect that is important to recognize at birth. The newborn should not be circumcised because surgical correction may use foreskin tissue to extend urethral length.

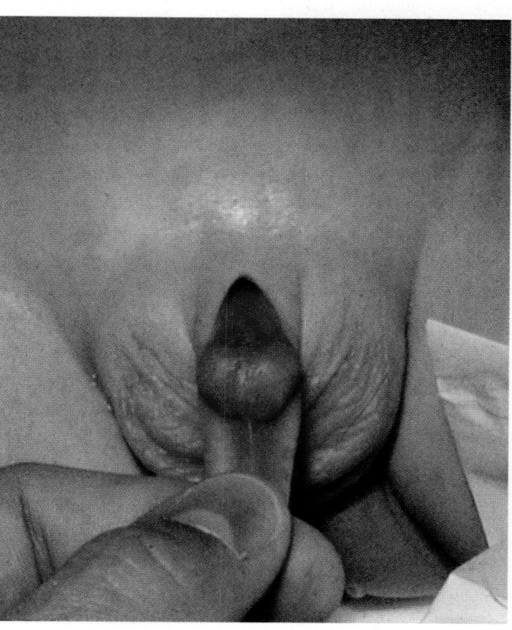

Epispadias

Meatus opens on the dorsal (upper) side of glans or shaft above a broad, spadelike penis. Rare; less common than hypospadias but more disabling because of associated urinary incontinence and separation of pubic bones.

Priapism (not illustrated)

Prolonged painful erection of penis without sexual stimulation and unrelieved by intercourse or masturbation, most common in men in 30s and 40s. A rare condition but when lasting 4 hours or longer can cause ischemia of penis, fibrosis of tissue, erectile dysfunction. Can occur as a side effect of some medications and street drugs and with sickle-cell trait or disease; leukemia in which increased numbers of white blood cells produce engorgement; malignancy; or local trauma or spinal cord injuries with autonomic nervous system dysfunction.

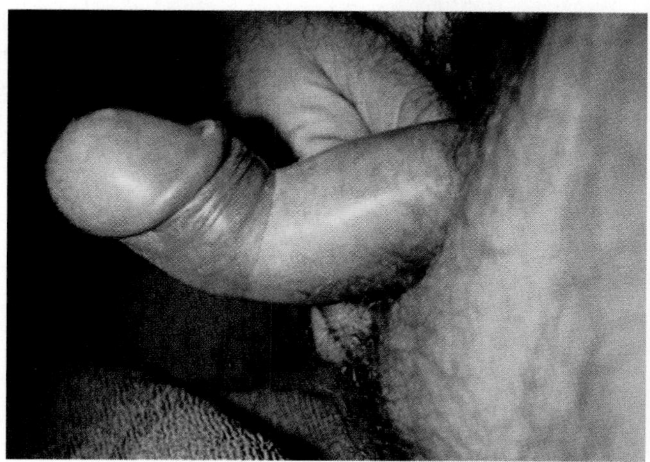

Peyronie Disease

Hard, nontender, subcutaneous plaques palpated on dorsal or lateral surface of penis. May be single or multiple and asymmetric. They are associated with painful bending of the penis during erection. Plaques are fibrosis of covering of corpora cavernosa. Usually occurs after 45 years. Its cause is trauma to the erect penis (e.g., unexpected change in angle during intercourse). More common in men with diabetes, gout, and Dupuytren contracture of the palm.

TABLE 24-6 **Abnormalities in the Scrotum**

Disorder	Clinical Findings	Discussion
Absent Testis, Cryptorchidism 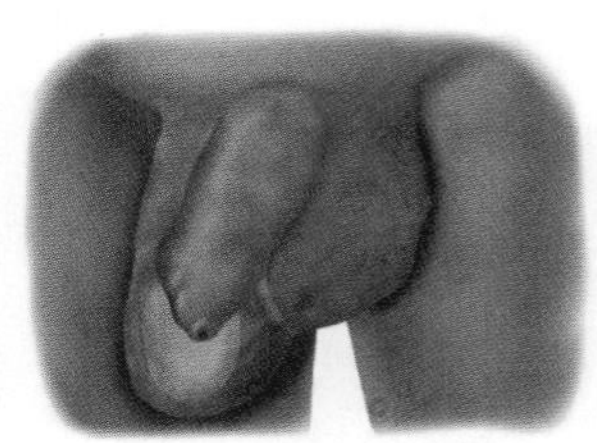	S: Empty scrotal half O: Inspection—in true maldescent, atrophic scrotum on affected side Palpation—no testis A: Absent testis	True cryptorchidism—testes that have never descended. Incidence at birth is 3% to 4%; one half of these descend in first month. Incidence with premature infants is 30%; in the adult, 0.7% to 0.8%. True undescended testes have a histologic change by 6 years, causing decreased spermatogenesis and infertility.
Small Testis 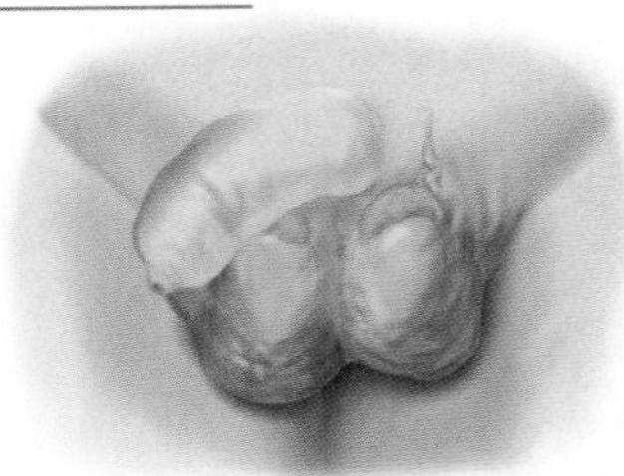	S: (None) O: Palpation—small and soft (rarely may be firm) A: Small testis	Small and soft (<3.5 cm) indicates atrophy as with cirrhosis, hypopituitarism, following estrogen therapy, or as a sequelae of orchitis. Small and firm (<2 cm) occurs with Klinefelter's syndrome (hypogonadism).
Testicular Torsion 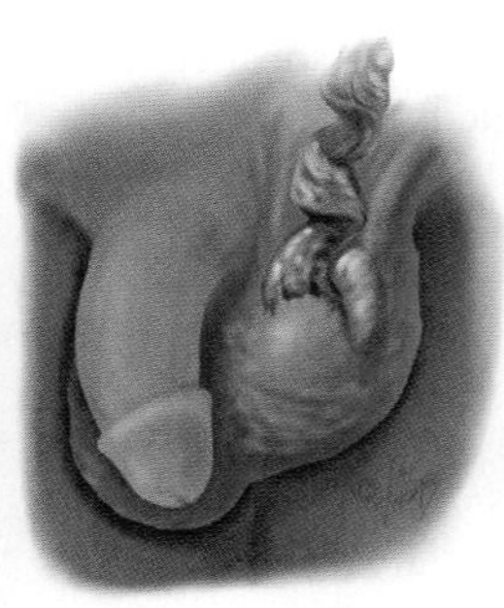	S: Excruciating pain in testicle of sudden onset, often during sleep or following trauma. May also have lower abdominal pain, nausea and vomiting, no fever O: Inspection—red, swollen scrotum, one testis (usually left) higher owing to rotation and shortening Palpation—cord feels thick, swollen, tender; epididymis may be anterior; cremasteric reflex is absent on side of torsion	Sudden twisting of spermatic cord. Occurs in late childhood, early adolescence, rare after age 20 years. Torsion usually on the left side; faulty anchoring of testis on wall of scrotum allows testis to rotate. The anterior part of the testis rotates medially toward the other testis. Blood supply is cut off, resulting in ischemia and engorgement. This is an emergency requiring surgery; testis can become gangrenous in a few hours.
Epididymitis 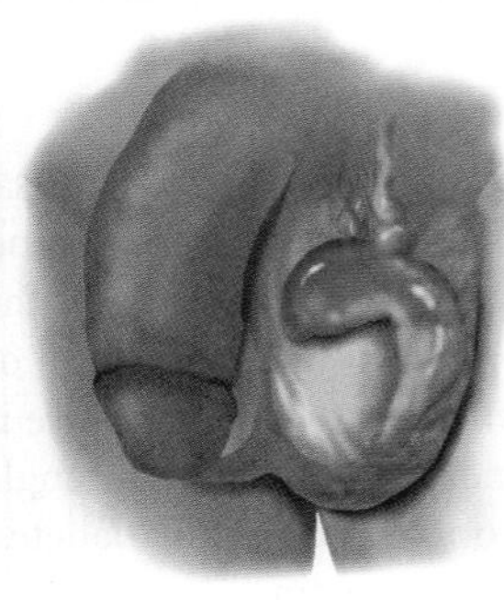	S: Severe pain of sudden onset in scrotum, somewhat relieved by elevation (a positive Prehn sign); also rapid swelling, fever O: Inspection—enlarged scrotum; reddened Palpation—exquisitely tender; epididymis enlarged, indurated; may be hard to distinguish from testis. Overlying scrotal skin may be thick and edematous Laboratory—white blood cells and bacteria in urine A: Tender swelling of epididymis	Acute infection of epididymis commonly caused by prostatitis, after prostatectomy because of trauma of urethral instrumentation, or due to chlamydia, gonorrhea, or other bacterial infection. Often difficult to distinguish between epididymitis and testicular torsion.

TABLE 24-6 Abnormalities in the Scrotum—cont'd

Disorder	Clinical Findings	Discussion
Varicocele 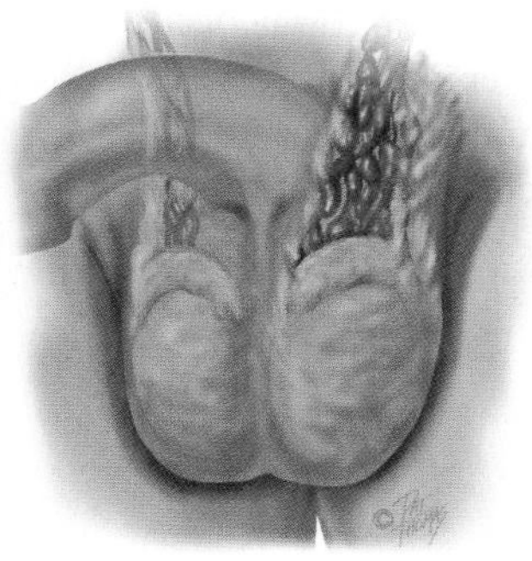	S: Dull pain; constant pulling or dragging feeling; or may be asymptomatic O: Inspection—usually no sign. May show bluish color through light scrotal skin Palpation—when standing, feel soft, irregular mass posterior to and above testis; collapses when supine, refills when upright. Feels distinctive, like a "bag of worms" The testis on the side of the varicocele may be smaller owing to impaired circulation A: Soft mass on spermatic cord	A varicocele is dilated, tortuous varicose veins in the spermatic cord due to incompetent valves within the vein, which permit reflux of blood. Most often on left side, perhaps because left spermatic vein is longer and inserts at a right angle into left renal vein. Common in young males. Screen at early adolescence; early treatment important to prevent potential infertility when an adult.
Spermatocele 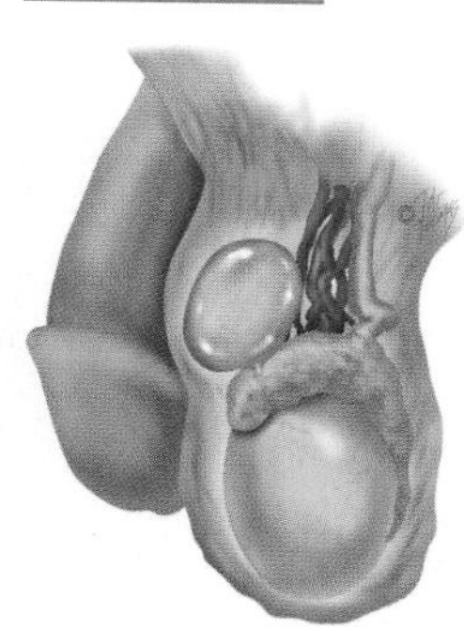	S: Painless, usually found on examination O: Inspection—does transilluminate higher in the scrotum than a hydrocele, and the sperm may fluoresce Palpation—round, freely movable mass lying above and behind testis. If large, feels like a third testis A: Free cystic mass on epididymis	Retention cyst in epididymis. Cause unclear but may be obstruction of tubules. Filled with thin, milky fluid that contains sperm. Most spermatoceles are small (<1 cm); occasionally, they may be larger and then mistaken for hydrocele.
Early Testicular Tumor 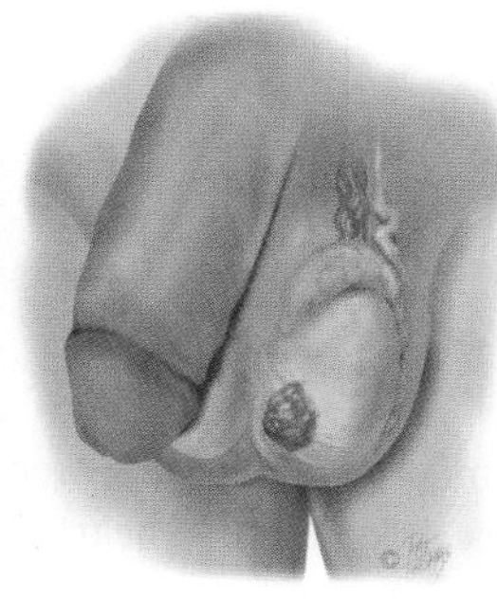	S: Painless, found on examination O: Palpation—firm nodule or harder than normal section of testicle A: Solitary nodule	Most testicular tumors occur between the ages of 18 and 35. Practically all are malignant. Occur in whites; relatively rare in Blacks, Mexican Americans, and Asians. Must biopsy to confirm. Most important risk factor is undescended testis, even those surgically corrected. Early detection important in prognosis, but practice of testicular self-examination is currently low.
Diffuse Tumor 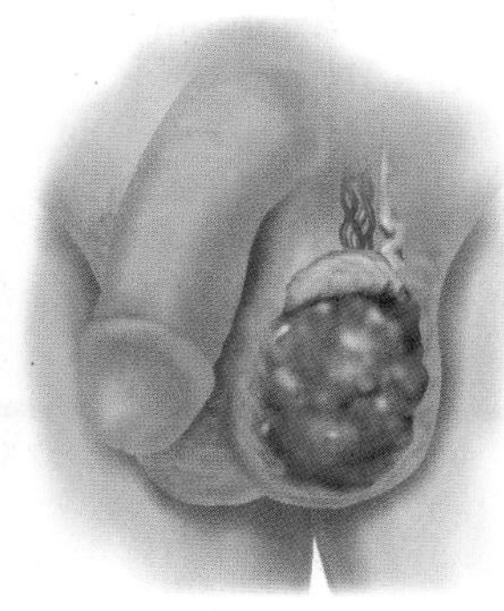	S: Enlarging testis (most common symptom). When enlarges, has feel of increased weight O: Inspection—enlarged, does not transilluminate Palpation—enlarged, smooth, ovoid, firm Important—firm palpation does *not* cause usual sickening discomfort as with normal testis A: Nontender swelling of testis	Diffuse tumor maintains shape of testis.

Continued

TABLE 24-6 Abnormalities in the Scrotum—cont'd

Disorder	Clinical Findings	Discussion
Hydrocele 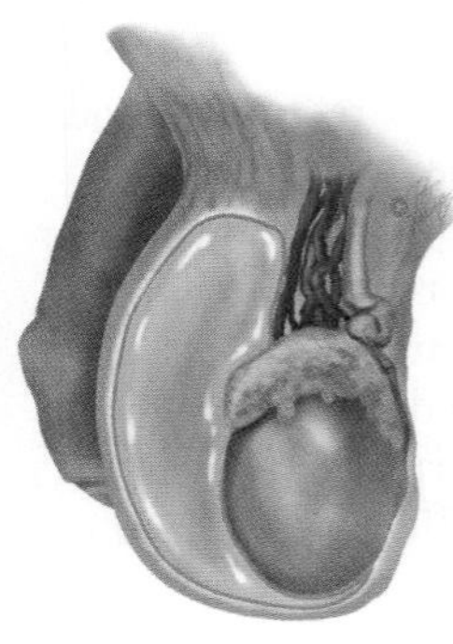	S: Painless swelling, although person may complain of weight and bulk in scrotum O: Inspection—enlarged, mass does transilluminate with a pink or red glow (in contrast to a hernia) Palpation—nontender mass, able to get fingers above mass (in contrast to scrotal hernia) A: Nontender swelling of testis	Cystic. Circumscribed collection of serous fluid in tunica vaginalis, surrounding testis. May occur following epididymitis, trauma, hernia, tumor of testis, or spontaneously in the newborn.
Scrotal Hernia 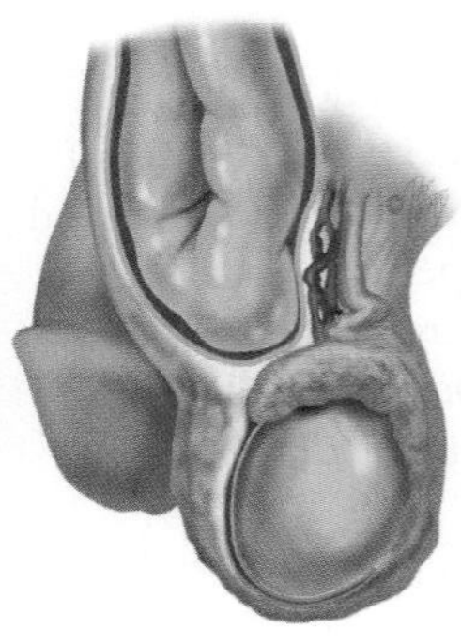	S: Swelling, may have pain with straining O: Inspection—enlarged, may reduce when supine, does not transilluminate Palpation—soft, mushy mass; palpating fingers cannot get above mass. Mass is distinct from testicle that is normal A: Nontender swelling of scrotum	Scrotal hernia usually due to indirect inguinal hernia (see Table 24-7).
Orchitis 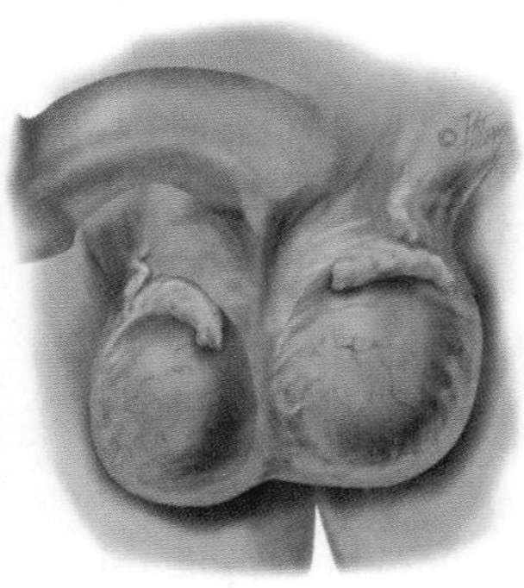	S: Acute or moderate pain of sudden onset, swollen testis, feeling of weight, fever O: Inspection—enlarged, edematous, reddened; does not transilluminate Palpation—swollen, congested, tense, and tender; hard to distinguish testis from epididymis A: Tender swelling of testis	Acute inflammation of testis. Most common cause is mumps; can occur with any infectious disease. May have associated hydrocele that does transilluminate.
Scrotal Edema 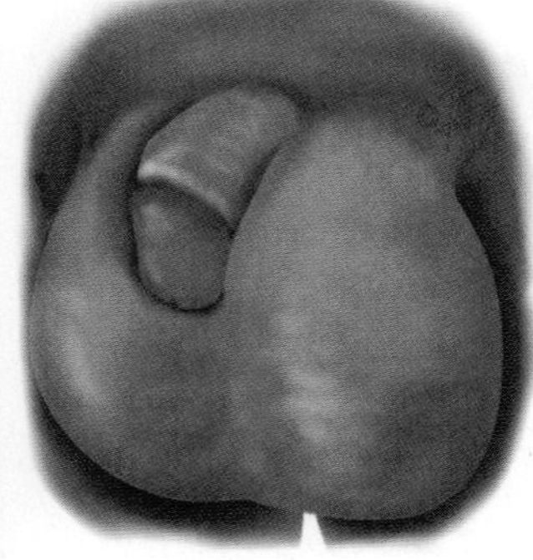	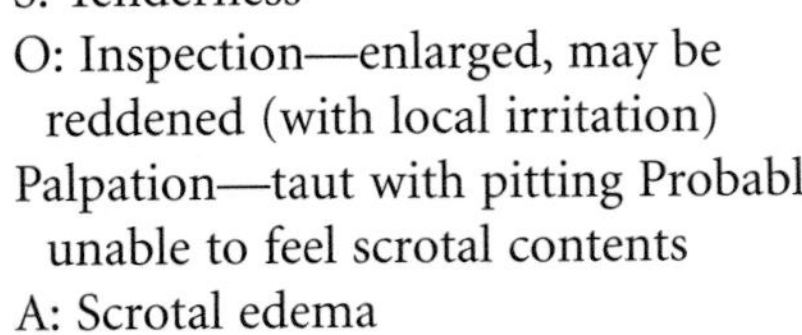 S: Tenderness O: Inspection—enlarged, may be reddened (with local irritation) Palpation—taut with pitting Probably unable to feel scrotal contents A: Scrotal edema	Accompanies marked edema in lower half of body (e.g., congestive heart failure, renal failure, and portal vein obstruction). Occurs with local inflammation: epididymitis, torsion of spermatic cord. Also, obstruction of inguinal lymphatics produces lymphedema of scrotum.

S, Subjective data; *O*, objective data; *A*, assessment.

TABLE 24-7 **Inguinal and Femoral Hernias**

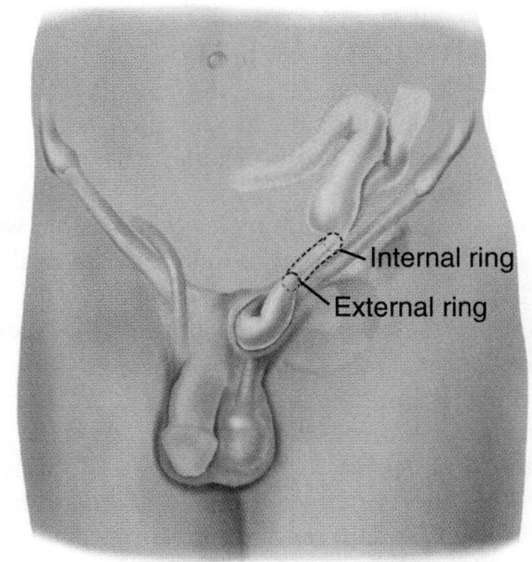

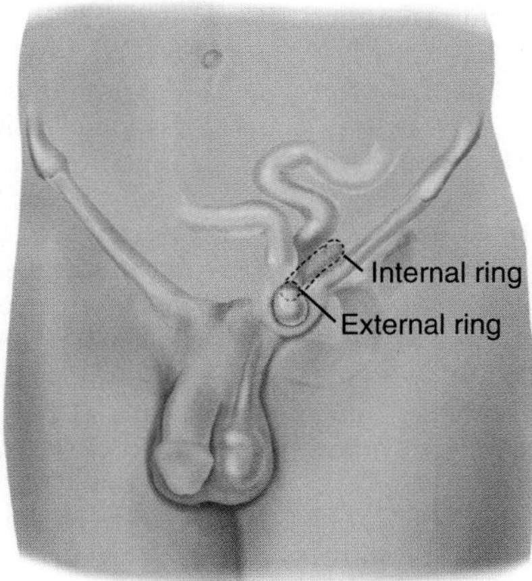

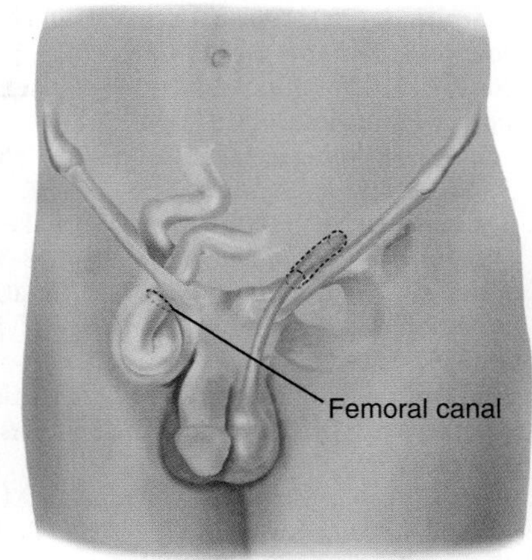

	Indirect Inguinal	Direct Inguinal	Femoral
Course	Sac herniates through internal inguinal ring; can remain in canal or pass into scrotum	Directly behind and through external inguinal ring, above inguinal ligament; rarely enters scrotum	Through femoral ring and canal, below inguinal ligament, more often on right side
Clinical Symptoms and Signs	Pain with straining; soft swelling that increases with increased intra-abdominal pressure; may decrease when lying down	Usually painless; round swelling close to the pubis in area of internal inguinal ring; easily reduced when supine*	Pain may be severe; may become strangulated
Frequency	Most common; 60% of all hernias. More common in infants <1 year and in males 16 to 20 years of age	Less common; occurs most often in men older than 40 years, rare in women	Least common, 4% of all hernias; more common in women
Cause	Congenital or acquired	Acquired weakness; brought on by heavy lifting, muscle atrophy, obesity, chronic cough, or ascites	Acquired; due to increased abdominal pressure, muscle weakness, or frequent stooping

***Reducible**—contents will return to abdominal cavity by lying down or gentle pressure. **Incarcerated**—herniated bowel cannot be returned to abdominal cavity. **Strangulated**—blood supply to hernia is shut off. Accompanied by nausea, vomiting, and tenderness.

BIBLIOGRAPHY

1. American Cancer Society. (2009). *What are the risk factors for testicular cancer?* Retrieved June 15, 2010, from www.cancer.org/docroot/cri/content/cri_2_4_2x_what_are_the_risk_factors_for_testicular_cancer_41.asp.
2. Baumann, B. M., Welsh, B. E., Rogers, C. J., et al. (2008). Nurses using volumetric bladder ultrasound in the pediatric ED. *American Journal of Nursing, 108*(4), 73-76.
3. Bohnenkamp, S., & Yoder, L. H. (2009). The medical-surgical nurse's guide to testicular cancer. *Medsurg Nursing, 18*(2), 116-123.
4. Bradway, C., & Rodgers, J. (2009). Evaluation and management of genitourinary emergencies. *Nurse Practitioner, 34*(5), 37-44.
5. Brady, M. T. (2010). Newborn circumcision. *Archives of Pediatrics & Adolescent Medicine, 164*(1), 94-96.
6. Cochran, S. D., & Mays, V. M. (2007). Physical health complaints among lesbians, gay men, and bisexual and homosexually experienced heterosexual individuals: results from the California quality of life survey. *American Journal of Public Health, 97*(11), 2048-2055.

6a. Copstead, L. C., & Banasik, J. L. (2010). *Pathophysiology* (4th ed.). St. Louis: Saunders.

7. Crestodina, L. R. (2007). Assessment and management of urinary incontinence in the elderly male. *Nurse Practitioner, 32*(9), 27-35.
8. Fitzgerald, M., & Walker, S. M. (2009). Infant pain management: a developmental neurobiological approach. *Nature Clinical Practice. Neurology, 5*(1), 35-50.
9. Golden, M. R., & Wasserheit, J. N. (2009). Prevention of viral sexually transmitted infections. *New England Journal of Medicine, 360*(13), 1349-1351.
10. Gray, R. H., Wawer, M. J., Serwadda, D., et al. (2009). The role of male circumcision in the prevention of human papillomavirus and HIV infection. *Journal of Infectious Diseases, 199*(1), 1-3.
11. Hayes-Lattin, B., & Nichols, C. R. (2009). Testicular cancer: a prototypic tumor of young adults. *Seminars in Oncology, 36*(5), 432-438.
12. Heidelbaugh, J. J. (2010). Management of erectile dysfunction. *American Family Physician, 81*(3), 305-312.

13. Herman-Giddens, M. E., Wang, L., & Koch, G. (2001). Secondary sexual characteristics in boys. *Archives of Pediatrics & Adolescent Medicine, 155*(1), 1022-1028.
14. Hornor, G. (2004). Sexual behavior in children: normal or not? *Journal of Pediatric Health Care, 18*(2), 57-64.
15. Joffe, A. (2009). Should we teach testicular self-exam? *Contemporary Pediatrics, 26*(8), 33-34.
16. Jones, L., Felblinger, D., & Cooper, L. (2009). *Mycoplasma genitalium. Nurse Practitioner, 34*(8), 50-52.
17. Leung-Chen, P. (2008). Syphilis makes another comeback. *American Journal of Nursing, 108*(2), 28-30.
18. Marshall, W., & Tanner, J. (1970). Variations in the pattern of pubertal changes in boys. *Archives of Disease in Childhood, 45*(239), 13.
19. Pearson, M. Z. (2008). Racial disparities in chronic kidney disease: current data and nursing roles. *Nephrology Nursing Journal, 35*(5), 485-489.
20. Ries, L. A. G., Melbert, D., Krapcho, M., et al. (2008). *SEER cancer statistics reviews, 1975-2005*. Bethesda, MD: National Cancer Institute. Retrieved June 15, 2010, from http://seer.cancer.gov/csr/1975_2005/.
21. Sobngwi-Tambekou, J., Talijaard, D., Nieuwoudt, M., et al. (2009). Male circumcision and *Neisseria gonorrhoeae, Chlamydia trachomatis,* and *Trichomonas vaginalis*: observation after a randomized controlled trial for HIV prevention. *Sexually Transmitted Infections, 85*(1), 116-120.
22. Tobian, A. A. R., Serwadda, D., Quinn, T. C., et al. (2009). Male circumcision for the prevention of HSV-2 and HPV infections and syphilis. *New England Journal of Medicine, 360*(13), 1298-1309.
23. U.S. Renal Data System (USRDS). (2007). *USRDS 2007 annual data report: atlas of end-stage renal disease in the United States.* National Institutes of Health, National Institute of Diabetes and Digestive and Kidney Diseases, Chronic Kidney Disease, Economic Costs, Clinical Indicators.
24. Viscidi, R. P., & Shah, K. V. (2010). Adult male circumcision: will it reduce disease caused by human papillomavirus? *Journal of Infectious Diseases, 201*(10), 1447-1449.
25. Wallace, M. A. (2008). Assessment of sexual health in older adults. *The American Journal of Nursing, 108*(7), 52-61.
26. Ward, M. M. (2008). Socioeconomic status and the incidence of ESRD. *American Journal of Kidney Diseases, 51*(4), 563-572.
27. Wawer, M. J., Makumbi, F., Kigozi, G., et al. (2009). Circumcision in HIV-infected men and its effect on HIV transmission to female partners in Rakai, Uganda: a randomized controlled trial. *Lancet, 374*(1), 229-237.
28. Weiss, H. A., Larke, N., Halperin, D., et al. (2010). Complications of circumcision in male neonates, infants and children: a systematic review. *BMC Urology, 10*(1), 2.
29. Yamada, J., Stinson, J., Lamba, J., et al. (2008). A review of systematic reviews on pain interventions in hospitalized infants. *Pain Research & Management, 13*(5), 413-420.

Summary Checklist: Male Genitalia Examination

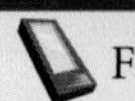 For a PDA-downloadable version, go to http://evolve.elsevier.com/Jarvis/.

1. Inspect and palpate the penis.
2. Inspect and palpate the scrotum.
3. If a mass exists, transilluminate it.
4. Palpate for an inguinal hernia.
5. Palpate the inguinal lymph nodes.

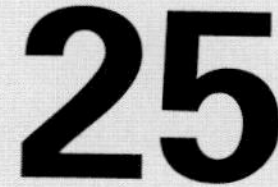

Anus, Rectum, and Prostate

evolve WEBSITE

http://evolve.elsevier.com/Jarvis/

- Animations
- Audio Key Points
- Bedside Assessment Summary Checklist
- Case Study
  Rectal Cancer
- Health Promotion Guide
  Colon and Rectal Cancer
  Prostate Cancer
- NCLEX Review Questions
- Physical Examination Summary Checklist
- Quick Assessment for Common Conditions
  Benign Prostatic Hypertrophy

OUTLINE

Structure and Function, 709

Anus and Rectum
Prostate

Subjective Data, 712

Health History Questions

Objective Data, 713

Preparation
The Perianal Area
The Anus and Rectum

Documentation and Critical Thinking, 718

Abnormal Findings, 720

Abnormal Findings for Advanced Practice, 723

STRUCTURE AND FUNCTION

ANUS AND RECTUM

The **anal canal** is the outlet of the gastrointestinal (GI) tract, and it is about 3.8 cm long in the adult. It is lined with modified skin (having no hair or sebaceous glands) that merges with rectal mucosa at the anorectal junction. The canal slants forward toward the umbilicus, forming a distinct right angle with the rectum, which rests back in the hollow of the sacrum. Although the rectum contains only autonomic nerves, numerous somatic sensory nerves are present in the anal canal and external skin, so a person feels sharp pain from any trauma to the anal area.

The anal canal is surrounded by two concentric layers of muscle, the **sphincters** (Fig. 25-1). The internal sphincter is under involuntary control by the autonomic nervous system. The external sphincter surrounds the internal sphincter but also has a small section overriding the tip of the internal sphincter at the opening. It is under voluntary control. Except for the passing of feces and gas, the sphincters keep the anal canal tightly closed. The **intersphincteric groove** separates the internal and external sphincters and is palpable.

The **anal columns** (or columns of Morgagni) are folds of mucosa. These extend vertically down from the rectum and end in the **anorectal junction** (also called the *mucocutaneous junction, pectinate,* or *dentate line*). This junction is not palpable, but it is visible on proctoscopy. Each anal column contains an artery and a vein. Under conditions of chronic increased venous pressure, the vein may enlarge, forming a hemorrhoid. At the lower end of each column is a small crescent fold of mucous membrane, the **anal valve.** The space above the anal valve (between the columns) is a small recess, the **anal crypt.**

The **rectum,** which is 12 cm long, is the distal portion of the large intestine. It extends from the sigmoid colon, at the level of the third sacral vertebra, and ends at the anal canal. Just above the anal canal, the rectum dilates and turns posteriorly, forming the rectal ampulla. The rectal interior has three semilunar transverse folds called the **valves of Houston.**

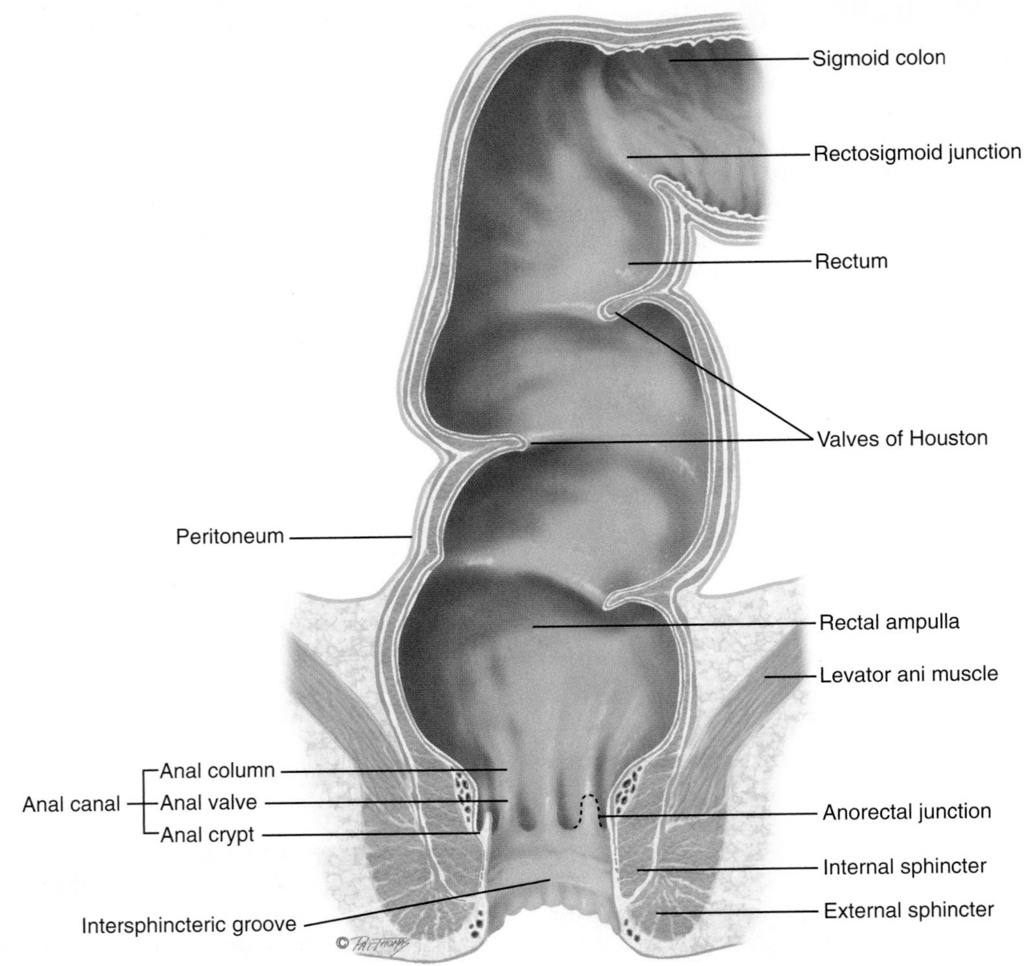

25-1

These cross one-half the circumference of the rectal lumen. Their function is unclear, but they may serve to hold feces as the flatus passes. The lowest is within reach of palpation, usually on the person's left side, and must not be mistaken for an intrarectal mass.

Peritoneal Reflection. The peritoneum covers only the upper two thirds of the rectum. In the male, the anterior part of the peritoneum reflects down to within 7.5 cm of the anal opening, forming the **rectovesical pouch** (Fig. 25-2) and then covers the bladder. In the female, this is termed the **recto-uterine pouch** and extends down to within 5.5 cm of the anal opening.

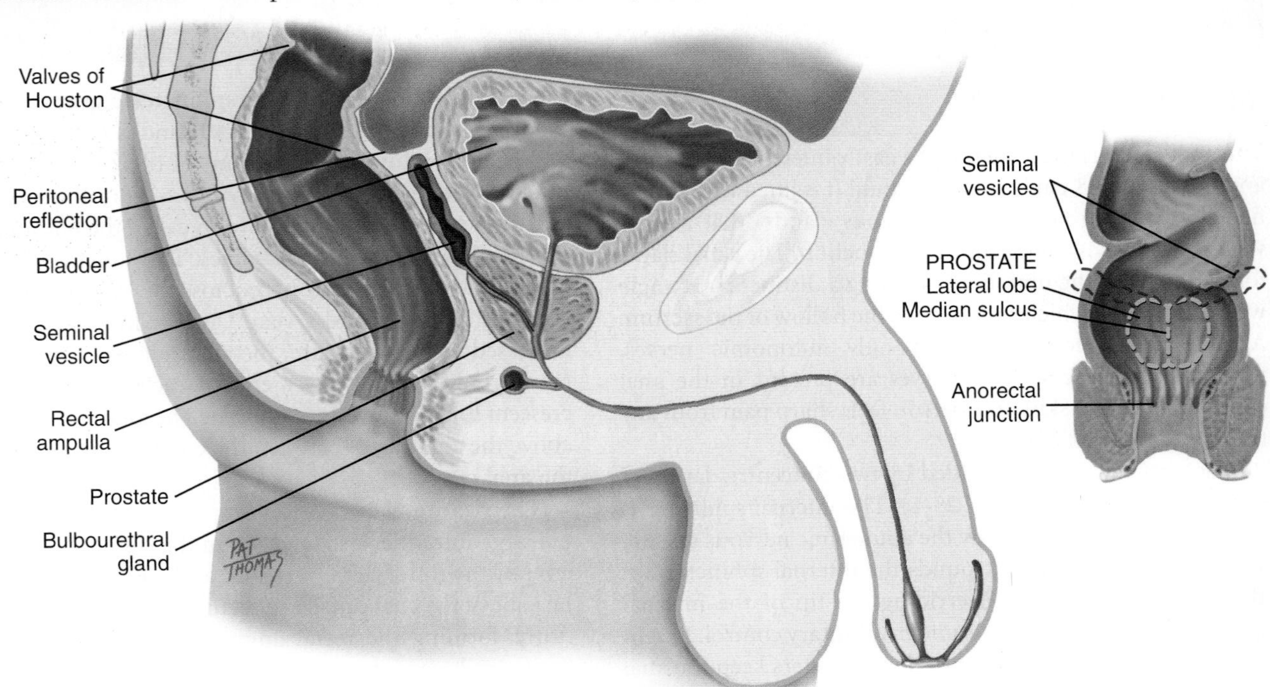

25-2

PROSTATE

In the male, the **prostate gland** lies in front of the anterior wall of the rectum and 2 cm behind the symphysis pubis. It surrounds the bladder neck and the urethra and has 15 to 30 ducts that open into the urethra. The prostate secretes a thin, milky, alkaline fluid that helps sperm viability. It is a bilobed structure with a round or heart shape. It measures 2.5 cm long and 4 cm in diameter. The two lateral lobes are separated by a shallow groove called the **median sulcus.**

The two **seminal vesicles** project like rabbit ears above the prostate. The seminal vesicles secrete a fluid that is rich in fructose, which nourishes the sperm and contains prostaglandins. The two **bulbourethral** (Cowper) glands are each the size of a pea and are located inferior to the prostate on either side of the urethra (also see Fig. 25-5). They secrete a clear, viscid mucus.

Regional Structures

In the female, the uterine cervix lies in front of the anterior rectal wall and may be palpated through it.

The combined length of the anal canal and the rectum is about 16 cm in the adult. The average length of the examining finger is from 6 cm to 10 cm, bringing many rectal structures within reach.

The sigmoid colon is named from its S-shaped course in the pelvic cavity. It extends from the iliac flexure of the descending colon and ends at the rectum. It is 40 cm long and is accessible to examination only through the colonoscope. The flexible fiberoptic scope in current use provides a view of the entire mucosal surface of the sigmoid, as well as the colon.

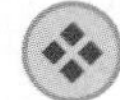

DEVELOPMENTAL COMPETENCE

The first stool passed by the newborn is dark green meconium and occurs within 24 to 48 hours of birth, indicating anal patency. From that time on, the infant usually has a stool after each feeding. This response to eating is a wave of peristalsis called the *gastrocolic reflex.* It continues throughout life, although children and adults usually produce no more than one or two stools per day.

The infant passes stools by reflex. Voluntary control of the external anal sphincter cannot occur until the nerves supplying the area have become fully myelinated, usually around 1½ to 2 years of age. Toilet training usually starts after age 2 years.

At male puberty, the prostate gland undergoes a very rapid increase to more than twice its prepubertal size. During young adulthood, its size remains fairly constant.

The prostate gland commonly starts to enlarge during the middle adult years. This **benign prostatic hypertrophy (BPH)** is present in 1 of 10 males at the age of 40 years and grows larger with age. It is thought that the hypertrophy is caused by hormonal imbalance that leads to the proliferation of benign adenomas. These gradually impede urine output because they obstruct the urethra.

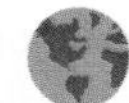

CULTURE AND GENETICS

Prostate cancer (PC) is more common in North America and northwestern Europe and is less common in Central and South America, Africa, and Asia. The incidence of PC is higher for African-American men than for men of other racial groups; African-American men are more likely to be diagnosed at an advanced stage of the disease, and mortality rates are two times higher for African-American men than for white men.[2]

What are the risk factors? Family history is positively associated; men with one first-degree relative (father or brother) are 2 to 3 times more likely to develop PC.[2] Genetic factors contribute some risk: men with BRCA2 mutations have increased risk for developing a more aggressive form of PC and at a younger age. Environmental factors may account for more risk than genetics because migration studies show men of Asian and African heritage living in the United States have a higher risk for PC than their counterparts living in Asia and Africa.[2,9] Environmental factors include diet, a potentially modifiable risk factor. Diets high in red meat and processed meat, animal and saturated fats, and dairy products may increase risk,[2] whereas diets high in fiber, fruits, and vegetables may lower risk.[23]

Of the men who have PC, those more likely to have an advanced disease at diagnosis include men who were uninsured or Medicaid-insured and men of racial/ethnic minority groups.[24] This has implications for screening and culturally appropriate health education. Screening guidelines were updated in 2010[2] and state the ages at which men should receive health information about benefits and risks of PC tests. Men at average risk for PC should receive information at 50 years; at higher risk (African Americans and positive family history) at 45 years; and at very high risk (multiple family members with PC) at 40 years. Screening includes the blood test for prostate-specific antigen (PSA) and a physical examination (i.e., a digital rectal exam [DRE]).[32]

Colorectal cancer has a racial variation as well. The incidence rates are almost 20% higher for African-American women and men than for whites, and the mortality rates are almost 50% higher for African Americans than for whites.[10] Because colorectal cancer can largely be prevented by removal of adenomatous polyps, guidelines for average-risk adults start at age 50 years and include health teaching about options for screening. Options include a colonoscopy every 10 years with bowel preparation and conscious sedation, and an annual guaiac-based fecal occult blood test or fecal immunochemical test.[22]

SUBJECTIVE DATA

1. Usual bowel routine
2. Change in bowel habits
3. Rectal bleeding, blood in the stool
4. Medications (laxatives, stool softeners, iron)
5. Rectal conditions (pruritus, hemorrhoids, fissure, fistula)
6. Family history
7. Self-care behaviors (diet of high-fiber foods, most recent examinations)

Examiner Asks	Rationale
1. **Usual bowel routine.** Bowels move regularly? How often? Usual color? Hard or soft?	Assess usual bowel routine. Constipation is ≤3 stools/week and is a common concern among aging adults.
• Any straining at stool, incomplete evacuation, urge to have bowel movement but nothing comes?	
• Eat breakfast? (This increases colon motility and prompts a bowel movement in many.)	
• Pain while passing a bowel movement?	**Dyschezia.** Pain due to a local condition (hemorrhoid, fissure) or constipation.
2. **Change in bowel habits.** Any **change** in usual **bowel habits?** Loose stools or diarrhea? When did this start? Is the diarrhea associated with nausea and vomiting, abdominal pain, something you ate recently?	Diarrhea occurs with gastroenteritis, colitis, irritable colon syndrome.
• Eaten at a restaurant recently? Anyone else in your group or family have the same symptoms?	Consider food poisoning.
• Traveled to a foreign country during the past 6 months?	Consider parasitic infection.
• Stools have a hard consistency? When did this start?	Constipation.
3. **Rectal bleeding, blood in the stool.** Ever had black or bloody stools? When did you first notice blood in the stools? What is the color, bright red or dark red-black? How much blood: spotting on the toilet paper or outright passing of blood with the stool? Do the bloody stools have a particular smell?	**Melena.** Black stools may be tarry due to occult blood (melena) from GI bleeding or nontarry from ingestion of iron medications. Red blood in stools occurs with GI bleeding or local bleeding around the anus and with colon and rectal cancer.
• Ever had clay-colored stools?	Clay color indicates absent bile pigment.
• Ever had mucus or pus in stool?	
• Frothy stool?	**Steatorrhea** is excessive fat in the stool as in malabsorption of fat.
• Need to pass gas frequently?	Flatulence.
4. **Medications.** What **medications** do you take—prescription and over-the-counter? Laxatives or stool softeners? Which ones? How often? Iron pills? Do you ever use enemas to move your bowels? How often?	
5. **Rectal conditions.** Any problems in rectal area: itching, pain or burning, hemorrhoids? How do you treat these? Any hemorrhoid preparations? Ever had a fissure or fistula? How was this treated?	Pruritus.
• Ever had a problem controlling your bowels?	Fecal incontinence. Mucoid discharge and soiled underwear occur with prolapsed hemorrhoids.
6. **Family history.** Any **family history:** polyps or cancer in colon or rectum, inflammatory bowel disease, prostate cancer?	Risk factors for colon cancer, rectal cancer, prostate cancer.

Examiner Asks	Rationale
7. **Self-care behaviors.** What is the usual amount of **high-fiber foods** in your daily diet: cereals, apples or other fruits, vegetables, whole-grain breads? How many glasses of water do you drink each day?	High-fiber foods of the soluble type (beans, prunes, barley, carrots, broccoli, cabbage) lower cholesterol, whereas insoluble fiber foods (cereals, wheat germ) reduce risk for colon cancer. Also, fiber foods fight obesity, stabilize blood sugar, and help some GI disorders.
• Date of last: digital rectal examination, stool blood test, colonoscopy, (for men) prostate-specific antigen blood test.	Early detection for cancer: DRE performed annually after age 50 years; fecal occult blood test annually after age 50 years; sigmoidoscopy every 5 years or colonoscopy every 10 years after age 50 years; PSA blood test annually for men older than 50 years, except Black men beginning at age 45 years.[2]
Additional History for Infants and Children	
1. Have you ever noticed any irritation in your child's anal area: redness, raised skin, frequent itching?	In children, pinworms are a common cause of intense itching and irritated anal skin.
2. How are your child's bowel movements? Frequency? Any problems? Any pain or straining with BM?	Assess usual stooling pattern. Constipation is a decrease in BM frequency, with difficult passing of very hard, dry stools. **Encopresis** is persistent passing of stools into clothing in a child older than 4 years, at which age continence would be expected.

OBJECTIVE DATA

PREPARATION

Perform a rectal examination on all adults and particularly those in middle and late years. Help the person assume one of the following positions (Fig. 25-3):

Examine the male in the left lateral decubitus or standing position. Instruct the standing male to point his toes together; this relaxes the regional muscles, making it easier to spread the buttocks.

Place the female in the lithotomy position if examining genitalia as well; use the left lateral decubitus position for the rectal area alone.

EQUIPMENT NEEDED

Penlight
Lubricating jelly
Glove
Guaiac test container

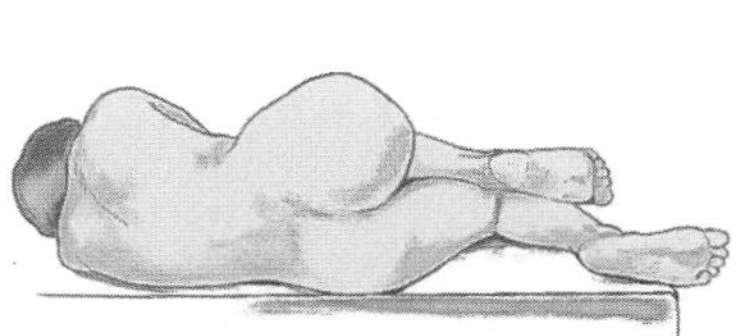

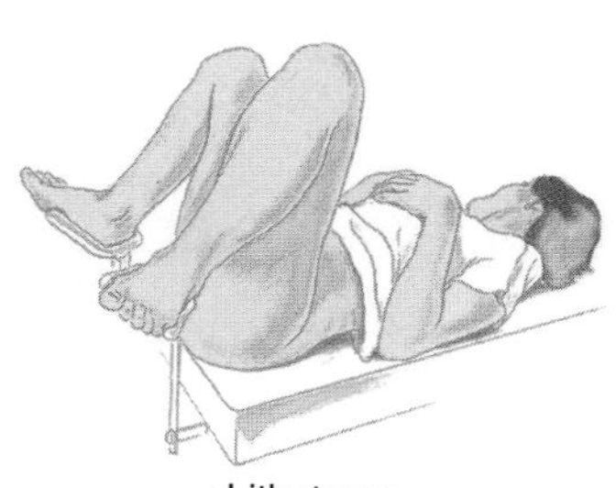

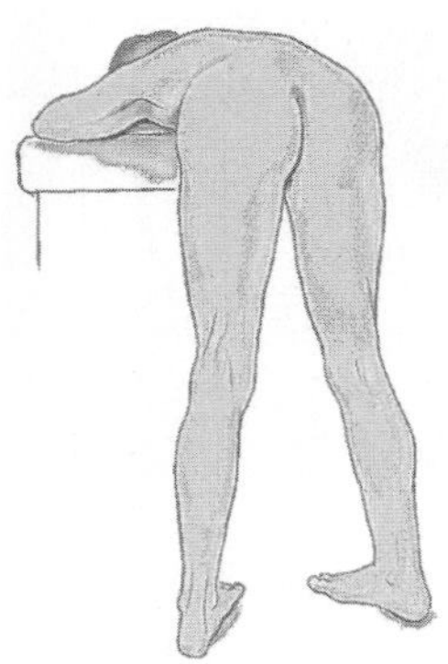

25-3 Positions for rectal examination.

Objective Data

Normal Range of Findings	Abnormal Findings
INSPECT THE PERIANAL AREA	
Spread the buttocks wide apart and observe the perianal region. The anus normally looks moist and hairless, with coarse, folded skin that is more pigmented than the perianal skin. The anal opening is tightly closed. No lesions are present.	Inflammation. Lesions or scars. Linear split—fissure. Flabby skin sac—hemorrhoid. Shiny blue skin sac—thrombosed hemorrhoid. Small round opening in anal area—fistula (see Table 25-1, Abnormalities of the Anal Region, p. 720).
Inspect the sacrococcygeal area. Normally, it appears smooth and even.	Inflammation or tenderness, swelling, tuft of hair, or dimple at tip of coccyx may indicate pilonidal cyst (see Table 25-1).
Instruct the person to hold the breath and bear down by performing a Valsalva maneuver. No break in skin integrity or protrusion through the anal opening should be present. Describe any abnormality in clock-face terms, with the 12 o'clock position as the anterior point toward the symphysis pubis and the 6 o'clock position toward the coccyx.	Appearance of fissure or hemorrhoids. Circular red doughnut of tissue—rectal prolapse.
PALPATE THE ANUS AND RECTUM	
Drop lubricating jelly onto your gloved index finger. Instruct the person that palpation is not painful but may feel like needing to move the bowels. Place the pad of your index finger gently against the anal verge (Fig. 25-4). You will feel the sphincter tighten and then relax. As it relaxes, flex the tip of your finger and slowly insert it into the anal canal in a direction toward the umbilicus. *Never* approach the anus at right angles with your index finger extended. Such a jabbing motion does not promote sphincter relaxation and is painful.	

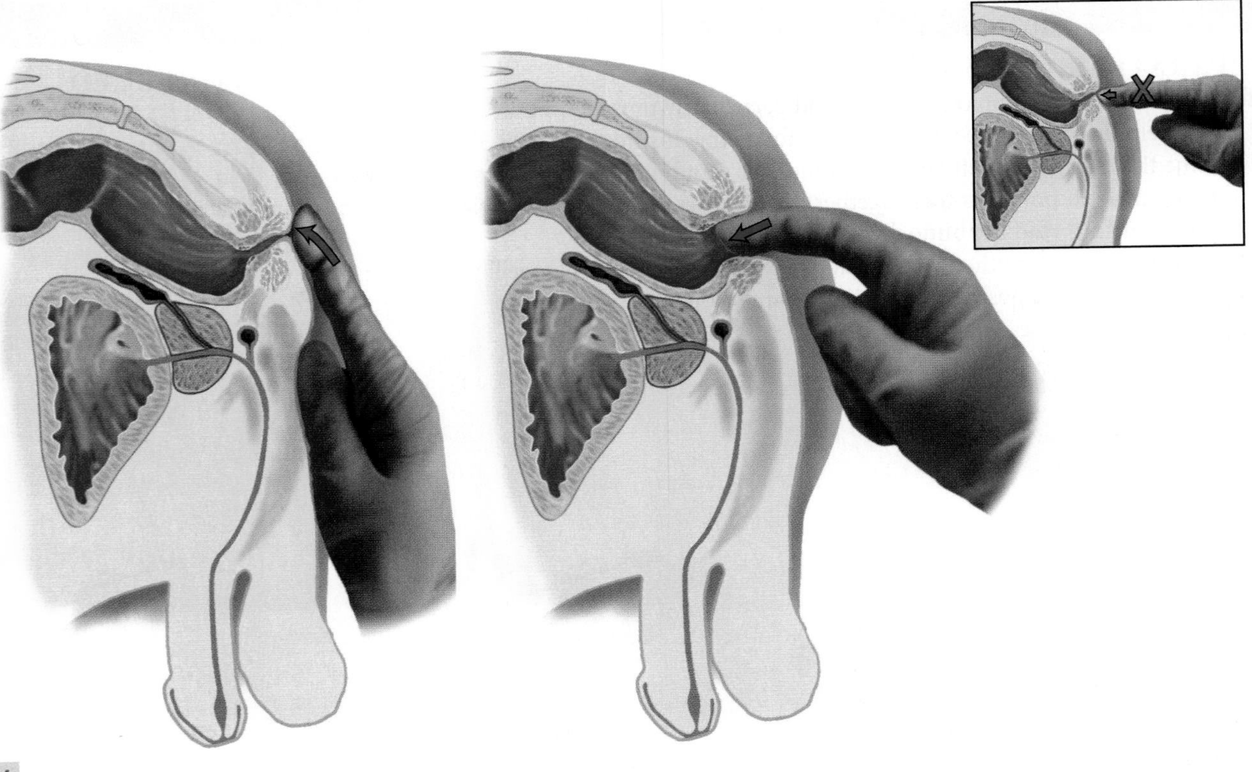

25-4

Normal Range of Findings

Rotate your examining finger to palpate the entire muscular ring. The canal should feel smooth and even. Note the intersphincteric groove circling the canal wall. To assess tone, ask the person to tighten the muscle. The sphincter should tighten evenly around your finger with no pain to the person.

Use a bi-digital palpation with your thumb against the perianal tissue (Fig. 25-5). Press your examining finger toward it. This maneuver highlights any swelling or tenderness and helps assess the bulbourethral glands.

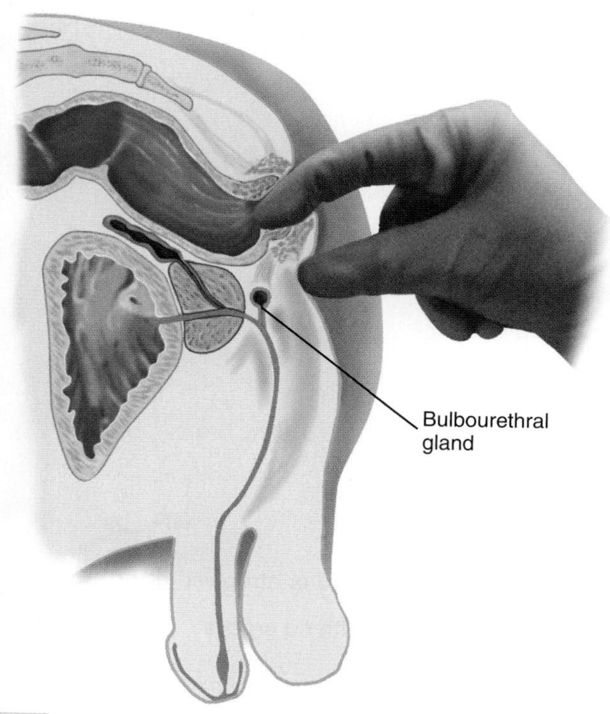

25-5

Above the anal canal, the rectum turns posteriorly, following the curve of the coccyx and sacrum. Insert your finger farther and explore all around the rectal wall. It normally feels smooth with no nodularity. Promptly report any mass you discover for further examination.

Prostate Gland. On the anterior wall in the male, note the elastic, bulging prostate gland (Fig. 25-6). Palpate the entire prostate in a systematic manner, but note that only the superior and part of the lateral surfaces are accessible to examination. Press *into* the gland at each location, because when a nodule occurs, it will not project into the rectal lumen. The surface should feel smooth and muscular; search for any distinct nodule or diffuse firmness. Note these characteristics:

Abnormal Findings

Decreased tone.

Increased tone occurs with inflammation and anxiety.

Tenderness.

Internal hemorrhoid above anorectal junction is not palpable unless thrombosed.

A soft, slightly movable mass may be a polyp.

A firm or hard mass with irregular shape or rolled edges may signify carcinoma (see Table 25-2, Abnormalities of the Rectum, p. 722).

Normal Range of Findings	Abnormal Findings

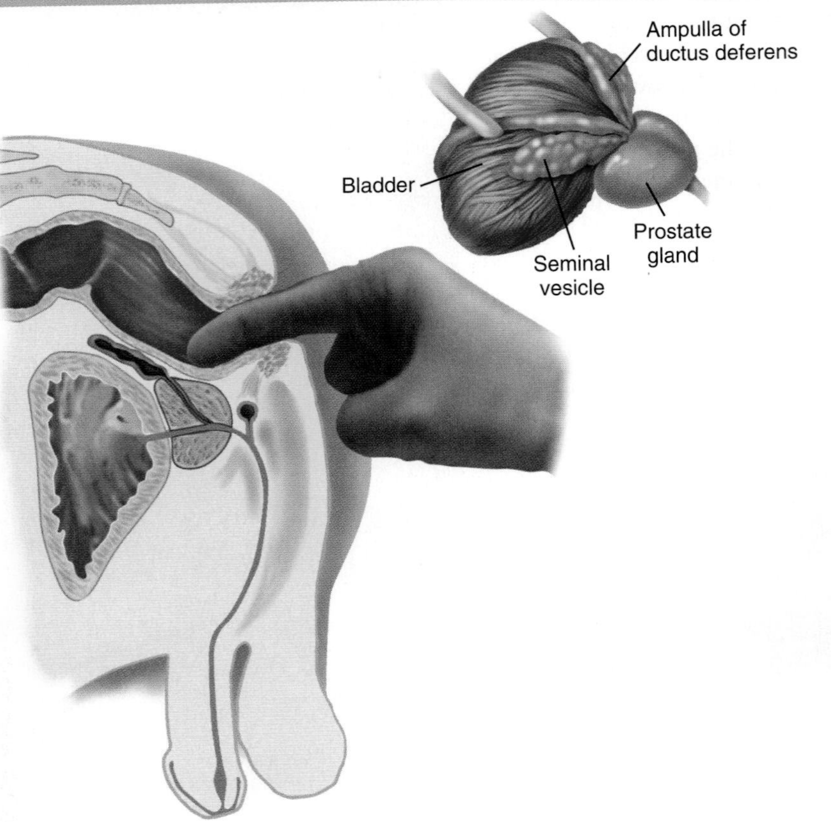

25-6

Size—2.5 cm long by 4 cm wide; should not protrude more than 1 cm into the rectum

Enlarged or atrophied gland.

Shape—heart shape, with palpable central groove

Flat with no groove.

Surface—smooth

Nodular.

Consistency—elastic, rubbery

Hard; or boggy, soft, fluctuant.

Mobility—slightly movable

Fixed.

Sensitivity—nontender to palpation

Tender.

Enlarged, firm, smooth gland with central groove obliterated suggests benign prostatic hypertrophy.

Swollen, exquisitely tender gland accompanies prostatitis.

Any stone-hard, irregular, fixed nodule indicates carcinoma (see Table 25-3).

In the female, palpate the cervix through the anterior rectal wall. It normally feels like a small, round mass. You also may palpate a retroverted uterus or a tampon in the vagina. Do not mistake the cervix or a tampon for a tumor.

Withdraw your examining finger; normally, no bright red blood or mucus is on the glove. To complete the examination, offer the person tissues to remove the lubricant and help the person to a more comfortable position.

Examination of Stool. Inspect any feces remaining on the glove. Normally, the color is brown and the consistency is soft.

Jelly-like mucus shreds mixed in stool indicate inflammation.

Bright red blood on stool surface indicates rectal bleeding. Bright red blood mixed with feces indicates possible colonic bleeding.

Normal Range of Findings

Test any stool on the glove for **occult blood** using the specimen container that your agency directs. A negative response is normal. If the stool is *Hematest* positive, it indicates occult blood. Note that a false-positive finding may occur if the person has ingested significant amounts of red meat within 3 days of the test.

Enhance self-care by providing the average-risk patient an at-home collection kit to screen for asymptomatic colorectal cancer and precancerous lesions (high-risk adenomas). A patient collects the stool specimen at home and mails it to the laboratory. The guaiac-based fecal occult blood test has long been in use but it requires three separate stool samples to yield a sensitivity of 92%.[16] Also, false positives can occur due to ingestion of red meat and other foods and certain medications. Evidence shows the newer fecal immunochemical test is easier and requires only one stool sample. It detects antibodies specific for human hemoglobin and is sensitive to invasive cancers and precancerous lesions.[14]

Abnormal Findings

Black tarry stool with distinct malodor indicates upper GI bleeding with blood partially digested. (Must lose more than 50 mL from upper GI tract to be considered melena.)

Black stool—also occurs with ingesting iron or bismuth preparations.

Gray, tan stool—absent bile pigment (e.g., obstructive jaundice).

Pale yellow, greasy stool—increased fat content (steatorrhea), as occurs with malabsorption syndrome.

Occult bleeding usually indicates cancer of the colon.

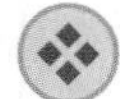

DEVELOPMENTAL COMPETENCE

Infants and Children

For the newborn, hold the feet with one hand and flex the knees up onto the abdomen. Note the presence of the anus. Confirm a patent rectum and anus by noting the first meconium stool passed within 24 to 48 hours of birth. To assess sphincter tone, check the *anal reflex.* Gently stroke the anal area and note a quick contraction of the sphincter.

Imperforate anus.

For each infant and child, note that the buttocks are firm and rounded with no masses or lesions. Recall that the *mongolian spot* is a common variation of hyperpigmentation in Black, American Indian, Mediterranean, and Asian newborns (see Chapter 12).

Flattened buttocks in cystic fibrosis or celiac syndrome.

Coccygeal mass.

Meningocele (sac containing meninges that protrude through a defect in the bony spine).

Tuft of hair or pilonidal dimple.

The perianal skin is free of lesions. However, diaper rash is common in children younger than 1 year and is exhibited as a generalized reddened area with papules or vesicles.

Pustules indicate secondary infection of diaper rash.

Signs of physical or sexual abuse (e.g., anal abrasions, perianal tears).

Fissure—common cause of constipation or rectal bleeding in child. (Painful, so the child does not defecate.)

Omit palpation unless the history or symptoms warrant. When internal palpation is needed, position the infant or child on the back with the legs flexed and gently insert a gloved, well-lubricated finger into the rectum. Your fifth finger usually is long enough, and its smaller size is more comfortable for the infant or child. However, you may need to use the index finger because of its better control and increased tactile sensitivity. On withdrawing the finger, scant bleeding or protruding rectal mucosa may occur.

Inspect the perianal region of the school-age child and adolescent during examination of the genitalia. Internal palpation is not performed routinely.

The Aging Adult

As an aging person performs the Valsalva maneuver, you may note relaxation of the perianal musculature and decreased sphincter control. Otherwise, the full examination proceeds as that described earlier for the younger adult.

PROMOTING A HEALTHY LIFESTYLE: COLORECTAL CANCER SCREENING

Screen for Life: National Colorectal Cancer Action Campaign

Colorectal cancer (CRC), or colon cancer for short, is currently the second leading cancer killer in the United States. However, it should not be, because it is preventable. The Centers for Disease Control and Prevention (CDC) *Screen for Life: National Colorectal Cancer Action Campaign* is focused on informing adults 50 years of age and older about the importance of having regular colorectal screening tests, because an estimated 40% of these adults, the age-group at greatest risk, have not been screened. Screening tests can actually prevent some colorectal cancers from occurring because they identify precancerous polyps and remove them before they turn into cancer. Screening can also find CRC early, when treatment can be effective. If everyone age 50 years or older had regular screening tests, it is estimated that at least one third of deaths from this cancer could be avoided. The *Screen for Life* educational campaign has a number of materials (available in English and Spanish and easily downloaded) for patients and health care professionals.

CRC is most often found in people age 50 years and older. The older a person is, the higher his or her risk. Both men and women get CRC. However, the risk for CRC may be increased if the individual or a close relative has had colorectal polyps or inflammatory bowel disease (*ulcerative colitis* or *Crohn disease*) or if a close relative has or had CRC. These individuals may need to be screened earlier and will need to talk with their health care provider. Whereas some people with colorectal polyps or CRC are asymptomatic, others have symptoms that include blood in stools, pain, aches, abdominal cramping, a change in bowel habits, iron deficiency anemia, or unexplained weight loss. Several tests are used to screen for CRC. Each is used alone or in combination with each other. Individuals need to be encouraged to discuss with their health care provider the option that is right for them. The CDC *Screening Tests at a Glance* is an excellent reference for health care providers.

When an individual's family history includes two or more relatives with CRC, the possibility of a genetic syndrome, such as *hereditary nonpolyposis colon cancer (HNPCC)*, is increased substantially. A detailed review of the family history is done to determine the number of relatives affected, the age at which the colorectal cancer was diagnosed, and the presence of any other cancers consistent with an inherited colorectal cancer syndrome. HNPCC families may need to begin colorectal screening as early as age 20 to 25 years. Some other red flags for HNPCC include a colorectal and/or endometrial cancer diagnosis younger than age 50 years and two or more HNPCC-related cancers, such as endometrial, ovarian, and gastric cancer, in one individual or family. More information on the genetics of CRC is available at www.cancer.gov/cancertopics/pdq/genetics/colorectal/healthprofessional.

Resources

Screen for Life: National Colorectal Cancer Action Campaign. Website: www.cdc.gov/cancer/colorectal/sfl/.

Screening Tests at a Glance. Website: www.cdc.gov/cancer/colorectal/pdf/SFL_inserts_screening.pdf.

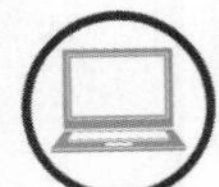

DOCUMENTATION AND CRITICAL THINKING

Sample Charting

SUBJECTIVE

Has one BM daily, soft, brown, no pain, no change in bowel routine. On no medications. Has no history of pruritus, hemorrhoids, fissure, or fistula. Diet includes one to two servings daily each of fresh fruits and vegetables but no whole-grain cereals or breads.

OBJECTIVE

No fissure, hemorrhoids, fistula, or skin lesions in perianal area. Sphincter tone good, no prolapse. Rectal walls smooth, no masses or tenderness. Prostate not enlarged, no masses or tenderness. Stool brown, Hematest negative.

ASSESSMENT

Rectal structures intact, no palpable lesions

Focused Assessment: Clinical Case Study

C.M. is a 62-year-old white male with chronic obstructive pulmonary disease for 15 years, who today has "diarrhea for 3 days."

SUBJECTIVE

7 days PTA—C.M. seen at this agency for acute respiratory infection that was diagnosed as acute bronchitis and treated with oral ampicillin. Took medication as directed.

3 days PTA—symptoms of respiratory infection improved. Ingesting usual diet. Onset of four to five loose, unformed, brown stools a day. No abdominal pain or cramping. No nausea.

Now—diarrhea continues. No blood or mucus noticed in stool. No new foods or restaurant food in past 3 days. Wife not ill.

OBJECTIVE

Vital signs: 37° C-88-18. BP 142/82.

Respiratory: Respirations unlabored. Barrel chest. Hyperresonant to percussion. Lung sounds clear but diminished. No crackles or rhonchi today.

Abdomen: Flat. Bowel sounds present. No organomegaly or tenderness to palpation.

Rectal: No lesions in perianal area. Sphincter tone good. Rectal walls smooth, no mass or tenderness. Prostate smooth and firm, no median sulcus palpable, no masses or tenderness. Stool brown, Hematest negative.

ASSESSMENT

Diarrhea R/T effects of antibiotic medication

ABNORMAL FINDINGS

TABLE 25-1 Abnormalities of the Anal Region

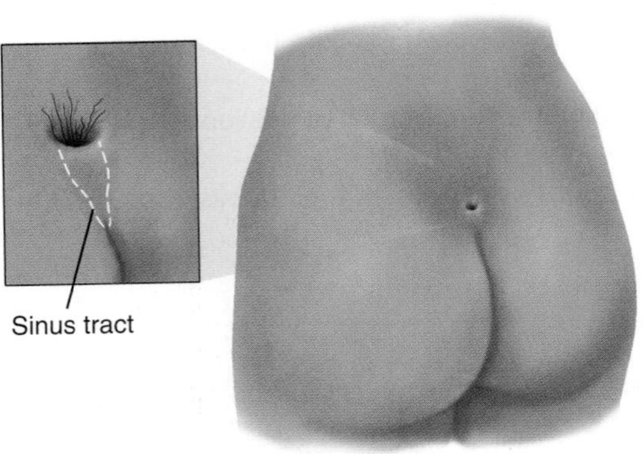

Pilonidal Cyst or Sinus

A hair-containing cyst or sinus located in the midline over the coccyx or lower sacrum. Often opens as a dimple with visible tuft of hair and, possibly, an erythematous halo. Or, may appear as a palpable cyst. When advanced, has a palpable sinus tract. Although it is a congenital disorder, the lesion is first diagnosed between the ages of 15 and 30 years.

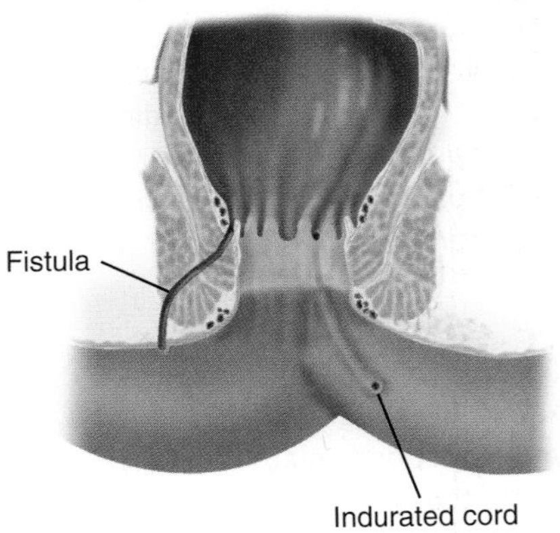

Anorectal Fistula

A chronically inflamed gastrointestinal tract creates an abnormal passage from inner anus or rectum out to skin surrounding anus. Usually originates from a local abscess. The red, raised tract opening may drain serosanguineous or purulent matter when pressure is applied. Bi-digital palpation may reveal an indurated cord.

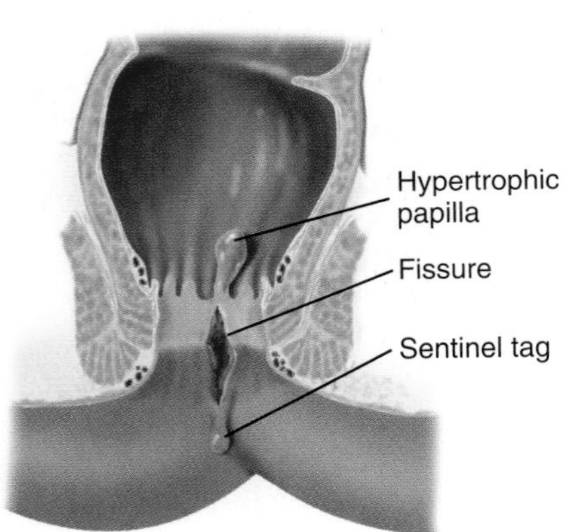

Fissure

A painful longitudinal tear in the superficial mucosa at the anal margin. Most fissures (>90%) occur in the posterior midline area. They are frequently accompanied by a papule of hyperplastic skin, called a *sentinel tag,* on the anal margin below. Fissures often result from trauma (e.g., passing a large, hard stool) or from irritant diarrheal stools. The person has itching, bleeding, and exquisite pain. A resulting spasm in the sphincters makes the area painful to examine; local anesthesia may be indicated.

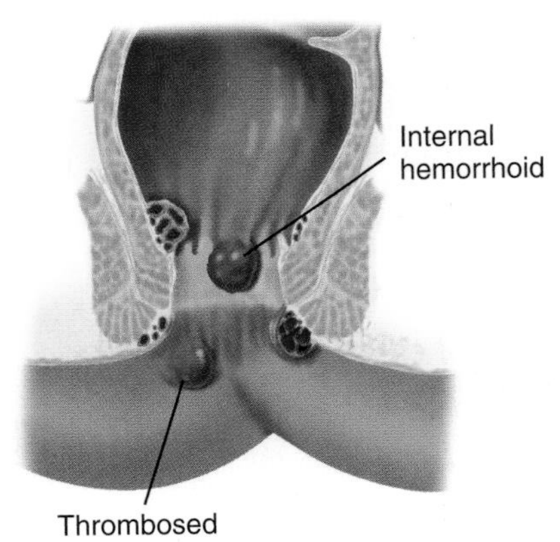

Hemorrhoids

These painless, flabby papules are due to a varicose vein of the hemorrhoidal plexus. An *external hemorrhoid* originates below the anorectal junction and is covered by anal skin. When *thrombosed,* it contains clotted blood and becomes a painful, swollen, shiny blue mass that itches and bleeds with defecation. When it resolves, it leaves a painless, flabby skin sac around the anal orifice. An *internal hemorrhoid* originates above the anorectal junction and is covered by mucous membrane. When the person performs a Valsalva maneuver, it may appear as a red mucosal mass. It is not palpable. All hemorrhoids result from increased portal venous pressure, as occurs with straining at stool, chronic constipation, pregnancy, obesity, chronic liver disease, or the low-fiber diet common in Western society.

TABLE 25-1 Abnormalities of the Anal Region—cont'd

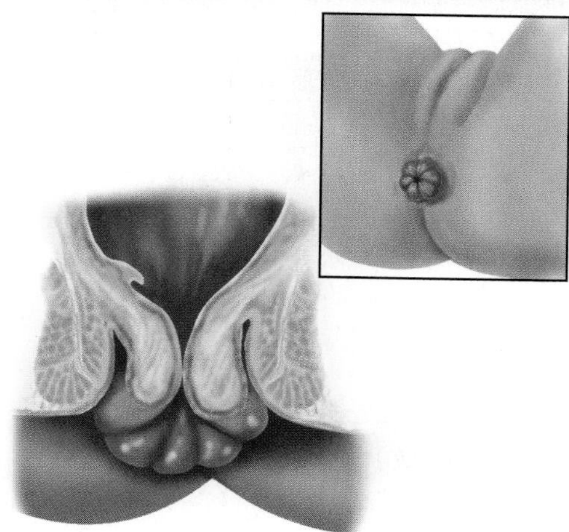

Rectal Prolapse

The rectal mucous membrane protrudes through the anus, appearing as a moist red donut with radiating lines. When prolapse is incomplete, only the mucosa bulges. When complete, it includes the anal sphincters. Occurs following a Valsalva maneuver, such as straining at stool, or with exercise.

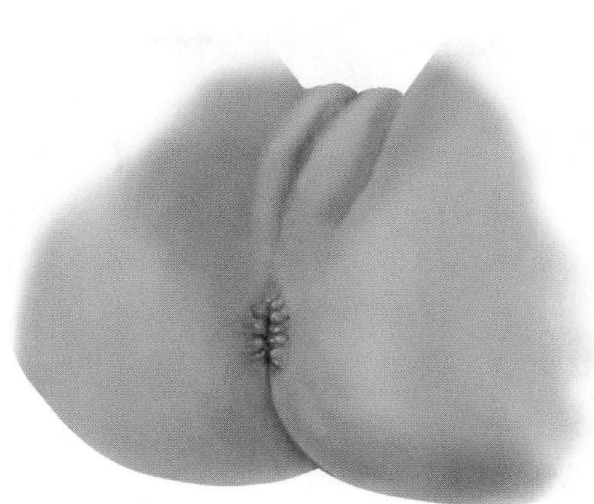

Pruritus Ani

Intense perianal itching is manifested by red, raised, thickened, excoriated skin around the anus. Common causes are pinworms in children and fungal infections in adults. The area is swollen and moist, and with a fungal infection, it appears dull grayish pink. The skin is dry and brittle with psychosomatic itching.

TABLE 25-2 Abnormalities of the Rectum

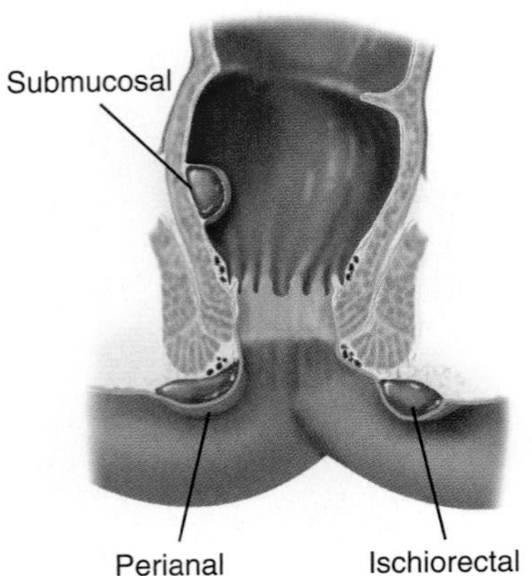

Abscess

A localized cavity of pus from infection in a pararectal space. Infection usually extends from an anal crypt. Characterized by persistent throbbing rectal pain. Termed by the space it occupies (e.g., a perianal abscess is superficial around the anal skin) and appears red, hot, swollen, indurated, and tender. An ischiorectal abscess is deep and tender to bi-digital palpation. It occurs laterally between the anus and ischial tuberosity and is uncommon.

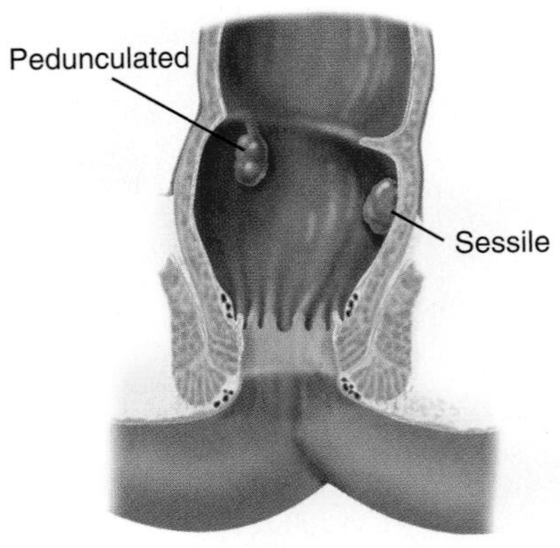

Rectal Polyp

A protruding growth from the rectal mucous membrane that is fairly common. The polyp may be *pedunculated* (on a stalk) or *sessile* (a mound on the surface, close to the mucosal wall). The soft nodule is difficult to palpate. Proctoscopy is needed as well as biopsy to screen for a malignant growth.

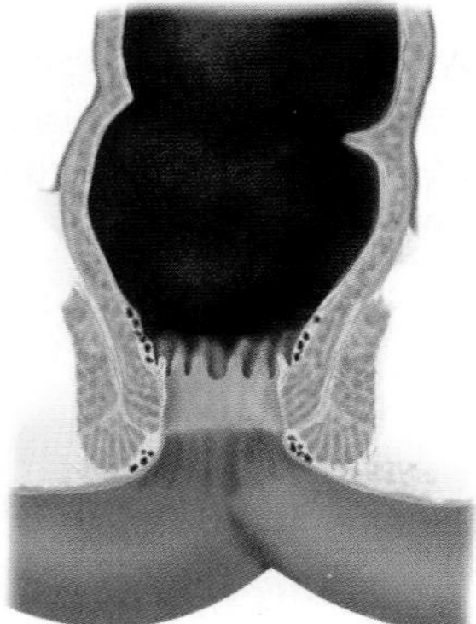

Fecal Impaction

A collection of hard, desiccated feces in the rectum. The obstruction often results from decreased bowel motility, in which more water is reabsorbed from the stool. Also occurs with retained barium from gastrointestinal x-ray examination. The person may complain of constipation or of diarrhea as a fecal stream passes around the impaction.

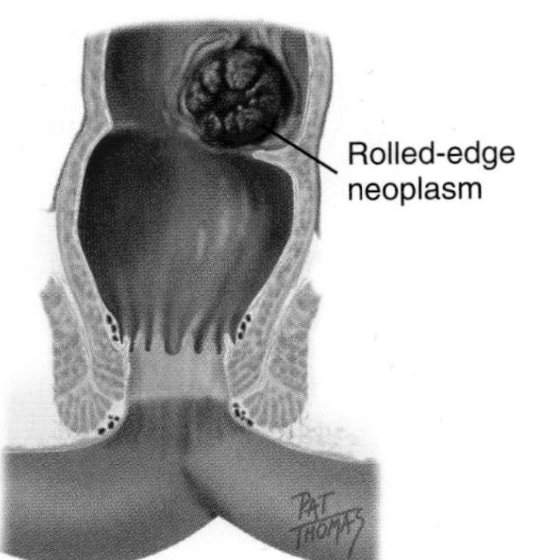

Carcinoma

A malignant neoplasm in the rectum is asymptomatic, thus the importance of routine rectal palpation. An early lesion may be a single firm nodule. You may palpate an ulcerated center with rolled edges. As the lesion grows, it has an irregular cauliflower shape and is fixed and stone-hard. Refer a person with any rectal lesion for further study because about half are malignant.

ABNORMAL FINDINGS FOR ADVANCED PRACTICE

TABLE 25-3 Abnormalities of the Prostate Gland

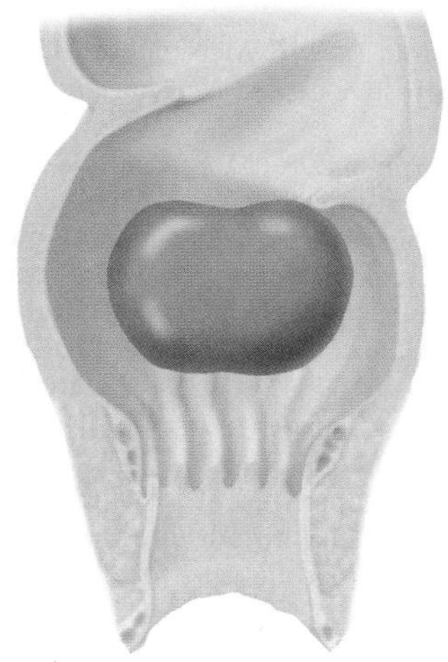

Benign Prostatic Hypertrophy (BPH)

S: Urinary frequency, urgency, hesitancy, straining to urinate, weak stream, intermittent stream, sensation of incomplete emptying, nocturia.

O: A symmetric nontender enlargement, commonly occurs in males beginning in the middle years. The prostate surface feels smooth, rubbery, or firm (like the consistency of the nose), with the median sulcus obliterated.

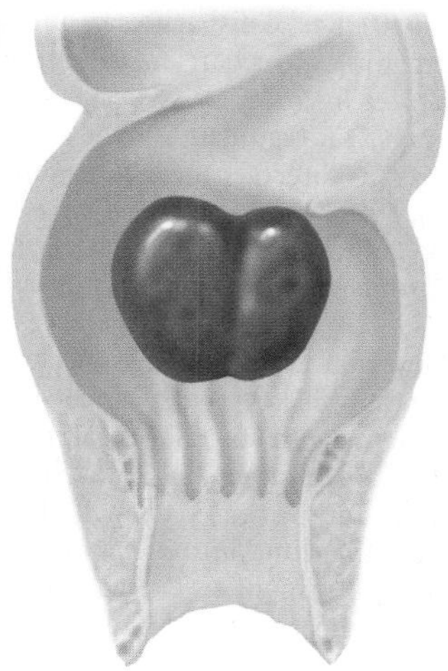

Prostatitis

S: Fever, chills, malaise, urinary frequency and urgency, dysuria, urethral discharge; dull, aching pain in perineal and rectal area.

O: An exquisitely tender enlargement is *acute* inflammation of the prostate gland yielding a swollen, slightly asymmetric gland that is quite tender to palpation.

With a chronic inflammation, the signs can vary from tender enlargement with a boggy feel to isolated firm areas due to fibrosis. Or the gland may feel normal.

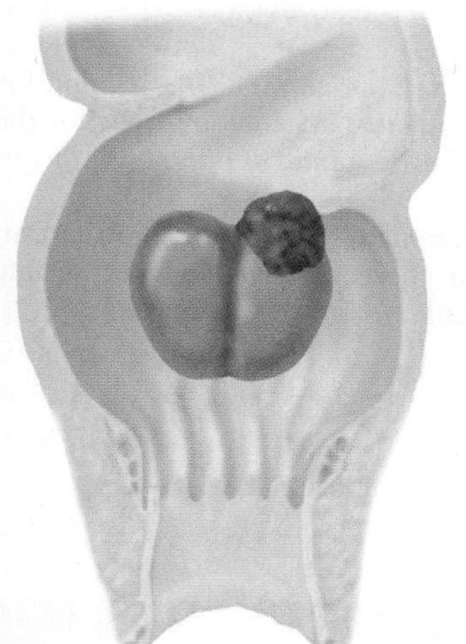

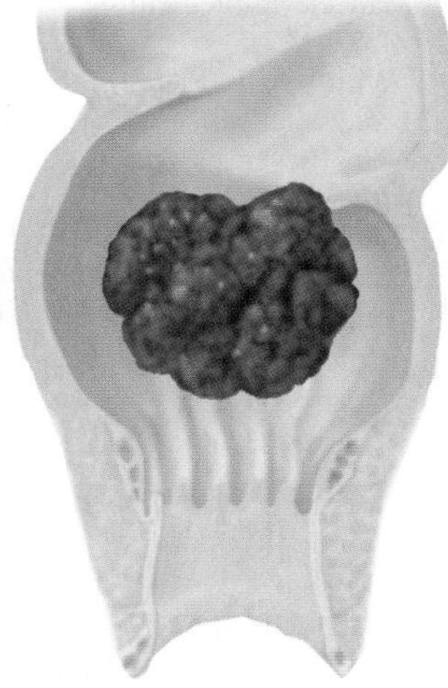

Carcinoma

S: Frequency, nocturia, hematuria, weak stream, hesitancy, pain or burning on urination; continuous pain in lower back, pelvis, thighs.

O: A malignant neoplasm often starts as a single hard nodule on the posterior surface, producing asymmetry and a change in consistency. As it invades normal tissue, multiple hard nodules appear, or the entire gland feels stone-hard and fixed. The median sulcus is obliterated.

S, Subjective data; *O*, objective data.

BIBLIOGRAPHY

1. American Cancer Society. (2010). *Cancer facts and figures 2010.* Atlanta: Author.
2. American Cancer Society. (2010). *Cancer facts and figures 2010 (Special section: Prostate cancer, pp. 23-36).* Atlanta: Author.
3. Arras-Boyd, R. E., Boyd, R. E., & Gaehle, K. (2009). Reaching men at highest risk for undetected prostate cancer. *International Journal of Men's Health, 8*(2), 116-128.
4. Ayanian, J. Z. (2010). Racial disparities in outcomes of colorectal cancer screening: biology or barriers to optimal care? *Journal of the National Cancer Institute, 102*(8), 511-513.
5. Berry, J., Bumpers, K., Ogunlade, V., et al. (2009). Examining racial disparities in colorectal cancer care. *Journal of Psychosocial Oncology, 27*(1), 59-83.
6. Bouras, E. P., & Tangalos, E. G. (2009). Chronic constipation in the elderly. *Gastroenterology Clinics of North America, 38*(3), 463-480.
7. Chan, J. A., Meyerhardt, J. A., Niedzwiecki, D., et al. (2008). Association of family history with cancer recurrence and survival among patients with stage III colon cancer. *Journal of the American Medical Association, 229*(21), 2515-2523.
8. Daly, J. M., Merchant, M. L., & Levy, B. T. (2009). Colorectal cancer screening. *American Journal of Nursing, 109*(10), 60-62.
9. Delongchamps, N. B., Singh, A., & Haas, G. P. (2007). Epidemiology of prostate cancer in Africa: another step in the understanding of the disease? *Current Problems in Cancer, 31*(3), 226-236.

9a. Dunivan, G. C., Heymen, S., Palsson, O. S., et al. (2010). Fecal incontinence in primary care: Prevalence, diagnosis, and health care utilization. *American Journal of Obstetrics and Gynecology, 202*, 493.e1-e6.

10. Edwards, B. K., Ward, E., Kohler, B. A., et al. (2010). Annual report to the nation on the status of cancer, 1975-2006, featuring colorectal cancer trends and impact of interventions (risk factors, screening, and treatment) to reduce future rates. *Cancer, 116*(3), 544-573.
11. Fried, R. G. (2010). Performing digital rectal examination can detect cancers. *American Family Physician, 31*(9), 1073.
12. Gray, M., & Sims, T. (2006). Prostate cancer: prevention and management of the localized disease. *Nurse Practitioner, 31*(9), 14-31.
13. Greene, M. D. (2009). Diagnosis and management of HPV-related anal dysplasia. *Nurse Practitioner, 34*(5), 45-51.
14. Guittet, L., Bouvier, V., Mariotte, N., et al. (2009). Comparison of a guaiac and an immunochemical faecal occult blood test for the detection of colonic lesions according to lesion type and location. *British Journal of Cancer, 100*(8), 1230-1235.
15. Holcomb, S. S. (2008). Colorectal cancer: new screening guideline. *Nurse Practitioner, 33*(9), 13-18.
16. Imperiale, T. F., Ransohoff, D. F., Itzkowitz, S. H., et al. (2004). Fecal DNA versus fecal occult blood for colorectal-cancer screening in an average-risk population. *New England Journal of Medicine, 351*(26), 2704-2714.
17. Jones, R. A., Steeves, R., & Williams, I. (2009). How African American men decide whether or not to get prostate cancer screening. *Cancer Nursing, 32*(2), 166-172.
18. Knight, D. (2004). Health care screening for men who have sex with men. *American Family Physician, 69*(9), 2149-2156.
19. Kong, A. P., & Stamos, M. J. (2005). Anorectal complications: office diagnosis and treatment, Part 1. *Consultant, 45*(7), 731-734.
20. Kong, A. P., & Stamos, M. J. (2005). Anorectal complications: office diagnosis and treatment, Part 2. *Consultant, 45*(7), 735-738.
21. Lee, T. H., Kantoff, P. W., & McNaughton-Collins, M. F. (2009). Screening for prostate cancer. *New England Journal of Medicine, 360*(13), e18.
22. Levin, B., Lieberman, D. A., McFarland, B., et al. (2008). Screening and surveillance for the early detection of colorectal cancer and adenomatous polyps, 2008: a joint guideline from the American Cancer Society, the U.S. Multi-Society Task force on Colorectal Cancer, and the American College of Radiology. *CA: A Cancer Journal for Clinicians, 58*(3), 130-156.
23. Lewis, J. E., Soler-Vilá, H., Clark, P. E., et al. (2009). Intake of plant foods and associated nutrients in prostate cancer risk. *Nutrition and Cancer, 61*(2), 216-224.
24. Marlow, N. M., Halpern, M. T., Pavluck, A. L., et al. (2010). Disparities associated with advanced prostate cancer stage at diagnosis. *Journal of Health Care for the Poor and Underserved, 21*(1), 112-131.
25. Moses, K. A., Paciorek, A. T., Penson, D. F., et al. (2010). Impact of ethnicity on primary treatment choice and mortality in men with prostate cancer: data from CaPSURE. *Journal of Clinical Oncology, 28*(6), 1069-1074.
26. Peters, D. P. (2008). Colon cancer screening: recommendations and barriers to patient participation. *Nurse Practitioner, 33*(12), 14-21.

26a. Philichi, L. (2008). Pediatric constipation and encopresis. *Gastroenterology Nursing, 31*(2), 121-130.

27. Sanford, K. W., & McPherson, R. A. (2009). Fecal occult blood testing. *Clinics in Laboratory Medicine, 29*(3), 523-541.
28. Walia, R., Mahajan, L., & Steffen, R., (2009). Recent advances in chronic constipation. *Current Opinion in Pediatrics, 21*(5), 661-666.
29. Wallace, M., Bailey, D. E., & Brion, J. (2009). Shedding light on prostate cancer. *Nurse Practitioner, 34*(10), 25-34.
30. Ward-Smith, P. (2009). Screening and preventing prostate cancer: implementing the evidence. *Urologic Nursing, 29*(6), 437-443.
31. Whitlock, E. P., Lin, J. S., Liles, E., et al. (2008). Screening for colorectal cancer: a targeted, updated systematic review for the U.S. Preventive Services Task Force. *Annals of Internal Medicine, 149*(9), 638-658.
32. Wolf, A. M., Wender, R. C., Etzioni, R. B., et al. (2010). American Cancer Society guideline for the early detection of prostate cancer: update 2010. *CA: A Cancer Journal for Clinicians, 60*(2), 70-98.

Summary Checklist: Anus, Rectum, and Prostate Examination

For a PDA-downloadable version, go to http://evolve.elsevier.com/Jarvis/.

1. **Inspect anus** and perianal area.
2. Inspect during Valsalva maneuver.
3. **Palpate anal canal** and rectum on all adults.
4. **Test stool** for occult blood.

CHAPTER

26

Female Genitourinary System

evolve WEBSITE

http://evolve.elsevier.com/Jarvis/

- Animations
- Audio Key Points
- Bedside Assessment Summary Checklist
- Health Promotion Guide
  Cervical Cancer
  Sexually Transmitted Infections (STIs)
- NCLEX Review Questions
- Physical Examination Summary Checklists
- Quick Assessment for Common Conditions
  Premenstrual Syndrome (PMS)
  Renal Calculus (Urolithiasis)
  Urinary Tract Infection
- Video—Assessment
  Female Genitalia and Rectum

OUTLINE

Structure and Function, 725

External Genitalia
Internal Genitalia

Subjective Data, 729

Health History Questions

Objective Data, 732

Preparation
Position
External Genitalia
Internal Genitalia

Documentation and Critical Thinking, 750

Abnormal Findings for Advanced Practice, 752

STRUCTURE AND FUNCTION

EXTERNAL GENITALIA

The external genitalia are called the **vulva,** or pudendum (Fig. 26-1). The **mons pubis** is a round, firm pad of adipose tissue covering the symphysis pubis. After puberty, it is covered with hair in the pattern of an inverted triangle. The **labia majora** are two rounded folds of adipose tissue extending from the mons pubis down and around to the perineum. After puberty, hair covers the outer surfaces of the labia, whereas the inner folds are smooth and moist and contain sebaceous follicles.

Inside the labia majora are two smaller, darker folds of skin, the **labia minora.** These are joined anteriorly at the clitoris where they form a hood, or prepuce. The labia minora are joined posteriorly by a transverse fold, the **frenulum,** or fourchette. The **clitoris** is a small, pea-shaped erectile body, homologous with the male penis and highly sensitive to tactile stimulation.

The labial structures encircle a boat-shaped space, or cleft, termed the **vestibule.** Within it are numerous openings. The **urethral meatus** appears as a dimple 2.5 cm posterior to the clitoris. Surrounding the urethral meatus are the tiny, multiple **paraurethral (Skene's) glands.** Their ducts are not visible but open posterior to the urethra at the 5 and 7 o'clock positions.

The **vaginal orifice** is posterior to the urethral meatus. It appears either as a thin median slit or as a large opening with irregular edges, depending on the presentation of the membranous **hymen.** The hymen is a thin, circular or

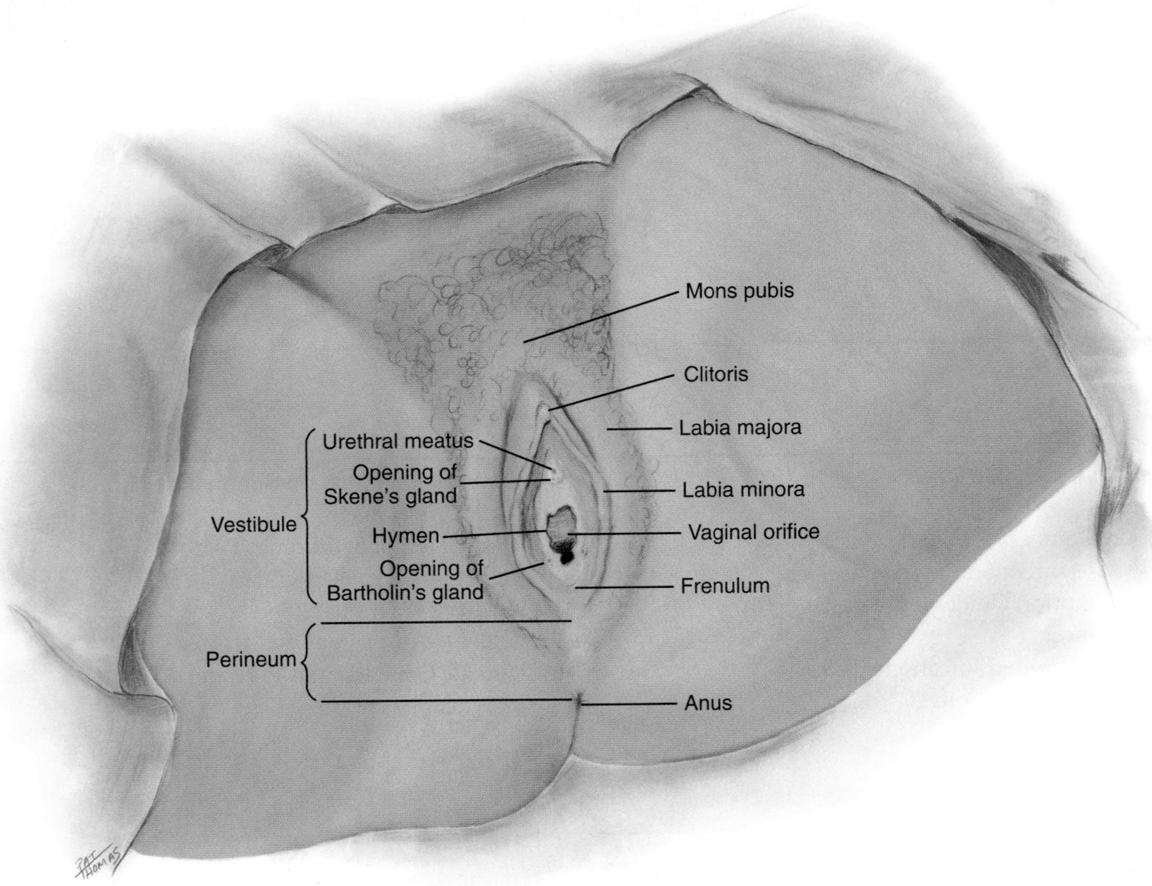

26-1

crescent-shaped fold that may cover part of the vaginal orifice or may be absent completely. On either side and posterior to the vaginal orifice are two **vestibular (Bartholin's) glands,** which secrete a clear lubricating mucus during intercourse. Their ducts are not visible but open in the groove between the labia minora and the hymen.

INTERNAL GENITALIA

The internal genitalia include the **vagina,** a flattened, tubular canal extending from the orifice up and backward into the pelvis (Fig. 26-2). It is 9 cm long and sits between the rectum posteriorly and the bladder and urethra anteriorly. Its walls are in thick transverse folds, or **rugae,** enabling the vagina to dilate widely during childbirth.

At the end of the canal, the uterine **cervix** projects into the vagina. In the nulliparous female, the cervix appears as a smooth doughnut-shaped area with a small circular hole, or **os.** After childbirth, the os is slightly enlarged and irregular. The cervical epithelium is of two distinct types. The vagina and cervix are covered with smooth, pink, stratified squamous epithelium. Inside the os, the endocervical canal is lined with columnar epithelium that looks red and rough. The point where these two tissues meet is the **squamocolumnar junction** and is not visible.

A continuous recess is present around the cervix, termed the **anterior fornix** in front and the **posterior fornix** in back. Behind the posterior fornix, another deep recess is formed by the peritoneum. It dips down between the rectum and cervix to form the **rectouterine pouch,** or **cul-de-sac of Douglas.**

The **uterus** is a pear-shaped, thick-walled, muscular organ. It is flattened anteroposteriorly, measuring 5.5 to 8 cm long by 3.5 to 4 cm wide and 2 to 2.5 cm thick. It is freely movable, not fixed, and usually tilts forward and superior to the bladder (a position labeled as *anteverted* and *anteflexed,* see p. 745).

The **fallopian tubes** are two pliable, trumpet-shaped tubes, 10 cm in length, extending from the uterine fundus laterally to the brim of the pelvis. There they curve posteriorly, their fimbriated ends located near the **ovaries.** The two ovaries are located one on each side of the uterus at the level of the anterior superior iliac spine. Each is oval-shaped, 3 cm long by 2 cm wide by 1 cm thick, and serves to develop ova (eggs) and the female hormones.

DEVELOPMENTAL COMPETENCE

Infants and Adolescents

At birth, the external genitalia are engorged because of the presence of maternal estrogen. The structures recede in a few weeks, remaining small until puberty. The ovaries are located in the abdomen during childhood. The uterus is small with a straight axis and no anteflexion.

At puberty, estrogens stimulate the growth of cells in the reproductive tract and the development of secondary sex characteristics. The first signs of puberty are breast and pubic hair development, beginning between the ages of 8½ and 13 years. These signs are usually concurrent, but it is not abnormal if they do not develop together. They take about 3 years to complete.

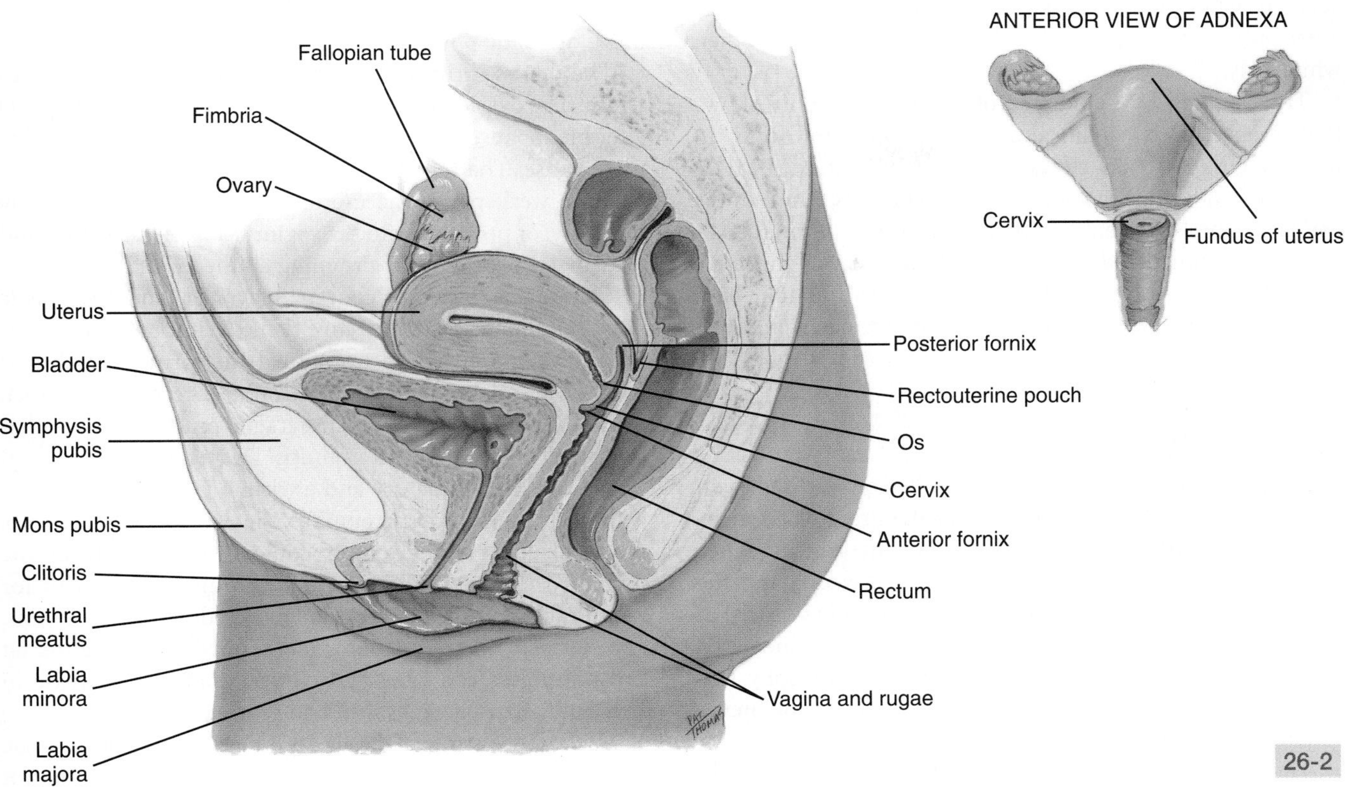

26-2

Menarche occurs during the latter half of this sequence, just after the peak of growth velocity. Irregularity of the menstrual cycle is common during adolescence because of the girl's occasional failure to ovulate. With menarche, the uterine body flexes on the cervix. The ovaries now are in the pelvic cavity.

Tanner's table on the five stages of pubic hair development (sexual maturity rating [SMR]) is helpful in teaching girls the expected sequence of sexual development (Table 26-1). These data may not generalize to all racial groups; mature Asian women normally have fine, sparse pubic hair.

Data from NHANES III found that contemporary U.S. girls' development is consistent with Tanner's findings.[40] However, African-American and Mexican-American girls had pubic hair and achieved menarche at younger ages than white girls. The mean age at onset of pubic hair and menarche was 9.5 and 12.1 years for African-American girls; 10.3 and 12.2 years for Mexican-American girls; and 10.5 and 12.7

TABLE 26-1 Sexual Maturity Ratings (SMR) in Girls

Stage 1 Preadolescent. No pubic hair. Mons and labia covered with fine vellus hair as on abdomen.

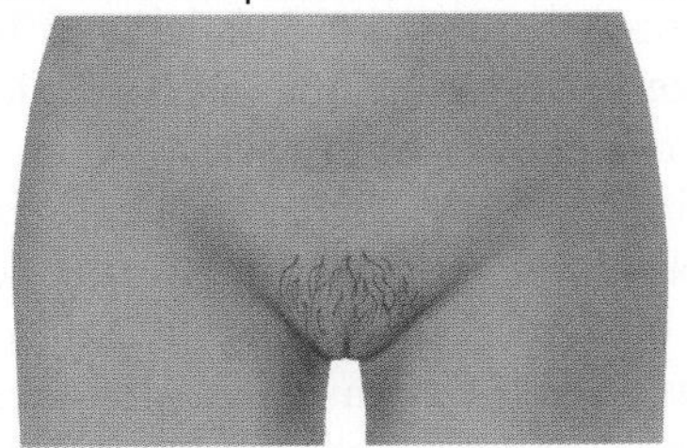

Stage 2 Growth sparse and mostly on labia. Long, downy hair, slightly pigmented, straight or only slightly curly.

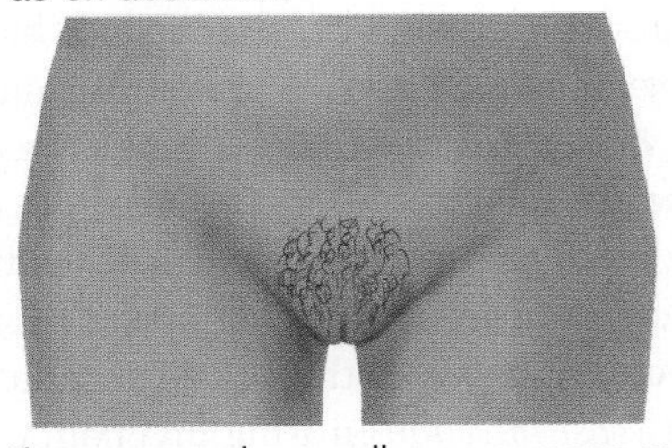

Stage 3 Growth sparse and spreading over mons pubis. Hair is darker, coarser, curlier.

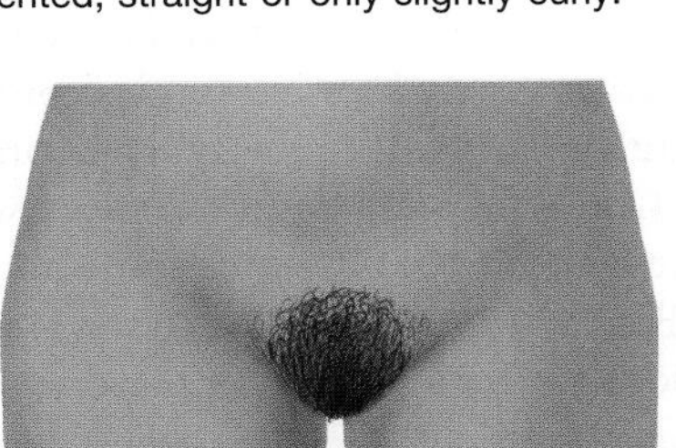

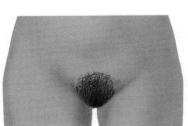

Stage 4 Hair is adult in type but over smaller area; none on medial thigh.

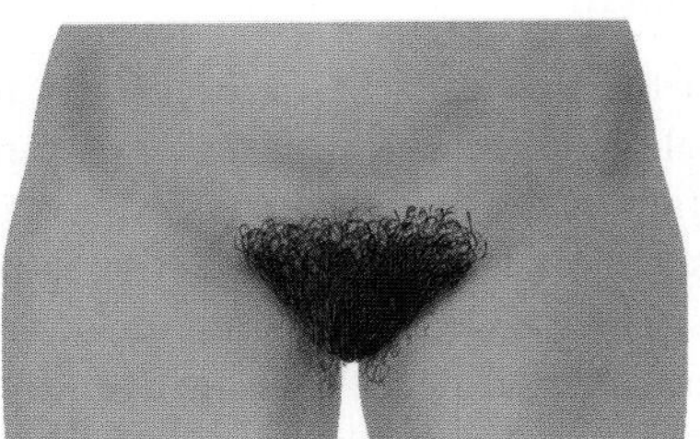

Stage 5 Adult in type and pattern; inverse triangle. Also on medial thigh surface.

Adapted from Tanner, J.M. (1962). *Growth at adolescence.* Oxford, England: Blackwell Scientific.

years for white girls. Thus African-American girls on average enter puberty first, followed by Mexican-American and then white girls.[34,40]

The ongoing U.S. epidemic of childhood obesity shows that menarche is significantly more likely to occur in preteen girls with an elevated body mass index (BMI).[34] The median age of achieving menarche was 5.4 months earlier in obese preteen girls than in girls with normal BMI. The association of adiposity with menarche was independent of race or ethnicity. In conclusion, BMI should be a major consideration when a clinician evaluates pubertal development.[34]

The Pregnant Woman

A complete discussion of the pregnant woman follows in Chapter 29. In summary, shortly after the first missed menstrual period, the genitalia show signs of the growing fetus. The cervix softens *(Goodell sign)* at 4 to 6 weeks, and the vaginal mucosa and cervix look cyanotic *(Chadwick sign)* at 8 to 12 weeks. These changes occur because of increased vascularity and edema of the cervix and hypertrophy and hyperplasia of the cervical glands. The isthmus of the uterus softens *(Hegar sign)* at 6 to 8 weeks.

The greatest change is in the uterus itself. It increases in capacity by 500 to 1000 times its nonpregnant state, at first because of hormone stimulation and then because of the increasing size of its contents.[12] The nonpregnant uterus has a flattened pear shape. Its early growth encroaches on the space occupied by the bladder, producing the symptom of urinary frequency. By 10 to 12 weeks' gestation, the uterus becomes globular in shape and is too large to stay in the pelvis. At 20 to 24 weeks, the uterus has an oval shape. It rises almost to the liver, displacing the intestines superiorly and laterally.

A clot of thick, tenacious mucus forms in the spaces of the cervical canal (the mucus plug), which protects the fetus from infection. The mucus plug dislodges when labor begins at the end of term, producing a sign of labor called "bloody show." Cervical and vaginal secretions increase during pregnancy and are thick, white, and more acidic. The increased acidity occurs because of the action of *Lactobacillus acidophilus,* which changes glycogen into lactic acid. The acidic pH keeps pathogenic bacteria from multiplying in the vagina, but the increase in glycogen increases the risk for candidiasis (commonly called a *yeast infection*) during pregnancy.

The Aging Woman

In contrast to the slowly declining hormones in the aging male, the female's hormonal milieu decreases rapidly. *Menopause* is cessation of the menses. Usually this occurs around 48 to 51 years, although a wide variation of ages from 35 to 60 years exists. The stage of menopause includes the preceding 1 to 2 years of decline in ovarian function, shown by irregular menses that gradually become farther apart and produce a lighter flow. Ovaries stop producing progesterone and estrogen. Because cells in the reproductive tract are estrogen dependent, decreased estrogen levels during menopause bring dramatic physical changes.

The uterus shrinks in size because of decreased myometrium. The ovaries atrophy to 1 to 2 cm and are not palpable after menopause. Ovulation still may occur sporadically after menopause. The sacral ligaments relax and the pelvic musculature weakens, so the uterus droops. Sometimes it may protrude, or prolapse, into the vagina. The cervix shrinks and looks paler with a thick, glistening epithelium.

The vagina becomes shorter, narrower, and less elastic because of increased connective tissue. Without sexual activity, the vagina atrophies to one-half its former length and width. The vaginal epithelium atrophies, becoming thinner, drier, and itchy. This results in a fragile mucosal surface that is at risk for bleeding and vaginitis. Decreased vaginal secretions leave the vagina dry and at risk for irritation and pain with intercourse (dyspareunia). The vaginal pH becomes more alkaline, and glycogen content decreases from the decreased estrogen. These factors also increase the risk for vaginitis because they create a suitable medium for pathogens.

Externally, the mons pubis looks smaller because the fat pad atrophies. The labia and clitoris gradually decrease in size. Pubic hair becomes thin and sparse.

Declining estrogen levels produce some physiologic changes in the female sexual response cycle: reduced amount of vaginal secretion and lubrication during excitement; shorter duration of orgasm; and rapid resolution. However, these changes do not affect sexual pleasure and function. As with the male, the older female is capable of sexual expression and function given reasonably good health and an interested partner. Aging women greatly outnumber their male counterparts, and aging women are more likely to be single, whereas males their same age are more likely to be married.

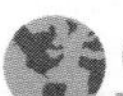

CULTURE AND GENETICS

The increased use of the Papanicolaou (Pap) test in the United States has resulted in a 74% decline in the cervical cancer death rate between 1955 and 1992.[2] Today, however, cervical cancer occurs most often in Hispanic women; their incidence is over twice that of white women. African-American women have a 50% higher incidence rate than white women. Relative to white women, Hispanic women are less likely to die of cervical cancer despite their lower socioeconomic status (SES), known as the "Hispanic paradox."[11] Reasons are unclear but include differences in comorbid conditions, social support, cultural influences, and religion/faith.

Female circumcision, known as *infibulation* or *female genital mutilation,* is an invasive surgical procedure that is performed on girls before puberty. It is practiced within Aboriginal, Christian, and Muslim families who have emigrated to the United States from western and southern Asia, the Middle East, and large areas of Africa. It is a social custom, not a religious practice. This procedure involves removal, partial or total, of the clitoris and is believed to inhibit sexual pleasure. There are about 130 to 140 million women alive today who have had this procedure.[22] The procedure is outlawed in the United States.

SUBJECTIVE DATA

1. Menstrual history
2. Obstetric history
3. Menopause
4. Self-care behaviors
5. Urinary symptoms
6. Vaginal discharge
7. Past history
8. Sexual activity
9. Contraceptive use
10. Sexually transmitted infection (STI) contact
11. STI risk reduction

Examiner Asks	Rationale
1. Menstrual history. Tell me about your menstrual periods:	**Menstrual history** is usually nonthreatening; thus it is a good place to start.
• Date of your last menstrual period?	LMP—last menstrual period.
• Age at first period?	Menarche—mean age at onset at 12 to 13 years; delayed onset suggests endocrine or underweight problem.
• How often are your periods?	Cycle—normally every 18 to 45 days. Amenorrhea—absent menses.
• How many days does your period last? • Usual amount of flow: light, medium, heavy? How many pads or tampons do you use each day or hour?	Duration—average 3 to 7 days. Menorrhagia—heavy menses.
• Any clotting?	Clotting indicates heavy flow or vaginal pooling.
• Any pain or cramps before or during period? How do you treat it? Interfere with daily activities? Any other associated symptoms: bloating, breast tenderness, moodiness? Any spotting between periods?	Dysmenorrhea.
2. Obstetric history. Have you ever been pregnant? • How many times? • How many babies have you had? • Any miscarriage or abortion?	Gravida—number of pregnancies. Para—number of births. Abortions—interrupted pregnancies, including elective abortions and spontaneous miscarriages.
• For each pregnancy, describe: duration, any complication, labor and delivery, baby's sex, birth weight, condition. • Do you think you may be pregnant now? What symptoms have you noticed?	
3. Menopause. Have your periods slowed down or stopped? • Any associated symptoms of menopause (e.g., hot flash, night sweats, numbness and tingling, headache, palpitations, drenching sweats, mood swings, vaginal dryness, itching)? Any treatment?	**Menopause**—cessation of menstruation. Perimenopausal period from 40 to 55 years has hormone shifts, resulting in vasomotor instability.
• If hormone replacement, how much? How is it working? Any side effects?	Side effects of HRT include fluid retention, breast pain, vaginal bleeding, and breast cancer risk.
• How do you feel about going through menopause?	Although a normal life stage, reaction varies from acceptance to feelings of loss.
4. Self-care behaviors. How often do you have a gynecologic checkup?	Begin cervical cancer screening within 3 years after first vaginal intercourse or age 21 years, and continue annually until age 30. After age 30, if have three consecutive normal Pap tests, women may be screened every 2 to 3 years.[37]
• Last Pap smear? Results? • Has your mother ever mentioned taking hormones while pregnant with you?	Maternal ingestion of diethylstilbestrol (DES) causes cervical and vaginal abnormalities in female offspring requiring frequent follow-up.

Examiner Asks	Rationale
5. Urinary symptoms. Any problems with urinating? Frequently and small amounts? Cannot wait to urinate?	Urgency.
• Any burning or pain on urinating?	Dysuria.
• Awaken during night to urinate?	Nocturia.
• Blood in the urine?	Hematuria.
• Urine dark, cloudy, foul smelling?	Bile in urine or urinary tract infection.
• Any difficulty controlling urine or wetting yourself?	**Urge** incontinence—involuntary urine loss from overactive detrusor muscle in bladder. It contracts, causing urgent need to void.
• Urinate with a sneeze, laugh, cough, bearing down?	**Stress** incontinence—involuntary urine loss with physical strain, sneezing, or coughing.
6. Vaginal discharge. Any unusual **vaginal discharge?** Increased amount?	Normal discharge is small, clear or cloudy, and always nonirritating.
• Character or color: white, yellow-green, gray, curdlike, foul smelling?	Suggests vaginal infection; character of discharge often suggests causative organism (see Table 26-5 on p. 756).
• When did this begin?	Acute versus chronic problem.
• Is the discharge associated with vaginal itching, rash, pain with intercourse?	Rash is result of irritation from discharge. Dyspareunia occurs with vaginitis of any cause.
• Taking any medications?	Factors that increase risk for vaginitis: • Oral contraceptives increase glycogen content of vaginal epithelium, providing fertile medium for some organisms. • Broad-spectrum antibiotics alter balance of normal flora.
• Family history of diabetes?	• Diabetes increases glycogen content.
• What part of your menstrual cycle are you in now?	• Menses, postpartum, menopause have a more alkaline vaginal pH.
• Use a vaginal douche? How often?	• Frequent douching alters pH.
• Use feminine hygiene spray?	• Spray has risk for contact dermatitis.
• Wear nonventilating underpants, pantyhose?	• Local irritation.
• Treated the discharge with anything? Result?	
7. Past history. Any other problems in the genital area? Sores or lesions—now or in the past? How were these treated? • Any abdominal pain?	
• Any past surgery on uterus, ovaries, vagina?	Assess feelings. Some fear loss of sexual response after hysterectomy, which may cause problems in intimate relationships.
8. Sexual activity. Often women have a question about their **sexual relationship** and how it affects their health. Do you? • Are you in a relationship involving sex now? • Are aspects of sex satisfactory to you and your partner? • Satisfied with the way you and partner communicate about sex? • Satisfied with your ability to respond sexually? • Do you have more than one sexual partner?	Begin with open-ended question to assess individual needs. Include appropriate questions as a routine: • Communicates that you accept individual's sexual activity and believe it is important. • Your comfort with discussion prompts person's interest and possibly relief that the topic has been introduced. • Establishes a database for comparison with any future sexual activities. • Provides opportunity to screen sexual problems.

Examiner Asks	Rationale
• What is your sexual preference: relationship with a man, with a woman, both?	The practice environment must be welcoming and respectful of lesbians and bisexual women to discuss their health concerns.
9. **Contraceptive use.** Currently planning a pregnancy, or avoiding pregnancy? • Do you and your partner use a **contraceptive?** Which method? Is this satisfactory? Do you have any questions about method?	Assess smoking history. Oral contraceptives, together with cigarette smoking, increase the risk for vascular problems.
• Which methods have you used in the past? Have you and partner discussed having children? • Have you ever had any problems becoming pregnant?	Infertility is considered after 1 year of engaging in unprotected sexual intercourse without conceiving.
10. **Sexually transmitted infection (STI) contact.** Any sexual contact with partner having an STI, such as gonorrhea, herpes, HIV/AIDS, chlamydial infection, venereal warts, syphilis? When? How was this treated? Were there any complications?	An STI includes all conditions that can be transmitted during intimate sexual contact with an infected partner.
11. **STI risk reduction.** Any precautions to reduce risk for STIs? Use condoms at each episode of sexual intercourse?	

Additional History for Infants and Children

Examiner Asks	Rationale
1. Does your child have any problem urinating? Pain with urinating, crying, holding genitals? Urinary tract infection? • (If the child is older than 2 to 2½ years) Has toilet training started? How is it progressing? • Does the child wet bed at night? Is this a problem for child or you (parents)? What have you (parents) done?	
2. Problem with genital area: itching, rash, vaginal discharge?	Occurs with poor perineal hygiene or insertion of foreign body in vagina.
3. (To child) Has anyone ever touched you in between your legs and you did not want them to? Sometimes that happens to children. They should remember they have not been bad. They should try to tell a big person about it. Can you tell me three different big people you trust who you could talk to?	Screen for sexual abuse (see Chapter 7). For prevention, teach the child that it is not okay for someone to look at or touch her private parts while telling her it is a secret. Naming three trusted adults will include someone outside the family—important because most molestation is by a parent.

Additional History for Preadolescents and Adolescents

Use the following questions to assess sexual growth and development and sexual behavior. First:

- Ask questions that seem appropriate for girl's age, but norms vary widely. When in doubt, ask too many questions rather than omit something. Children obtain information, often misinformation, from the media and from peers at surprisingly early ages. You can be sure your information will be more thoughtful and accurate.
- Ask direct, matter-of-fact questions. Avoid sounding judgmental.
- Start with a *permission statement:* "Often girls your age experience …." This conveys that it is normal to think or feel a certain way.

Subjective Data

Examiner Asks	Rationale
• Try the open-ended question: "When did you ...." rather than "Do you ...." This is less threatening because it implies that the topic is normal and unexceptional.	
1. Around age 9 or 10 years, girls start to develop breasts and pubic hair. Have you ever seen charts and pictures of normal growth patterns for girls? Let us go over these now.	
2. Have your periods started? How did you feel? Were you prepared or surprised?	Assess attitude of girl and parents. Note inadequate preparation or attitude of distaste.
3. To who in your family do you talk about your body changes and about sex information? How do these talks go? Do you think you get enough information? What about sex education classes at school? Is there a teacher, a nurse or doctor, a minister, a counselor to whom you can talk? Often girls your age have questions about sexual activity. Do you have questions? Are you dating? Someone steady? Do you and your boyfriend have intercourse? Are you using condoms? What kind of protection did you use the last time you had sex?	Avoid the term "sexually active," which is ambiguous.
4. Has anyone ever talked to you about sexually transmitted infections, such as chlamydia, herpes, gonorrhea, or HIV/AIDS?	Teach STI risk reduction.
5. Have you and your parents discussed the human papillomavirus (HPV) vaccine (Gardasil, Cervarix)? It is recommended before girls become sexually active.	The HPV vaccines are approved for girls and women ages 9 to 26 for prevention of cervical cancer. They cannot protect against established infections.[2]
6. Sometimes a person touches a girl in a way that she does not want them to. Has that ever happened to you? If that happens, the girl should remember it is not her fault. She should tell another adult about it.	Screen for sexual abuse.
Additional History for the Aging Adult	
1. After menopause, noted any vaginal bleeding?	Postmenopausal bleeding warrants further workup and referral.
2. Any vaginal itching, discharge, pain with intercourse?	Associated with atrophic vaginitis.
3. Any pressure in genital area, loss of urine with cough or sneeze, back pain, or constipation?	Occurs with weakened pelvic musculature and uterine prolapse.
4. Are you in a relationship involving sex now? Are aspects of sex satisfactory to you and your partner? Is there adequate privacy for a sexual relationship?	

OBJECTIVE DATA

PREPARATION

Assemble the equipment before helping the woman into position. Arrange within easy reach. Familiarize yourself with the vaginal speculum before the examination. Practice opening and closing the blades, locking them into position, and releasing them. Try both metal and plastic types. Note that the plastic speculum locks and unlocks with a resounding click that can be alarming to the uninformed woman.

EQUIPMENT NEEDED

Gloves
Gooseneck lamp with a strong light
Vaginal speculum of appropriate size (Fig. 26-3):
- Graves speculum—useful for most adult women, available in varying lengths and widths

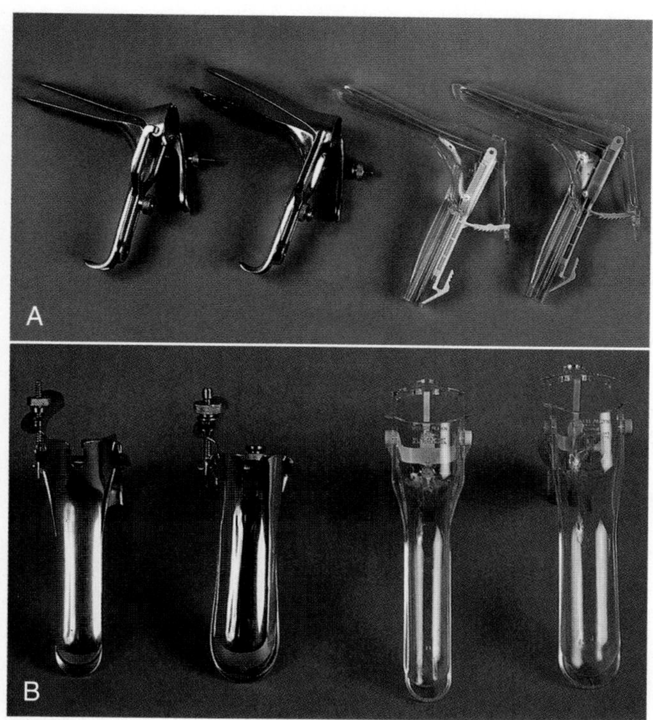

26-3

POSITION

Initially, the woman should be sitting up. An equal-status position is important to establish trust and rapport before the vaginal examination.

For the examination, the woman should be placed in the lithotomy position, with the examiner sitting on a stool. Help the woman into lithotomy position, with the body supine, feet in stirrups and knees apart, and buttocks at edge of examining table (Fig. 26-4). Ask the woman to lift her hips as you guide them to the edge of the table. Some women prefer to leave their shoes or socks on. Or, you can place an examination glove over each of the stirrups to warm the stirrups and keep her feet from slipping.

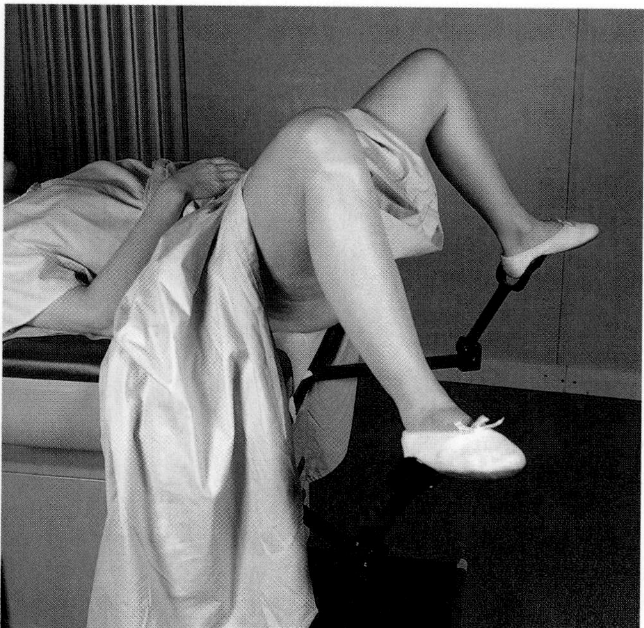
26-4

EQUIPMENT NEEDED—cont'd

- Pederson speculum—narrow blades, useful for young or postmenopausal women with narrowed introitus
- Large cotton-tipped applicators (rectal swabs)
- Materials for cytologic study:
  - Glass slide with frosted end
  - Sterile cytobrush or cotton-tipped applicator
  - Liquid-based cytology vial
  - Ayre spatula
  - Spray fixative
  - Specimen container for gonorrhea culture (GC)/chlamydia
  - Small bottle of normal saline solution, potassium hydroxide (KOH), and acetic acid (white vinegar)
- Lubricant

Place her arms at her sides or across the chest, not over the head, because this position only tightens the abdominal muscles. The traditional mode is to drape the woman fully, covering the stomach and legs, exposing only the vulva to your view. Be sure to push down the drape between the woman's legs and elevate her head so that you can see her face.

The lithotomy position leaves many women feeling helpless and vulnerable. Indeed, many women tolerate the pelvic examination because they consider it basic for health care, yet they find it embarrassing and uncomfortable. Previous examinations may have been painful or the previous examiner's attitude hurried and patronizing.

The examination need not be this way. You can help the woman relax, decrease her anxiety, and retain a sense of control by using these measures:

- Have her empty the bladder before the examination.
- Position the examination table so that her perineum is not exposed to an inadvertent open door.
- Ask if she would like a friend, family member, or chaperone present. Position this person by the woman's head to maintain privacy.
- Elevate her head and shoulders to a semisitting position to maintain eye contact.
- Place the stirrups so that the legs are not abducted too far.
- Explain each step in the examination before you do it.
- Assure the woman she can stop the examination at any point should she feel any discomfort.
- Use a gentle, firm touch and gradual movements.
- Communicate throughout the examination. Maintain a dialogue to share information.

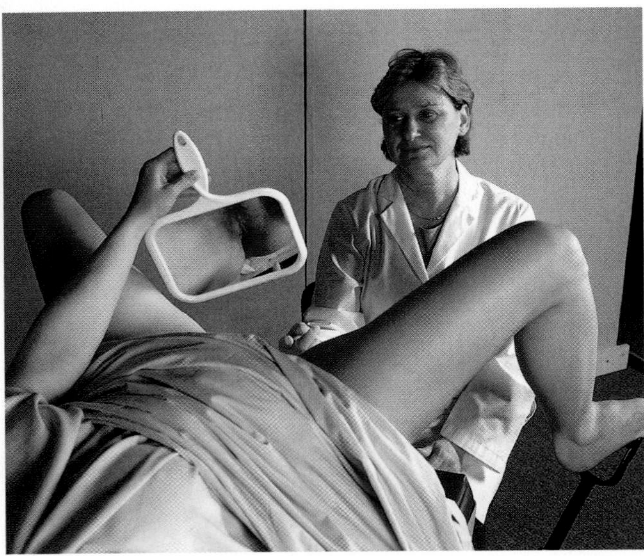

26-5

- Use the techniques of the *educational* or *mirror pelvic examination* (Fig. 26-5). This is a routine examination with some modifications in attitude, position, and communication. First, the woman is considered an active participant, one who is interested in learning and in sharing decisions about her own health care. The woman props herself up on one elbow, or the head of the table is raised. Her other hand holds a mirror between her legs, above the examiner's hands. The woman can see all that the examiner is doing and has a full view of her genitalia.

The mirror works well for teaching normal anatomy and its relationship to sexual behavior. Even women who are in a sexual relationship or who have had children may be surprisingly uninformed about their own anatomy. You will find the woman's enthusiasm on seeing her own cervix is rewarding too.

The mirror pelvic examination also works well when abnormalities arise, because the woman can see the rationale for treatment and can monitor progress at the next appointment. She is more willing to comply with treatment when she shares in the decision.

Normal Range of Findings	Abnormal Findings

EXTERNAL GENITALIA

Inspection

Note:

- Skin color is even; labia minora are a darker pink (Fig. 26-6).

Note any pigmented nevus or lesion that the woman cannot see. Refer any suspicious lesion for biopsy.

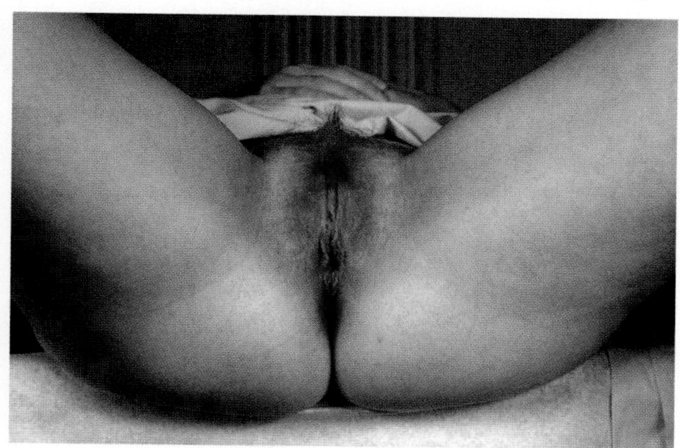

26-6

- Hair distribution is in the usual female pattern of inverted triangle, although it normally may trail up the abdomen toward the umbilicus.

Consider delayed puberty if no pubic hair or breast development has occurred by age 13 years.

Nits or lice at the base of pubic hair.

- Labia majora normally are symmetric, plump, and well formed. In the nulliparous woman, labia meet in the midline; after a vaginal delivery, the labia are gaping and slightly shriveled.

Swelling.

- No lesions should be present, except for occasional sebaceous cysts. These are yellowish, 1-cm nodules that are firm, nontender, and often multiple.

Excoriation, nodules, rash, or lesions (see Table 26-2, Abnormalities of the External Genitalia, p. 752).

With your gloved hand, separate the labia majora to inspect:

- Clitoris (Fig. 26-7).

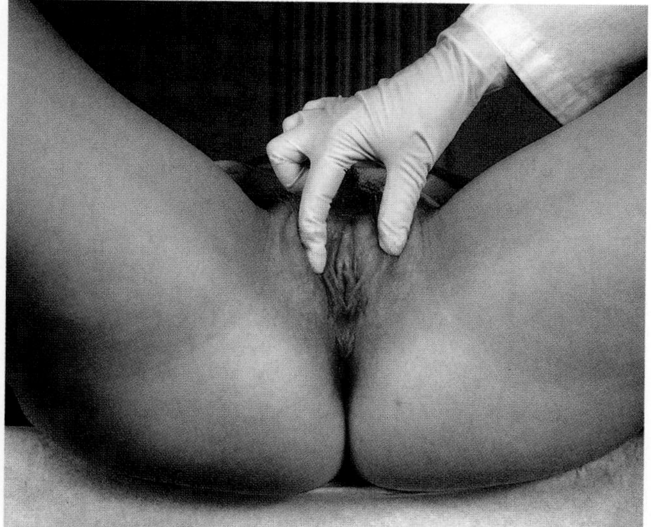

26-7

Normal Range of Findings	Abnormal Findings
• Labia minora are dark pink and moist, usually symmetric.	Inflammation or lesions.
• Urethral opening appears stellate or slitlike and is midline.	Polyp.
• Vaginal opening, or introitus, may appear as a narrow vertical slit or as a larger opening.	Foul-smelling, irritating discharge.
• Perineum is smooth. A well-healed episiotomy scar, midline or mediolateral, may be present after a vaginal birth.	
• Anus has coarse skin of increased pigmentation (see Chapter 25 for assessment).	

Palpation

Assess the urethra and Skene's glands (Fig. 26-8). Dip your gloved finger in a bowl of warm water to lubricate. Then insert your index finger into the vagina, and gently milk the urethra by applying pressure up and out. This procedure should produce no pain. If any discharge appears, culture it.

Tenderness.
Induration along urethra.
Urethral discharge.

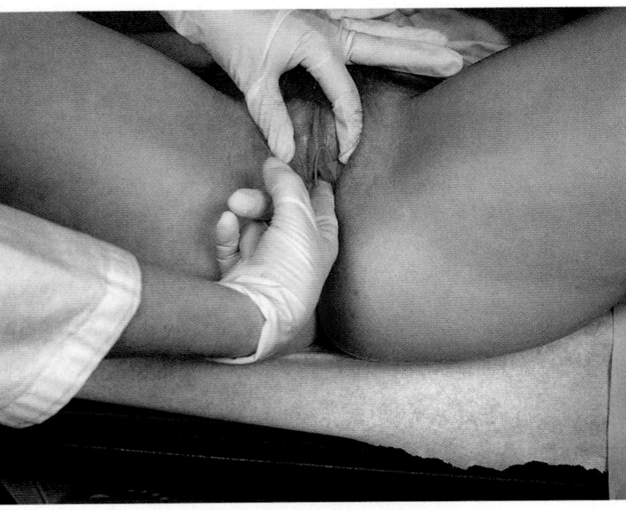

26-8

Assess Bartholin's glands. Palpate the posterior parts of the labia majora with your index finger in the vagina and your thumb outside (Fig. 26-9). Normally, the labia feel soft and homogeneous.

Swelling (see Table 26-2).
Induration.
Pain with palpation.
Erythema around or discharge from duct opening.

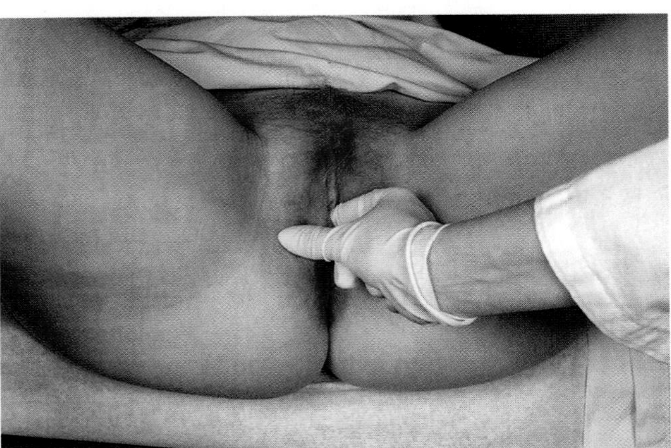

26-9

Objective Data

Normal Range of Findings	Abnormal Findings
Assess the support of pelvic musculature by using these maneuvers:	
1. Palpate the perineum. Normally, it feels thick, smooth, and muscular in the nulliparous woman and thin and rigid in the multiparous woman.	Tenderness. Paper-thin perineum.
2. Ask the woman to squeeze the vaginal opening around your fingers; it should feel tight in the nulliparous woman and have less tone in the multiparous woman.	Absent or decreased tone may diminish sexual satisfaction.
3. Using your index and middle fingers, separate the vaginal orifice and ask the woman to strain down. Normally, no bulging of vaginal walls or urinary incontinence occurs.	Bulging of the vaginal wall indicates cystocele, rectocele, or uterine prolapse (see Table 26-3, p. 754). Urinary incontinence.

INTERNAL GENITALIA

Speculum Examination

Select the proper-size speculum. Warm and lubricate the speculum under warm running water. Regarding Pap test cytology, evidence shows applying a small amount (dime size) of water-soluble gel lubricant on the outer inferior blade increases patient comfort and yields no more unsatisfactory slides than does water-only lubricant.[3,17] However, the effect of gel lubricant on interference with bacterial or viral cultures has not been tested.

A good technique is to dedicate one hand to the patient and the other hand to picking up equipment in the room. For example, hold the speculum in your left hand (the equipment hand), with the index and the middle fingers surrounding the blades and your thumb under the thumbscrew. This prevents the blades from opening painfully during insertion. With your right index and middle fingers (the patient hand), push the introitus down and open to relax the pubococcygeal muscle (Fig. 26-10). Tilt the width of the blades obliquely and insert the speculum past your right fingers, applying any pressure *downward.* This avoids pressure on the sensitive urethra above it.

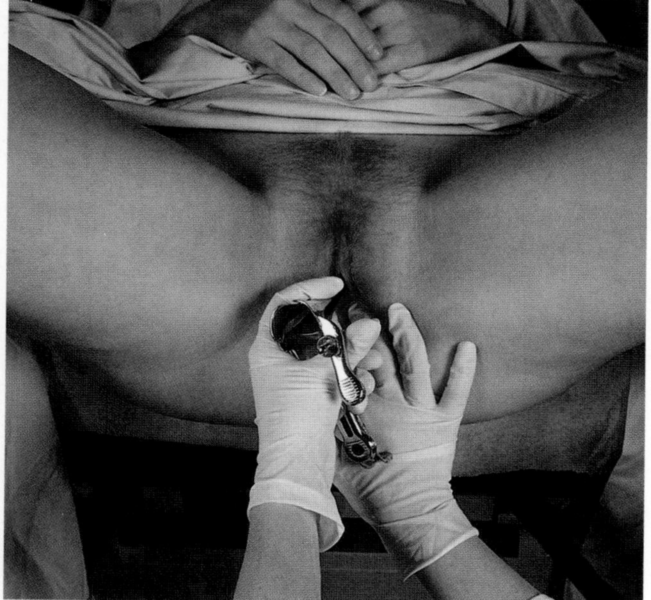

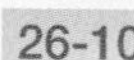
26-10

Objective Data

Normal Range of Findings

Ease insertion by asking the woman to bear down. This method relaxes the perineal muscles and opens the introitus. (With experience, you can combine speculum insertion with assessing the support of the vaginal muscles.) As the blades pass your right fingers, withdraw your fingers. Now change the hand holding the speculum to your right hand and turn the width of the blades horizontally. Continue to insert in a 45-degree angle *downward* toward the small of the woman's back (Fig. 26-11). This matches the natural slope of the vagina.

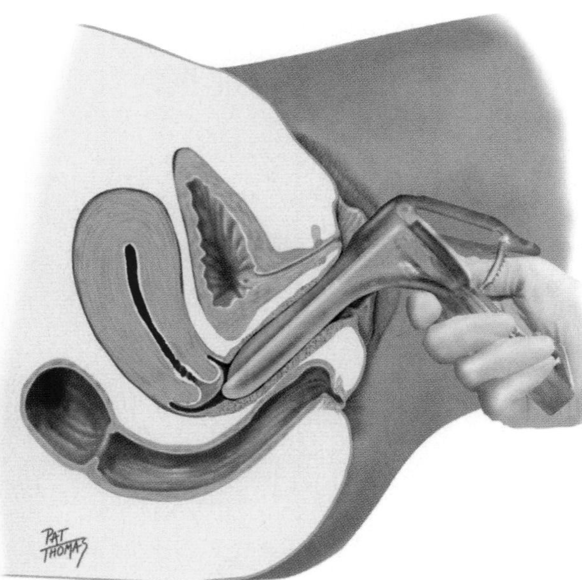

26-11

After the blades are fully inserted, open them by squeezing the handles together (Fig. 26-12). The cervix should be in full view. Sometimes this does not occur (especially with beginning examiners) because the blades are angled above the location of the cervix. Try closing the blades, withdrawing about halfway, and reinserting in a more *downward* plane. Then slowly sweep upward. Once you have the cervix in full view, lock the blades open by tightening the thumbscrew.

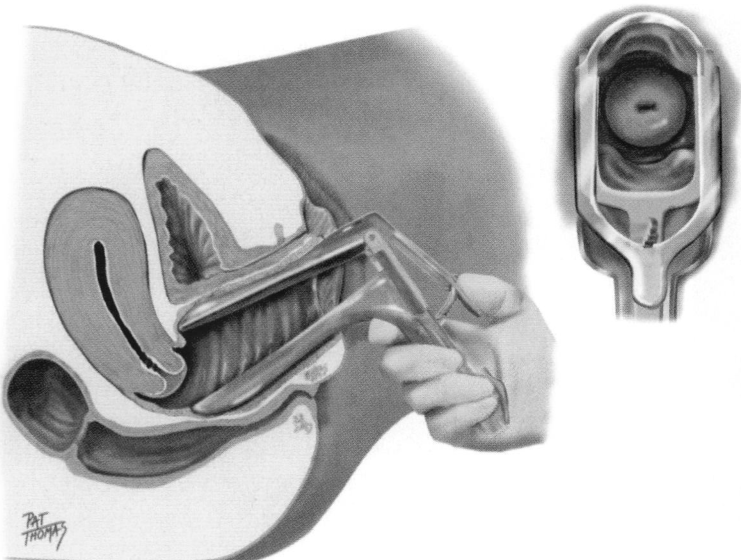

26-12

Abnormal Findings

Normal Range of Findings	Abnormal Findings

Inspect the Cervix and Its Os

Note:

- **Color.** Normally the cervical mucosa is pink and even (Fig. 26-13, *A*). During the 2nd month of pregnancy, it looks blue (Chadwick sign), and after menopause, it is pale.

Redness, inflammation.

Pallor with anemia.

Cyanotic other than with pregnancy (see Table 26-4, p. 754).

- **Position.** Midline, either anterior or posterior. Projects 1 to 3 cm into the vagina.

Lateral position may be due to adhesion or tumor. Projection of more than 3 cm may be a prolapse.

- **Size.** Diameter is 2.5 cm (1 inch).

Hypertrophy of more than 4 cm occurs with inflammation or tumor.

- **Os.** This is small and round in the nulliparous woman. In the parous woman, it is a horizontal, irregular slit and also may show healed lacerations on the sides (Fig. 26-13, *A* and *B*).

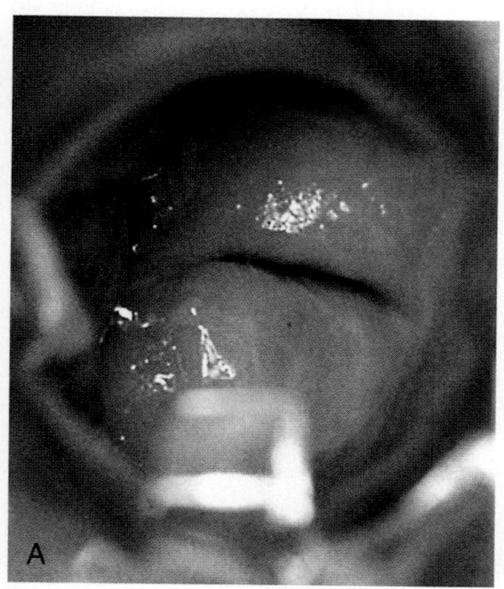

NORMAL VARIATIONS OF THE CERVIX

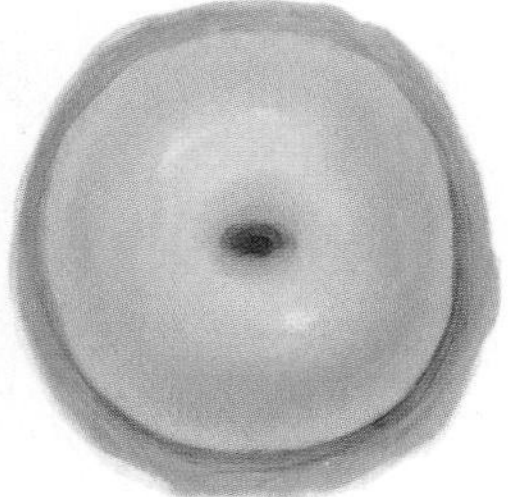

Nulliparous

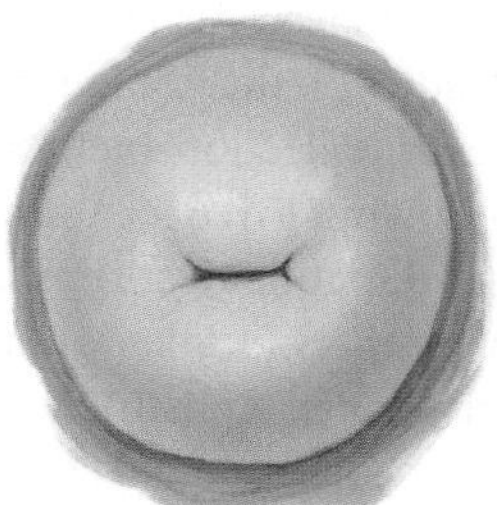

Parous (after childbirth)

LACERATIONS

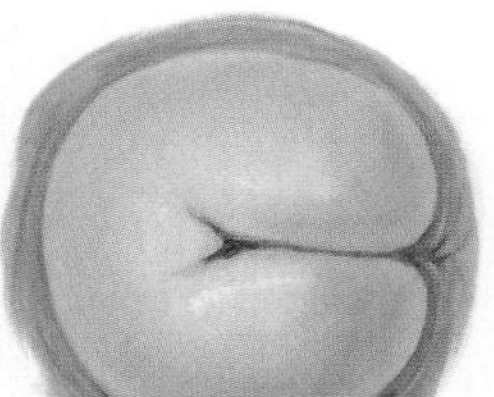

B Unilateral transverse

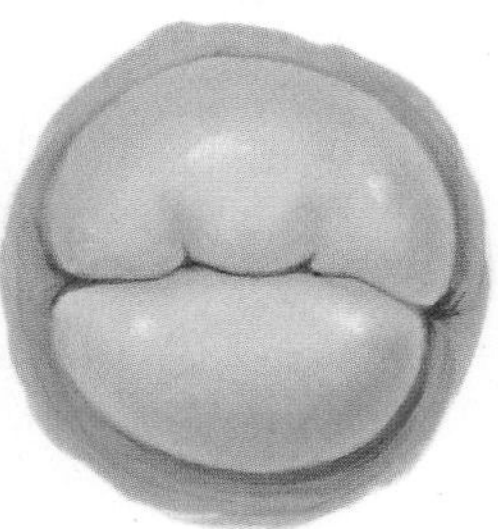

Bilateral transverse

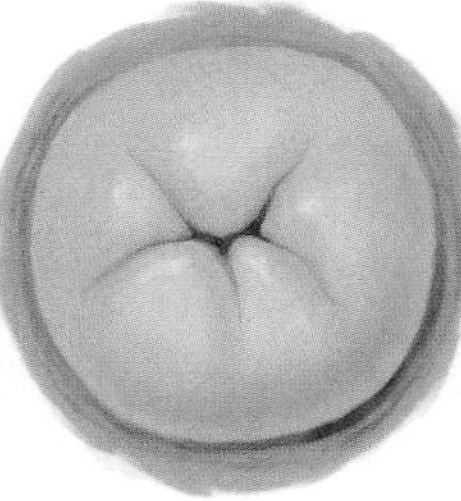

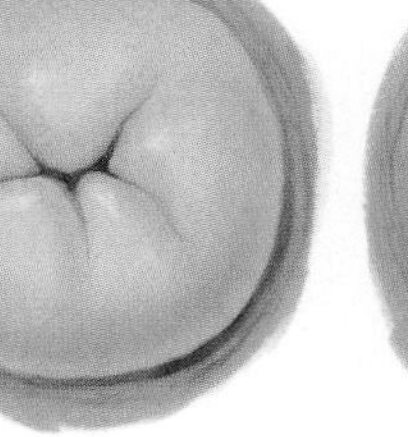

Stellate

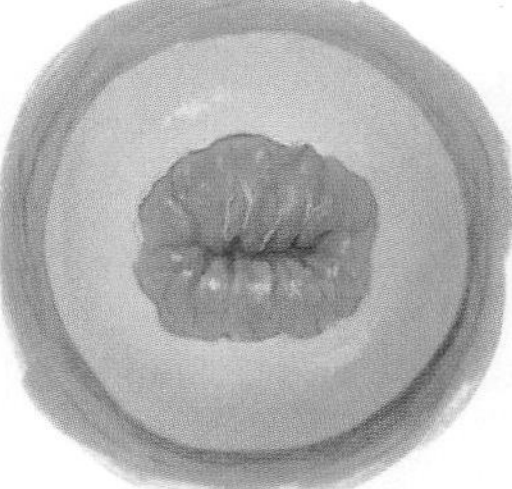

Cervical eversion

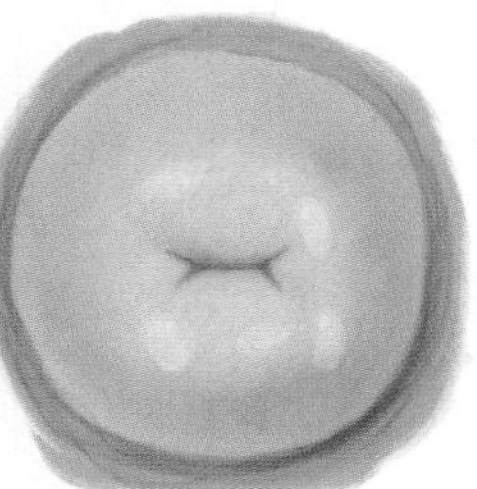

Nabothian cysts

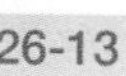

26-13

Normal Range of Findings

- **Surface.** This is normally smooth, but **cervical eversion,** or ectropion, may occur normally after vaginal deliveries (Fig. 26-13, *B*). The endocervical canal is everted or "rolled out." It looks like a red, beefy halo inside the pink cervix surrounding the os. It is difficult to distinguish this normal variation from an abnormal condition (e.g., erosion or carcinoma), and biopsy may be needed.

Nabothian cysts are benign growths that commonly appear on the cervix after childbirth. They are small, smooth, yellow nodules that may be single or multiple. Less than 1 cm, they are retention cysts caused by obstruction of cervical glands.

- **Note the cervical secretions.** Depending on the day of the menstrual cycle, secretions may be clear and thin, or thick, opaque, and stringy. Always they are odorless and nonirritating.

If secretions are copious, swab the area with a thick-tipped rectal swab. This method sponges away secretions, and you have a better view of the structures.

Obtain Cervical Smears and Cultures

The Papanicolaou, or Pap, test screens for cervical cancer and not for endometrial or ovarian cancer. Do not obtain during the woman's menses or if a heavy infectious discharge is present. Instruct the woman to not douche, have intercourse, or put anything into the vagina within 24 hours before collecting the specimens.

Obtain the Pap smear before other specimens so you will not disrupt or remove cells. Most U.S. clinics have changed from conventional cytology collection using glass slides to liquid-based cytology vials. Using liquid-based cytology, the cervical specimens are dipped into a vial with preservative rather than being smeared on a slide. Conventional glass slides can come back from the laboratory as "unsatisfactory" because of obscuring by blood or inflammation or clumped distribution of cells. Thus evidence shows that just stirring off the cells into the liquid vial results in fewer unsatisfactory tests and is more sensitive in detecting cervical neoplasia.[7] Using liquid-based cytology, microscopic evaluation is made clearer by the uniform spread of epithelial cells in a thin layer. Also, after cytology examination, pathologists can perform further studies on the liquid remnant such as testing for high-risk HPV types.[4,36] Whichever collection method you are using, collect the cellular specimens from the following three locations.

Vaginal Pool. Gently rub the blunt end of an Ayre spatula over the vaginal wall under and lateral to the cervix (Fig. 26-14). Wipe the specimen on a glass slide or dip into a liquid vial. If the mucosa is very dry (as in a postmenopausal woman), moisten a sterile swab with normal saline solution to collect this specimen.

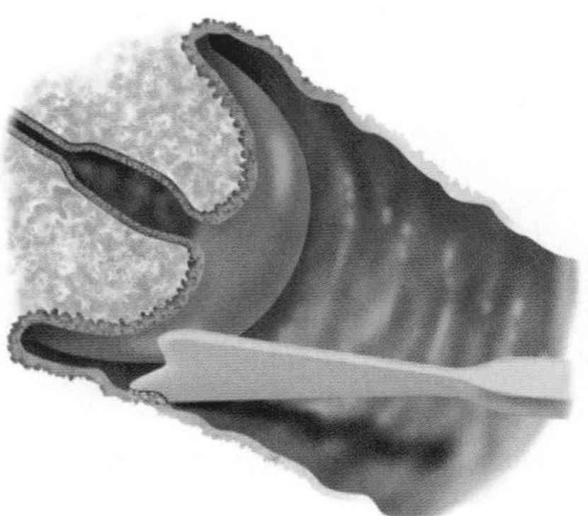

26-14

Abnormal Findings

Surface reddened, granular, and asymmetric, particularly around os.

Friable, bleeds easily.

Any lesions: white patch on cervix; strawberry spot.

Refer any suspicious red, white, or pigmented lesion for biopsy (see Erosion and Carcinoma sections in Table 26-4).

Cervical polyp—bright red growth protruding from the os (see Table 26-4).

Foul-smelling, irritating, with yellow, green, white, or gray discharge (see Table 26-5, Vulvovaginal Inflammations, p. 756).

Objective Data

Normal Range of Findings	Abnormal Findings

Cervical Scrape (Fig. 26-15). Insert the bifid end of the Ayre spatula into the vagina with the more pointed bump into the cervical os. Rotate it 360 to 720 degrees, using firm pressure. The rounded cervix fits snugly into the spatula's groove. The spatula scrapes the surface of the squamocolumnar junction (SCJ) and cervix as you turn the instrument. Spread the specimen from both sides of the spatula onto a glass slide. Use a single stroke to thin out the specimen, not a back-and-forth motion. This specimen is important for the adolescent whose endocervical cells have not yet migrated into the endocervical canal.

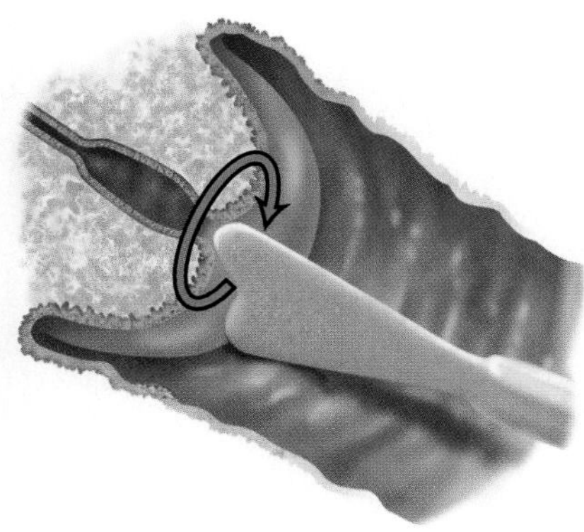

26-15

Endocervical Specimen (Fig. 26-16). Insert a cytobrush (instead of a cotton applicator) into the os. A cytobrush gives a higher yield of endocervical cells at the SCJ and is safe for use during pregnancy.[38] The woman may feel a slight pinch with the brush, and scant bleeding may occur. For this reason, collect the endocervical specimen last so that bleeding will not obscure cytologic evaluation.

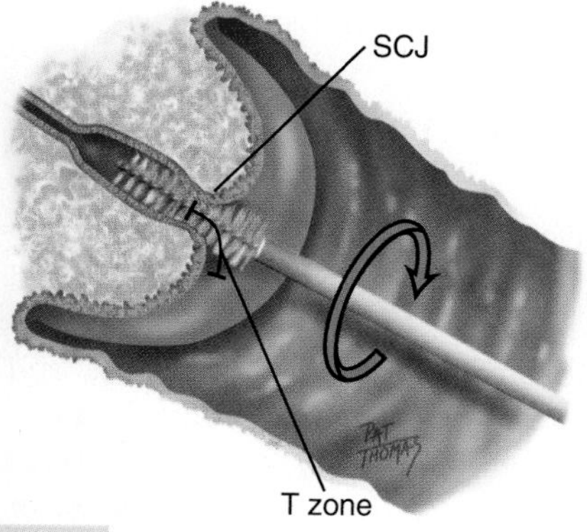

26-16

Rotate the brush 720 degrees in ONE direction in the endocervical canal, either clockwise or counterclockwise. Then rotate the brush gently on a slide to deposit all the cells. Rotate in the opposite direction from the one in which you obtained the specimen. Avoid leaving a thick specimen that would be hard to read under the microscope. Immediately (within 2 seconds) spray the slide with fixative to avoid drying. Or stir the cytobrush gently into the liquid vial.

For the woman after hysterectomy whose cervix has been removed, collect a scrape from the end of the vagina and a vaginal pool.

Normal Range of Findings	Abnormal Findings

Label the frosted ends of the slides or the vial with the woman's name. Send specimens to the laboratory with the following necessary data:

- Date of specimen
- Woman's date of birth
- Date of last menstrual period
- Any hormone medication
- If pregnant, estimated date of delivery
- Known infections
- Prior surgery or radiation
- Prior abnormal cytology
- Abnormal findings on physical examination

These data are important for accurate interpretation (e.g., a specimen may be interpreted as positive unless the laboratory technicians know the woman has had prior radiation treatment).

To screen for STIs and if you note any abnormal vaginal discharge, obtain the **gonorrhea (GC)/chlamydia** culture. Insert a sterile cotton applicator into the os, rotate it 360 degrees, and leave it in place 10 to 20 seconds for complete saturation. Insert into labeled container.

Occasionally you will need the following samples:

Saline Mount, or "Wet Prep." Spread a sample of the discharge onto a glass slide and add one drop of normal saline solution and a coverslip.

KOH Prep. To a sample of the discharge on a glass slide, add one drop of potassium hydroxide and a coverslip.

Anal Culture. Insert a sterile cotton swab into the anal canal about 1 cm. Rotate it, and move it side to side. Leave in place 10 to 20 seconds. If the swab collects feces, discard it and begin again. Insert into specimen container.

Acetic Acid Wash. Acetic acid (white vinegar) screens for asymptomatic human papillomavirus (HPV), which causes genital warts. After all other specimens are gathered, soak a thick-tipped cotton rectal swab with acetic acid and "paint" the cervix. Acetic acid dissolves mucus and temporarily causes intracellular dehydration and coagulation of protein. A normal response (indicating no HPV infection) is no change in the cervical epithelium.

Rapid acetowhitening or blanching, especially with irregular borders, suggests HPV infection (see Table 26-2).

Inspect the Vaginal Wall

Loosen the thumbscrew but continue to hold the speculum blades open. Slowly withdraw the speculum, rotating it as you go, to fully inspect the vaginal wall. Normally, the wall looks pink, deeply rugated, moist and smooth, and free of inflammation or lesions. Normal discharge is thin and clear or opaque and stringy but always odorless.

Inflammation or lesions.

Leukoplakia, appears as spot of dried white paint.

Vaginal discharge: thick, white, and curdlike with candidiasis; profuse, watery, gray-green, and frothy with trichomoniasis; or any gray, green-yellow, white, or foul-smelling discharge (see Table 26-5).

When the blade ends are near the vaginal opening, let them close, but be careful not to pinch the mucosa or catch any hairs. Turn the blades obliquely to avoid stretching the opening. Place the metal speculum in a basin to be cleaned later and soaked in a sterilizing and disinfecting solution; discard the plastic variety. Discard your gloves, and wash hands.

Bimanual Examination

Rise to a stand, and have the woman remain in lithotomy position. Drop lubricant onto the first two fingers of your gloved intravaginal hand (Fig. 26-17).

Normal Range of Findings	Abnormal Findings

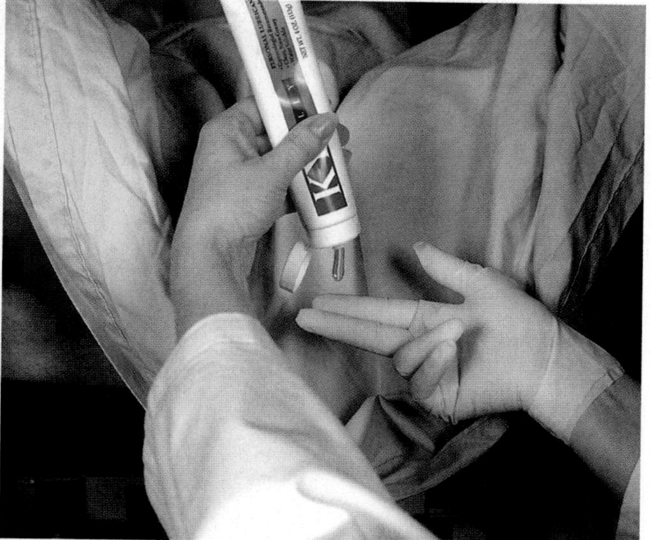

26-17

Assume the "obstetric" position with the first two fingers extended, the last two flexed onto the palm, and the thumb abducted. Insert your fingers into the vagina, with any pressure directed posteriorly. Wait until the vaginal walls relax, and then insert your fingers fully.

You will use both hands to palpate the internal genitalia to assess their location, size, and mobility and to screen for any tenderness or mass. One hand is on the abdomen while the other hand (often the dominant, more sensitive hand) inserts two fingers into the vagina (Fig. 26-18). It does not matter which you choose as the intravaginal hand; try each way, and settle on the most comfortable method for you.

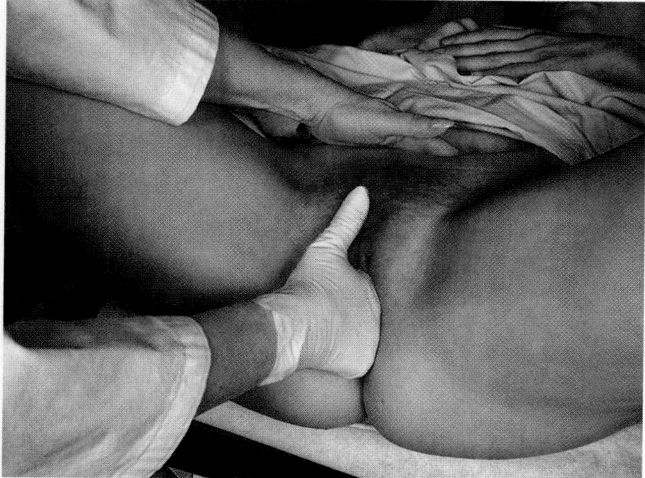

26-18

Palpate the vaginal wall. Normally, it feels smooth and has no area of induration or tenderness.

Nodule.
Tenderness.

Normal Range of Findings

Cervix. Locate the cervix in the midline, often near the anterior vaginal wall. The cervix points in the opposite direction of the fundus of the uterus. Palpate using the palmar surface of the fingers. Note these characteristics of a normal cervix:

- **Consistency**—feels smooth and firm, as the consistency of the tip of the nose. It softens and feels velvety at 5 to 6 weeks of pregnancy (Goodell sign).
- **Contour**—evenly rounded.
- **Mobility**—with a finger on either side, move the cervix gently from side to side. Normally, this produces no pain (Fig. 26-19).

Palpate all around the fornices; the wall should feel smooth.

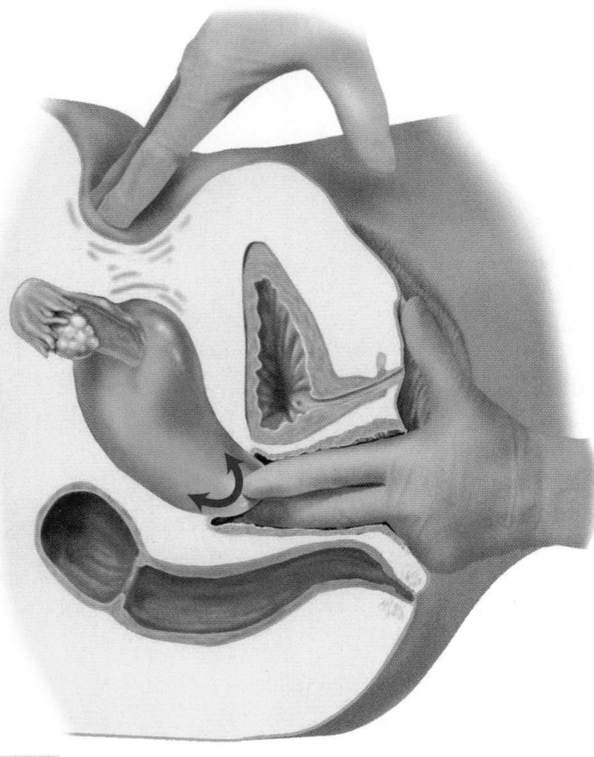

26-19

Next, use your abdominal hand to push the pelvic organs closer for your intravaginal fingers to palpate. Place your hand midway between the umbilicus and the symphysis; push down in a slow, firm manner, fingers together and slightly flexed. Brace the elbow of your pelvic arm against your hip, and keep it horizontal. The woman must be relaxed.

Uterus. With your intravaginal fingers in the anterior fornix, assess the uterus. Determine the position, or *version*, of the uterus (Fig. 26-20). This compares the long axis of the uterus with the long axis of the body. In many women, the uterus is anteverted; you palpate it at the level of the pubis with the cervix pointing posteriorly. Two other positions occur normally (midposition and retroverted), as well as two aspects of flexion, in which the long axis of the uterus is not straight but is flexed.

Abnormal Findings

Hard with malignancy.
Nodular.
Irregular.
Immobile with malignancy.

Painful with inflammation or ectopic pregnancy.

Normal Range of Findings

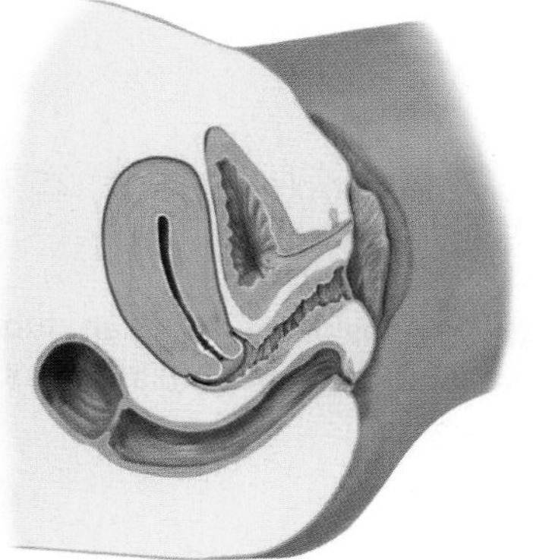

Anteverted

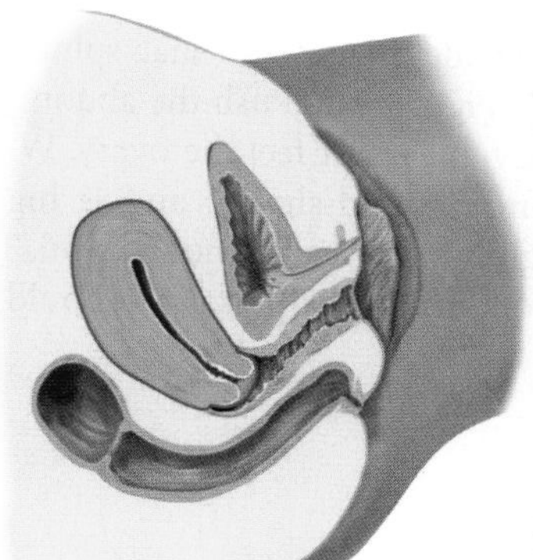

Midposition

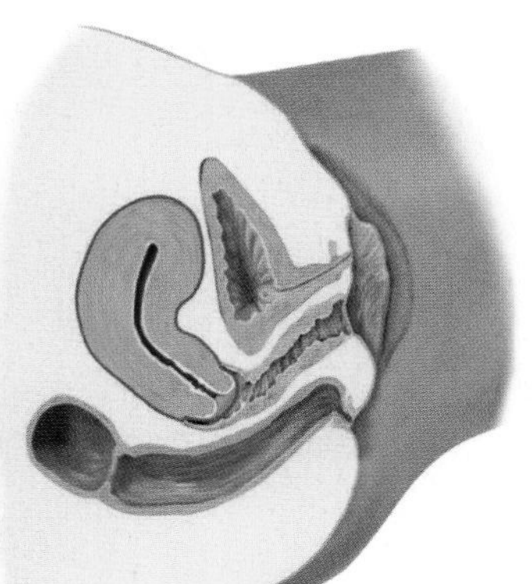

Anteflexed

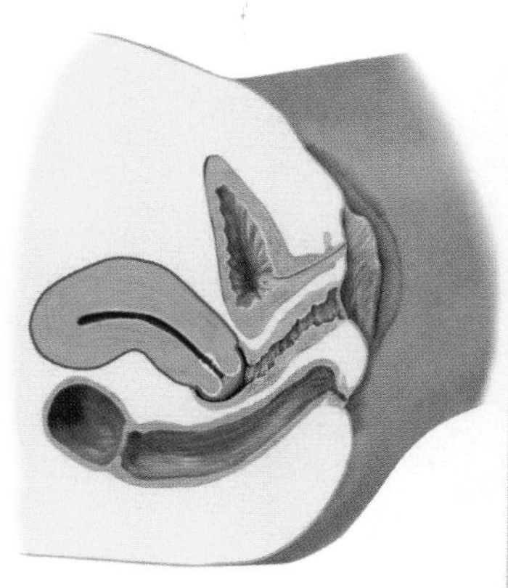

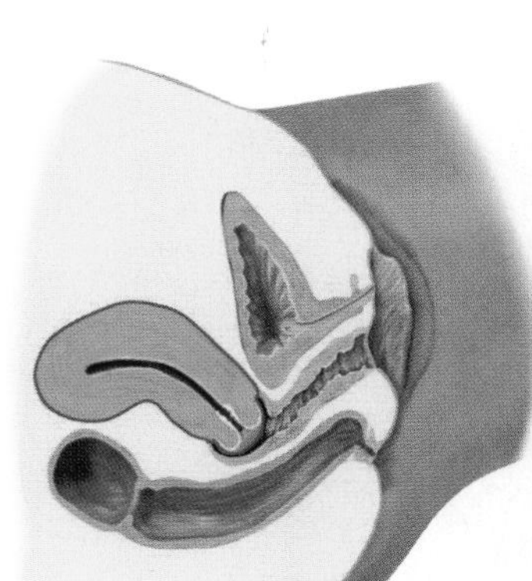

Retroflexed

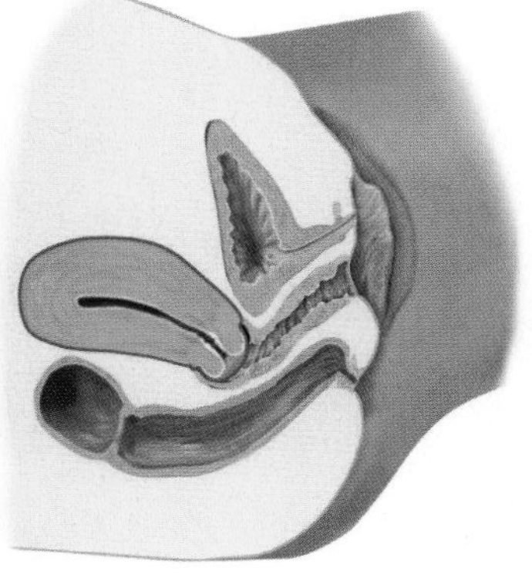

Retroverted

26-20

Palpate the uterine wall with your fingers in the fornices. Normally, it feels firm and smooth, with the contour of the fundus rounded. It softens during pregnancy. Bounce the uterus gently between your abdominal and intravaginal hand. It should be freely movable and nontender.

Abnormal Findings

Enlarged uterus (see Table 26-6, pp. 757-758).

Lateral displacement.

Nodular mass. Irregular, asymmetric uterus.

Fixed and immobile.

Tenderness.

Normal Range of Findings

Adnexa. Move both hands to the right to explore the adnexa. Place your abdominal hand on the lower quadrant just inside the anterior iliac spine and your intravaginal fingers in the lateral fornix (Fig. 26-21). Push the abdominal hand in and try to capture the ovary. Often, you cannot feel the ovary. When you can, it normally feels smooth, firm, and almond-shaped and is highly movable, sliding through the fingers. It is slightly sensitive but not painful. The fallopian tube is not palpable normally. No other mass or pulsation should be felt.

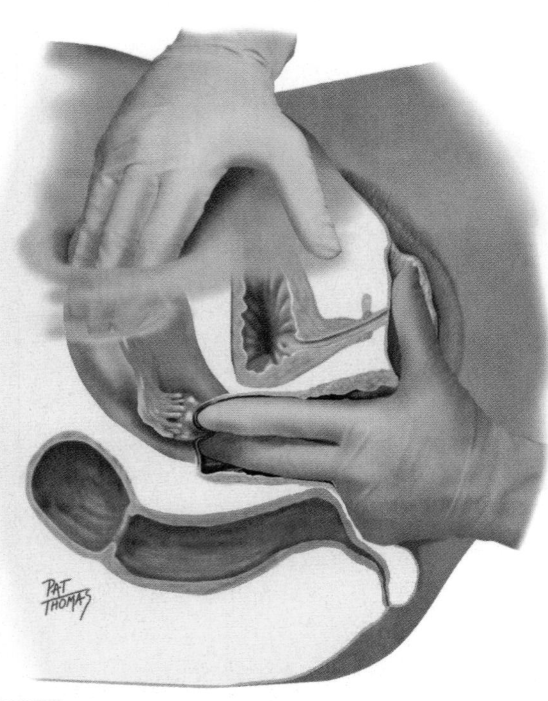

26-21

A note of caution—normal adnexal structures often are not palpable. Be careful not to mistake an abnormality for a normal structure. To be safe, consider abnormal any mass that you cannot *positively* identify, and refer the woman for further study.

Move to the left to palpate the other side. Then, withdraw your hand and check secretions on the fingers before discarding the glove. Normal secretions are clear or cloudy and odorless.

Rectovaginal Examination

Use this technique to assess the rectovaginal septum, posterior uterine wall, cul-de-sac, and rectum. Change gloves to avoid spreading any possible infection. Lubricate the first two fingers. Instruct the woman that this may feel uncomfortable and will mimic the feeling of moving her bowels. Ask her to bear down as you insert your index finger into the vagina and your middle finger gently into the rectum (Fig. 26-22).

Abnormal Findings

Enlarged adnexa. Nodules or mass in adnexa.

Immobile.

Markedly tender (see Table 26-7, Adnexal Enlargement, p. 759).

Pulsation or palpable fallopian tube suggests ectopic pregnancy; this warrants immediate referral.

Normal Range of Findings	Abnormal Findings

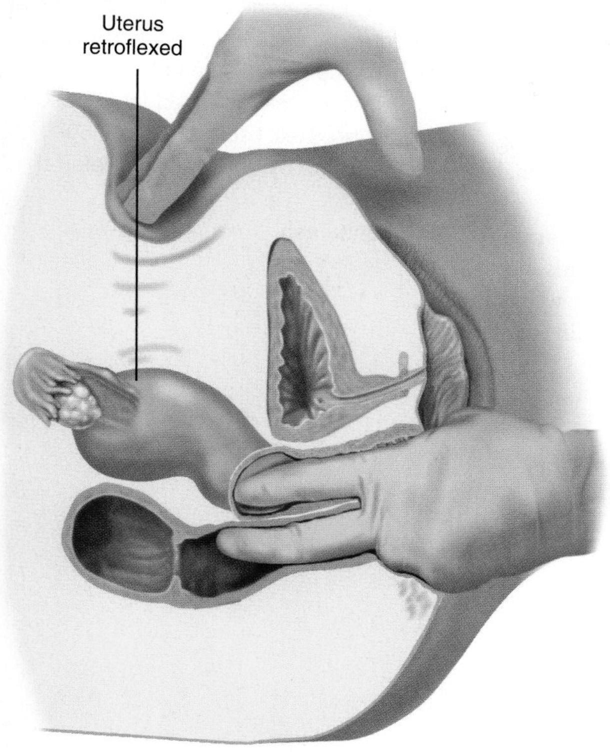

RECTOVAGINAL PALPATION 26-22

While pushing with the abdominal hand, repeat the steps of the bimanual examination. Try to keep the intravaginal finger on the cervix so the intrarectal finger does not mistake the cervix for a mass. Note:

- Rectovaginal septum should feel smooth, thin, firm, and pliable.
- Rectovaginal pouch, or cul-de-sac, is a potential space and usually not palpated.
- Uterine wall and fundus feel firm and smooth.

Abnormal Findings: Nodular or thickened.

Rotate the intrarectal finger to check the rectal wall and anal sphincter tone. (See Chapter 25 for assessment of anus and rectum.) Check your gloved finger as you withdraw; test any adherent stool for occult blood.

Give the woman tissues to wipe the area, and help her up. Remind her to slide her hips back from the edge before sitting up so she will not fall.

DEVELOPMENTAL COMPETENCE

Infants and Children

Preparation

- **Infant**—place on examination table.
- **Toddler/preschooler**—place on parent's lap.
  - Frog-leg position—hips flexed, soles of feet together and up to bottom.
  - Preschool child may want to separate her own labia.
  - No drapes—the young girl wants to see what you are doing.
- **School-age child**—place on examination table, frog-leg position, no drapes.

During childhood, a routine screening is limited to inspection of the external genitalia to determine that (1) the structures are intact, (2) the vagina is present, and (3) the hymen is patent (open).

Normal Range of Findings

The newborn's genitalia are somewhat engorged. The labia majora are swollen, the labia minora are prominent and protrude beyond the labia majora, the clitoris looks relatively large, and the hymen appears thick. Because of transient engorgement, the vaginal opening is more difficult to see now than it will be later. Place your thumbs on the labia majora. Push laterally while pushing the perineum down, and try to note the vaginal opening above the hymenal ring. Do not palpate the clitoris because it is very sensitive.

A sanguineous vaginal discharge or leukorrhea (mucoid discharge) is normal during the first few weeks because of the maternal estrogen effect. (This also may cause transient breast engorgement and secretion.) During the early weeks, the genital engorgement resolves and the labia minora atrophy and remain small until puberty (Fig. 26-23).

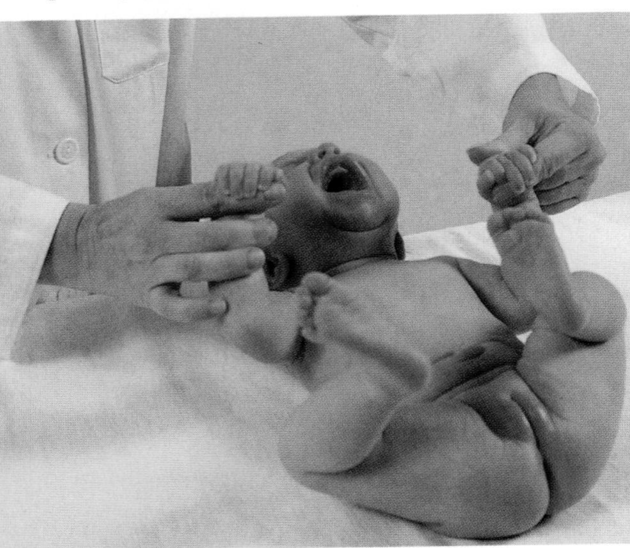

26-23

Between the ages of 2 months and 7 years, the labia majora are flat, the labia minora are thin, the clitoris is relatively small, and the hymen is tissue-paper thin. Normally, no irritation or foul-smelling discharge is present.

In the young school-age girl (7 to 10 years), the mons pubis thickens, the labia majora thicken, and the labia minora become slightly rounded. Pubic hair appears beginning around age 11 years, although sparse pubic hair may occur as early as age 8 years. Normally, the hymen is perforate.

Almost always in these age-groups, an external examination will suffice. If needed, an internal pelvic examination is best performed by a pediatric gynecologist using specialized instruments.

The Adolescent

The adolescent girl has special needs during the genitalia examination. Examine her alone, without the mother present. Assure her of privacy and confidentiality. Allow plenty of time for health education and discussion of pubertal progress. Assess her growth velocity and menstrual history, and use the SMR charts to teach breast and pubic hair development. Assure her that increased vaginal fluid (physiologic *leukorrhea*) is normal because of the estrogen effect.

Perform a pelvic examination when contraception is desired, when the girl's sexual activity includes intercourse, or at 21 years of age. Start Pap smears within 3 years after intercourse begins. Although the techniques of the

Abnormal Findings

Ambiguous genitalia are rare but are suggested by a markedly enlarged clitoris, fusion of the labia (resembling scrotum), and palpable mass in fused labia (resembling testes) (see Table 26-8, p. 760).

Imperforate hymen warrants referral.

Lesions, rash.

Poor perineal hygiene.

Pest inhabitants. Excoriations.

During and after toddler age, foul-smelling discharge occurs with lodging of foreign body, pinworms, or infection.

Absence of pubic hair by 13 years indicates delayed puberty.

Amenorrhea in adolescent, together with bluish and bulging hymen, indicates imperforate hymen and warrants referral.

Objective Data

Normal Range of Findings | **Abnormal Findings**

examination are listed in the adult section, you will need to provide additional time and psychological support for the adolescent having her first pelvic examination.

The experience of the first pelvic examination determines how the adolescent will approach future care. Your accepting attitude and gentle, unhurried approach are important. You have a unique teaching opportunity here. Take the time to teach, using the girl's own body as illustration. Your frank discussion of anatomy and sexual behavior communicates that these topics are acceptable to discuss and not taboo with health care providers. This affirms the girl's self-concept.

During the bimanual examination, note that the adnexa are not palpable in the adolescent.

Pelvic or adnexal mass.

The Pregnant Woman

Depending on the week of gestation of the pregnancy, inspection shows the enlarging abdomen (see Fig. 29-1 on p. 796). The height of the fundus ascends gradually as the fetus grows. At 16 weeks, the fundus is palpable halfway between the symphysis and umbilicus; at 20 weeks, at the lower edge of the umbilicus; at 28 weeks, halfway between the umbilicus and the xiphoid; and at 34 to 36 weeks, almost to the xiphoid. Then, close to term, the fundus drops as the fetal head engages in the pelvis.

The external genitalia show hyperemia of the perineum and vulva because of increased vascularity. Varicose veins may be visible in the labia or legs. Hemorrhoids may show around the anus. Both are caused by interruption in venous return from the pressure of the fetus.

Internally, the walls of the vagina appear violet or blue (Chadwick sign) because of hyperemia. The vaginal walls are deeply rugated, and the vaginal mucosa thickens. The cervix looks blue, feels velvety, and feels softer than in the nonpregnant state, making it a bit more difficult to differentiate from the vaginal walls.

During bimanual examination, the isthmus of the uterus feels softer and is more easily compressed between your two hands (Hegar sign). The fundus balloons between your two hands; it feels connected to, but distinct from, the cervix because the isthmus is so soft.

Search the adnexal area carefully during early pregnancy. Normally, the adnexal structures are not palpable.

An ectopic pregnancy has serious consequences (see Table 26-7).

The Aging Adult

Natural lubrication is decreased; to avoid a painful examination, take care to lubricate instruments and the examining hand adequately. Use the Pedersen speculum (rather than the Graves) because its narrower, flatter blades are more comfortable in women with vaginal stenosis or dryness.

Menopause and the resulting decrease in estrogen production cause numerous physical changes. Pubic hair gradually decreases, becoming thin and sparse in later years. The skin is thinner and fat deposits decrease, leaving the mons pubis smaller and the labia flatter. Clitoris size also decreases after age 60 years.

Internally, the rugae of the vaginal walls decrease and the walls look pale pink because of the thinned epithelium. The cervix shrinks and looks pale and glistening. It may retract, appearing to be flush with the vaginal wall. In some, it is hard to distinguish the cervix from the surrounding vaginal mucosa. Or, the cervix may protrude into the vagina if the uterus has prolapsed.

Refer any suspicious red, white, or pigmented lesion for biopsy.

Vaginal atrophy increases the risk for infection and trauma.

With the bimanual examination, you may need to insert only one gloved finger if vaginal stenosis exists. The uterus feels smaller and firmer, and the ovaries are not palpable normally.

Refer any mass for prompt evaluation.

Be aware that older women may have special needs and will appreciate the following plans of care: for those with arthritis, taking a mild analgesic or

Normal Range of Findings	Abnormal Findings
anti-inflammatory before the appointment may ease joint pain in positioning; schedule appointment times when joint pain or stiffness is at its least; allow extra time for positioning and "unpositioning" after the examination; and be careful to maintain dignity and privacy. Women should continue cervical cancer screening up to age 70 years if they have an intact cervix and are in good health.[37] After age 70, women may decide to stop screening if (1) they have had no abnormal cytology tests in the previous 10 years and (2) if the three most recent Pap tests are documented as technically satisfactory and with normal results.[37] Women who have had a total hysterectomy for benign gynecologic disease do not need cervical cancer screening. But if the hysterectomy was for cervical neoplasia, Pap tests should continue until a 10-year history of no abnormal results.[37]	

PROMOTING A HEALTHY LIFESTYLE: NEW HPV VACCINE

A Breakthrough Vaccine in Cancer Prevention

In June 2006, the Advisory Committee on Immunization Practices (ACIP) voted to recommend the first vaccine developed to prevent cervical cancer. The ACIP is a national group of experts that advises the Centers for Disease Control and Prevention (CDC) on vaccine issues. This represents one of the most important advances in women's health in recent years.

The vaccine targets human papilloma virus (HPV), the virus responsible for most cases of cervical cancer. HPV is the most common sexually transmitted infection (STI). Most people who have become infected with HPV do not even know they had it because the virus usually does not cause any symptoms and in 90% of the cases, the body's immune system can fight it off. However, sometimes the virus lingers in a woman's cervix and can cause changes that may eventually lead to cervical cancer.

The HPV vaccine is recommended for girls ages 11 to 12 but can be started as early as 9 years of age. Catch-up vaccination is recommended for 13- to 26-year-old females who did not receive the vaccine series. Ideally, the HPV vaccine is recommended *before* they become sexually active because it is not effective if the individual is already infected with HPV. However, sexually active females may still benefit, since few women are infected by all four HPV types (6, 11, 16, 18) targeted by the vaccines. It is contraindicated during pregnancy and lactation.

The HPV vaccine is given in three separate injections over a 6-month period. The second and third doses are 2 and 6 months after the first dose. The vaccine can be administered at the same visit as other age-appropriate vaccines, such as the Tdap, Td, and hepatitis B vaccines.

It is important to remind women that obtaining the vaccine does not mean that they can forget about routine pelvic examinations and Papanicolaou (Pap) tests. The vaccine will protect against major types of HPV that cause cervical cancer, but not all types. Pap tests can detect cell changes in the cervix *before* they turn into cancer, at an early, curable stage. Other than the vaccine, the only way to prevent HPV is to abstain from all sexual activity. Using protection, such as a condom, may not be enough because areas not covered by a condom can be exposed to the virus.

Resources

HPV Vaccination. Website: www.cdc.gov/vaccines/vpd-vac/hpv/.

For clinicians. Website: www.cdc.gov/std/HPV/STDFact-HPV-vaccine-hcp.htm#vaccrec.

HPV Fact Sheet. Website: www.cdc.gov/std/HPV/STDFact-HPV.htm.

DOCUMENTATION AND CRITICAL THINKING

Sample Charting

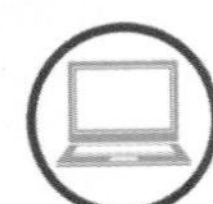

SUBJECTIVE

Menarche age 12 years, cycle usually q 28 days, duration 5 days, flow moderate, no dysmenorrhea, LMP April 3. Grav 0/Para 0/Ab 0. Gyne checkups yearly. Last Pap test 1 year PTA, negative.

No urinary problems, no irritating or foul-smelling vaginal discharge, no sores or lesions, no history pelvic surgery. Satisfied with sexual relationship with husband, uses vaginal diaphragm for birth control, no plans for pregnancy at this time. Not aware of any STI contact to herself or husband.

OBJECTIVE

External genitalia: No swelling, lesions, or discharge. No urethral swelling or discharge.
Internal: Vaginal walls have no bulging or lesions, cervix pink with no lesions, scant clear mucoid discharge.
Bimanual: No pain on moving cervix, uterus anteflexed and anteverted, no enlargement or irregularity.

Adnexa: Ovaries not enlarged.

Rectal: No hemorrhoids, fissures, or lesions; no masses or tenderness; stool brown with guaiac test negative.

ASSESSMENT

Genital structures intact and appear healthy

Focused Assessment: Clinical Case Study 1

J.K., 27-year-old white married newspaper reporter, Grav 0/Para 0/Ab 0. Presents at clinic with "urinary burning, vaginal itching, and discharge × 4 days."

SUBJECTIVE

3 weeks PTA—treated at clinic for bronchitis with erythromycin. Improved within 5 days.

4 to 5 days PTA—noted burning on urination; intense vaginal itching; thick, white, "smelly" discharge. Warm water douche—no relief.

No previous history vaginal infection, urinary tract infection, or pelvic surgery. Monogamous sexual relationship, has used low-estrogen birth control pills for 3 years with no side effects.

OBJECTIVE

Vulva and vagina erythematous and edematous. Thick, white, curdlike discharge clinging to vaginal walls. Cervix pink, no lesions.

Bimanual examination: No pain on palpating cervix, uterus not enlarged, ovaries not enlarged.

Specimens: Pap smear, GC/chlamydia to lab. KOH prep shows mycelia and spores of *Candida albicans.*

ASSESSMENT

Candida vaginitis

Pain R/T infectious process

Focused Assessment: Clinical Case Study 2

Brenda, 17-year-old white high school student, comes to clinic for pelvic examination.

SUBJECTIVE

Menarche 12 years, cycle q 30 days, duration 6 days, mild cramps relieved by acetaminophen. LMP March 10. No dysuria, vaginal discharge, vaginal itching. Relationship involving intercourse with one boyfriend for 8 months PTA. For birth control, boyfriend uses condoms "sometimes." Wants to start birth control pills. Never had pelvic examination. Never had teaching about breast self-examination or STIs except AIDS. Smokes cigarettes, ½ PPD, started age 11 years.

OBJECTIVE

Breasts: Symmetric, no lesions or discharge, palpation reveals no mass or tenderness.

External genitalia: No redness, lesions, or discharge.

Internal genitalia: Vaginal walls and cervix pink with no lesions or discharge. Specimens obtained. Acetic acid wash shows no acetowhitening.

Bimanual: No tenderness to palpation, uterus anteverted with no enlargement, ovaries not enlarged.

Rectum: No masses, fissure, or tenderness. Stool brown and guaiac test negative.

Specimens: GC, chlamydia, Pap smear to lab.

ASSESSMENT

Breast and pelvic structures appear healthy

Deficient knowledge regarding: breast self-examination; birth control measures; STI prevention; cigarette smoking R/T lack of exposure

ABNORMAL FINDINGS FOR ADVANCED PRACTICE

TABLE 26-2 Abnormalities of the External Genitalia

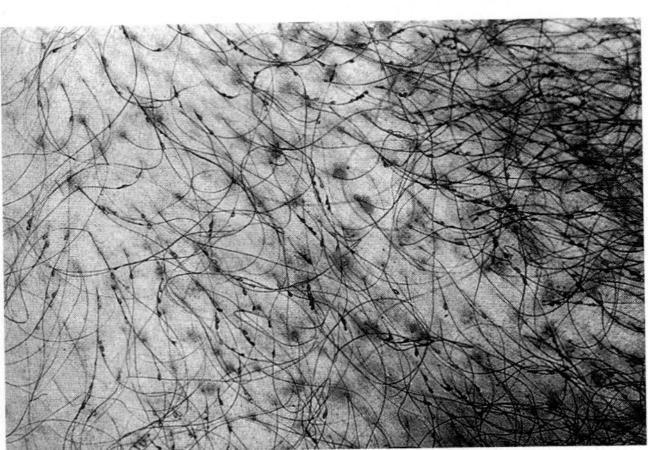

Pediculosis Pubis (Crab Lice)

S: Severe perineal itching.

O: Excoriations and erythematous areas. May see little dark spots (lice are small), nits (eggs) adherent to pubic hair near roots. Usually localized in pubic hair, occasionally in eyebrows or eyelashes.

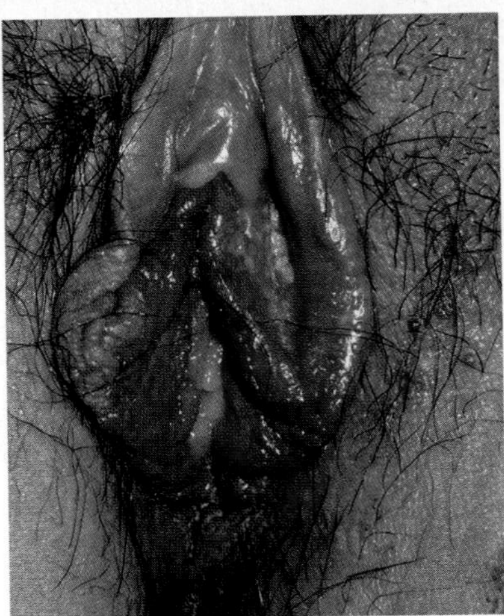

Herpes Simplex Virus—Type 2 (Herpes Genitalis)

S: Episodes of local pain, dysuria, fever.

O: Clusters of small, shallow vesicles with surrounding erythema; erupt on genital areas and inner thigh. Also, inguinal adenopathy, edema. Vesicles on labia rupture in 1 to 3 days, leaving painful ulcers. Initial infection lasts 7 to 10 days. Virus remains dormant indefinitely; recurrent infections last 3 to 10 days with milder symptoms.

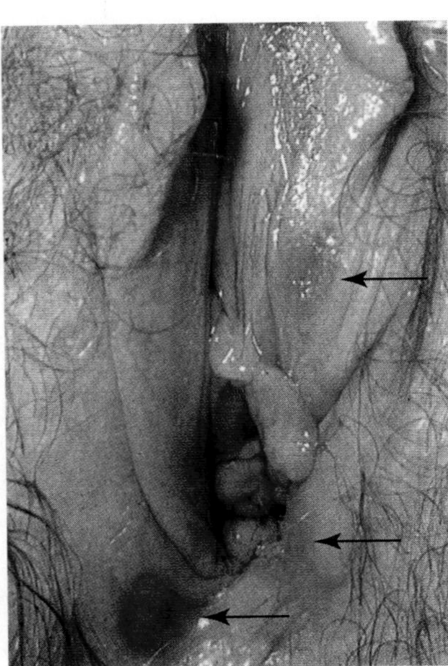

Syphilitic Chancre

O: Begins as a small, solitary silvery papule that erodes to a red, round or oval, superficial ulcer with a yellowish serous discharge. Palpation—nontender indurated base; can be lifted like a button between thumb and finger. Nontender inguinal lymphadenopathy.

Reprinted from Edmond, R. (1995). *Colour atlas of infectious diseases* (3rd ed., p. 173). St. Louis: Mosby.

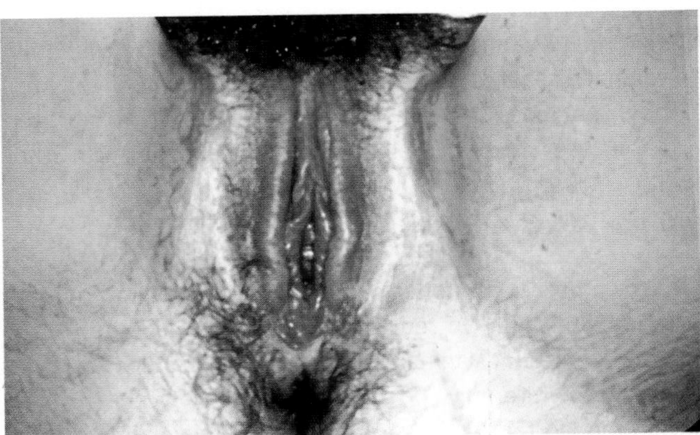

Red Rash—Contact Dermatitis

S: History of skin contact with allergenic substance in environment, intense pruritus.

O: Primary lesion—red, swollen vesicles. Then may have weeping of lesions, crusts, scales, thickening of skin, excoriations from scratching. May result from reaction to feminine hygiene spray or synthetic underclothing.

TABLE 26-2 **Abnormalities of the External Genitalia—cont'd**

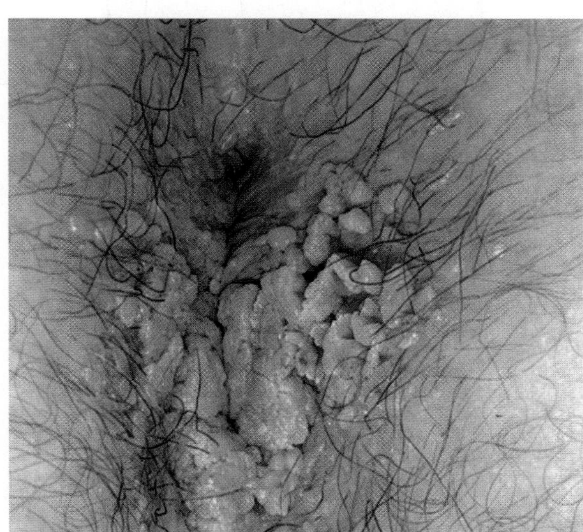

Human Papillomavirus (HPV) Genital Warts

S: Painless warty growths, may be unnoticed by woman.
O: Pink or flesh-colored, soft, pointed, moist, warty papules. Single or multiple in a cauliflower-like patch. Occur around vulva, introitus, anus, vagina, cervix. (NOTE: Advanced case shown here.)

HPV infection is common among sexually active women, especially adolescents, regardless of ethnicity or socioeconomic status. Risk factors include early age at menarche and multiple sexual partners. The long incubation period (6 weeks to 8 months) makes it difficult to establish history of exposure.

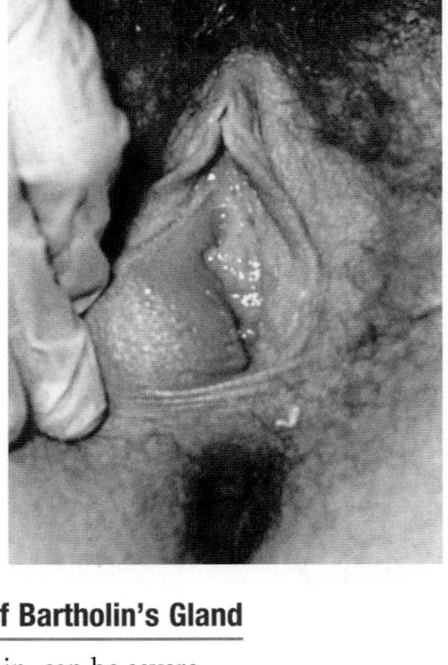

Abscess of Bartholin's Gland

S: Local pain, can be severe.
O: Overlying skin red, shiny, and hot. Posterior part of labia swollen; palpable fluctuant mass and tenderness. (Compare with wrinkled skin on the other, normal side.) Mucosa shows red spot at site of duct opening. Requires incision and drainage, antibiotic therapy.

Reprinted from Edmond, R. (1995). *Colour atlas of infectious diseases* (3rd ed., p. 161). St. Louis: Mosby.

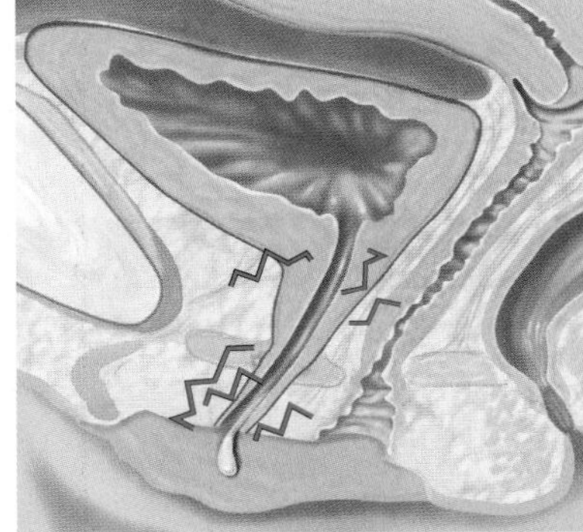
Urethritis

Urethritis

S: Dysuria, burning sensation.
O: Palpation of anterior vaginal wall shows erythema, tenderness, induration along urethra, purulent discharge from meatus. Caused by *Neisseria gonorrhoeae,* chlamydia, or staphylococcus infection.

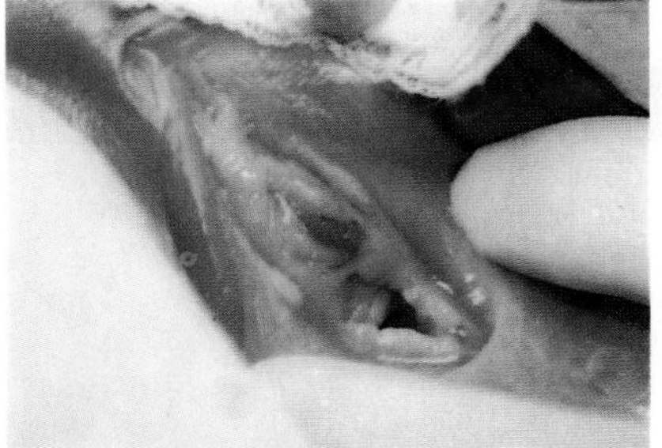

Urethral Caruncle

S: Tender, painful with urination, urinary frequency, hematuria, dyspareunia, or asymptomatic.
O: Small, deep red mass protruding from meatus; usually secondary to urethritis or skenitis; lesion may bleed on contact.

S, Subjective data; *O,* objective data.

TABLE 26-3 Abnormalities of the Pelvic Musculature

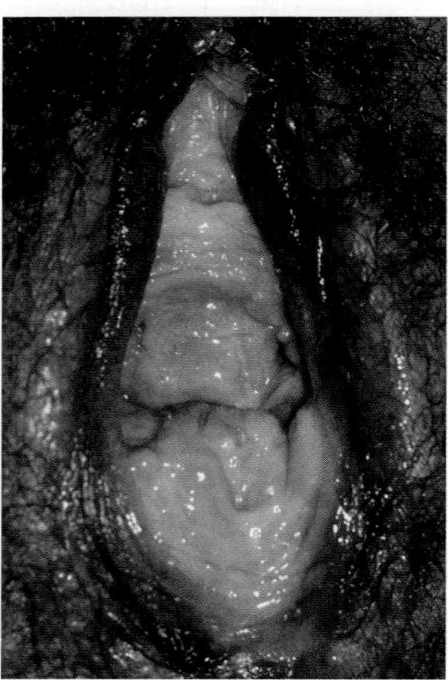

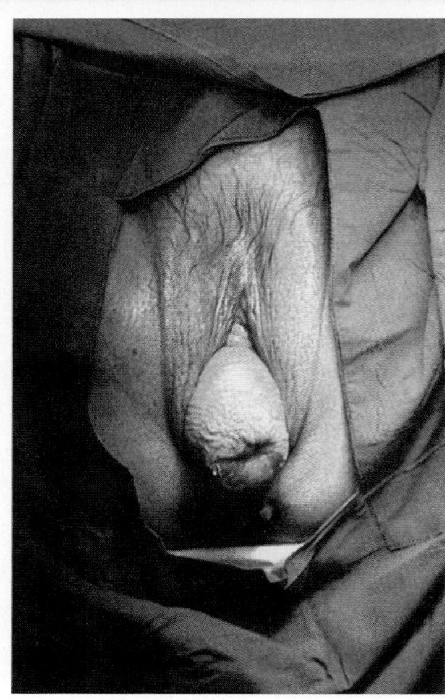

Cystocele

S: Feeling of pressure in vagina, stress incontinence.
O: With straining, note introitus widening and the presence of a soft, round *anterior* bulge. The bladder, covered by vaginal mucosa, prolapses into vagina.

Rectocele

S: Feeling of pressure in vagina, possibly constipation.
O: With straining, note introitus widening and the presence of a soft, round bulge from *posterior*. Here, part of the rectum, covered by vaginal mucosa, prolapses into vagina.

Uterine Prolapse

O: With straining or standing, uterus protrudes into vagina. Nontender, non-fluctuant, smooth hemisphere; may cause a broad-based gait. Prolapse is graded: 1st degree, cervix appears at introitus with straining; 2nd degree, cervix bulges outside introitus with straining; 3rd degree (in this case), whole uterus protrudes even without straining—essentially, uterus is inside out.

S, Subjective data; *O*, objective data.

TABLE 26-4 Abnormalities of the Cervix

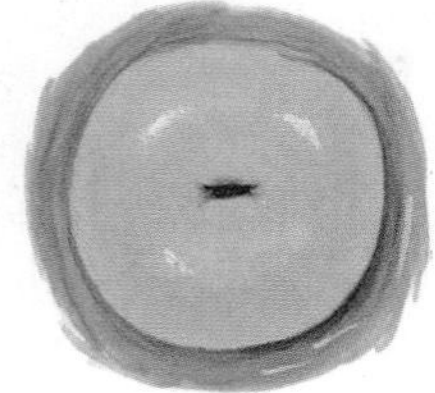

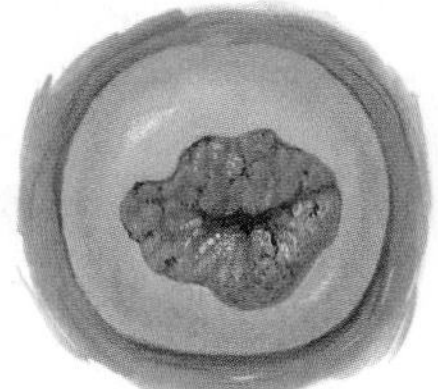

Bluish Cervix—Cyanosis

O: Bluish discoloration of the mucosa occurs normally in pregnancy (Chadwick sign at 6 to 8 weeks' gestation) and with any other condition causing hypoxia or venous congestion (e.g., heart failure, pelvic tumor).

Erosion

O: Cervical lips inflamed and eroded. Reddened granular surface is superficial inflammation, with no ulceration (loss of tissue). Usually secondary to purulent or mucopurulent cervical discharge. Biopsy needed to distinguish erosion from carcinoma; cannot rely on inspection.

TABLE 26-4 Abnormalities of the Cervix—cont'd

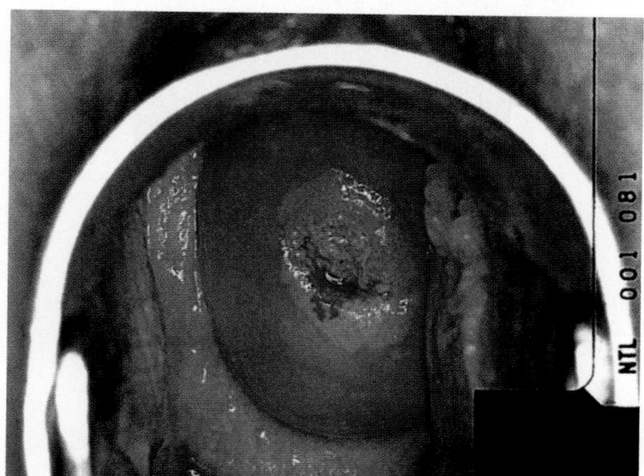

Human Papillomavirus (HPV, Condylomata)

O: Virus can appear in various forms when affecting cervical epithelium. Here, warty growth appears as abnormal thickened white epithelium. Visibility of lesion is enhanced by acetic acid (vinegar) wash, which dissolves mucus and temporarily causes intracellular dehydration and coagulation of protein.

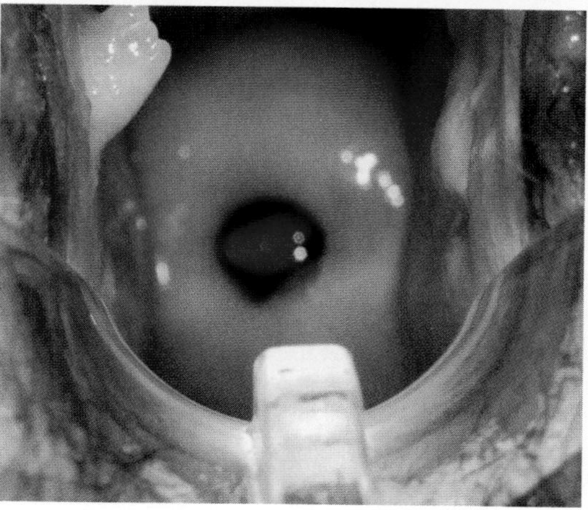

Polyp

S: May have mucoid discharge or bleeding.

O: Bright red, soft, pedunculated growth emerges from os. It is a benign lesion, but this must be determined by biopsy. May be lined with squamous or columnar epithelium.

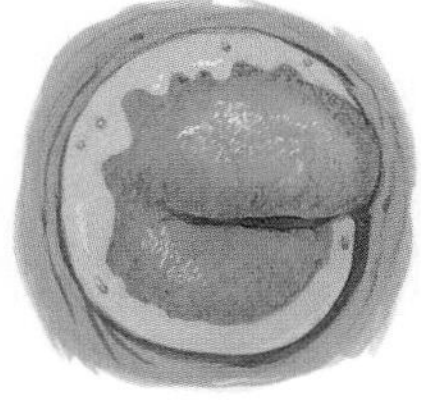

Diethylstilbestrol (DES) Syndrome

S: Prenatal exposure to DES causes cervical and vaginal abnormalities not apparent until adolescence.

O: Red, granular patches of columnar epithelium extend beyond normal squamocolumnar junction onto cervix and into fornices (vaginal adenosis). Also cervical abnormalities: circular groove, transverse ridge, protuberant anterior lip, "cockscomb" formation.

Structural abnormalities cause infertility, ectopic pregnancy, spontaneous abortion, and preterm labor.

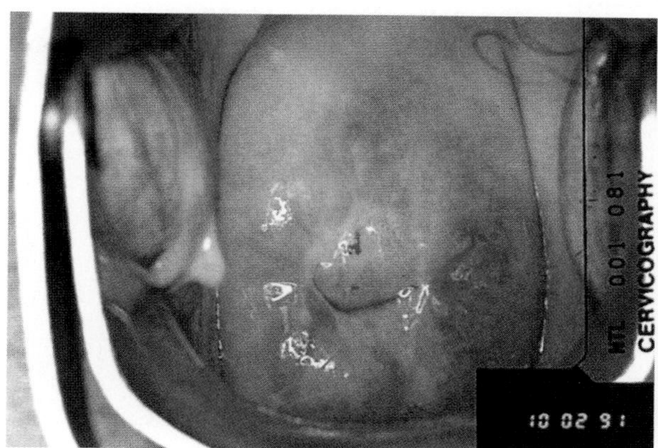

Carcinoma

S: Bleeding between menstrual periods or after menopause, unusual vaginal discharge.

O: Chronic ulcer and induration are early signs of carcinoma, although the lesion may or may not show on the exocervix. (Here, lesion is mostly around the external os.)

Diagnosed by Pap smear and biopsy. Risk factors for cervical cancer are early age at first intercourse, multiple sex partners, cigarette smoking, certain sexually transmitted infections.

S, Subjective data; *O,* objective data.

TABLE 26-5 Vulvovaginal Inflammations

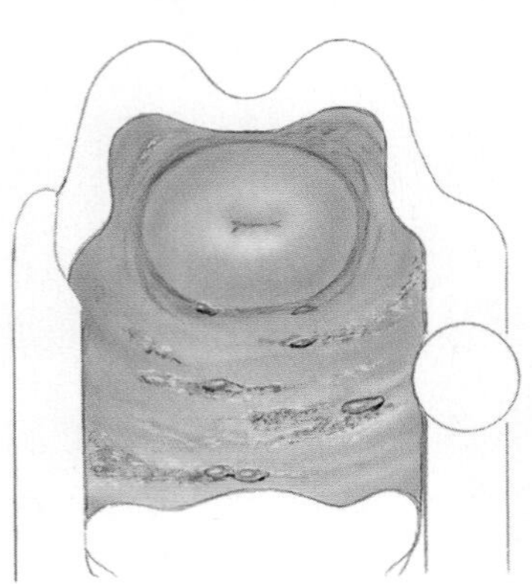

Atrophic Vaginitis

S: Postmenopausal vaginal itching, dryness, burning sensation, dyspareunia, mucoid discharge (may be flecked with blood).

O: Pale mucosa with abraded areas that bleed easily; may have bloody discharge.

An opportunistic infection related to chronic estrogen deficiency.

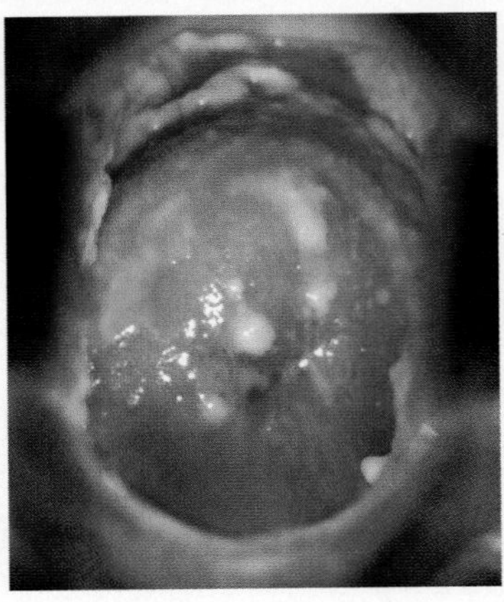

Candidiasis (Moniliasis)

S: Intense pruritus, thick whitish discharge.

O: Vulva and vagina are erythematous and edematous. Discharge is usually thick, white, curdy, "like cottage cheese." Diagnose by microscopic examination of discharge on potassium hydroxide wet mount.

Predisposing causes—use of oral contraceptives or antibiotics, more alkaline vaginal pH (as with menstrual periods, postpartum, menopause), also pregnancy from increased glycogen and diabetes.

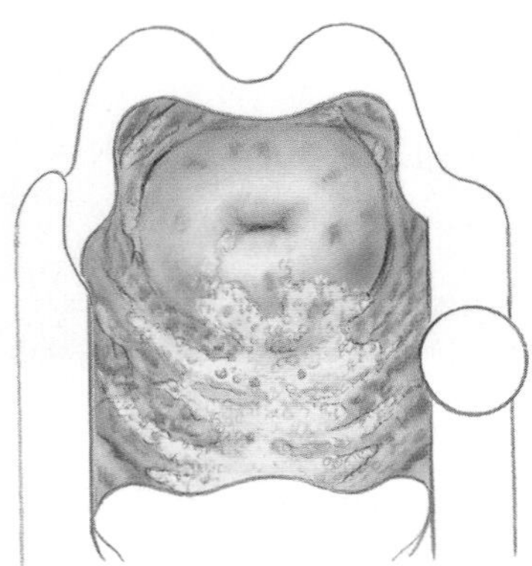

Trichomoniasis

S: Pruritus, watery and often malodorous vaginal discharge, urinary frequency, terminal dysuria, itching. Symptoms are worse during menstruation when the pH becomes optimal for the organism's growth.

O: Vulva may be erythematous. Vagina diffusely red, granular, occasionally with red, raised papules and petechiae ("strawberry" appearance). Frothy, yellow-green, foul-smelling discharge. Microscopic examination of saline wet mount specimen shows characteristic flagellated cells.

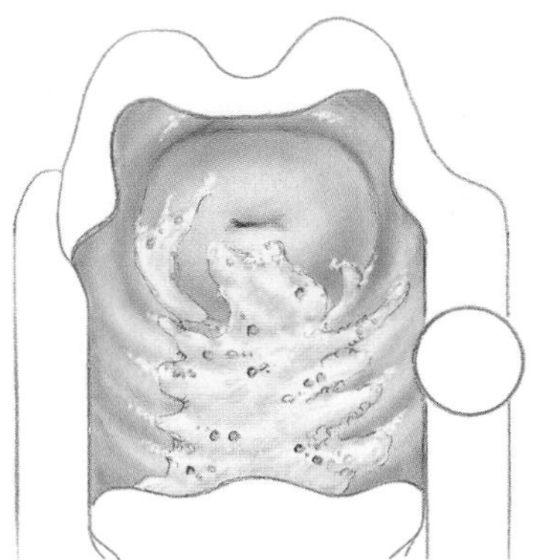

Bacterial Vaginosis (*Gardnerella vaginalis, Haemophilus vaginalis,* or Nonspecific Vaginitis)

S: Profuse discharge, "constant wetness" with "foul, fishy, rotten" odor.

O: Thin, creamy, gray-white, malodorous discharge. No inflammation on vaginal wall or cervix because this is a surface parasite. Vaginal pH >4.5. Microscopic view of saline wet mount specimen shows typical "clue cells" (epithelial cells with stippled borders). Sniff for fishy odor after adding KOH to slide ("whiff test").

TABLE 26-5 Vulvovaginal Inflammations—cont'd

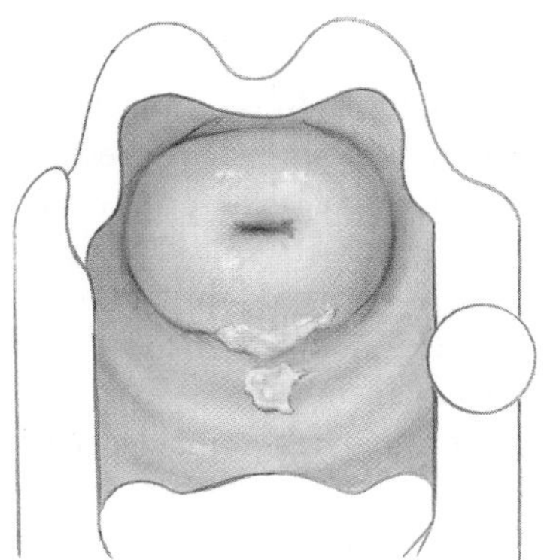

Chlamydia

S: Minimal or no symptoms. May have urinary frequency, dysuria, or vaginal discharge, postcoital bleeding.

O: May have yellow or green mucopurulent discharge, friable cervix, cervical motion tenderness.

Signs are subtle, easily mistaken for gonorrhea. The two are important to distinguish because antibiotic treatment is different; if the wrong drug is given or if untreated, chlamydia can ascend to cause pelvic inflammatory disease (PID) and result in infertility. This is the most common STI; the highest prevalence is among sexually active adolescent girls. Now, urine chlamydia testing using nucleic acid amplification tests (NAAT) is a noninvasive method to screen. Use a single urine specimen to detect both pregnancy and chlamydia.

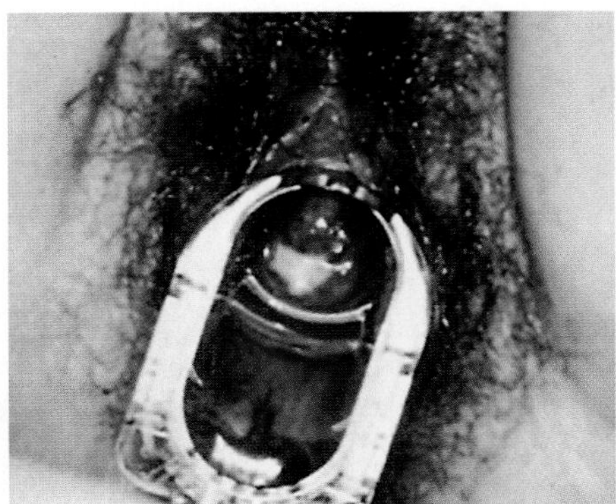

Gonorrhea

S: Variable: vaginal discharge, dysuria, abnormal uterine bleeding, abscess in Bartholin's or Skene's glands; the majority of cases are asymptomatic.

O: Often no signs are apparent. May have purulent vaginal discharge. Diagnose by positive culture of organism. If the condition is untreated, it may progress to acute salpingitis, PID.

S, Subjective data; *O,* objective data.

TABLE 26-6 Uterine Enlargement

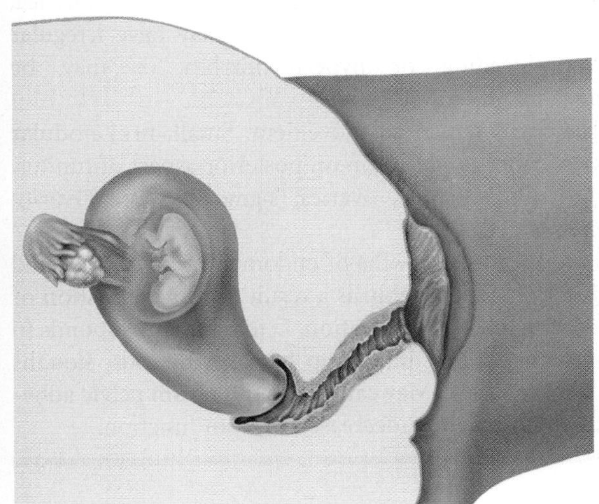

◀ Pregnancy

Obviously a normal condition, pregnancy is included here for comparison.

S: Amenorrhea, fatigue, breast engorgement, nausea, change in food tolerance, weight gain.

O: Early signs: cyanosis of vaginal mucosa and cervix (Chadwick sign). Palpation—soft consistency of cervix, enlarging uterus with compressible fundus and isthmus (Hegar sign at 10 to 12 weeks).

Continued

TABLE 26-6 Uterine Enlargement—cont'd

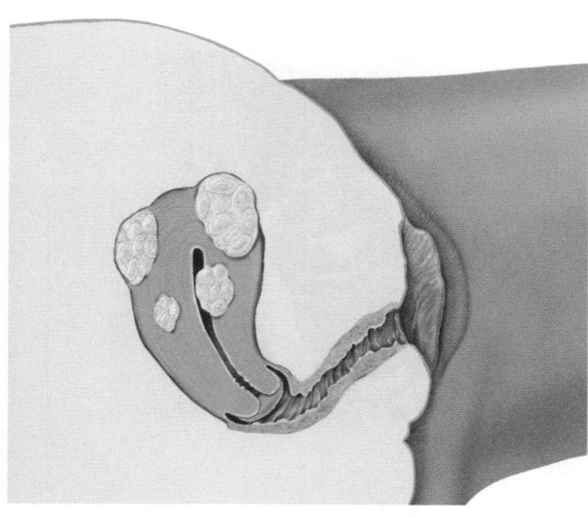

◀ Myomas (Leiomyomas, Uterine Fibroids)

S: Varies, depending on size and location. Often no symptoms. When symptoms do occur, include vague discomfort, bloating, heaviness, pelvic pressure, dyspareunia, urinary frequency, backache, or hypermenorrhea if myoma disturbs endometrium.

O: Uterus irregularly enlarged, firm, mobile, and nodular with hard, painless nodules in the uterine wall. Heavy bleeding produces anemia.

They are usually benign. Highest incidence between the ages of 30 and 45 years and in Blacks. Myomas are estrogen dependent; after menopause, the lesions usually regress but do not disappear. Surgery may be indicated.

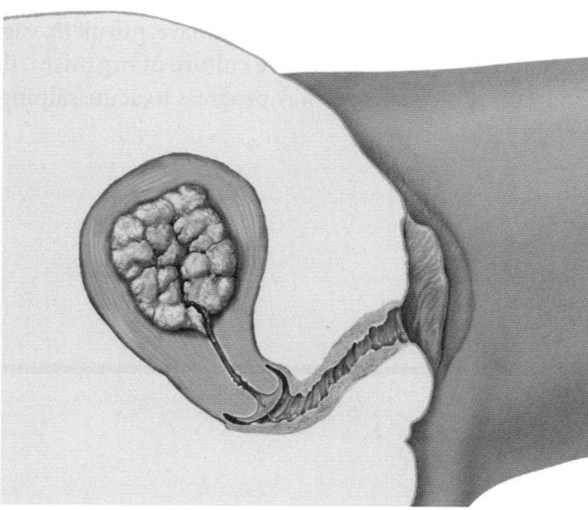

Carcinoma of the Endometrium

S: Abnormal and intermenstrual bleeding before menopause; postmenopausal bleeding or mucosanguineous discharge. Pain and weight loss occur late in the disease.

O: Uterus may be enlarged.

The Pap smear is rarely effective in detecting endometrial cancer. Women with abnormal vaginal bleeding or at high risk should have an endometrial tissue sample. Risk factors for endometrial cancer are early menarche, late menopause, history of infertility, failure to ovulate, tamoxifen, unopposed estrogen therapy (which continually stimulates the endometrium, causing hyperplasia), and obesity (which increases endogenous estrogen).

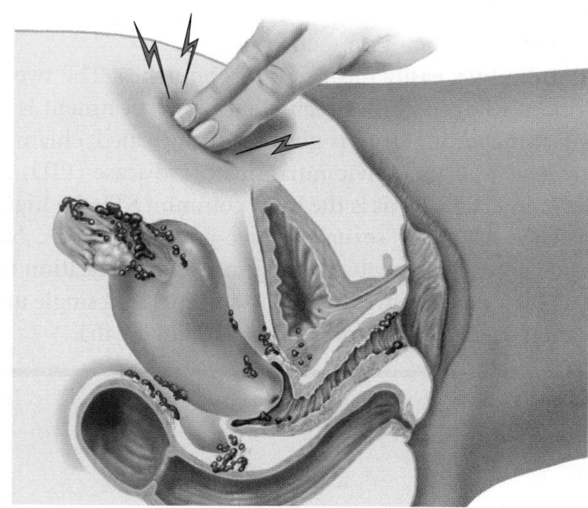

Endometriosis

S: Cyclic or chronic pelvic pain, occurring as dysmenorrhea, or dyspareunia, low backache. Also may have irregular uterine bleeding or hypermenorrhea or may be asymptomatic.

O: Uterus fixed, tender to movement. Small, firm nodular masses tender to palpation on posterior aspect of fundus, uterosacral ligaments, ovaries, sigmoid colon. Ovaries often enlarged.

Masses are aberrant growths of endometrial tissue scattered throughout pelvis, probably as a result of transplantation of tissue by retrograde menstruation. Ectopic tissue responds to hormone stimulation; builds up between periods, sloughs during menstruation. May cause infertility from pelvic adhesions, tubal obstruction, decreased ovarian function.

S, Subjective data; *O,* objective data.

TABLE 26-7 Adnexal Enlargement

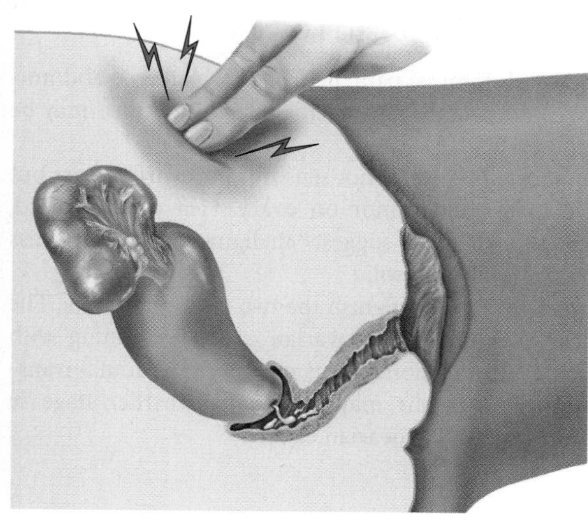

Fallopian Tube Mass—Acute Salpingitis (Pelvic Inflammatory Disease [PID])

S: Sudden fever >38° C or 100.4° F, suprapubic pain and tenderness.

O: Acute—rigid, boardlike lower abdominal musculature. May have purulent discharge from cervix. Movement of uterus and cervix causes intense pain. Pain in lateral fornices and adnexa. Bilateral adnexal masses difficult to palpate because of pain and muscle spasm. Chronic—bilateral, tender, fixed adnexal masses.

Complications include ectopic pregnancy, infertility, and reinfection. PID usually caused by *Neisseria gonorrhoeae* and *Chlamydia trachomatis.*

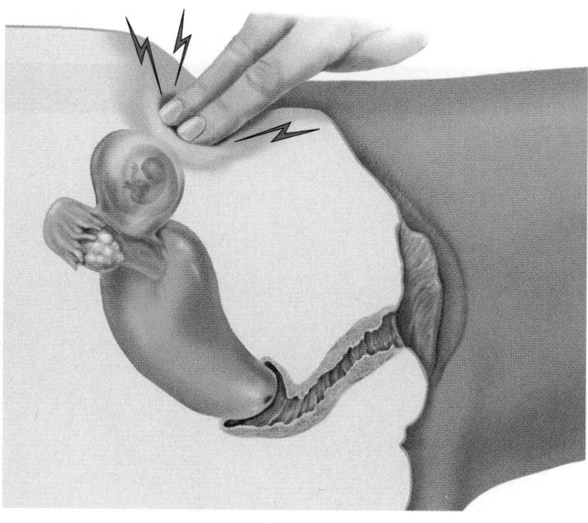

Fallopian Tube Mass—Ectopic Pregnancy

S: Amenorrhea or irregular vaginal bleeding, pelvic pain.

O: Softening of cervix and fundus; movement of cervix and uterus causes pain; palpable tender pelvic mass, which is solid, mobile, unilateral.

This has potential for serious sequelae; seek gynecologic consultation immediately, before the mass ruptures or shows signs of acute peritonitis.

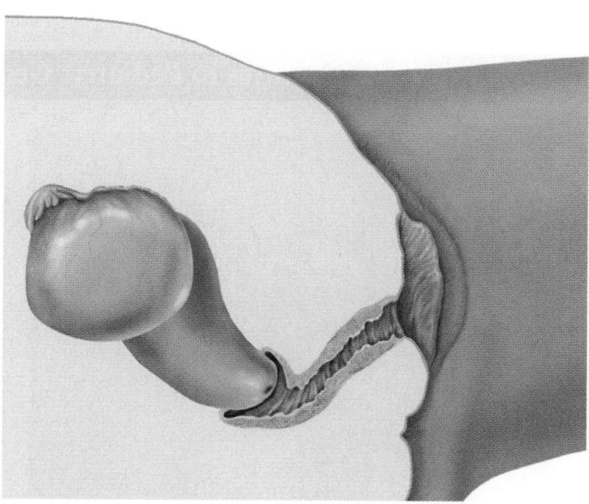

Fluctuant Ovarian Mass—Ovarian Cyst

S: Usually asymptomatic.

O: Smooth, round, fluctuant, mobile, nontender mass on ovary. Some cysts resolve spontaneously within 60 days but must be followed closely.

Continued

TABLE 26-7 Adnexal Enlargement—cont'd

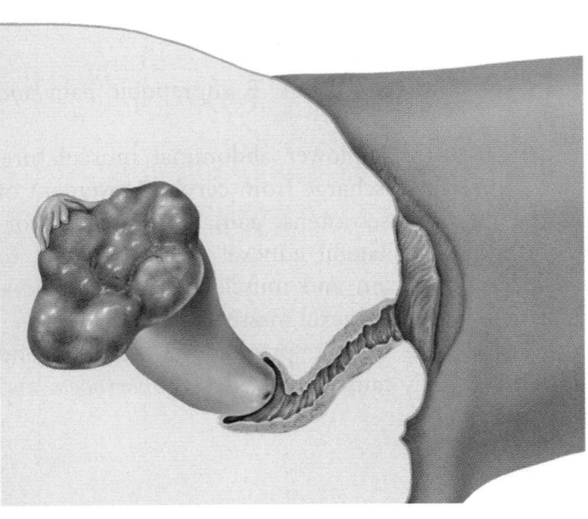

◀ Solid Ovarian Mass—Ovarian Cancer

S: May have abdominal pain, pelvic pain, increased abdominal size, bloating, or nonspecific GI symptoms or may be asymptomatic.

O: Physical examination is not sensitive for ovarian mass but may palpate solid tumor on ovary. Heavy, solid, fixed, poorly defined mass suggests malignancy; benign mass may feel mobile and solid.

Biopsy necessary to distinguish the two types of masses. The Pap smear does not detect ovarian cancer. Screening with serum CA 125 test is done but is not specific. Annual transvaginal ultrasonography may detect at an earlier stage in women at high risk for ovarian cancer.[33]

S, Subjective data; *O,* objective data.

TABLE 26-8 Abnormalities in Pediatric Genitalia

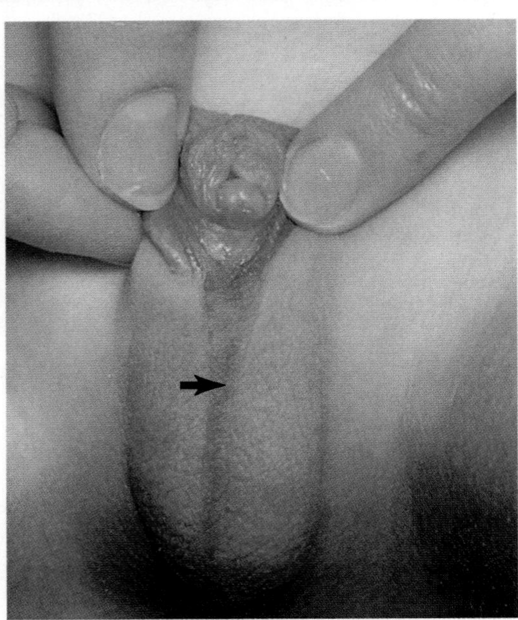

Ambiguous Genitalia

Female pseudohermaphroditism is a congenital anomaly resulting from hyperplasia of the adrenal glands, which exposes the female fetus to excess amounts of androgens. This causes masculinized external genitalia, here shown as enlargement of the clitoris and fusion of the labia. *Ambiguous* means the enlarged clitoris here may look like a small penis with hypospadias, and the fused labia look like an incompletely formed scrotum with absent testes. Other forms of intersexual conditions occur, and the family must be referred for diagnostic evaluation.

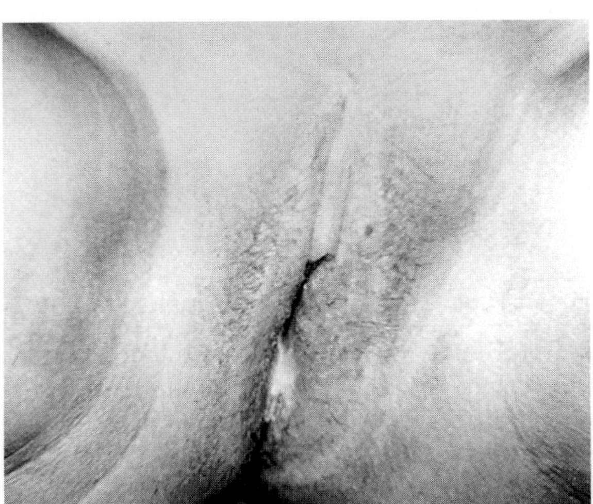

Vulvovaginitis in Child

This infection is caused by *Candida albicans* in a diabetic child. Symptoms include pruritus and burning when urine touches excoriated area. Examination shows red, shiny, edematous vulva; vaginal discharge; excoriated area from scratching.

Other, more common causes of vulvovaginitis in the prepubertal child include infection from a respiratory or bowel pathogen, sexually transmitted infection, or presence of a foreign body.

BIBLIOGRAPHY

1. Ackerson, K. (2010). Personal influences that affect motivation in Pap smear testing among African American women. *Journal of Obstetric, Gynecologic, and Neonatal Nursing, 39*(2), 136-146.
2. American Cancer Society. (2010). *Cancer facts & figures 2010.* Atlanta: Author.
3. Amies, A. M., Miller, L., & Lee, S. K. (2002). The effect of vaginal speculum lubrication on the rate of unsatisfactory cervical cytology diagnosis. *Obstetrics and Gynecology, 100*(5), 889-892.
4. Arbyn, M., Bergeron, C., Klinkhamer, P., et al. (2008). Liquid compared with conventional cervical cytology. *Obstetrics and Gynecology, 111*(1), 167-177.
5. Banikarim, C., & Chacko, M. (2005). Pelvic inflammatory disease in adolescents. *Seminars in Pediatric Infectious Diseases, 16,* 175-180.
6. Bartoszek, M. P. (2009). Recognizing polycystic ovary syndrome in the primary care setting. *Nurse Practitioner, 34*(7), 23-29.
7. Beerman, H., van Dorst, E. B. L., Kuenen-Boumeester, V. et al. (2009). Superior performance of liquid-based versus conventional cytology in a population-based cervical cancer screening program. *Gynecologic Oncology, 112*(3), 572-576.
8. Berecki-Gisolf, J., Begum, N., & Dobson, A. J. (2009). Symptoms reported by women in midlife: menopausal transition or aging? *Menopause, 16*(5), 1021-1029.
9. Bruce, M. L., & Baril, C. (2008). Save the date: screening tips and new vaccines for female HPV. *Nurse Practitioner, 33*(9), 29-34.
10. Burns, N., Briggs, P., & Gaudet, C. A. (2007). Chlamydia screening in teenage girls. *Nurse Practitioner, 32*(6), 41-43.
11. Coker, A. L., DeSimone, C. P., Eggleston, K. S., et al. (2009). Ethnic disparities in cervical cancer survival among Texas women. *Journal of Women's Health, 18*(10), 1577-1582.
12. Cunningham, F. G., Leveno, K. J., Bloom, S. L., et al. (2010). *Williams' obstetrics* (23rd ed.). New York: McGraw-Hill.
13. Daley, A. (2009). Exercise and premenstrual symptomatology: a comprehensive review. *Journal of Women's Health, 18*(6), 895-899.
14. Daley, A. M., & Cromwell, P. F. (2002). How to perform a pelvic exam for the sexually active adolescent. *Nurse Practitoner, 27,* 28-45.
15. Dowling-Castronovo, A., & Specht, J. K. (2009). Assessment of transient urinary incontinence in older adults. *American Journal of Nursing, 109*(2), 62-72.
16. Espindola, D., Kennedy, K. A., & Fischer, E. G. (2007). Management of abnormal uterine bleeding and the pathology of endometrial hyperplasia. *Obstetrics and Gynecology Clinics of North America, 34*(4), 717-737.
17. Harer, W. B., Valenzuela, G., & Lebo, D. (2002). Lubrication of the vaginal introitus and speculum does not affect Papanicolaou smears. *Obstetrics and Gynecology, 100*(5), 887-888.
18. Jones, S. (2006). A step-by-step approach to HIV/AIDS. *Nurse Practitioner, 31,* 26-41.
19. Kelsey, B. (2010). Contraceptive considerations for obese women. *The Nurse Practitioner, 35*(3), 25-32.
20. Kimberlin, D. W., & Rouse, D. J. (2004). Genital herpes. *New England Journal of Medicine, 350,* 1970-1977.
21. Kirkland, L. G. (2006). New developments in the management of STDs. *Nurse Practitioner, 31*(12), 12-23.
22. Kontoyannis, M., & Katsetos, C. (2010). Female genital mutilation. *Health Science Journal, 4*(1), 31-36.
23. Kulp, J. L., & Taylor, H. S. (2009). New theories on the causes and treatment of endometriosis. *Contemporary Ob/Gyn, 54*(4), 34-41.
24. Likes, W. M. (2009). Vulvar cancer in the wake of increasing incidence. *Nurse Practitioner, 34*(2), 45-50.
25. Lockwood-Rayermann, S., Donovan, H. S., Rambo, D. et al. (2009). Women's awareness of ovarian cancer risks and symptoms. *American Journal of Nursing, 109*(9), 36-46.
26. Mao, A. J., & Anastasi, J. K. (2010). Diagnosis and management of endometriosis: the role of the advanced practice nurse in primary care. *Journal of the American Academy of Nurse Practitioners, 22*(2), 109-116.
27. Marshall, W. A., & Tanner, J. M. (1969). Variations in pattern of pubertal changes in girls. *Archives of Disease in Childhood, 44,* 291-303.
28. McCloskey, C. (2010). Updated office testing skills for vaginal infections. *Nurse Practitioner, 35*(2), 46-52.
29. Miller, M. M., Wilson, J. M., & Waldrop, J. (2008). Current acceptance of the HPV vaccine. *Nurse Practitioner, 33*(4), 18-23.
30. Nelson, W., Moser, R. P., Gaffey, A., et al. (2009). Adherence to cervical cancer screening guidelines for U.S. women aged 25-64: data from the 2005 Health Information National Trends Survey (HINTS). *Journal of Women's Health, 18*(11), 1759-1768.
31. Noone, J. (2007). Strategies for contraceptive success. *Nurse Practitioner, 32*(6), 29-36.
32. Norton, P., & Brubaker, L. (2006). Urinary incontinence in women. *Lancet, 367*(9504), 57-67.
33. Roett, M. A., & Evans, P. (2009). Ovarian cancer: an overview. *American Family Physician, 80*(6), 609-616.
34. Rosenfield, R. L., Lipton, R. B., & Drum, M. L. (2009). Thelarche, pubarche, and menarche attainment in children with normal and elevated body mass index. *Pediatrics, 123*(1), 84-88.
35. Scarinci, I. C., Garcés-Palacio, I. C., & Partridge, E. E. (2007). An examination of acceptability of HPV vaccination among African American women and Latina immigrants. *Journal of Women's Health, 16*(8), 1224-1233.
36. Siebers, A. G., Klinkhamer, P. J. J. M., Grefte, J. M. M., et al. (2009). Comparison of liquid-based cytology with conventional cytology for detection of cervical cancer precursors: a randomized controlled trial. *Journal of the American Medical Association, 302*(16), 1757-1764.
37. Smith, R. A., Cokkinides, V., & Brawley, O.W. (2008). Cancer screening in the United States, 2008: a review of current American Cancer Society guidelines. *CA: A Cancer Journal for Clinicians, 58,* 161-179.
38. Stillson, T., Knight, A. L., & Elswick, R. K. (1997). The effectiveness and safety of two cervical cytologic techniques during pregnancy. *Journal of Family Practice, 45*(2), 159-163.
39. Warman, J. (2010). Cervical cancer screening in young women: saving lives with prevention and detection. *Oncology Nursing Forum, 37*(1), 33-38.
40. Wu, T., Mendola, P., & Buck, G. M. (2002). Ethnic differences in the presence of secondary sex characteristics and menarche among U.S. girls: the NHANES III, 1988-1994. *Pediatrics,110,* 752-757.

Summary Checklist: Female Genitalia Examination

For a PDA-downloadable version, go to http://evolve.elsevier.com/Jarvis/.

1. **Inspect external genitalia.**
2. **Palpate labia,** Skene's and Bartholin's glands.
3. Using **vaginal speculum,** inspect cervix and vagina.
4. Obtain **specimens** for cytologic study.
5. Perform **bimanual examination:** cervix, uterus, adnexa.
6. Perform **rectovaginal** examination.
7. **Test stool** for occult blood.

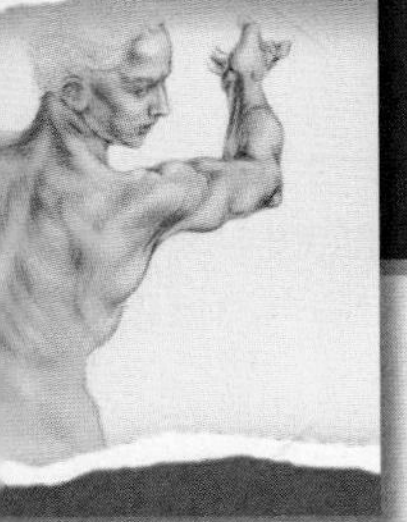

CHAPTER

27

The Complete Health Assessment: Putting It All Together

evolve WEBSITE

http://evolve.elsevier.com/Jarvis/

- Audio Key Points
- Complete Physical Examination Form
- Head-to-Toe Examination of the Adult
- Head-to-Toe Examination of the Child
- Head-to-Toe Examination of the Neonate
- NCLEX Review Questions
- Quick Assessment for Common Conditions
  Sepsis

The choreography of the complete history and physical examination is the art of arranging all the separate steps you have learned so far into a fluid whole. Your first examination may seem awkward and contrived; you may have to pause and think of what comes next rather than just gather data. Repeated rehearsals will make the choreography smoother. You will come to the point at which the procedure flows naturally, and even if you forget a step, you will be able to insert it gracefully into the next logical place.

The following examination sequence is one suggested route. It is intended to minimize the number of position changes for the patient and for you. With experience, you may wish to adapt this and arrange a sequence that feels natural for you.

A complete examination is performed at a patient's first entry in an outpatient setting or initial admission to the hospital. Perform all the steps listed here for a complete examination. With experience, you will learn to strike a balance between which steps you must retain to be thorough and which corners you may safely cut when time is pressing. The steps for the follow-up or shift assessment are described in the next chapter.

Have all equipment prepared and accessible before the examination. Review Chapter 8 for the list of necessary equipment, the setting, the patient's emotional state, your demeanor, and the preparation of the patient considering his or her age.

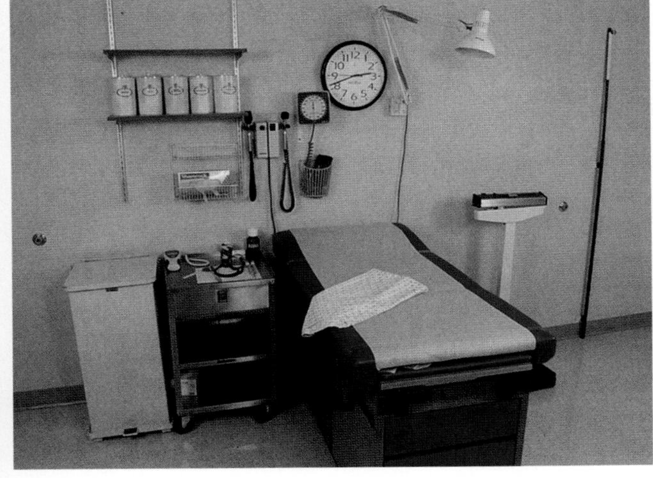

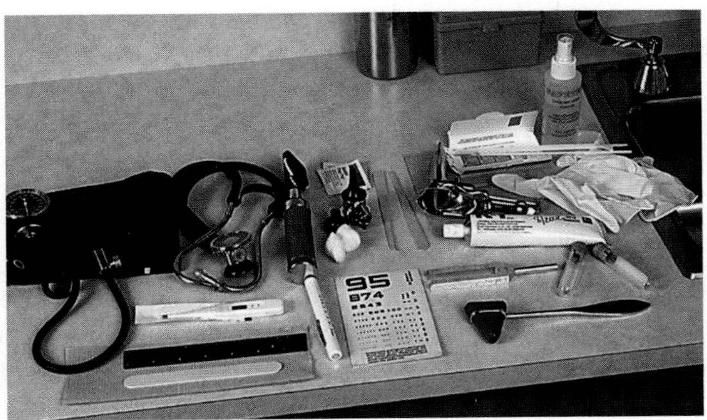

Sequence	Selected Photos

The patient walks into the room, sits; the examiner sits facing the patient; the patient remains in street clothes. (Note: Position changes are in **bold** letters.)

THE HEALTH HISTORY

Collect the history, complete or limited as visit warrants. While obtaining the history and throughout the examination, note data on the person's general appearance.

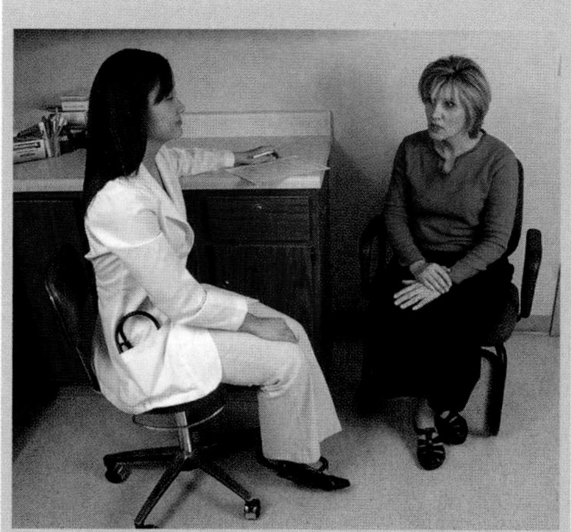

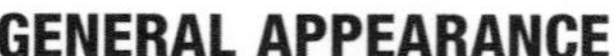

GENERAL APPEARANCE

1. Appears stated age
2. Level of consciousness
3. Skin color
4. Nutritional status
5. Posture and position comfortably erect
6. Obvious physical deformities
7. Mobility
   Gait
   Use of assistive devices
   Range of motion (ROM) of joints
   No involuntary movement
   Able to rise from a seated position easily
8. Facial expression
9. Mood and affect
10. Speech: articulation, pattern, content appropriate, native language
11. Hearing
12. Personal hygiene

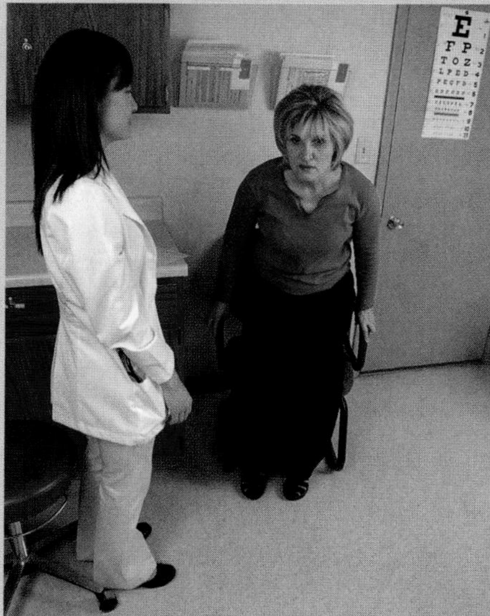

MEASUREMENT

1. Weight
2. Height
3. Waist circumference
4. Compute body mass index
5. Vision using Snellen eye chart

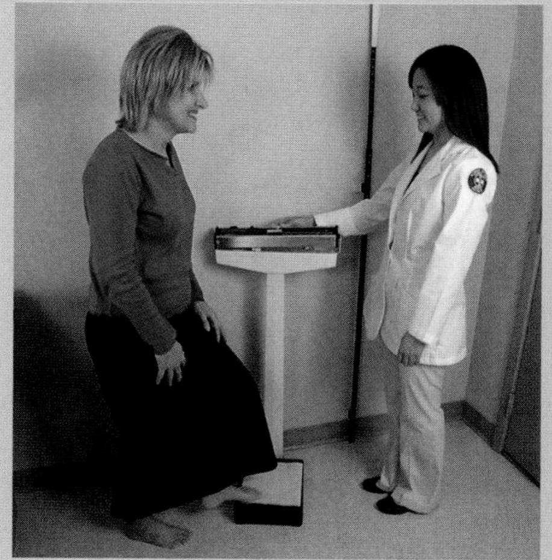

Ask the person to empty the bladder (save specimen, if needed), to disrobe except for underpants, and to put on a gown. The person **sits with legs dangling** off the side of the bed or table; you stand in front of the person.

SKIN

1. Examine both hands, and inspect the nails.
2. For the rest of the examination, examine the skin with the corresponding regional examination.

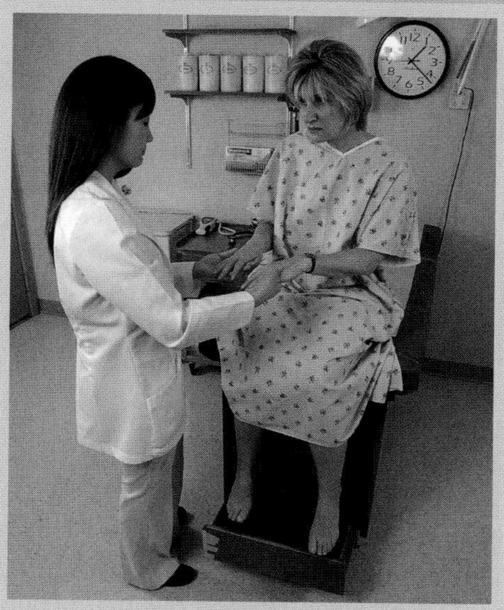

VITAL SIGNS

1. Radial pulse
2. Respirations
3. Blood pressure (BP) in arm(s)
4. BP in lower leg; compute ankle/brachial index (if indicated)
5. Temperature (if indicated)

HEAD AND FACE

1. Inspect and palpate scalp, hair, and cranium.
2. Inspect face: expression, symmetry (cranial nerve VII).
3. Palpate the temporal artery, then the temporomandibular joint as the person opens and closes the mouth.
4. Palpate the maxillary sinuses and the frontal sinuses.

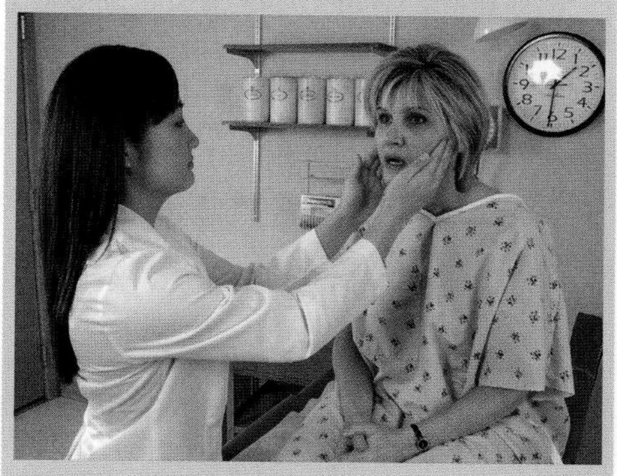

EYES

1. Test visual fields by confrontation (cranial nerve II).
2. Test extraocular muscles: corneal light reflex, six cardinal positions of gaze (cranial nerves III, IV, VI).
3. Inspect external eye structures.
4. Inspect conjunctivae, sclerae, corneas, irides.
5. Test pupil: size, response to light and accommodation.

Darken room.

6. Using an ophthalmoscope, inspect ocular fundus: red reflex, disc, vessels, and retinal background.

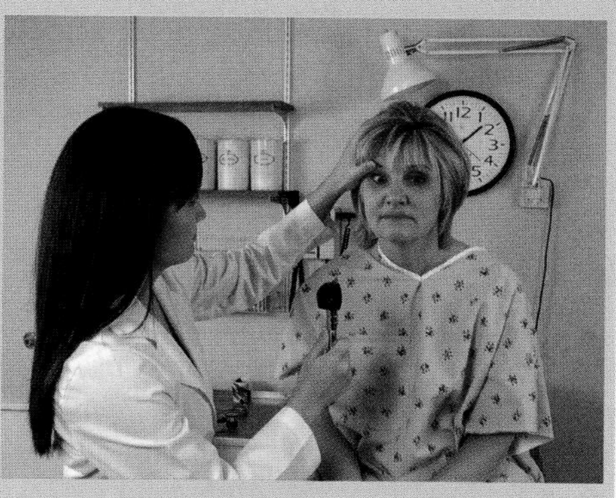

EARS

1. Inspect the external ear: position and alignment, skin condition, and auditory meatus.
2. Move auricle and push tragus for tenderness.
3. With an otoscope, inspect the canal, then the tympanic membrane for color, position, landmarks, and integrity.
4. Test hearing: whispered voice test.

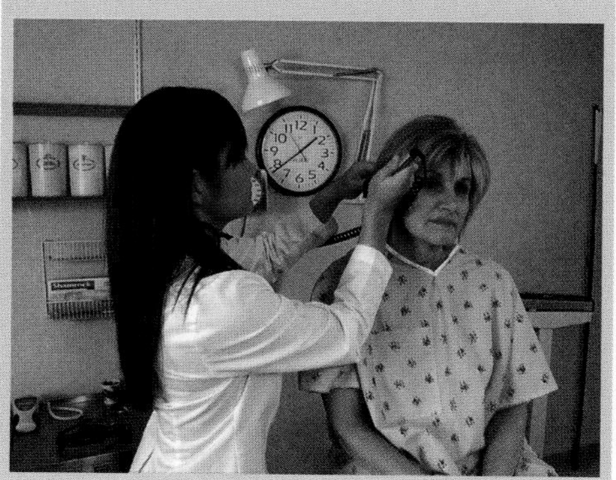

Sequence	Selected Photos

NOSE

1. Inspect the external nose: symmetry, lesions.
2. Inspect facial symmetry (cranial nerve VII).
3. Test the patency of each nostril.
4. With a speculum, inspect the nares: nasal mucosa, septum, and turbinates.

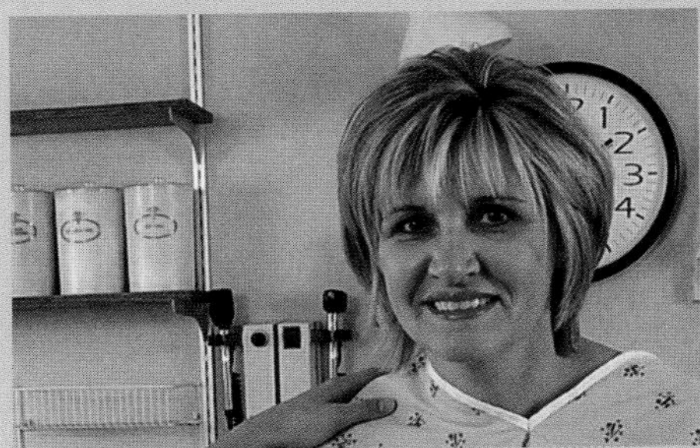

MOUTH AND THROAT

1. With a penlight, inspect the mouth: buccal mucosa, teeth and gums, tongue, floor of mouth, palate, and uvula.
2. Grade tonsils, if present.
3. Note mobility of uvula as the person phonates "ahh," and test gag reflex (cranial nerves IX, X).
4. Ask the person to stick out the tongue (cranial nerve XII).
5. With a gloved hand, bimanually palpate the mouth, if indicated.

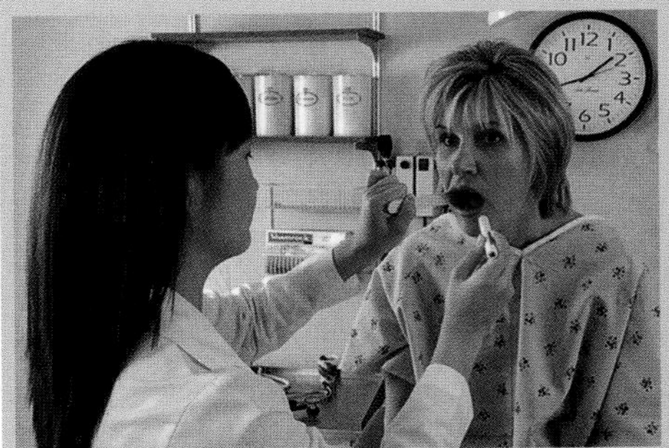

NECK

1. Inspect the neck: symmetry, lumps, and pulsations.
2. Palpate the cervical lymph nodes.
3. Inspect and palpate the carotid pulse, one side at a time. If indicated, listen for carotid bruits.
4. Palpate the trachea in midline.
5. Test ROM and muscle strength against your resistance: head forward and back, head turned to each side, and shoulder shrug (cranial nerve XI).

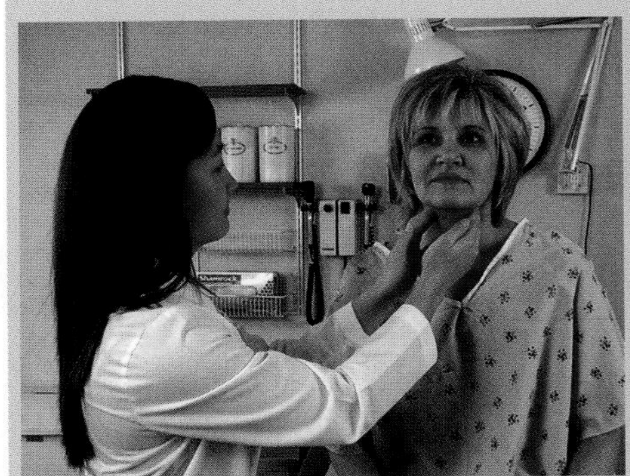

Step behind the person, taking your stethoscope, ruler, and marking pen with you.

6. Palpate thyroid gland, posterior approach.

Open the person's gown to expose all of the back for examination of the thorax, but leave gown on shoulders and anterior chest.

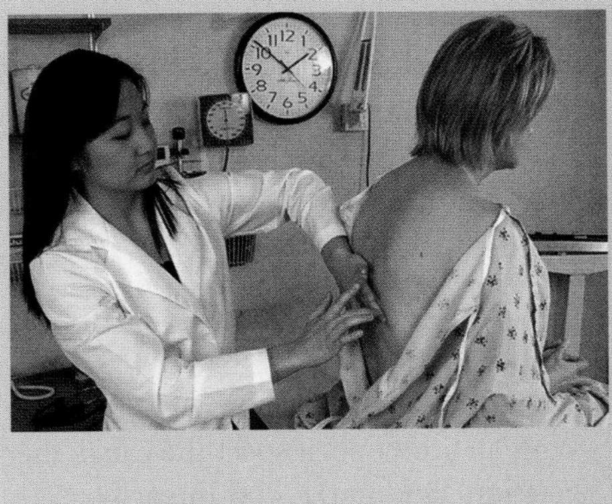

Sequence	Selected Photos

CHEST, POSTERIOR AND LATERAL

1. Inspect the posterior chest: configuration of the thoracic cage, skin characteristics, and symmetry of shoulders and muscles.
2. Palpate: symmetric expansion; tactile fremitus; lumps or tenderness.
3. Palpate length of spinous processes.
4. Percuss over all lung fields; percuss diaphragmatic excursion.
5. Percuss costovertebral angle, noting tenderness.
6. Auscultate breath sounds, comparing side to side in upper and lower lung fields; note any adventitious sounds.

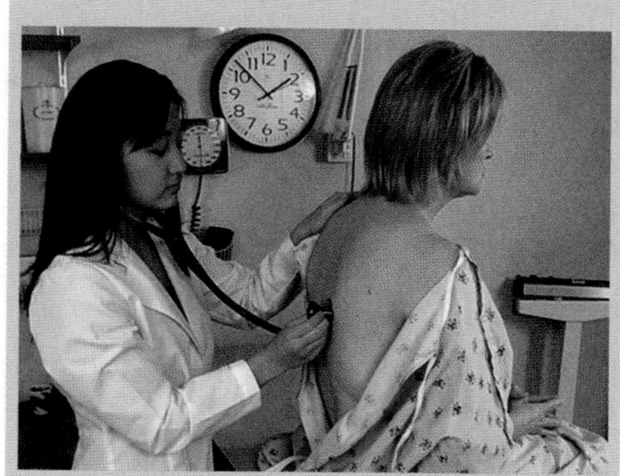

Move around to face the patient; the patient remains sitting. For a female breast examination, ask permission to lift gown to drape on the shoulders, exposing the anterior chest; for a male, lower the gown to the lap.

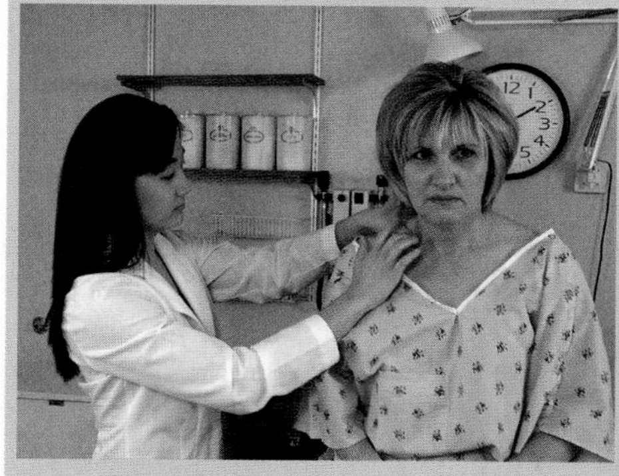

CHEST, ANTERIOR

1. Inspect: respirations and skin characteristics.
2. Palpate: tactile fremitus, lumps, or tenderness.
3. Percuss anterior lung fields.
4. Auscultate breath sounds, comparing side to side in upper and lateral lung fields.

HEART

1. Ask the person to lean forward and exhale briefly; auscultate cardiac base for any murmurs.

UPPER EXTREMITIES

1. Test ROM and muscle strength of hands, arms, and shoulders.
2. Palpate the epitrochlear nodes.

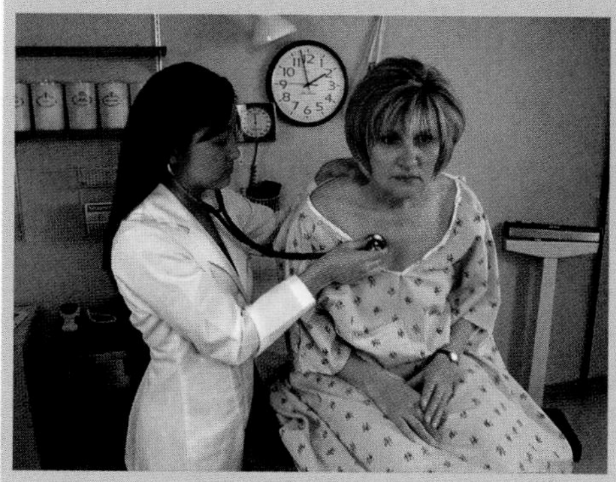

FEMALE BREASTS

1. Inspect for symmetry, mobility, and dimpling as the woman lifts arms over the head, pushes the hands on the hips, and leans forward.
2. Inspect supraclavicular and infraclavicular areas.

Help the woman to **lie supine with head at a flat** to 30-degree angle. Stand at the person's *right* side. Drape the gown up across shoulders, and place an extra sheet across lower abdomen.

3. Palpate each breast, lifting the same-side arm up over head. Include the tail of Spence and areola.
4. Palpate each nipple for discharge.
5. Support the person's arm, and palpate axilla and regional lymph nodes.
6. Teach breast self-examination.

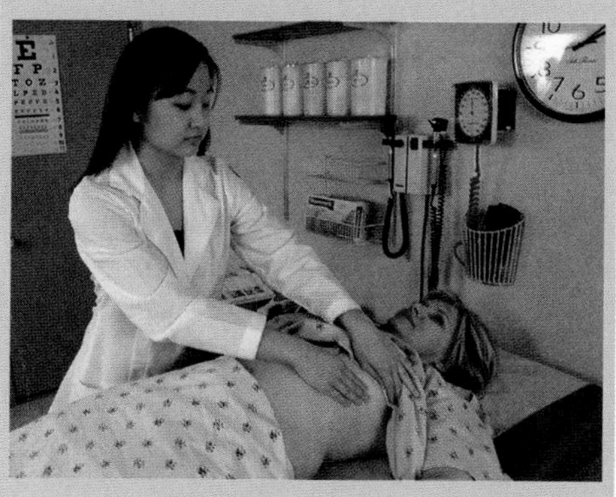

Objective Data

Sequence

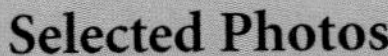

Selected Photos

MALE BREASTS

1. Inspect and palpate while palpating the anterior chest wall.
2. Supporting each arm, palpate the axilla and regional nodes.

NECK VESSELS

1. Inspect each side of neck for a jugular venous pulse, turning the person's head slightly to the other side.
2. Estimate jugular venous pressure, if indicated.

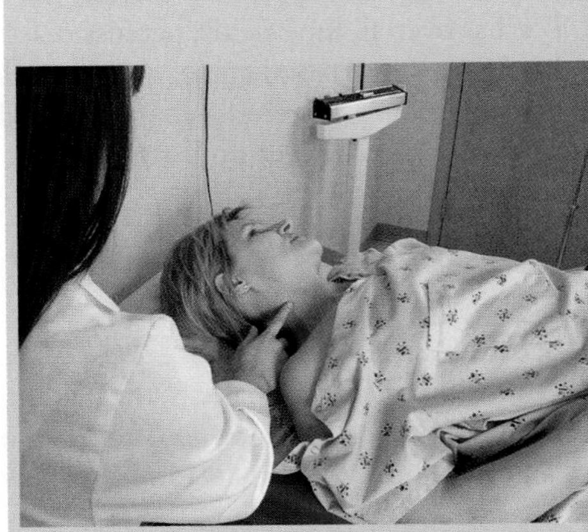

HEART

1. Inspect the precordium for any pulsations or heave (lift).
2. Palpate the apical impulse and note the location.
3. Palpate the precordium for any abnormal thrill.
4. Auscultate apical rate and rhythm.
5. Auscultate with the diaphragm of the stethoscope to study heart sounds, inching from the apex up to the base, or vice versa.
6. Auscultate the heart sounds with the bell of the stethoscope, again inching through all locations.
7. Turn the person over to left side while again auscultating apex with the bell.

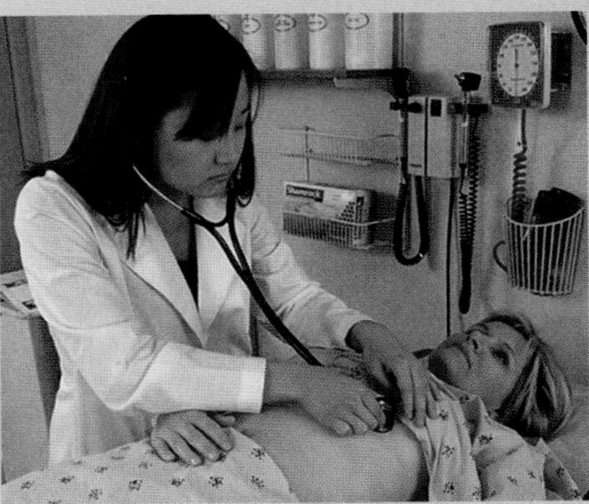

The person should be **supine,** with the bed or table flat; arrange drapes to expose the abdomen from the chest to the pubis.

ABDOMEN

1. Inspect: contour, symmetry, skin characteristics, umbilicus, and pulsations.
2. Auscultate bowel sounds.
3. Auscultate for vascular sounds over the aorta and renal arteries.
4. Percuss all quadrants.
5. Percuss height of the liver span in right midclavicular line.
6. Percuss the location of the spleen.

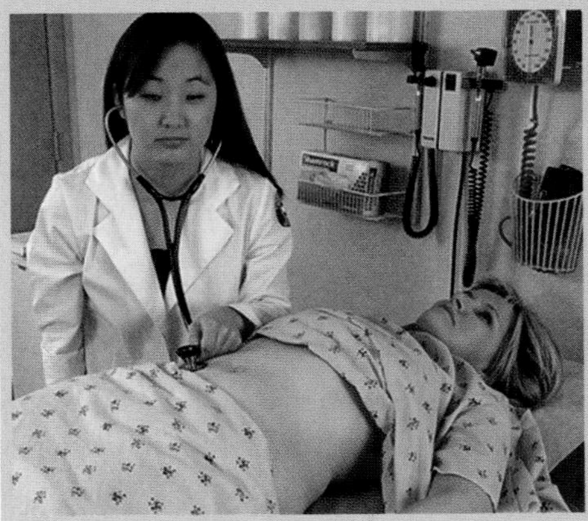

7. Palpate: light palpation in all quadrants, then deep palpation in all quadrants.
8. Palpate for liver, spleen, and kidneys.
9. Palpate aortic pulsation, if indicated.

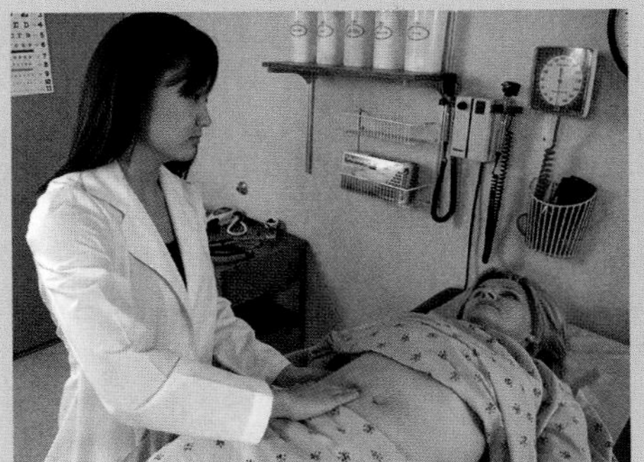

INGUINAL AREA

1. Palpate each groin for the femoral pulse and the inguinal nodes. Lift the drape to expose the legs.

Sequence	Selected Photos

LOWER EXTREMITIES

1. Inspect: symmetry, skin characteristics, and hair distribution.
2. Palpate pulses: popliteal, posterior tibial, dorsalis pedis.
3. Palpate for temperature and pretibial edema.
4. Separate toes and inspect.
5. Test ROM and muscle strength of hips, knees, ankles, and feet.

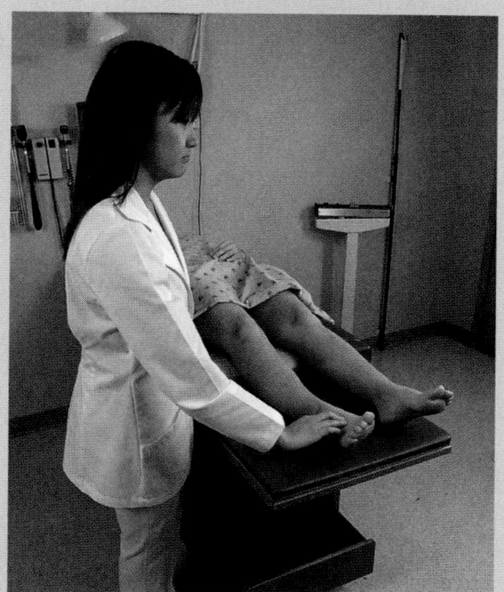

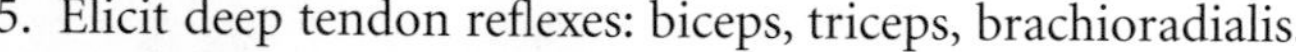

Ask the person to **sit up and to dangle** the legs off the bed or table. Keep the gown on and the drape over the lap.

MUSCULOSKELETAL

1. Note muscle strength as person sits up.

NEUROLOGIC

1. Test sensation in selected areas on face, arms, hands, legs, and feet: superficial pain, light touch, and vibration.
2. Test position sense of finger, one hand.
3. Test stereognosis, using a familiar object.
4. Test cerebellar function of the upper extremities using finger-to-nose test or rapid-alternating-movements test.

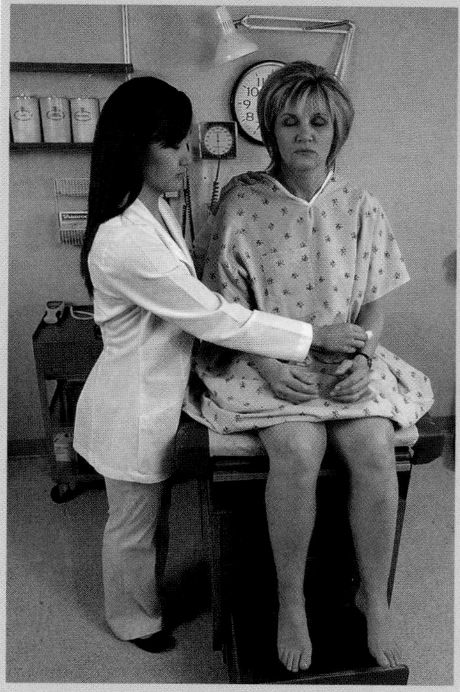

5. Elicit deep tendon reflexes: biceps, triceps, brachioradialis.

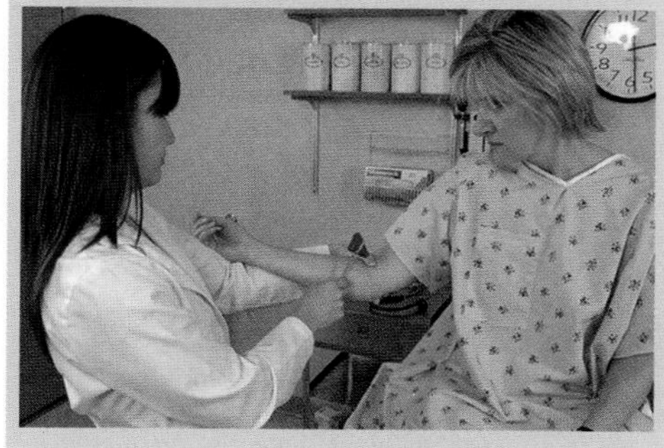

Sequence	Selected Photos

6. Test the cerebellar function of the lower extremities by asking the person to run each heel down the opposite shin.
7. Elicit deep tendon reflexes: patellar and Achilles.
8. Test the Babinski reflex.

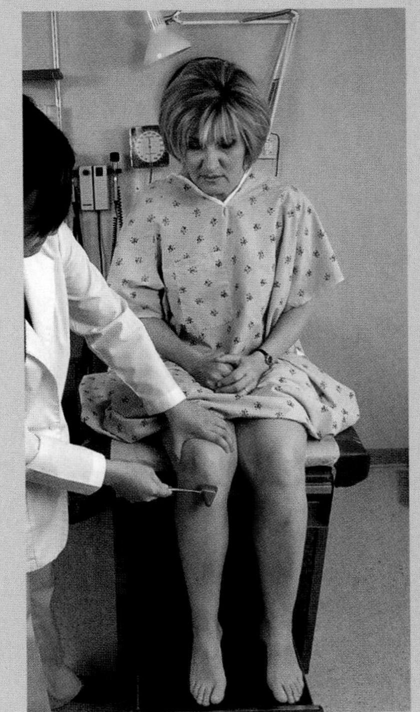

Ask the person to **stand** with the gown on. Stand close to the person.

LOWER EXTREMITIES

1. Inspect legs for varicose veins.

MUSCULOSKELETAL

1. Ask the person **to walk** across the room in his or her regular walk, turn, and then walk back toward you in heel-to-toe fashion.
2. Ask the person to walk on the toes for a few steps, then to walk on the heels for a few steps.
3. Stand close and check Romberg's sign.

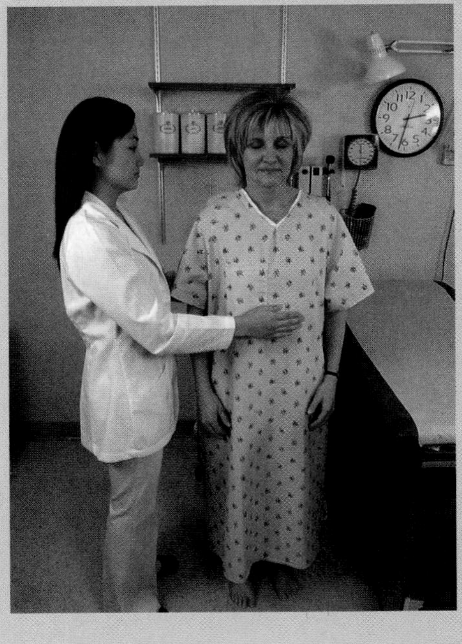

Sequence	Selected Photos

4. Ask the person to hold the edge of the bed and to perform a shallow knee bend, one for each leg.
5. Stand behind and check the spine as the person touches the toes.
6. Stabilize the pelvis and test the ROM of the spine as the person hyperextends, rotates, and laterally bends.

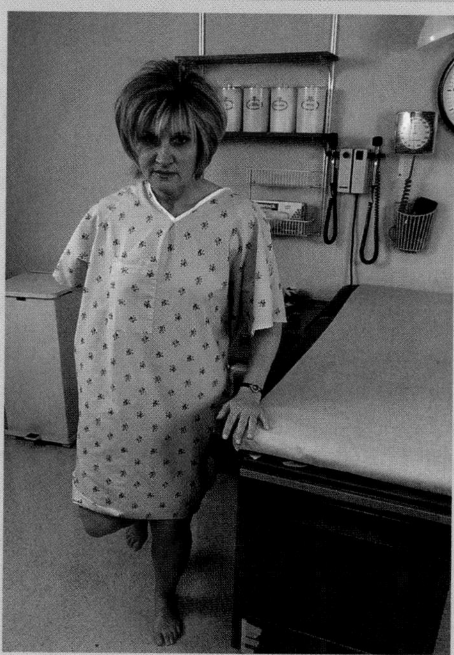

For the male patient, sit on a stool in front of him. The person stands.

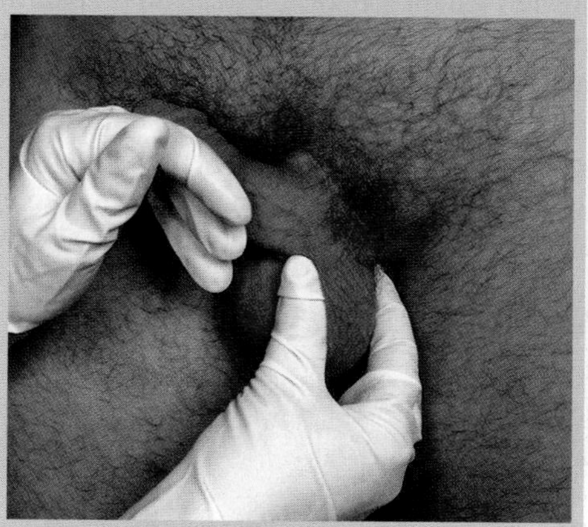

MALE GENITALIA

1. Inspect the penis and scrotum.
2. Palpate the scrotal contents. If a mass exists, transilluminate.
3. Check for inguinal hernia.
4. Teach testicular self-examination.

For an adult male, ask him to bend over the examination table, supporting the torso with forearms on the table. Assist the bedfast male to a left lateral position, with the right leg drawn up.

MALE RECTUM

1. Inspect the perianal area.
2. With a gloved lubricated finger, palpate the rectal walls and prostate gland.
3. Save a stool specimen for an occult blood test.

Assist the female back to the examination table, and help her assume **the lithotomy position.** Drape her appropriately. You sit on a stool at the foot of the table for the speculum examination, and then stand for the bimanual examination.

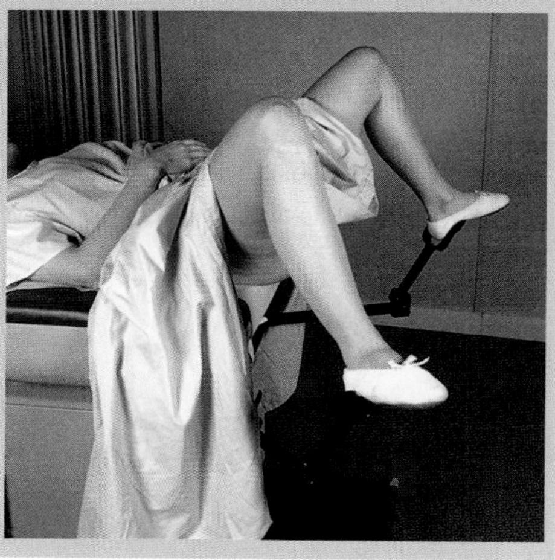

Sequence

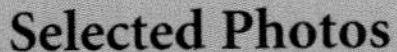

Selected Photos

FEMALE GENITALIA

1. Inspect the perineal and perianal areas.
2. With a vaginal speculum, inspect the cervix and vaginal walls.
3. Procure specimens.
4. Perform a bimanual examination: cervix, uterus, and adnexa.
5. Continue the bimanual examination, checking the rectum and rectovaginal walls.
6. Save a stool specimen for an occult blood test.
7. Provide tissues for the female to wipe the perineal area, and help her up to a **sitting position**.

Tell the patient you are finished with the examination and that you will leave the room as he or she gets dressed. Return to discuss the examination and further plans and to answer any questions. Thank the person for his or her time.

For the hospitalized person, return the bed and any room equipment to the way you found it. Make sure the call light and telephone are within easy reach.

THE NEONATE AND INFANT

Review Chapter 8 for the steps on preparation and positioning and on developmental principles of the infant. The 1-minute and 5-minute Apgar results will give important data on the neonate's immediate response to extrauterine life. The following sequence will expand these data. You may reorder this sequence as the infant's sleep and wakefulness state or physical condition warrants.

The infant is **supine** on a warming table or examination table with an overhead heating element. The infant may be nude except for a diaper over a boy.

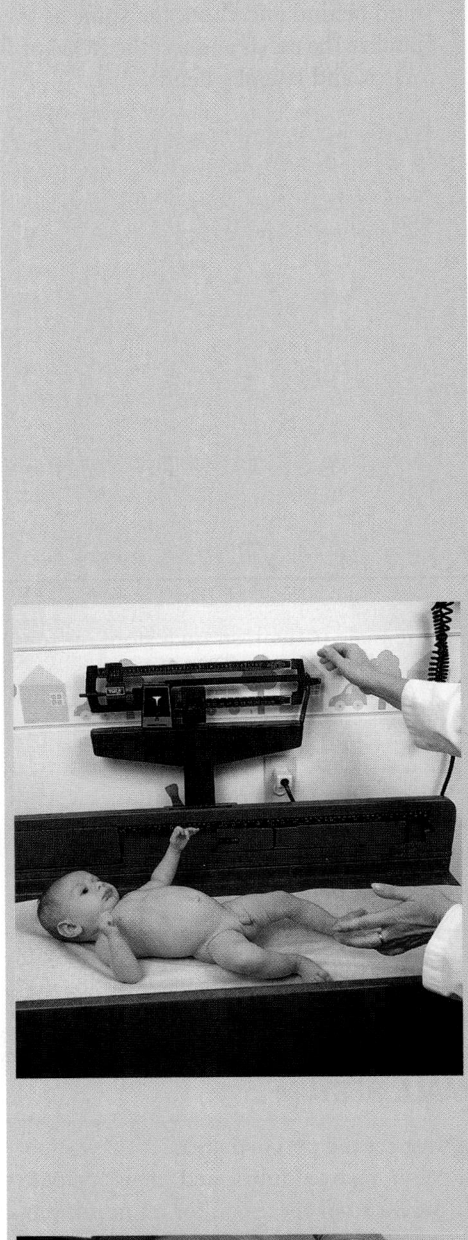

Vital Signs

Note pulse, respirations, and temperature.

Measurement

Weight, length, and head circumference are measured and plotted on growth curves for the infant's age.

General Appearance

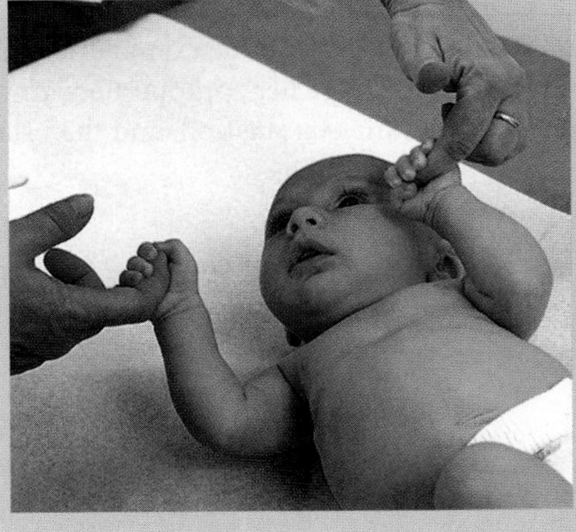

1. Body symmetry, spontaneous position, flexion of head and extremities, and spontaneous movement.
2. Skin color and characteristics, any obvious deformities.
3. Symmetry and positioning of the facial features.
4. Alert, responsive affect.
5. Strong, lusty cry.

Sequence

Selected Photos

Chest and Heart

1. Inspect the skin condition over the chest and abdomen, chest configuration, and nipples and breast tissue.
2. Note movement of the abdomen with respirations, and note any chest retraction.
3. Palpate apical impulse and note its location; chest wall for thrills; tactile fremitus if the infant is crying.
4. Auscultate breath sounds, heart sounds in all locations, and bowel sounds in the abdomen and in the chest.

Abdomen

1. Inspect the shape of the abdomen and skin condition.
2. Inspect the umbilicus; count vessels; note condition of cord or stump, any hernia.
3. Palpate skin turgor.
4. Palpate lightly for muscle tone, liver, spleen tip, and bladder.
5. Palpate deeply for kidneys, any mass.
6. Palpate femoral pulses, inguinal lymph nodes.
7. Percuss all quadrants.

Head and Face

1. Note molding after delivery, any swelling on cranium, bulging of fontanel with crying or at rest.
2. Palpate fontanels, suture lines, and any swellings.
3. Inspect positioning and symmetry of facial features at rest and while the infant is crying.

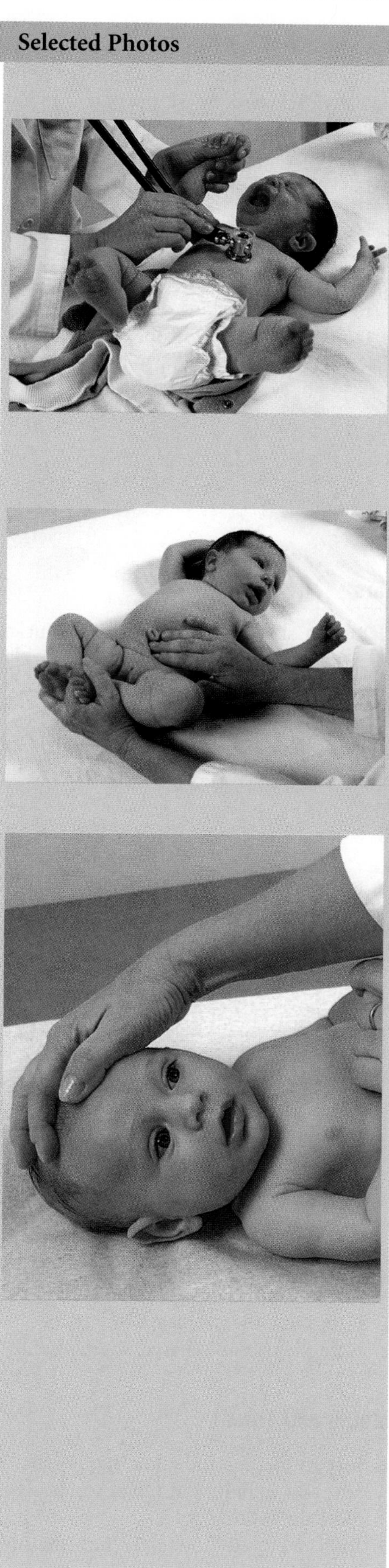

Sequence	Selected Photos

To open the neonate's eyes, support the head and shoulders and gently lower the baby backward, or ask the parent to hold the baby over his or her shoulder while you stand behind the parent.

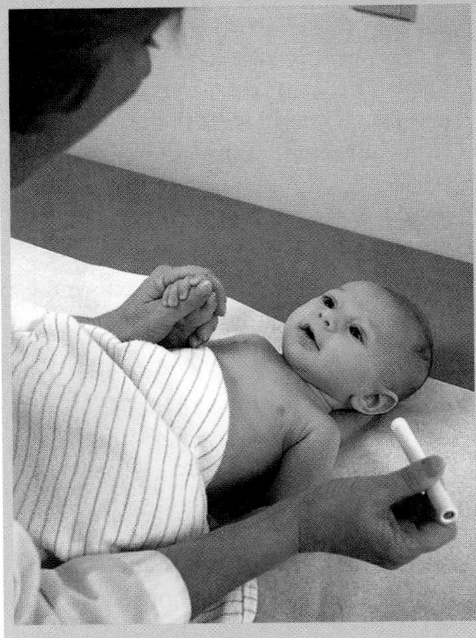

Eyes

1. Inspect the lids (edematous in the neonate), palpebral slant, conjunctivae, any nystagmus, and any discharge.
2. Using a penlight, elicit the pupillary reflex, blink reflex, and corneal light reflex; assess tracking of moving light.
3. Using an ophthalmoscope, elicit the red reflex.

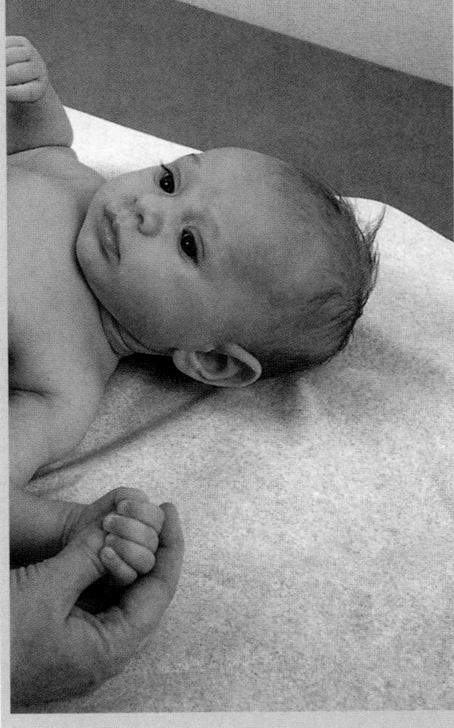

Ears

1. Inspect size, shape, alignment of auricles, patency of auditory canals, any extra skin tags or pits.
2. Note the startle reflex in response to a loud noise.
3. Palpate flexible auricles.

(Defer otoscopic examination until the end of the complete examination.)

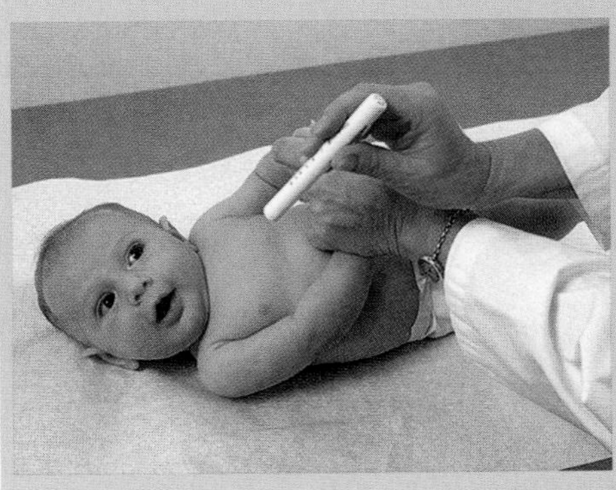

Nose

1. Determine the patency of the nares.
2. Note the nasal discharge, sneezing, and any flaring with respirations.

Mouth and Throat

1. Inspect the lips and gums, high-arched intact palate, buccal mucosa, tongue size, and frenulum of tongue; note absent or minimal salivation in neonate.
2. Note the rooting reflex.
3. Insert a gloved little finger, note the sucking reflex, and palpate the palate.

Sequence	Selected Photos

Neck

1. Lift the shoulders and let the head lag to inspect the neck: note midline trachea, any skinfolds, and any lumps.
2. Palpate the lymph nodes, the thyroid, and any masses.
3. While the infant is supine, elicit the tonic neck reflex; note a supple neck with movement.

Upper Extremities

1. Inspect and manipulate, noting ROM, muscle tone, and absence of scarf sign (elbow should not reach midline).
2. Count fingers, count palmar creases, and note color of hands and nail beds.
3. Place your thumbs in the infant's palms to note the grasp reflex; then wrap your hands around infant's hands to pull up, and note the head lag.

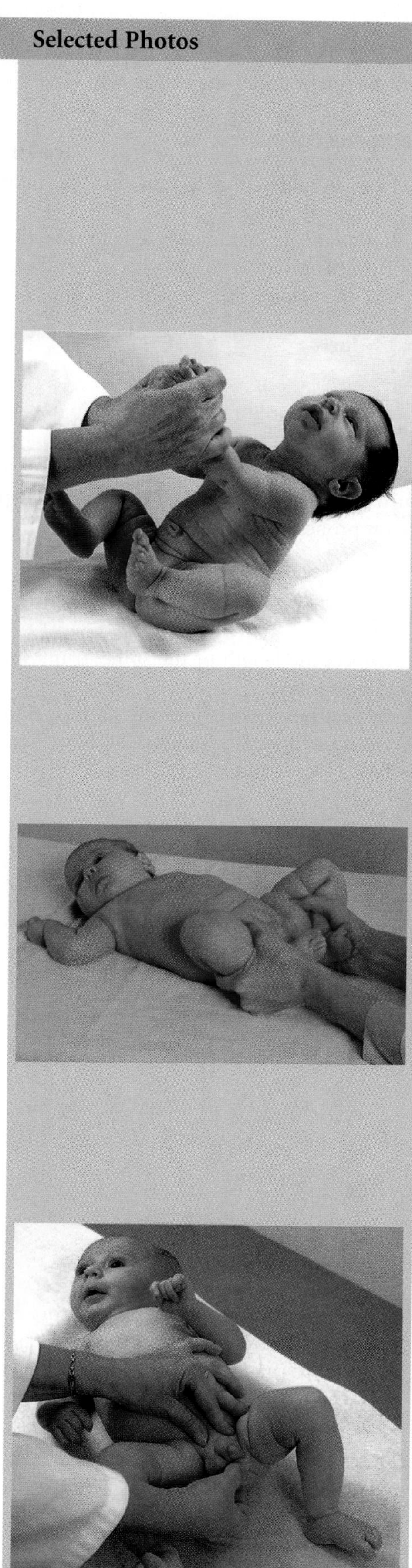

Lower Extremities

1. Inspect and manipulate the legs and feet, noting ROM, muscle tone, and skin condition.
2. Note alignment of feet and toes, look for flat soles, and count toes; note any syndactyly.
3. Test Ortolani sign for hip stability.

Genitalia

1. *Females.* Inspect labia and clitoris (edematous in the newborn), vernix caseosa between labia, and patent vagina.
2. *Males.* Inspect position of urethral meatus (do not retract foreskin), strength of urine stream if possible, and rugae on scrotum.
3. Palpate the testes in the scrotum.

Sequence	Selected Photos

Lift the infant under the axillae, and hold the infant facing you at eye level.

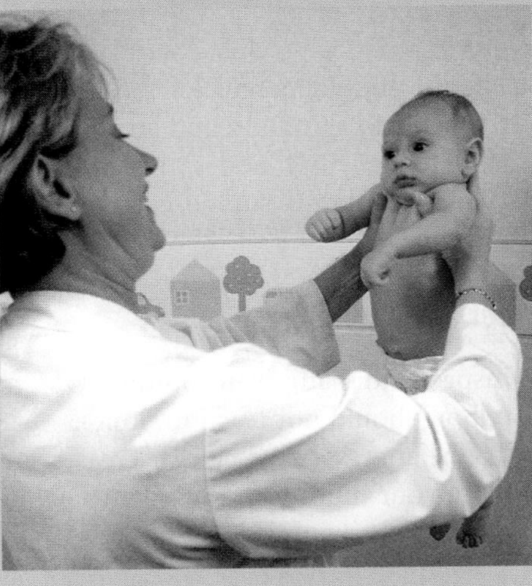

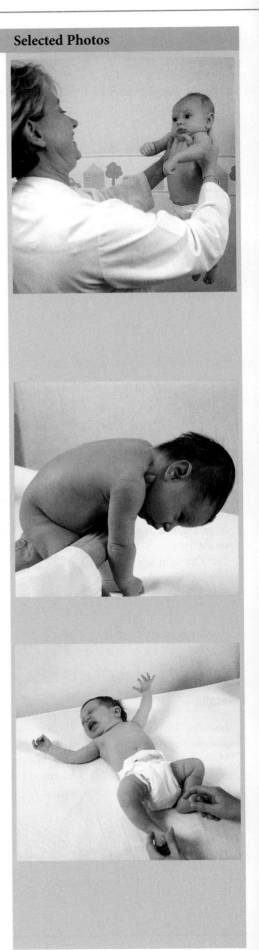

Neuromuscular

1. Note shoulder muscle tone and the infant's ability to stay in your hands without slipping.
2. Rotate the neonate slowly side to side; note the doll's eye reflex.
3. Turn the infant around so his or her back is to you; elicit the stepping reflex and the placing reflex against the edge of the examination table.

Turn the infant over and hold him or her prone in your hands, or place the infant prone on the examination table.

Spine and Rectum

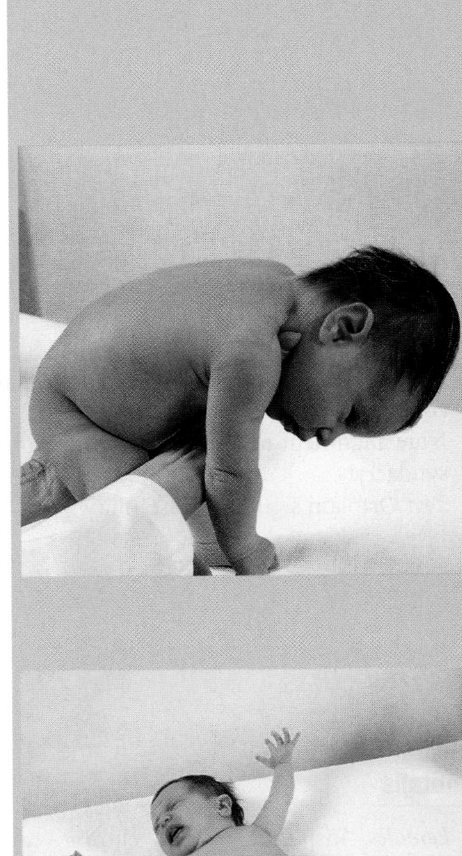

1. Inspect the length of the spine, trunk incurvation reflex, and symmetry of gluteal folds.
2. Inspect intact skin; note any sinus openings, protrusions, or tufts of hair.
3. Note patent anal opening. Check for passage of meconium stool during the first 24 to 48 hours.

Final Procedures

1. With an otoscope, inspect the auditory canals and the tympanic membranes.
2. Elicit the Moro reflex by letting the infant's head and trunk drop back a short way, by jarring crib sides, or by making a loud noise.

Sequence

Selected Photos

THE YOUNG CHILD

Review the developmental considerations in preparing for an examination of the toddler and the young child in Chapter 8. A young child during this time is beset with independence and dependence needs on the parent, is aware of and fearful of a new environment, has a fear of invasive procedures, dislikes being restrained, and may be attached to a security object.

Focus on the parent as the child plays with a toy.

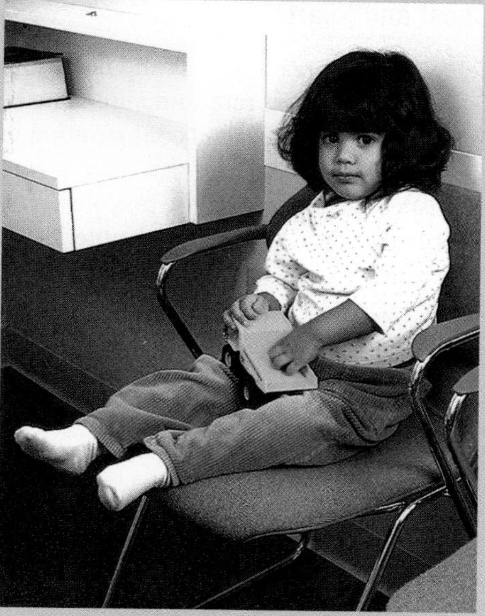

The Health History

1. Collect the history, including developmental data.
2. During the history, note data on general appearance.

General Appearance

1. Note child's ability to amuse himself or herself while the parent speaks.
2. Note parent and child interaction.
3. Note gross motor and fine motor skills as the child plays with toys.

Gradually focus on and involve yourself with the child, at first in a "play" period.

4. Evaluate developmental milestones by using a Denver II test: gait, jumping, hopping, building a tower, and throwing a ball.
5. Evaluate posture while the child is sitting and standing. Evaluate alignment of the legs and feet while the child is walking.
6. Evaluate speech acquisition.
7. Evaluate vision, hearing ability.
8. Evaluate social interaction.

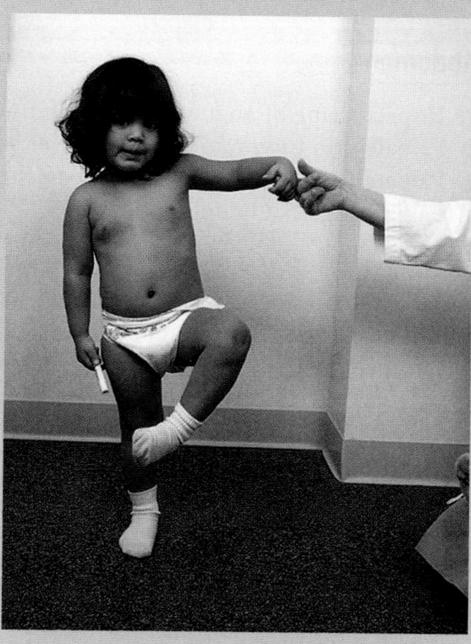

Ask the parent to undress the child to the diaper or the underpants. Position the older infant and young child, 6 months to 2 or 3 years, in the parent's lap. Move your chair to sit knee-to-knee with the parent. A 4- or 5-year-old child usually feels comfortable on the examination table.

Measurement

Height, weight, head circumference (may need to defer head circumference until later in the examination).

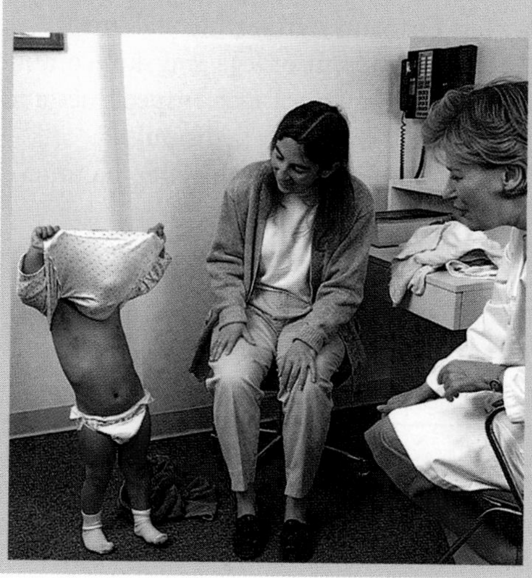

Sequence	Selected Photos

Chest and Heart

1. Auscultate breath sounds and heart sounds in all locations, count respiratory rate, count heart rate, and auscultate bowel sounds.
2. Inspect size, shape, and configuration of chest cage. Assess respiratory movement.
3. Inspect pulsations on the precordium. Note nipple and breast development.
4. Palpate apical impulse and note location, chest wall for thrills, any tactile fremitus.

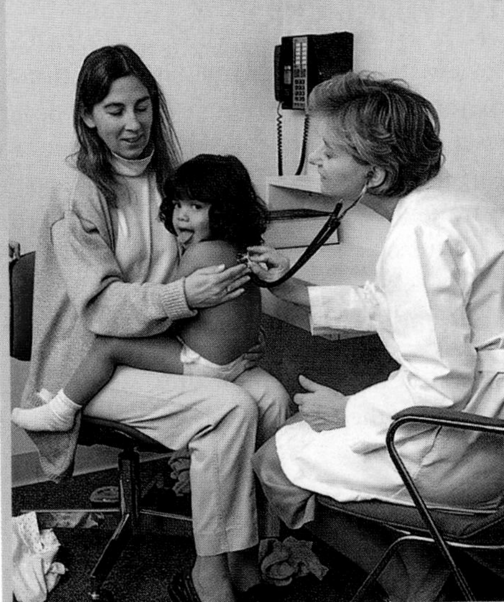

The child should be sitting up in the parent's lap or on the examination table, diaper or underpants in place.

Abdomen

1. Inspect shape of abdomen, skin condition, and periumbilical area.
2. Palpate skin turgor, muscle tone, liver edge, spleen, kidneys, and any masses.
3. Palpate the femoral pulses. Compare strength with radial pulses.
4. Palpate inguinal lymph nodes.

Genitalia

1. Inspect the external genitalia.
2. On males, palpate the scrotum for testes. If masses are present, transilluminate.

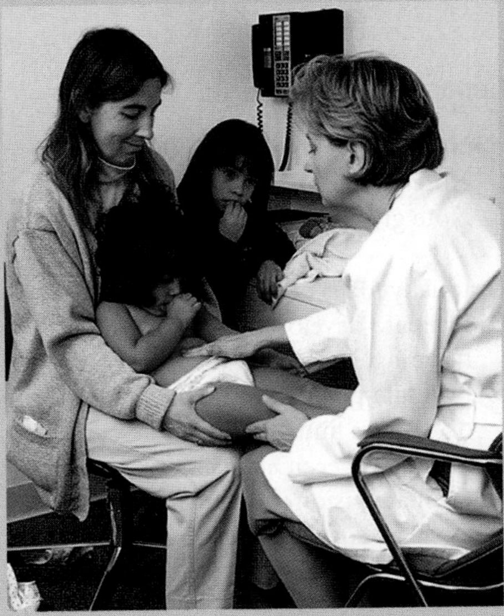

Lower Extremities

1. Test Ortolani sign for hip stability.
2. Note alignment of legs and skin condition.
3. Note alignment of feet. Inspect toes and longitudinal arch.
4. Palpate the dorsalis pedis pulse.
5. Gain cooperation with reflex hammer. Elicit plantar, Achilles, and patellar reflexes.

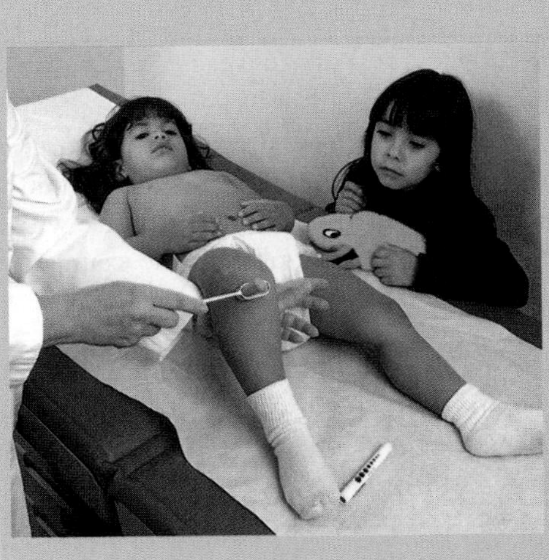

Sequence	Selected Photos

The child should be sitting up in the parent's lap or on the examination table, diaper or underpants in place.

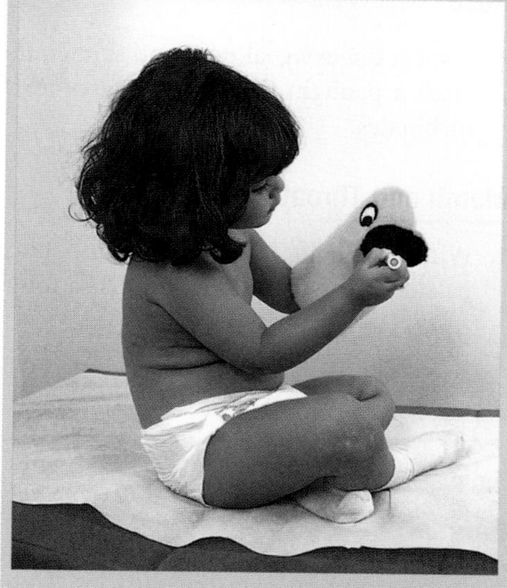

Upper Extremities

1. Inspect arms and hands for alignment, skin condition; inspect fingers, and note palmar creases.
2. Palpate and count the radial pulse.
3. Test biceps and triceps reflexes with a reflex hammer.
4. Measure blood pressure.

Head and Neck

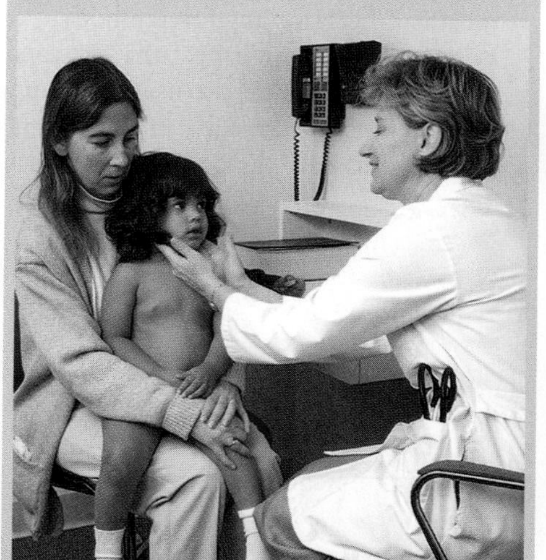

1. Inspect the size and shape of the head and symmetry of facies.
2. Palpate the fontanels and cranium. Palpate the cervical lymph nodes, trachea, and thyroid gland.
3. Measure the head circumference.

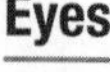

Eyes

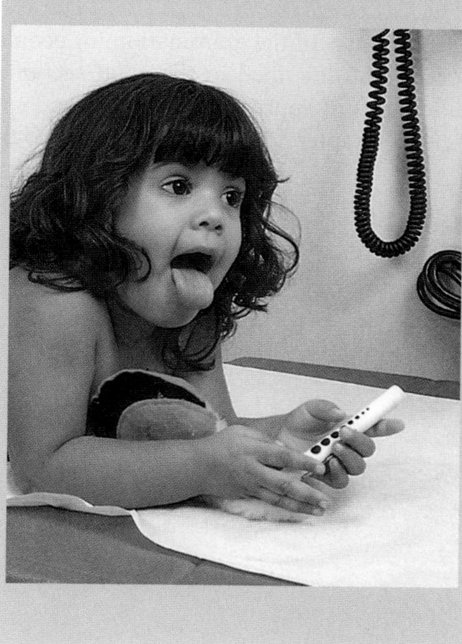

1. Inspect the external structures. Note any palpebral slant.
2. With a penlight, test the corneal light and pupillary light reflexes.
3. Direct a moving penlight for cardinal positions of gaze.
4. If indicated, perform the cover test, covering the eye with your thumb in a young child or using an index card.
5. Inspect conjunctivae and sclerae.
6. With an ophthalmoscope, check the red reflex. Inspect the fundus as much as possible.

Sequence	Selected Photos

Nose

1. Inspect the external nose and skin condition.
2. With a penlight, inspect the nares for foreign body, mucosa, septum, and turbinates.

Mouth and Throat

1. With a penlight, inspect the mouth, buccal mucosa, teeth and gums, tongue, palate, and uvula in midline. Use a tongue blade as the last resort.

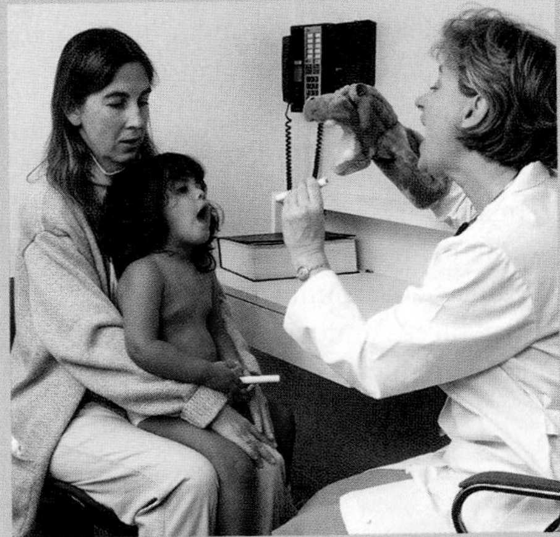

Ears

1. Inspect and palpate the auricles. Note any discharge from the auditory meatus. Check for any foreign body.
2. With an otoscope, inspect the ear canals and tympanic membranes. Gain cooperation through the use of a puppet, encouraging the child to handle the equipment or to look in the parent's ear as you hold the otoscope. You may need to have the parent help restrain the child.

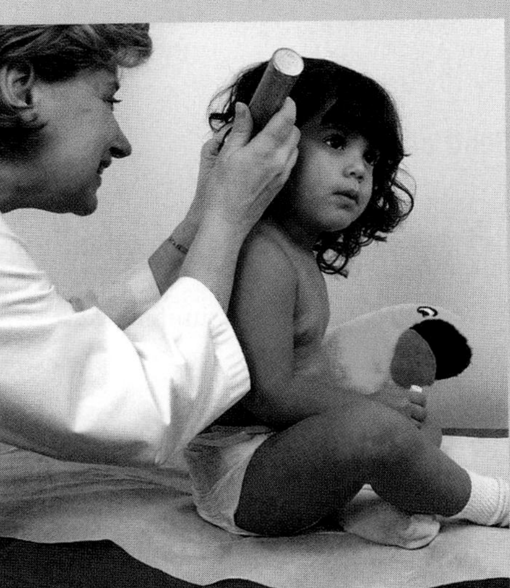

THE SCHOOL-AGE CHILD, THE ADOLESCENT, AND THE AGING ADULT

The sequence of the examination for people in these age-groups is the head-to-toe format described in the adult section. However, you should be aware of differences in approach and timing and special developmental considerations. Review Chapter 8 for a full discussion of these factors.

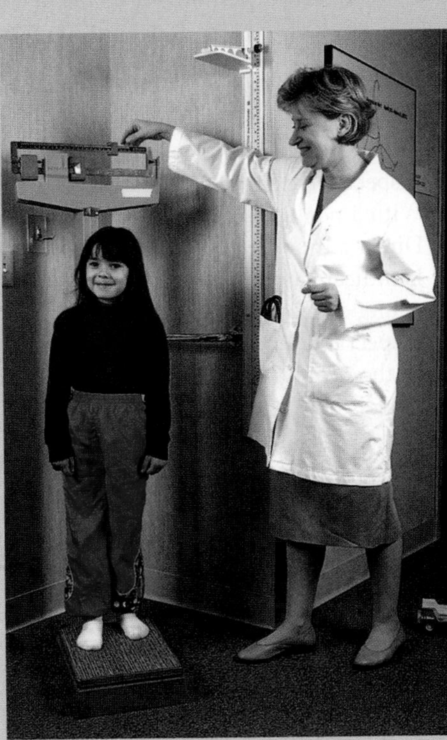

DOCUMENTATION AND CRITICAL THINKING

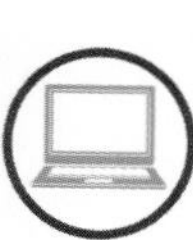

Recording the Data

Record the data from the history and physical examination as soon after the event as possible. Memory fades as the day develops, especially when you are responsible for the care of more than one person.

It is difficult to strike a balance between recording too much data and recording too little. It is important to remember that, from a legal perspective, if it is not documented, it was not done. Data important for the diagnosis and treatment of the person's health should be recorded, as well as data that contribute to your decision-making process. This includes charting relevant normal or negative findings.

On the other hand, a listing of every assessment parameter described in this text yields an unwieldy, unworkable record. One way to keep your record complete yet succinct is to study your writing style. Use short, clear phrases. Avoid redundant introductory phrases such as "The patient states that…." Avoid redundant descriptions such as "No inguinal, femoral, or umbilical hernias." Just write, "No hernias."

Use simple line drawings to describe your findings. You do not need artistic talent; draw a simple sketch of a tympanic membrane, breast, abdomen, or cervix, and mark your findings on it. A clear picture is worth many sentences of words.

Study the following complete history and physical examination for a sample write-up. Note that the subject is the same young woman introduced in Chapter 1 of this text.

Health History

BIOGRAPHIC DATA

Name: Ellen K.
Address: 123 Center St.
Marital Status: Single

Birth date: 1/18/
Birthplace: Springfield
Race: White

Ellen K. is a 23-year-old single white female cashier at a tavern, currently unemployed for 6 months.

Source. Ellen, seems reliable.

Reason for Seeking Care. "I'm coming in for alcohol treatment."

History of Present Illness. First alcoholic drink, age 16. First intoxication, age 17, drinking one or two times per week, a 6-pack per occasion. Attending high school classes every day, but grades slipping from A–/B+ average to C– average. At age 20, drinking two times per week, six to nine beers per occasion. At age 22, drinking two times per week, a 12-pack per occasion, and occasionally a 6-pack the next day to "help with the hangover." During this year, experienced blackouts, failed attempts to cut down on drinking, was physically sick the morning after drinking, and was unable to stop drinking once started. Also, incurred three driving-under-the-influence (DUI) legal offenses. Last DUI 1 month PTA; last alcohol use just before DUI, 18 beers that occasion. Abstinent since that time.

PAST HEALTH

Childhood Illnesses. Chickenpox at age 6. No measles, mumps, croup, pertussis. No rheumatic fever, scarlet fever, or polio.

Accidents. (1) Auto accident, age 12; father driving, Ellen thrown from car, right leg crushed. Hospitalized at Memorial; surgery for leg pinning to repair multiple compound fractures. (2) Auto accident, age 21; head hit dashboard, no loss of consciousness, treated and released at Memorial Hospital ED. (3) Auto accident, age 23; "car hit median strip," no injuries, not seen at hospital.

Chronic Illnesses. None.

Hospitalizations. Age 12, Memorial Hospital, surgery to repair right leg as described; Dr. M.J. Carlson, surgeon.

Obstetric History. Gravida 0/Para 0/Abortion 0.

Immunizations. Childhood immunizations up to date. Last tetanus "probably high school." No TB skin test.

Last Examinations. Yearly pelvic examinations at health department since age 15, told "normal." High school sports physical as sophomore. Last dental examination as high school junior; last vision test for driver's license age 16; never had ECG, chest x-ray study.

Allergies. No known allergies.

Current Medications. Birth control pills, low-estrogen type, 1/day, for 5 years. No other prescription or over-the-counter medications.

FAMILY HISTORY

Ellen is second youngest child, parents divorced 8 years, father has chronic alcoholism. See Family genogram below.

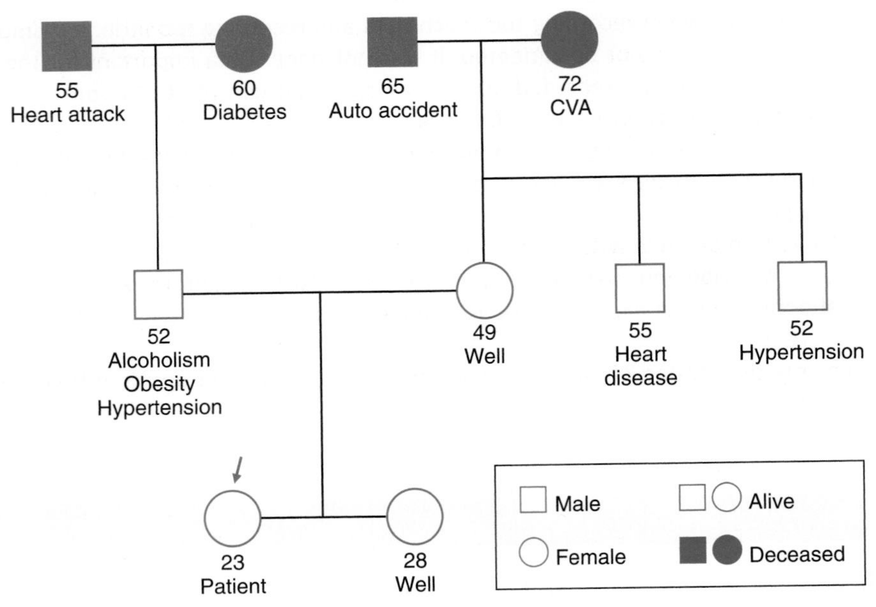

REVIEW OF SYSTEMS

General Health. Reports usual health "OK." No recent weight change; no fatigue, weakness, fever, sweats.

Skin. No change in skin color, pigmentation, or nevi. No pruritus, rash, lesions. Has bruise now over right eye, struck by boyfriend 1 week PTA. No history skin disease. Hair: no loss, change in texture. Nails: no change. Self-care: Stays in sun "as much as I can." No use of sunscreen. Goes to tanning beds at hair salon twice/week during winter.

Head. No unusually frequent or severe headaches; no head injury, dizziness, syncope, or vertigo.

Eyes. No difficulty with vision or double vision. No eye pain, inflammation, discharge, lesions. No history glaucoma or cataracts. Wears no corrective lenses.

Ears. No hearing loss or difficulty. No earaches; no infections now or as child; no discharge, tinnitus, or vertigo. Self-care: No exposure to environmental noise; cleans ears with washcloth.

Nose. No discharge; has two or three colds per year; no sinus pain, nasal obstruction, epistaxis, or allergy.

Mouth and Throat. No mouth pain, bleeding gums, toothache, sores or lesions in mouth, dysphagia, hoarseness, or sore throat. Has tonsils. Self-care: Brushes teeth twice/day, no flossing.

Neck. No pain, limitation of motion, lumps, or swollen glands.

Breasts. No pain, lump, nipple discharge, rash, swelling, or trauma. No history breast disease in self, mother, or sister. No surgery. Self-care: Does not do breast self-examination.

Respiratory. No history of lung disease; no chest pain with breathing; no wheezing or shortness of breath. Colds sometimes "go to my chest"; treats with over-the-counter cough medicine and aspirin. Occasional early-morning cough, nonproductive. Smokes cigarettes 2 PPD × 2 years; prior use 1 PPD × 4 years. Never tried to quit. Works in poorly ventilated tavern; "Everybody smokes."

Cardiovascular. No chest pain, palpitation, cyanosis, fatigue, dyspnea with exertion, orthopnea, paroxysmal nocturnal dyspnea, nocturia, edema. No history of heart murmur, hypertension, coronary artery disease, or anemia.

Peripheral Vascular. No pain, numbness or tingling, swelling in legs. No coldness, discoloration, varicose veins, infections, or ulcers. Legs are unequal in length as sequelae of accident age 12. Self-care: Usual work as cashier involves standing for 8-hour shifts; no support hose.

Gastrointestinal. Appetite good with no recent change. No food intolerance, heartburn, indigestion, pain in abdomen, nausea, or vomiting. No history of ulcers, liver or gallbladder disease, jaundice, appendicitis, or colitis. Bowel movement 1/day, soft, brown; no rectal bleeding or pain. Self-care: No use of vitamins, antacids, laxatives. Diet recall—see Functional Assessment.

Urinary. No dysuria, frequency, urgency, nocturia, hesitancy, or straining. No pain in flank, groin, suprapubic region. Urine color yellow; no history kidney disease.

Genitalia. Menarche age 11. Last menstrual period April 18. Cycle usually q 28 days, duration 4 to 5 days, flow moderate, no dysmenorrhea. No vaginal itching, discharge, sores, or lesions.

Sexual health. In relationship now that includes intercourse. This boyfriend has been her only sexual partner for 2 years; had one other partner before that. Uses birth control pills to prevent pregnancy; partner uses no condoms. Concerned that boyfriend may be having sex with other women but has not confronted him. Not aware of any STI contact. Never been tested for AIDS. History of sexual abuse by father from ages 12 to 16 years; abuse did not include intercourse. Ellen is unwilling to discuss further at this time.

Musculoskeletal. No history of arthritis, gout. No joint pain, stiffness, swelling, deformity, or limitation of motion. No muscle pain or weakness. Bone trauma at age 12; has sequela of unequal leg lengths, right leg shorter, walks with limp. Self-care: No walking or running for sport or exercise "because of leg." Able to stand as cashier. Uses lift pad in right shoe to equalize leg length.

Neurologic. No history of seizure disorder, stroke, fainting. Has had blackouts with alcohol use. No weakness, tremor, paralysis, problems with coordination, difficulty speaking or swallowing. No numbness or tingling. Not aware of memory problem, nervousness or mood change, depression. Had counseling for sexual abuse in the past. Denies any suicidal ideation or intent during adolescent years or now.

Hematologic. No bleeding problems in skin, no excessive bruising. Not aware of exposure to toxins, never had blood transfusion, never used needles to shoot drugs.

Endocrine. Paternal grandmother with diabetes. No increase in hunger, thirst, or urination; no problems with hot or cold environments; no change in skin or appetite; no nervousness.

FUNCTIONAL ASSESSMENT

Self-Concept. Graduated from high school. Trained "on-the-job" as bartender; also worked as cashier in tavern. Unemployed now, on public aid, does not perceive she has enough money for daily living. Lives with older sister. Raised as Presbyterian, believes in God, does not attend church. Believes self to be "honest, dependable." Believes limitations are "smoking, weight, drinking."

Activity-Exercise. Typical day: Arises 9 AM, light chores or TV, spends day looking for work, running errands, with friends, bedtime at 11 PM. No sustained physical exercise. Believes self able to perform all ADLs; limp poses no problem in bathing, dressing, cooking, household tasks, mobility, driving a car, or work as cashier. No mobility aids. Hobbies are fishing, boating, snowmobiling; however, currently has no finances to engage in most of these.

Sleep-Rest. Bedtime 11 PM. Sleeps 8 to 9 hours. No sleep aids.

Nutrition. 24-hour recall: Breakfast—none; lunch—bologna sandwich, chips, diet soda; dinner—hamburger, French fries, coffee; snacks—peanuts, pretzels, potato chips, "bar food." This menu is typical of most days. Eats lunch at home alone. Most dinners at fast-food restaurants or in tavern. Shares household grocery expenses and cooking chores with sister. No food intolerances.

Alcohol. See History of Present Illness. Denies use of street drugs. Cigarettes: Smokes 2 PPD × 2 years; prior use 1 PPD × 4 years. Never tried to quit. Boyfriend smokes cigarettes.

Interpersonal Relationships. Describes family life growing up as chaotic. Father physically abusive toward mother and sexually abusive toward Ellen. Parents divorced because of father's continual drinking. Few support systems currently. Estranged from mother; "Didn't believe me about my father." Father estranged from entire family. Gets along "OK" with sister. Relationship with boyfriend chaotic; has hit her twice in the past. Ellen has never pressed legal charges. No close women friends. Most friends are "drinking buddies" at tavern.

Coping and Stress Management. Believes housing adequate, adequate heat and utilities, and neighborhood safe. Believes home has no safety hazards. Does not use seat belts. No travel outside 60 miles of hometown.

Identifies current stresses to be drinking, legal problems with DUIs, unemployment, financial worries. Considers her drinking to be problematic.

PERCEPTION OF HEALTH

Identifies alcohol as a health problem for herself; feels motivated for treatment. Never been interested in physical health and own body before; "Now I think it's time I learned." Expects health care providers to "Help me with my drinking. I don't know beyond that." Expects to stay at this agency for 6 weeks; "Then, I don't know what."

Physical Examination

MEASUREMENT

Height: 163 cm (5′4″); Weight: 68.6 kg (151 lb); Waist circumference: 32 inches
BP: 142/100 mm Hg right arm, sitting
140/96 mm Hg right arm, lying
138/98 mm Hg left arm, lying
Temp: 37° C; Pulse: 76 bpm, regular; Respirations: 16 per min, unlabored

General Survey. Ellen K. is a 23-year-old white female, not currently under the influence of alcohol or other drugs, who articulates clearly, ambulates without difficulty, and is in no distress.

HEAD-TO-TOE EXAMINATION

Skin. Uniformly tan-pink in color, warm, dry, intact; turgor good. No lesions, birthmarks, edema. Resolving 2-cm yellow-green hematoma present over right eye; no swelling; ocular structures not involved. Hair: normal distribution and texture, no pest inhabitants. Nails: no clubbing, biting, or discolorations. Nail beds: pink and firm with prompt capillary refill.

Head. Normocephalic, no lesions, lumps, scaling, parasites, or tenderness. Face: symmetric, no weakness, no involuntary movements.

Eyes. Acuity by Snellen chart: right eye 20/20; left eye 20/20–1. Visual fields full by confrontation. EOMs intact, no nystagmus. No ptosis, lid lag, discharge, or crusting. Corneal light reflex symmetric; no strabismus. Conjunctivae clear. Sclerae white; no lesion or redness. Pupils: 3 mm resting, 2 mm constricted, and = bilaterally. PERRLA.

Fundi: discs flat with sharp margins. Vessels present in all quadrants without crossing defects. Background has even color, no hemorrhage or exudates.

Ears. Pinna: no mass, lesions, scaling, discharge, or tenderness to palpation. Canals clear. Tympanic membrane: pearly gray, landmarks intact, no perforation. Whispered words heard bilaterally.

Nose. No deformities or tenderness to palpation. Nares patent. Mucosa pink, no lesions. Septum midline, no perforation. No sinus tenderness.

Mouth. Mucosa and gingivae pink, no lesions or bleeding. Right lower 1st molar missing, multiple dark spots on most teeth, gums receding on lower incisors. Tongue symmetric, protrudes midline, no tremor. Pharynx pink, no exudate. Uvula rises midline on phonation. Tonsils 1+. Gag reflex present.

Neck. Neck supple with full ROM. Symmetric; no masses, tenderness, lymphadenopathy. Trachea midline. Thyroid nonpalpable, not tender. Jugular veins flat @ 45 degrees. Carotid arteries 2+ and = bilaterally; no bruits.

Spine and Back. Normal spinal profile; no scoliosis. No tenderness over spines; no CVA tenderness.

Thorax and Lungs. AP < transverse diameter. Chest expansion symmetric. Tactile fremitus equal bilaterally. Lung fields resonant. Diaphragmatic excursion 4 cm and = bilaterally. Breath sounds diminished. Expiratory wheeze in posterior chest at both bases, scattered rhonchi in posterior chest at both bases, do not clear with coughing.

Breasts. Symmetric; no retraction, discharge, or lesions. Contour and consistency firm and homogeneous. No masses or tenderness, no lymphadenopathy.

Heart. Precordium: no abnormal pulsations, no heaves. Apical impulse at 5th ICS in left MCL, no thrills. S_1–S_2 are not diminished or accentuated, no S_3 or S_4. Systolic murmur, grade ii/vi, loudest at left lower sternal border, no radiation, present supine and sitting.

Abdomen. Flat, symmetric. Skin smooth with no lesions, scars, or striae. Bowel sounds present, no bruits. Tympany predominates in all quadrants. Liver span 7 cm in right MCL. Abdomen soft, no organomegaly, no masses or tenderness, no inguinal lymphadenopathy.

Extremities. Color tan-pink; no redness, cyanosis, lesions other than surgical scar. Scar right lower leg, anterior, 28 cm × 2 cm wide, well healed. No edema, varicosities. No calf tenderness. All peripheral pulses present, 2+ and = bilaterally. Asymmetric leg length—right leg 3 cm shorter than left.

Musculoskeletal. Temporomandibular joint: no slipping or crepitation. Neck: full ROM, no pain. Vertebral column: no tenderness, no deformity or curvature; full extension, lateral bending, rotation. Arms symmetric, legs measure as described, extremities have full ROM, no pain or crepitation. Muscle strength: able to maintain flexion against resistance and without tenderness.

Neurologic. Mental status: Appearance, behavior, speech appropriate. Alert and oriented to person, place, time. Thought coherent. Remote and recent memories intact. Cranial nerves II through XII intact. Sensory: Pinprick, light touch, vibration intact. Stereognosis: Able to identify key. Motor: No atrophy, weakness, or tremors. Gait: Has limp, able to tandem walk with shoes on. Negative Romberg's sign. Cerebellar: Finger-to-nose smoothly intact. DTRs: See *stick gram.*

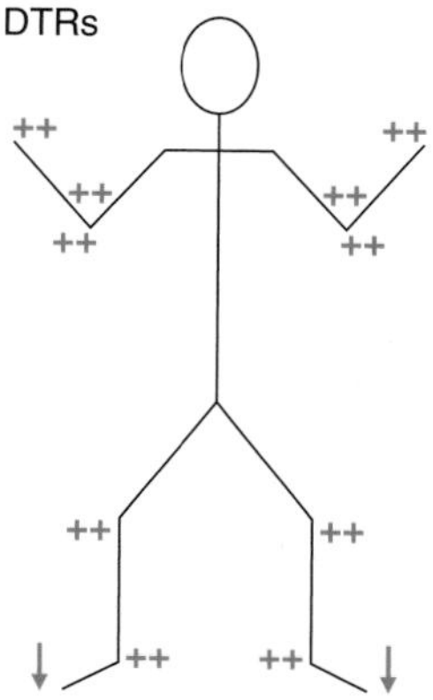

Genitalia. External genitalia: no lesion, discharge. Internal genitalia: vaginal walls pink, no lesion. Cervix: pink, nulliparous os, no lesions, small amount nonodorous clear discharge. Specimens for Pap test, GC/chlamydia, trichomoniasis, moniliasis obtained. Swabbing mucosa with acetic acid shows no acetowhitening.

Bimanual: no pain on moving cervix; uterus midline; no enlargement, masses, or tenderness. Adnexa—ovaries not enlarged, no tenderness. Anus—no hemorrhoids, fissures, or lesions. Rectal wall intact, no masses or tenderness. Stool soft, brown; hematest negative.

ASSESSMENT

Alcohol dependence, severe, with physiologic dependence
Nicotine dependence with physiologic dependence
Hypertension
Systolic heart murmur
Ineffective airway clearance R/T tracheobronchial secretions and obstruction
Right orbital contusion (resolving)
Risk for trauma
Self-care deficit: oral hygiene R/T lack of motivation
Deficient knowledge about alcoholism disease process, treatment options, support systems R/T lack of exposure
Deficient knowledge about balanced diet R/T lack of exposure and substance abuse
Dysfunctional family processes: alcoholism
Chronic low self-esteem R/T effects of alcoholism, sexual abuse, physical abuse

28

Bedside Assessment of the Hospitalized Adult

evolve WEBSITE

http://evolve.elsevier.com/Jarvis/

- Audio Key Points
- NCLEX Review Questions
- Quick Assessment for Common Conditions Sepsis

In a hospital setting, the patient does not require a complete head-to-toe physical examination during every 24-hour stay. The patient *does* require a consistent specialized examination at least every 8 hours that focuses on certain parameters. Note that some measurements, such as daily weights, abdominal girth, or the circumference of a limb, must be taken very carefully. The utility of such measurements depends entirely on the consistency of the procedure from nurse to nurse.

Also remember that many assessments must be done frequently throughout the course of a shift. This chapter outlines the initial assessment that will allow you to get to know your patient. As you perform this sequence, take note of anything that will need continuous monitoring, such as a blood pressure or pulse oximetry reading that is not what you expect or breath sounds that suggest a difficult respiratory effort. If there is no protocol in place for a particular assessment situation, then decide for yourself how often you need to check on the person's status—it is very easy to be distracted by ringing bells and alarms as the shift progresses, but your own judgment about a patient's needs is just as important as any electronic alert or alarm.

The need for multiple assessments of each patient highlights the need for efficiency in the hospital setting. Your assessments must be thorough and accurate, yet you must be able to complete them rapidly without seeming hurried. The only solution to this paradox is practice. Remember that practicing in a laboratory setting, with simulated patients or with classmates, may feel artificial but it is the quickest route to feeling confident in the presence of hospitalized patients.

The basic reassessment applies to adults in medical, surgical, and cardiac step-down care areas. Each assessment must then be specialized to each adult, and the findings must be integrated into your complete knowledge base regarding the patient. This includes what you read in the chart, what you hear in report, and the results of any laboratory tests and diagnostic imaging that are available.

Sequence | **Selected Photos**

Assist the person into bed. The patient is in bed with the bed at a comfortable level for the examiner.

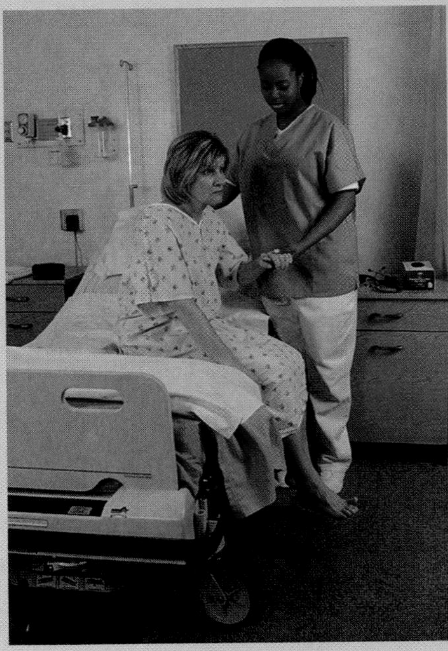

THE HEALTH HISTORY

On your way into the room, verify that any necessary markers or flags are in place at the doorway regarding such conditions as isolation precautions, latex allergies, or fall precautions. Once in the room, introduce yourself as the patient's nurse for the next 8 (or 12) hours.

Make direct eye contact, and do not allow yourself to be distracted by intravenous (IV) pumps or other equipment as you ask how he or she is feeling, how he or she spent the previous shift. Refer to what you have heard from the previous shift in the process of your own questioning—this alleviates the person's frustration at answering the same questions every time with a new staff member. Assess for pain: "Are you currently having any pain or discomfort?" You should know when the last pain medication was given and what physician orders are written. Determine if further dosing is needed or if you need to contact the physician. Knowing the written orders, confirm settings on the patient-controlled analgesia (PCA) pump or epidural setting if in place. Confirm IV solution hanging matches orders for rate and type.

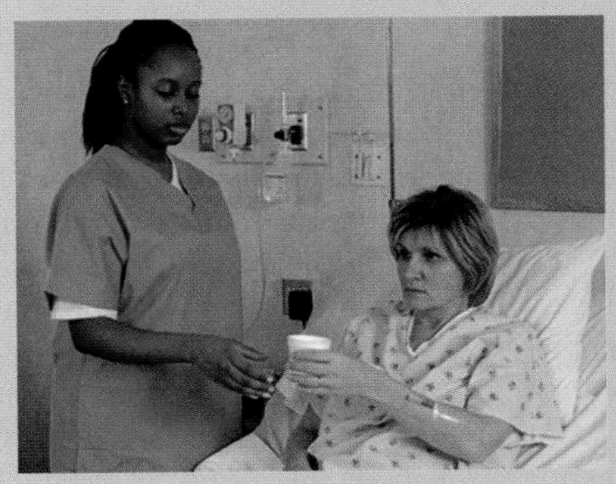

Wash your hands in the patient's presence. Offer water as a courtesy but also note the physical data this gives you: the person's ability to hear, to follow directions, to cross the midline, and especially, to swallow. As you collect this and subsequent history, note data on the General Appearance listed below. Complete your initial overview by verifying that the correct name band has been applied to the wrist.

GENERAL APPEARANCE

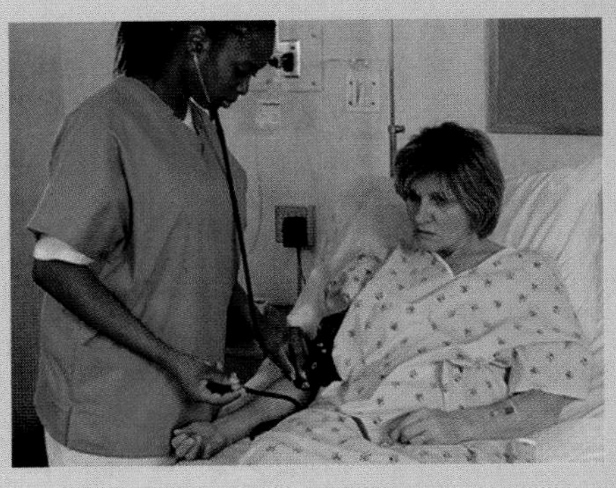

1. Facial expression: appropriate to the situation.
2. Body position: relaxed and comfortable or tense, in pain.
3. Level of consciousness: alert and oriented, attentive to your questions, responds appropriately.
4. Skin color: even tone consistent with racial heritage.
5. Nutritional status: weight appears in healthy range, even fat distribution, hydration appears healthy.
6. Speech: articulation clear and understandable, pattern fluent and even, content appropriate.
7. Hearing: responses and facial expression consistent with what you have said.
8. Personal hygiene: ability to attend to hair, makeup, shaving.

MEASUREMENT

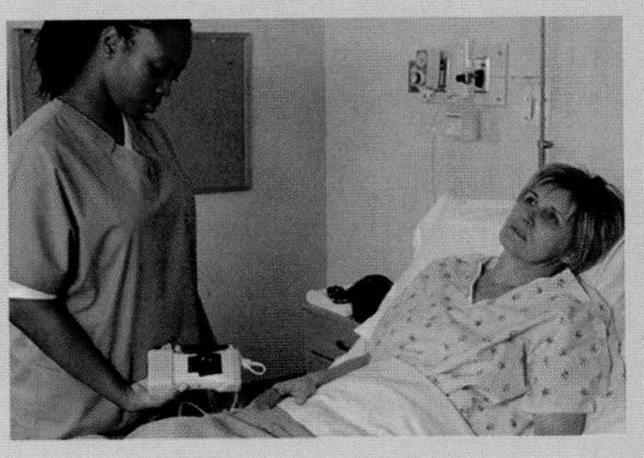

1. Measure baseline vital signs (VS) now—temperature, pulse, respirations, blood pressure (BP). Note which arm to avoid for BP because of surgery, IV access. Collect and document VS more frequently if patient is unstable or if patient condition changes. Know that VS are the ultimate responsibility of the nurse—the nursing assistant is not responsible for interpretation.
2. Pulse oximetry—maintain ≥92%. Check oxygen use at least first 24 hours after surgery or as ordered. May need to monitor continuously if patient is lethargic or on a PCA or epidural.

Sequence	Selected Photos

3. Rate pain level on a 1-to-10 scale at this and every subsequent visit or VS measure. Note patient's ability to tolerate pain.
4. If pain medication given, note response in 15 minutes for IV administration or 1 hour for oral dosing.

NEUROLOGIC SYSTEM

1. Eyes open spontaneously to name.
2. Motor response is strong and equal bilaterally.
3. Verbal response makes sense; speech is clear and articulate.
4. Pupil size in mm and reaction, R and L.
5. Muscle strength, R and L upper, using hand grips.
6. Muscle strength, R and L lower, pushing feet against your palms.
7. Any ptosis, facial droop.
8. Sensation (omit unless indicated).
9. Communication.
10. Ability to swallow.

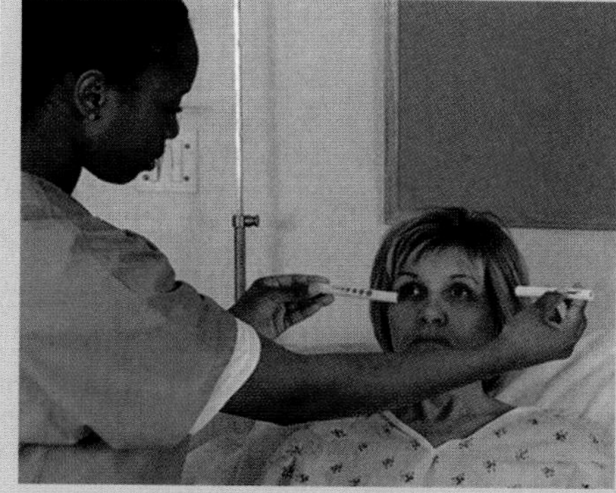

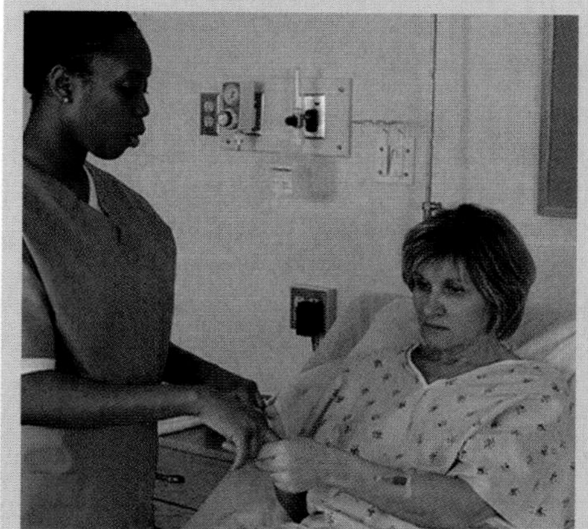

RESPIRATORY SYSTEM

1. Oxygen by mask, nasal prongs, check fitting.
2. Note FIo_2.
3. Respiratory effort.
4. Auscultate breath sounds, comparing side to side:
   Posterior lobes: left upper, right upper, left lower, right lower.
   Note: If not able to sit up, have another nurse hold patient side to side.
   Anterior lobes: right upper, left upper, right middle and lower, left lower.
5. Cough and deep breathe. Any mucus? Check color and amount.
6. Incentive spirometer if ordered—encourage patient to use every hour for 10 inspirations. If pulse oximetry % or respiratory rate drops, encourage use every 15 minutes.

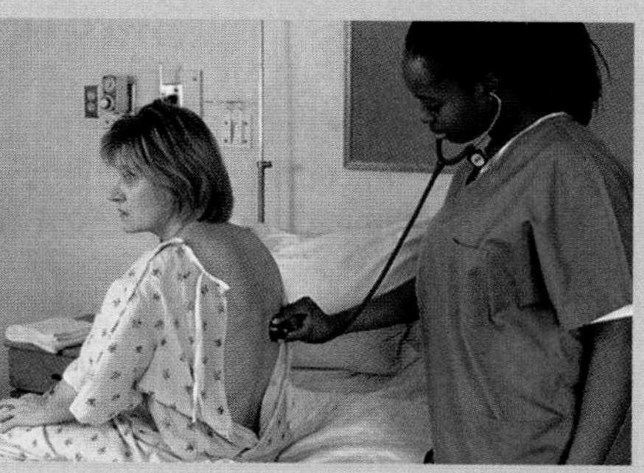

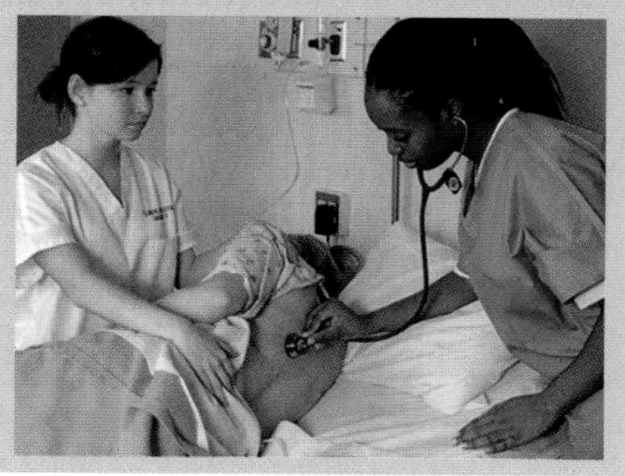

Sequence	Selected Photos

CARDIOVASCULAR SYSTEM

1. Auscultate rhythm at apex: regular, irregular? (Do NOT listen over gown.)
2. Check apical pulse against radial pulse, noting perfusion of all beats.
3. Assess heart sounds in all auscultatory areas: first with diaphragm, repeat with bell.
4. Check capillary refill for prompt return.

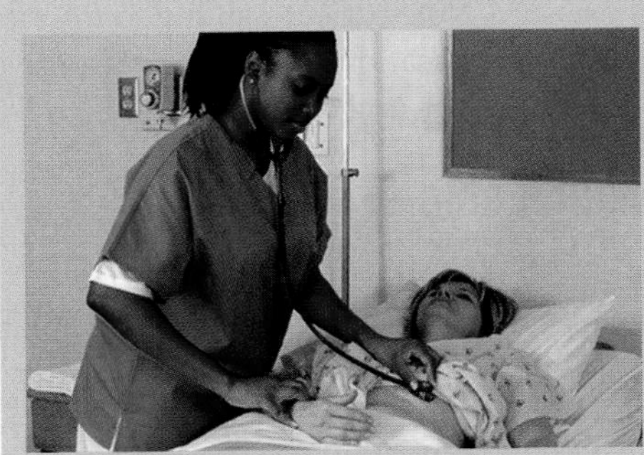

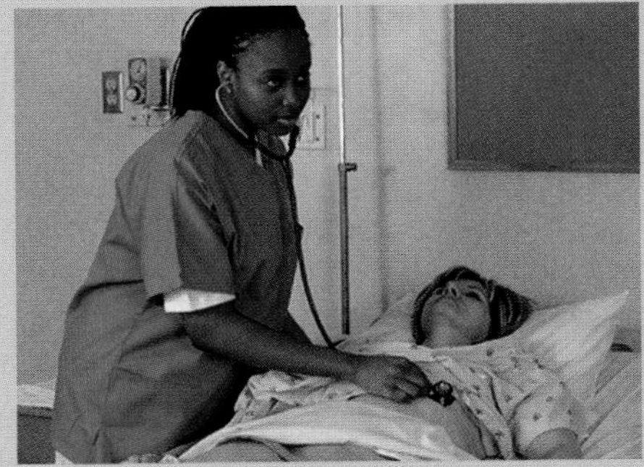

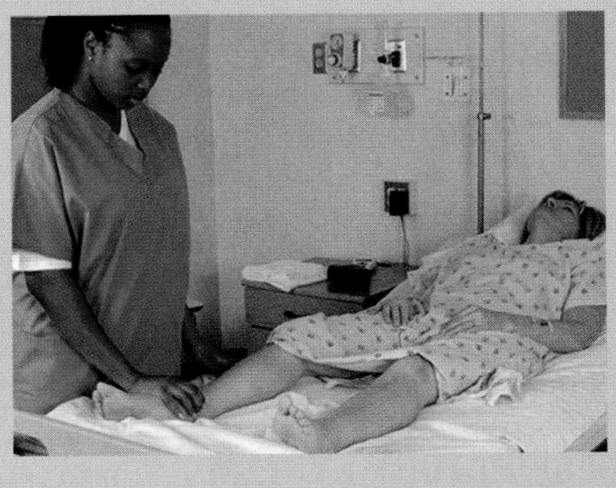

5. Check pretibial edema.
6. Palpate posterior tibial pulse, right and left.
7. Palpate dorsalis pedis pulse, right and left.
   Note: Be prepared to assess pulses in the lower extremities by Doppler imaging if you cannot find them by palpation.
8. Verify that the proper IV solution is hanging and flowing at the proper rate according to the physician's orders and your own assessment of the patient's needs.

SKIN

1. Note skin color, consistent with person's racial or ethnic heritage.
2. Palpate skin temperature; expect warm and dry.
3. Pinch up a fold of skin under the clavicle or on the forearm to note mobility and turgor.
4. Note skin integrity, any lesions, and the condition of any dressings. Note any bleeding or infection, but do not change dressing until after physical examination.
5. Date IV site, and note surrounding skin condition.
6. Complete any standardized scales used to quantify the risk for skin breakdown.
7. Verify that any air loss or pressure loss surfaces being used are properly applied and operating at the correct settings.

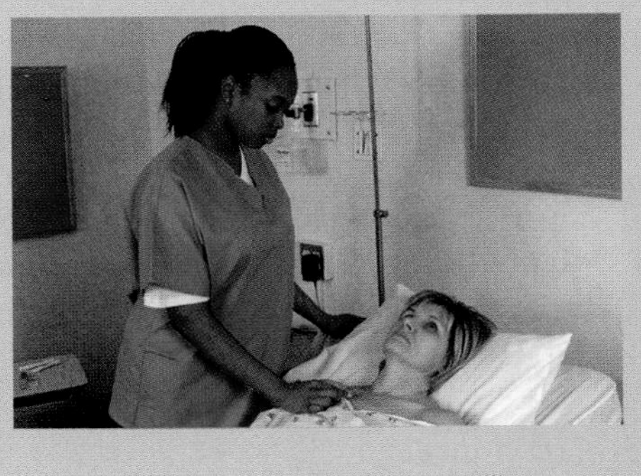

Sequence	Selected Photos

ABDOMEN

1. Assess contour of abdomen: flat, rounded, protuberant.
2. Listen to bowel sounds in all four quadrants.
3. Check any drainage tube placement for color and amount of drainage and insertion site integrity.
4. Inquire whether passing flatus or stool.
5. Knowing diet orders, determine if patient is tolerating ice chips, liquids, solids. Order correct diet as it is advanced. Note if patient is high risk for nutrition deficit.

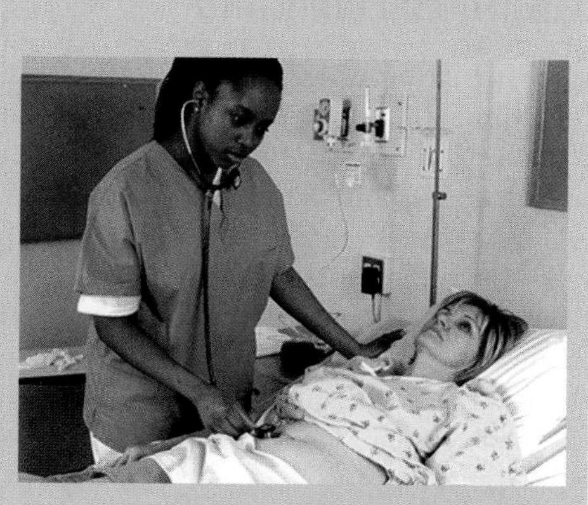

GENITOURINARY

1. Inquire whether voiding regularly. Note: Needs to void within 4 to 6 hours after surgery.
2. Check urine for color, clarity.
3. If Foley catheter in place, check color, quantity, clarity of urine with every VS check.
4. If urine output is below the expected amount, perform a bladder scan according to agency protocol. Is the problem in the production of urine or its retention?

ACTIVITY

1. Knowing activity orders, if on bedrest, head of bed should be ≥15 degrees. Is patient at high risk for skin breakdown?
2. SCDs, TED hose, foot pumps need to be hooked up and turned on. Must be on patient 22 out of 24 hours to be effective.
3. If ambulatory, assist patient to sitting up level and move to chair.
4. Note any assistance needed, how tolerates movement, distance walked to chair, ability to turn.
5. Need for any ambulatory aid or equipment.
6. Complete any standardized scales used to quantify the patient's risk for falling.
7. Initiate or continue appropriate Plan of Care. Check if any core measures apply, such as heart failure. Implement core measures as appropriate.
8. Complete initial assessment to document into computer when finished.
9. Note examination findings requiring immediate attention:
    - High or low BP (≤90 or ≥160 mm Hg systolic)
    - High or low temp (≤97° or ≥100° F)
    - High or low heart rate (≤60 or ≥90 bpm)
    - High or low respirations (≤12 or ≥28/min)
    - O_2 saturations ≤92%
    - Low or no urine output (≤30 mL/hr or ≤240 mL/8 hr)
    - Dark amber or bloody urine (except for urology patients)
    - Post-op nausea and/or vomiting
    - Surgical pain not controlled with medication. Any other unusual pain, such as chest pain
    - Bleeding
    - Altered level of consciousness (LOC), confusion, or difficult to arouse
    - Sudden restlessness and/or anxiety

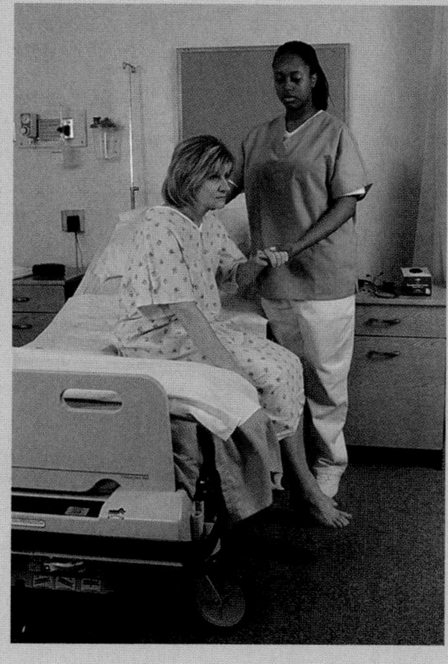

Sequence

ELECTRONIC CHARTING

Charting in most hospitals is at least partially computerized. Although this can be intimidating at first, it has several advantages. First, for new clinicians, the structure imposed by the computerized database can serve as a prompt to guide one through a complete assessment. Second, it decreases the chances that nurses will waste time waiting to gain access to a paper chart or searching for it when it is not in the proper location. Finally, charting in a computer system rarely depends on writing or typing in narrative form—check boxes and drop-down menus are much more common. When you avoid the temptation to write everything on paper first and learn to use all the functions programmed into the hospital's system, you will find that computer charting is faster than its paper equivalent.

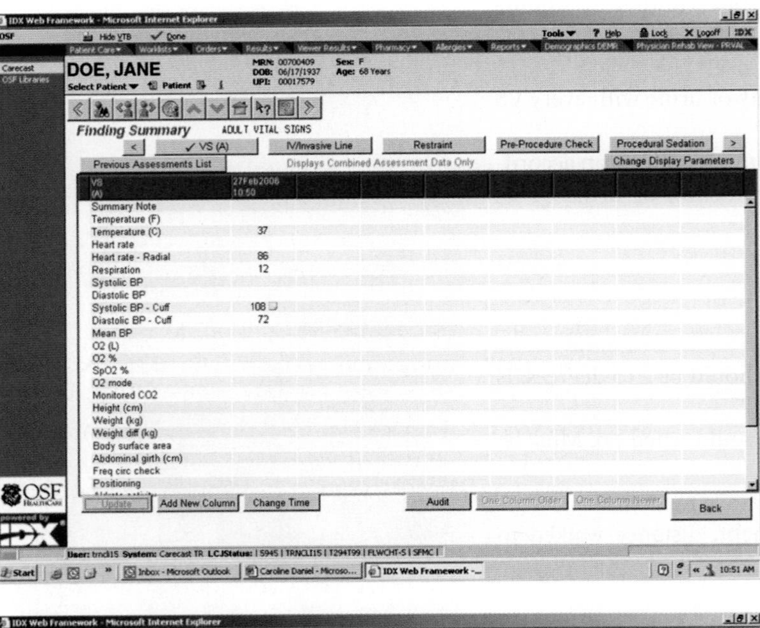

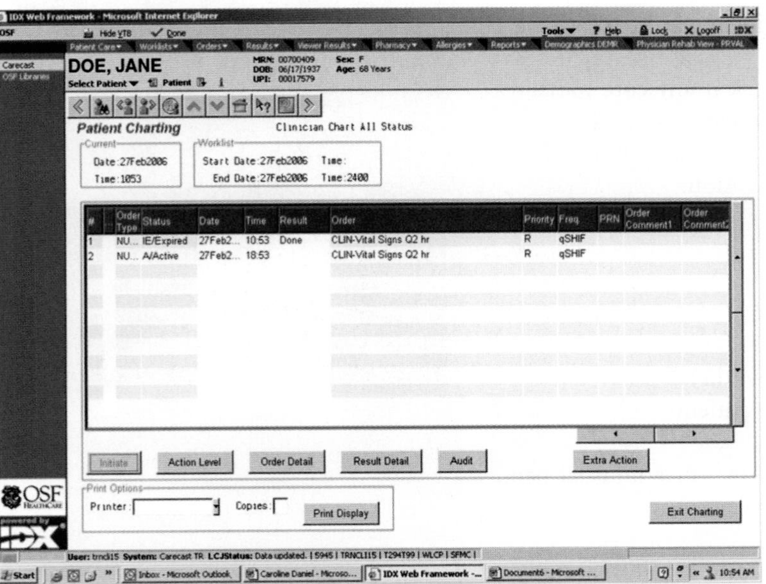

Selected Photos

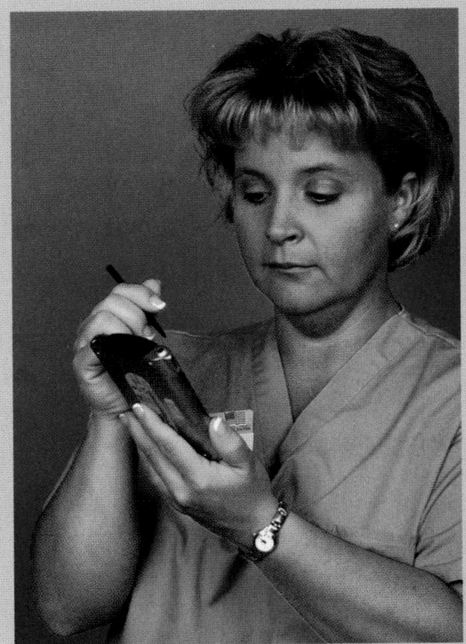

USING SBAR FOR STAFF COMMUNICATION

Throughout this text we have used the SOAP acronym (**S**ubjective, **O**bjective, **A**ssessment, **P**lan) to organize assessment findings into written or charted communication. Now we turn to organizing assessment data for *verbal* communication (e.g., calls to physicians, nursing shift reports, patient transfers to other units). For all these verbal reports, we use the SBAR framework: **S**ituation, **B**ackground, **A**ssessment, **R**ecommendation.

SBAR was first developed in the U.S. military to standardize communication and prevent misunderstandings. In the hospital, communications errors contribute to most sentinel events that are reported.[3] Thus SBAR is used at health care facilities all over the country to improve verbal communication and reduce medical errors.[2,4] SBAR is a standardized framework to transmit important in-the-moment information. Using SBAR will keep your message concise and focused on the immediate problem yet give your colleague enough information to grasp the current situation and make a decision. To formulate your verbal message, use these four points:

Situation. What is happening right now? What are you calling about? State your name, your unit, patient's name, room number, patient's problem, when it happened or when it started, how severe it is.

Background. Do not recite the patient's full history since admission. Do state the data pertinent to this moment's problem: admitting diagnosis, when admitted, and appropriate immediate assessment data (e.g., vital signs, pulse oximetry, change in mental status, allergies, current medications, IV fluids, laboratory results).

Assessment. What do YOU think is happening in regard to the current problem? If you do not know, at least state which body system you think is involved. How severe is the problem?

Recommendation. What do you want the physician to do to improve the patient's situation? Here you offer probable solutions. Order more pain medication? Come and assess the patient?

Review the following examples of SBAR communication.

Situation 1

S: This is Bill on the Oncology Unit. I'm calling about Daniel Meyers in room 8417. He is refusing all oral medications as of now.

B: Daniel is a 59 y.o. male with multiple myeloma. He was admitted for an autologous stem cell transplant and received chemotherapy 10 days ago. Now he is 5 days post–auto transplant. Vital signs are stable, alert and oriented, IVs are dextrose 5% water. As of 1 hour ago, he is feeling extreme nausea and vomiting, refusing all food and oral meds.

A: I think the chemo he had pre-transplant is hitting him now. His uncontrolled nausea isn't going away in next few days.

R: I'm concerned he cannot stay hydrated and he needs his meds. I need you to please change the IV rate and change all scheduled oral meds to IV. I also think we need to add an additional PRN antiemetic. If he continues to refuse food, we may have to consider starting him on TPN/lipids.

Situation 2

S: This is Andrea. I'm the nurse taking care of Max Goodson in 6443. His condition has changed and his most recent vital signs show a significant drop in blood pressure.

B: Max is 40 years old with a history of alcoholism. He was admitted through the ED last night with abdominal pain and a suspected GI bleed. His BPs have been running in the 130s/80s. He just had a large amount of liquid maroon stool and reported feeling dizzy. I rechecked his vitals, and his BP is 88/50 and heart rate is 104.

A: I'm worried his GI bleed is getting worse.

R: Will you order a STAT complete blood count and place an order to transfuse red blood cells if his hemoglobin is below 8 g? Also, can you please come and assess? I think we may need to drop an NG tube and lavage him.

BIBLIOGRAPHY

1. Rodgers, K. L. (2007). Using the SBAR communication technique to improve nurse-physician phone communication: a pilot study. *AAACN Viewpoint, 29*(2), 7-10.
2. Safer Healthcare. (2008). *SBAR: a communication technique for today's healthcare professional.* Retrieved July 15, 2010, from www.saferhealthcare.com/index2.php?option=com_content&task=view&id=33&pop=1&page=0&itemid=84&print=1.
3. The Joint Commission. (2008). *Hand-off communications: standardized approach.* Retrieved July 15, 2010, from www.jointcommission.org/AccreditationAmbulatoryCare/Standards/09_FAQs/NPSG/Communication/NPSG.02.05.01/.
4. Thomas, C. M., Bertram, E., & Johnson, D. (2009). The SBAR communication technique. *Nurse Educator 34*(4):176-180.

29

The Pregnant Woman

evolve WEBSITE

http://evolve.elsevier.com/Jarvis/

- Animations
- Audio Key Points
- Bedside Assessment Summary Checklist
- Case Study
  Assessing the Pregnant Woman
- Head-to-Toe Examination of the Pregnant Woman
- NCLEX Review Questions
- Physical Examination Summary Checklist
- Quick Assessment for Common Conditions
  Iron Deficiency Anemia

OUTLINE

Structure and Function, 795

Pregnancy and the Endocrine Placenta
Changes During Normal Pregnancy

Subjective Data, 799

Health History Questions

Objective Data, 806

Preparation
General Survey
Skin
Mouth
Neck
Breasts
Heart
Lungs
Peripheral Vasculature
Neurologic
Abdomen
Fetal Heart Tones
Pelvic Examination
Routine Laboratory and Radiologic Imaging Studies

Documentation and Critical Thinking, 820

Abnormal Findings for Advanced Practice, 822

STRUCTURE AND FUNCTION

PREGNANCY AND THE ENDOCRINE PLACENTA

The first day of the menses is day 1 of the menstrual cycle. For the first 14 days of the cycle, one or more follicles in the ovary develop and mature. One follicle grows faster than the others, and on day 14 of the menstrual cycle, this dominant follicle ruptures and ovulation occurs. If the ovum meets viable sperm, fertilization occurs somewhere in the oviduct (fallopian tube). The remaining cells in the follicle form the **corpus luteum,** or "yellow body," which makes important hormones. Chief among these is progesterone, which prevents the sloughing of the endometrial wall, ensuring a rich vascular network into which the fertilized ovum will implant.

The fertilized ovum, now called the **blastocyst,** continues to divide, differentiate, and grow rapidly. Specialized cells in the blastocyst produce human chorionic gonadotropin (hCG), which stimulates the corpus luteum to continue making progesterone. Between days 20 and 24, the blastocyst implants into the wall of the uterus, which may cause a small amount of vaginal bleeding. A specialized layer of cells around the blastocyst becomes the **placenta.** The placenta starts to produce progesterone to support the pregnancy at 7 weeks and takes over this function completely from the corpus luteum at about 10 weeks.

The placenta functions as an endocrine organ and produces several hormones. These hormones help in the growth and maintenance of the fetus, and they direct changes in the woman's body to prepare for birth and lactation. The hCG stimulates the rise in progesterone during pregnancy. Progesterone maintains the endometrium around the fetus, increases the alveoli in the breast, and keeps the uterus in a quiescent state. Estrogen stimulates the duct formation in the breasts, increases the weight of the uterus, and increases certain receptors in the uterus that are important at birth.

The average length of pregnancy is 280 days from the first day of the last menstrual period (LMP), which is equal to 40 weeks, 10 lunar months, or 9 calendar months. Note that this includes the 2 weeks when the follicle was maturing but before conception actually occurred. Pregnancy is divided into three trimesters: (1) the first 12 weeks, (2) from 13 to 27 weeks, and (3) from 28 weeks to delivery.

A woman who is pregnant for the first time is called a **primigravida.** After she delivers, she is called a **primipara.** The **multigravida** is a pregnant woman who has previously carried a fetus to the point of viability. She is a **multipara** after delivery. Any pregnant woman might be called a *gravida.* Commonly used terminology is G (gravida), P (para), T (term), PT (preterm deliveries), A (abortion—missed, therapeutic, voluntary), L (living children). It may be written as G5 T3 PT0 A2 L3.

CHANGES DURING NORMAL PREGNANCY

Pregnancy is diagnosed by three types of signs and symptoms. **Presumptive signs** are those the woman experiences, such as amenorrhea, breast tenderness, nausea, fatigue, and increased urinary frequency. **Probable signs** are those detected by the examiner, such as an enlarged uterus. **Positive signs** of pregnancy are those that are direct evidence of the fetus, such as the auscultation of fetal heart tones (FHTs) or positive cardiac activity on ultrasound (US).

First Trimester

Conception occurs on approximately the 14th day of the menstrual cycle. The blastocyst (developing fertilized ovum) implants in the uterus 6 to 10 days after conception, sometimes accompanied by a small amount of painless bleeding, which may be interpreted as a menstrual period.[14] The serum hCG becomes positive after implantation when it is first detectable in maternal serum at approximately 8 to 11 days after conception.

The following menstrual period is missed. At the time of the missed menses, hCG can be detected in the urine. Breast tingling and tenderness begin as the rising estrogen levels promote mammary growth and development of the ductal system; progesterone stimulates the alveolar system as well as the mammary growth. Chorionic somatomammotropin (also called *human placental lactogen* or *hPL*), also produced by the placenta, stimulates breast growth and exerts lactogenic properties.[40] More than half of all pregnant women have nausea and vomiting. The cause is unclear but may involve the hormonal changes of pregnancy, low blood sugar, gastric overloading, slowed peristalsis, an enlarging uterus, and emotional factors. Fatigue is common and may be related to the initial fall in metabolic rate that occurs in early pregnancy.[40]

Estrogen and possibly progesterone cause hypertrophy of the uterine muscle cells, and uterine blood vessels and lymphatics enlarge. The uterus becomes globular in shape, softens, and flexes easily over the cervix (**Hegar sign**). This causes compression of the bladder, which results in urinary frequency. Increased vascularity, congestion, and edema cause the cervix to soften (**Goodell sign**) and become bluish purple (**Chadwick sign**).

Early first-trimester blood pressures (BPs) reflect prepregnancy values. In the 7th gestational week, BP begins to drop until mid-pregnancy as a result of falling peripheral vascular resistance. The BP gradually returns to the nonpregnant baseline by term. Systemic vascular resistance decreases from the vasodilatory effect of progesterone and prostaglandins and possibly because of the low resistance of the placental bed.[13]

At the end of 9 weeks, the embryonic period ends and the fetal period begins, at which time major structures are present.[40] FHTs can be heard by Doppler US between 9 and 12 weeks. The uterus may be palpated just above the symphysis pubis at about 12 weeks. See Fig. 29-1 for growth of the uterine fundus during the first trimester.

When the pregnancy is viable, a gestational sac should be visible on transvaginal ultrasound by 5 weeks gestation or

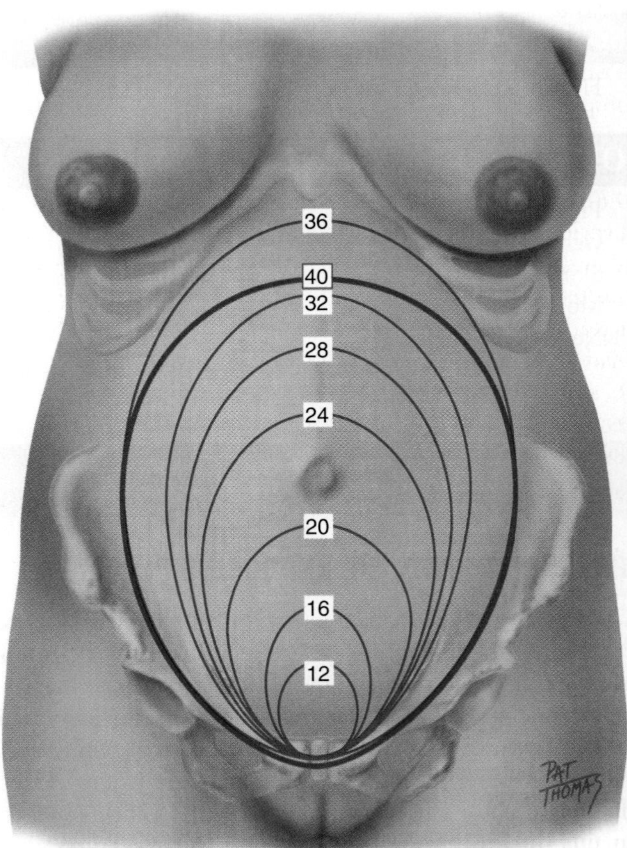

HEIGHT OF FUNDUS AT WEEKS OF GESTATION

29-1

when the maternal serum hCG level is between 1100 and 1500 mU/mL.[13] When a fertilized egg develops a placenta and membranes but no embryo, this is called a *blighted ovum.* With this, the hCG levels will rise early on, then begin to drop, and vaginal bleeding ensues. Some women will not be aware that they were pregnant.

Second Trimester

By weeks 12 to 16, the nausea, vomiting, fatigue, and urinary frequency of the first trimester improve. The woman recognizes fetal movement ("quickening") at approximately 18 to 20 weeks (the multigravida earlier). As breast enlargement continues, the veins of the breast enlarge and are more visible through the skin of lightly pigmented women. **Colostrum,** the precursor of milk, may be expressed from the nipples. Colostrum is yellow in color and contains more minerals and protein but less sugar and fat than mature milk. Colostrum also contains antibodies, which are protective for the newborn during its first days of life until mature milk production begins.[14]

The areolae and nipples darken, it is thought, because estrogen and progesterone have a melanocyte-stimulating effect, and melanocyte-stimulating hormone levels escalate from the second month of pregnancy until delivery. For the same reason, the midline of the abdominal skin becomes pigmented and is called the **linea nigra.** You may note **striae gravidarum** ("stretch marks") on the breast, abdomen, and areas of weight gain.

During the second trimester, systolic BP may be 2 to 8 mm Hg lower and diastolic BP 5 to 15 mm Hg lower than prepregnancy levels.[14] This drop is most pronounced at 20 weeks and may cause symptoms of dizziness and faintness, particularly after rising quickly. Stomach displacement from the enlarging uterus and altered esophageal sphincter and gastric tone as a result of progesterone predispose the woman to heartburn. Intestines are also displaced by the growing uterus, and tone and motility are decreased because of the action of progesterone, often causing constipation. The gallbladder, possibly resulting from the action of progesterone on its smooth muscle, empties sluggishly and may become distended. The stasis of bile, together with the increased cholesterol saturation of pregnancy, predisposes some women to gallstone formation.

Progesterone and, to a lesser degree, estrogen cause increased respiratory effort during pregnancy by increasing tidal volume. Hemoglobin, and therefore oxygen-carrying capacity, also increases. Increased tidal volume causes a slight drop in partial pressure of arterial carbon dioxide ($Paco_2$), causing the woman to occasionally have dyspnea.[14]

With the rise of hCG in the first trimester, there is a transient decrease in thyroid-stimulating hormone (TSH) levels between 8 and 14 weeks' gestation. Plasma iodine levels decrease, allowing a transient increase in thyroid gland size in approximately 15% of pregnant women.

Cutaneous blood flow is augmented during pregnancy, caused by decreased vascular resistance, presumably helping to dissipate heat generated by increased metabolism. Gums may hypertrophy and bleed easily. This condition is called **gingivitis** or **epulis of pregnancy** due to growth of the capillaries of the gums.[14] For the same reason, nosebleeds may occur more frequently than usual. Pregnant women with periodontal disease, a chronic local oral infection, are at risk for preterm delivery.

FHTs are audible by fetoscope (as opposed to Doppler imaging) at approximately 17 to 19 weeks. The fetal outline is palpable through the abdominal wall at approximately 20 weeks. Fig. 29-1 illustrates the growth of the uterine fundus during the second trimester.

Third Trimester

Blood volume, which increased rapidly during the second trimester, peaks in the middle of the third trimester at approximately 45% greater than the prepregnancy level and plateaus thereafter. This volume is greater in multiple gestations.[13] Erythrocyte mass increases by 20% to 30% (caused by an increase in erythropoiesis, mediated by progesterone, estrogen, and placental chorionic somatomammotropin). However, plasma volume increases slightly more, causing a slight hemodilution and a small drop in hematocrit. BP slowly rises again to approximately the prepregnancy level.[14]

Uterine enlargement causes the diaphragm to rise and the shape of the rib cage to widen at the base. Decreased space for lung expansion may cause a sense of shortness of breath. The rising diaphragm displaces the heart up and to the left. Cardiac output, stroke volume, and force of contraction are increased. The pulse rate rises 15 to 20 beats per minute.[13] Because of the increase in blood volume, a functional systolic murmur, grade ii/iv or less, can be heard in more than 95% of pregnant women.[13]

Edema of the lower extremities may occur as a result of the enlarging fetus impeding venous return and from lower colloid osmotic pressure. The edema worsens with dependency, such as prolonged standing. Varicosities, which have a familial tendency, may form or enlarge from progesterone-induced vascular relaxation. Also causing varicosities is the engorgement caused by the weight of the full uterus compressing the inferior vena cava and the vessels of the pelvic area, resulting in venous congestion in the legs, vulva, and rectum. Hemorrhoids are varicosities of the rectum that are worsened by constipation, which occurs from relaxation of the large bowel by progesterone.

Progressive lordosis (an inward curvature of the lumbar spine) occurs to compensate for the shifting center of balance caused by the anteriorly enlarging uterus, predisposing the woman to backaches. Slumping of the shoulders and anterior flexion of the neck from the increasing weight of the breasts may cause aching and numbness of the arms and hands as a result of compression of the median and ulnar nerves in the arm,[40] commonly referred to as *carpal tunnel syndrome.*

Approximately 2 weeks before going into labor, the primigravida experiences engagement (also called "lightening" or "dropping"), when the fetal head moves down into the pelvis. Symptoms include a lower-appearing and smaller-measuring fundus, urinary frequency, increased vaginal secretions from increased pelvic congestion, and increased lung capacity. In the multigravida, the fetus may move down at any time in late pregnancy or often not until labor. The cervix, in preparation for labor, begins to thin (efface) and open (dilate). A thick **mucous plug,** formed in the cervix as a mechanical barrier during pregnancy, is expelled at variable times before or during labor. Between 37 and 42 weeks, the pregnancy is considered *term.* After 42 weeks, the pregnancy is considered *postdates.*

Determining Weeks of Gestation

The expected date of delivery, or EDD, being 280 days from the first day of the LMP, may be calculated by using **Nägele's rule.** That is, determine the first day of the last normal menstrual period (normal in timing, length, premenstrual symptoms, and amount of flow and cramping). Using the first day of the LMP, add 7 days and subtract 3 months. This date is the EDD. This date can then be used with a pregnancy wheel on which the EDD arrow is set, and then the present date will be pointing to the present week's gestation (Fig. 29-2). The number of weeks of gestation also can be estimated by physical examination (bimanual and pelvic examination), by measurement of the maternal serum hCG, by US, and by signs such as the first perceived fetal movement.

Weight Gain in Pregnancy

The amount of weight gained by term represents a baby, amniotic fluid, placenta, increased uterine size, increased blood volume, increased extravascular fluid, maternal fat stores, and increased breast size. Weight gain during pregnancy reflects both the mother and fetus; approximately 25% of the total gain is attributed to the fetus, 11% to the placenta and amniotic fluid, and the remainder to the mother.[11]

The Institute of Medicine, based on the World Health Organization guidelines, recommends the following weight gain in pregnancy based on initial body mass index (BMI). *Underweight* (<18.5 kg/m^2)—total weight gain range: 28-40 pounds; *normal weight* (18.5-24.9 kg/m^2)—total weight gain range: 25-35 pounds; *overweight* (25.0-29.9 kg/m^2)—total weight gain range: 15-25 pounds; *obese* (≥30.0 kg/m^2)—total weight gain range: 11-20 pounds. For *twin gestation and normal weight women*—total weight gain range: 37-54 pounds; *overweight*—31-50 pounds; and *obese*—25-42 pounds.[41]

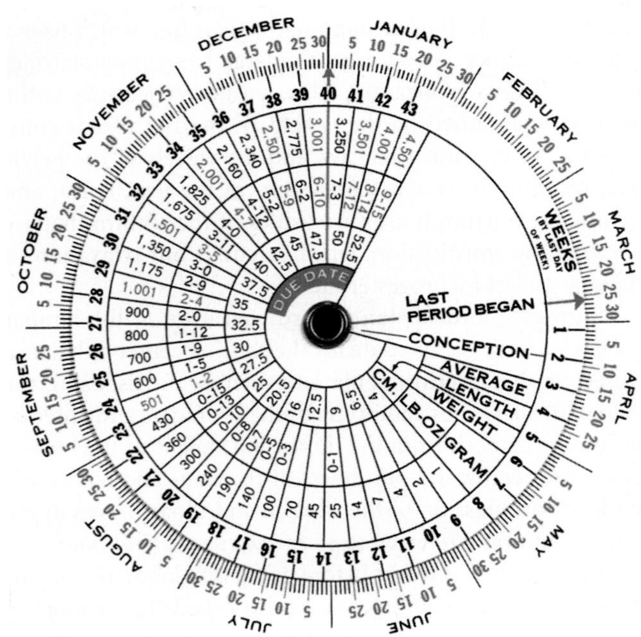

29-2 Pregnancy wheel.

DEVELOPMENTAL COMPETENCE

Each year in the United States, almost one million teenage women, ages 15 to 19 years, become pregnant and 78% are unplanned. Many of these pregnancies pose serious medical risks for both mother and fetus, such as toxemia and low-birth-weight infants; it is unclear whether these risks are due to biologic or social factors, prolonged labor, or postpartum complications.[18] Other risks for the pregnant adolescent are psychosocial. This young woman is at risk for the downward cycle of poverty beginning with an incomplete education, failure to limit family size, and continuing with failure to establish a vocation and become independent. She may be unprepared emotionally to be a mother. Her social situation may be stressful. She may not have the support of her family, her partner, or his family. Medical risks for the pregnant adolescent are generally related to poverty, inadequate nutrition, substance abuse, and sometimes sexually transmitted infections (STIs), poor health before pregnancy, and emotional and physical abuse from her partner, family, and peers.

The adolescent, for social reasons, often seeks health care later and is noncompliant with ongoing prenatal care, although early prenatal care has been shown to provide optimal management. In developing countries, maternal mortality for pregnant teenagers is a major concern because of hypertension, embolism, ectopic pregnancy, and complications from pregnancy termination where abortion is illegal.[14]

On the other hand, many Baby Boomers have delayed childbearing, and since the advent of assisted fertility, more women older than 35 years are now becoming pregnant. Women of "advanced maternal age" (after age 35 years) are often more prepared emotionally and financially to parent; however, they are more at risk for infertility and age-related anomalies. Fertility declines with advancing maternal age due to a decrease in the number and health of eggs to be ovulated, a decrease in ovulation, endometriosis, and early-onset menopause.

The risk for Down syndrome increases from about 1 in 1250 at age 25 to 1 in 1000 at age 30, 1 in 400 at age 35, 1 in 100 at age 40, and 1 in 30 at age 45.[26a]

Women ages 35 years and older or with a history of a genetic abnormality are offered genetic counseling and the options of both prenatal diagnostic screening tests. Two prenatal diagnostic options are chorionic villi sampling (CVS) performed between weeks 11 and 13 in which a small sample of chorionic villi is removed, and amniocentesis between weeks 15 and 20 in which a small amount of amniotic fluid is removed to analyze genetic makeup. Both are associated with a small risk for complications and miscarriage. Prenatal screening involves a fetal anatomy US scan and serum screening.

Carrier screening for cystic fibrosis (CF) is offered to check the inherited genetic disease affecting breathing and digestion. Both parents need to be carriers to pass the condition on to the fetus (a 25% chance [1 in 4] that the child will have CF).

Because the incidence of chronic diseases increases with age, women older than 35 years who are pregnant more often have medical complications such as diabetes, obesity, and hypertension.[14] The increased incidence of hypertension causes an increase in placental abruption and preeclampsia. Hypertension, in turn, increases intrauterine growth restriction (IUGR). More women of advanced maternal age have placenta previa, placental abruption, uterine rupture, and cesarean deliveries. They have more spontaneous abortions, in part because of the increase in genetically abnormal embryos.

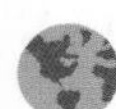

CULTURE AND GENETICS

Some complications of pregnancy occur more frequently in certain racial groups. Women who live in underdeveloped nations do not have the advantages of advanced technology. More than 500,000 women die in childbirth each year. According to the United Nations Populations Fund, this number remains globally high in an age in which these deaths are preventable. Of these maternal deaths, 90% occur in Africa and Asia and occur from severe bleeding, sepsis, eclampsia, obstructed labor, and unsafe abortions. Many women who survive pregnancy and childbirth may suffer a lifetime of physical and emotional complications such as vaginal/rectal fistula.[39a]

The Hispanic population within the United States between 1990 and 2000 grew by more than 40%. It is projected that between 2000 and 2010 that will increase by another 34%. Hispanics had the highest birth rate in 2003, with 82.2 births per 1000 teen females ages 15 to 19.[32] Still there are disparities in adequate access to preventive, prenatal, and dental care with these cultural groups along with Asian/Pacific Islander and American Indian/Alaska Native population.[32] Nonwhite pregnant women have an increased risk for gestational diabetes mellitus (GDM), pregnancy-induced hypertension (PIH), and preterm labor and delivery (PTL/PTD).

Pregnancy is not only a medical event but also one with profound psychological and social meaning for the woman and for her family and community. All cultures recognize pregnancy as a unique period in a woman's life that surrounds special customs and beliefs that have been developed throughout the ages. The spiritual practices and beliefs provide her either with or without support. Understanding what role these beliefs and practices play in the woman's pregnancy helps you acknowledge the cultural differences. Pregnancy is intensely personal and involves such charged issues as sexuality, relationships, contraception, nutritional practices, maternal weight gain, gender of the fetus, and abortion. You may begin by inquiring whether the woman or her significant others have any special requests. This communicates your intention to respect cultural differences and preferences. A continuing rapport will help enable the woman to bring up issues as they develop.

A woman's resistance to an action or a suggestion by the clinician may represent a cultural, social, or financial issue. Such issues may also be held differently by the woman and her significant others. Examples of culturally charged issues are dietary practices, sexuality during and after pregnancy, preference for gender of care provider, preference for gender of infant, and contraceptive usage. Use your skill to understand such preferences within a cultural context and accept rather than judge the person. Whenever safe and possible, respect such wishes. This enhances the success of the birth in its psychological and social dimensions.

SUBJECTIVE DATA

1. Menstrual history
2. Gynecologic history
3. Obstetric history
4. Current pregnancy
5. Medical history
6. Family history
7. Review of systems
8. Nutritional history
9. Environment/hazards

Examiner Asks	Rationale
1. Menstrual history • When was the first day of your last menstrual period that was normal in timing, premenstrual symptoms, length, amount of flow, cramping? • Number of days in cycle? • Age at menarche?	Using Nägele's rule, calculate the EDD with this date. With a pregnancy wheel, determine the current number of weeks of gestation.

Examiner Asks	Rationale
2. Gynecologic history	
• Ever had surgery of the cervix? Uterus? Fallopian tubes?	Cervical surgery may affect the integrity of the cervix during pregnancy and increases the risk for cervical insufficiency, preterm cervical dilation, and preterm delivery. Uterine surgery increases the risk for uterine rupture during pregnancy and labor.
• Any known history of or exposure to genital herpes?	Onset during pregnancy is potentially *teratogenic* (i.e., causing physical defects in the developing fetus), and a lesion at delivery precludes vaginal birth.
• Papanicolaou (Pap) tests: When was your last one? Any history of abnormal? If so, when? Have you ever had a colposcopy? Cervical biopsy?	Because more women delay childbearing, there may be an increase in diagnosing gynecologic cancers during pregnancy. Cancer is the second most common cause of maternal death in the reproductive years.[19]
• Any history of infertility, fibroids, or uterine abnormalities?	May increase risk for ectopic pregnancy, miscarriage, PTL/PTD.
• Any history of gonorrhea, chlamydia, syphilis, trichomoniasis, pelvic inflammatory disease (PID)?	STIs increase the risk for premature rupture of membranes, PTL/PTD, postpartum maternal and fetal infections.
• Do you or does your partner have more than one sexual partner?	Increases the risk for STIs and human immunodeficiency virus (HIV) infection.
• Were you a preterm infant?	Patients who themselves were preterm infants are at increased risk for PTD.
• Have you had a mammogram, breast biopsy, breast implants, lumpectomy, or mastectomy?	Breast cancer is the most common cancer in pregnancy, affecting approximately 1 in 3000 pregnancies, occurring between the ages of 32 and 38 years.[28]
3. Obstetric history	
• Number of times pregnant? Number of term or preterm deliveries? Number of spontaneous miscarriages, elective abortions, or ectopic pregnancies? Any fetal or neonatal deaths?	An obstetric history helps provide care during the current pregnancy.
• In earlier pregnancies, any history of gestational hypertension, preeclampsia, eclampsia, HELLP (**H**emolysis, **E**levated **L**iver enzymes, **L**ow **P**latelets) syndrome, diabetes, β-hemolytic *Streptococcus* infection, IUGR, congenital anomalies, premature labor, postpartum hemorrhage, or postpartum depression?	The woman who has experienced these complications in the past is at increased risk for them in subsequent pregnancies.
• How did you experience previous pregnancies and deliveries?	The subjective quality of previous experiences affects current pregnancy.
• Ever had a cesarean section? If so, what was the indication? At how many centimeters of dilation, if any, was the surgery performed? What type of uterine incision was made? (Confirming records of this surgery must be obtained.) Have you ever had a vaginal birth after a cesarean section (VBAC)?	The vertical, or "classical," incision carries a higher risk for rupture and mandates that all subsequent deliveries be by cesarean section. The "low transverse" or horizontal incision carries a low risk, and subsequent deliveries may be vaginal. Note that the direction of the skin scar does not necessarily tell how the uterus was incised.
• Any history of infertility? Have you used assisted reproductive technology?	With donor eggs, the age of the egg donor is used in calculating genetic testing.
• Any history of preterm labor or preterm rupture of membranes?	Requires close observation during the current pregnancy. Previous PTD is associated with recurrence.

Examiner Asks	Rationale
• Have you been told you have cervical insufficiency? Incompetency? Have you had a cervical cerclage placed in previous pregnancies?	A cervical cerclage is a stitch placed surgically to hold the cervix closed during the pregnancy and normally placed between weeks 12 and 15.
• Tell me the gestational ages and weights of your babies at birth.	A small infant may indicate prematurity or IUGR—complications that are repeatable. A large infant may indicate GDM (also repeatable). Conversely, birth weights of other children may indicate a "constitutional size" (e.g., the tendency of a couple to conceive smaller but normal children). Also, the woman's pelvis has been "proven" to the weight of the largest baby born vaginally; bear this number in mind as labor begins, estimating and comparing the weight of the baby about to be born.
• Did you breastfeed the previously born infants? How was that experience for you?	Her experience and knowledge base will shape your teaching and support.
• Any history of mastitis?	A poor or painful previous experience increases breastfeeding support after this pregnancy.
4. **Current pregnancy.** (Having calculated the current number of weeks of gestation, you can reassess the probable accuracy of that date when eliciting the following history.)	
• What method of contraceptive did you use most recently, and when did you discontinue it?	Recent use of birth control pills or other hormonal contraceptives causes delayed ovulation and irregular menses—consider when establishing the EDD. An intrauterine device (IUD) that is still in place requires removal; it threatens the pregnancy. Also, this opens topic of whether pregnancy was planned.
• Was the pregnancy planned? How do you feel about it?	Even a planned pregnancy represents loss—perhaps a loss of freedom, compromise of goals, loss of time with other children or partner. The first trimester is known as the "trimester of ambivalence," and encouraging acceptance and expression of these feelings helps resolution.
• How does the baby's father feel about the pregnancy? Other family members?	The woman may need assistance in gathering her support group. Inviting significant others to future visits affirms their importance and supports involvement.
• Experienced any vaginal bleeding? When? How much? What color? Accompanied by any pain?	Vaginal bleeding may indicate threatened abortion, cervicitis, or ectopic pregnancy in 1st trimester and must be investigated.
• Are you experiencing any nausea and/or vomiting?	Nausea and vomiting usually begin between weeks 4 and 5, peak between weeks 8 and 12, and resolve between weeks 14 and 16. Persistent and severe nausea and vomiting lead to hyperemesis.

Examiner Asks	Rationale
• Experienced abdominal pain? When? Where in your abdomen? Accompanied by vaginal bleeding?	Common causes of abdominal pain in early pregnancy are spontaneous abortion, ectopic pregnancy, urinary tract infection (UTI), and round ligament discomfort. Late pregnancy causes are premature labor, placental abruption, and HELLP syndrome (see Table 29-2, Preeclampsia, p. 822). Also consider other medical and surgical causes for abdominal pain.
• Experienced any illnesses since being pregnant? Any recent fever(s), unexplained rash, or infections?	Helps establish any possible exposures to infectious agents.
• Had any x-rays? Taken any medications?	Discuss the potential effect of any teratogenic exposure. Refer for expert counseling if necessary.
• Experiencing any visual changes such as the new onset of blurred vision or spots before your eyes?	In the third trimester, may be a sign of preeclampsia. Evaluate for other signs and symptoms of preeclampsia (see Table 29-2).
• Experiencing any edema? Where and under what circumstances?	In the third trimester, differentiate the normal weight-dependent edema of pregnancy from the edema of preeclampsia.
• Any frequency or burning with urination? Any blood in your urine? Do you void in small amounts? Any history of UTIs, pyelonephritis, or kidney stones?	Differentiate the normal urinary frequency of the first and third trimesters from UTI, for which pregnant women are at increased risk. Confirm by urinalysis. UTIs increase the rate of PTD.
• Any vaginal burning or itching? Any foul-smelling or colored discharge?	To rule out vaginal infection, add cultures or a wet mount to the pelvic examination. Explain the normal increase in vaginal secretions during pregnancy.
• What date did you first feel the baby move?	This sign is compared with the EDD to evaluate the accuracy of that date.
• How does the baby move on a daily basis?	Fetal movement is an excellent indicator of fetal health. Clinicians assign women to count fetal movements starting at 28 weeks of pregnancy.
• Do you have cats in the home?	Explain toxoplasmosis, a teratogenic disease transmitted through cat feces. To avoid exposure, another person should empty cat litter at frequent intervals.
• What are your plans for breastfeeding this baby?	Arrange reading, classes, and other support for the woman who is breastfeeding for the first time or for the woman with an unsuccessful earlier experience.
5. Medical history	
• Do you have allergies to medications or foods? If so, what type of reaction?	Prevents prescribing error.
• Any personal or family history of cancer?	Advanced maternal age during pregnancy increases risk for breast, ovarian, uterine, and colon cancers.
• Do you have a history of asthma? If yes, have you ever had an attack in which you needed a breathing tube placed?	Poor control and frequent exacerbations of asthma during pregnancy may result in maternal hypoxia and decrease in fetal oxygenation.

Examiner Asks	Rationale
• Ever had German measles (rubella)?	This mild childhood disease is highly teratogenic, especially during the first trimester. Instruct the woman who has not had rubella to avoid small children who are ill. Check immunity status in the serum prenatal panel. The nonimmune woman will be offered immunization after delivery.
• Ever had chickenpox?	Rarely, varicella causes congenital anomalies. The nonimmune woman should avoid exposure.
• Any history of injury to the back or another weight-bearing part?	The localized and overall weight gain of pregnancy and the joint-softening property of progesterone cause lordosis and will aggravate such injuries with increasing gestational age.
• Have you been tested for HIV? When? What was the result? Ever had a blood transfusion? Used a needle to take street drugs? Had a sexual partner who had any HIV risk factors?	HIV screening *must* be offered to all pregnant women to decrease the risk for transmission of the virus across the placenta to the fetus. Breastfeeding is contraindicated for the HIV-positive mother because the virus is present in the breast milk.
• Do you smoke cigarettes? How many? For how many years? Ever tried to quit? Drink any alcohol? How many times per week? Use any street drugs?	Explain the danger of these substances in pregnancy. Smoking increases the risk for ectopic pregnancy, spontaneous abortion, low birth weight, prematurity, preterm premature rupture of membranes, pregnancy-induced hypertension, placental abruption, and sudden infant death syndrome. Alcohol increases the risk to the fetus for fetal alcohol syndrome (see Table 13-4). Cocaine use during pregnancy is associated with congenital anomalies, a fourfold increased risk for abruptio placentae, and the risk for fetal addiction. Narcotic-addicted infants may have developmental delays or behavioral disturbances.[14] Refer to a counseling/support program and periodic toxicology screening. Refer to a smoking cessation program.
• Do you take any prescribed, over-the-counter, or herbal medications?	Screen all medications to establish safety during pregnancy.
• Do you have a regular exercise program? What type?	Regular exercise in pregnancy may reduce risk for pregnancy-induced hypertension.
• Has your vitamin D level been checked?	Vitamin D is essential for maternal response to the calcium demands of the fetus for growth and bone development. Maternal anorexia and malaise often are associated with vitamin D deficiency[22] and should be evaluated when these symptoms occur.

Examiner Asks	Rationale
6. Family history	
• Anyone in your family have hypertension?	Increases the risk for chronic hypertension and for preeclampsia.
• Diabetes? If so, of juvenile or adult onset? Insulin dependent?	Increases risk for GDM. A heavy family history might prompt early screening and dietary interventions.
• Mental illness, including depressive, anxiety, eating, personality, and psychotic disorders?	Maternal depression is associated with low birth weight, preterm delivery, and stillbirth[20] and postpartum depression.
• Kidney disease?	Increases risk for renal disease, hypertension, and preeclampsia.
• Fraternal twins?	The tendency to ovulate twice in one month is familial, increasing the incidence of twinning.
• Anyone in your family or in the family of the baby's father had congenital anomalies?	Some anomalies, such as heart conditions, are familial. Offer genetic counseling if needed.
• Is your racial or ethnic descent Mediterranean?	Increased risk for β-thalassemia.
African American?	Increased risk for sickle-cell disease.
Ashkenazi Jewish?	Increased risk for Tay-Sachs disease.
Irish?	Increased risk for spinal malformations.
7. Review of systems	
• Your weight before pregnancy?	Baseline needed to evaluate changes.
• Wear glasses?	A transient change in visual correction may occur during pregnancy.
• When did you last see the dentist? Need any dental work?	Gums may be puffy and bleed easily during pregnancy, predisposing caries. Poor dental hygiene can lead to PTD, low-birth-weight babies, and neonatal death. Dental care is an important part of prenatal care; notify the dentist that she is pregnant.
• Been exposed to tuberculosis (TB) or had a positive PPD skin test or chest x-ray examination?	Consider TB screening; positive result requires chest x-ray examination even in pregnancy.
• Any cardiovascular disease, heart disease, or disease of a heart valve?	The woman with cardiac disease is monitored carefully for signs of cardiac compromise. Blood volume increases by 40%, and the demand on the heart is significantly increased.
• Any anemia? What kind? When? Was it treated? How? Did it improve?	Pregnancy worsens any preexisting anemia because iron is used extensively by the fetus. Identify the need for early supplementation. Sickle-cell anemia may worsen during pregnancy, whereas sickle-cell carriers have more UTIs. Screen the latter periodically for bacteriuria.
• Had thrombophlebitis, pulmonary embolus (PE), or deep venous thrombosis (DVT)? Or known clotting disorder?	Pregnancy itself is a hypercoagulable state because of increases in coagulation factors. This increases the risk for phlebitis, DVTs, or PEs.[14]

Subjective Data

Examiner Asks	Rationale
• Have you had hypertension or kidney disease?	Renal disease or chronic hypertension increases risk for preeclampsia. Know the baseline BP and renal function to evaluate any changes.
• Any history of hepatitis B or C?	Confirm with serum testing. Perinatal transmission occurs by exposure to infected blood and genital secretions during delivery and by cracked and bleeding nipples during feeding.
• Any history of thyroid disease?	Uncontrolled hyperthyroidism is associated with increased neonatal morbidity resulting from preterm birth and low birth weight. Uncontrolled hypothyroidism is related to delayed mental development in children.
• Any history of seizures? On any medications?	Women with epilepsy taking medications have increased incidence of stillbirths and IUGR and a 4% to 8% risk for birth defects, such as cleft lip or palate, heart abnormalities, and spina bifida.[17]
• Have you had urinary tract infections?	The hormonal milieu of pregnancy predisposes the woman to UTIs, indicating periodic screening. Pregnancy may also mask the symptoms of UTIs. Further, a serious UTI may cause irritability of the uterus, threatening preterm labor. Educate the woman in measures to prevent UTIs.
• Have you had depression or any other mental illness?	This woman will be at risk for postpartum depression. Assist her to prepare a support network. Counseling may help her navigate the developmental challenges of becoming a mother.
• Do you feel safe in your relationship or home environment?	Violence during pregnancy is common. Questioning the safety of the woman is part of prenatal care.
• Are you in a relationship with someone who physically or emotionally abuses or threatens you?	Most women will not freely offer this information. You must ask these questions at the appropriate time and in a nonthreatening manner.
• Has anyone forced you to have sexual activities against your will?	Incest or other abuse increases risk for dysfunctional labor and cesarean delivery.
• Do you have diabetes? On oral hypoglycemics, insulin injection, or insulin pump? Did you have diabetes during a previous pregnancy?	Diabetes is carefully managed during pregnancy to avoid serious complications, such as a macrosomic infant and operative delivery. Consider early screening and nutritional interventions.
8. Nutritional history	
• Do you follow a special diet? Are you vegetarian?	A special diet may have nutritional risk. Help achieve adequate nutrition within the confines of her diet. Refer for dietary counseling.
• Any food intolerance?	A food intolerance might affect the woman's and fetus's nutrition, such as lactose intolerance limiting calcium intake.

Examiner Asks	Rationale
9. Environment/hazards • What is your occupation? What are the physical demands of the work? Are you exposed to any strong odors, chemicals, radiation, or other harmful substances? Or potentially harmful physical contact?	Hazards? Possible teratogenic exposures? The woman who is rubella nonimmune may be advised not to continue working in a daycare center. Suitability for pregnancy? The woman whose job requires long hours of standing may be disabled early if signs of PTL occur.
• Do you consider your food and housing adequate?	Refer for state and federal programs to assist with food, housing, or other needs.
• How do you wear your seatbelt when driving?	For maternal and fetal safety, instruct the woman to place the lap belt below the uterus and to use the shoulder strap.
• Other questions or concerns?	Encourage the woman to write down questions between visits.

OBJECTIVE DATA

PREPARATION

The initial examination for pregnancy is often a woman's first pelvic examination, and many women are extremely anxious. Alternatively, the woman may not know for certain whether she is pregnant, and she may be anxious about the findings. Verbally prepare the woman for what will happen during the examination before touching her. Save the pelvic examination for last—by that time, the woman will be more comfortable with your gentle, informing manner. Communicate all findings as you go along to demonstrate your respectful affirmation of her control and responsibility in her own health and health care and that of her child.

Ask the woman to empty her bladder before the examination, reserving a clean-catch specimen for dipping for protein and glucose, and for urinalysis, if required. Before the examination, ask her to weigh herself on the office scale. Provide the woman with an escort or chaperone during examinations.

Give the woman a gown and drape. Begin the examination with the woman sitting on the examination table, wearing the gown, her lap covered by a drape. During the breast examination, help her lie down. She remains recumbent for the abdominal and extremity examination. Use the lithotomy position for the pelvic examination (see Chapter 26). Help her to a seated position to check her BP. Recheck after the examination if BP is elevated.

EQUIPMENT NEEDED

Stethoscope, BP cuff
Centimeter measuring tape
Fetoscope and Doppler sonometer
Reflex hammer
Urine collection containers
Dipstix for checking urine for glucose and protein
Equipment needed for pelvic examination as noted in Chapter 26.

Normal Range of Findings	Abnormal Findings
GENERAL SURVEY	
Observe the woman's state of nourishment and her grooming, posture, mood, and affect, which reflect her mental state. Throughout the examination, observe her maturity and ability to attend and learn so that you can plan your teaching of the information she needs to successfully complete a healthy pregnancy.	Undernourished or obese. Poor grooming, a slumped posture, and a flat affect may be signs of depression and risk for postpartum depression. Poor grooming may reflect a lack of resources and a need for a social service referral.

Normal Range of Findings

Abnormal Findings

A lack of attention may indicate some preoccupation with a concern. The woman with learning difficulties benefits from written and verbal information, special classes, and a support person to accompany her. A flat, unclear affect may indicate depression or the influence of drugs.

SKIN

Note any scars (particularly those of previous cesarean delivery). Many women have skin changes during pregnancy that may spontaneously resolve after the pregnancy, such as acne or skin tags. Vascular spiders may be present on the upper body. Some women have **chloasma,** known as the "mask of pregnancy," which is a butterfly-shaped pigmentation of the face. Note the presence of the **linea nigra,** a hyperpigmented line that begins at the sternal notch and extends down the abdomen through the umbilicus to the pubis (Fig. 29-3). Also note **striae,** or stretch marks, in areas of weight gain, particularly on the abdomen and breasts of multiparous women. These marks are bright red when they first form, but they will shrink and lighten to a silvery color (in the lightly pigmented woman) after the pregnancy (see Fig. 29-3).

Multiple bruises suggest physical abuse.

Tracks (scars along easily accessed veins) may indicate intravenous drug use.

Complaints of nasal irritation, nasal crusting, nasal stuffiness, or recurrent nosebleeds may indicate drug sniffing.

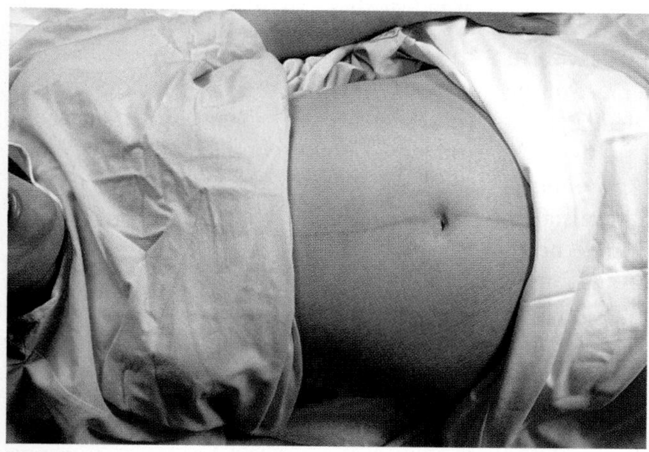

29-3

MOUTH

Mucous membranes should be red and moist. Gum hypertrophy (surface looks smooth, and stippling disappears) may occur normally during pregnancy (pregnancy gingivitis). Bleeding gums may be from estrogen stimulation, which causes increased vascularity and fragility.

Pale mucous membranes are indicative of anemia.

Poor dental hygiene during pregnancy may lead to PTD or low-birth-weight infants.

NECK

The thyroid may be palpable and feel full but smooth during the normal pregnancy of a euthyroid woman.

Solitary nodules indicate neoplasm; multiple nodules usually indicate inflammation or a multinodular goiter. Significant diffuse enlargement occurs with hyperthyroidism, thyroiditis, and hypothyroidism.

Normal Range of Findings

Abnormal Findings

BREASTS

The breasts are enlarged (Fig. 29-4), perhaps with resulting striae, and may be very tender. The areolae and nipples enlarge and darken in pigmentation, the nipples become more erect, and "secondary areolae" (mottling around the areolae) may develop. The blood vessels of the breasts enlarge and may shine blue through a seemingly more translucent than usual chest wall. When auscultating, blood flow through these blood vessels can be heard and may be mistaken for a cardiac murmur. This sound is called the *mammary souffle* (SOO-FL). Montgomery's tubercles, located around the areolae and responsible for skin integrity of the areolae, enlarge. Colostrum, a thick yellow fluid, may be expressed from the nipples.

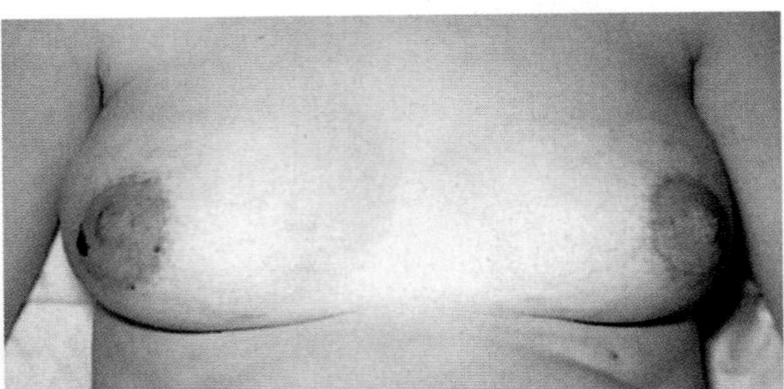

29-4

The breast tissue feels nodular as the mammary alveoli hypertrophy. Take this opportunity to teach or reinforce breast self-examination (BSE). The woman should expect changes in the breast tissue during the pregnancy. Because of the lack of menses, instruct her to perform BSE according to the calendar on a monthly basis, on a date familiar to her such as her birth date.

Note any abnormal mass within the breast, and refer to a breast specialist for further evaluation. Ultrasound of the breast(s) is used in lieu of mammograms during pregnancy and lactation.

Recall that some women have an embryologic remnant called a *supernumerary nipple,* which may or may not have breast tissue beneath it. Possibly mistaken previously for a mole, these occur under the arm or in a line directly underneath each nipple on the abdominal wall (see Chapter 17). This nipple and breast tissue may show the same changes of pregnancy. Instruct the woman to check these areas as well during BSE.

HEART

The pregnant woman often has a functional, soft, blowing, systolic murmur that occurs as a result of increased volume. The murmur requires no treatment and will resolve after pregnancy.

Note any other murmur and refer. Valvular disease may necessitate the use of prophylactic antibiotics at delivery. Pregnancy places a large hemodynamic burden on the heart, and the woman with cardiac disease is managed closely.

LUNGS

The lungs are clear bilaterally to auscultation with no crackles or wheezing. Shortness of breath is common in the third trimester from pressure on the diaphragm from the enlarged uterus.

Women with asthma exacerbations during pregnancy may have expiratory (and possibly inspiratory) wheeze.

PERIPHERAL VASCULATURE

The legs may show diffuse, symmetric, bilateral pitting edema, particularly if the examination is occurring later in the day when the woman has been on her feet and in the third trimester. Varicose veins in the legs are common in the third trimester. The Homan sign is negative.

Edema, together with increased BP and proteinuria, is a sign of preeclampsia. Edema and pain in one leg occur with DVT. Carefully evaluate any redness or

Normal Range of Findings	Abnormal Findings
	red, hot, tender swelling to rule out phlebitis. Varicosities increase the risk for thrombophlebitis; she should not wear restrictive clothing or sit without moving legs for a long period. Varicosities will worsen with the weight and volume of pregnancy; support hose help minimize them.

NEUROLOGIC

Using the reflex hammer, check the biceps, patellar, and ankle deep tendon reflexes (DTRs). Normally, these are 1+ and 2+ and equal bilaterally.

Brisk or greater than 2+ DTRs and clonus may be associated with elevated BP and cerebral edema in the preeclamptic woman.

INSPECT AND PALPATE THE ABDOMEN

Observe the shape and contours of the abdomen to discern signs of fetal position. As the woman lifts her head, you may see the **diastasis recti,** the separation of the abdominal muscles, which occurs during pregnancy, with the muscles returning together after pregnancy with abdominal exercise. When palpating, note the abdominal muscle tone, which grows more relaxed with each subsequent pregnancy. Note any tenderness; the uterus is normally nontender.

The fundus should be palpable abdominally from 12 weeks' gestation on. Use the side of your hand and begin palpating centrally on the abdomen higher than you expect the uterus to be. Palpate down until you feel the fundus (the top of the uterus). Alternatively, stand at the woman's right side facing her head (Fig. 29-5). Place the palm of your right hand on the curve of the uterus in the left lower quadrant and your left palm on the curve of the uterus in the right lower quadrant. Moving from hand to hand, allowing the curve of the uterus to guide you, "walk" your hands to where they meet centrally at the fundus.

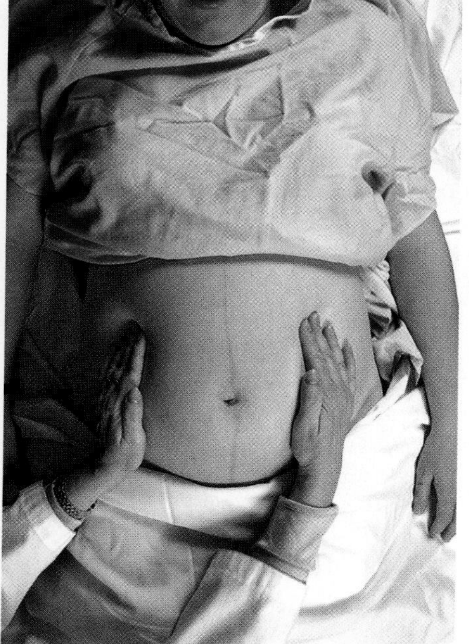

29-5

Objective Data

Normal Range of Findings

Note the fundal location by landmarks and fingerbreadths, as described in Fig. 29-1. Note that individual women's variations in location of landmarks and examiner's variations in fingerbreadths make this measurement inexact. It is more accurate to use the centimeter measuring tape and measure the height of the fundus in centimeters from the superior border of the symphysis to the fundus (Fig. 29-6). After 20 weeks, the number of centimeters should approximate the number of weeks of gestation.

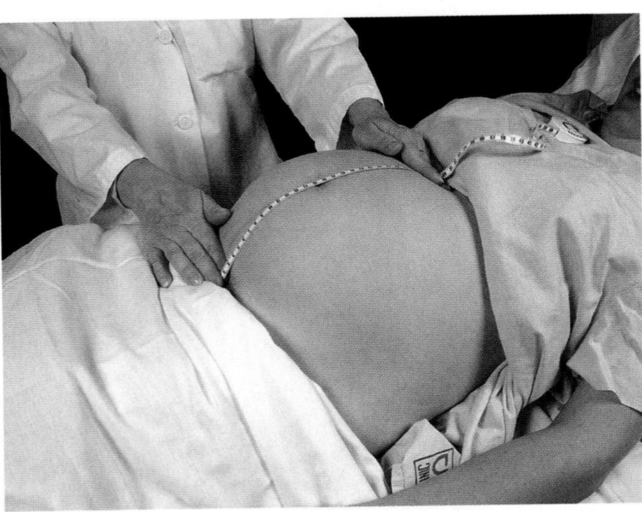

29-6

Beginning at 20 weeks, you may feel fetal movement and the fetus's head can be ballotted. A gentle, quick palpation with the fingertips can locate a head that not only is hard when you push it away but also is hard as it bobs or bounces back against your fingers.

If you suspect the woman to be in labor, palpate for uterine contractions. Palpate the uterus over its entire surface to familiarize yourself with its "indentability." Then rest your hand lightly on the uterus with fingers opened. When the uterus contracts, it rises and pulls together, drawing your fingers closer together.

During the contraction, notice that the uterus is firm and less "indentable." When the uterus relaxes, your fingers relax open again. In this way, contractions can be monitored for frequency (from the beginning of one contraction to the beginning of the next), length, and quality.

Note that a mild contraction feels like the firmness of the tip of your nose; a moderate contraction feels like your chin; and a hard contraction feels like your forehead. (Make allowance for the amount of soft tissue between your fingers and the uterus.)

Leopold's Maneuvers

In the third trimester, perform Leopold's maneuvers to determine fetal lie, presentation, attitude, position, variety, and engagement. **Fetal lie** is the orientation of the fetal spine to the maternal spine and may be longitudinal, transverse, or oblique. **Presentation** describes the part of the fetus that is entering the pelvis first (i.e., vertex [head], breech, foot). **Attitude,** the position of fetal parts in relation to each other, may be flexed, military (straight), or extended. **Position** designates the location of a fetal part to the right or left of the maternal pelvis. **Variety** is the location of the fetal back to the anterior, lateral, or posterior part of the maternal pelvis. **Engagement** occurs when the widest diameter of the presenting part has descended into the pelvic inlet—specifically, to the imagined plane at the level of the ischial spines.

Abnormal Findings

A lagging fundal height ≥2 cm may indicate IUGR, transverse lie, or oblique presentation of the fetus.

An abnormal uterine contraction is dystonic in nature; the contraction begins in the lower uterine segment and may delay cervical dilation.

Normal Range of Findings

Leopold's first maneuver is performed by facing the gravida's head and placing your fingertips around the top of the fundus (Fig. 29-7). Note its size, consistency, and shape. Imagine what fetal part is in the fundus. The breech feels large and firm. Moving it between the thumb and fingers of the hand, because it is attached to the fetus at the waist, results in moving it slowly and with difficulty. In contrast, the fetal head feels large, round, and hard. When it is ballotted, it feels hard as you push it away and hard again as it bobs back against your fingers in an "answer." Note that the "bobbing" or "ballotting" sensation of the movement occurs because the head is attached at the neck and moves easily. If there is no part in the fundus, the fetus is in the transverse lie.

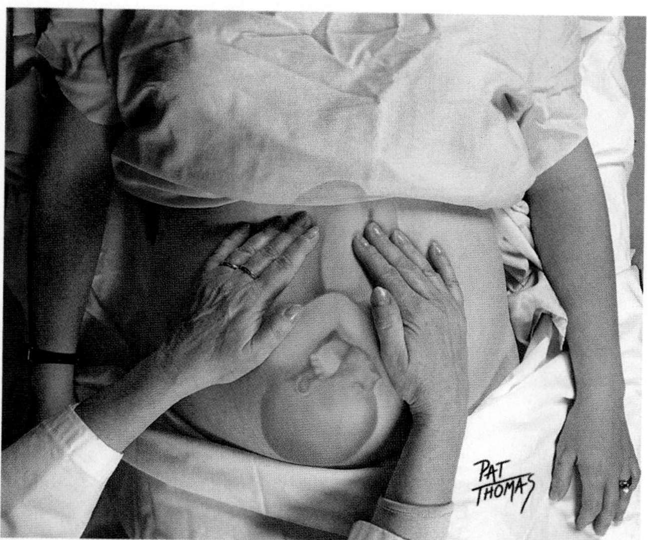

29-7 Leopold's first maneuver.

For **Leopold's second maneuver,** move your hands to the sides of the uterus (Fig. 29-8). Note whether small parts or a long, firm surface are palpable on the woman's left or right side. The long, firm surface is the back. Note whether the back is anterior, lateral, or out of reach (posterior). The small parts, or limbs, indicate a posterior position when they are palpable all over the abdomen.

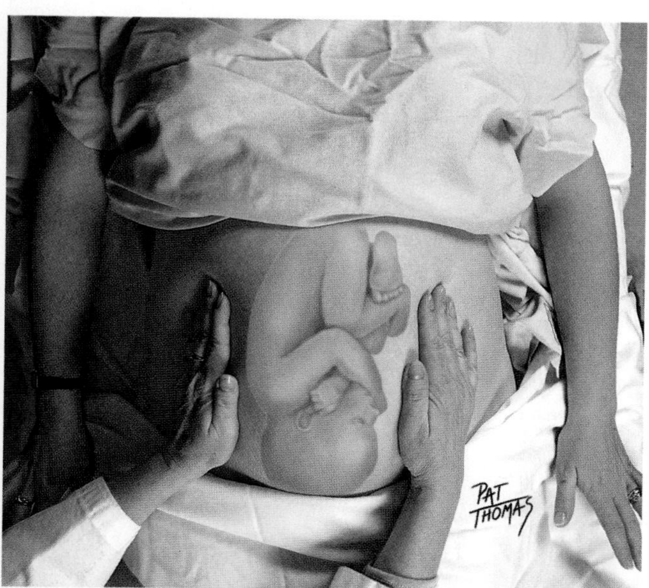

29-8 Leopold's second maneuver.

Abnormal Findings

Normal Range of Findings

Leopold's third maneuver, also called *Pawlik's maneuver,* requires the woman to bend her knees up slightly (Fig. 29-9). Grasp the lower abdomen just above the symphysis pubis between the thumb and fingers of one hand to determine what part of the fetus is there. If the presenting part is beginning to engage, it will feel "fixed." With this maneuver alone, it may be difficult to differentiate the shoulder from the vertex.

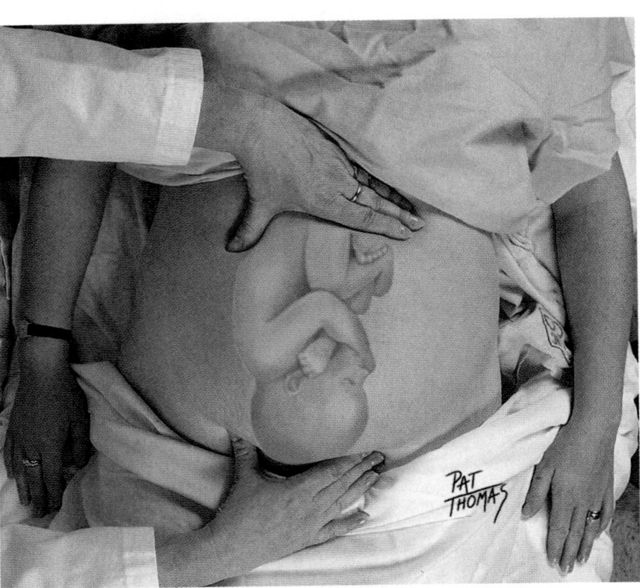

29-9 Leopold's third maneuver.

The **fourth maneuver** assists in determining engagement and, in the vertex presentation, to differentiate shoulder from vertex (Fig. 29-10). The woman's knees are still bent. Facing her feet, place your palms, with fingers pointing toward the feet, on either side of the lower abdomen. Pressing your fingers firmly, move slowly down toward the pelvic inlet. If your fingers meet, the presenting part is not engaged. If your fingers diverge at the pelvic rim meeting a hard prominence on one side, this prominence is the occiput. This indicates the vertex is presenting with a deflexed head (the face presenting). If your fingers meet hard prominences on both sides, the vertex is engaged in either a military or a flexed position. If your fingers come to the pelvic brim diverged but with no prominences palpable, the vertex is "dipping" into the pelvis, or is engaged. In this case, the firm object felt above the symphysis pubis in the third maneuver is the shoulder.

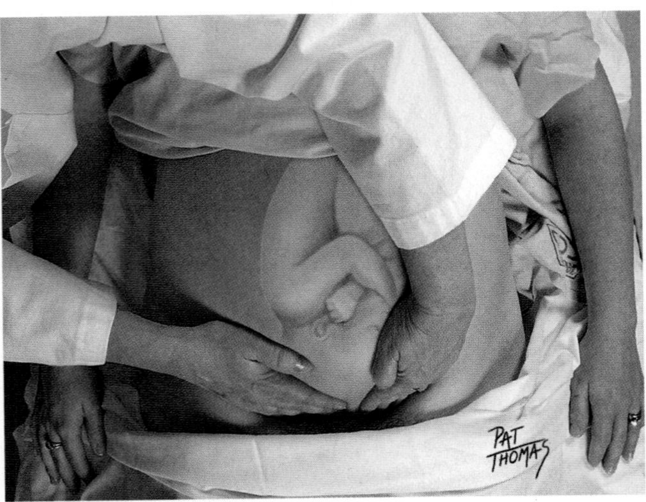

29-10 Leopold's fourth maneuver.

Abnormal Findings

Normal Range of Findings	Abnormal Findings
See Fig. 29-11 for various fetal positions and where to auscultate the FHTs for each. At the end of pregnancy, about 96% of fetal presentations are vertex, 3.3% are breech, 0.3% are face, and 0.4% are shoulder.[14]	

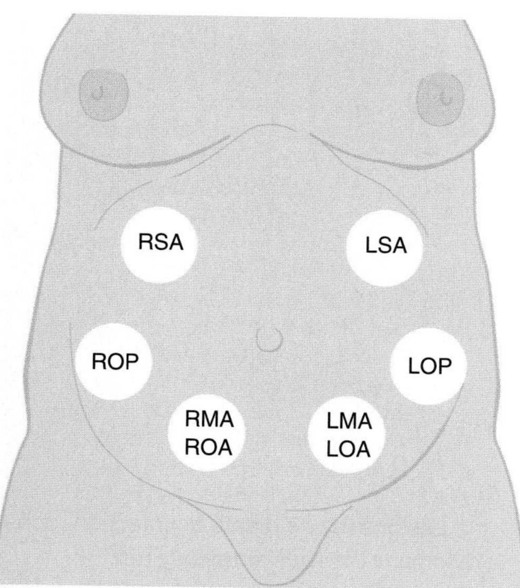

RSA and LSA = right and left sacral anterior (breech)
RMA and LMA = right and left mentum anterior (face)
ROA and LOA = right and left occiput anterior (vertex)
ROP and LOP = right and left occiput posterior (vertex)

29-11 Location of FHTs for various fetal positions.

AUSCULTATE THE FETAL HEART TONES

FHTs are a positive sign of pregnancy. They can be heard by Doppler US at 8 to 10 weeks' gestation and with a fetoscope at 20 weeks. This use of the fetoscope assists in dating the pregnancy. FHTs are auscultated best over the shoulder of the fetus. After identifying the position of the fetus (see Fig. 29-11), use the heart tones to confirm your findings. Count the FHTs for 15 seconds and multiply by four to obtain the rate (Fig. 29-12). The normal rate is between 120 and 160 beats per minute. Spontaneous accelerations of FHTs indicate fetal well-being.

If no FHTs are heard, verify fetal cardiac activity with US.

Further investigate any decelerations of FHTs.

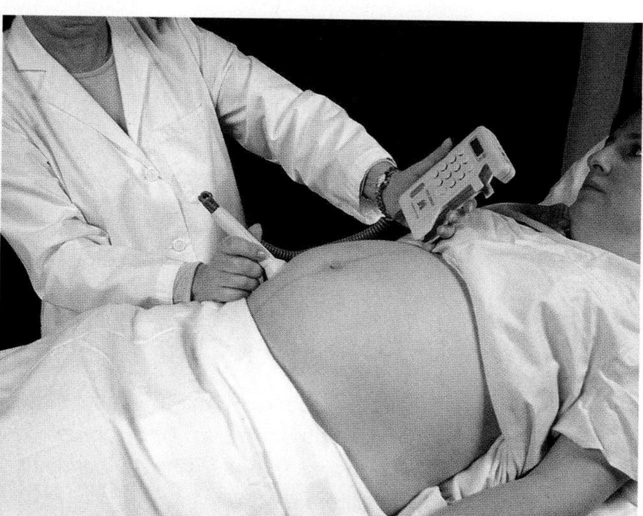

29-12

Objective Data

Normal Range of Findings	Abnormal Findings

Differentiate the FHTs from the slower rate of the maternal pulse and the uterine souffle (the soft, swishing sound of the placenta receiving the pulse of maternal arterial blood) by palpating the mother's pulse while you listen. Also, distinguish FHTs from the funic souffle (blood rushing through the umbilical arteries at the same rate as the FHTs). The FHTs are a double sound, like the tick-tock of a watch under a pillow, whereas the funic souffle is a sharp, whistling sound that is heard only 15% of the time.[14]

All the abdominal findings are of interest to the woman—share them with her. Often she will want to listen to FHTs with her significant others. For the hearing-impaired pregnant woman, place her hand on the fetal monitor to feel the fetal heart vibrating.

PELVIC EXAMINATION

Genitalia

Use the procedure for the pelvic examination described in Chapter 26. Note the following characteristics. The enlargement of the labia minora is common in multiparous women. Labial varicosities may be present. The perineum may be scarred from a previous episiotomy or from lacerations. Note any hemorrhoids of the rectum. Note any lesions on the symphysis pubis, labia, or perianal area.

Lesions may indicate an infection, condyloma, or herpes simplex virus.

Speculum Examination

When examining the vagina, you may see **Chadwick sign,** the bluish purplish discoloration and congested look of the vaginal wall and cervix from increased vascularity and engorgement (Fig. 29-13). Note the vaginal discharge. Vaginal discharge in pregnancy may be heavier in amount but should be similar in description to the woman's nonpregnant discharge and should not be associated with itching, burning, or an unusual odor (except that, occasionally, chapping of the vaginal area may be seen due to excessive moisture). Perform a wet mount or culture of the discharge when you are uncertain of its normalcy.

Many cervical infections or STIs are asymptomatic. Any cervical secretions that are purulent or mucopurulent (chlamydia or gonorrhea); yellow or green frothy (trichomoniasis); thin, white, gray, or milky, with a "fishy" odor (bacterial vaginosis); or thick, white, and clumpy (candidiasis) should be treated appropriately during the pregnancy. Bacterial vaginosis can lead to PTL and rupture of membranes.

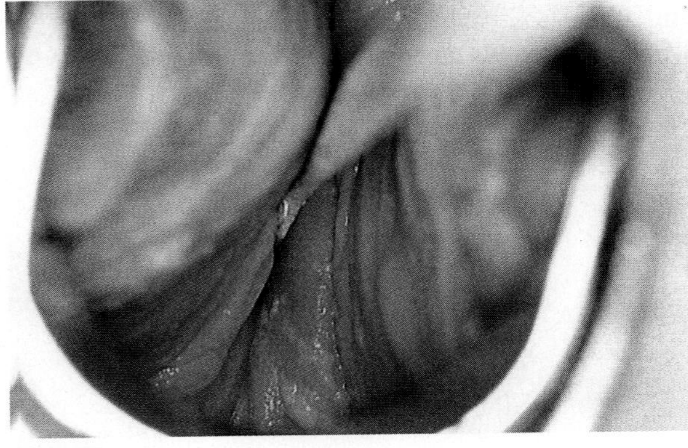

29-13

Note whether the cervix appears open. Note whether it is the smooth, round cervix with a dotlike external os of the nulliparous woman or the irregular multiparous cervix with an external os that appears more like a crooked line, the result of cervical dilation and possibly lacerations in a previous pregnancy.

A friable cervix bleeds easily when touched with a cotton swab, cytobrush, or speculum and may be due to cervicitis. Obtain cultures.

Objective Data

Normal Range of Findings	Abnormal Findings

Bimanual Examination

As described in Chapter 26, palpate the uterus between your internal and external hands. Note its position. The pregnant uterus may be rotated toward the right side as it rises out of the pelvis because of the presence of the descending colon on the left. This is called **dextrorotation.** Irregular enlargement of the uterus may be noted at 8 to 10 weeks and occurs when implantation occurs close to a cornual area of the uterus. This is called **Piskacek sign.** Also, you may note **Hegar sign,** when the enlarged uterus bends forward on its softened isthmus between the 4th and 6th weeks of pregnancy.

Note the size and consistency of the uterus. In a singleton pregnancy, the 6-week gestation uterus may seem only slightly enlarged and softened. The 8-week gestation uterus is approximately the size of an avocado, approximately 7 to 8 cm across the fundus. The 10-week gestation uterus is about the size of a grapefruit and may reach to the pelvic brim, but it is narrow and does not fill the pelvis from side to side; the 12-week gestation uterus will fill the pelvis. After 12 weeks, the uterus is sized from the abdomen. The multigravid uterus may be larger initially, and early sizing of this uterus may be less reliable for dating.

Uterine fibroids (leiomyomas) may also be felt during a bimanual examination.

Softening of the cervix is called **Goodell sign.** When examining the cervix, note its position (anterior, midposition, or posterior), degree of effacement (or thinning, expressed in percentages assuming a ≥2-cm–long cervix initially), dilation (opening, expressed in centimeters), consistency (soft or firm), and the station of the presenting part (centimeters above or below the ischial plane) (Fig. 29-14).

A shortened cervix is <2 cm.

Objective Data

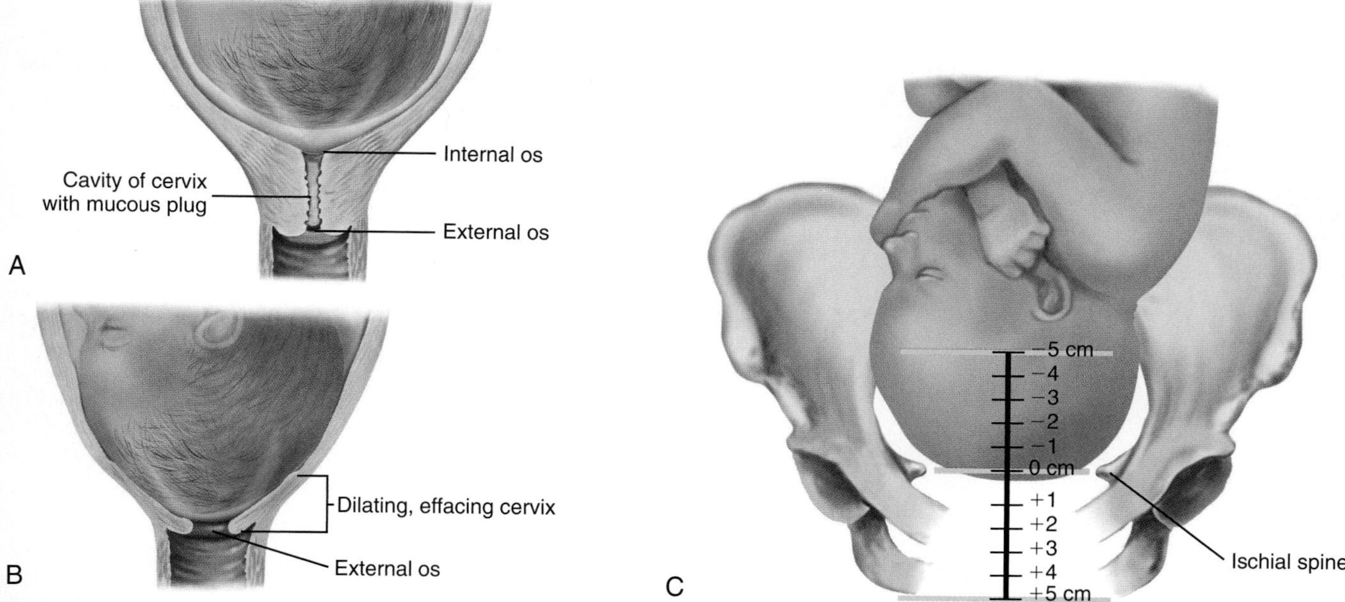

29-14 A, Cervix before labor. **B,** Cervix begins to efface and dilate. **C,** Station height of presenting part in relation to ischial spines.

The ovaries rise with the growing uterus. Always examine the adnexa to rule out the presence of a mass, such as an ectopic pregnancy.

Adnexal enlargement and pain with palpation occur with ectopic pregnancy or ovarian mass.

To determine tone, ask the woman to squeeze your fingers as they rest in the vagina. Take this opportunity to teach Kegel exercise, the squeezing of the vagina, which the woman can do to prepare for and to recover from birth. (The woman can also identify the exercise of these muscles by stopping the flow of urine midstream, although she should do this only once and should usually let urine flow freely.) Direct the woman to squeeze slowly to a peak at the count of eight and then release slowly to the count of eight. You can prescribe this exercise to be performed 50 to 100 times a day.

Normal Range of Findings	Abnormal Findings

Pelvimetry

Assess the bones of the pelvis for shape and size. The dimensions may indicate the favorableness of the bony structure for vaginal delivery. However, the relaxation of the pelvic joints, the widening of the pelvis in the squatting position, and the capacity of the fetal head to mold to the shape of the pelvis may enable a vaginal birth despite seemingly unfavorable measurements.

To aid in visualizing the pelvis, imagine three planes: the pelvic inlet (from the sacral promontory to the upper edge of the pubis), the midpelvis, and the pelvic outlet (from the coccyx to the lower edge of the pubis) (Fig. 29-15). Assessment of each of these pelvic planes, as described in the following techniques, allows you to estimate the adequacy of the pelvis for vaginal delivery.

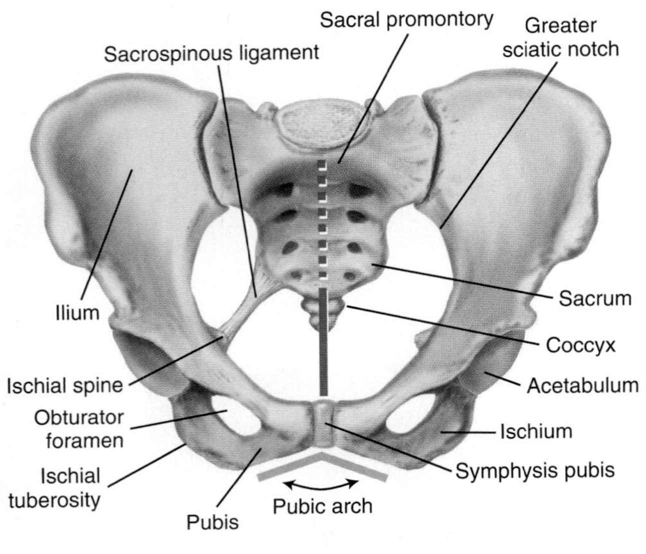

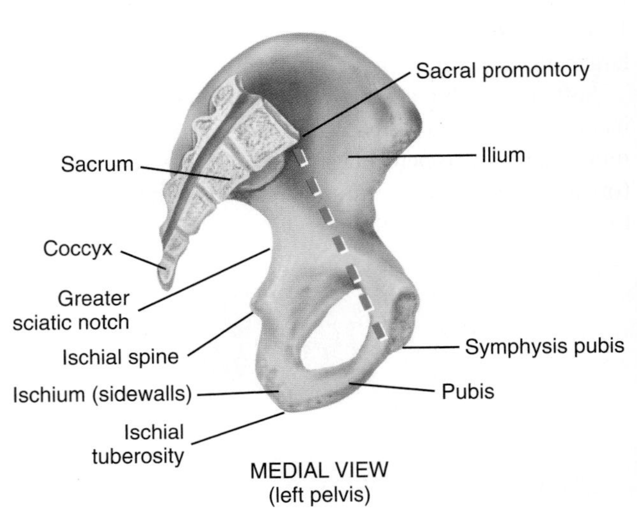

29-15

There are four general types of pelves: gynecoid, anthropoid, android, and platypelloid (Table 29-1). You may postpone examination of the bony pelvis until the third trimester when the vagina is more distensible. With your two fingers still in the vagina, note the shape and width of the pubic arch (a 90-degree arch, or 2 fingerbreadths, is desirable). If you are right-handed, move your hand to the woman's right pelvis. If you are left-handed, move it to the left side of the woman's pelvis. Assess the inclination and curve of the side walls and the prominence of the ischial spine (refer to Fig. 29-15 for location of these landmarks). Move your fingers back and forth between the spines to get an impression of the transverse diameter—10 cm is desirable. Sweep your fingers down the sacrum, noting its shape and inclination (hollow, J-shaped, or straight). Assess the coccyx for prominence and mobility. From the sacrum, locate the sacrospinous ligament. Assess the length of the ligament—2½ to 3 fingerbreadths is adequate. Assess the shape and width of the sacrospinous notch. Shift to the other side of the pelvis and assess it for similarity to the first.

TABLE 29-1 The Four Pelvic Types

The Gynecoid Pelvis

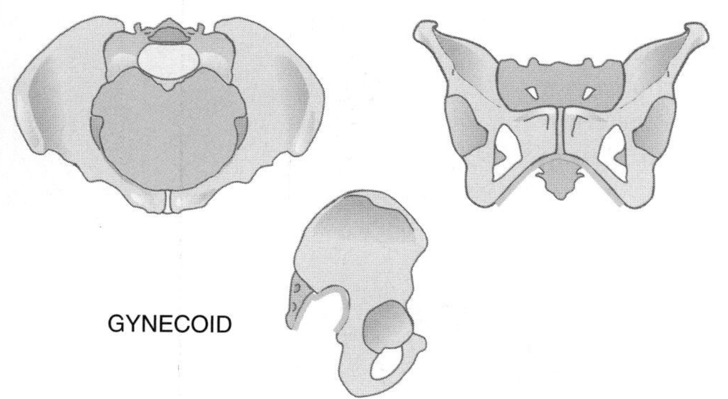

Inlet round or oval.
Posterior sagittal diameter of inlet only slightly less than anterior sagittal diameter.
Pubic arch wide (90 degrees or more).
Spines are not prominent, allowing a transverse diameter at spines 10 cm or more.
Sacrosciatic notch round and wide.
Straight side walls.
Posterior pelvis round and wide.
Sacrum is parallel with the symphysis pubis; hollow and concave.
Favors vaginal delivery.
Seen in 50% of all women.

The Android Pelvis

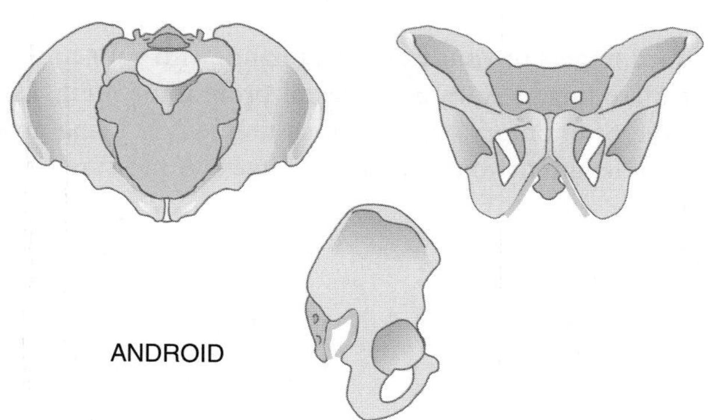

Inlet heart-shaped.
Posterior sagittal diameter of inlet less than the anterior sagittal diameter.
Pubic arch narrow (less than 90 degrees).
Spines are prominent, decreasing transverse diameter at spines.
Sacrosciatic notch is narrow and highly arched.
Side walls converge.
Posterior sagittal diameter decreases from inlet to outlet as sacrum inclines forward.
Sacrum is straight and prominent; coccyx may be prominent.
Anterior of pelvis is narrow and triangular.
The "male" pelvis.
Poor prognosis for vaginal delivery.
Seen more frequently in white women.

The Anthropoid Pelvis

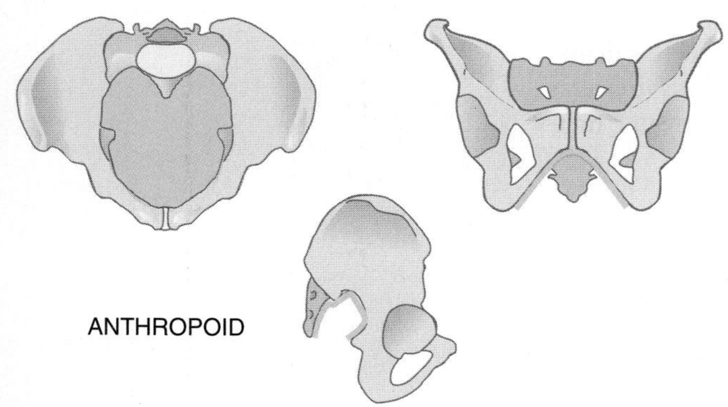

Inlet oval in shape.
Pubic arch may be somewhat narrow.
Spines usually prominent but not encroaching because of the spaciousness of the posterior segment.
Sacrosciatic notch average height but wide (about 4 fingerbreadths).
Side walls somewhat convergent.
Sacrum posteriorly inclined, with posterior sagittal diameters long throughout the pelvis.
Occurs in 40.5% nonwhite women; 23.5% white women.
If pelvis somewhat large, adequate for vaginal delivery because posterior pelvis is generous.

The Platypelloid Pelvis

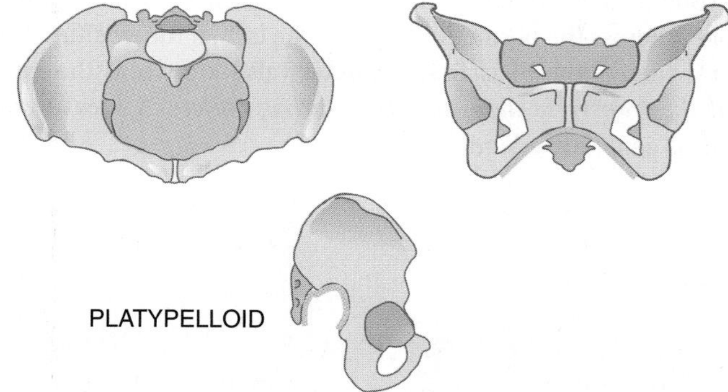

Inlet shaped like a flattened gynecoid pelvis.
Pubic arch wide.
Spines usually prominent but not encroaching because of the already wide interspinous diameter.
Sacrosciatic notch wide and flat.
Side walls slightly convergent.
Sacrum inclined posteriorly and hollow, making a short and shallow pelvis.
Occurs in fewer than 3% of all women.
Not conducive to vaginal delivery.

Data from Varney, H. (1997). *Varney's midwifery* (3rd ed.). Sudbury, MA: Jones & Bartlett.

Normal Range of Findings

The pelvic inlet cannot be reached by clinical examination, but you can estimate it by the measure of the **diagonal conjugate,** which indicates the anteroposterior diameter of the pelvic inlet. Having measured the length of the second and third fingers of your examining hand, with your fingers still in the vagina, point these fingers toward the sacral promontory (Fig. 29-16). If you cannot reach the promontory, note the measurement as being greater than the centimeters of length of your examining fingers. A measurement of 11.5 to 12.0 cm is desirable.

Abnormal Findings

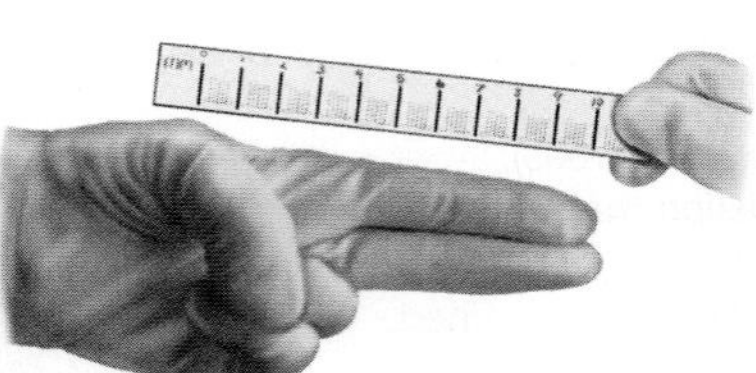

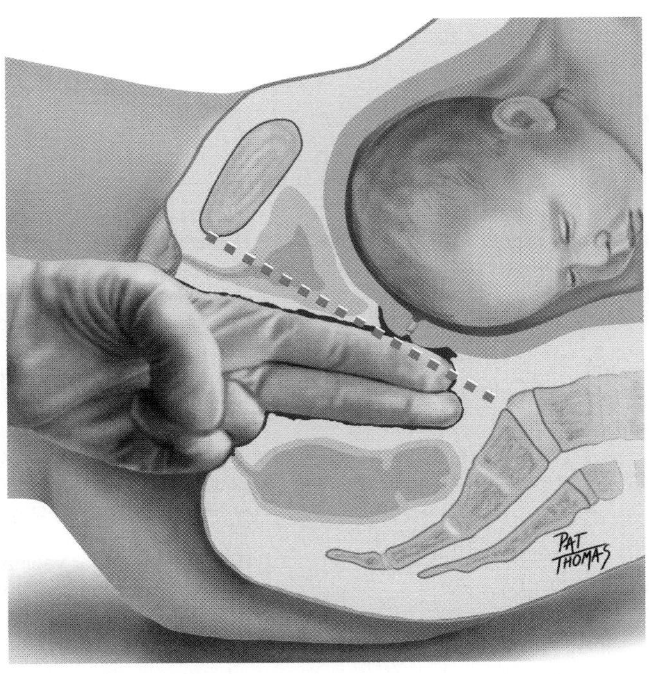

29-16 Diagonal conjugate.

Remove your fingers from the vagina. Having previously measured the width of your own hand across the knuckles, form your hand into a closed fist and place it across the perineum between the ischial tuberosities. Estimate this diameter, which is the **bi-ischial diameter** (also known as the *intertubous diameter and the transverse diameter of the pelvic outlet*). A measurement greater than 8 cm is generally adequate (Fig. 29-17).

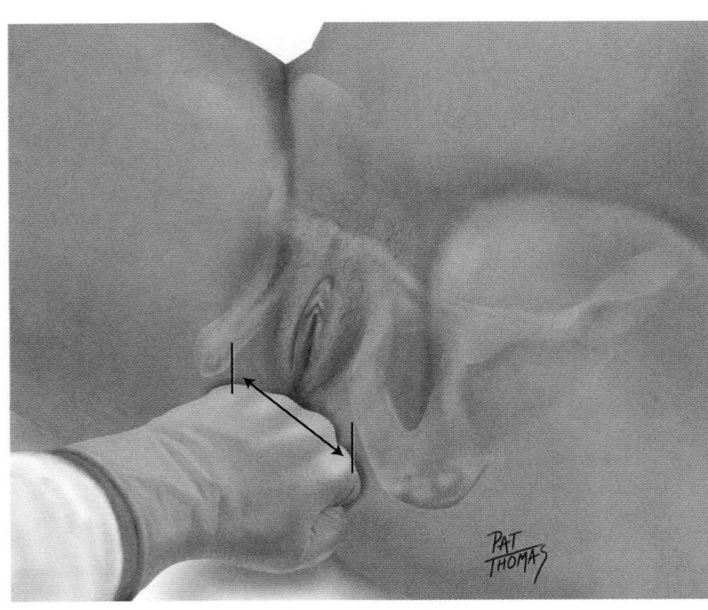

29-17 Bi-ischial diameter.

Normal Range of Findings	Abnormal Findings
When describing pelvimetry, note all the just-mentioned measurements and state the pelvic type. The pelvis may be described as being "proven" to the number of pounds of the largest vaginally born infant. Alternatively, to describe a small pelvis, you may make the assessment, for example, "adequate for a 7-lb baby."	

Blood Pressure

After the examination, take the blood pressure when the woman is the most relaxed, in the semi-Fowler's or upright position. Recheck an elevated pressure.

Chronic hypertension: a documented history of high BP before pregnancy or a persistent elevation of at least 140/90 mm Hg on two occasions more than 24 hours apart before the 20th week of gestation.[19]

ROUTINE LABORATORY AND RADIOLOGIC IMAGING STUDIES

At the first prenatal visit, order a routine prenatal panel, which usually includes a complete blood cell count, serology, rubella antibodies, hepatitis B screening, blood type and Rhesus factor, and antibody screening. Some providers screen for herpes simplex viruses I and II and thyroid function. A vitamin D level is helpful. Sickle-cell or thalassemia screening may be indicated. For some populations, a PPD/tine test may be indicated to rule out active or exposure to tuberculosis. Offer the woman HIV screening and cystic fibrosis screening. Obtain a Pap smear at the initial visit along with cervical cultures.

Collect a clean-catch urinalysis at the initial prenatal visit to rule out cystitis. At each prenatal visit, check the urine for protein and glucose. A clean-catch specimen is ideal for this dip because a random specimen may include vaginal secretions, which contain protein, skewing the results. For women with active substance abuse, a urine toxicology screen is beneficial.

Each clinic has a policy regarding the frequency of ultrasound (US) examinations. Some providers prefer to do US for dating when the maternal serum alpha-fetoprotein or "quad" screening is drawn because accurate dating is essential. Others will do it later (11 to 14 weeks' gestation), when measuring for fetal nuchal translucency (another fetal risk screening tool), which is best done at this gestation. Some providers use US only when there is a medical indication; others routinely order US to confirm dates and fetal normalcy (insofar as US is able to determine normalcy) and for any specific medical indication, such as the fundus measuring small or large for dates. The US shows placental and fetal location and fetal gender.

Antepartum fetal testing's ultimate goal is to improve the perinatal outcome by decreasing stillbirth and long-term neurologic impairments (of the fetus).[34] This testing consists of monitoring fetal growth, amniotic fluid volume, biophysical profiling, and other potential fetal/maternal markers using ultrasonography. Fetal testing (non-stress test [NST] or contraction stress test [CST]) using electronic fetal monitors to graph and audibly hear the fetal heart rate and determine uterine activity is another method. The American College of Obstetricians and Gynecologists (ACOG) most recently recommended that the NST be performed at least twice weekly. Fetal movement counting is something the mother can actively participate in and gives good indication of fetal well-being.[34]

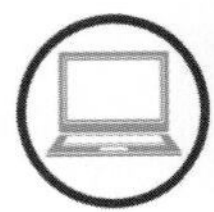

DOCUMENTATION AND CRITICAL THINKING

Focused Assessment: Clinical Case Study 1

Rosa is a 27-year-old Latina woman, gravida 2 para 1, who presents with her husband and daughter for her first prenatal visit.

SUBJECTIVE

Rosa is a full-time homemaker who completed 2 years of college. Last normal menstrual period (LNMP) was April 4 of this year (certain of date), with an expected date of delivery (EDD) of January 11 of next year, making her 10 weeks' gestation today. Her obstetric history includes a normal spontaneous vaginal delivery (NSVD) 3 years ago of a viable 7 lb, 12 oz female infant after an 8-hour labor without anesthesia, with a midline episiotomy. No complications of pregnancy, delivery, or the postpartum. She breastfed her daughter, Ana, for 1 year. Present pregnancy was planned, and Rosa and her husband are pleased. Rosa is having breast tenderness and nausea on occasion, which resolves with crackers. No past medical or surgical conditions are present. She denies allergies. Family history is significant only for diet-controlled adult-onset diabetes in two maternal aunts.

OBJECTIVE

General: Appears well nourished and is carefully groomed. English is second language, and Rosa is fluent.

Skin: Light tan in color, surface smooth with no lesions, small tattoo noted on left forearm.

Mouth: Good dentition and oral hygiene. Oral mucosa pink, no gum hypertrophy. Thyroid gland small and smooth.

Chest: Expansion equal, respirations effortless. Lung sounds clear bilaterally with no adventitious sounds. No CVA tenderness.

Heart: Rate 76 bpm, regular rhythm, S_1 and S_2 are normal, not accentuated or diminished, with soft, blowing systolic murmur Gr ii/vi at 2nd left interspace.

Breasts: Tender, without masses; with supple, everted nipples. Breast self-exam reviewed.

Abdomen: No masses, bowel sounds present. No hepatosplenomegaly. Uterus nonpalpable. No inguinal lymphadenopathy noted.

Extremities: No varicosities, redness, or edema. Homan sign negative. DTRs 2+ and equal bilaterally.

BP 110/68 mm Hg, sitting.

Pelvic: Bartholin's, urethra, and Skene's glands (BUS) negative for discharge. Vagina: pink, with white, creamy, non-odorous discharge. Cervix: pink, closed, multiparous, 2 cm long, firm.

Uterus: 10-week size, consistent with dates, nontender, dextrorotated. FHTs heard with Doppler, rate 140s.

Pelvis: Pubic arch wide; side walls straight, spines blunt, interspinous diameter >10 cm.

Sacrum hollow; coccyx mobile. Sacrospinous ligament 3 fingerbreadths (FBs) wide. Diagonal conjugate >12 cm, bituberous diameter >8 cm. Spacious gynecoid pelvis proven to 7 lb, 12 oz.

ASSESSMENT

Intrauterine pregnancy 10 weeks by good dates, size = dates.

Rosa and husband happy with pregnancy; she feels well.

PLAN

Begin prenatal vitamins.

Prenatal blood screen and urinalysis.

HIV screening offered and accepted.

Reviewed comfort measures for nausea.

Reviewed warning signs—vaginal bleeding and abdominal pain.

Return visit in 4 weeks.

Focused Assessment: Clinical Case Study 2

Kadija is a 30-year-old Ethiopian woman, gravida 9 para 7, who presents with an interpreter and her eldest daughter for her first prenatal visit.

SUBJECTIVE

Kadija is a full-time homemaker and runs a daycare facility within her home. She immigrated to the United States 5 years ago with her husband and children. Her husband is employed. She lives in a one-bedroom apartment with her family. Her last menstrual period was May 28th of this year, with an EDD of March 5th of next year, making her 11 weeks' gestation today. She is a poor historian for her deliveries in Ethiopia other than one child "died in childbirth." She delivered her last child vaginally, here in the United States without complications after 5 hours of labor. She is unsure of the baby's weight. She had a female circumcision as a child. She is having nausea with occasional vomiting, has breast tenderness, and 1 week ago experienced "pink" vaginal spotting. She is unsure of her family history. Both parents are deceased as well as all but one of her seven siblings. This pregnancy is unexpected, but okay. She is concerned about transportation to her appointments since her husband works days and she does not drive.

OBJECTIVE

General: Appears well nourished and is carefully groomed. English is second language, but she understands some. Daughter who is present with her mom is well groomed and speaks English.

Skin: Dark tan in color, surface smooth, Small scarring on left arm and both legs. No lesions or tattoos.

Mouth; Poor dentition. Oral mucosa pink, some gum hypertrophy. Thyroid gland small and smooth.

Chest: Expansion equal, respiration effortless. Lung sounds clear bilaterally with no adventitious sounds. No CVA tenderness.

Heart: Rate 84 bpm, regular rhythm, S_1 and S_2 are normal, not accentuated or diminished, with soft, blowing systolic murmur Gr ii/vi at 2nd left interspace.

Breasts: Tender, no masses, large everted nipples. No drainage present. Breast self-exam reviewed.

Abdomen: No masses, bowel sounds present in four quadrants. No hepatomegaly or splenomegaly. Uterus non-palpable. No inguinal lymphadenopathy noted. No healed incision(s) noted.

Extremities: No lower extremity varicosities, edema, or redness noted. Negative Homan sign. 1+ DTRs. BP 124/76 mm Hg.

Pelvic: Female circumcision present without infibulated scarring. Bartholin's, urethra, and Skene's glands (BUS) negative for discharge. Vagina pink, with white, creamy, non-odorous discharge. Cervix pink, non-friable, closed, and approximately 3 cm long and soft. Vaginal wall muscles lax. No evidence of a cystocele or rectocele.

Uterus: Approximately 11-week size and nontender. Dextrorotated. FHTs not heard with Doppler. Confirmed on ultrasound along with dating.

Pelvis: Pubic arch wide; side walls straight, spines blunt, interspinous diameter >12 cm, bituberous diameter >8 cm. Spacious, proven, gynecoid pelvis to ≈8 pounds.

ASSESSMENT

Intrauterine pregnancy at 11 weeks' gestation by ultrasound today with positive fetal cardiac activity. Size = dates. Aware of potential language and cultural issues. Via interpreter, understands advised prenatal testing, clinic routine, and warning signs and symptoms in pregnancy. Physical examination within normal limits (WNL)

PLAN

Begin prenatal vitamins.
Routine prenatal blood screening, plus check thyroid function tests, vitamin D level, Sickle cell, and thalassemia screen.
HIV and CF screening discussed, offered, and accepted.
Reviewed prenatal screening (Seq 1 and 2, US for NT). Will discuss with her husband and let us know.
Reviewed clinic routing and how to contact clinic personal after hours.
Reviewed comfort measures for nausea and vomiting. Offered medication; declined at this time.
Reviewed warning signs: vaginal bleeding, abdominal pain, pain with urination.
Return to clinic in 2 weeks if desires prenatal screening, or 4 weeks if does not.
Refer to social worker and transportation services.
Obtain records from previous pregnancy and delivery in United States.

ABNORMAL FINDINGS FOR ADVANCED PRACTICE

TABLE 29-2 Preeclampsia

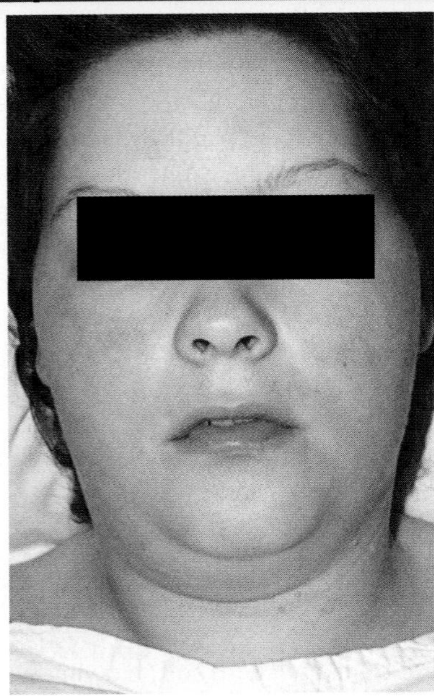

Preeclampsia is a condition specific to pregnancy that is rarely seen before 20 weeks' gestation except in the presence of a molar (gestational trophoblastic) pregnancy. It occurs in 5% to 8% of pregnancies. Its etiology remains unknown, but theories include coagulation abnormalities, vascular endothelial damage, cardiovascular maladaptation, immunologic phenomena, dietary deficiencies or excess, and genetic predisposition. In addition, much literature focus is on trophoblastic invasion by the placenta. Predisposing factors include preeclampsia in a previous pregnancy, multifetal gestation, chronic hypertension, pregestational diabetes, vascular and connective tissue disease, nephropathy, antiphospholipid antibody syndrome, obesity, age 35 years or older, and African American race.[5]

Preeclampsia's classic symptoms are hypertension and proteinuria. Hypertension is a systolic BP of ≥140 mm Hg or higher or a diastolic BP of ≥90 mm Hg that occurs after 20 weeks' gestation in a woman with previously normal blood pressure.[5]

The BP should be compared with the woman's first prenatal BP (before 20 weeks' gestation). Hypertension is necessary for the diagnosis of preeclampsia, but preeclampsia may be seen without the edema or proteinuria.

Onset and worsening symptoms may be sudden. Subjective signs may include headaches and visual changes (spots, blurring, or flashing lights) caused by cerebral edema or may include right upper quadrant/epigastric pain from liver enlargement where it becomes enlarged, necrotic, and hemorrhagic. Liver enzyme levels become elevated. Hematocrit usually increases, and the platelets drop. Serum creatinine and blood urea nitrogen elevate. Hemolysis occurs, in part at least, as a result of vasospasm. A serious variant of preeclampsia, the **HELLP** syndrome, involves **H**emolysis, **E**levated **L**iver enzymes, and **L**ow **P**latelets and represents an ominous clinical picture. Untreated preeclampsia may progress to eclampsia, which is manifested by generalized tonic-clonic seizures. Eclampsia may develop as late as 10 days postpartum.

Before the syndrome becomes clinically manifested, it is affecting the placenta through vasospasm and a series of small infarctions. The placenta's capacity to deliver oxygen and nutrients may be seriously diminished, and fetal growth may be restricted.

TABLE 29-3 Fetal Size Inconsistent with Dates

SIZE SMALL FOR DATES	Fundal height measures smaller than expected for dates.
Inaccuracy of Dates	Conception may have occurred later than originally thought. Reconsider the woman's menstrual history, sexual history, contraceptive use, early pregnancy testing, early sizing of the uterus, US results, timing of pregnancy symptoms including the date of quickening, and the fundal height measurements. If, after this review, the EDD is correct, then further investigation is required.
Preterm Labor	When preterm labor engages the presenting part of the fetus into the pelvis for delivery, the fundus may shorten. Preterm birth occurs before 37 weeks' gestation. Other than delivery, preterm labor is the leading cause of hospital admission during pregnancy.[43] Preterm birth occurs in 18.4% of African Americans, 11.7% of whites, 13.7% of American Indians, 10.6% of Asians, and 12.1% of Hispanics.[35] Risk indicators for preterm birth include abdominal surgery during the current pregnancy, age of <18 years or >35 years, chronic urinary tract infections, conization of the cervix, hydramnios, hypertensive disorders, low socioeconomic status, low prepregnancy weight, African-American race, multiple gestation, woman was herself a preterm infant, poor nutrition, previous preterm delivery, cigarette smoking, strenuous work, substance/drug abuse (especially cocaine and alcohol), two or more second-trimester terminations, uterine anomalies, and uterine infections.[39]
Intrauterine Growth Restriction (IUGR) or Fetal Growth Restriction	IUGR, a syndrome in which the neonate fails to meet its growth potential, is associated with an increase in fetal and neonatal mortality and morbidity. Its origin may be fetoplacental, as with chromosomal abnormalities, genetic syndromes, congenital malformations, infectious diseases, and placental pathology. Or its origin may be maternal, as with decreased uteroplacental blood flow as seen with hypertensive disorders, poor maternal weight gain, poor maternal nutrition, and a previous pregnancy with an IUGR infant. Other factors include infectious diseases (rubella, cytomegalovirus); multiple gestations; and environmental toxins such as smoking, maternal drug ingestion, and alcohol.
Fetal Position	Fetal position varies until about 34 weeks, when the vertex should settle into the pelvis and remain there. The fetus occupying a transverse lie, or shoulder presentation, results in the maternal abdomen widening from side to side and the fundal height diminishing. Fetal malposition may occur with lax maternal abdominal musculature (simply not holding the baby in close), an abnormality in the fetus (e.g., the enlarged head of the hydrocephalic infant), placenta previa (the placenta being implanted over the cervix, blocking fetal descent), or a restricted maternal pelvis.
SIZE LARGE FOR DATES	Fundal height measures larger than expected for dates.
Inaccuracy of Dates	Review the same findings as listed above.
Hydatidiform Mole	Also termed *gestational trophoblastic neoplasia,* it is a result of abnormal proliferation of trophoblastic tissue associated with pregnancy. In 50% of cases, uterine size is excessive; in these cases, the gestational age and uterine size do not coincide.
Multiple Fetuses	The frequency of multiple fetuses increases with advanced maternal age and is enhanced by the increasing use of fertility drugs. The uterus enlarges where the fundal height may be beyond the calculated/expected gestational age. US examination confirms the diagnosis.
Polyhydramnios	An amniotic fluid volume is a maximum volume pocket above 8 cm or an amniotic fluid index (AFI) above the 95th percentile or ≥20 cm. The cause is usually idiopathic but may be due to fetal anomalies, insulin-dependent diabetes, GDM, and multiple fetuses.[13]

Continued

TABLE 29-3 **Fetal Size Inconsistent with Dates—cont'd**

Oligohydramnios	Oligohydramnios is a reduction in amniotic fluid volume or an AFI less than 5 cm at term. An acceptable AFI is between 10 and 20.[19]
Leiomyoma (Myoma or "Fibroids")	These are preexisting benign tumors of the uterine wall, which then are stimulated to enlarge by the estrogen levels of pregnancy. Myomata may be located anywhere in the uterine wall (see Table 26-6). When they grow in the outer uterine wall, the myometrium, they may affect the clinician's judgment of where the fundus of the uterus should be measured. A myoma may grow just underneath the endometrial surface into the uterine cavity, displacing the fetus or preventing its descent into the pelvis.
Fetal Macrosomia 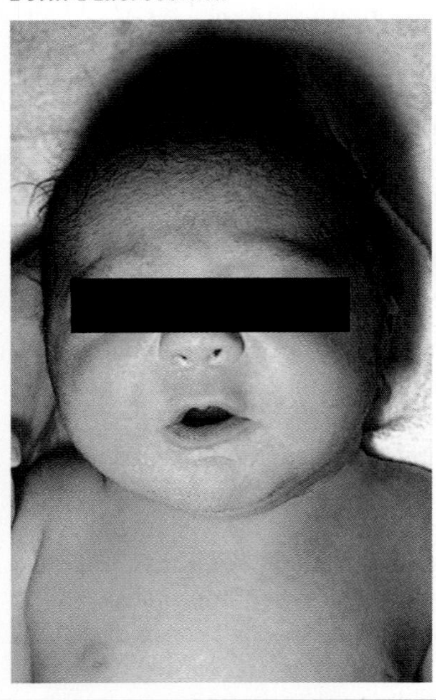	This is a condition in which the infant's weight is beyond 4000 g or 4500 g regardless of the gestational age. 1998 data from the National Center for Health Statistics showed that 10% of all live-born infants in the United States weighed more than 4000 g.[2] Maternal risk factors for macrosomia include a prior history of a macrosomic infant, maternal obesity, weight gain during the pregnancy, multiparity, male fetus, gestational age >40 weeks, ethnicity, maternal birth weight, maternal height, maternal age <17 years, and a positive 50-g glucose screen with a negative 3-hour glucose tolerance test. Birth risks to the mother include labor abnormalities, an increased incidence for cesarean delivery, bladder trauma, and vaginal tissue trauma. Fetal risks include birth trauma such as fractured clavicle and brachial plexus nerve damage from shoulder dystocia, depressed Apgar scores, extended hospitalizations, and possible fetal mortality.

TABLE 29-4 Disorders of Pregnancy

Disorder/Condition	Description
Anemia	The most common cause of anemia in pregnancy is iron deficiency. Women should be tested at their prenatal visit and again between 24 and 28 weeks' gestation.[27] This is usually done at the same time as the gestational diabetes screening. The fetus uses maternal red blood cells for growth and development, which increases around week 20. Women at risk for iron deficiency anemia are those with persistent nausea and vomiting and are unable to eat a healthy diet rich in iron, those with multiple gestation, those having two pregnancies relatively close together, and those with poor nutrition before pregnancy. Iron deficiency anemia during pregnancy increases risk for low birth weight, preterm delivery, and perinatal mortality. Severe anemia with maternal hemoglobin (Hgb) less than 6 g/dL is associated with abnormal fetal oxygenation, which shows as a nonreassuring fetal heart rate pattern during fetal monitoring.[6] Oral iron supplementation is usually sufficient, but some women cannot tolerate this and require intravenous iron administration.
Vaginal Bleeding	Some women will have bright red, pink, or dark brown spotting at some time during the first trimester. This is not always a sign of pending pregnancy loss but may be from a blighted ovum, friable cervix, ectopic pregnancy, perigestational hemorrhage, or cervical lesions. In the second and third trimesters, vaginal bleeding may be indicative of abruptio placentae, placenta previa, uterine rupture, cervical dilation, or a friable cervix. Risk factors for increased risk for vaginal bleeding include pregnancy-induced hypertension, chronic hypertension, cocaine use, abdominal trauma, uterine anomalies, premature rupture of membranes, prior placental abruption, and cervical infection such as chlamydia, gonorrhea, bacterial vaginosis, and candidiasis.
Incompetent Cervix	Cervical incompetence is marked by gradual and painless premature dilation and effacement of the cervix that can lead to fetal loss if not detected early enough to have a cervical cerclage placed. Its cause may be congenital, as seen in some women after DES exposure, or it may be acquired after cervical trauma or a cone biopsy.
Hyperemesis	Hyperemesis is excessive vomiting in pregnancy that may last well into the second trimester and beyond. It can interfere with electrolytes, acid-base balance, and nutritional status. Dehydration and starvation may ensue and lead to fetal IUGR. Nausea and vomiting are not uncommon in pregnancy, usually resolve between weeks 16 and 20, and may be controlled with dietary and lifestyle changes or oral antiemetics. Hyperemesis is the extreme of vomiting and may require home infusion therapy or hospitalization. Risk factors include a previous history of hyperemesis, molar pregnancy, multiple gestation, emotional stress, history of gastrointestinal reflux, uncontrolled thyroid disease, primigravida, and obesity.
Preterm Labor	Preterm labor is labor occurring after 20 weeks' and before completion of 37 weeks' gestation. Preterm labor is a major factor for fetal morbidity and mortality. Some risk factors include chronic urinary tract infections, polyhydramnios, multiple gestation, previous PTL/PTD, smoking, substance abuse, poor prenatal care, poor weight gain after 20 weeks' gestation, history of cervical conization, low socioeconomic status, nonwhite race, uterine infections, and cases in which the patient herself was a preterm infant.
Decreased Fetal Movement	Fetal movement is one indicator of fetal well-being and should begin from 28 weeks' gestation. Various methods are used; the important thing is to be consistent and count every day. A decrease in fetal movement should be reported and followed by a non-stress test (fetal monitoring). Cessation of fetal movement may be indicative of fetal distress or impending fetal death.
Psychological Illness	Mental illness during pregnancy has significant effects on fetal well-being. Research reports that as many as 18% of pregnant women experience depression during pregnancy. Depression is a risk factor for low fetal birth weight and premature delivery. Anxiety disorders, eating disorders, and psychotic illness present during pregnancy are additional predictors of adverse perinatal outcomes. It is important to understand these disorders and their effect on pregnancy in order to weigh the potential risks from psychiatric medications used to treat these disorders.[20]

TABLE 29-5 Malpresentations

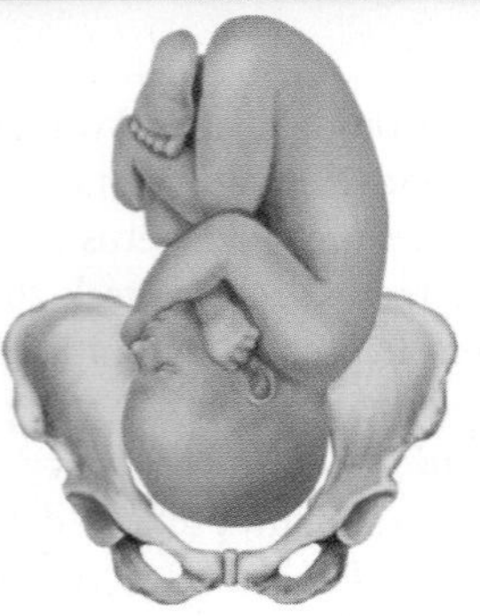

Vertex (for comparison)

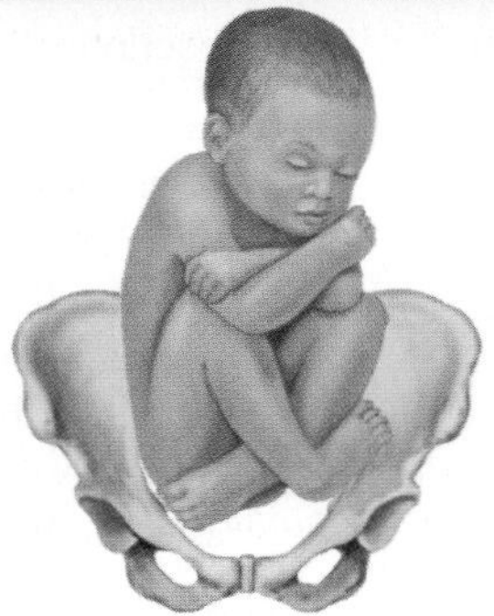

Complete breech

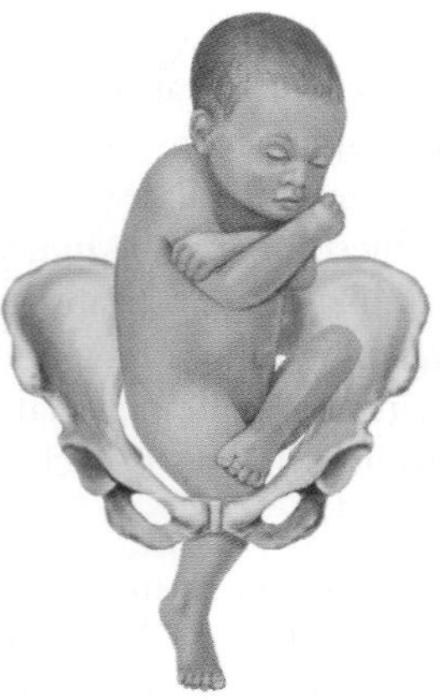

Footling breech

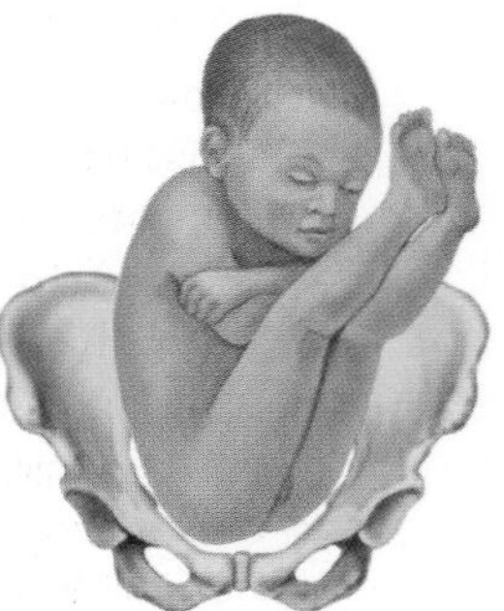

Frank breech

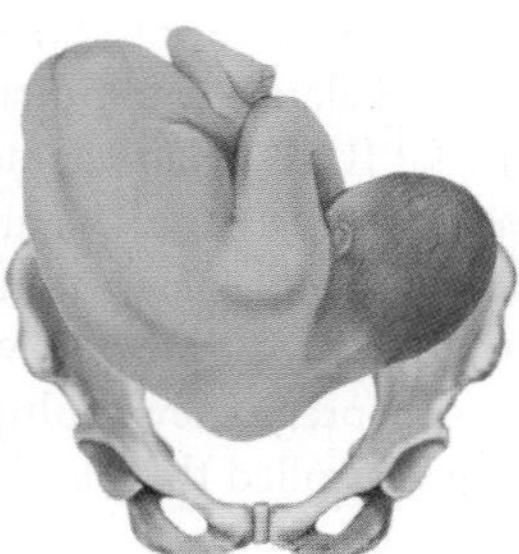

Transverse lie and shoulder presentation

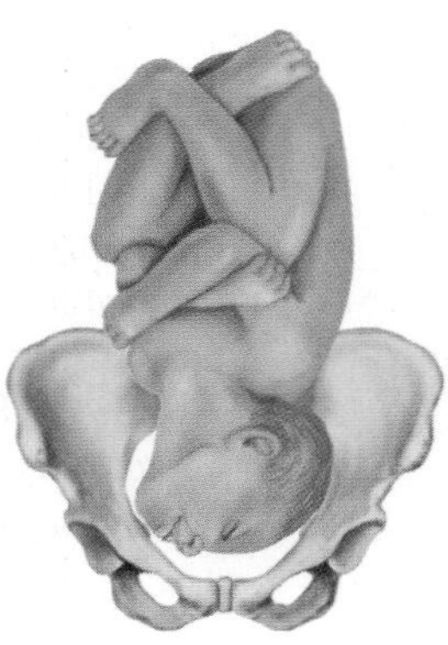

Face presentation

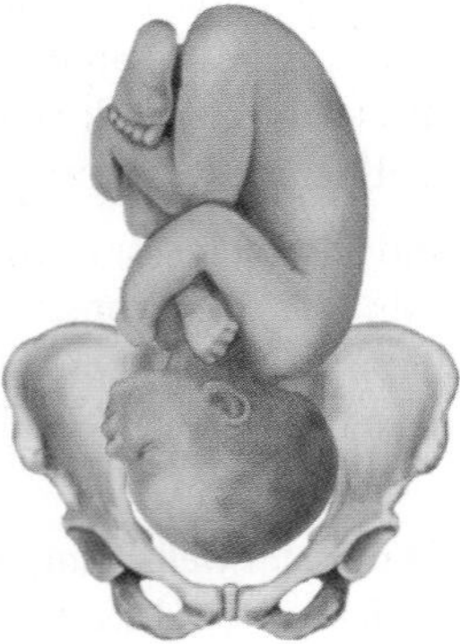

Brow presentation

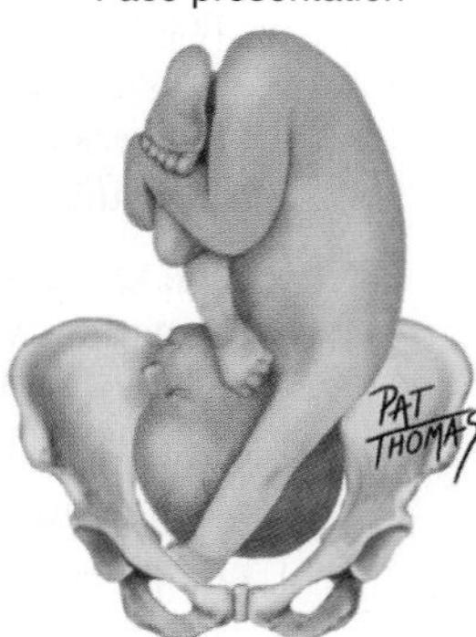

Compound presentation

Malpresentations may be detected by the hands of an experienced examiner, confirmed by the FHT location, and further confirmed by US. Before 34 weeks' gestation, any position is normal. The vertex presentation is desirable thereafter because spontaneous turning becomes less likely as the fetus grows in proportion to the amount of space and fluid in the uterus and pelvis.

BIBLIOGRAPHY

1. American College of Obstetricians and Gynecologists (ACOG). (1999). *Antepartum fetal surveillance* (Technical Bulletin No. 9). Washington, DC: Author.
2. American College of Obstetricians and Gynecologists (ACOG). (2000). *Fetal macrosomia* (Technical Bulletin No. 22). Washington, DC: Author.
3. American College of Obstetricians and Gynecologists (ACOG). (2001). *Prenatal diagnosis of fetal chromosomal abnormalities* (Practice Bulletin No. 27). Washington, DC: Author.
4. American College of Obstetricians and Gynecologists (ACOG). (2002). *Thyroid disease in pregnancy* (Technical Bulletin No. 37). Washington, DC: Author.
5. American College of Obstetricians and Gynecologists (ACOG), (2004). *Special problems of multiple gestation* (Educational Bulletin No. 56). Washington, DC: Author.
6. American College of Obstetricians and Gynecologists (ACOG). (2008). *Anemia in pregnancy* (Practice Bulletin No. 95). Washington, DC: Author.
7. American Society of Clinical Oncology. (2009). *Pregnancy and cancer*. Author. Retrieved July 10, 2009, from www.cancer.net.

7a. Anderson, C. L., & Brown, C. E. L. (2009). Fetal chromosomal abnormalities: antenatal screening and diagnosis. *American Family Physician, 79*(2), 117-123.

7b. Aruda, M. M., Waddicor, K., Frese, L., et al. (2010). Early pregnancy in adolescents: diagnosis, assessment, options counseling, and referral. *Journal of Pediatric Health Care, 24*(1), 4-13.

8. Barclay, L. (March 20, 2009). CDC reports slight increase in U.S. teen birthrates in 2007 for second consecutive year. *Medscape Medical News*. Retrieved July 4, 2009, from www.medscape.com/viewarticle/589912_print.
9. Barclay, L. (June 1, 2009). Vitamin D deficiency linked to bacterial vaginosis. *Medscape Medical News*. Retrieved June 16, 2009, from www.medscape.com/viewarticle//703582_print.
10. Beamer, L. C. (2001). Fetal nuchal translucency: a prenatal screening tool. *Journal of Obstetric, Gynecologic, and Neonatal Nursing, 30*, 376-385.

10a. Benninger, C., & McCallister, J. (2010). Asthma in pregnancy: reading between the lines. *Nurse Practitioner, 35*(4), 10-20.

11. Blackburn, S. T. (2007). *Maternal, fetal & neonatal physiology: a clinical perspective* (3rd ed.). St. Louis: Saunders.
12. Chin, H. G. (2001). *On call obstetrics and gynecology* (2nd ed.). Philadelphia: Saunders.
13. Creasy, R. K., Resnick, R., Iams, J. D., et al. (2009). *Creasy and Resnik's maternal-fetal medicine: principles and practice* (6th ed.). Philadelphia: Saunders.
14. Cunningham, F. G., Leveno, K., Bloom, S., et al. (2010). *Williams' obstetrics* (23rd ed.). Stamford, CT: Appleton & Lange.
15. Dasanayake, A. P., Gennaro, S., Henddricks-Munoz, K. D., et al. (2008). Maternal periodontal disease, pregnancy, and neonatal outcomes. *MCN. American Journal of Maternal Child Nursing, 33*(1), 45-49.
16. Ebrahim, S. H., Anderson, J. E., Correa-de-Araujo, R., et al. (2009). Overcoming social and health inequalities among U.S. women of reproductive age: challenges to the nation's health in the 21st century. *Health Policy, 90*(2), 196-205.
17. Epilepsy Foundation. *Pregnancy and parenting: pregnancy issues*. Retrieved July 11, 2009, from www.epilepsyfoundation.org/living/women/pregnancy/welpregnancy.cfm.

17a. Farley, D., & Dudley, D. J. (2009). Fetal assessment during pregnancy. *Pediatric Clinics of North America, 56*(3), 489-504.

18. Fiebach, N. H., Kern, D. E., Thomas, P. A., et al. (2007). *Principles of ambulatory medicine* (7th ed.). Philadelphia: Lippincott Williams & Wilkins.
19. Gabbe, S. G., Niebyl, J. R., Simpson, J. L., et al. (2007). *Obstetrics: normal and problem pregnancies* (5th ed.). New York: Churchill Livingstone.
20. Gold, K. J., & Marcus, S. M. (June 26, 2008). Effect of maternal mental illness on pregnancy outcomes. *Expert Review of Obstetrics & Gynecology*. Retrieved July 11, 2009, from www.medscape.com/viewarticle/573947_print.
21. Hamilton, B. E., Martin, J. A., & Ventura, S. J. (2009). Births: preliminary data for 2007. *National Vital Statistics Reports, 57*(12), 1-23.
22. Hollis, B. W., & Wagner, C. L. (2004). Assessment of dietary vitamin D requirements during pregnancy and lactation. *American Journal of Clinical Nutrition, 79*, 717-726.

22a. Howland, R. H. (2009). Categorizing the safety of medications during pregnancy and lactation. *Journal of Psychosocial Nursing, 47*(4), 17-20.

23. Jacobson, B., Ladfors, L., & Milsom, I. (2004). Advanced maternal age and adverse perinatal outcome. *Obstetrics and Gynecology, 104*(4), 727-733.
24. Kaiser Daily Health Policy Report. (August 29, 2007). Maternal mortality rate in U.S. highest in decades, experts say. *Medical News Today*. Retrieved July 5, 2009, from www.medicalnewstoday.com.

24a. Keegan, J., Parva, M., Finnegan, M., et al. (2010). Addiction in pregnancy. *Journal of Addictive Diseases, 29*(2), 175-191.

25. Lichtman, R., & Papera, S. (1990). *Gynecology: well-woman care*. East Norwalk, CT: Appleton & Lange.
26. March of Dimes. (2006). *Carrier screening for cystic fibrosis*. White Plains, NY: March of Dimes Birth Defects Foundation.

26a. March of Dimes. (2009). *Birth defects, Down syndrome*. White Plains, NY: March of Dimes Birth Defects Foundation.

27. March of Dimes Foundation. (2009). *Anemia during pregnancy*. Author. Retrieved July 5, 2009, from www.marchofdimes.com/printableArticles/188_1049.asp.
28. National Cancer Institute. (2009). *Breast cancer treatment and pregnancy*. U.S. National Institutes of Health. Retrieved June 16, 2009, from www.cancer.gov/cancertopics/pdg/treatment/breast-cancer-and-pregnancy/Patient.
29. Neal, D. M., Cootauco, A. C., & Burrow, G. (2007). Thyroid disease in pregnancy. *Clinics in Perinatology, 34*(4), 543-557.
30. Nour, N. M. (2004). Female genital cutting: clinical and cultural guidelines. *Obstetrical & Gynecological Survey, 59*(4), 272-279.
31. Pawley, N., & Bishop, N. J. (2004). Prenatal and infant predictors of bone health: the influence of vitamin D. *American Journal of Clinical Nutrition, 80*(Suppl.), 1748S-1751S.
32. Ryan, S., Franzetta, K., & Manlove, J. (2005). Hispanic teen pregnancy and birth rates: looking behind the numbers. *Child Trends*, Publication No. 2005-2001.
33. Seely, E. W., & Maxwell, C. (2007). Chronic hypertension in pregnancy. *Circulation, 115*, e188-e190.
34. Signore, C., Freeman, R. K., & Spong, C. Y. (2009). Antenatal testing—a reevaluation: executive summary of a Eunice Kennedy Shriver National Institute of Child Health and Human Development Workshop. *Obstetrics and Gynecology, 113*(3), 687-701.
35. Simpson, R. K., & Creehan, P. A. (2008). *AWHONN's perinatal nursing* (3rd ed.). Philadelphia: Lippincott Williams & Wilkins.
36. Specker, B. (2004). Vitamin D requirements during pregnancy. *American Journal of Clinical Nutrition, 80*(Suppl.), 1740S-1747S.
37. Star, W. L., Shannon, M. T., Lommelet, L. L., et al. (1999). *Ambulatory obstetrics* (3rd ed.). San Francisco: UCSF Nursing Press.
38. Surbone, A., Peccatori, F., & Pavlidis, N. (2008). *Cancer in pregnancy* (vol. 178). New York: Springer Berlin Heidelberg Publishers.
39. Swenson, D. (2001). *Telephone triage for the obstetric patient: a nursing guide*. Philadelphia: Saunders.

39a. United Nations Population Fund. (2007). *State of world population*. Retrieved July 5, 2009, from www.unfpa.org/public/others.
40. Varney, H. (2004). *Varney's midwifery* (4th ed.). Sudbury, MA: Jones & Bartlett.
41. Vega, C. (May 29, 2009). Institute of Medicine sets new guidelines for weight gain during pregnancy. *Medscape Medical News*. Retrieved June 14, 2009, from www.cme.medscape.com/viewarticle/703521.
42. World Health Organization. (2007). *Executive summary: maternal mortality in 2005*. Geneva: Author.
43. Yost, N. P., Bloom, S. L., McIntire, D. D., et al. (2005). Hospitalization for women with arrested preterm labor: a randomized trial. *Obstetrics and Gynecology, 106*(1), 14-18.

Summary Checklist: The Pregnant Woman

For a PDA-downloadable version, go to http://evolve.elsevier.com/Jarvis/.

1. Collect historical information.
2. Determine EDD and current number of weeks of gestation.
3. Instruct the woman to undress and empty her bladder, saving her urine to dip it for protein and glucose.
4. Measure weight.
5. Perform a physical examination, starting with general survey.
6. Inspect skin for pigment changes, scars.
7. Check oral mucous membranes.
8. Palpate thyroid gland.
9. Inspect breast changes, and palpate for masses.
10. Auscultate breath sounds, heart sounds, heart rate, and any murmurs.
11. Check lower extremities for edema, varicosities, and reflexes.
12. The abdomen: Measure fundal height, perform Leopold's maneuvers, auscultate FHTs.
13. The pelvic examination: Note signs of pregnancy, the condition of the cervix, and the size and position of the uterus.
14. Perform pelvimetry.
15. Measure the BP.
16. Obtain appropriate laboratory work.

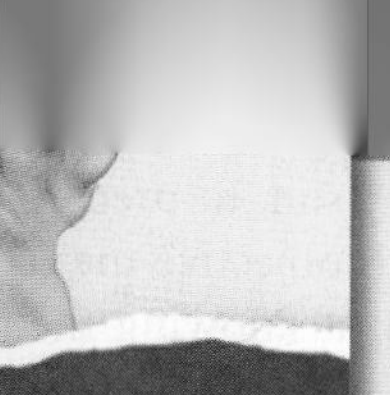

30

Functional Assessment of the Older Adult

evolve WEBSITE

http://evolve.elsevier.com/Jarvis/

- Audio Key Points
- Head-to-Toe Examination of the Older Adult
- Health Promotion Guide
  Aging Macular Degeneration
- NCLEX Review Questions
- Quick Assessment for Common Conditions
  Alzheimer Disease

The United States has a large and expanding population of older adults. The implications of the graying of America are staggering for all health care systems (Fig. 30-1). In 2006, persons 65 years of age and older represented 12.6% (over one in every eight) of the U.S. population.[3] They also accounted for 38% of non-federal short-stay hospitalizations, with those ages 75 years and older totaling 24% of all inpatients.[26] In 2005, older adults averaged more office visits than younger adults (7.7 visits for those ages 75 years and older vs. 3.9 visits for those 45 to 65 years of age). Older Americans also had higher out-of-pocket health care expenditures than younger Americans (12.7% of total expenditures on health care for older Americans vs. 5.7% for all other consumers).[3]

Older adults also make up 80% of home care visits and 90% of those in nursing homes.[34] Many older Americans live with disabilities or have activity limitations, often a result of having multiple chronic conditions that may include sensory, physical, or mental impairments. Approximately 37% of older adults reported a severe disability in 2005 requiring some type of assistance.[3]

In 2007, 1.57 million older Americans lived in nursing homes, with 15% of these residents being ages 85 years and older. In addition, between 2% and 5% of older adults lived in senior housing and had access to at least one assistive service.

Personal caregiving can be formal (hired, paid caregivers) or informal (family, friends). In 1999, 3.7 million older Medicare enrollees received either formal or informal care and two thirds of these persons were receiving informal care only.[27a] In addition, *aging* or *older adult* cannot be defined only by the chronologic age of an individual as it is for Social Security (ages 65 years and older). Older adults are truly heterogeneous, and differences exist among biological, social, physical, and emotional rates of aging.[69] Older age-groups are often categorized as young-old (65-74 years), middle-old (75-84 years), and old-old (85 years and older). Although the number of chronic diseases does increase with aging, it is important to remember that a substantial number of older adults both enjoy aging and report good to excellent health.[60]

The comprehensive assessment of an older adult requires knowledge of not only normal aging changes but also the consequences of chronic diseases, genetic makeup, and lifestyle. A comprehensive geriatric assessment is multidimen-

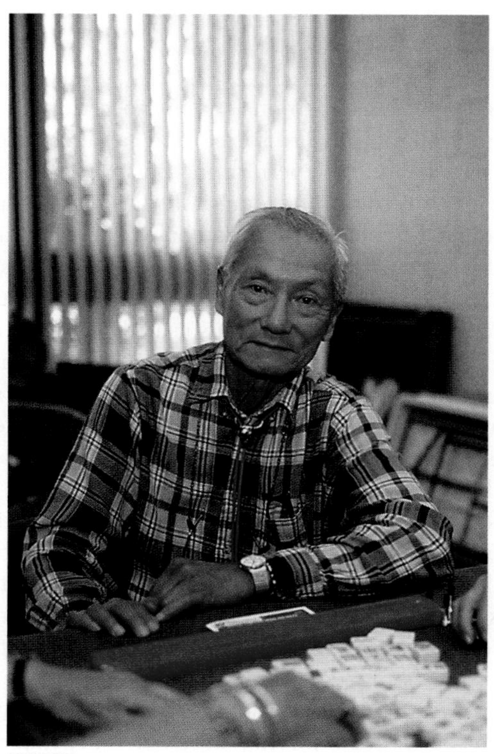

30-1

sional and incorporates the physical examination as well as assessments of mental status, functional status, social and economic status, pain, and examination of the physical environment for safety concerns. Multiple disciplines may participate in this assessment, including physicians; nurses; physical, occupational, and speech therapists; social workers; case managers; nutritionists; and pharmacists. Early recognition of disabilities and treatable conditions is instrumental in preserving function and quality of life for older adults.

The normal changes of aging presented in previous chapters do not necessarily represent pathology, but with the imposition of acute and chronic illnesses, including hospitalization, an older adult may be predisposed to disability. Older adults may arrive in clinics or hospitals not only with an acute illness such as pneumonia but also with ongoing chronic "geriatric syndromes," such as urinary incontinence, fragile skin, confusion, problems with eating or feeding, falls, and sleep disorders.[46] If these syndromes are not identified early, an older adult may develop functional decline.

Normal aging changes and the development of disease may precipitate transitions from home to a variety of settings, where nursing-focused assessments are performed. Care may be provided in hospitals; in skilled nursing, long-term care, assisted living, and acute rehabilitation facilities; and in hospice, senior centers, homes, and clinics. The setting where care is provided usually determines the types of assessment and instruments used. However, the goal of the functional assessment remains the same (i.e., to identify an older adult's strengths and any limitations) so that appropriate interventions will promote independence and prevent functional decline.

FUNCTIONAL ABILITY

Functional ability refers to one's ability to perform activities necessary to live in modern society and can include driving, using the telephone, or performing personal tasks such as bathing and toileting. Functional ability also incorporates an older adult's physiologic and psychological status and the physical and social environment.[86] Functional status, as defined by Richmond et al.,[91] is "the individuals' actual performance of activities and tasks associated with their current life roles" and depends on motivation, sensory capacity such as vision and hearing, degree of assistance needed to accomplish the tasks, and cognition.[54] For example, the effect that arthritis might have on a person's ability to exercise may affect physical function. A condition such as Alzheimer disease may affect problem solving, safety concerns, and motivation, which in turn affect function. Lack of social support or a safe physical setting is an environmental issue that affects functional status and possibly the ability to live independently. The interaction of these components provides a *snapshot* of an older adult's functional status at a given point in time.[86] Functional status is not static; older adults may move continuously through varying stages of independence and disability.

The assessment of function is an important geriatric tenet to provide a baseline for continuing comparison, to predict prognosis, and to assist the practitioner with objective measures to determine efficacy of treatments. Just knowing the person's medical diagnosis is not sufficient to predict functional abilities. Older adults may not experience the usual symptoms of an acute illness. Often a decline in functional status may herald the presence of another process such as an infection.

A functional assessment of an older adult is the basis for care planning, goal setting, and discharge planning. A functional assessment also is needed for eligibility to obtain many services such as durable medical equipment, home modifications, and inpatient or outpatient rehabilitation services. For the older adult and family, a functional assessment can identify areas for current and future planning, such as the most appropriate living situation.

A functional assessment includes three overarching domains: **activities of daily living (ADLs), instrumental activities of daily living (IADLs),** and **mobility.**[86] A functional evaluation should be systematic, with attention paid to the particular needs of the person, such as the presence of pain, fatigue, shortness of breath, or memory problems. There are two approaches to use for performing a functional assessment: (1) *asking individuals* about their abilities to perform the tasks (using self-reports) or (2) actually *observing* their ability to perform the tasks. For persons with memory problems, the use of surrogate reporters (proxy reports) such as family members or caregivers may be necessary, keeping in mind that they may either overestimate or underestimate the actual abilities.

Activities of Daily Living

ADLs are those tasks necessary for self-care. Typically, ADLs measure domains of eating/feeding, bathing, grooming (the individual tasks of washing face, combing hair, shaving, cleaning teeth), dressing (lower body and upper body), toileting (bowel and bladder), walking (including propelling a wheelchair), using stairs (ascending and descending), and transferring (e.g., bed to chair). The ADL instruments are designed as either self-report, observation of tasks, or proxy/surrogate report.

The Katz Index of Independence in ADL

The Katz Index of ADL[51] is based on the concept of physical disability and was intended to measure physical function in older adults and the chronically ill. It is one of the few functional assessment instruments to provide a theoretical framework for its domains of measurement,[70] and it is the foundation for most of the newer functional assessment instruments.[86] It is widely used in both clinical practice and research to measure performance, evaluate treatment outcomes, and predict the need for continuing supervised care.

The Index of ADL was developed as a hierarchical structure. Katz believed that physical functions were lost in the most complex activities first, then were lost in descending

Katz Activities of Daily Living

Activities

Points (1 or 0)

Independence
(1 Point)
NO supervision, direction, or personal assistance

Dependence
(0 Points)
WITH supervision, direction, personal assistance, or total care

Bathing
Points _____
(1 Point) Bathes self completely or needs help in bathing only a single part of the body such as the back, genital area, or disabled extremity
(0 Point) Needs help with bathing more than one part of the body or with getting in or out of the tub or shower; requires total bathing

Dressing
Points _____
(1 Point) Gets clothes from closet and drawers and puts on clothes and outer garments complete with fasteners; may have help tying shoes
(0 Point) Needs help with dressing self or needs to be completely dressed

Toileting
Points _____
(1 Point) Gets to toilet, gets on and off, arranges clothes, cleans genital area without help
(0 Point) Needs help transferring to the toilet or cleaning self, or uses bedpan or commode

Transferring
Points _____
(1 Point) Moves into and out of bed or chair unassisted; mechanical transferring aides are acceptable
(0 Point) Needs help in moving from bed to chair or requires a complete transfer

Continence
Points _____
(1 Point) Exercises complete self-control over urination and defecation
(0 Point) Is partially or totally incontinent of bowel or bladder

Feeding
Points _____
(1 Point) Gets food from plate into mouth without help; preparation of food may be done by another person
(0 Point) Needs partial or total help with feeding or requires parenteral feeding

Total Points = _____
6 = High (patient independent)
0 = Low (patient very dependent)

Adapted from Gerontological Society of America. Katz S., et al. (1970). Progress in the development of the index of ADL. *Gerontologist* 10:20-30.

30-2

order, and were regained again in order of ascending complexity.[70] Activities assessed are bathing, dressing, toileting, transferring from bed to chair, continence, and feeding. This instrument has been modified over the years since its development. A simplified method for scoring the instrument is to use a dichotomous rating of independence or dependence in the six activities (Fig. 30-2). One point is given for each independent item. Only those activities that can be performed without help are rated as independent.

The Katz ADL is a useful instrument in many settings. The tool takes approximately 5 minutes to administer, but its use has limitations. In an outpatient setting or clinic visit, the provider cannot observe the older adult perform the activity and must rely on a self-report or surrogate report. In the hospital, nursing staff may be assisting with transferring or grooming activities and may underestimate ability for self-care. In addition, small changes in the ability to perform these activities may not be identified.

Remember that the instrument is measuring function at the current point in time and is valuable for planning specific types of assistance the older person may need. For example, a person may be unable to bathe independently on hospital discharge but can feed himself or herself and transfer to a commode safely and independently. In this case, plan for a home health aide to go twice a week to the home to assist the older adult with bathing.

Additional Activity-of-Daily-Living Instruments

Additional tools used to assess ADL ability are the Barthel Index,[64] the Functional Independence Measure (FIM),[39] and the Rapid Disability Rating Scale-2 (RDS-2).[62,63] The Barthel Index includes definitions of each task to facilitate ease of scoring and has a more comprehensive assessment of mobility than the Katz instrument. The Barthel Index is often used to follow progress in rehabilitation settings.[86]

The FIM was developed by a consensus panel of physical medicine and rehabilitation staff, has been widely tested on older adults, and has a telephone, an in-person, and a proxy version of the instrument. It is more sensitive to change than the other ADL instruments but takes formal training and is more time consuming.[86]

The RDS-2 is completed by a family member or professional caregiver familiar with the abilities of the older adult. It is designed to measure what the person can *actually do* versus what he or she could do. You should conduct a training session to orient the observer to this instrument.

Instrumental Activities of Daily Living

Many IADL instruments have been developed since the 1960s, with the goal of measuring functional abilities necessary for independent community living. Typically, IADL tasks include shopping, meal preparation, housekeeping, laundry, managing finances, taking medications, and using transportation. Tasks such as yard work or home maintenance and leisure activities such as reading and other hobbies are included in some but not all IADL instruments. These instruments may have cultural and gender biases, especially in older cohorts.[86] IADL instruments measure tasks (doing laundry, cooking, housework) historically done by women, and most do not address activities done primarily by men, such as home repairs and working in the yard.

Lawton Instrumental Activities of Daily Living

IADL measures were first developed by Lawton and Brody in 1969 to address higher-order components of the Katz ADL scale and to measure the more complex ADLs required for a person to adapt to the environment.[86] The instrument was originally developed to determine the most suitable living situation for an older adult. The theory was that determining competence and maintenance of life skills such as shopping, cooking, and managing finances is a meaningful way to assess function because these abilities are a prerequisite for independent living. As with the Katz Index, the IADL instrument assumes a hierarchical nature of skill acquisition and loss. The Lawton IADL scale contains eight items (Fig. 30-3): use of telephone, shopping, meal preparation, housekeeping, laundry, transportation, self-medication, and management of finances. Women are scored in all eight domains, whereas men are scored in five, omitting laundry, housekeeping, and preparing food.

The Lawton IADL instrument is designed as a self-report measure of performance rather than ability. Direct testing is often not feasible, such as demonstrating the ability to prepare food while a hospital inpatient. Attention to the final score is less important than identifying a person's strengths and areas where assistance is needed. The instrument is useful in acute hospital settings for discharge planning and ongoing in outpatient settings. It would not be useful for those residing in institutional settings because many of these tasks are already being managed for the resident.

Additional IADL Instruments

Other IADL instruments available are the Older Americans Resources and Services Multidimensional Functional Assessment Questionnaire-IADL (OARS-IADL)[31] and the Direct Assessment of Functional Abilities (DAFA).[50] The OARS-IADL assesses five areas of personal function: social, economic, mental health, physical health, and self-care capacity; it is administered either as a self-report or trained observer instrument. The questions are the same for men and women. The DAFA is a 10-item observational instrument for use with adults with dementia. It requires the person to demonstrate tasks of money management, shopping, hobbies, meal preparation, awareness, reading, and transportation.[86] The obvious strength of this instrument is the direct observation versus self-reporting or proxy reporting; however, it can take up to an hour and a half to complete, so it would not be feasible to use in an acute hospital setting.

Advanced Activities of Daily Living

Advanced activities of daily living (AADLs) are activities that an older adult performs as a family member, a member of society, and community, including occupational and recreational activities.[38] Various AADL instruments commonly include self-care, mobility, work (either paid or volunteer), recreational activities/hobbies, and socialization. Occupational therapists often perform assessment of AADLs. The older adult sets priorities for these activities so that interventions can be individualized.

Measuring Physical Performance

A disadvantage of many of the ADL and IADL instruments is the self-report or proxy report of functional activities. Incorporating an objective standardized measure of performance prevents overestimation or underestimation of abilities. Many of the physical performance measures also incorporate balance, gait, motor coordination, and endurance. Many of the tests are timed. Although there are clear advantages to directly observing the older adult perform the activities, there are some disadvantages. The instruments can be very time consuming, require training and special equipment, and have the possibility that the individual might fall or sustain an injury during the testing.

The Physical Performance Test (PPT)[90] is appropriate for use with community-dwelling older adults. Administered by a trained observer, the test requires approximately 15 minutes to complete and assesses upper body fine motor and coarse motor activities, balance, mobility, coordination, and endurance. Activities such as eating, dressing, transferring, and stair climbing are simulated and timed.

The Performance Activities of Daily Living (PADL)[56] uses a trained observer and specific props. Examples of activities tested are drinking from a cup, combing hair, shaving, lifting food with a spoon and into mouth, putting on and removing slippers, making a phone call, and turning a key in

The Lawton Instrumental Activities of Daily Living Scale

Item	Score
A. Ability to Use Telephone	
1. Operates telephone on own initiative; looks up and dials numbers	1
2. Dials a few well-known numbers	1
3. Answers telephone, but does not dial	1
4. Does not use telephone at all	0
B. Shopping	
1. Takes care of all shopping needs independently	1
2. Shops independently for small purchases	0
3. Needs to be accompanied on any shopping trip	0
4. Completely unable to shop	0
C. Food Preparation	
1. Plans, prepares, and serves adequate meals independently	1
2. Prepares adequate meals if supplied with ingredients	0
3. Heats and serves prepared meals or prepares meals, but does not maintain adequate diet	0
4. Needs to have meals prepared and served	0
D. Housekeeping	
1. Maintains house alone with occasional assistance (heavy work)	1
2. Performs light daily tasks such as dishwashing, bed making	1
3. Performs light daily tasks, but cannot maintain acceptable level of cleanliness	1
4. Needs help with all home maintenance tasks	1
5. Does not participate in any housekeeping tasks	0
E. Laundry	
1. Does personal laundry completely	1
2. Launders small items, rinses socks, stockings, etc	1
3. All laundry must be done by others	0
F. Mode of Transportation	
1. Travels independently on public transportation or drives own car	1
2. Arranges own travel via taxi, but does not otherwise use public transportation	1
3. Travels on public transportation when assisted or accompanied by another	1
4. Travel limited to taxi or automobile with assistance of another	0
5. Does not travel at all	0
G. Responsibility for Own Medications	
1. Is responsible for taking medication in correct dosages at correct time	1
2. Takes responsibility if medication is prepared in advance in separate dosages	0
3. Is not capable of dispensing own medication	0
H. Ability to Handle Finances	
1. Manages financial matters independently (budgets, writes checks, pays rent and bills, goes to bank); collects and keeps track of income	1
2. Manages day-to-day purchases, but needs help with banking, major purchases, etc	1
3. Incapable of handling money	0

Scoring: For each category, circle the item description that most closely resembles the client's highest functional level (either 0 or 1).

From Lawton, M.P., & Brody, E.M. (1969). Assessment of older people: Self-maintaining and instrumental activities of daily living. *Gerontologist 9*:179-186.

a lock. The older adult has 2 minutes to complete each task before moving on to the next one. The instrument has demonstrated high correlations with proxy reports and has a high predictive validity for future hospitalizations and mortality.[86]

The Get Up and Go Test[67] is a reliable and valid test to quantify functional mobility. The test is quick, requires little training and no special equipment, and is appropriate to use in many settings, including hospitals and clinics. This instrument can predict a person's ability to go outside alone safely. As the practitioner observes, the person rises from a chair, walks 10 feet, turns, walks back to the chair, and sits down. Factors to note are sitting balance, transferring from sitting to standing (e.g., does the person need to push off the armrest to rise), pace and stability of walking, ability to turn without staggering, and sitting back down in the chair. Another instrument to assess gait and balance is the Tinetti Gait and Balance Evaluation,[98] a 28-point tool that is performed by trained observers and takes approximately 20 minutes to complete. Both of these instruments also provide useful information about falls risk.

Assessment of Risk for Functional Decline During Hospitalization

Losing the ability to perform ADLs and IADLs as a result of acute illness and hospitalization is common in older adults and can have significant negative consequences, including nursing home discharge and death.[20,32] This functional decline is attributable to the imposition of acute illness on an aging body with diminished physiologic reserve and to limited mobility commonly experienced during a hospital admission.[23] Because hospital-acquired functional decline has been noted to occur within 2 days of a hospital admission,[44] it is

Hospital Admission Risk Profile (HARP)

1. Scoring range 0-5

A. Age

Age Category	Risk Score	Score =
<75	0	
75-84	1	
≥85	2	

B. Cognitive function (abbreviated MMSE*)

MMSE Score	Risk Score	Score =
15-21	0	
0-14	1	

C. IADL function prior to admission†

Independent IADLS	Risk Score	Score =
6-7	0	
0-5	2	

2. Risk categories

Total Score	Risk of Decline in ADL Function	TOTAL =
4 or 5	High risk	
2 or 3	Intermediate risk	
0 or 1	Low risk	

*Abbreviated MMSE includes only the following 21 components of the original 30-item test: orientation (10 items: year, season, month, date, day, city, county, state, hospital, floor), registration (3 unrelated items, such as hat, ball, tree), attention (5 items, such as spelling WORLD backwards), and recall (same 3 items as in registration). Each correct answer is scored one point.

† A person is judged independent in an activity if he or she is able to perform the activity without assistance. A person is scored dependent if he or she either does not perform an activity, requires the assistance of another person, or is unable to perform an activity. IADL activities include telephoning, shopping, cooking, doing housework, taking medications, using transportation, and managing finances.

30-4

important to identify older adults who are at greatest risk for loss of ADLs or mobility at this critical time.

One easy-to-use assessment instrument is the Hospital Admission Risk Profile (HARP)[92] (Fig. 30-4). The HARP was developed based on three predictive variables for ADL loss during and after hospitalization for an acute medical illness and includes (1) older age, (2) impaired cognitive functioning, and (3) reduced IADL ability within 2 weeks before admission.[92] The HARP instrument assesses patients using age, an abbreviated 21-point Folstein Mini-Mental State Exam (MMSE), and IADL preadmission status.[92] The MMSE portion of the instrument consists of 10 orientation questions, registration (3 items), attention (5 items), and recall (previous 3 registration items). Depending on the score, patients are then identified as low, medium, or high risk for loss of ADLs and can be referred early for restorative interventions such as in-hospital rehabilitation, care on a geriatric unit, and multidisciplinary discharge planning.[37]

Assessment of Cognition

The assessment of cognitive status in older adults is an important part of the functional assessment. Cognitive impairment resulting from disease may be attributed by patients, families, and health care providers to normal changes with aging and can delay diagnostic workup. In general, a gradual and mild to moderate decline in short-term memory may be attributable to aging; an older adult may need more time to learn new material or a new task or may need a system for reminders. Domains of cognition included in most mental status assessments are attention, memory, orientation, language, visuospatial skills, and higher cognitive functions, such as the ability to plan and execute functioning.

Altered cognition in older adults is commonly attributed to three disorders—**dementia, delirium,** or **depression**—although other disorders, such as normal pressure hydrocephalus, also may contribute. Depressed persons often complain of memory impairment. Delirium presents as an acute change in cognition, affecting the domain of attention. Delirium is usually attributable to an acute illness, such as an infection, or a medication side effect, whereas persons with Alzheimer dementia have alterations in word finding and naming objects in addition to memory problems. These disorders commonly occur simultaneously and can complicate assessments. For example, persons with dementia are at higher risk for delirium and, in the early stages of dementia, may also be depressed.

For nurses in various settings, cognitive assessments provide continuing comparisons with the individual's baseline to detect any acute changes, such as with delirium. The assessments are not diagnostic but, rather, are for screening purposes and identify the need for a more comprehensive workup. Cognitive assessments are important for discharge planning (e.g., will the person remember to take the prescribed medications) and to assess for readiness for learning. As with screening for ADLs and IADLs, assessment of cognition helps with determining the best discharge plan. Common assessment instruments are listed in Table 30-1.

Depression and Function

Depression is common in older adults although, contrary to popular belief, it is not a normal part of aging or a natural reaction to acute illness or hospitalization. Although aging is often accompanied by loss and unwanted change, most older adults do not suffer from depression. Emotional experiences of sadness, grief, response to loss, and temporary "blue" moods are considered normal. Persistent depression that interferes significantly with ability to function is not. Fortunately, mood disorders including depression are the most common reversible psychiatric conditions in later life.

TABLE 30-1 Common Cognitive Assessment Instruments

Name of Instrument	Type of Test	Domains Covered	Administration Time
Mini-Mental State Examination (Folstein et al, 1975)	Mental status	Orientation, immediate and delayed recall, working memory, language, visuospatial ability	10 minutes
Short Portable Mental Status Questionnaire (Pfeiffer, 1975)	Mental status	Orientation, general/personal information, working memory	5-10 minutes
Mini-Cog (Borson et al, 2003)	Mental status	Immediate and delayed recall, visuospatial ability	5-10 minutes
Blessed Orientation-Memory-Concentration Test (BOMC) (Katzman et al, 1983)	Mental status	Orientation, immediate and delayed recall, working memory	3-6 minutes
Geriatric Depression Scale, Short Form (Yesavage and Brink, 1983)	Depression	Depression and changes in level of depression	5-10 minutes
Confusion Assessment Method (Inouye et al, 1990)	Delirium		
Neecham Confusion Scale (Neelon et al, 1996)	Delirium		

Estimates of major depression in older people living in the community range from less than 1% to about 5% but rise to 13.5% in those who require home health care and to 11.5% in hospitalized older patients.[45]

Functional impairment in both ADLs and IADLs has been associated with higher levels of depressive symptoms.[24] Although older adults with physical impairments are at greater risk for depression, depression is not an inevitable consequence of functional impairment.

Prevention and treatment of depression may be two of the most effective targets for interventions aimed at reducing functional decline and increasing the number of years an older adult maintains independence.[12,87] Therefore it is vital to screen and identify those who have depressive symptoms. Several short screening instruments have been developed and validated for depression screening in the older adult. One example of a screening tool is the Geriatric Depression Scale, Short Form (Fig. 30-5).[92a,101a] This basic screening tool consists of 15 *yes/no* questions easily used in a variety of care settings spanning from the community to acute care hospitals and long-term care settings. The Geriatric Depression Scale, Short Form can be used with both cognitively intact patients and patients who have mild to moderate cognitive impairments. Typically it takes 5 to 7 minutes to complete. Each question can equal one point. A score of 0 to 5 is considered normal; scores above 5 warrant further clinical assessment.[57,92a,101a]

Depression tends to be long lasting and can recur. Because of these two factors, a wait-and-see approach to treatment is not desirable and timely treatment is necessary. Common treatment options are psychotherapy, antidepressant medications, and electroconvulsive therapy.

Social Domain

The quality of life an older person experiences is closely linked to the success of social function. The social domain focuses on relationships within family, social groups, and the community and comprises multiple dimensions including the sources of formal and informal assistance available from those relationships. Knowledge of the day-to-day routines can give you baseline information and a reference point to detect functional decline during future encounters.

A comprehensive social assessment is spread over several evaluation periods. Because more than 80% of all care provided is by family members, the social assessment also addresses assessment of caregivers.[14,94] By use of a multidimensional approach, potential risks such as elder mistreatment may be identified (Table 30-2).

Social networks consist of informal supports that are accessed by the older adult.[74] Informal support is based on cultural beliefs regarding who should be providing care, prior relationships, and location and availability of the caregiver. Informal support includes family and close long-time friends and is usually provided free of charge. The total economic value of informal caregiving in the United States for all diseases is estimated to be at least $306 billion annually, more than twice the amount paid for nursing home care.[5,75] Services provided include tasks such as shopping, bathing, feeding, and paying bills. An example of informal support is a neighbor who has daily contact with the client and shares food and company.

Formal supports include programs such as social welfare and other social service and health care delivery agencies such as home health care. Semiformal supports such as church societies, neighborhood groups, and senior centers also form an important role in social support.[21,102]

The availability of assistance from family or friends frequently determines whether a functionally dependent older adult remains at home or is institutionalized. Several studies conclude that the presence of a caregiver is the most important factor in the discharge plan of older adults from an acute care hospital.[10] Knowing who would be available to help the

Geriatric Depression Scale (Short Form)

1. Are you basically satisfied with your life?	Yes	No
2. Have you dropped many of your activities and interests?	Yes	No
3. Do you feel that your life is empty?	Yes	No
4. Do you often get bored?	Yes	No
5. Are you in good spirits most of the time?	Yes	No
6. Are you afraid that something bad is going to happen to you?	Yes	No
7. Do you feel happy most of the time?	Yes	No
8. Do you often feel helpless?	Yes	No
9. Do you prefer to stay at home rather than go out and do new things?	Yes	No
10. Do you feel you have more problems with memory than most?	Yes	No
11. Do you think it is wonderful to be alive now?	Yes	No
12. Do you feel pretty worthless the way you are now?	Yes	No
13. Do you feel full of energy?	Yes	No
14. Do you feel that your situation is hopeless?	Yes	No
15. Do you think that most people are better off than you are?	Yes	No

*Score:*____/15. One point for "no" to questions 1, 5, 7, 11, 13; one point for "yes" to other questions. Normal: 3 ± 2; mildly depressed: 7 ± 3; very depressed: 12 ± 2.

30-5

TABLE 30-2 Components of Social Assessment
• Social network (formal, semiformal, informal)
• Caregiver assessment
• Elder mistreatment
• Environment
• Spiritual

person if he or she becomes ill is important to document, even for healthy older adults.

Gather your assessment of social support in a systematic manner. Several standardized assessment instruments are available to provide structured assessment. The Norbeck Social Support Questionnaire[79,80] was developed to measure the multiple components of social support.* It allows the individual to rate his or her own social network and perceived social support from the network. The Norbeck Social Support Questionnaire can also be used to measure social support with caregivers. Primary caregivers (especially spouse and adult children) often face high levels of demand and limitations on personal freedom that can result in increased stress, burden, and impaired physical health.

CAREGIVER ASSESSMENT

Most older adults with functional impairment live in the community with the help of informal support (commonly a spouse or other family member, often a daughter). Many spousal caregivers are as frail as the person they are caring for, or many adult children are themselves older than 65 years and may be having to cope with their own chronic illnesses. Although many caregivers experience satisfaction from providing care, great mental and physical stressors may also be linked with caregiving.[53,89] High levels of functional dependency place a burden on the caregiver and may result in caregiver burnout, sleep disturbances, depression, morbidity, and even increased mortality.[6,83]

An older person's need for institutionalization often is better predicted from assessment of the caregiver characteristics and stress than from the severity of the patient's illness.[95] The health and well-being of the patient and caregiver are closely linked. For these reasons, part of caring for a frail older adult involves paying attention to the well-being of the caregiver. For the stressed caregiver, a health care provider may help identify programs such as caregiver support groups, respite programs, adult day care, or hired home health aides.

Assessment of Caregiver Burden

All caregivers should be screened for caregiver burden; for individuals caring for a frail, frequently cognitively impaired older adult, the demands can be overwhelming. The level of care the older adult requires may exceed caregiver ability. Caregiver burden is the perceived strain by the person who cares for an elderly, chronically ill, or disabled person. Caregiver burden is linked to the caregiver's ability to cope and handle stress. Signs of possible caregiver burnout include multiple somatic complaints, increased stress and anxiety, social isolation, depression, and weight loss.

One formal screening tool is the Modified Caregiver Strain Index, which identifies caregivers of any age needing a more comprehensive assessment (Fig. 30-6). It is a brief tool with 13 questions addressing potential strain in employment, financial, physical, social, and time domains.[82,97] Caregiver stress can potentially lead to elder mistreatment; therefore a thorough assessment may identify opportunities to prevent and stop elder mistreatment (see Chapter 7).

CONTEXTS OF CARE

Older adults reside and enter the health care system along multiple levels or contexts of care. Nurses, as part of the health care team, care for older adults along a continuum of these contexts including acute care hospitalization, inpatient nursing facilities, in the community, and at home providing home health care. Some common threads shared by these care settings are the focus on functionally impaired older adults and optimizing the functional status and quality of life through the involvement of a team of care providers. The comprehensive functional assessment aids in determining the type and level of services an older adult may need and the most appropriate match to the needs and wants of the individual.

The location of the care setting contributes to the ability to perform a comprehensive functional assessment. It may be more difficult to perform a complete assessment in the acute care setting while the older adult is experiencing an acute illness and the length of stay may be short versus in a nursing facility where an assessment may be achieved over time. In addition, if a resident resides in the home environment, the parameters of assessment will be broader than if he or she is in an inpatient long-term living situation. For example, older adults who live at home require an assessment of the home environment and community resources available, caregiver assessment if needed, and the ability to self-perform ADLs and IADLS.

Acute Care Setting

For older adults, acute hospitalization offers the hope of relief of symptoms and treatment of illness and disease. But it also puts them at risk for adverse consequences of hospitalization including functional decline, iatrogenic complications, and subsequent discharge to a nursing facility.[35,71]

Researchers have found that older adults admitted to a hospital for acute illness will lose independent function in one or more ADLs.[21,40,99]

In the past decade, a few hospital-based models of care have emerged designed to enhance patient functioning during hospitalization and improve outcomes for older adults

*Norbeck Social Support Questionnaire is available online at http://evolve.elsevier.com/Jarvis.

Modified Caregiver Strain Index

Directions: Here is a list of things that other caregivers have found to be difficult. Please put a checkmark in the columns that apply to you. We have included some examples that are common caregiver experiences to help you think about each item. Your situation may be slightly different, but the item could still apply.

	Yes, on a regular basis = 2	Yes, sometimes = 1	No = 0
My sleep is disturbed (For example, *the person I care for* is in and out of bed or wanders around at night)			
Caregiving is inconvenient (For example, helping takes so much time or it's a long drive over to help)			
Caregiving is a physical strain (For example, lifting in or out of a chair; effort or concentration is required)			
Caregiving is confining (For example, helping restricts free time or *I* cannot go visiting)			
There have been family adjustments (For example, helping has disrupted *my* routine; there has been no privacy)			
There have been changes in personal plans (For example, *I* had to turn down a job; *I* could not go on vacation)			
There have been other demands on my time (For example, other family members *need me)*			
There have been emotional adjustments (For example, severe arguments *about caregiving)*			
Some behavior is upsetting (For example, incontinence; *the person cared for* has trouble remembering things; or *the person I care for* accuses people of taking things)			
It is upsetting to find the person I care for has changed so much from his or her former self (For example, he or she is a different person than he or she used to be)			
There have been work adjustments (For example, *I* have to take time off *for caregiving duties)*			
Caregiving is a financial strain			
I feel completely overwhelmed (For example, *I* worry about *the person I care for; I* have concerns about how *I* will manage)			

Total Score =

Words appearing in *italics* represent modifications from the original Caregiver Strain Index from Robinson, B.C. (1983). Validation of a caregiver strain index. *J Gerontol 38*:344-348. Copyright © The Gerontological Society of America.

30-6

post-discharge. Hospitals have come to appreciate the increased risk for functional decline and adverse outcomes, and targeted interventions to prevent decline have shown to be successful. One popular model of care is the Acute Care for Elders (ACE) unit, which is a dedicated unit within a hospital setting focused toward preventing functional decline in older adults through the design of the physical environment (e.g., bright lights, flooring to help prevent falls), collaboration among interdisciplinary teams, patient-centered care, and nursing protocols for clinical care (e.g., indwelling urinary catheter removal, reduction of restraint use, early mobilization).[19,84] Acute care nurses equipped with specialized knowledge and skills can have an impact on improving outcomes for the hospitalized older adult.

Community

The vast majority of older adults reside in the community, and misconceptions about nursing homes statistics are common. Fewer than 5% of older adults live in nursing homes on any given day. The percentage of those who live in a long-term care facility at any point in time increases from 1% of those ages 65 to 74 years to about 17% of those older than 85 years.[3] Since the mid-1980s, the rate of nursing home residence for people older than 65 years has been declining.[3] This decline can be contributed partly to the increase in assistive living facilities and popularity and availability of home health care services.

One of the goals of community-based services is to assist the older adult to remain at home. Assessment of functional status assists in determining the type of services an older adult needs to maintain independence and living at home. A low or negative result on a screening tool during assessment does not necessarily lead to the need for institutionalization. It may mean the older adult requires increased services to maintain home living. The availability of support through community services is a factor helping older adults maintain their independence and avoid institutionalization.

Home Care

Home care refers to a range of supportive social and health services provided in the home environment. Services include skilled nursing care, primary care, therapy (physical, occupational, and speech), social work, nutrition, case management, ADL assistance, and some durable medical equipment. Physical, psychosocial, and functional assessments are all part of the home care nurse's responsibility. The home care nurse is tending not only to the illness of the older adult but also to the home safety considerations, family dynamics, and functional ability. Because of advances in health care technology, equipment is smaller and more portable. As a result, people who once were limited to hospitalization can now be treated or managed at home. In addition to cost advantages with home care versus hospitalization, older adults have been shown to recover faster when at home in familiar settings than when placed in institutions and also can avoid the risk for infection exposure.

Nursing Facilities

Nursing facilities include a broad range of services from minimal support to maximal assistance. The length of stay at nursing facilities also varies from short stays after hospitalization for rehabilitation to long-term residential living.

Assistive Living

Assistive living facilities are a popular choice for older adults and typically are considered between home care and long-term care. There is great diversity in the services provided. Most assistive living facilities provide apartment-style living, although there are some single-family dwellings that are licensed to provide care. Facilities offer homelike environments where residents have the opportunity for social interaction through group dining and activities. All provide room, meals, and housekeeping. Some offer assistance with personal care and/or support with ADLs, transportation, and recreational activities as part of an overall package; others offer services that can be added on separately.

Continuing Care Retirement Communities

The unique feature of continuing care retirement communities is that all care needs for the older adult can be met in one community, supporting the concept of aging in place. These facilities feature independent living arrangements and homes that offer a variety of social and recreational activities. But they also have assisted-living and skilled nursing level of care. In these types of communities, residents can progress through the continuum of care while residing in the same community. An older adult can enter the community at the independent level of living, and as illness and/or functional limitations occur, they can move to a higher level of support to the assisted living locations and then the skilled nursing level if needed. Some older adults may not ever leave the independent living level, whereas others may progress to skilled nursing as the need for care arises.

MAINTAINING INDEPENDENCE

Exercise

Exercise and activity are essential for health promotion and maintenance in the older adult and to assist in achieving an optimal level of functioning. A sedentary lifestyle is an important contributor to the loss in the ability to independently perform ADLs. Exercise does not prevent the process of aging, but it increases functional ability, helping to maximize the older adult's independence.

Exercise has positive health effects in older adults, including those with impairments.[43,48] The positive effects of exercise include improving cardiovascular function, postural stability, flexibility and range of motion, and strength and muscle mass; decreasing body fat; and possibly helping to reduce pain and discomfort. Because of these positive effects, fall risk and fractures may be decreased. In addition, participation in physical exercise has shown to reduce depressive symptoms and improve feelings of psychosocial well-being.[42,61,72,88]

The American Heart Association and the American College of Sports Medicine both provide recommendations for different types of activity and steps to implement exercise programs for those older than 65 years.[78] Physical exercise is separated into four categories: aerobic, muscle strengthening, flexibility, and balance. Aerobic activity guidelines suggest a minimum of 30 minutes of moderate-intensity exercise 5 days a week or a minimum of 20 minutes of vigorous-intensity exercise 3 days a week, or a combination of both moderate and vigorous exercise. The definitions for moderate and vigorous intensity depend on the older adult's baseline physical condition.[78] Muscle strengthening includes resistance and weight training and is recommended to be performed 2 days a week. Weight training has been shown to be beneficial in the older adult for muscle strength and endurance.[7] Flexibility training to maintain range of motion is recommended 2 days a week for at least 10 minutes. Balance training to improve stability is important to help prevent falls. Tai chi has been shown to improve range of motion, balance, and flexibility.[7]

To help with compliance, physical activities should be readily available and have minimal cost associated with participation. Because pathology, both known and undiscovered, may be present in older adults (e.g., osteoporosis), the physical activity chosen should not present excessive stress on the skeletal system. Walking is a popular mode of exercise for cardiovascular endurance, is accessible, and is associated with minimal cost. Water activities or stationary cycling may be alternative exercise modes for individuals where walking is not feasible. The American Heart Association and the American College of Sports Medicine guidelines emphasize a graduated and step-wise approach to initiating exercise.[78] Developing an activity plan, particularly for older adults with chronic health conditions, may warrant clearance and input from a health care provider or referral to a specialty program (e.g., cardiac rehabilitation).

Health Care Maintenance

Functional decline and a loss of independence are not inevitable consequences of aging. Although the prevalence of chronic disease increases with age, most older people remain functionally independent. But given the presence of chronic disease among older adults, evidence-based interventions for screening and detection of health conditions and disease are important to maximize quality of life. The Agency for Healthcare Research and Quality (AHRQ) in partnership with AARP provides recommendations on daily steps to promote good health, screening tests, and medications to help in disease prevention in the publication "Staying Healthy at 50+." It provides a guide for older adults to follow to ensure they are receiving screening appropriate for their age and health status. Multiple age-related conditions are amenable to prevention or improvement with screening and appropriate and timely intervention.

ENVIRONMENTAL ASSESSMENT

The physical environment of the older person includes the home environment and community system and is critical to maintaining independence. Environmental hazards within the home can be a potential constraint on the older adult's day-to-day functioning. Common environmental hazards include inadequate lighting, loose throw rugs, curled carpet edges, obstructed hallways, cords in walkways, lack of grab bars in tub and shower, and low and loose toilet seats.[15,28,52] These hazards increase the risk for falls and fractures. Environmental modification can promote mobility and reduce the likelihood of the older adult's falling.

The functional assessment should inquire about the safety of the neighborhood and ask whether older persons have transportation or transportation services available in geographic proximity to where they live (Fig. 30-7). The community needs to possess access to basic services such as food and clothing stores, pharmacists, financial institutions, health care facilities, and social service agencies. The community environment needs to provide safety conditions such as street lamps, sidewalks, and police and fire protection.[15] Both the home and community environment affect the safety of the older adult.[13] These are especially important for older adults dependent in IADLs and still living within the community.

Older persons often have problems not easily detected during an office visit. A home visit can reveal challenges in the living situation, such as household and bathing hazards, social isolation, family/caregiver stress, and nutrition issues.[52] For example, a walk through the kitchen can assist the health care provider in assessing the nutritional status and food preferences of the older adult. An empty refrigerator and/or kitchen cabinets may give clues to previously unrecognized functional impairment, such as dementia, mobility challenges, or a decline in the ability to perform IADLs, which would warrant further assessment. Interventions such as home health assistance, transportation, and shopping services may support the older adult to maintain community living. The U.S. Consumer Product Safety Commission website (www.cpsc.gov/CPSCPUB/PUBS/705.pdf) has a safety checklist an older person or family member can use for a self-assessment. See also Table 30-3.

Older Adult Drivers

Older adult drivers account for 15% of all licensed drivers in the United States, 8% of all traffic crash injuries, and 19% of all pedestrian fatalities.[76] Safe driving requires intact cognitive functioning, sensory perception, good physical abilities (e.g., strength to turn the steering wheel and use pedals; enough range of motion to turn head and neck), alertness, and suitable reflexes.[55] Early and routine attention to health care maintenance activities such as vision and hearing checks, exercise to maintain flexibility and range of motion, and workup of any cognitive abnormalities may allow the older adult to continue to drive safely for longer periods.

Driving represents independence, freedom, and control and is often a necessary part of functioning in daily life, such as getting to work or shopping for groceries. Driving also facilitates remaining connected socially with family and friends. Driving cessation can be devastating to an older adult and can lead to intensified and prolonged symptoms of depression[66] and steep declines in physical functioning.[27b]

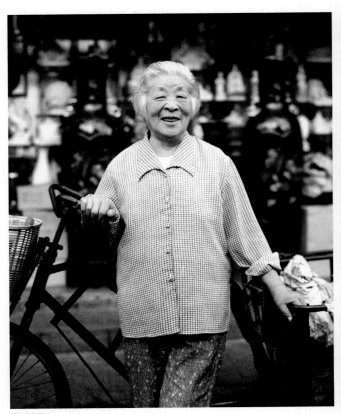

30-7

TABLE 30-3 National Safety Council Home Safety Checklist

Make your home a safer place. Use this checklist to evaluate home hazards.

OUTSIDE THE HOUSE:

- Problem areas have been leveled or marked to prevent a fall.
- Ice melt, salt, or sand for icy driveways, sidewalks, and porches is readily available.
- Power tools and hazardous substances such as weed killers, fertilizers, or grease-removing solvents are locked inside a cabinet, out of children's reach.
- Flammable materials such as gasoline or oil-soaked rags are stored in manufacturer-recommended containers.
- The garage door is down and locked at all times.
- The automatic reverse mechanism on the garage door is working properly and tested monthly.
- If you have a swimming pool, there is a locked barrier at least four feet high or taller to keep out children when there is no adult supervision.

INSIDE THE HOUSE:

- Smoke alarms are tested monthly and batteries are changed when the clocks change each spring and fall.
- A home fire escape route has been identified and practiced with the whole family.
- Any frayed wires have been replaced, wires under carpets and loose plugs have been secured, and gas odors around pipes or appliances have been reported.
- All throw rugs have nonskid padding.
- Staircases have handrails and slip-resistant floor coverings.
- There is a bath mat near the bathtub or shower.
- Household cleaning products and medications are kept out of children's reach and have childproof caps.
- Carbon monoxide detectors are in place, especially near sleeping areas.
- The local poison control center number is posted near every phone.

If driving must be limited or cease altogether, it is important to establish a plan of action to enhance independence and maintain normal activity levels. This might mean accessing public transportation, carpooling, or increased involvement of family and friends for activities that require motor transportation. The decision to allow an older adult to continue driving is generally made by local state licensing agencies. Many states, either by statute or regulation, have identified mandated physician reporting obligations for conditions such as sensory impairments or neurodegenerative illnesses.

Older adults often recognize that their driving abilities have changed and adjust their driving habits accordingly, such as limiting to daytime, good weather conditions, or only local driving. However, when this is not the case, family members, friends, or health care providers may be concerned enough about the safety of the older driver and others in the community that they need to intervene. Several resources are available to assist with either self-assessment of driving skills or for use by caregivers and health care providers. One practical approach is published by The American Association of Retired Persons (AARP) and is a checklist of warning signs of when to stop driving (Table 30-4). In addition, the American Automobile Association (AAA) and AARP provide online driver self-assessment tests, and local departments of motor vehicles and area agencies on aging can provide additional resources to assist older adults and their families with ongoing assessment and planning. The National Highway Traffic Safety Administration (NHTSA) has published a brochure that outlines assessment, critical conversations, planning and evaluation, and resources for older adults, their families, or health care providers related to safe driving (www.nhtsa.dot.gov/people/injury/olddrive/UnderstandOlderDrivers/pages/Preface.html).

Sleep

Sufficient sleep is a necessary part of health. Sleep architecture does change with aging, such as more difficulty falling and staying asleep; however, significantly altered sleep patterns are not a normal part of aging, and the prevalence of insomnia is low in healthy older adults.[4] Most adults of all ages need about 8 hours of sleep per night to feel alert and rested. Medical and psychiatric illnesses, such as cardiac and pulmonary disease, osteoarthritis, dementia, delirium, and depression, as well as side effects of the medications to treat these disorders (beta-blockers corticosteroids, bronchodilators, decongestants, diuretics) are contributing factors to insomnia. In addition, other causes of insomnia are intake of alcohol, nicotine, and caffeine; sleep apnea; restless leg syndrome; and circadian rhythm disturbances.[4,18] Detrimental consequences of poor sleep in older adults are poor health

TABLE 30-4 Warning Signs for When to Stop Driving

1. Almost crashing, with frequent close calls
2. Finding dents and scrapes on the car, fences, mailboxes, garage doors, curbs, or the like
3. Getting lost
4. Having trouble seeing or following traffic signals, road signs, and pavement markings
5. Responding more slowly to unexpected situations, having trouble moving your foot from the gas to the brake pedal; confusing the two pedals
6. Misjudging gaps in traffic at intersections and on highway entrance and exit ramps
7. Experiencing road rage or having other drivers frequently honk at you
8. Easily becoming distracted or having difficulty concentrating while driving
9. Having a hard time turning around to check over your shoulder while backing up or changing lanes
10. Receiving traffic tickets or warnings from traffic or law enforcement officers in the last year or two

Adapted from AARP. (2010). What are the warning signs that indicate someone should begin to limit driving or to stop altogether? Retrieved January 5, 2011, from www.aarp.org/home-garden/transportation/info-05-2010/Warning_Signs_Stopping.print.html.

outcomes such as obesity,[81] altered physical functioning,[25] falls,[58] impaired cognition,[81] and increased risk for death.[27]

Sleep is disrupted very often in the hospital; the need for tests, vital signs, and pain assessments occurs 24 hours a day. Bright lights, pagers, inability to maintain a cool environment, and staff conversation all contribute to sleep disruption. In addition, delirium, an acute and fluctuating change in mental status, is common in older hospitalized adults. Delirium contributes to disruption in sleep-wake cycles, in which patients are awake all night and difficult to keep awake during the day.

Because medications such as sedatives and hypnotics, often used to treat insomnia, have many side effects for older adults, such as falls and delirium, a nonpharmacologic approach to managing sleep in the hospital is recommended (Table 30-5). In the home, use of relaxing music; exposure to sunlight during the day; consistent bedtime routines; limiting food and drink after early evening; reduced light, noise, and room temperature; and whole-body relaxation may improve sleep.[55]

One instrument useful for measurement of the quality and patterns of sleep in older adults is the Pittsburgh Sleep Quality Index (PSQI). The PSQI can be used across health care settings and can be used for initial and ongoing assessments.[93]

SPIRITUAL ASSESSMENT

Spirituality provides personal answers about the meaning and purpose of one's own life[41] and how to interpret life events and regard them as "bigger than oneself." Spiritual health may improve with age, even as physical and mental health deteriorate. The aging process is a part of one's journey

TABLE 30-5 Nonpharmacologic Interventions to Promote Sleep

Category	Intervention	Rationale
Dietary	Limit caffeine (coffee, tea, soft drinks, and chocolate) to 2 caffeinated drinks per day, none after lunch.	Caffeine promotes wakefulness by blocking adenosine receptors in the brain.
	Restrict alcohol to 1 drink per day, none after dinner.	Alcohol may shorten the time it takes to fall asleep, but it is metabolized quickly and withdrawal occurs in the last half of the night, producing lighter sleep and aggravating obstructive sleep apnea, restless legs syndrome, sympathetic arousal, and sweating.
	Restrict fluid intake in the evening.	This reduces nighttime awakening resulting from a full bladder.
	Avoid heavy, spicy meals near bedtime.	This reduces nighttime awakening caused by heartburn.
	Have a light bedtime snack of milk or cheese and crackers.	This promotes sleep by reducing hypoglycemia.
Schedule	Adhere to a regular schedule for meals and sleep, using an alarm, if necessary, to ensure rising at a regular time. Limit naps to one 30-minute, early-afternoon nap.	Maintaining temporal patterns of rest and activity enhances synchrony with circadian rhythms. Excessive daytime napping weakens the homeostatic drive to sleep.
Environment	Maintain daytime light and nighttime dark. Open drapes and blinds, increase the wattage in lamps. Increase sunlight exposure to at least ½ hour per day. Keep the sleep environment dark.	Circadian rhythms are established primarily by patterns of light and dark.
	Use the bed only for sleep or sex, not for work or watching television. Limit time spent in bed to the average time spent asleep. If not asleep after 30 minutes, get up and engage in a relaxing activity until the need to sleep is felt.	The bed becomes an environmental cue for sleep.
	Promote uninterrupted sleep by, for example, controlling the noise level and limiting or consolidating nighttime interventions.	Limiting noise minimizes sleep disruption.
Activities	Maintain an active physical and social daytime schedule. Avoid passive activities such as watching television.	Vigorous activity promotes daytime arousal, prevents napping, and lessens depression, which can disrupt sleep.
	Keep to a relaxing bedtime ritual using, for example, massage, reading, prayer, music, and warm baths.	Relaxing activities augment one's readiness for sleep. A warm bath enhances a drop in core temperature.
Delirium	Frequently reorient the patient by keeping a clock and calendar in the room and maintaining a regular schedule and associated light and dark patterns.	These measures decrease anxiety.

From Cole, C., & Richards, K. (2007). Sleep disruption in older adults. *American Journal of Nursing, 107*(5), 40-49.

with capability for growth.[8] Views on spirituality vary greatly from one adult to another and among people of the same faith or belief system. It is important to acknowledge spirituality as a powerful coping mechanism during stressful life events and illness through to the end of life.[73]

Spiritual assessment is highly individual and may be delayed until a provider-client relationship has been developed. Open-ended questions provide a foundation for future dialogue. A sample question posed during the initial assessment may be "Do you consider yourself to be a spiritual person?" If the person says "yes," a follow-up question could be "How does that spirituality relate to your health or health care decisions?" Involving chaplains or clergy members when possible and appropriate can provide the older adult with support and can serve as a resource to the clinician.

SPECIAL CONSIDERATIONS

Assessment of the functional status of an older adult can be more time consuming than for younger adults. It may take longer for him or her to understand and process the questions and to respond. The presence of physical disabilities, anxiety, depression, pain, or fatigue may necessitate several sessions to complete the assessment (Fig. 30-8). The older adult may need assistance with clothing and may prefer that a family member be present for all or parts of the examination. For hospitalized or institutionalized older adults, consider assessing function during normal activities such as grooming, at mealtime, or during toileting.

Understand that a person with multiple medical problems may tire early and easily and that many medications have side effects that contribute to fatigue or affect the attention span. Again, assessments may need to be done incrementally, such as positioning for comfort and clustering similar tasks to prevent fatigue. Having the person use glasses or hearing aids can mitigate communication difficulties resulting from vision or hearing loss. Provide directions in written format if necessary, and have hearing amplifiers and page magnifiers available. Face the person as much as possible, speak slowly in a lower-pitched voice, and enunciate words clearly. Be prepared to use interpreters rather than family members for non–English-speaking clients.

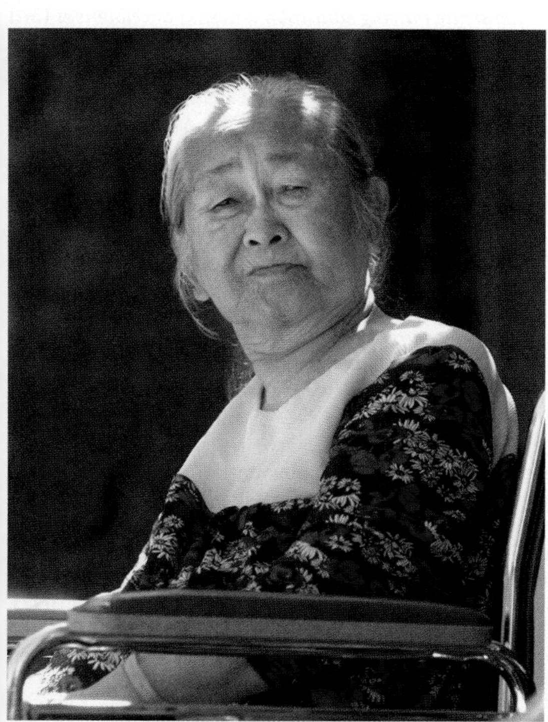

30-8

Older adults are a heterogeneous group. You must be aware of your own attitudes and beliefs about older adults to ensure that the functional assessment is truly reflecting abilities and not the myth that functional decline is a normal outcome of aging. Demonstrating respect and interest and treating the client as an individual are imperative. Ask how the older adult would like to be addressed. Maximize communication by using terminology understandable to the person rather than using medical jargon. Including the older adult in decision making about how the interview or testing is to be done will establish rapport and promote self-esteem. Be aware of body language and behaviors, and be prepared to modify your approach. Touch can also help in establishing rapport and can reduce anxiety.

A functional assessment can be intimidating for older adults. Frustration or embarrassment may arise if some physical maneuvers cannot be performed or questions cannot be answered during cognitive testing. They may also be fearful about the consequences of functional testing, such as losing independent living or having a caregiver move into the home. Try to provide reassurance that not everyone can complete all of the tasks or answer all of the questions and that, to the extent possible, confidentiality will be honored.

Ensure adequate space if doing tests of mobility. An aging adult may need room to maneuver an assistive device. When testing mobility, stand close to him or her to prevent a fall. The environment should be well lighted with increased illumination; avoid high-gloss, shiny, slippery surfaces. Minimize extraneous noise such as those from intercoms, televisions, or high-traffic areas. Warm rooms, access to fluids, proximity to a bathroom, and privacy are important.

Cultural Considerations

Be aware that cultural influences are parts of the person's life (review Chapter 2). Food habits and dietary beliefs may conflict with dietary recommendations made by health care providers. The response to pain, including how it is perceived, how much is considered tolerable, and the reaction to pain experienced, varies among and within different cultures. How the person interprets the symptoms, meaning, and causes of illness can be defined by his or her culture. It also plays a part in when the older adult seeks care and may influence how the illness is treated. He or she may want to try traditional/alternative practices to prevent or treat certain conditions.

Wide differences appear among individuals in every culture. Learn how the person's culture fits together with suggested interventions. Culture also influences whether the older adult relies on family for care or the approach to decision making (i.e., involvement of family and friends), disclosure of medical information (e.g., cancer diagnosis), and end-of-life care (i.e., advance directives, resuscitation preferences, and nutrition).[16,33,101]

Assessing Those in Pain

If the older adult is feeling pain or discomfort, the depth of knowledge gathered through the assessments will suffer. Alleviating pain should be a priority over other aspects of the assessment. It may be necessary to administer premedication before portions of the assessment, especially if the assessment requires movement. Another strategy is to use positioning to decrease pain. Ask what position is most comfortable. Providing comfort can help maximize the information gathered. It is paramount to remember older adults with cognitive impairment do *not* experience less pain. This population suffers from conditions typically associated with pain (e.g., arthritis, osteoporosis, cancer, shingles) just as frequently as cognitively intact persons.

A variety of pain assessment scales are available to use in the cognitively impaired older adult population. The "gold standard" continues to be a person's self-report. Several studies have demonstrated that those with cognitive impairment can provide self-report pain, which must be taken seriously.[85]

Assessing Older Adults with Altered Cognition

Cognitive impairment poses unique challenges. The older adult may not be able to actively participate in the evaluation and/or provide consistent answers. Gathering information from the older adult firsthand is always the best but is not always feasible. To ensure the collection of reliable information, one strategy is to interview the caregiver and/or family to obtain subjective assessment data. Another is to arrange opportunities to assess the person during different times of the day, when he or she may be more clear-headed. If possible, split the assessment into smaller sections at a time. Be flexible.

Adults with cognitive impairment may need questions or directions broken down into single commands, repeated word for word, with ongoing verbal cueing or a physical cue. For example, after getting the person's attention, the interviewer might say "sit here" and pat the chair. Never assume that he or she cannot respond to questions even when there is known cognitive impairment. Using *yes* or *no* questions may prevent frustration. Be relaxed and patient because a person with dementia may mirror your emotions. If a family member or caregiver does need to provide collateral information, avoid doing this in front of the person.

BIBLIOGRAPHY

1. AARP. (2010). *Know when to limit or stop driving.* Retrieved January 5, 2010, from www.aarp.org/home-garden/transportation/info-05-2010/Warning_Signs_Stopping.print.html.
2. Reference deleted in proofs.
3. Administration on Aging. (2008). *Aging statistics.* Retrieved August 31, 2009, from www.aoa.gov/AoARoot/Aging_Statistics/index.aspx.
4. Ancoli-Israel, S. (2009). Sleep and its disorders in aging populations. *Sleep Medicine, 10*(Suppl. 1), S7-S11, 2009.
5. Arno, P. S., Levine, C., & Memmott, M. M. (1999). The economic value of informal caregiving. *Health Affairs, 18,* 182-188.
6. Beach, S. R., Schulz, R., Williamson, G. M., et al. (2005). Risk factors for potentially harmful informal caregiver behavior. *Journal of the American Geriatrics Society, 53,* 255-261.
7. Bellew, J. W., Symons, T. B., & Vandervoort, A. A. (2005). Geriatric fitness: effects of aging and recommendations for exercise in older adults. *Cardiopulmonary Physical Therapy Journal, 16*(1), 20-31.
8. Berggren-Thomas, P., & Griggs, M. J. (1995). Spirituality in aging: spiritual need or spiritual journey? *Journal of Gerontological Nursing, 21*(3), 5-10.
9. Reference deleted in proofs.
10. Brown, L. J., Potter, J. F., & Foster, B. G. (1990). Caregiver burden should be evaluated during geriatric assessment. *Journal of the American Geriatrics Society, 38,* 455-460.
11. Buhr, GT., & Kuchibhatla, M. (2006). Caregivers' reasons for nursing home placement: cues for improving discussions with families prior to transition. *The Gerontologist, 46*(1), 52-61.
12. Callahan, C. M., Kroenke, K., Counsell, S. R., et al. (2005). Treatment of depression improves physical functioning in older adults. *Journal of the American Geriatrics Society, 53,* 367-373.
13. Carol, W. (1996). Socioeconomic and environmental influences. In A. G. Lueckenotte (Ed.), *Gerontological nursing* (pp. 180-191). St. Louis: Mosby.
14. Chichin, E., et al. (2001). Caregiving/mistreatment. In M. Mezey, T. Fulmer, & C. Mariano (Eds.), *Best nursing practices for older adults: incorporating essential gerontological content into baccalaureate nursing education and staff development* (3rd ed.). New York: American Association of Colleges of Nursing Washington DC & The John A. Hartford Foundation Institute for Geriatric Nursing.
15. Chu, N. (1998). Environment/home. In A. S. Luggen, S. S. Travis, & S. Meiner (Eds.), *NGNA core curriculum for gerontological advanced practice nurses.* Thousand Oaks, CA: SAGE.
16. Chu, N. L. (1998). Culture, race, and ethnicity. In A. S. Luggen, S. S. Travis, & S. Meiner (Eds.), *NGNA core curriculum for gerontological advanced practice nurses.* Thousand Oaks, CA: SAGE.
17. Cole, C., & Richards, K. (2007). Sleep disruption in older adults. *American Journal of Nursing, 107*(5), 40-50.
18. Cooke, J. R., & Ancoli-Israel, S. (2006). Sleep and its disorders in older adults. *Psychiatric Clinics of North America, 29*(4), 177-193.
19. Counsell, S. R., Holder, C. M., Liebenauer, L. L., et al. (2000). Effects of a multicomponent intervention on functional outcomes and process of care in hospitalized older patients: a randomized controlled trial of acute care for elders (ACE) in a community hospital. *Journal of the American Geriatrics Society, 48*(12), 1572-1581.
20. Covinsky, K. E., Justice, A. C., Rosenthal, G. E., et al. (1997). Measuring prognosis and case mix in hospitalized elders: the importance of functional status. *Journal of General Internal Medicine, 12*(4), 203-208.
21. Covinsky, K. E., Newcomer, R., Fox, P., et al. (2003). Patient and caregiver characteristics associated with depression in

caregivers on patients with dementia. *Journal of General Internal Medicine, 18*(12), 1006-1014.
22. Reference deleted in proofs.
23. Creditor, M. C. (1993). Hazards of hospitalization of the elderly. *Annals of Internal Medicine, 18*(3), 219-223.
24. Cummings, S. M., Neff, J. A., & Husaini, B. A. (2003). Functional impairment as a predictor of depressive symptomatology: the role of race, religiosity, and social support. *Health & Social Work, 29*(1), 23-32.
25. Dam, T. T. , Ewing, S., Ancoli-Israel, S., et al. (2008). Association between sleep and physical function in older men: the osteoporotic fractures in men sleep study. *Journal of the American Geriatrics Society, 56*(9), 1665-1673.
26. DeFrances, C. J., Lucas, C. A., Buie, V. C., et al. (2008). 2006 National hospital discharge survey. *National Health Statistics Reports, 30*(5), 1-20.
27. Dew, M. A., Hoch, C. C., Busse, D. J., et al. (2003). Healthy older adults' sleep predicts all-cause mortality at 4 to 19 years of follow-up. *Psychosomatic Medicine, 65*(1), 63-73.
27a. Duke University and the National Institute on Aging. (1999). *National Long Term Care Survey*. Retrieved January 5, 2011, from: http://www.nltcs.aas.duke.edu/index.htm.
27b. Edwards J. D., Lunsman, M., Perkins, M., et al. (2009). Driving cessation and health trajectories in older adults. *Journal of Gerontology: A Biological Science, 64*(12), 1290-1295.
28. Eliopoulis, C. (1997). *Gerontological nursing* (4th ed.). Philadelphia: Lippincott.
29. Reference deleted in proofs.
30. Reference deleted in proofs.
31. Fillenbaum, G. G., & Smyer, M. A. (1981). The development, validity, and reliability of the OARS multidimensional functional assessment questionnaire. *Journal of Gerontology, 36(4)*, 428-434.
32. Fortinsky, R. H., Covinsky, K. E., Palmer, R. M., et al. (1999). Effects of functional status changes before and during hospitalization on nursing home admission of older adults. *The Journals of Gerontology. Series A, Biological Sciences and Medical Sciences, 54*(10), M521-M526.
33. Reference deleted in proofs.
34. GeroNurse Online. (2009). *Why gerontological nursing certification?* Retrieved January 5, 2011, from www.geronurseonline.com/.
35. Gillis, A., & MacDonald, B. (2005). Deconditioning in the hospitalized elderly. *Canadian Nurse, 101*(6), 16-20.
36. Reference deleted in proofs.
37. Graf, C. (2008). The hospital admission risk profile. *American Journal of Nursing, 108*(8), 62-72.
38. Guse, L. W. (2006). Assessment of the older adult. In K. L. Mauk (Ed.), *Gerontological nursing competencies for care* (pp. 265-292). Sudbury, MA: Jones & Bartlett.
39. Hamilton, B. B., Granger, C. V., Sherwin, F. S., et al. (1987). A uniform national data system for medical rehabilitation. In M. J. Fuher (Ed.), *Rehabilitation outcomes: analysis and measurement*. Baltimore: Brooks.
40. Hart, B. D., Birkas, J., Lachmann, M., et al. (2002). Promoting positive outcomes for elderly persons in the hospital: prevention and risk factor modification. *AACN Clinical Issues, 13*(1), 22-33.
41. Heriot, C. S. (1992). Spirituality and aging. *Holistic Nursing Practice, 7*(1), 22-31.
42. Hessert, M. J., Gugliucci, M. R., & Pierce, H. R. (2005). Functional fitness: maintaining or improving function for elders with chronic diseases. *Family Medicine, 37*(7), 472-476.
43. Heyn, P., Abreu, B. C., & Ottenbacher, K. J. (2004). The effects of exercise training on elderly persons with cognitive impairment and dementia: a meta-analysis. *Archives of Physical Medicine and Rehabilitation, 85*(10), 1694-1704.
44. Hirsch, C. H., Sommers, L., Olsen, A., et al. (1990). The natural history of functional morbidity in hospitalized patients. *Journal of the American Geriatrics Society, 38*(12), 1296-1303.
45. Hybels, C. F., & Blazer, D. G. (2003). Epidemiology of late-life mental disorders. *Clinics in Geriatric Medicine, 19*(4), 663-696.
46. Inouye, S. K., van Dyck, C. H., Alessi, C. A., et al. (1990). Clarifying confusion: the confusion assessment method. *Annals of Internal Medicine, 113*, 941-948.
47. Reference deleted in proofs.
48. Jette, A. M., & Keysor, J. J. (2003). Disability models: implications for arthritis exercise and physical activity interventions. *Arthritis and Rheumatism, 49*, 114-120.
49. Reference deleted in proofs.
50. Karagiozis, H., Gray, S., Sacco, J., et al. (1998). The direct assessment of functional abilities (DAFA): a comparison to an indirect measure of instrumental activities of daily living. *The Gerontologist, 38*, 113-121.
51. Katz, S., Ford, A. B., Moskowitz, R. W., et al. (1963). Studies of illness in the aged: the index of ADL, a standardized measure of biological and psychosocial functioning. *Journal of the American Medical Association, 185*, 94-101.
52. Kim, L. C., & Dyer, C. B. (2006). Assessment of older adults in their homes. In J. J. Gallo (Ed.), *Handbook of geriatric assessment* (4th ed.). Sudbury, MA: Jones & Bartlett.
53. Kramer, B. (1997). Gain in the caregiving experience: Where are we? What next? *The Gerontologist, 37*, 218-232.
54. Kresevic, D. M., & Mezey, M. (2003). Assessment of function. In M. Mezey et al (Eds.), *Geriatric nursing protocols for best practice* (2nd ed., pp. 31-46). New York: Springer Publishing.
55. Krieger-Blake, L. S. (2006). Changes that affect independence in later life. In K. L. Mauk (Ed.), *Gerontological nursing: competencies for care* (pp. 321-354). Boston: Jones & Bartlett.
56. Kuriansky, J. B., & Gurland, B. (1976). Performance test of activities of daily living, *International Journal of Aging & Human Development, 7*, 343-352.
57. Kurlowicz, L., & Greenberg, S. A. (Revised 2007). The Geriatric Depression Scale, *Try this: best practices in nursing care to older adults*. Issue #4. Retrieved September 1, 2009, from http://consultgerirn.org/uploads/File/trythis/try_this_4.pdf.
58. Latimer, Hill E., Cumming, R. G., Lewis, R., et al. (2007). Sleep disturbances and falls in older people. *The Journal of Gerontology. Series A, Biological Sciences and Medical Sciences, 62*(1), 62-66.
59. Lawton, M. P., & Brody, E. M. (1969). Assessment of older people: self-maintaining and instrumental activities of daily living. *The Gerontologist, 9*, 179-186.
60. Lehman, C. A., & Poindexter, A. (2006). The aging population. In K. L. Mauk (Ed.)., *Gerontological nursing: competencies for care* (pp. 29-56). Boston: Jones & Bartlett.
61. Lin, S., & Woollacott, M. (2002). Postural muscle responses following changing balance threats in young, stable older, and unstable older adults. *Journal of Motor Behavior, 34*(1), 37-44.
62. Linn, M. (1988). Rapid Disability Rating Scale-2 (RDRS-2). *Psychopharmacology Bulletin, 24*, 799-800.
63. Linn, M., & Linn, B. (1982). The Rapid Disability Rating Scale-2. *Journal of the American Geriatrics Society, 30*, 378-382.
64. Mahoney, F. I., & Barthel, D. W. (1965). Functional evaluation: the Barthel Index. *Maryland State Medical Journal, 14*, 61-65.
65. Reference deleted in proofs.
66. Marottoli, R. A., Mendes de Leon, C. F., Glass, T. A., et al. (1997). Driving cessation and increased depressive symptoms: prospective evidence from the New Haven Established Populations for Epidemiologic Studies of the Elderly (EPESE). *Journal of the American Geriatrics Society, 45*, 202-206.
67. Mathias, S., Nayak, U. S., & Isaacs, B. (1986). Balance in elderly patients: the "Get Up and Go" test. *Archives of Physical Medicine and Rehabilitation, 67*, 387-389.
68. Reference deleted in proofs.

69. Mauk, K. L. (2006). Introduction to gerontological nursing. In K. L. Mauk (Ed.), *Gerontological nursing: competencies for care* (pp. 5-28). Boston: Jones & Bartlett.
70. McDowell, I., & Newell, C. (1996). *Measuring health: a guide to rating scales and questionnaires* (2nd ed., pp. 47-121). New York: Oxford University Press.
71. Mezey, M. D., Fulmer, T., & Abraham, I. (2003). *Geriatric nursing protocols for best practice* (2nd ed.). New York: Springer Publishing.
72. Milton, D., Porcari, J. P., Foster, C., et al. (2008). The effect of functional exercise training on functional fitness levels of older adults. *Gundersen Lutheran Medical Journal, 5*(1), 4-8.
73. Moore, S. (1998). Spirituality. In A. S. Luggen, S. S. Travis, & S. Meiner (Eds.), *NGNA core curriculum for gerontological advanced practice nurses.* Thousand Oaks, CA: SAGE.
74. Morano, C., & Morano, B. (2006). Social assessment. In J. J. Gallo et al (Eds.), *Handbook of geriatric assessment* (4th ed.). Sudbury, MA: Jones & Bartlett.
75. National Family Caregivers Association (NFCA) and Family Caregiver Alliance (FCA). (2006). *Prevalence, hours and economic value of family caregiving: updated state-by-state analysis of 2004 national estimates.* Kensington, MD: NFCA; and San Francisco: FCA.
76. National Highway Traffic Safety Administration National Center for Statistics and Analysis. (2007). *2007 data—traffic safety facts: older adults* (DOT HS 810 992). Washington, DC: National Highway Traffic Safety Administration.
77. Reference deleted in proofs.
78. Nelson, M. E., Rejeski, J., Blair, S. N., et al. (2007). Physical activity and public health in older adults: recommendations from the American College of Sports Medicine and the American Heart Association. *Circulation, 116*, 1094-1105.
79. Norbeck, J. S., Lindsey, A. M., & Carrieri, V. L. (1980). The development of an instrument to measure social support. *Nursing Research, 30*, 264-269.
80. Norbeck, J. S., Lindsey, A. M., & Carrieri, V. L. (1983). Further development of the Norbeck Social Support Questionnaire: normative data and validity testing. *Nursing Research, 32*, 4-9.
81. Ohayon, M. M., & Vecchierini, M. F. (2005). Normative sleep data, cognitive function and daily living activities in older adults in the community. *Sleep, 289*(8), 981-989.
82. Onega, L. L. (2008). How to try this—helping those who help others: the modified caregiver strain index. *American Journal of Nursing, 108*(9), 62-70.
83. O'Rourke, N., & Tuokko, H. (2000). The psychological and physical costs of caregiving: the Canadian Study of Health and Aging. *Journal of Applied Gerontology, 19*, 389-404.
84. Palmer, R. M., Counsell, S. R., & Landefeld, S. C. (2003). Acute care for elders unit: practical considerations for optimizing health outcomes. *Disease Management and Health Outcomes, 11*(8), 507-517.
85. Pautex, S., & Gold, G. (2006). Assessing pain intensity in older adults. *Geriatrics & Aging, 9*, 399-402.
86. Pearson, V. (2000). Assessment of function. In R. Kane & R. Kane (Eds.), *Assessing older persons: measures, meaning and practical applications* (pp. 17-48). New York: Oxford University Press.
87. Penninx, B. W., Deeg, D. J., van Eijk, J. T., et al. (2000). Changes in depression and physical decline in older adults: a longitudinal perspective. *Journal of Affective Disorders, 61*, 1-12.
88. Penninx, B. W., Rejeski, W. J., Pandya, J., et al. (2002). Exercise and depressive symptoms: a comparison of aerobic and resistance exercise effects on emotional and physical function in older persons with high and low depressive symptomatology. *The Journal of Gerontology. Series B, Psychological Sciences and Social Sciences, 57*, P124-P132.
89. Pinquart, M., & Sorensen, S. (2007). Correlates of physical health of informal caregivers: a meta-analysis. *The Journal of Gerontology. Series B, Psychological Sciences and Social Sciences, 62*(2), 126-137.
89a. Reuben, D. B., et al (Eds.). (2009). *Geriatrics at your fingertips.* New York: The American Geriatrics Society.
90. Reuben, D. B., & Siu, A. L. (1990). An objective measure of physical function of elderly outpatients: the physical performance test. *Journal of the American Geriatrics Society, 38*(10), 1105-1112.
91. Richmond, T., Tang, S. T., Tulman, L., et al. (2004). Measuring function. In M. Frank-Stromberg, & S. J. Olsen (Eds.). *Instruments for clinical health-care research* (3rd ed.). Sudbury, MA: Jones & Bartlett.
92. Sager, M. A., Rudberg, M. A., Jalaluddin, M., et al. (1996). Hospital admission risk profile (HARP): identifying older patients at risk for functional decline following acute medical illness and hospitalization. *Journal of the American Geriatrics Society, 44*(3), 251-257.
92a. Sheikh J. I., & Yesavage J. A. (1986). Geriatric depression scale: Recent evidence and development of a shorter version. *Clinical Gerontology, 5*, 165-172.
93. Smyth, C. A. (2008). Evaluating sleep quality in older adults. *The American Journal of Nursing, 108*(5), 42-51.
94. Stone, R., Cafferate, G. L., & Sangl, J. (1987). Caregivers of the frail elderly: a national profile. *The Gerontologist, 27*, 616-626.
95. Reference deleted in proofs.
96. Sullivan, M. T. (Revised 2007). The modified caregiver strain index (CSI), Try this: best practices in nursing care to older adults. Issue # 14. Retrieved January 5, 2011 from http://consultgerirn.org/uploads/File/trythis/try_this_14.pdf.
97. Thornton, M., & Travis, S. S. (2003). Analysis of the reliability of the modified caregiver strain index. *The Journals of Gerontology. Series B, Psychological Sciences and Social Sciences, 58B*(2), 127-132.
98. Tinetti, M. E. (1986). Performance-oriented assessment of mobility problems on elderly patients. *Journal of the American Geriatrics Society, 34*, 119-126.
99. Tucker, D., Molsberger, S. C., & Clark, A. (2004). Walking for wellness: a collaborative program to maintain mobility in hospitalized older adults. *Geriatric Nursing, 25*(4), 242-245.
100. Reference deleted in proofs.
101. Welch, A. (1996). Cultural influences. In A. G. Lueckenotte (Ed.), *Gerontological nursing.* St. Louis: Mosby.
101a. Yesavage J. A., Brink T. L., & Rose T. L., et al. (1983). Development and validation of a geriatric depression rating scale: a preliminary report. *Journal of Psychiatric Research, 17*, 27.
102. Zarit, S., & Pearlin, L. (1993). Family caregiving: integrating informal and formal systems for care. In S. Zarit, L. Pearlin, & K. Schaie (Eds.), *Caregiving systems: informal and formal helpers* (pp. 303-316). Hillsdale, NJ: L. Erlbaum Associates.

ILLUSTRATION CREDITS

Chapter 1

Figure 1-2: Modified from Alfaro-LeFevre, R. (2009). *Critical thinking and clinical judgment: a practical approach* (4th ed.). Philadelphia: Saunders.

Figure 1-4: From Potter, P.A., & Perry, A.G. (2009). *Fundamentals of nursing* (7th ed.). St. Louis: Mosby.

Chapter 2

Figures 2-2 and 2-3, A-D: Courtesy Rachel E. Spector, 2006.

Figure 2-4: Heritage assessment. From Spector, R.E. (2009). *Cultural diversity in health and illness* (7th ed.). Upper Saddle River, NJ: Prentice Hall.

Figures 2-5, 2-6, A-D, and 2-7, A-D: Courtesy Rachel E. Spector, 2006.

Chapter 4

Figure 4-2: Adapted from The American Society of Human Genetics. (2004). www.ashg.org.

Figure 4-4: The HEEADSSS Psychosocial Interview for Adolescents. Goldenring, J.M., & Rosen, D.S. (2004). Getting into adolescent heads: an essential update. *Contemporary Pediatrics, 21*(1), 64-68, 70, 73-74.

Chapter 5

Figure 5-1: GAD-7. From Kroenke, K. et al. (2007). Anxiety disorders in primary care: prevalence, impairment, comorbidity, and detection. *Annals of Internal Medicine, 146*(5), 317-325.

Chapter 7

Figure 7-1: From Nursing Research Consortium on Violence and Abuse (NRCVA). (1988).

Figure 7-2: From Family Violence Prevention Fund. Retrieved September 2007, from http://endabuse.org/.

Figures 7-3, 7-4, 7-5, 7-6, 7-7, 7-8, and 7-9: Courtesy Daniel J. Sheridan, PhD, RN, CNS. Hanover, MD.

Figure 7-10: Courtesy Jacquelyn C. Campbell, PhD, RN. © 1985, 1988, 2001.

Chapter 8

Figure 8-14: Courtesy *The Pantagraph.* (August 10, 1998). Bloomington, IL.

Chapter 9

Figure 9-2: © Pat Thomas, 2010.

Figure 9-5: © Pat Thomas, 2006.

Figure 9-18: From Rossman, I. (1986). *Clinical geriatrics* (3rd ed.). Philadelphia: Lippincott.

Figure 9-19: From Potter, P.A., & Perry, A.G. (2005). *Fundamentals of nursing* (6th ed.). St. Louis: Mosby.

Art for Table 9-5: (hypopituitary dwarfism) from Hall, R., & Evered, D.C. (1990). *Color atlas of endocrinology* (2nd ed.). London: Mosby; (gigantism) from Hall, R., & Evered, D.C. (1990). *Color atlas of endocrinology* (2nd ed.). London: Mosby; (acromegaly [hyperpituitarism]) reprinted from the Collection on the Rheumatic Diseases. © 1991, 1995, 1997. Used by permission of the American College of Rheumatology; (Marfan's syndrome) from Manusov, E.G., & Martucci, E. (1994). The Marfan syndrome. *Archives of Family Medicine, 3,* 824. © 1994, American Medical Association; (achondroplastic dwarfism) from Jones, A., & Owen, R. (1995). *Color atlas of clinical orthopedics* (2nd ed.). London: Mosby; (anorexia nervosa) courtesy George D. Comerci, MD; (endogenous obesity—Cushing's syndrome) from Wenig, B.M., Heffess, C.S., & Adair, C.F. (1997). *Atlas of endocrine pathology.* Philadelphia: Saunders.

Chapter 10

Figures 10-4, 10-5, and 10-6: From McCaffery, M., & Pasero, C. (1999). *Pain: clinical manual* (2nd ed.). St. Louis: Mosby.

Figure 10-7: From Hicks, C.L. et al. (2001). Faces pain scale—revised: toward a common metric in pediatric pain measurement. *Pain, 93,* 173-183. © 2001 the International Association for the Study of Pain (IASP).

Figure 10-8: From Rick Brady, Riva, MD.

Figure 10-9: From Krechel, S.W., & Bildner, J. (1995). CRIES—a new neonatal postoperative pain measurement score: initial testing of validity and reliability. *Pediatric Anesthesia, 5,* 53-61.

Figure 10-10: Pain Assessment in Advanced Dementia (PAINAD) Scale. Source: Warden, V., Hurley, A.C., & Voticer, L. (2003). Development and psychometric evaluation of the Pain Assessment in Advanced Dementia (PAINAD) Scale. *Journal of the American Medical Directors Association, 4,* 9-15.

Chapter 11

Figure 11-1: Courtesy *The Pantagraph.* (July 15, 2001). Bloomington, IL.

Figure 11-2: Mini Nutritional Assessment (MNA). ®Société des Produits Nestlé S.A., Vevey, Switzerland, Trademark Owners.

Figure 11-3: From U.S. Department of Health and Human Services. (2006). www.MyPyramid.gov.

Art for Table 11-6: (marasmus) from Hall, R., & Evered, D.C. (1990). *Color atlas of endocrinology* (2nd ed.). London: Mosby.

Art for Table 11-7: (pellagra) from Latham, M.C. et al. (1980). *Scope manual on nutrition.* Kalamazoo: The Upjohn Company, © Thomas Spies, MD; (follicular hyperkeratosis) from Taylor, K.B., & Anthony, L.E. (1983). *Clinical nutrition.* New York: McGraw-Hill, © Harold H. Sandstead; (scorbutic gums) from Taylor, K.B., & Anthony, L.E. (1983). *Clinical nutrition.* New York: McGraw-Hill, © The Upjohn Company; (kwashiorkor) from Hall, R., & Evered, D.C. (1990). *Color atlas of endocrinology* (2nd ed.). London: Mosby; (magenta tongue) from McLaren, D.S. (1981). *Color atlas of nutritional disorders.* London: Wolfe Medical, © C.E. Butterworth, Jr; (rickets) from Latham, M.C. et al. (1980). *Scope manual on nutrition.* Kalamazoo: The Upjohn Company, © Rosa Lee Nemir, MD; (HIV infection discordant twins) from Friedman-Kien, A.E. (1989). *Color atlas of AIDS.* Philadelphia: Saunders; (Bitot's spots) from Taylor, K.B., & Anthony, L.E. (1983). *Clinical nutrition.* New York: McGraw-Hill, © Helen Keller International, Inc.

Chapter 12

Figure 12-3, B: From Lookingbill, D.P., & Marks, J.G. (1993). *Principles of dermatology* (2nd ed.). Philadelphia: Saunders.

Figure 12-4, A and B: From Hurwitz, S. (1993). *Clinical pediatric dermatology: a textbook of skin disorders of childhood and adolescence* (2nd ed.). Philadelphia: Saunders.

Figure 12-4, C: From Lookingbill, D.P., & Marks, J.G. (1993). *Principles of dermatology* (2nd ed.). Philadelphia: Saunders.

Figures 12-6, 12-9, 12-10, and 12-12: Courtesy Lemmi & Lemmi, 2011.

Figure 12-13: From Bowden, V.R., Dickey, S.B., & Greenburg, C.S. (1998). *Children and their families: the continuum of care.* Philadelphia: Saunders.

Figures 12-14 and 12-15: From Hurwitz, S. (1993). *Clinical pediatric dermatology: a textbook of skin disorders of childhood and adolescence* (2nd ed.). Philadelphia: Saunders.

Figure 12-16: Courtesy Lemmi & Lemmi, 2011.

Figure 12-17: From Hurwitz, S. (1993). *Clinical pediatric dermatology: a textbook of skin disorders of childhood and adolescence* (2nd ed.). Philadelphia: Saunders.

Figure 12-18: From Murray, S.S., & McKinney, E.S. (2010). *Foundations of maternal-newborn and women's health nursing* (5th ed.). St. Louis: Saunders.

Figure 12-19, A and B: From Habif, T.P. et al. (2005). *Skin disease: diagnosis and treatment* (2nd ed.). Philadelphia: Mosby.

Figure 12-20: From Lookingbill, D.P., & Marks, J.G. (1993). *Principles of dermatology* (2nd ed.). Philadelphia: Saunders.

Figure 12-21: Courtesy Lemmi & Lemmi, 2011.

Figure 12-22: From Habif, T.P. et al. (2001). *Skin disease: diagnosis and treatment.* St. Louis: Mosby.

Figure 12-23: From Lookingbill, D.P., & Marks J.G. (1993). *Principles of dermatology* (2nd ed.). Philadelphia: Saunders.

Figure 12-24: From Callen, J.P. et al. (1993). *Color atlas of dermatology.* Philadelphia: Saunders.

Art for Table 12-4: Line drawings © Pat Thomas, 2010; (macule), (patch), (papule), (plaque), (nodule), (tumor), (wheal), (vesicle), (bulla), (cyst), and (pustule) courtesy Lemmi & Lemmi, 2011; (urticaria) from Fireman, P. (1996). *Atlas of allergies* (2nd ed.). London: Mosby.

Art for Table 12-5: Line drawings © Pat Thomas, 2010; (crust), (scale), (fissure), (erosion), (ulcer), (excoriation), (scar), (atrophic scar), (lichenification), and (keloid) courtesy Lemmi & Lemmi, 2011.

Art for Table 12-6: (pressure ulcers) from Potter, P.A., & Perry, A.G. (2009). *Fundamentals of nursing* (7th ed.). St. Louis: Mosby.

Art for Table 12-8: (port-wine stain [nevus flammeus]) from Paller, A.S., & Mancini, A.J. (2011). *Hurwitz clinical pediatric dermatology: a textbook of skin disorders of childhood and adolescence* (4th ed.). Philadelphia: Saunders; (strawberry mark [immature hemangioma]) from Lookingbill, D.P., & Marks, J.G. (1993). *Principles of dermatology* (2nd ed.). Philadelphia: Saunders; (cavernous hemangioma [mature]) from Habif, T.P. et al. (2005). *Skin disease: diagnosis and treatment* (2nd ed.). St. Louis: Mosby; (telangiectasia) and (spider or star angioma) courtesy Lemmi & Lemmi, 2011; (venous lake) from Habif, T.P. et al. (2001). *Skin disease: diagnosis and treatment.* St. Louis: Mosby; (petechiae) from Dockery, G.L. (1997). *Cutaneous disorders of the lower extremity.* Philadelphia: Saunders; (ecchymosis) courtesy Lemmi & Lemmi, 2011; (purpura) from Paller, A.S., & Mancini, A.J. (2011). *Hurwitz clinical pediatric dermatology: a textbook of skin disorders of childhood and adolescence* (4th ed.). Philadelphia: Saunders.

Art for Table 12-9: (diaper dermatitis) from Paller, A.S., & Mancini, A.J. (2011). *Hurwitz clinical pediatric dermatology: a textbook of skin disorders of childhood and adolescence* (4th ed.). Philadelphia: Saunders; (intertrigo [candidiasis]) and (impetigo) courtesy Lemmi & Lemmi, 2011; (atopic dermatitis [eczema]) from Paller, A.S., & Mancini, A.J. (2011). *Hurwitz clinical pediatric dermatology: a textbook of skin disorders of childhood and adolescence* (4th ed.). Philadelphia: Saunders; (measles [rubeola] in dark skin) from Feigin, R.D. et al. (2009). *Feigin and Cherry's textbook of pediatric infectious diseases* (6th ed.). Philadelphia: Saunders; (measles [rubeola] in light skin) courtesy Lemmi & Lemmi, 2011; (German measles [rubella]) from Paller, A.S., & Mancini, A.J. (2011). *Hurwitz clinical pediatric dermatology: a textbook of skin disorders of childhood and adolescence* (4th ed.). Philadelphia: Saunders; (chickenpox [varicella]) from Callen, J.P. et al. (1993). *Color atlas of dermatology.* Philadelphia: Saunders.

Art for Table 12-10: (primary contact dermatitis) and (allergic drug reaction) from Lookingbill, D.P., & Marks, J.G.

(1993). *Principles of dermatology* (2nd ed.). Philadelphia: Saunders; (tinea corporis [ringworm of the body]) from Paller, A.S., & Mancini, A.J. (2011). *Hurwitz clinical pediatric dermatology: a textbook of skin disorders of childhood and adolescence* (4th ed.). Philadelphia: Saunders; (tinea pedis [ringworm of the foot]), (labial herpes simplex [cold sores]), (tinea versicolor), and (herpes zoster [shingles]) courtesy Lemmi & Lemmi, 2011; (erythema migrans of Lyme disease) from Swartz, M.H. (2005). *Textbook of physical diagnosis: history and examination* (5th ed.). Philadelphia: Saunders; (psoriasis) from Lookingbill, D.P., & Marks, J.G. (1993). *Principles of dermatology* (2nd ed.). Philadelphia: Saunders.

Art for Table 12-11: (basal cell carcinoma) from Lookingbill, D.P., & Marks, J.G. (1993). *Principles of dermatology* (2nd ed.). Philadelphia: Saunders; (squamous cell carcinoma) from Habif, T.P. et al. (2001). *Skin disease: diagnosis and treatment.* St. Louis: Mosby; (malignant melanoma) from Lookingbill, D.P., & Marks, J.G. (1993). *Principles of dermatology* (2nd ed.). Philadelphia: Saunders; (metastatic malignant melanoma) courtesy Lemmi & Lemmi, 2011.

Art for Table 12-12: (AIDs-related Kaposi sarcoma: patch stage) from Friedman-Kien, A.E. (1989). *Color atlas of AIDS.* Philadelphia: Saunders; (toxic alopecia) from Hurwitz, S. (1993). *Clinical pediatric dermatology: a textbook of skin disorders of childhood and adolescence* (2nd ed.). Philadelphia: Saunders; (tinea capitis [scalp ringworm]) from Lookingbill, D.P., & Marks, J.G. (1993). *Principles of dermatology* (2nd ed.). Philadelphia: Saunders; (alopecia areata), (traumatic alopecia: traction alopecia), and (seborrheic dermatitis [cradle cap]) from Hurwitz, S. (1993). *Clinical pediatric dermatology: a textbook of skin disorders of childhood and adolescence* (2nd ed.). Philadelphia: Saunders; (pediculosis capitis [head lice]) and (trichotillomania) from Callen, J.P. et al. (1993). *Color atlas of dermatology.* Philadelphia: Saunders; (hirsutism) from Wenig, B.M., Heffess, C.S., & Adair, C.F. (1997). *Atlas of endocrine pathology.* Philadelphia: Saunders; (furuncle and abscess) from Lookingbill, D.P., & Marks, J.G. (1993). *Principles of dermatology* (2nd ed.). Philadelphia: Saunders.

Art for Table 12-13: (scabies) and (paronychia) courtesy Lemmi & Lemmi, 2011; (Beau's line) and (splinter hemorrhages) from Callen, J.P. et al. (1993). *Color atlas of dermatology.* Philadelphia: Saunders; (onycholysis) courtesy Lemmi & Lemmi, 2011; (late clubbing) reprinted from the Clinical Slide Collection on the Rheumatic Diseases. ©1991, 1995, 1997. Used by permission of the American College of Rheumatology; (pitting) and (habit-tic dystrophy) courtesy Lemmi & Lemmi, 2011.

Chapter 13

Figure 13-8: © Pat Thomas, 2006.

Figure 13-14, B: Courtesy Lemmi & Lemmi, 2011.

Figures 13-16 and 13-17, A: From Murray, S.S., & McKinney, E.S. (2010). *Foundations of maternal-newborn and women's health nursing* (5th ed.). St. Louis: Saunders.

Art for Table 13-2: (hydrocephalus) from Bowden, V.R., Dickey, S.B., & Greenburg, C.S. (1998). *Children and their families: the continuum of care.* Philadelphia: Saunders; (Paget's disease of bone [osteitis deformans]) reprinted from the Clinical Slide Collection on the Rheumatic Diseases. © 1991, 1995, 1997. Used by permission of the American College of Rheumatology; (acromegaly) from Damjanov, I. (1996). *Pathology for the health-related professions.* Philadelphia: Saunders.

Art for Table 13-3: (torticollis [wryneck]) from Zitelli, B.J., & Davis, H.W. (2007). *Atlas of pediatric physical diagnosis* (5th ed.). St. Louis: Mosby; (goiter) courtesy Lemmi & Lemmi, 2011; (thyroid—multiple nodules) from Swartz, M.H. (2005). *Textbook of physical diagnosis: history and examination* (5th ed.). Philadelphia: Saunders; (pilar cyst [wen]) from Callen, J.P. et al. (1993). *Color atlas of dermatology.* Philadelphia: Saunders; (parotid gland enlargement) from Swartz, M.H. (2005). *Textbook of physical diagnosis: history and examination* (5th ed.). Philadelphia: Saunders.

Art for Table 13-4: (fetal alcohol syndrome) from Streissguth, A.P. et al. (1980). Teratogenic effects of alcohol in humans and laboratory animals. *Science, 209,* 353-361. Illustration © Pat Thomas, 2006; (congenital hypothyroidism) from Zitelli, B.J., & Davis, H.W. (2007). *Atlas of pediatric physical diagnosis* (5th ed.). St. Louis: Mosby, courtesy Dr. Thomas P. Foley, Jr.; (Down syndrome), (atopic [allergic] facies), and (allergic salute and crease) from Zitelli, B.J., & Davis, H.W. (2007). *Atlas of pediatric physical diagnosis* (5th ed.). St. Louis: Mosby.

Art for Table 13-5: (Cushing's syndrome) from Zitelli, B.J., & Davis, H.W. (2007). *Atlas of pediatric physical diagnosis* (5th ed.). St. Louis: Mosby; (hyperthyroidism) from Swartz, M.H. (2005). *Textbook of physical diagnosis: history and examination* (5th ed.). Philadelphia: Saunders; (myxedema [hypothyroidism]) from Hall R., & Evered, D.C. (1990). *Color atlas of endocrinology* (2nd ed.). London: Mosby; (Bell's palsy [right side]) from Swartz, M.H. (2005). *Textbook of physical diagnosis: history and examination* (5th ed.). Philadelphia: Saunders; (cachectic appearance) courtesy Lemmi & Lemmi, 2011; (scleroderma) reprinted from the Clinical Slide Collection on the Rheumatic Diseases. © 1991, 1995, 1997. Used by permission of the American College of Rheumatology.

Chapter 14

Figures 14-1, 14-3, 14-4, and 14-19: © Pat Thomas, 2006.

Figures 14-23: Courtesy Heather Boyd-Monk and Wills Eye Hospital, Philadelphia.

Figures 14-24 and 14-25: Courtesy Lemmi & Lemmi, 2011.

Figure 14-30: From Zitelli, B.J., & Davis, H.W. (2007). *Atlas of pediatric physical diagnosis* (5th ed.). St. Louis: Mosby.

Figure 14-31: From Albert, D.M., & Jakobiec, F.A. (1994). *Principles and practice of ophthalmology.* Philadelphia: Saunders.

Figure 14-32: Courtesy Lemmi & Lemmi, 2011.

Figure 14-33: From Swartz, M.H. (2005). *Textbook of physical diagnosis: history and examination* (5th ed.). Philadelphia: Saunders.

Figure 14-34: Courtesy Lemmi & Lemmi, 2011.

Figure 14-35: From Friedman, N., & Pineda, R. (1998). *The Massachusetts eye and ear infirmary illustrated manual of ophthalmology.* Philadelphia: Saunders.

Art in Table 14-1: (**A,** pseudostrabismus), (**B,** esotropia), and (**C,** exotropia) from Zitelli, B.J., & Davis, H.W. (2007). *Atlas of pediatric physical diagnosis* (5th ed.). St. Louis: Mosby.

Art in Table 14-2: (periorbital edema) from Ibsen, O.A.C., & Phelan, J.A. (1992). *Oral pathology for the dental hygienist* (2nd ed.). Philadelphia: Saunders; (exophthalmos [protruding eye]) and (ptosis [drooping upper lip]) courtesy Lemmi & Lemmi, 2011; (upward palpebral slant) from Zitelli, B.J., & Davis, H.W. (2007). *Atlas of pediatric physical diagnosis* (5th ed.). St. Louis: Mosby; (ectropion) and (entropion) from Albert, D.M., & Jakobiec, F.A. (1994). *Principles and practice of ophthalmology* (vol. 3). Philadelphia: Saunders.

Art in Table 14-3: (blepharitis [inflammation of the eyelids]) from Friedman, N., & Pineda, R. (1998). *The Massachusetts eye and ear infirmary illustrated manual of ophthalmology.* Philadelphia: Saunders; (chalazion) courtesy Heather Boyd-Monk and Wills Eye Hospital, Philadelphia; (hordeolum [stye]) courtesy Lemmi & Lemmi, 2011; (dacryocystitis [inflammation of the lacrimal sac]) from Friedman, N., & Pineda, R. (1998). *The Massachusetts eye and ear infirmary illustrated manual of ophthalmology.* Philadelphia: Saunders; (basal cell carcinoma) from Scheie, H.G., & Albert, D.M. (1977). *Textbook of ophthalmology* (9th ed.). Philadelphia: Saunders.

Art in Table 14-6: (conjunctivitis) and (subconjunctival hemorrhage) courtesy Lemmi & Lemmi, 2011; (iritis [circumcorneal redness]) and (acute glaucoma) from Scheie, H.G., & Albert, D.M. (1977). *Textbook of ophthalmology* (9th ed.). Philadelphia: Saunders.

Art in Table 14-7: (pterygium) courtesy Lemmi & Lemmi, 2011; (corneal abrasion) courtesy Heather Boyd-Monk and Wills Eye Hospital, Philadelphia; (hyphema) courtesy Lemmi & Lemmi, 2011; (hypopyon) from Scheie, H.G., & Albert, D.M. (1977). *Textbook of ophthalmology* (9th ed.). Philadelphia: Saunders.

Art in Table 14-8: (central gray opacity—nuclear cataract) and (star-shaped opacity—cortical cataract) from Friedman, N., & Pineda, R. (1998). *The Massachusetts eye and ear infirmary illustrated manual of ophthalmology.* Philadelphia: Saunders.

Art in Table 14-9: (optic atrophy [disc pallor]), (papilledema [choked disc]), and (excessive cup-disc ratio) from Friedman, N., Kaiser, P.K., & Pineda, R. (2009). *The Massachusetts eye and ear infirmary illustrated manual of ophthalmology* (3rd ed.). Philadelphia: Saunders.

Art in Table 14-10: (arteriovenous crossing [nicking]) from Friedman, N., Kaiser, P.K., & Pineda, R. (2009). *The Massachusetts eye and ear infirmary illustrated manual of ophthalmology* (3rd ed.). Philadelphia: Saunders; (narrowed [attenuated] arteries, 14 years and 61 years) and (microaneurysms) courtesy Lemmi & Lemmi, 2011; (intraretinal hemorrhages) from Friedman, N., Kaiser, P.K., & Pineda, R. (2009). *The Massachusetts eye and ear infirmary illustrated manual of ophthalmology* (3rd ed.). Philadelphia: Saunders; (exudates) courtesy Lemmi & Lemmi, 2011.

Chapter 15

Figure 15-1: Courtesy Lemmi & Lemmi, 2011.

Figure 15-2: © Pat Thomas, 2010

Figure 15-4: © Pat Thomas, 2006.

Figure 15-9: Courtesy Lemmi & Lemmi, 2011.

Figure 15-10: © Pat Thomas, 2006.

Art for Table 15-1: (frostbite) reprinted from the Clinical Slide Collection on the Rheumatic Diseases. © 1991, 1995, 1997. Used by permission of the American College of Rheumatology; (otitis externa—swimmer's ear) courtesy Lemmi & Lemmi, 2011; (branchial remnant and ear deformity) from Liebert, P.S. (1996). *Color atlas of pediatric surgery* (2nd ed.). Philadelphia: Saunders; (cellulitis) courtesy Lemmi & Lemmi, 2011.

Art for Table 15-2: (sebaceous cyst) from Liebert, P.S. (1996). *Color atlas of pediatric surgery* (2nd ed.). Philadelphia: Saunders; (tophi) reprinted from the Clinical Slide Collection on the Rheumatic Diseases. © 1991, 1995, 1997. Used by permission of the American College of Rheumatology; (chondrodermatitis nodularis helicis) from Habif, T.P. et al. (2005). *Skin disease: diagnosis and treatment* (2nd ed.). St. Louis: Mosby; (keloid) courtesy Lemmi & Lemmi, 2011; (carcinoma) from Callen, J.P. et al. (1993). *Color atlas of dermatology.* Philadelphia: Saunders.

Art for Table 15-3: © Pat Thomas, 2010.

Art for Table 15-5: (retracted drum) from Adams, G.L., Boies, L.R., & Hilger, P.A. (1989). *Boies fundamentals of otolaryngology: a textbook of ear, nose, and throat diseases* (6th ed.). Philadelphia: Saunders; (otitis media with effusion [OME]) from Swartz, M.H. (2005). *Textbook of physical diagnosis: history and examination* (5th ed.). Philadelphia: Saunders; (acute purulent otitis media—early stage) and (acute purulent otitis media—later stage) from Adams, G.L., Boies, L.R., & Hilger, P.A. (1989). *Boies fundamentals of otolaryngology: a textbook of ear, nose, and throat diseases* (6th ed.). Philadelphia: Saunders; (perforation) from Swartz, M.H. (2005). *Textbook of physical diagnosis: history and examination* (5th ed.). Philadelphia: Saunders; (insertion of tympanostomy tubes) from Fireman, P. (1996). *Atlas of allergies* (2nd ed.). London: Mosby; (cholesteatoma) and (bullous myringitis) from Swartz, M.H. (2005). *Textbook of physical diagnosis: history and examination* (5th ed.). Philadelphia: Saunders; (scarred drum), (blue drum), and (fungal infection) © Pat Thomas, 2010.

Chapter 16

Figures 16-1, 16-2, and 16-3: © Pat Thomas, 2006.
Figures 16-4 and 16-5: © Pat Thomas, 2010.
Figure 16-6: © Pat Thomas, 2006.
Figure 16-9: From Fireman, P. (1996). *Atlas of allergies* (2nd ed.). London: Mosby.
Figure 16-16: From Ibsen, O.A.C., & Phelan, J.A. (1996). *Oral pathology for the dental hygienist* (2nd ed.). Philadelphia: Saunders.
Figure 16-17: Courtesy Lemmi & Lemmi, 2011.
Figure 16-18: © Pat Thomas, 2006.
Figure 16-22: From Zitelli, B.J., & Davis, H.W. (2007). *Atlas of pediatric physical diagnosis* (5th ed.). St. Louis: Mosby.
Figures 16-23 and 16-24: Courtesy Lemmi & Lemmi, 2011.
Art for Table 16-1: (foreign body) from Fireman, P. (1996). *Atlas of allergies* (2nd ed.). London: Mosby; (perforated septum) from Hawke, M. (1998). *Diagnostic handbook of otorhinolaryngology.* London: Martin Dunitz; (acute rhinitis), (allergic rhinitis), and (nasal polyps) from Fireman, P. (1996). *Atlas of allergies* (2nd ed.). London: Mosby.
Art for Table 16-2: (cleft lip) from Ibsen, O.A.C., & Phelan, J.A. (1996). *Oral pathology for the dental hygienist* (2nd ed.). Philadelphia: Saunders; (herpes simplex 1) and (angular cheilitis [stomatitis, perlèche]) from Callen, J.P. et al. (1993). *Color atlas of dermatology.* Philadelphia: Saunders; (carcinoma) and (retention "cyst" [mucocele]) from Hawke, M. (1998). *Diagnostic handbook of otorhinolaryngology.* London: Martin Dunitz.
Art for Table 16-3: (baby bottle tooth decay) courtesy F. Ferguson, Department of Children's Dentistry, School of Dental Medicine, SUNY at Stony Brook, Stony Brook, NY 11733; (dental caries) courtesy A. McWhorter, Pediatric Dentistry, Baylor College of Dentistry, The Texas A & M University System, Dallas, TX; (epulis) and (gingival hyperplasia) from Ibsen, O.A.C., & Phelan, J.A. (1996). *Oral pathology for the dental hygienist* (2nd ed.). Philadelphia: Saunders; (gingivitis) from Callen, J.P. et al. (1993). *Color atlas of dermatology.* Philadelphia: Saunders; (meth mouth) from Neville, B.W. et al. (2009). *Oral and maxillofacial pathology* (3rd ed.). St. Louis: Saunders.
Art for Table 16-4: (aphthous ulcers) courtesy Lemmi & Lemmi, 2011; (Koplik spots) from Feigin, R.D., & Cherry, J.D. (1998). *Textbook of pediatric infectious diseases* (4th ed.). Philadelphia: Saunders; (leukoplakia) from Sleisinger, M.H., & Fordtran, J.S. (1993). *Gastrointestinal diseases: pathophysiology, diagnosis, and management* (5th ed., vol. 1). Philadelphia: Saunders; (candidiasis or monilial infection) from Callen, J.P. et al. (1993). *Color atlas of dermatology.* Philadelphia: Saunders (herpes simplex 1) courtesy Lemmi & Lemmi, 2011.
Art for Table 16-5: (ankyloglossia) from Ibsen, O.A.C., & Phelan, J.A. (1996). *Oral pathology for the dental hygienist* (2nd ed.). Philadelphia: Saunders; (geographic tongue [migratory glossitis]) courtesy Lemmi & Lemmi, 2011; (smooth, glossy tongue [atrophic glossitis]) from Adams, G.L., Boies, L.R., & Hilger, P.A. (1989). *Boies fundamentals of otolaryngology: a textbook of ear, nose, and throat diseases* (6th ed.). Philadelphia: Saunders; (black hairy tongue) from Callen, J.P. et al. (1993). *Color atlas of dermatology.* Philadelphia: Saunders; (fissured or scrotal tongue) courtesy Lemmi & Lemmi, 2011; (carcinoma) from Wenig, B.M., Heffess, C.S., & Adair, C.F. (1997). *Atlas of endocrine pathology.* Philadelphia: Saunders; (enlarged tongue [macroglossia]) from Zitelli, B.J., & Davis, H.W. (2002). *Atlas of pediatric physical diagnosis* (4th ed.). St. Louis: Mosby, courtesy Dr. Christine Williams.
Art for Table 16-6: (cleft palate) from Zitelli, B.J., & Davis, H.W. (2002). *Atlas of pediatric physical diagnosis* (4th ed.). St. Louis: Mosby, courtesy Dr. Michael Sherlock; (bifid uvula) from Hawke, M. (1998). *Diagnostic handbook of otorhinolaryngology,* London: Martin Dunitz; (oral Kaposi's sarcoma) from Friedman-Kien, A.E. (1989). *Color atlas of AIDS.* Philadelphia: Saunders; (acute tonsillitis and pharyngitis) courtesy Lemmi & Lemmi, 2011.

Chapter 17

Figures 17-1 and 17-2: © Pat Thomas, 2010.
Figure 17-6: Redrawn from Tanner, J.M. (1962). *Growth at adolescence.* Oxford: Blackwell Scientific.
Figure 17-8: From Callen, J.P. et al. (1993). *Color atlas of dermatology.* Philadelphia: Saunders.
Figure 17-21: From Moore, K.L., & Persaud, T.V.N. (2008). *Before we are born: essentials of embryology and birth defects* (7th ed.). Philadelphia: Saunders.
Art for Table 17-3: (dimpling) from Evans, A.J. et al. (1998). *Atlas of breast disease management: 50 illustrative cases.* Philadelphia: Saunders; (edema [peau d'orange]) from Mansel, R. (1995). *Color atlas of breast diseases.* London: Mosby; (fixation) and (deviation in nipple pointing) from Mansel, R. (1995). *Color atlas of breast diseases.* London: Mosby.
Art for Table 17-6: (mammary duct ectasia) from Mansel, R. (1995). *Color atlas of breast diseases.* London: Mosby; (carcinoma) from Evans, A.J. et al. (1998). *Atlas of breast disease management: 50 illustrative cases.* Philadelphia: Saunders; (intraductal papilloma) and (Paget's disease [intraductal carcinoma]) from Mansel, R. (1995). *Color atlas of breast diseases.* London: Mosby.
Art for Table 17-7: (mastitis) and (breast abscess) from Mansel, R. (1995). *Color atlas of breast diseases.* London: Mosby.
Art for Table 17-8: (gynecomastia) courtesy Lemmi & Lemmi, 2011; (male breast cancer) from Haagensen, C.D. (1986). *Diseases of the breast* (3rd ed.). Philadelphia: Saunders.

Chapter 18

Figures 18-1, 18-2, and 18-10: © Pat Thomas, 2010.
Figure 18-11: © Pat Thomas, 2006.
Figure 18-12: From Nichols, F.H., & Zwelling, E. (1997). *Maternal-newborn nursing: theory and practice.* Philadelphia: Saunders.

Chapter 19

Figures 19-2, 19-3, 19-4, 19-8, and 19-9: © Pat Thomas, 2006.
Figure 19-15: From Lakatta, E.G. (1985). Cardiovascular function in later life. *Cardiovascular Medicine, 10,* 37-40.
Art for Promoting a Healthy Lifestyle box: From *The heart truth: awareness and prevention.* www.4women.gov/hearttruth.
Art for Tables 19-8, 19-9, and 19-10: © Pat Thomas, 2006.

Chapter 20

Figures 20-1, 20-2, 20-3, and 20-5: © Pat Thomas, 2010.
Figure 20-7: From Kliegman, R.M. et al. (2007). *Nelson textbook of pediatrics* (18th ed.). Philadelphia: Saunders.
Figure 20-20, B: From Bloom, A., Watkins, P.H., & Ireland, J. (1992). *Color atlas of diabetes* (2nd ed.). St. Louis: Mosby.
Figure 20-21: © Pat Thomas, 2006.
Figure 20-23, B: Courtesy Lemmi & Lemmi, 2011.
Art for Table 20-2: (Raynaud's phenomenon) and (hand cyanosis) courtesy Lemmi & Lemmi, 2011; (lymphedema) from Walsh, T.D. et al. (2009). *Palliative medicine.* Philadelphia: Saunders.
Art for Table 20-4: (arterial-ischemic ulcer) from Dockery, G.L. (1997). *Cutaneous disorders of the lower extremity.* Philadelphia: Saunders; (venous [stasis] ulcer) from Lookingbill, D.P., & Marks, J.G. (1993). *Principles of dermatology.* (2nd ed.). Philadelphia: Saunders; (diabetes) courtesy Lemmi & Lemmi, 2011.
Art for Table 20-5: (superficial varicose veins) courtesy Lemmi & Lemmi, 2011; (deep vein thrombophlebitis [DVT]) from Dockery, G.L. (1997). *Cutaneous disorders of the lower extremity.* Philadelphia: Saunders.

Chapter 21

Figures 21-1, 21-2, 21-3, and 21-4: © Pat Thomas, 2006.
Art for Table 21-2: © Pat Thomas, 2006.
Art for Table 21-3: (umbilical hernia) from Zitelli, B.J., & Davis, H.W. (2007). *Atlas of pediatric physical diagnosis* (5th ed.). St. Louis: Mosby, courtesy Dr. Thomas P. Foley, Jr; (incisional hernia) courtesy Lemmi & Lemmi, 2011.

Chapter 22

Figure 22-2: © Pat Thomas, 2006.
Figures 22-32, C and 22-33, B: From Dieppe, P.A., Cooper, C., & McGill, N. (1991). *Arthritis and rheumatism in practice.* London: Gower Medical Publishing.
Figure 22-37: Courtesy Lemmi & Lemmi, 2011.
Figure 22-50: From Zitelli, B.J., & Davis, H.W. (2007). *Atlas of pediatric physical diagnosis* (5th ed.). St. Louis: Mosby.
Figures 22-51, B and 22-54: Courtesy Lemmi & Lemmi, 2011.
Art for Table 22-2 (atrophy), (dislocated shoulder), and (joint effusion) from Bunker, T., & Schranz, P.J. (1998). *Clinical challenges in orthopaedics: the shoulder.* London: Martin Dunitz; (tear of rotator cuff) and (frozen shoulder—adhesive capsulitis) from Polley, H.F., & Hunder, G.G. (1978). *Physical examination of the joints* (2nd ed.). Philadelphia: Saunders.
Art for Table 22-3: (olecranon bursitis) from Dieppe, P.A., Cooper, C., & McGill, N. (1991). *Arthritis and rheumatism in practice.* London: Gower Medical Publishing; (gouty arthritis) from Polley, H.F., & Hunder, G.G. (1978). *Physical examination of the joints* (2nd ed.). Philadelphia: Saunders; (subcutaneous nodules) from Callen, J.P. et al. (1983). *Color atlas of dermatology.* Philadelphia: Saunders; (epicondylitis—tennis elbow) from Jones, A., & Owen, R. (1995). *Color atlas of clinical orthopedics* (2nd ed.). London: Mosby.
Art for Table 22-4: (ganglion cyst) from Callen, J.P. et al. (1993). *Color atlas of dermatology.* Philadelphia: Saunders; (carpal tunnel syndrome with atrophy of thenar eminence) reprinted from the Clinical Slide Collection on the Rheumatic Diseases. © 1991, 1995, 1997. Used by permission of the American College of Rheumatology; (ankylosis) from Polley, H.F., & Hunder, G.G. (1978). *Physical examination of the joints* (2nd ed.). Philadelphia: Saunders; (Dupuytren's contracture) and (swan-neck and boutonnière deformity) reprinted from the Clinical Slide Collection on the Rheumatic Diseases. © 1991, 1995, 1997. Used by permission of the American College of Rheumatology; (ulnar deviation or drift) and (degenerative joint disease or osteoarthritis) from Walker, J.M., & Helewa, A. (1996). *Physical therapy in arthritis.* Philadelphia: Saunders; (syndactyly) and (polydactyly) from Liebert, P.S. (1996). *Color atlas of pediatric surgery* (2nd ed.). Philadelphia: Saunders; (gout in thumb) courtesy Lemmi & Lemmi, 2011.
Art for Table 22-5: (swelling of menisci) from Jones, A., & Owen, R. (1995). *Color atlas of clinical orthopedics* (2nd ed.). London: Mosby; (mild synovitis) and (prepatellar bursitis) from Dieppe, P.A., Cooper, C., & McGill, N. (1991). *Arthritis and rheumatism in practice.* London: Gower Medical Publishing; (Osgood-Schlatter disease) from Zitelli, B.J., & Davis, H.W. (2002). *Atlas of pediatric physical diagnosis* (4th ed.). St. Louis: Mosby; (post polio muscle atrophy) courtesy Lemmi & Lemmi, 2011.
Art for Table 22-6: (Achilles tenosynovitis) from Dieppe, P.A., Cooper, C., & McGill, N. (1991). *Arthritis and rheumatism in practice.* London: Gower Medical Publishing; (tophi with chronic gout) from Dockery, G.L. (1997). *Cutaneous disorders of the lower extremity.* Philadelphia: Saunders; (acute gout) from Dieppe, P.A., Cooper, C., & McGill, N. (1991). *Arthritis and rheumatism in practice.* London: Gower Medical Publishing; (hallux valgus with bunion and hammertoes) from Walker, J.M., & Helewa, A. (1996). *Physical therapy in arthritis.* Philadelphia: Saunders; (callus), (ingrown toenail), and (plantar wart) courtesy Lemmi & Lemmi, 2011.
Art for Table 22-7: (scoliosis [*top*]) courtesy Lemmi & Lemmi, 2011; (scoliosis [*bottom*]) from Zitelli, B.J., & Davis, H.W. (2002). *Atlas of pediatric physical diagnosis* (4th ed.). St. Louis: Mosby; (herniated nucleus pulposus) from Polley,

H.F., & Hunder, G.G. (1978). *Physical examination of the joints* (2nd ed.). Philadelphia: Saunders.

Art for Table 22-8: (congenital dislocated hip) from Zitelli, B.J., & Davis, H.W. (2002). *Atlas of pediatric physical diagnosis* (4th ed.). St. Louis: Mosby; (talipes equinovarus [clubfoot]) from A.E. Chudley, MD; (spina bifida) from Walsh, P.C. et al. (1986). *Campbell's urology* (5th ed.). Philadelphia: Saunders.

Art for Table 22-9: © Pat Thomas, 2010.

Chapter 23

Figures 23-1, 23-2, 23-3, and 23-4: © Pat Thomas, 2006.

Figure 23-5: © Pat Thomas, 2010.

Figure 23-7: © Pat Thomas, 2006.

Figure 23-53, B: From Fenichel, G.M. (1988). *Clinical pediatric neurology.* Philadelphia: Saunders.

Figure 23-59: From Hickey, J.V. (1986). *Neurological and neurosurgical nursing* (2nd ed.). Philadelphia: Lippincott.

Art for Tables 23-10 and 23-12: © Pat Thomas, 2006.

Chapter 24

Figures 24-1, 24-2, and 24-3: © Pat Thomas, 2010.

Figure 24-4: Redrawn from Marshall, W.A., & Tanner, J.M. (1970). Variations in the pattern of pubertal changes in boys. *Archives of Disease in Childhood, 45,* 22.

Unnumbered figure of urine color changes: Courtesy Connie Cooper.

Figure 24-10, B: Courtesy Lemmi & Lemmi, 2011.

Art for Table 24-3: (urethritis [urethral discharge and dysuria]) from Edmond, R. (1995). *Colour atlas of infectious diseases* (3rd ed., p. 161). St. Louis: Mosby.

Art for Table 24-4: (tinea cruris) courtesy Lemmi & Lemmi, 2011; (genital herpes—HSV-2 infection) courtesy Pfizer Laboratories Division, Pfizer Inc, New York. From *A close look at VD: a slide presentation produced as a public service;* (genital warts) from Habif, T.P. et al. (2005). *Skin disease: diagnosis and treatment* (2nd ed.). St. Louis: Mosby; (syphilitic chancre) from Emond, R.T., Rowl, H.A.K., & Welsby, P. (1995). *Color atlas of infectious diseases* (3rd ed.). London: Mosby; (carcinoma) from Callen, J.P. et al. (1993). *Color atlas of dermatology.* Philadelphia: Saunders.

Art for Table 24-5: (phimosis) and (hypospadias) from Liebert, P.S. (1996). *Color atlas of pediatric surgery* (2nd ed.). Philadelphia: Saunders; (epispadias) from Zitelli, B.J., & Davis, H.W. (2002). *Atlas of pediatric physical diagnosis* (4th ed.). St. Louis: Mosby; (Peyronie's disease) courtesy Dr. Hans Stricker, Department of Urology, Henry Ford Hospital, Detroit, MI.

Art for Tables 24-6 and 24-7: © Pat Thomas, 2006.

Chapter 25

Figure 25-1: © Pat Thomas, 2010.

Chapter 26

Figure 26-13, A: Courtesy Lemmi & Lemmi, 2011.

Art for Table 26-2: (pediculosis pubis [crab lice]) from Callen, J.P. et al. (1993). *Color atlas of dermatology.* Philadelphia: Saunders; (herpes simplex virus—type 2 [herpes genitalis]) courtesy Lemmi & Lemmi, 2011; (syphilitic chancre) from Emond, R.T., Rowl, H.A.K., & Welsby, P. (1995). *Colour atlas of infectious diseases* (3rd ed.). London: Mosby; (red rash—contact dermatitis) courtesy Pfizer Laboratories Division, Pfizer Inc, New York. From *A close look at VD: a slide presentation produced as a public service;* (human papillomavirus [HPV] genital warts]) from Habif, T.P. et al. (2001). *Skin disease: diagnosis and treatment.* St. Louis: Mosby; (abscess of Bartholin's gland) from Emond, R.T., Rowl, H.A.K., & Welsby, P. (1995). *Color atlas of infectious diseases* (3rd ed.). London: Mosby; (urethral caruncle) from Rimsza, M.E. (1989). An illustrated guide to adolescent gynecology. *Pediatric Clinics of North America, 36*(3), 641.

Art for Table 26-3: (cystocele) courtesy Lemmi & Lemmi, 2011; (uterine prolapse) from Symonds, E.M., & McPherson, M.B.A. (1997). *Diagnosis in color: obstetrics and gynecology.* London: Mosby-Wolfe.

Art for Table 26-4: (human papillomavirus [HPV, condylomata]) from Symonds, E.M., & McPherson, M.B.A. (1997). *Diagnosis in color: obstetrics and gynecology.* London: Mosby-Wolfe; (polyp) courtesy Lemmi & Lemmi, 2011; (carcinoma) from Symonds, E.M., & McPherson, M.B.A. (1997). *Diagnosis in color: obstetrics and gynecology.* London: Mosby-Wolfe.

Art for Table 26-5: (candidiasis [moniliasis]) courtesy Lemmi & Lemmi, 2011; (gonorrhea) courtesy Pfizer Laboratories Division, Pfizer Inc, New York. From *A close look at VD: a slide presentation produced as a public service.*

Art for Table 26-8: (ambiguous genitalia) from Moore, K.L., & Persaud, T.V.N. (1998). *Before we are born: essentials of embryology and birth defects* (5th ed.). Philadelphia: Saunders; (vulvovaginitis in child) from Feigin, R.D., & Cherry, J.D. (1998). *Textbook of pediatric infectious diseases* (4th ed.). Philadelphia: Saunders.

Chapter 28

Art for unnumbered figures, center and bottom page 792 from Sorrentino, S.A. (2011). *Mosby's textbook for long-term care nursing assistants* (6th ed.). St. Louis: Mosby.

Chapter 29

Figures 29-4 and 29-13: From Symonds, E.M., & McPherson, M.B.A. (1997). *Diagnosis in color: obstetrics and gynecology.* London: Mosby-Wolfe.

Art for Table 29-2: (preeclampsia) from Symonds, E.M., & McPherson, M.B.A. (1997). *Diagnosis in color: obstetrics and gynecology.* London: Mosby-Wolfe.

Art for Table 29-3: (fetal macrosomia) from Symonds, E.M., & McPherson, M.B.A. (1997). *Diagnosis in color: obstetrics and gynecology.* London: Mosby-Wolfe.

Chapter 30

Figure 30-2: Adapted from Gerontological Society of America, Katz, S. et al. (1970). Progress in the development of the index of ADL. *Gerontologist, 10,* 20-30.

Figure 30-3: From Lawton, M.P., & Brody, E.M. (1969). Assessment of older people: self-maintaining and instrumental activities of daily living, *Gerontologist, 9,* 179-186. © The Gerontological Society of America.

Figure 30-4: Hospital Admission Risk Profile (HARP). From Sager, M.A. et al. (1996). Hospital admission risk profile (HARP): identifying older patients at risk for functional decline following acute medical illness and hospitalization. *Journal of the American Geriatrics Society, 44*(3), 251-257.

Figure 30-5: Geriatric Depression Scale (Short Form). Adapted from Sheikh, J.I., & Yesavage, J.A. (1986). Geriatric depression scale (GDS): recent evidence and development of a shorter version. In T.L. Brink, *Clinical gerontology: a guide to assessment and intervention* (pp. 165-173). Binghamton, NY: Haworth Press.

Figure 30-6: Modified Caregiver Strain Index. Words appearing in *italics* represent modifications from the original Caregiver Strain Index from Robinson, B.C. (1983). Validation of a caregiver strain index, *Journal of Gerontology, 38,* 344-348. © The Gerontological Society of America.

INDEX

A

A delta fiber, 160, 160f
A wave of jugular venous pulse, 463
ABCDE mnemonic for skin lesions, 212-213
Abdomen, 527-564
  abdominal friction rubs and vascular sounds and, 562t
  abnormal bowel sounds and, 561t
  of aging adult, 531
  bedside assessment of, 791
  cultural and genetic considerations in, 531-532
  distention of, 557-558t
  enlarged organs and, 562-563t
  health history of, 532-535
  hepatitis risk and, 554
  incisional hernia and, 560t
  of infants and children, 531
  internal anatomy of, 527-530, 528-530f
  physical examination of, 536-556
    in aging adult, 554
    aorta palpation in, 550, 550f
    auscultation of bowel and vascular sounds in, 539f, 539-540, 540f
    in child, 553, 553f
    contour and, 536, 536f
    costovertebral angle tenderness and, 543, 543f
    demeanor and, 539
    documentation and critical thinking in, 555-556
    fluid wave and, 543f, 543-544
    hair distribution and, 538
    iliopsoas muscle test in, 551, 551f
    in infant, 552f, 552-553
    inspiratory arrest in, 551
    kidney palpation in, 550, 550f
    light and deep palpation in, 545-547, 545-547f
    liver palpation in, 548, 548f
    liver span percussion in, 541f, 541-542
    percussion of general tympany in, 540, 540f
    pulsation or movement and, 538
    rebound tenderness and, 551, 551f
    shifting dullness and, 544f, 544-545
    skin and, 537f, 537-538, 538f
    spleen palpation in, 549, 549f
    splenic dullness and, 542, 542f
    symmetry and, 537, 537f
    umbilicus and, 537
  of pregnant woman, 531, 809f, 809-810, 810f
  quadrants of, 530, 530f
  sequence in health assessment, 768, 773, 778
  surface landmarks of, 527, 528f
  umbilical hernia and, 560t
Abdominal aortic aneurysm, 524t
Abdominal bruit, 562t
Abdominal friction rub, 562t
Abdominal pain, 168
  costovertebral angle tenderness and, 543, 543f
  history of, 532-533
  in infants and children, 534
  during pregnancy, 802
  rebound tenderness and, 551, 551f
  referred, 559, 559t
Abdominal reflexes, 650, 650f
Abducens nerve, 627f
  abnormalities of, 668t
  infant reflexes and, 651t
  testing of, 633
Abduction, 566, 567f
ABI; *See* Ankle-brachial index
Abrasion
  corneal, 295, 318t
  forensic term, 109t
Abscess, 248t
  Bartholin's gland, 753t
  of breast, 408t
  rectal, 722t
Absent breath sounds, 428
Absent testis, 704t
Abstract reasoning, 72

Page numbers followed by "b" indicates boxes, "f" indicates figures, "t" indicates tables.

Abuse
  child, 103-114
    documentation of, 111
    health effects of, 105
    pattern injury in, 237t
    physical examination in, 109-110
    screening for, 108
  elder, 103-114, 104t
    assessing for, 107, 107t
    documentation of, 110f, 110-111, 111f
    health effects of, 105
    physical examination in, 108-109, 109t
  intimate partner, 105-107, 106f, 107f
  lesions caused by, 237t
  substance
    alcohol and, 93, 94t, 95t
    clinical signs of, 100-101t
    defining of, 94
    diagnosis of, 95t, 95-96
    functional assessment and, 58
    interview and, 41
    nutritional assessment and, 183
    prescription medications and, 100
Abuse Assessment Screen, 106, 106f
Accident
  in adult health history, 52
  in child health history, 60
  in older adult health history, 66
Accommodation, 284, 296, 296f
Acculturation, 16
Acetic acid wash, 742
Achilles reflex, 646-647, 647f
Achilles tenosynovitis, 615t
Achondroplastic dwarfism, 155t
Acinus, 415f, 416
Acne, 223, 224f
Acoustic nerve abnormalities, 669t
Acquired immunodeficiency syndrome
  circumcision and, 683
  Kaposi sarcoma in, 246t
  nutritional deficiencies in, 199t
  pregnant woman and, 803
Acrochordon, 225, 225f
Acrocyanosis, 221
Acromegaly, 154t, 271t
Acromion process, 570, 570f
Actinic keratosis, 225, 225f
Active listening, 30
Active range of motion, 578
Activities of daily living
  adult and, 57
  child and, 63
  depression and, 836
  musculoskeletal examination and, 575, 605
  older adult and, 67-69, 830-832, 831f
Activity
  adolescent psychosocial interview and, 65f
  adult and, 57
  bedside assessment of, 791
  child and, 64
  older adult and, 68, 839-840
Actual diagnoses, 5
Acute care setting, functional assessment of older adult and, 837-838
Acute closed-angle glaucoma, 308
Acute confusional state, 83t
Acute gout, 615t
Acute narrow-angle glaucoma, 317t
Acute otitis media, 347t
Acute pain, 163, 168
Acute respiratory distress syndrome, 453t
Acute rheumatoid arthritis, 612t
Acute rhinitis, 374t
Acute salpingitis, 759t
Acute tonsillitis, 381t
Acute urinary retention, 700t
Acute venous disease, 523t
Acutely ill person
  interview of, 41
  physical examination of chest and lungs of, 437
Adam's apple, 255
Adderall; *See* Dextroamphetamine
Adduction, 566, 567f
Adhesive capsulitis, 609t
Adie's pupil, 315t
Adipose tissue, 204, 204f
  of aging adult, 574
  aging-related changes in, 531
  of breast, 384f, 385
Adnexa, 727f
  bimanual examination of, 746, 746f
  enlargement of, 759-760t
Adolescent
  abdomen of, 534-535
  breast of, 386, 386f, 387t
    health history of, 391
    physical examination of, 401
  female genitourinary system of, 726-728, 727t
    health history of, 731-732
    physical examination of, 748-749
  health history of, 64, 65f
  interview of, 39-40
  male genitourinary system of, 681-683, 682t, 683f
    health history of, 686-687
    physical examination of, 697
  musculoskeletal system of
    health history of, 576
    physical examination of, 603, 603f
  noise-induced hearing loss and, 338
  nutritional assessment and, 176
    health history in, 184
    laboratory tests in, 193
    physical examination in, 191
  positioning for physical examination, 125
  pregnancy and, 798
  preparation for physical examination, 125
  respiratory rate of, 135t
  sequence of health assessment, 125, 780
  skin of
    health history of, 210
    physical examination of, 223, 224f
    secondary sex characteristics and, 206
  substance abuse and, 94
Advanced activities of daily living, 832
Adventitious lung sounds, 429-430, 444-445t
Advice giving, 35
Affect, 72
  abnormalities of, 85t
  general survey and, 129
  mental status and, 74
African heritages
  asthma and, 418
  bone mineral density and, 574
  breast development and disease in, 388
  culture-bound syndromes in, 26t
  diabetes mellitus and, 467
  female genitourinary development and, 727-728
  glaucoma and, 285
  health and illness beliefs and practices, 25t
  lactose intolerance and, 531
  male genital development and, 682-683
  nose, mouth, and throat differences in, 356
  obesity and, 532
  prostate and colorectal cancer and, 711
  skin conditions and, 207
  stroke and, 629
Afterload, 462, 462f
Age
  blood pressure and, 136
  general survey and, 127
Age-related changes
  in cardiovascular function, 465
  dental, 355
  in hair, 206
  in sensory perception, 72
  in taste and smell, 356
Aging adult; *See* Older adult
Agoraphobia, 90t
AIDS; *See* Acquired immunodeficiency syndrome
Air conduction pathway of hearing, 325f, 326
Air in abdomen, 557t
Ala, 351, 351f

Alaska native heritages
culture-bound syndromes in, 26t
glaucoma and, 285
health and illness beliefs and practices, 25t
stroke and, 629
Alcohol use and abuse, 93
appearance and behavior in, 101t
categories and patterns of, 95t
defining standard drink, 94t
functional assessment and, 58
gamma glutamyl transferase and, 99
nutritional assessment and, 183
older adult and, 96
oral cavity health history and, 358
pregnant woman and, 96, 803
Alcohol Use Disorders Identification Test, 96-97, 97t
Alert level of consciousness, 83t
Allergic drug reaction, 243t
Allergic facies, 275t
Allergic rhinitis, 374t
Allergic salute and crease, 275t
Allergy, 357
in adult health history, 52
in child health history, 61
food, 183
skin eruption in, 208, 243t
Allis test, 599f, 599-600
Alopecia, 208, 226, 246t
Alopecia areata, 246t
Altered cognition in older adult, 844
Alzheimer disease, 75, 632, 667t
Ambiguous genitalia, 760t
Ambivalence, 85t
American Indian heritages
culture-bound syndromes in, 26t
glaucoma and, 285
health and illness beliefs and practices, 25t
nose, mouth, and throat differences in, 356
stroke and, 629
Amnestic disorders, 88t
Amphetamines
appearance and behavior in abuse of, 101t
use in attention-deficit hyperactivity disorder, 100
Amulet, 21-22, 22f
Anabolic steroids, 184
Anal canal, 709, 710f
Anal column, 709, 710f
Anal crypt, 709
Anal culture and sensitivity, 742
Anal sphincter, 709, 710f
Anal valve, 709
Analgesia, 642
Anasarca, 215
Android pelvis, 816, 817t
Anemia during pregnancy, 825t
Anesthesia, 642
Aneurysm, 524t
aortic, 563t
vascular sounds in, 562t
Anger during interview, 42
Angina, 467
Angle of Louis, 412, 412f
Angular cheilitis, 375t
Animistic thinking, 38-39
Anisocoria, 295, 315t
Ankle, 572-573, 573f
abnormalities of, 615-616t
dermatomes of, 628f
physical examination of, 592-594, 593f, 594f
Ankle-brachial index, 516
Ankle jerk, 646-647, 647f
Ankyloglossia, 369, 379t
Ankylosing spondylitis, 608t
Ankylosis, 577, 611t
Annular skin lesion, 230t
Annulus, 324, 325f
Anorectal fissure, 720t
Anorectal fistula, 720t
Anorectal junction, 709, 710f
Anorexia nervosa, 155t, 535
Anteflexed uterus, 745f
Anterior axillary line, 413, 414f
Anterior chamber, 280f, 282, 282f, 318t
Anterior fontanel, 256, 256f
Anterior fornix, 726, 727f
Anterior palpation of thyroid gland, 264, 264f
Anterior spinothalamic tract, 624, 624f
Anterior superior iliac spine, 528f, 571, 571f
Anterior thorax
auscultation of, 433
inspection of, 430-431, 473
landmarks of, 412, 412f
lobes of lung and, 414, 414f
palpation of, 431f, 431-432, 432f
percussion of, 432f, 432-433
sequence in health assessment, 767
Anterior tibial artery, 500f
Anterior tibial vein, 501f
Anterior triangle, 253, 254f
Anterolateral spinothalamic tract, 160, 160f
Anteverted uterus, 745f
Anthropoid pelvis, 816, 817t
Anthropometric measures, 187-190f, 187-191
Antihelix, 324f
Antitragus, 324f
Anus, 709-724
abnormalities of, 720-721t
female, 726f
health history of, 712-713
of infants and children, 711
physical examination of, 713-719
documentation and critical thinking in, 718-719
in infants and children, 717
inspection of perianal area in, 713
palpation in, 714f, 714-715, 715f
patient positioning for, 713, 713f
stool examination in, 716-717
structure and function of, 709-710, 710f
Anxiety, 85t
in heart failure, 486t
during interview, 42
Anxiety disorders, 77, 77f, 90-91
Aorta, 456, 457f, 529f, 529-530
palpation of, 550, 550f
pulsation of, 538
Aortic aneurysm, 562t, 563t
Aortic arch aneurysm, 524t
Aortic area for heart auscultation, 475f
Aortic prosthetic valve sounds, 489t
Aortic regurgitation, 497t
Aortic stenosis, 494t
Aortic valve, 457f, 458
Apex
of heart, 455, 456f, 457f
of lung, 414
Apgar scoring system, 435, 435t
Aphasia, 73, 75, 84t
Aphthous ulcer, 378t
Apical impulse, 473, 474, 474f
Apocrine sweat gland, 204f, 205
Appearance
bedside assessment of, 788
cultural considerations in, 152-153
in mental status assessment, 73-74
sequence in health assessment, 764, 772, 777
in substance use disorders, 101t
Appendicitis, 559t
Appendix, 528f
Appetite, 532
Arcus senilis, 284, 307, 307f
ARDS; *See* Acute respiratory distress syndrome
Areola, 383, 384f
Argyll Robertson pupil, 315t
Arm
anthropometric measures of, 189f, 189-190, 190f
arteries in, 500, 500f
dermatomes of, 628f
inspection and palpation of, 506-509, 507-509f
musculoskeletal examination of, 581-587
elbow and, 582-584, 583f, 584f
shoulder and, 581f, 581-582, 582f
wrist and hand and, 584-586, 584-586f
peripheral vascular disease of, 520t
skin changes of, 505
swelling of, 505
veins in, 501
Arm pressure, 138f, 138-140, 139t
Arm span, 190
Arrector pili muscle, 204, 204f
Arterial bruit, 562t
Arterial leg ulcer, 522t
Arterial occlusion, 524t
Arterial ulcer, 522t
Arteries, 499-500, 500f
Arteriosclerosis, 504
Arteriovenous crossing, 320t
Arthritis
gouty, 610t
osteoarthritis, 608t, 612t
rheumatoid, 574-575, 608t, 612t
Articular process, 569f
Articulation, 565
Artificial tanning, 227
Ascending colon, 528f
Ascites, 543-544, 557t
in heart failure, 486t
ASD; *See* Atrial septal defect
Asian heritages
culture-bound syndromes in, 26t
health and illness beliefs and practices, 25t
nose, mouth, and throat differences in, 356
Aspartate aminotransferase, 99
Assessment; *See also* Health assessment
evidence-based, 1f, 1-10
critical thinking and, 2-6, 3f, 5t
cultural competence and, 9, 9f
data collection in, 7-8
diagnostic reasoning and, 2
evidence-based practice and, 6, 6f
expanding concept of health and, 8, 8f
of health-related beliefs and practices, 24t
heritage, 17-19, 18f
techniques for, 115-126
auscultation in, 118, 118f
inspection in, 115
palpation in, 115-116
percussion in, 116f, 116-117, 117f, 117t
Assimilation, 16
Assistive living, 839
Association auditory cortex, 84t
AST; *See* Aspartate aminotransferase
Astereognosis, 644
Asthma, 418, 449t
Asymmetric corneal light reflex, 311t
Atelectasis, 447t
Atelectatic crackles, 430, 444t
Atherosclerosis, 504
Athetosis, 671t
Athlete's foot, 243t
Atlas, 252f
Atopic dermatitis, 241t
Atopic facies, 275t
Atresia, choanal, 373t
Atrial gallop, 478, 491t
Atrial kick, 458
Atrial septal defect, 493t
Atrial systole, 458
Atrioventricular node, 461, 461f
Atrioventricular valves, 457f, 458
diastolic rumbles of, 496t
Atrium, 457
Atrophic glossitis, 379t
Atrophic scar, 235t
Atrophic vaginitis, 756t
Atrophy
optic, 320t
of shoulder, 609t
of thenar eminence, 611t
Attention, 72
mental status and, 75
Attention-deficit hyperactivity disorder, 100
Attic perforation of tympanic membrane, 347t
Attitude of fetus, 810
AUDIT questionnaire, 96-97, 97t
Aura, 630
Auricle, 323
Auscultation, 118, 118f
of anterior chest, 433
of bowel and vascular sounds, 539f, 539-540, 540f
of carotid artery, 471f, 471-472
of fetal heart tones, 813, 813f
of heart, 475-480, 475-480f
of infant abdomen, 552
of infant skull, 267
of neonatal chest, 436
of posterior chest, 427f, 427-430, 428t, 429f
of thyroid gland, 264
Auscultatory gap, 138
Automaticity of heart, 461
Autonomic nervous system, 628-629
Avoidance language, 35

Avulsion, 109t
Axilla
health history of, 55, 391
palpation of, 395, 395f
Axillary artery, 500f
Axillary lymph node, 503
Axillary temperature measurement, 147
Axis, 252f

B

Babbling, 651
Babinski reflex, 655, 655f, 677t
Baby bottle tooth decay, 376t
Back
of infant, 600, 600f
of preschool and school-age children, 601
Bacterial vaginosis, 756t
Balance tests, 637-639, 638f, 639f
Ballottement of patella, 590, 590f
Bariatric surgery, 200t
Barrel chest, 440t
Barthel Index, 831
Bartholin's gland, 726, 726f
abscess of, 753t
Basal cell carcinoma, 245t
of eyelid, 314t
Basal cell layer, 203, 204f
Basal ganglia, 622, 623f
Base
of heart, 455, 456f
of lung, 414
Basilar membrane, 325, 325f
Beau's line, 249t
Bed wetting, 686
Bednar aphthae, 369
Bedside assessment, 787-793
abdomen and, 791
activity level and, 791
cardiovascular system and, 790
electronic charting and, 792
general appearance and, 788
genitourinary system and, 791
health history in, 788
neurologic system and, 789
respiratory system and, 789
SBAR framework for staff communication and, 793
skin and, 790
vital signs measurement in, 788-789
Behavior
of aging adult, 80
general survey and, 129
of infants and children, 142
in mental status assessment, 74
pain and, 168-169, 169f
in substance use disorders, 101t
Behavioral Checklist, 79t
Bell endpiece of stethoscope, 118, 118f
Bell's palsy, 276t
Benign breast disease, 405t, 406t
Benign prostatic hypertrophy, 711, 723t
Benzodiazepines abuse, 101t
Bi-ischial diameter, 818, 818f
Biased questions, 36
Biceps reflex, 646, 646f
Biculturalism, 16
Bicycle helmet safety, 267
Bifid uvula, 356, 366, 381t
Biliary colic, 559t
Bimanual pelvic examination, 742-746, 743-746f
of pregnant woman, 815, 815f
Binaural interaction, 325
Binge eating, 185
Bioelectrical impedance analysis, 189
Biographic data
in adult health history, 49-50
in child health history, 59
Biomedical theory of illness, 21
Biot's respiration, 442t
Bipolar disorder, 89t
Birthmark, 209, 222, 223f
Bitot's spots, 199t
Black hairy tongue, 380t
Black tarry stool, 717
Blackhead, 223, 224f
Bladder, 528f, 529, 529f
female, 727f
male, 680f
Blastocyst, 795
Bleeding
gastrointestinal, 717
of gums, 357
rectal, 712
vaginal, 801, 825t
Blepharitis, 314t
Blessed Orientation-Memory-Concentration Test, 835t
Blindness
monocular, 315t
pediatric, 303
racial and ethnic variations in, 285
visual field loss and, 316t
Blocking, 86t
Blood
in stool, 712
venous, 501-502, 502f
Blood flow, 458, 458f
Blood pressure
abnormalities in, 156-157t
aging-related changes in, 465
cardiovascular heart disease and, 466
heart failure and, 486t
lifestyle modifications and, 152
measurement of, 136f, 136-142
aging adult and, 150
arm for, 138f, 138-140
common errors in, 141t
factors affecting, 136-137, 137f
in infants and children, 148
Korotkoff sounds and, 139t
thigh for, 142, 142f
metabolic syndrome and, 200t
preeclampsia and, 822t
during pregnancy, 796, 797, 819
Blood pressure cuff, 137-138, 138f
Blood urea nitrogen, 694
Blood vessels
arteries in, 499-500, 500f
effects of elasticity on blood pressure, 137, 137f
veins in, 501, 501f
Blood volume
blood pressure and, 137, 137f
during pregnancy, 464-465, 797
Blue drum, 348t
Blumberg sign, 551, 551f
Blunted affect, 85t
BMD; *See* Bone mineral density
BMI; *See* Body mass index
Body language, 30
Body mass index, 130-132, 131t
of aging adult, 149
breast development and, 388
calculation of, 187
of child, 191
menarche and, 728
obesity and, 195t
overnutrition and, 175-176
Body movements, mental status assessment and, 73
Body odor, 206
Body structure
abnormalities of, 154-155t
general survey and, 128
Body temperature measurement, 132-134
in aging adult, 149
in infants and children, 146-147, 147f
Bone(s), 565
of elbow, 570, 570f
of foot, 573f
of hip, 571, 571f
Paget's disease of, 271t
remodeling of, 573
of shoulder, 570, 570f
of wrist and hand, 570, 571f
Bone conduction pathway of hearing, 325f, 326
Bone mineral density, 574
Bone pain, 575
Bony labyrinth, 325
Bony orbit, 280f
Borborygmus, 539, 561t
Bossing, 264
Botanica, 22, 22f, 23f
Bottle caries, 376t
Bottle-feeding, infant health history and, 534
Bouchard node, 612t
Bounding pulse, 519t
Boutonniere deformity, 612t
Bowel habits, 533
anus, rectum, and prostate examination and, 712
of older adult, 535
Bowel sounds
abnormal, 561t
auscultation of, 539f, 539-540, 540f
of pregnant woman, 531
Bowlegged stance, 601, 601f
BPH; *See* Benign prostatic hypertrophy
Brachial artery, 500, 500f
Brachial pulse, 508, 508f
Brachiocephalic artery, 500f
Brachioradialis reflex, 647, 647f
Bradycardia, 134
in infant, 481
Bradypnea, 442t
Brain
cerebral cortex of, 621-622, 622f
lesions of, 73
pain and, 159-160, 160f
role in body temperature regulation, 132
Brain injury
history of, 257-258
prevention of, 267
Brainstem, 623, 623f
in control of respiration, 416
hearing and, 325
Branchial remnant of ear, 327t
Breakthrough pain, 163
Breast, 383-410
abnormal nipple discharge from, 407t
of adolescent girl, 386, 386f, 387t
of aging woman, 387-388
cultural and genetic considerations of, 388
disorders occurring during lactation, 408t
health history of, 389-391
adult, 55
pediatric, 62, 391
internal anatomy of, 384f, 384-385, 385f
lump in, 405-406t
male, 388
physical examination of, 392-401
adolescent and, 401
aging woman and, 401
breast self-examination education and, 398-399, 399f
documentation and critical thinking in, 402-403
infants and children and, 400-401
inspection and palpation of axillae in, 395, 395f
inspection of breast in, 392-394, 392-394f
lactating woman and, 401
male breast and, 400, 400f
palpation of breast in, 395-398, 395-398f
pregnant woman and, 401
of pregnant woman, 386, 808, 808f
retraction and inflammation of, 404t
sequence in health assessment, 767
surface anatomy of, 383, 384f
Breast cancer, 388, 405t
abnormal discharge from nipple in, 407t
history of, 390
lymphedema after, 520t
male, 409t
risk factors for, 391, 391t
screening for, 402
Breast self-examination, 390, 398-399, 399f
Breastfeeding, 176
infant health history and, 534
Breath alcohol analysis, 100
Breath odor, 367
Breath sounds, 427t, 427-429, 428t, 429f, 433
Brief Pain Inventory, 166, 166f
Broca's aphasia, 84t
Broca's area, 84t, 622, 622f
Bronchial sounds, 428, 428t
Bronchitis, 448t
Bronchophony, 446t
Bronchovesicular sounds, 428, 428t
Bronzed skin, 230t
Brow presentation, 826t
Brown-S[ac]equard syndrome, 675t
Brudzinski reflex, 677t
Bruise, forensic term, 109t
Bruising, 216, 216f, 237t, 240t
in abuse and neglect, 108-109, 209
birth-related, 220
health history of, 208

Bruit, 264
abdominal, 540, 562t
carotid artery, 471
Brushfield's spots, 305
Buccal mucosa
abnormalities of, 378-379t
mucocele of, 375t
physical examination of, 365, 365f
snuff and, 370
Buccinator muscle, 252f
Buddhism, dietary practices of, 178t
Bulb matrix of hair, 204
Bulbar conjunctiva, 280, 280f
Bulbourethral gland, 680f, 710f, 711
Bulge sign, 590, 590f
Bulla, 232t
Bullous myringitis, 348t
BUN; *See* Blood urea nitrogen
Bundle of His, 461f
Bunion, 616t
Bursa
hip, 571, 571t
prepatellar, 572, 572f
Bursitis
olecranon, 610t
prepatellar, 614t
subacromial, 609t

C

C fiber, 160, 160f
C-reactive protein, 192
C wave of jugular venous pulse, 463
Cachetic appearance, 277t
Caf[ac]e-au-lait spot, 220, 220f
CAGE questionnaire, 58, 98
Calf pain, 511
Calf pump, 501
Callus, 616t
Cancer
breast, 388, 405t
abnormal discharge from nipple in, 407t
history of, 390
lymphedema after, 520t
male, 409t
risk factors for, 391, 391t
screening for, 402
cervical
cultural considerations in, 728
human papillomavirus vaccine and, 750
older female and, 750
screening for, 729
colon, 722t
genetic factors in, 711
screening for, 718
endometrial, 758t
oral, 356
ovarian, 760t
pharyngeal, 356
prostate, 723t
genetic factors in, 711
screening for, 697
skin, 227, 245t
smokeless tobacco and, 370
Cancer pain, 163, 172t
Candidiasis, 241t
oral, 378t
pregnant woman and, 728
vulvovaginal, 756t
Canker sore, 378t
Cannabis, 101t
Canthus, 279, 280f
Capacitance vessels, 501
Capillary refill, 219, 506
Caput succedaneum, 264, 265f
Carcinoma
of breast, 407t
cervical, 755t
of ear, 343t
endometrial, 758t
of eyelid, 314t
of lip, 375t
penile, 702t
rectal, 722t
of tongue, 380t
Cardiac cycle, 458-460, 459f
Cardiac enlargement, 475, 482
Cardiac history, 468
Cardiac output
blood pressure and, 137, 137f
in heart failure, 486t
stroke volume and, 462
Cardiac tamponade, 519t
Cardinal positions of gaze, 312t
Cardiovascular assessment, 455-498
bedside, 790
clinical manifestations of heart failure and, 486t
congenital heart defects and, 492-493t
diastolic extra heart sounds and, 490-491t
extracardiac sounds and, 491-492t
first heart sound variations and, 487t
health history in, 467-470
adult, 55
child, 62
older adult, 67
heart structure and function and, 455-498
aging adult and, 465, 465f
cardiac cycle and, 458-460, 459f
cardiovascular heart disease and, 466-467
direction of blood flow and, 458, 458f
electrical conduction system and, 461f, 461-462
heart sounds and, 460f, 460-461
of infants and children, 464, 464f, 465f
position and surface landmarks in, 455-456, 456f, 457f
of pregnant woman, 464-465
pulmonary and systemic circulations and, 455, 456f
pumping ability in, 462, 462f
wall, chambers, and valves in, 456-458, 457t
neck vessels and, 462-463, 463f
physical examination in, 470-485
aging adult and, 483
anterior chest inspection in, 473
apical impulse palpation in, 474, 474f
auscultation of heart in, 474-480f, 475-480
carotid artery auscultation in, 471, 471f
carotid artery palpation in, 470-471, 471f
documentation and critical thinking in, 484-485
estimation of jugular venous pressure in, 473, 473f
in infants and children, 480-482, 481f, 482f
jugular venous pulse and, 472, 472t
palpation across precordium in, 474, 474f
patient preparation for, 470
percussion in, 475
pregnant woman and, 483
second heart sound variations and, 488t
sequence in health assessment, 767, 768, 773, 778
split second heart sound and, 488t
systolic extra heart sounds and, 489t
valvular defect-related murmurs and, 494-497t
women and heart attacks and, 484
Cardiovascular heart disease, 466-467
obesity and, 532
risk factors for, 468-469
Caregiver assessment, 837, 838f
Caries, 376t
Carotene, 204
Carotenemia, 222, 229t
Carotid artery, 253f, 462, 463f, 500
auscultation of, 471f, 471-472
palpation of, 470-471, 471f
Carotid artery pulse, 462, 463f, 472t
Carotid bruit, 471
Carotid sinus hypersensitivity, 471
Carpal tunnel syndrome, 587, 611t
during pregnancy, 797
Carpals, 570, 571t
Carrier screening for cystic fibrosis, 799
Cartilage, 566
Caruncle, 279, 280f
Cataract, 285, 319t
Catholicism, dietary practices of, 178t
Cavernous hemangioma, 238t
Cecum, 528f
Cellulitis of ear, 327t
Central American heritages
culture-bound syndromes in, 26t
health and illness beliefs and practices of, 25t
Central axillary lymph node, 385, 385f
Central nervous system, 621-626; *See also* Neurologic system
changes from poorly controlled pain, 169t
malnutrition and, 186t
Central nervous system (*Continued*)
motor pathways of, 624-625, 625f
pain and, 159-160, 160f
sensory pathways of, 623-624, 624f
structures in, 621-623, 622f, 623f
upper and lower motor neurons of, 626, 626f
Central perforation of tympanic membrane, 347t
Central sulcus, 622f
Central venous pressure, 472
Cephalhematoma, 265, 265f
Cerebellar ataxia, 672t
Cerebellar function assessment, 637-639, 638f, 639f
Cerebellar lesion, 674t
Cerebellar system, 625
Cerebellum, 622f, 622-623, 623f
Cerebral blood flow, 629
Cerebral cortex, 621-622, 622f
lesion of, 676t
Cerebral palsy, 674t
Cerebrovascular accident
abnormal facies in, 277t
mental status assessment in, 73
Cerumen, 323
impaction of, 327, 344t
Ceruminolytics, 327
Cervarix; *See* Human papillomavirus vaccine
Cervical cancer, 755t
cultural considerations in, 728
human papillomavirus vaccine and, 750
older female and, 750
screening for, 729
Cervical eversion, 740
Cervical lymph node, 255, 255f, 503
Cervical os, 727f, 739f, 739-740
Cervical scrape, 741, 741f
Cervical secretions, 740
during pregnancy, 728, 814
Cervical smear and culture, 740f, 740-742, 741f
Cervical spinal nerves, 628f
Cervical spine, 252f, 580, 580f, 628f
Cervix, 726, 727f
abnormalities of, 754-755t
bimanual examination of, 744, 744f
examination during pregnancy, 814f, 814-815, 815f
incompetent, 825t
inspection of, 739f, 739-740
Chadwick sign, 728, 796, 814, 814f
Chalazion, 314t
Chambers of heart, 456-458, 457t
Chancre, 702t, 752t
Charting
electronic, 792
of mental status assessment, 82
Cheilitis, 362, 375t
Cherry angioma, 216, 216f
Chest, 411-454
abnormal tactile fremitus and, 443t
of aging adult, 418
biocultural differences in lung diseases and, 418
common respiratory conditions and, 447-453t
configurations of, 440-441t
health history of, 418-421
of infants and children, 416-417, 417f
mechanics of respiration and, 416, 417f
physical examination of, 421-439, 473
of acutely ill person, 437
adventitious lung sounds and, 429-430, 444-445t
of aging adult, 437
auscultation of anterior chest in, 433
breath sounds and, 427t, 427-429, 428t, 429f
diaphragmatic excursion and, 426, 426f
documentation and critical thinking in, 438-439
of infants and children, 434-437, 435f, 435t, 436f
inspection of anterior chest in, 430-431
inspection of thoracic cage in, 422
measurement of pulmonary function status in, 433-434
palpation of anterior chest in, 431f, 431-432, 432f
percussion of anterior chest in, 432f, 432-433
percussion of lung fields in, 424-426, 425f
of pregnant woman, 437
symmetric chest expansion and, 422f, 422-423
tactile fremitus and, 423f, 423-424
voice sounds and, 430, 446t
position and surface landmarks of, 411-413, 412f, 413f
of pregnant woman, 418

Chest (*Continued*)
respiration patterns and, 441-442t
sequence in health assessment, 767, 773, 778
thoracic cavity and, 414f, 414-416, 415f
Chest circumference, 146, 146f
Chest pain, 467
with breathing, 420
Chewing tobacco, 370
Cheyne-Stokes respiration, 442t
Chickenpox, 242t, 803
Child
abdomen of, 531
health history of, 534
physical examination of, 553, 553f
anus, rectum, and prostate of
health history of, 713
physical examination of, 717
blood pressure measurement in, 148
body temperature measurement in, 146-147, 147f
breast examination in, 400-401
congenital musculoskeletal abnormalities of, 618t
ear of, 326, 326f
health history of, 329
otitis media and, 327
physical examination of, 334-336f, 334-337
eye of, 284
health history of, 62, 287
physical examination of, 302-305f, 302-306
female genitourinary system of, 726-728, 727t
abnormalities of, 760t
health history of, 731
physical examination of, 747-748
general survey of, 142-143
head and neck of, 256, 256f
facial abnormalities and, 274-275t
health history of, 259
physical examination of, 266
size and contour abnormalities of, 271t
swelling of, 272t
health history of, 59f, 59-64
heart of, 464, 464f, 465f
health history of, 469
physical examination of, 481-482, 482f
height measurement in, 144f, 144-145
lungs of, 416-418, 417f
health history of, 420-421
physical examination of, 434-437, 435f, 435t, 436f
male genitourinary system of
health history of, 686
physical examination of, 695f, 695-697, 696f
mental status assessment of, 72, 79f, 79-80
musculoskeletal system of, 573
health history of, 576
physical examination of, 601f, 601-603, 602f
neurologic system of
frontal release signs and, 677t
health history of, 631-632
physical examination of, 657-660, 658f
nose, mouth, and throat of, 355
health history of, 358
physical examination of, 367-369, 367-369f
nutritional assessment and, 176
health history in, 183-184
laboratory tests in, 193
physical examination in, 191, 193
pain and, 167, 167f
parent interview and, 37-38, 38f
peripheral vascular system and lymphatics of, 504, 504f
physical examination of, 516-517
positioning for physical examination, 125, 125f
preparation for physical examination, 125
respirations measurement in, 148
sequence of examination of, 125
skin of, 205-206
health history of, 209-210
lesions and, 241-242t
physical examination of, 220-223, 220-223f
weight measurement in, 143, 143f
Child abuse and neglect, 103-114
documentation of, 111
health effects of, 105
lesions caused by, 237t
physical examination in, 109-110
screening for, 108, 686
Childhood illnesses
adult health history and, 51
child health history and, 60
Chinese medicine, 21
Chlamydia, 742, 757t
Chloasma, 206, 224, 267, 807
Choanal atresia, 373t
Choked optic disc, 320t
Cholecystitis, 559t
Cholesteatoma, 348t
Cholesterol
cardiovascular heart disease and, 466
nutritional assessment and, 192
Chondrodermatitis nodularis helicus, 342t
Chordae tendineae, 457f, 458
Chorea, 671t
Chorionic somatomammotropin, 796
Choroid, 281, 282f
Chronic gout, 615t
Chronic illness
in adult health history, 52
in child health history, 60
in older adult health history, 66
Chronic kidney disease, 683-684
Chronic obstructive pulmonary disease, 442t
Chronic pain, 163, 169
Chronic venous disease, 523t
Ciliary body, 282, 282f
Circulation, 455, 456f
fetal, 464, 464f
Circumcision, 683
female, 728
Circumcorneal redness, 317t
Circumduction, 566, 567f
Circumlocution, 86t
Circumstantiality, 86t
Cirrhosis, 93
Cisterna chyli, 503f
Clanging, 86t
Clarification in interview, 34
Claudication distance, 505
Clavicle, 253f, 254f, 412f
infant fracture of, 600
Clean field, 120
Cleft lip and palate, 356, 375t, 381t
Clinical breast examination, 390
Clinical evidence, 2
Clinical setting for physical examination, 118-119, 119f
patient approach in, 121
safety of, 120-121, 121t
Clitoris, 725, 726f, 727f, 735, 735f
Clonus, 645, 647, 647f
Closed-angle glaucoma, 308
Closed questions, 33, 33t
Clubbing, 218, 218f, 249t
Clubfoot, 618t
Cluster headache, 270t
CNS; *See* Central nervous system
Coarctation of aorta, 142, 493t
Cocaine, 101t
Coccygeal spinal nerve, 628f
Coccyx, 628f
Cochlea, 324f, 325
Cognitive function
in mental status assessment, 74-76
older adult and, 80-81, 835, 835t, 844
Cogwheel rigidity, 669t
Cold, 357
Cold sore, 244t, 375t
Collaborative problems, 6
Collagen, 204
Collateral ligament, 572, 572f
Colles fracture, 611t
Colon, 529
referred abdominal pain and, 559t
Colon cancer, 722t
genetic factors in, 711
screening for, 718
Color
of hair, 217
of nails, 218, 218f
of skin, 212f, 212-214, 213f
of aging adult, 224, 224f
changes in legs and feet, 514-515, 515f
detecting changes in, 229-230t
determination of, 204
of ear, 330
Color (*Continued*)
external variables influencing, 211t
general survey and, 128
of infant, 220
of posterior chest, 422
of stool, 717
of urine, 684-685, 685f
Color blindness, 303
Color vision, 303
Colostrum, 386, 401, 797
Columella, 351, 351f
Coma, 83t
Comedone, 223, 224f
Common carotid artery, 253f, 457f
Common cold, 357
Common iliac artery, 500f, 529f
Common iliac vein, 501f, 529f
Communication
assisting narrative in, 33-34, 34f
cross-cultural, 42-45, 43f, 44t
nonverbal, 30, 36-37, 37t
child interview and, 38
cross-cultural, 47-48
open-ended questions and, 32-33, 33t
overcoming barriers in, 45f, 45-48, 46t, 47t
process of, 29-32, 31f
SBAR framework for, 793
traps in, 35
Community-based services, functional assessment of older adult and, 838
Competency, 3
Complementary and alternative medicine, 26-27
Complete breech presentation, 826t
Complete database, 7
Complete neurologic examination, 632
Complex regional pain syndrome, 172
Compound nevus, 212, 213f
Compound presentation, 826t
Comprehensive nutritional assessment, 180, 180t
Compulsion, 87t
Conception, 796
Concerta; *See* Methylphenidate
Conduction system of heart, 461f, 461-462
Conductive hearing loss, 326
Condylomata, 755t
Confabulation, 86t
Confluent skin lesion, 230t
Confrontation in interview, 34
Confrontation test, 289f, 289-290, 290f
Confusion Assessment Method, 835t
Congenital abnormalities
of musculoskeletal system, 618t
pilonidal cyst in, 720t
Congenital dislocation of hip, 599, 599f, 618t
Congenital heart defects, 492-493t
Congenital hypothyroidism, 274t
Conjugate movement of eye, 281
Conjunctiva, 280, 280f, 282f
inspection of, 293, 293f
of newborn, 304
Conjunctivitis, 317t
Connective tissue, 204, 204f
Consciousness, mental status and, 72
Consensual light reflex, 283, 284f, 295
Constipation
aging adult and, 531
in infants and children, 534
Contact dermatitis, 243t
of female external genitalia, 752t
Contact lenses, 286
Continuing care retirement community, 839
Contour of abdomen, 536, 536f
Contraceptives, 731
male history of, 685-686
use before pregnancy, 801
Contract, interview as, 29
Contraction stress test, 819
Contracture, 577
Dupuytren, 611t
Contusion, 109t, 237t
Cooper's ligaments, 384t, 385
Coordination
child and, 659
history of problems of, 631
testing of, 640f, 640-641, 641f

Coping
adult and, 58
child and, 64
older adult and, 68
Coracoid process, 570, 570f
Cornea, 280f, 281, 282f
abnormalities of, 318-319t
inspection of, 295
Corneal abrasion, 295, 318t
Corneal light reflex, 281, 290, 311t, 634
child and, 304, 304f
Corona of penis, 679, 680f
Coronal suture, 251, 252f, 256f
Coronary artery disease, 468-469
Corpus callosum, 623f
Corpus cavernosum, 679, 680f
Corpus luteum, 795
Corpus spongiosum, 679, 680f
Corrigan's pulse, 519t
Cortical cataract, 319t
Corticospinal tract, 624-625, 625f
Costal angle, 412f
Costal cartilage, 412f
Costal facet, 569f
Costal margin, 412f, 528f
Costochondral junction, 411, 412f
Costodiaphragmatic recess, 415f, 416
Costovertebral angle, 530
Costovertebral angle tenderness, 543, 543f
Cotton wool spots, 321t
Cough
cardiovascular assessment and, 468
history of, 418-419
Coughing, Standard Precautions and, 121t
Cover test, 290, 291f
child and, 304
extraocular muscle dysfunction and, 311t
Cowper's gland, 710f, 711
Coxa plana, 618t
Crab lice, 752t
Crack cocaine, 101t
Crackles, 430, 444t, 486t
Cradle cap, 247t
Cramping of muscle, 575
Cranial bones, 251
molding in newborn, 265
Cranial nerves, 627, 627f
abnormalities of, 668-669t
extraocular muscle movement and, 281
of infant, 651t
testing of, 633-636, 634-636f
Cranial suture, 251
Craniosynostosis, 265
Cranium, 251
Creatinine, 694
Cremaster muscle, 680, 680f, 681f
Cremasteric reflex, 650, 696
Crepitation, 578
Crepitus, 424
Cricoid cartilage, 254
CRIES Neonatal Postoperative Pain Measurement Score, 169, 170f
Critical thinking, 2-6, 3f, 5t
in abdominal examination, 555-556
in anus, rectum, and prostate examination, 718-719
in breast examination, 402-403
in cardiovascular assessment, 484-485
in chest examination, 438-439
in ear examination, 338-340
in examination of pregnant woman, 820-821
in eye examination, 309-310
in female genitourinary examination, 750-751
in head and neck examination, 268-269
in male genitourinary examination, 698
in mental status assessment, 82
in musculoskeletal examination, 607
in neurologic examination, 665-666
in nose, mouth, and throat examination, 371-372
in nutritional assessment, 195
in pain assessment, 171
in peripheral vascular and lymphatic examination, 518
sequence of health assessment and, 781-785
in skin examination, 227-228
in vital signs, 153
Critically ill person, interview of, 41
Cross-cultural communication, 42-45, 43f, 44t
nonverbal, 47-48
Crossed representation, 623
Cruciate ligaments, 572, 572f
Crust, 233t
Crying during interview, 42
Cryptorchidism, 696, 704t
Cuff, 137-138, 138f
Cul-de-sac of Douglas, 726, 727f
Cultural care, 14
Cultural competence, 11-28
demographic profile of United States and, 11-12
developmental competence and, 20-21
health history and, 54
health-related beliefs and practices and, 19-20
heritage and, 14-16, 15f, 17f
heritage assessment and, 17-19, 18f
immigration and, 12
national standards for, 12f, 12-14, 13t
steps to, 27, 27t
traditional causes of illness and, 21-24, 22f, 23f, 24t, 25t
transcultural expression of illness and, 25-27, 26t
Cultural considerations
in abdominal disorders, 531-532
in breast development and disease, 388
in cardiovascular heart disease, 466
in differences of skin, 206-207
in domestic violence assessment, 113
in ear variations, 327
in eye disorders, 285
in female genitourinary issues, 728
in functional assessment of older adult, 843-844
in general appearance, 152-153
in interview, 42-45, 43f, 44t
in lung diseases, 418
in male genitourinary system, 683
in nose, mouth, and throat examination, 356
in nutritional assessment, 177f, 177-178, 178t
in pain assessment, 163
in pregnancy, 799
in prostate and colorectal cancer, 711
in skin and hair differences, 206-207
Cultural stereotyping, 178
Cultural taboos, 20
Culture, 14
Culture-bound syndromes, 26, 26t
Culture shock, 20-21
Cushing reflex, 663
Cushing syndrome
abnormal facies in, 275t
obesity in, 155t
Cutaneous pain, 162
Cutaneous reflexes, 648, 648f
Cuticle, 205, 205f
Cutis marmorata, 221, 221f
Cyanosis, 214, 229t
cardiovascular assessment and, 468
cervical, 754t
in Raynaud's phenomenon, 520t
Cyst, 233t
epididymal retention, 705t
ganglion, 611t
Nabothian, 740
ovarian, 557t, 759t
pilar, 266, 273t
pilonidal, 720t
retention, 375t
sebaceous, 342t
thyroglossal duct, 266
Cystic fibrosis, 799
Cystocele, 754t

D

Dacryocystitis, 314t
Daily Reference Intakes, 181
Dandruff, 217
Danger Assessment, 112f, 112-113
Dartos fascia, 680f
Darwin's tubercle, 330, 330f
Data collection
in evidence-based assessment, 7-8
interview as, 29
Database, 2, 7
Dead space, 416
Decerebrate rigidity, 676t
Deciduous teeth, 355, 355f
Decorticate rigidity, 676t
Decubitus ulcer, 236t
Deep cervical lymph node, 255, 255f, 261f
Deep palmar arch, 500, 500f
Deep palpation of abdomen, 545-547, 545-547f
Deep somatic pain, 162
Deep tendon reflexes, 626, 645-649, 646-649f
of aging adult, 659-660
Deep veins of leg, 501, 501f
Deep venous thrombophlebitis, 523t
Deformity of ear, 327t
Degenerative joint disease, 608t, 612t
Dehydration, 214
Delirium, 80, 83t, 88t, 835
Delirium tremens, 101t
Delusion, 87t
Dementia, 80, 88t, 835
pain and, 163, 170, 171f
Demographic profile of United States, 11-12
Denial of domestic violence, 113
Dental caries, 376t
Dentate line, 709, 710f
Denver II screening, 79
Dependence, term, 100t
Dependent rubor, 515
Depersonalization, 85t
Depression, 85t
adolescent and, 65f
of muscle movement, 566, 567f
older adult and, 835-836, 836f
pregnant woman and, 805
screening for, 77
suicide and, 78
Derived anthropometric measures, 189-190
Derived weight measures, 187
Dermal segmentation, 628
Dermatitis, 211
atopic, 241t
contact, 243t
diaper, 241t
of female external genitalia, 752t
seborrheic, 247t
Dermatome, 628, 628f
Dermis, 204, 204f
DES; *See* Diethylstilbestrol
Descending colon, 528f
Descriptor pain rating scales, 167
Developmental competence, 20-21
in abdominal examination, 552f, 552-554, 553f
in anus, rectum, and prostate examination, 717
in breast examination, 386f, 386-388, 387t
in cardiovascular assessment, 464-466, 465f
in chest examination, 416-418, 417f
in ear examination, 326-327
in examination of pregnant woman, 798-799
in eye examination, 302-308, 302-308f
in female genitourinary examination, 747-750, 748f
in head and neck examination, 256, 256f
in health history, 59, 59f
in interview, 37-40, 38f, 40f
in male genitourinary examination, 695f, 695-697, 696f
in mental status assessment, 72, 79f, 79-80
in musculoskeletal examination, 598-605
adolescent and, 603, 603f
aging adult and, 604-605, 605f
infant and, 598-600, 599f, 600f
pregnant woman and, 604, 604f
preschool and school-age children and, 601f, 601-602, 602f
in neurologic examination, 651-663
aging adult and, 659-660
infant and, 651t, 651-657, 652-657f
neurologic recheck and, 660-663, 661-663f
preschool and school-age children and, 657-659, 658f
in nose, mouth, and throat examination, 355f, 355-356
in nutritional assessment, 176-177, 191
in peripheral vascular and lymphatic examination, 516-517
in skin examination, 205-206
in substance use assessment, 96
Developmental history, 61
Deviated nasal septum, 360, 361f
DEXA; *See* Dual-energy x-ray absorptiometry
Dexedrine; *See* Dextroamphetamine

Dextroamphetamine, 100
Dextrorotation, 815
Diabetes mellitus, 522t
Diabetic ketoacidosis, 367
Diagnostic positions test, 291f, 291-292, 312t
Diagnostic reasoning, 2
Diagonal conjugate, 818, 818f
Diaper rash, 209, 241t
Diaphoresis, 214
Diaphragm, 411, 412f
Diaphragm of stethoscope, 118, 118f
Diaphragmatic excursion, 426, 426f
Diastasis recti, 552, 560t, 809
Diastole, 458, 459f
Diastolic extra heart sounds, 490-491t
Diastolic pressure, 136, 136t
Diet
  breast cancer risk and, 388
  MyPyramid Dietary Guidelines and, 181, 181f
  religious dietary practices and, 178t
  two thousand calories per day, 181t, 181-182
Diethylstilbestrol, 729, 755t
Digital arteries, 500f
Digital rectal examination, 697, 714f, 714-715, 715f
Dimpling of breast, 404t
Dinamap, 148
Diplopia, 286
Direct Assessment of Functional Abilities, 832
Direct inguinal hernia, 707t
Direct light reflex, 283, 284f, 295
Direct observation in nutritional assessment, 180-181
Direct questions, 33, 33t
Disc pallor, 320t
Discharge
  from ear, 328
  from eye, 286
  nasal, 356, 360
  from nipple, 407t
  penile, 685, 700t
  vaginal
    history of, 730
    newborn and, 748
    pregnant woman and, 728, 814
Discoloration of urine, 699t
Discrete skin lesion, 230t
Disease
  cultural considerations in, 27
  traditional causes of, 21-24, 22f, 23f, 24t, 25t
Dislocated shoulder, 609t
Disorientation, 75
Distance, cultural considerations in, 44, 44t
Distancing, 35
Distention of abdomen, 557-558t
Diurnal cycle of body temperature, 133
Diurnal rhythm of blood pressure, 136
Dizziness
  history of, 258, 630
  older adult and, 632
Documentation
  of abdominal examination, 555-556
  of anus, rectum, and prostate examination, 718-719
  of breast examination, 402-403
  of cardiovascular assessment, 484-485
  of chest examination, 438-439
  of domestic violence assessment, 110f, 110-111, 111f
  of ear examination, 338-340
  of examination of pregnant woman, 820-821
  of eye examination, 309-310
  of female genitourinary examination, 750-751
  of head and neck examination, 268-269
  of male genitourinary examination, 698
  of mental status assessment, 82
  of musculoskeletal examination, 607
  of neurologic examination, 665-666
  of nose, mouth, and throat examination, 371-372
  of nutritional assessment, 195
  of pain, 171
  of peripheral vascular and lymphatic examination, 518
  sequence of health assessment and, 781-785
  of skin examination, 227-228
  of vital signs, 153
Doll's eyes reflex, 304
Domestic violence assessment, 103-114
  assessment for risk of homicide in, 112, 112f
  child abuse and neglect and, 108
Domestic violence assessment (*Continued*)
  cultural considerations in, 113
  definitions in, 103-104, 104t
  denial in, 113
  documentation in, 110f, 110-111, 111f
  elder abuse and neglect and, 107, 107t
  health effects of violence and, 104-105
  history in, 108
  intimate partner violence and, 105-107, 106f, 107f
  physical examination in, 108-110, 109t
Doppler technique, 151f, 151-152
Doppler ultrasonic flowmeter, 151, 151f
Doppler ultrasonic stethoscope, 516, 516f
Dorsal arch, 500f
Dorsal column, 624, 624f
Dorsal venous arch, 501f
Dorsalis pedis artery, 500, 500f
Dorsalis pedis pulse, 512-513, 513f
Down syndrome, 274t
  maternal age and, 798-799
  simian crease and, 600
  tongue abnormalities in, 380t
Dress
  general survey and, 129
  interview and, 31
  mental status assessment and, 73
Driving, older adult and, 840-841, 841t
Drooping upper lid, 313t
Drug(s)
  adolescent and, 65f
  hepatitis risk and, 554
  for hypertension, 156t
  interactions with alcohol, 96
Drug abuse, 94, 100
Drug history
  in abdominal assessment, 533
  in allergic skin eruption, 208
  in anus, rectum, and prostate examination, 712
  in health history
    adult, 52
    child, 61
    older adult, 66
  in nutritional assessment, 183
Drug-induced disorders
  headache in, 257
  skin eruption in, 208
Drum hypomobility, 336
Drusen, 308, 308f
Dry mouth, 358
Dry skin, 207, 210, 225
Dry snuff, 370
Dual-energy x-ray absorptiometry, 189
Ductus arteriosus, 464, 464f
Dull percussion sound, 117t, 425
Duodenal ulcer, 559t
Duodenum, 529f
  referred abdominal pain and, 559t
Dupuytren contracture, 611t
Dwarfism, 154-155t
Dysarthria, 74, 84t, 631
Dyschezia, 712
Dysdiadochokinesia, 640
Dyskinesia, 659
Dysmetria, 631, 640
Dysphagia, 258, 358, 532
Dysphasia, 631
Dysphonia, 84t
Dysphoria, 74
Dyspnea, 467
  in heart failure, 486t
Dysrhythmias, 466
Dysthymic disorder, 89t
Dysuria
  male, 684
  in urethritis, 700t

E

Ear, 323-350
  abnormalities of
    ear canal, 344-345t
    external ear, 341t
    otoscopic findings in, 346t
    tympanic membrane, 346-348t
  of aging adult, 326-327
  external, 323-324, 324f, 325f
  genetic variations in, 327
Ear (*Continued*)
  health history of, 327-329
    adult, 55
    child, 62
    older adult, 67
  hearing and, 325-326, 326f
  inner, 325
  lumps and lesions on, 342-343t
  middle, 324
  noise-induced hearing loss and, 338
  otitis media and, 327
  pediatric, 326, 326f
  physical examination of, 330-340
    aging adult and, 337
    documentation and critical thinking in, 338-340
    external canal and, 332
    external ear and, 330f, 330-331
    hearing acuity test and, 333
    infants and children and, 334-336f, 334-337
    otoscopic inspection in, 331f, 331-332
    tympanic membrane and, 332f, 332-333
    vestibular apparatus and, 334
  sequence in health assessment, 765, 774, 780
  structure and function of, 323, 324f
Ear canal
  abnormalities of, 344-345t
  physical examination of, 332
Earache, 327
Earbuds, 338
Eardrum, 323-324, 324f, 325f
  abnormal otoscopic findings of, 346t
  abnormalities of, 346-348t
  physical examination of, 332f, 332-333
  vibratility of, 336
Early diastolic murmur, 497t
Eastern medicine, 21
Eating patterns
  of adolescent, 65f
  cultural considerations in, 177f, 177-178, 178t
  in health history, 182
Ecchymosis, 216, 216f, 237t, 240t
  in abuse and neglect, 108-109, 209
  birth-related, 220
  forensic term, 109t
  health history of, 208
Eccrine sweat gland, 204f, 205
ECG; *See* Electrocardiography
Echolalia, 86t
Eclampsia, 822t
Economic status, child functional assessment and, 64
Ectopic pregnancy, 759t
Ectropion, 313t
  cervical, 740
Eczema, 241t
Edema, 215
  of arm or leg, 505
  of breast, 390, 404t
  cardiovascular assessment and, 468
  in heart failure, 486t
  periorbital, 260, 312t
  pitting, 513f, 513-514
  during pregnancy, 797
  pretibial, 513, 513f
  scrotal, 706t
Effective care, 12
Effusion of joint, 609t
Egophony, 446t
EHR; *See* Electronic health recording
Ejaculatory duct, 681
Ejection click, 489t
Elation, 85t
Elbow, 570, 570f
  abnormalities of, 610t
  physical examination of, 582-584, 583f, 584f
Elder abuse and neglect, 103-114, 104t
  assessing for, 107, 107t
  documentation of, 110f, 110-111, 111f
  health effects of, 105
  physical examination in, 108-109, 109t
Elderly; *See* Older adult
Electrical conduction system of heart, 461f, 461-462
Electrocardiography
  age-related changes in, 466
  waveforms in, 461, 461f
Electronic charting, 792
Electronic health recording, 32
Electronic thermometer, 133

Electronic vital signs monitor, 150, 151f
Elevation, 566, 567f
Elimination
  adult and, 57
  older adult and, 68
Emergency database, 8
Emerging majority, 11
Emerging minority, 9
Emotional abuse, 103-104
Emotions, blood pressure and, 137
Empathy, interview and, 30, 34, 34f
Emphysema, 449t
  liver displacement in, 542
Encopresis, 713
Endocardium, 456, 457f
Endocervical specimen, 741f, 741-742
Endocrine system
  adult health history of, 56-57
  changes from poorly controlled pain, 169t
  child health history of, 63
Endogenous obesity, 155t
Endometrial carcinoma, 758t
Endometriosis, 758t
Energy-boosting drinks, 184
Engagement of fetus, 810
Enlarged organs, 562-563t
Enophthalmos, 313t
Entropion, 313t
Environment
  of examination room, 120-121, 121t
  functional assessment of older adult and, 840f, 840-842, 841t
  interview and, 31, 31f
Environmental hazards
  adult and, 58
  child and, 64
  history of exposure to, 420, 631
  older adult and, 68-69
  pregnant woman and, 806
  skin lesions and, 209
Environmental noise, 328-329
Ephelides, 212, 213f
Epicanthal fold, 304
Epicondyle, 583
Epicondylitis, 610t
Epidermal appendages, 204-205, 205f
Epidermis, 203-204, 204f
Epididymis, 680f, 681
Epididymitis, 704t
Epigastric area, 530, 530f
Epigastric hernia, 560t
Epiphyses, 573
Epispadias, 703t
Epistaxis, 357, 373t
Epitrochlear lymph node, 503, 503f, 508, 508f
Epstein's pearls, 369, 369f
Epulis, 376t
  of pregnancy, 797
Equal-status seating, 31, 31f
Equilibrium, 326
Equipment, 119f, 119-120, 120f
  for abdominal examination, 536
  for anus, rectum, and prostate examination, 713
  for breast examination, 392
  for cardiovascular assessment, 470
  for chest examination, 421
  for ear examination, 330
  for examination of pregnant woman, 806
  for eye examination, 287
  for female genitourinary examination, 732-733, 733f
  for male genitourinary examination, 688
  for musculoskeletal examination, 577
  for neurologic examination, 632
  for nose, mouth, and throat examination, 359
  for peripheral vascular and lymphatic examination, 506
  for skin examination, 211
Erb's point, 475f
Erosion, 234t
  cervical, 754t
Erythema, 213-214, 229t
Erythema migrans, 244t
Erythema toxicum, 221, 221f
Esophagus, referred abdominal pain and, 559t
Esotropia, 311t
Essential hypertension, 156t
Essential tremor, 671t
Estrogen
  aging woman and, 728
  pregnancy and, 796
  puberty and, 726
Ethmoid sinus, 352, 353f
Ethnicity, 14-15, 15f
Etiquette, cultural considerations in, 43-44
Euphoria, 85t
European heritages
  culture-bound syndromes in, 26t
  health and illness beliefs and practices of, 25t
Eustachian tube, 324, 324f, 352f
  of infant, 326, 326f
Eversion, 566, 567f
  cervical, 740
  of upper eyelid, 294, 294f
Evidence
  aging adult pain and, 163
  appendix location during pregnancy and, 531
  artificial ultraviolet tanning and, 227
  body mass index and, 130
  breast cancer risk and, 388
  breast-self examination and, 399
  of bruising, 108
  cardiac border and, 475
  cardiovascular disease risks and, 466
  chest percussion *versus* chest x-ray and, 475
  of child abuse, 109
  chronic pain and, 168
  corneal reflex test and, 634
  diabetes mellitus risks and, 467
  for growth potential, 145
  heart rate and, 134
  iliopsoas muscle test and, 551
  lymphedema after breast cancer and, 520
  of noise-induced hearing loss, 338
  of organic brain disease, 76
  of primary hypertension in children, 148
  of problem drinking, 99
  scratch test and, 542
  speculum examination and, 737
  stool samples and, 717
  testing for wheezing and, 430
  transillumination and, 361
  tuning fork tests and, 333
  tympanic thermometry and, 133
  women and heart attacks and, 484
Evidence-based assessment, 1f, 1-10
  critical thinking and, 2-6, 3f, 5t
  cultural competence and, 9, 9f
  data collection in, 7-8
  diagnostic reasoning and, 2
  evidence-based practice and, 6, 6f
  expanding concept of health and, 8, 8f
Evidence-based practice, 6f, 6-7
  in acute tonsillitis and pharyngitis, 381
Examination room, 118-119, 119f
  safety of, 120-121, 121t
Examination table, 119, 119f
Excessive cup-disc ratio, 320t
Excoriation, 234t
Exercise
  adolescent and, 535
  adult and, 57
  blood pressure and, 136
  nutritional assessment and, 183
  older adult and, 68, 839-840
Exophthalmos, 312t
Exostosis, 345t
Exotropia, 311t
Expected date of delivery, 798
Expiration, 416, 417f
Expiratory wheezing, 437
Expressive aphasia, 84t, 622
Extension, 566, 567f
External acoustic meatus, 252f
External anal sphincter, 709, 710f
External auditory canal, 323, 324f
  abnormalities of, 344t
  physical examination of, 332
External auditory meatus, 324f, 330-331
External carotid artery, 253f
External ear, 323-324, 324f, 325f
  abnormalities of, 341t
  physical examination of, 330f, 330-331
External genitalia of female, 725-726, 726f
  abnormalities of, 752-753t
  inspection of, 735f, 735-737, 736f
External hemorrhoid, 720t
External iliac artery, 500f, 529f
External iliac vein, 501f, 529f
External jugular vein, 253f, 462, 463f
External oblique muscle, 528f
Extinction test, 645
Extracardiac sounds, 491t
Extraocular muscles, 280-281, 281f
  of child, 304, 304f
  dysfunction of, 311-312t
  inspection of function of, 290-292, 291f
Extrapyramidal tract, 625, 625f
Exudate, retinal, 321t
Eye, 279-322
  abnormalities on cornea and iris, 318-319t
  of aging adult, 284-285
  Bitot's spots and, 199t
  external anatomy of, 279-281, 280f, 281f
  extraocular muscle dysfunction and, 311-312t
  eyelid abnormalities and, 312-313t
  eyelid lesions and, 314t
  glaucoma screening and, 308
  health history of, 285-297
    adult, 55
    child, 62
    older adult, 67
  of infants and children, 284
  internal anatomy of, 281-282, 282f
  malnutrition and, 186t
  opacities in lens and, 319t
  optic disc abnormalities and, 320t
  physical examination of, 287-310
    of aging adult, 306-308, 306-308f
    anterior eyeball structures inspection in, 295-296, 296f
    confrontation test in, 289f, 289-290, 290f
    cover test in, 290, 291f
    diagnostic positions test in, 291f, 291-292
    documentation and critical thinking in, 309-310
    external ocular structures inspection in, 292-294, 292-295f
    Hirschberg test in, 290
    of infants and children, 302-305f, 302-306
    near vision test in, 288, 289f
    ophthalmoscopy in, 296-302, 297-301f
    Snellen Eye Chart and, 287-288, 288f
  pupil abnormalities and, 315t
  racial differences in, 285
  retinal vessels abnormalities and, 320-321t
  sequence in health assessment, 765, 774, 779
  vascular disorders of external eye and, 317t
  visual field loss and, 316t
  visual pathways and visual fields of, 282-283, 283f
  visual reflexes of, 283-284, 284f
Eye contact
  cultural considerations in, 47-48
  nonverbal communication and, 37
Eye protection, Standard Precautions and, 121t
Eyebrow
  inspection of, 292, 292f
  of older adult, 306, 306f
Eyeglasses, 286
Eyelashes, 279, 280f
  of infant, 304
  inspection of, 292-293
Eyelid, 279-280, 280f
  abnormalities of, 312-313t
  eversion of, 294, 294f
  of infant, 304
  inspection of, 292-293
  lesions of, 314t

F

Face, 251-253, 252f
  abnormal appearance with chronic illness, 275-277t
  of child, 256, 266
  general survey and, 128
  pediatric abnormalities of, 274-275t
  physical examination of, 260
  sequence in health assessment, 765, 773-774
Face presentation, 826t
Face shield, Standard Precautions and, 121t
Faces Pain Scale-Revised, 167, 167f
Facial bones, 251, 252f
Facial expression
  general survey and, 129
  mental status assessment and, 74
  nonverbal communication and, 37

Facial nerve, 627f
abnormalities of, 668t
infant reflexes and, 651t
testing of, 635, 635f
Facilitation in interview, 33
Fallopian tube, 726, 727f
mass in, 759t
False assurance, 35
Family history
in adult health history, 52-54, 53f
in anus, rectum, and prostate examination, 712
cardiac, 468
in child health history, 62
in nutritional assessment, 183
in older adult health history, 67
pregnant woman and, 804
Family tree, 52, 53f
Family Violence Prevention Fund, 106, 107f
Far vision, 296, 296f
Farsighted, 299f
Fasciculation, 670t
Fasciculi, 566
Fatigue
cardiovascular assessment and, 468
in heart failure, 486t
Fear, 85t
Fecal impaction, 722t
Female
heart attack and, 484
pregnant; *See* Pregnant woman
rectum and anus of, 711
screening for alcohol problems, 98
Female circumcision, 728
Female genital mutilation, 728
Female genitourinary system, 725-762
abnormalities of external genitalia and, 752-753t
adnexal enlargement and, 759-760t
of aging woman, 728
cervical abnormalities and, 754-755t
culture and genetics and, 728
external genitalia in, 725-726, 726f
health history of, 729-732
adult, 56
child, 63
human papillomavirus vaccine and, 750
of infants and children, 726-728, 727t
internal genitalia in, 726, 727f
pediatric abnormalities of, 760t
pelvic musculature abnormalities and, 754t
physical examination of, 732-751
of adolescent, 748-749
of aging adult, 749-750
bimanual examination in, 742-746, 743-746f
documentation and critical thinking in, 750-751
of infants and children, 747-748
inspection of cervix and os in, 739f, 739-740
inspection of external genitalia in, 735f, 735-737, 736f
obtaining cervical smears and cultures in, 740f, 740-742, 741f
patient preparation and equipment for, 732-733, 733f
positioning for, 733f, 733-735, 734f
of pregnant woman, 749
rectovaginal examination in, 746-747, 747f
speculum examination in, 737f, 737-738, 738f
vaginal wall inspection in, 742
of pregnant woman, 728
sequence in health assessment, 772, 775
uterine enlargement and, 757-758t
vulvovaginal inflammations and, 756-757t
Female pseudohermaphroditism, 760t
Femoral aneurysm, 524t
Femoral artery, 500, 500f
occlusion of, 562t
Femoral canal, 681, 681f
Femoral hernia, 707t
Femoral pulse, 511, 511f
Femoral vein, 501, 501f
Femur, 571, 571f
Festinating gait, 672t
Fetal alcohol syndrome, 274t
Fetal circulation, 464, 464f
Fetal growth restriction, 823t
Fetal lie, 810
Fetal position, 810, 823t
Fetal testing, 819
Fetus
auscultation of fetal heart tones, 813, 813f
decreased movement of, 825t
determining weeks of gestation, 798, 798f
Leopold's maneuvers and, 810-813, 811-813f
malpresentations of, 826t
size inconsistent with dates, 823-824t
Fever, 133
Fibroadenoma of breast, 405t, 406t
Fibroids, 758t, 824t
Fibromyalgia, 619t
Financial abuse, 104t
Financial neglect, 104t
Fine crackles, 436
Fine touch test, 644
Finger
dermatomes of, 628f
Raynaud's phenomenon and, 520t
Finger-to-finger test, 640
Finger-to-nose test, 640f, 641
Fingernails, 205, 205f
abnormalities of, 248-250f
of aging adult, 226
health history of, 209
inspection and palpation of, 218f, 218-219, 219f
malnutrition and, 186t
First heart sound, 460, 460f, 476f, 476-477, 477f
variations in, 487t
First-level priority problems, 5
First trimester, 796f, 796-797
Fissure, 234t
anorectal, 720t
of lung, 414, 414f, 415f
Fissured tongue, 380t
Fistula, anorectal, 720t
Fixation of breast, 404t
Fixation reflex of eye, 283-284
Fixed split of second heart sound, 478, 488t
Flaccid quadriplegia, 676t
Flaccidity, 669t
Flat abdomen, 536f
Flat affect, 85t
Flat percussion sound, 117t
Flatfoot, 601
Flea bite, 221, 221f
Flight of ideas, 86t
Floater, 284, 285
Fluid wave, 543f, 543-544
Focused database, 7-8
Folk healer, 23-24
Follicular hyperkeratosis, 198t
Folliculitis, 247t
Follow-up database, 8
Fontanel, 256, 256f, 266
Food allergy, 183
Food diary, 180
Food frequency questionnaire, 180
Food intolerance, 532
Foot, 572-573, 573f
abnormalities of, 615-616t
arterial ulcer of, 522t
athlete's, 243t
care of, 517
clubfoot deformity of, 618t
dermatomes of, 628f
of infant, 598
physical examination of, 592-594, 593f, 594f
of preschool and school-age children, 601, 601f
Footdrop, 672t
Footling breech presentation, 826t
Foramen ovale, 464, 464f
Forced expiratory time, 433
Forced expiratory volume in 1 second, 434
Forced inspiration, 416
Forced vital capacity, 434
Fordyce's granule, 365, 365f
Foreign body
in ear, 344t
in nose, 373t
Forensic terminology, 109t
Foreskin, 679, 680f
abnormalities of, 702t
Forward bend test, 603, 603f
Four Unrelated Words Test, 75
Fourchette, 725, 726f
Fourth heart sound, 461, 491t
Fovea centralis, 282, 283f
Fracture
Colles, 611t
of infant clavicle, 600
Frame size, 190, 190f
Frank breech presentation, 826t
Freckles, 212, 213f
Frenulum, 354, 354f
labial, 725, 726f
penile, 679, 680f
tongue-tie and, 379t
Frequency, 684
Frontal bone, 252f
neonatal, 256f
Frontal lobe, 622, 622f
Frontal release signs, 677t
Frontal sinus, 352, 352f, 353f
palpation of, 361, 361f
Frontal suture of newborn, 256f
Frontalis muscle, 252f
Frostbite, 341t
Frozen shoulder, 609t
Full, bounding pulse, 519t
Functional ability, 830
Functional assessment
of adult, 57-59
of child, 63-64
in musculoskeletal examination, 575, 605
of older adult, 67-69, 829-847
activities of daily living and, 830-832, 831f
acute care setting and, 837-838
advanced activities of daily living and, 832
altered cognition and, 844
assistive living and, 839
caregiver assessment and, 837, 838f
cognitive evaluation in, 835, 835t
community-based services and, 838
continuing care retirement communities and, 839
cultural considerations in, 843-844
depression and, 835-836, 836f
driving and, 840-841, 841t
exercise and, 839-840
health care maintenance and, 840
home care and, 839
instrumental activities of daily living and, 832, 833f
measuring physical performance in, 832-834
nursing facilities and, 839
pain and, 844
risk for functional decline during hospitalization in, 834f, 834-835
sleep and, 841t, 841-842, 842t
social domain and, 836-837, 837t
spiritual assessment and, 842-843
Functional Independence Measure, 831-832
Functional murmur, 479, 482
Functional scoliosis, 617t
Fundus of uterus, 727f
Funduscopic examination, 296-302
of child, 306
macula and, 301-302
ophthalmoscope in, 296-297, 297f, 299f, 300f
optic disc and, 300f, 300-301, 301f
retinal vessels and, 301
Fungal infection
of ear, 348t
in jock itch, 701t
of nails, 226
in pruritus ani, 721t
Furuncle, 248t, 345t
nasal, 374t

G

GAD-7 scale, 77, 77f
Gag reflex, 367
Gait
abnormal, 672-673t
of aging adult, 149, 659
neurologic assessment of, 637-638, 638f
testing in child, 658, 658f
Galactorrhea, 389
Galea aponeurotica, 252f
Gallbladder, 528f, 529
enlarged, 563t
referred abdominal pain and, 559t
Gallstones, 531
Gamma glutamyl transferase, 99
Ganglion cyst, 611t

Gardasil; *See* Human papillomavirus vaccine
Gardnerella vaginalis, 756t
Gas in abdomen, 557t
Gastrocolic reflex, 711
Gastroesophageal reflux disease, 559t
Gastrointestinal bleeding, 717
Gastrointestinal system
  adult health history of, 55-56
  changes from poorly controlled pain, 169t
  child health history of, 63
Gaze, cardinal positions of, 312t
Gender
  blood pressure and, 136
  cultural considerations in, 44-45
  differences in pain behavior, 163
  general survey and, 127
General appearance
  bedside assessment of, 788
  cultural considerations in, 152-153
  in mental status assessment, 73-74
  sequence in health assessment, 764, 772, 777
  in substance use disorders, 101t
General overall health state
  in adult health history, 54
  in child health history, 62
  in older adult health history, 66
General survey, 127-129
  of infants and children, 142-143
  of pregnant woman, 806-807
Generalized anxiety disorder, 77, 91t
Genetics
  in breast development and disease, 388
  in ear variations, 327
  in eye variations, 285
  in female genitourinary issues, 728
  in nose, mouth, and throat differences, 356
  in prostate and colorectal cancer, 711
  in skin and hair differences, 206-207
Genital herpes, 701t
Genital lesion, 701-702t
Genital warts, 701t, 742, 753t
Genitourinary system
  bedside assessment of, 791
  changes from poorly controlled pain, 169t
  female, 725-762
    abnormalities of external genitalia and, 752-753t
    adnexal enlargement and, 759-760t
    of aging woman, 728
    cervical abnormalities and, 754-755t
    culture and genetics and, 728
    external genitalia in, 725-726, 726f
    health history of, 729-732
    human papillomavirus vaccine and, 750
    of infants and children, 726-728, 727t
    internal genitalia in, 726, 727f
    pediatric abnormalities of, 760t
    pelvic musculature abnormalities and, 754t
    of pregnant woman, 728
    uterine enlargement and, 757-758t
    vulvovaginal inflammations and, 756-757t
  male, 679-708
    of adolescent, 681-683, 682t, 683f
    of aging adult, 683, 697
    chronic kidney disease and, 683-684
    circumcision and, 683
    genital lesions and, 701-702t
    health history of, 684-688, 685f
    of infant, 681, 695f, 695-697, 696f
    inguinal and femoral hernias and, 692, 692f, 707t
    inguinal area in, f, 681
    inguinal lymph nodes and, 693, 693f
    penile abnormalities and, 702-703t
    penis in, 679, 680f, 689f, 689-690, 690f
    screening for prostate cancer and, 697
    scrotal abnormalities and, 704-706t
    scrotum in, 680-681, 690f, 690-692, 691f
    testicular self-examination and, 693-694, 694f
    urinary function assessment and, 694
    urinary problems and, 700t
    urine color and discolorations and, 699t
Genogram, 52, 53f
Genu valgum, 601, 601f
Genu varum, 601, 601f
Geographic tongue, 379t
GERD; *See* Gastroesophageal reflux disease
Geriatric Depression Scale, Short Form, 835t, 836, 836f
Geriatric patient; *See* Older adult
German measles, 242t, 803
Gestation, determining weeks of, 798, 798f
Gestational nutrition, 184
Gestures, nonverbal communication and, 36
Get Up and Go Test, 834
GFR; *See* Glomerular filtration rate
GGT; *See* Gamma glutamyl transferase
Gigantism, 154t
Gingival hyperplasia, 377t
Gingivitis, 377t
  during pregnancy, 369, 369f, 797
Glandular tissue of breast, 384, 384f
Glans penis, 679, 680f
Glasgow Coma scale, 80
  in neurologic recheck, 663, 663f
Glaucoma, 285
  excessive cup-disc ratio in, 320t
  history of, 286
  screening for, 308
Glenohumeral joint, 568-570, 569f, 570f
Global aphasia, 84t
Globe
  inspection of, 293
  lesion of, 316t
Glomerular filtration rate, 694
Glossitis, 379t
Glossopharyngeal nerve, 627f
  abnormalities of, 669t
  infant reflexes and, 651t
  testing of, 635
Gloves
  for inspection of tongue, 364, 364f
  safety and, 121
  Standard Precautions and, 121t
Glucose
  in metabolic syndrome, 200t
  plasma, 191
Glue ear, 346t
Goiter, 272t, 276t
Gonorrhea, 742, 757t
Goodell sign, 728, 796, 815
Gordon reflex, 677t
Gout, 615t
Gouty arthritis, 610t
Gower's sign, 658, 658f
Gown
  auscultation through, 118
  Standard Precautions and, 121t
Graphesthesia, 644, 644f
Grasp reflex, 677t
Graves' disease, 276t
Gravida, 796
Gray matter, 621
Great saphenous vein, 501, 501f
Great vessels, 456
Greater trochanter of femur, 571, 571f
Greater tubercle of humerus, 570, 570f
Groin, 681, 681f
Grooming, mental status assessment and, 74
Grouped skin lesions, 231t
Growth
  developmental history of, 61
  as index of child's general health, 145
Guaiac-based fecal occult blood test, 717
Guide to Clinical Preventive Services, 9
Gums
  abnormalities of, 376-377t
  bleeding, 357
  gingivitis and, 377t
  malnutrition and, 186t
  of older adult, 370, 370f
  physical examination of, 362, 363f
  of pregnant woman, 369, 369f, 807
  scorbutic, 198t
Gynecoid pelvis, 816, 817t
Gynecologic history, 800
Gynecomastia, 388, 400, 409t
Gyrate skin lesion, 231t
Gyrus, 622f

H

Habit-tic dystrophy, 250t
Habits
  adult and, 58
  child and, 64
Haemophilus vaginalis, 756t
Hair, 204-205, 205f
  abdominal, 538
  abnormalities of, 246-248t
  aging-related changes in, 206, 226
  biocultural differences in, 207
  health history of, 55
  inspection and palpation of, 217
  malnutrition and, 186t
  of newborn, 223, 223f
Hair follicle, 204f
  folliculitis and, 247t
Hair loss, 208-209, 226, 246t
Hair shaft, 204, 204f
Halal, dietary term, 178
Halitosis, 367
Hallucination, 87t
Hallux valgus, 593, 593f, 616t
Hammertoe, 616t
Hand
  abnormalities of, 611-613t
  dermatomes of, 628f
  physical examination of, 584-587, 584-587f
  Raynaud's phenomenon and, 520t
Handwashing, 120-121, 121t
Hard palate, 352f, 352-354, 353f, 365f, 365-366, 366f
Harlequin color change, 221
Harrison groove, 435
Hay fever, 357
Head, 251-278
  abnormal facies appearance with chronic illness, 275-277t
  brain injury prevention and, 267
  of child, 256, 256f
  dermatomes of, 628f
  head size and contour abnormalities and, 271t
  headaches and, 270t
  health history of, 256-259
    adult, 55
    child, 62
  infant posture and control of, 266
  lymphatics of, 255f, 255-256
  of older adult, 256
  pediatric facial abnormalities of, 274-275t
  physical examination of, 259-269
    aging adult and, 267
    documentation and critical thinking in, 268-269
    face and, 260
    lymph nodes and, 260-262, 261f, 262f
    pediatric, 264-267, 265f
    pregnant woman and, 267
    range of motion and, 260
    skull and, 259-260
    thyroid gland and, 263f, 263-264, 264f
    trachea and, 262, 263f
  sequence in health assessment, 765, 773, 779
  structure and function of, 251-255, 252-255f
  swelling of, 272-273t
Head circumference, 145, 145f
Head control in newborn, 652-653, 653f
Head injury
  history of, 257-258, 630
  prevention of, 267
Head lag, 266, 653
Head lice, 217, 247t
Headache, 256-257, 270t, 630
Healing, culture and, 22-23
Health, 11
  expanding concept of, 8, 8f
  perception of, 59
  role of religion and spirituality in, 15-16, 17f
Health assessment
  bedside, 787-793
    abdomen and, 791
    activity level and, 791
    cardiovascular system and, 790
    electronic charting and, 792
    general appearance and, 788
    genitourinary system and, 791
    health history in, 788
    neurologic system and, 789
    respiratory system and, 789
    SBAR framework for staff communication and, 793
    skin and, 790
    vital signs measurement in, 788-789

Health assessment (*Continued*)
cultural competence in, 9, 9f, 11-28
demographic profile of United States and, 11-12
developmental competence and, 20-21
health history and, 54
health-related beliefs and practices and, 19-20
heritage and, 14-16, 15f, 17f
heritage assessment and, 17-19, 18f
immigration and, 12
domestic violence, 103-114
assessment for risk of homicide in, 112, 112f
child abuse and neglect and, 108
cultural considerations in, 113
definitions in, 103-104, 104t
denial in, 113
documentation in, 110f, 110-111, 111f
elder abuse and neglect and, 107, 107t
health effects of violence and, 104-105
history in, 108
intimate partner violence and, 105-107, 106f, 107f
physical examination in, 108-110, 109t
evidence-based, 1f, 1-10
critical thinking and, 2-6, 3f, 5t
cultural competence and, 9, 9f
data collection in, 7-8
diagnostic reasoning and, 2
evidence-based practice and, 6, 6f
expanding concept of health and, 8, 8f
nutritional, 175-202
adolescent and, 176
adult and, 176
aging adult and, 176-177
anthropometric measures in, 187-190f, 187-191
cultural considerations in, 177f, 177-178
documentation and critical thinking in, 195
guidelines for two thousand calories per day, 181t, 181-182
health history in, 182-185
health promotion and, 193-194
infants and children and, 176, 191, 193
laboratory studies and, 191-192
malnutrition and, 186t, 196-197t
Malnutrition Screening Tool in, 178t, 179
metabolic syndrome and, 200t
Mini Nutritional Assessment in, 179, 179f
MyPyramid Dietary Guidelines and, 181, 181f
nutritional consequences of bariatric surgery and, 200t
nutritional deficiencies and, 198-199t
nutritional status and, 175
pregnancy and lactation and, 176
religious dietary practices and, 178t
serial assessment in malnourished individual and, 193
Subjective Global Assessment in, 180t, 180-181
sequence of, 763-785
abdomen and, 768
chest and, 767
documentation and critical thinking in, 781-785
ears and, 765
eyes and, 765
female breasts and, 767
female genitalia and, 772
general appearance and, 764
head and face and, 765
health history and, 764
heart and, 767, 768
inguinal area and, 768
lower extremities and, 769, 770
male breasts and, 768
male genitalia and, 771
male rectum and, 771
measurement and, 764
mouth and throat and, 766
musculoskeletal system and, 769, 770-771
neck and, 766
neck vessels and, 768
neurologic system and, 769-770
newborn and infant and, 772-776
nose and, 766
school-age child, adolescent, and aging adult and, 780
skin and, 765
toddler and preschool child and, 777-780
upper extremities and, 767
vital signs and, 765

Health assessment (*Continued*)
substance use, 93-102
aging adult and, 96
alcohol use and abuse and, 93, 94t
clinical signs of substance use disorders and, 100-101t
diagnosis of substance abuse and, 95t, 95-96
health history in, 96-99, 97t, 99t
illicit drug use and, 94
normal range of findings in, 99-100
pregnant woman and, 96
prescription medication abuse and, 100
Health care
maintenance by older adult, 840
national standards for, 12f, 12-14, 13t
Health disparity, 14
Health history, 49-69
of abdomen, 532-535
of adolescent, 64, 65f
of anus, rectum, and prostate, 712-713
bedside assessment and, 788
biographic data in, 49-50
of breast, 389-391, 391t
adult, 55
pediatric, 62, 391
in cardiovascular assessment, 467-470
of chest and lungs, 418-421
cultural competence and, 54
in ear assessment, 327-329
of eye, 285-297
family history in, 52-54, 53f
of female genitourinary system, 56, 63, 729-732
functional assessment in, 57-59
in head and neck assessment, 256-259
initial pain assessment and, 164
of male genitourinary system, 684-688, 685f
in mental status assessment, 72
of musculoskeletal system, 56, 574-577
aging adult and, 67
infants and children and, 63
of neurologic system, 630-632
in nose, mouth, and throat assessment, 356-369
in nutritional assessment, 182-185
of older adult, 66f, 66-69
past health in, 51-52
pediatric, 59f, 59-64, 777
perception of health in, 59
in peripheral vascular system assessment, 505-506
of pregnant woman, 799-806
present health or history of present illness in, 50-51
reason for seeking care in, 50
review of systems in, 54-57
sequence in health assessment, 764, 777
in skin assessment, 207-211
source of history in, 50
in substance use assessment, 96-99, 97t, 99t
Health promotion, 8, 8f
in artificial tanning and skin cancer risk, 227
child functional assessment and, 64
in colorectal cancer screening, 718
in foot care, 517
in glaucoma screening, 308
in helmet safety, 267
in hepatitis risk, 554
in human papillomavirus vaccine, 750
in noise-induced hearing loss, 338
in nutritional assessment, 193-194
in prescription medication abuse, 100
in prevention of osteoporosis, 606
in screening for prostate cancer, 697
in secondhand smoke, 438
in skin self-examination, 219, 219f
in smokeless tobacco and cancer risk, 370
in stroke prevention, 664
in vital signs, 152
in women and heart attacks, 484
Health-related beliefs and practices, 19-20, 24t, 25t
Hearing, 325-326, 326f
environmental noise and, 328-329
noise-induced hearing loss and, 338
Hearing acuity test, 333, 337
Hearing-impairment, interview and, 40-41
Hearing loss, 326
cerumen impaction-related, 331
child and, 337
health history of, 328
noise-induced, 338

Heart, 455-498
of aging adult, 465, 465f
auscultation of, 475-480, 475-480f
cardiac cycle and, 458-460, 459f
cardiovascular heart disease and, 466-467
changes from poorly controlled pain, 169t
direction of blood flow and, 458, 458f
electrical conduction system of, 461f, 461-462
enlargement of, 475, 482
health history of, 467-470
of infants and children, 464, 464f, 465f
position and surface landmarks of, 455-456, 456f, 457f
of pregnant woman, 464-465, 808
pulmonary and systemic circulations and, 455, 456f
pumping ability of, 462, 462f
sequence in health assessment, 767, 768
sounds of, 460f, 460-461
wall, chambers, and valves of, 456-458, 457t
Heart attack, woman and, 484
Heart disease
cultural considerations in, 466
risk factors for, 468-469
Heart failure, 450t, 486t
Heart murmur, 461, 494-497t
auscultation of heart and, 478-480, 478-480f
Heart rate, 476
of infant, 481
measurement of, 134
Heart rhythm, 476
Heart sounds, 460f, 460-461
of aging adult, 483
auscultation of, 476-478, 476-478f
diastolic extra, 490-491t
extracardiac, 491t
of pregnant woman, 483
systolic extra, 489t
Heart valves, 456-458, 457f, 457t
Heartburn, 532
Heave, 473, 492t
HEEADSSS method of interviewing, 64, 65f
Heel-to-shin test, 641, 641f
Hegar sign, 728, 796, 815
Height
abnormalities of, 154-155t
measurement of, 130
aging adult and, 149
child and, 144f, 144-145
of older adult, 191, 573-574
Helix, 324f
HELLP syndrome, 822t
Helmet safety, 267
Hemangioma, 238t
Hematocrit, 192
Hematologic health history
adult, 56
child, 63
Hematoma, 109t, 237t
Hemianopsia, 316t
Hemiplegia, 674t
Hemisection of spinal cord, 675t
Hemisphere, cerebral, 622
Hemoglobin, 192
Hemorrhage
forensic term, 109t
intraretinal, 321t
splinter, 249t
subconjunctival, 317t
Hemorrhoids, 720t
during pregnancy, 797
Hemotympanum, 348t
Hepatitis
pregnant woman and, 805
risk for, 554
Hepatojugular reflex, 473, 473f
Hepatomegaly, 541
Hepatosplenomegaly, 486t
Heritage, 14-16, 15f, 17f
Heritage assessment, 17-19, 18f
Heritage consistency, 14
Hernia
incisional, 560t
scrotal, 706t
umbilical, 560t
Herniated nucleus pulposus, 617t
Heroin, 101t
Herpes genitalis, 701t, 752t

- Herpes simplex virus, 375t, 379t
  - in Bell's palsy, 276t
  - in cold sore, 244t
- Herpes zoster, 244t
- Hesitancy, 684
- Heteronymous hemianopsia, 316t
- Heterosexism, 45
- Hiccup, 670t
- High-fiber foods, 713
- Higher intellectual function, 76
- Hinduism, dietary practices of, 178t
- Hip, 571f, 571-572
  - congenital dislocation of, 618t
  - of infant, 599, 599f
  - physical examination of, 588f, 588-589
- Hirschberg test, 290
- Hirsutism, 209, 217, 248t
- History of present illness
  - in adult health history, 50-51
  - in child health history, 60
- HIV; *See* Human immunodeficiency virus infection
- Hives, 232t
- Hoarseness, 357
- Hoffman reflex, 677t
- Holistic health, 8
- Holistic theory of illness, 21
- Hollow viscera, 527-529
- Holodiastolic murmur, 478
- Holosystolic/pandiastolic murmur, 478
- Homan sign, 511
- Home care, functional assessment of older adult and, 839
- Home environment
  - adolescent psychosocial interview and, 65f
  - child functional assessment and, 64
- Homicide risk in domestic violence, 112, 112f
- Homonymous hemianopsia, 316t
- Homunculus, 622f, 625
- Hooking technique, 548, 548f
- Hordeolum, 314t
- Horizontal fissure, 414, 414f
- Hormones, thyroid, 254
- Horner's syndrome, 315t
- Horny cell layer, 203, 204f
- Hospital Admission Risk Profile, 834f, 835
- Hospitalization
  - history of, 52, 60, 66
  - risk for functional decline during, 834f, 834-835
- Hospitalized adult
  - bedside assessment of, 787-793
    - abdomen and, 791
    - activity level and, 791
    - cardiovascular system and, 790
    - electronic charting and, 792
    - general appearance and, 788
    - genitourinary system and, 791
    - health history in, 788
    - neurologic system and, 789
    - respiratory system and, 789
    - SBAR framework for staff communication and, 793
    - skin and, 790
    - vital signs measurement in, 788-789
  - interview of, 41
- Hot/cold theory, 21
- Human chorionic gonadotropin, 795
- Human immunodeficiency virus infection
  - circumcision and, 683
  - Kaposi sarcoma in, 246t
  - nutritional deficiencies in, 199t
  - pregnant woman and, 803
- Human papillomavirus
  - acetic acid wash for, 742
  - circumcision and, 683
  - in condylomata, 755t
  - in genital warts, 701t, 753t
- Human papillomavirus vaccine, 732, 750
- Human placental lactogen, 796
- Hydatidiform mole, 823t
- Hydrocele, 696, 706t
- Hydrocephalus, 271t
- Hygiene
  - general survey and, 129
  - mental status assessment and, 74
- Hymen, 725-726, 726f
- Hyoid bone, 255
- Hyperactive bowel sounds, 539, 561t
- Hyperalgesia, 642
- Hypercapnia, 416
- Hyperemesis during pregnancy, 825t
- Hyperesthesia, 642
- Hyperopia, 299f
- Hyperpituitarism, 154t
- Hyperplasia
  - gingival, 377t
  - sebaceous, 226, 226f
- Hyperreflexia, 645
- Hyperresonance, 425
- Hyperresonant percussion sound, 117t
- Hypertension, 156t
  - alcohol consumption and, 93
  - cardiovascular heart disease and, 466
  - lifestyle modifications for, 152
  - during pregnancy, 799, 819, 822t
- Hyperthermia, 133, 214
- Hyperthyroidism, 276t
- Hypertonia, 669t
- Hyperventilation, 442t
- Hyphema, 319t
- Hypnotics, 101t
- Hypoactive bowel sounds, 539, 561t
- Hypoalgesia, 642
- Hypochondriasis, 87t
- Hypoesthesia, 642
- Hypogastric area, 530, 530f
- Hypoglossal nerve, 627f
  - abnormalities of, 669t
  - infant reflexes and, 651t
  - testing of, 636
- Hypopituitary dwarfism, 154t
- Hypopyon, 319t
- Hyporeflexia, 645
- Hypospadias, 703t
- Hypotension, 156t
- Hypothalamus, 132, 622, 623f
- Hypothermia, 133, 214
- Hypothesis, 2
- Hypothyroidism
  - abnormal facies in, 276t
  - congenital, 274t
- Hypotonia, 669t
- Hypoventilation, 442t
- Hypoxemia, 416

I

- Iberian heritages
  - culture-bound syndromes in, 26t
  - health and illness beliefs and practices of, 25t
- Icterus, scleral, 293
- Iliac crest, 571
- Iliopsoas muscle test, 551, 551f
- Illness, 11
  - in health history
    - adult, 52
    - child, 60
    - older adult, 66
  - health-related beliefs and practices and, 19-20, 25t
  - setting for physical examination and, 126
  - traditional causes of, 21-24, 22f, 23f, 24t, 25t
  - transcultural expression of, 25-27, 26t
- Illusion, 87t
- Imaging studies for pregnant woman, 819
- Immature hemangioma, 238t
- Immigration, 12
- Immune system, 502-503
  - changes from poorly controlled pain, 169t
- Immunization history
  - adult, 52
  - pediatric, 61
- Impaction
  - cerumen, 344t
  - fecal, 722t
- Impaired judgment, 76
- Impetigo, 241t
- Inappropriate affect, 85t
- Incision, forensic term, 109t
- Incisional hernia, 560t
- Incompetent cervix, 825t
- Incompetent valves, 501
- Incoordination, 631
- Incus, 324, 324f, 325f
- Indirect inguinal hernia, 707t
- Infant
  - abdomen of, 531
    - health history of, 534
    - physical examination of, 552f, 552-553
  - abuse and neglect of, 103-114
    - documentation of, 111
    - health effects of, 105
    - physical examination in, 109-110
    - screening for, 108
  - anus, rectum, and prostate of
    - health history of, 713
    - physical examination of, 717
  - blood pressure measurement in, 148
  - body temperature measurement in, 146-147, 147f
  - breast examination in, 400-401
  - chest circumference of, 146, 146f
  - developmental history of, 61
  - ear of
    - health history of, 329
    - otitis media and, 327
    - physical examination of, 334-336f, 334-337
  - eye of, 284
    - health history of, 62, 287
    - physical examination of, 302-305f, 302-306
  - female genitourinary system of, 726-728, 727t
    - abnormalities of, 760t
    - health history of, 731
    - physical examination of, 747-748, 748f
  - general survey of, 142-143
  - head and neck of, 256, 256f
    - health history of, 259
    - physical examination of, 264-266, 265f
    - size and contour abnormalities of, 271t
  - head circumference of, 145, 145f
  - heart of, 464, 464f, 465f
    - health history of, 469
    - physical examination of, 480-482, 481f, 482f
  - heart rate of, 481
  - interview of, 38
  - length measurement in, 144, 144f
  - lungs of, 416-418, 417f
    - health history of, 420-421
    - physical examination of, 434-437, 435f, 435t, 436f
  - male genitourinary system of, 681
    - health history of, 686
    - physical examination of, 695f, 695-697, 696f
  - mental status assessment of, 72, 79f, 79-80
  - musculoskeletal system of, 573
    - health history of, 576
    - physical examination of, 598-600, 599f, 600f
  - neurologic system of, 629
    - frontal release signs and, 677t
    - health history of, 631-632
    - physical examination of, 651t, 651-657, 652-657f
  - nose, mouth, and throat of, 355
    - health history of, 358
    - physical examination of, 367-369, 367-369f
  - nutritional assessment and, 176
    - health history in, 183-184
    - laboratory tests in, 193
    - physical examination in, 191, 193
  - pain and, 163, 167, 167f, 169, 170f
  - peripheral vascular system and lymphatics of, 504, 504f, 516-517
  - positioning for physical examination, 122-123, 123f
  - preparation for physical examination, 123
  - respirations measurement in, 148, 148f
  - respiratory rate of, 135t
  - sequence of health assessment in, 123, 772-776
  - skin of, 205-206
    - health history of, 209-210
    - lesions of, 241-242t
    - physical examination of, 220-223, 220-223f
  - weight measurement in, 143, 143f
- Infantile automatisms, 654
- Infection
  - in conjunctivitis, 317t
  - ear, 328, 329
    - acute otitis media in, 347t
    - fungal, 348t
    - otitis externa in, 341t
    - otitis media in, 327
    - otitis media with effusion in, 346t
  - of eyelid hair follicle, 314t

Infection (*Continued*)
fungal
of ear, 348t
in jock itch, 701t
of nails, 226
pruritus ani in, 721t
in hyphema, 319t
nosocomial, 120
in vaginosis, 756t
Inferior border of scapula, 412, 413f
Inferior oblique muscle, 281f
Inferior rectus muscle, 281f
Inferior turbinate and meatus, 352, 352f, 361
Inferior vena cava, 456, 457f, 529f
venous hum and, 562t
Infibulation, 728
Inflammation
of breast, 404t
of eyelid, 314t
of joints, 608t
of lacrimal sac, 314t
in prostatitis, 723t
in subacromial bursitis, 609t
vulvovaginal, 756-757t
Influenza vaccination, 420
Inframammary ridge, 397
Infrapatellar fat pad, 572, 572f
Ingrown toenail, 616t
Inguinal area, 681, 681f, 768
Inguinal canal, 680f, 681
Inguinal hernia, 692, 692f, 707t
Inguinal ligament, 528f, 681, 681f
Inguinal lymph node, 503f, 693, 693f
Initial Pain Assessment tool, 165, 165f
Injection, Standard Precautions and, 121t
Injury
in adult health history, 52
in child health history, 60
in older adult health history, 66
Inner ear, 324f, 325
Innocent murmur, 479, 482
Inspection, 115
of abdomen, 536-538f, 536-539
of pregnant woman, 809f, 809-810, 810f
of ankle and foot, 592-593, 593f
of anterior chest, 430-431, 473
of axilla, 395, 395f
of breast, 392-394, 392-394f
of pregnant woman, 401
of cervix and os, 739f, 739-740
of external ear, 330, 330f
of eye
anterior eyeball structures and, 295-296, 296f
external ocular structures and, 292-294, 292-295f
extraocular muscle function in, 290-292, 291f
ocular fundus and, 296-301f, 296-302
of face, 260
of female external genitalia, 735f, 735-737, 736f
of hair, 217
of hip, 588
of infant abdomen, 552, 552f
of infant thorax, 434-435, 435f
for inguinal hernia, 692, 692f
of jugular venous pulse, 472, 472t
of knee, 589
of mouth, 362-366, 362-366f
in musculoskeletal examination, 577
of nails, 218f, 218-219, 219f
of neck, 260-262, 261f, 262f
of nose, 359-361, 359-361f
of penis, 689f, 689-690, 690f
of perianal area, 714
of peripheral vascular system and lymphatics
of arm, 506-509, 507-509f
of leg, 509-516, 510-516f
of posterior chest, 422
of scrotum, 690f, 690-692, 691f
of skin, 212-217, 212-217f
of skull, 259-260
of spine, 594-595, 595f
of thoracic cage, 422
of throat, 366f, 366-367
of vaginal wall, 742
of wrist and hand, 584
Inspiration, 416, 417f
Inspiratory arrest, 551
Instrumental activities of daily living
adult and, 57
older adult and, 67, 832, 833f
Intention tremor, 671t
Intercostal space, 412f
Internal anal sphincter, 709, 710f
Internal carotid artery, 253, 253f
Internal genitalia of female, 726, 727f
bimanual examination of, 742-746, 743-746f
inspection of cervix and os, 739f, 739-740
obtaining cervical smears and cultures, 740f, 740-742, 741f
rectovaginal examination of, 746-747, 747f
speculum examination of, 737f, 737-738
vaginal wall inspection and, 742
Internal hemorrhoid, 720t
Internal jugular vein, 253f, 457f, 462, 463f
Internal oblique muscle, 528f
Interneuron, 160
Interpersonal relationships/resources
adult and, 57
child and, 63
older adult and, 68
Interphalangeal joint, 570, 571f, 585, 585f
Interpretation, interview and, 34
Interpreter, 45f, 45-47, 46t, 47t
Intersphincteric groove, 709
Intertrigo, 241t
Intertubous diameter, 818, 818f
Intervertebral disk, 568, 569f
Interview, 29-49
of acutely ill person, 41
of adolescent, 39-40
of angry person, 42
of anxious person, 42
closing of, 37
communication process and, 29-32, 31f
cross-cultural communication and, 42-45, 43f, 44t
crying during, 42
of hearing-impaired person, 40-41
HEEADSSS method of, 64, 65f
of infant, 38
introduction in, 32
nonverbal communication and, 36-37, 37t, 47-48
obstacles in, 35-36
of older adult, 40, 40f
of parent, 37-38, 38f
of person under influence of drugs or alcohol, 41
personal questions and, 41
of preschooler, 38-39
of school-age child, 39
sexually aggressive person and, 41-42
threat of violence in, 42
using interpreter in, 45f, 45-47, 46t, 47t
working phase of, 32-34, 33t, 34f
Intimate partner violence, 103-114
assessing for, 105-107, 106f, 107f
denial in, 113
documentation of, 110f, 110-111, 111f
functional assessment and, 58-59
health effects of, 104-105
history of, 108
physical examination in, 108-109, 109t
pregnant woman and, 805
risk of homicide in, 112f, 112-113
Intimate zone, 44t
Intoxication, 100t
Intraductal carcinoma of breast, 407t
Intraductal papilloma, 407t
Intraretinal hemorrhage, 321t
Intrauterine growth restriction, 823t
Intuition, 3
Inversion, 566, 567f
Involuntary movements, 637
Involuntary rigidity, 546
Iris, 280f, 282
abnormalities on, 318-319t
inspection of, 295-296, 296f
of newborn, 305
Iritis, 317t
Iron, 192
Irritability, 85t
Ischemia, 500
Ischemic ulcer, 522t
Ischial tuberosity, 571, 571f
Islam, dietary practices of, 178, 178t
Isometric contraction, 458, 459f
Isometric relaxation, 460
Isovolumic relaxation, 460
Itching, 207-208
in pruritus ani, 721t

J

Jargon, 35-36
Jaundice, 214, 229t
physiologic, 222
Jock itch, 701t
Joint, 565-566, 566f
abnormalities of, 608t
effusion of, 609t
pain in, 168, 574-575
palpation of, 578
of pregnant woman, 573
Joint Commission on documentation in health history, 50
Judaism, dietary practices of, 178, 178t
Judgment, mental status assessment and, 76
Jugular vein, 253f, 501
Jugular vein distention, 486t
Jugular venous pressure, 462, 473, 473f
Jugular venous pulse, 462, 463f, 472, 472t
Jugulodigastric lymph node, 255, 255f, 261f
Junctional nevus, 212, 213f

K

Kaposi sarcoma, 246t, 381t
Katz Index of Activities of Daily Living, 830-831, 831f
Keloid, 207, 235t, 343t
Keratin, 203
Keratomalacia, 199t
Keratoses, 225, 225f
Kernig reflex, 677t
Kidney, 529f, 530, 530f
enlarged, 563t
palpation of, 550, 550f
referred abdominal pain and, 559t
Kidney disease
male genitourinary examination and, 683-684
pregnant woman and, 805
Kidney stones, 700t
Kiesselbach plexus, 352
Kinesthesia, 643, 643f
Knee, 572, 572f
abnormalities of, 613-614t
dermatomes of, 628f
physical examination of, 589-592, 589-592f
Knee jerk, 648, 648f
Knock knees, 601, 601f
KOH prep, 742
Koplik spots, 365, 378t
Korotkoff sounds, 139t, 140
Kosher, dietary term, 178
Kwashiorkor, 197t
Kyphosis, 437, 441t, 574, 604-605, 605f

L

Labia majora, 725, 726f, 727f, 735, 735f
Labia minora, 725, 726f, 727f
Labial herpes simplex, 244t
Lability, 85t
Labor and delivery, child health history and, 60
Laboratory studies
in nutritional assessment, 191-192
during pregnancy, 819
in substance use assessment, 99-100
Labyrinth, 325, 326
Laceration, forensic term, 109t
Lacrimal apparatus, 280, 280f
inspection of, 294, 295f
of older adult, 306, 306f
Lacrimal bone, 252f
Lacrimal gland, 280f
Lacrimal sac, 280f
inflammation of, 314t
Lacrimation, 286
Lactation
disorders occurring during, 408t
inspection of breast during, 401
nutritional assessment and, 176, 185
Lactiferous duct, 384, 384f
plugged, 408t
Lactiferous sinus, 384f
Lactobacillus acidophilus, 728
Lactose intolerance, 531-532

Lambdoid suture, 251, 252f
Landau reflex, 653, 653f
Language, mental status and, 72
Language barriers, 13
Lanugo, 205, 223, 223f
Laségue's test, 597f, 597-598
Lateral axillary lymph node, 503f
Lateral canthus, 280f
Lateral epicondyle, 570, 570f
Lateral lymph node, 385, 385f
Lateral malleolus, 572, 573f
Lateral meniscus, 572, 572f
Lateral rectus muscle, 281f
Lateral spinothalamic tract, 624, 624f
Lateral sulcus, 622f
Lawton Instrumental Activities of Daily Living Scale, 832, 833f
Leading questions, 36
Left atrium, 457, 457t
Left subclavian vein, 503f
Left ventricle, 457, 457f
Leg
  arteries in, 500, 500f
  dermatomes of, 628f
  iliopsoas muscle test and, 551, 551f
  of infant, 598
  inspection and palpation of, 509-516, 510-516f
  length discrepancy of, 598, 598f, 673t
  pain in, 505
  peripheral vascular disease of, 523t
  of preschool and school-age children, 601, 601f
  skin changes on, 505
  swelling of, 505
  ulcer of, 522t
  veins in, 501, 502f
Legal resident, 12
Legg-Calv[ac]e-Perthes syndrome, 618t
Leiomyoma, 758t, 824t
Lens, 282, 282f
  inspection of, 295
  opacities in, 319t
Leopold's maneuvers, 810-813, 811-813f
Lesion
  of ear, 342-343t
  forensic term, 109t
  health history of, 208
  optic chiasm, 316t
  optic nerve, 316t
  oral, 357
  penile, 685
  of scalp, 217
  skin, 216-217, 217f, 230-245t
    ABCDE mnemonic for, 212-213
    in child, 241-242t
    common types of, 243-245t
    malignant, 245t
    pressure ulcer, 236t
    primary, 232-233t
    secondary, 233-235t
    shapes and configurations of, 230-231t
    trauma or abuse-related, 237t
    vascular, 238-240t
Lethargic level of consciousness, 83t
Leukoedema, 356, 365
Leukonychia striata, 218, 219f
Leukoplakia, 378t
Leukorrhea, 748
Levator ani muscle, 710f
Level of consciousness
  abnormal findings in, 83t
  of aging adult, 80
  general survey and, 128
  mental status assessment and, 74
  neurologic recheck of, 660
Lichenification, 235t
Lid lag, 292
Lifestyle modifications
  for breast cancer risk, 402
  for hypertension, 152, 157t
Lift, 473, 492t
Ligament, 566
Light palpation of abdomen, 545-547, 545-547f
Light touch, 642, 642f
Lighting in examination room, 118
Limbus, 279, 280f
Limited English proficiency, 12-13
Line-by-line translation, 47
Linea alba, 527, 528f, 537, 537t
Linea nigra, 206, 224, 797, 807, 807f
Linear skin lesion, 231t
Lingual tonsil, 504, 504f
Linguistic competence, 12-13, 13t
Lip
  abnormalities of, 375t
  carcinoma of, 375t
  cleft, 375t
  malnutrition and, 186t
  physical examination of, 362, 362f
Lip reading, 41
Listening, interview and, 30
Lithotomy position
  for anus, rectum, and prostate examination, 713, 713f
  for vaginal examination, 733f, 733-734
Liver, 528f
  enlarged, 562t
  palpation of, 548, 548f
  percussion of, 541f, 541-542
  peritoneal friction rub and, 562t
  prevention of disease of, 554
  referred abdominal pain and, 559t
Liver spots, 224, 224f
Lobar pneumonia, 448t
Lobe
  of brain, 622, 622f
  of breast, 384f, 384-385
  of lung, 414f, 414-416, 415f
Lobule
  of breast, 384, 384f
  of ear, 324f
Loosening associations, 86t
Lordosis during pregnancy, 573, 797
Low-density lipoprotein cholesterol, 192
Lower extremity examination, 588-594
  ankle and foot and, 592-594, 593f, 594f
  hip and, 588f, 588-589
  knee and, 589-592, 589-592f
  sequence in health assessment, 769, 770, 775, 778
Lower motor neuron, 625f, 626, 626f
  lesions of, 276t, 673t
Lumbar herniation, 617t
Lumbar lymph node, 503f
Lumbar spinal nerves, 628f
Lumbar vertebrae, 628f
Lump
  in axilla, 391
  in breast, 405-406t
    health history of, 389
    inspection of, 398, 398f
  on ear, 342-343t
Lung, 411-454
  abnormal tactile fremitus and, 443t
  of aging adult, 418
  biocultural differences in diseases of, 418
  common respiratory conditions and, 447-453t
  configurations of thorax and, 440-441t
  health history of, 418-421
  of infants and children, 416-417, 417f
  mechanics of respiration and, 416, 417f
  physical examination of chest and, 421-439
    of acutely ill person, 437
    adventitious lung sounds and, 429-430, 444-445t
    of aging adult, 437
    auscultation of anterior chest in, 433
    breath sounds and, 427t, 427-429, 428t, 429f
    diaphragmatic excursion and, 426, 426f
    documentation and critical thinking in, 438-439
    of infants and children, 434-437, 435f, 435t, 436f
    inspection of anterior chest in, 430-431
    inspection of thoracic cage in, 422
    measurement of pulmonary function status in, 433-434
    palpation of anterior chest in, 431f, 431-432, 432f
    percussion of anterior chest in, 432f, 432-433
    percussion of lung fields in, 424-426, 425f
    of pregnant woman, 437
    symmetric chest expansion and, 422f, 422-423
    tactile fremitus and, 423f, 423-424
    voice sounds and, 430, 446t
  position and surface landmarks of, 411-413, 412f, 413f
  of pregnant woman, 418, 808
  respiration patterns and, 441-442t
  thoracic cavity and, 414f, 414-416, 415f
Lunula, 205, 205f
Lyme disease, 244t
Lymph node, 503, 503f
  in child, 504
  enlargement of, 506
  inguinal, 693, 693f
Lymphadenopathy, 262
Lymphatic capillary, 503
Lymphatics, 502-504, 503f, 504f
  of breast, 385, 385f
  of head and neck, 255f, 255-256, 260-262, 261f, 262f
  of penis and scrotal surface, 681
Lymphedema, 520t
Lymphocyte, 503

M

Macewen's sign, 267
Machinery murmur, 492t
Macrocephalic, term, 264
Macroglossia, 380t
Macrosomia, 824t
Macula, 282, 282f, 283f
  ophthalmoscopic inspection of, 301f, 301-302
  retinal damage and, 316t
Macular degeneration, 285
Macule, 232t
Magenta tongue, 198t
Magicoreligious theory of illness, 21-22, 22f
Major depressive disorder, 89t
Major depressive episode, 89t
Malabsorption after bariatric surgery, 200t
Male breast, 388
  cancer of, 409t
  sequence in health assessment, 768
Male genitourinary system, 679-708
  of adolescent, 681-683, 682t, 683f
  of aging adult, 683
  chronic kidney disease and, 683-684
  circumcision and, 683
  genital lesions and, 701-702t
  health history of, 684-688, 685f
    adult, 56
    pediatric, 63
  of infant, 681
  inguinal and femoral hernias and, 707t
  inguinal area and, f, 681
  penile abnormalities and, 702-703t
  penis and, 679, 680f
  physical examination of, 688-698
    of adolescent, 697
    of aging adult, 697
    documentation and critical thinking in, 698
    of infant, 695f, 695-697, 696f
    inguinal lymph nodes and, 693, 693f
    palpation for inguinal hernia in, 692, 692f
    patient preparation for, 688-689
    penis and, 689f, 689-690, 690f
    scrotum and, 690f, 690-692, 691f
    testicular self-examination education and, 693-694, 694f
    urinary function assessment in, 694
  screening for prostate cancer, 697
  scrotal abnormalities and, 704-706t
  scrotum and, 680-681
  sequence in health assessment, 771, 775
  urinary problems and, 700t
  urine color and discolorations and, 699t
Male-pattern baldness, 226
Malignant lesion, 245t
Malignant melanoma, 245t
Malignant persistent pain, 163
Malleus, 324, 324f
Malnutrition
  classification of, 196-197t
  clinical signs of, 186t
  HIV-associated, 199t
  serial assessment in, 193
Malnutrition Screening Tool, 178t, 179
Malocclusion, 356, 369, 376t
Malpresentations, 826t
Mammary duct ectasia, 407t
Mammary souffle, 483, 808
Mammography, 390
Man; *See* Male
Mandible, 252f
Manic episode, 89t
Manual compression test, 514, 514f

Manubrium, 324, 324f
MAP; *See* Mean arterial pressure
Marasmus, 197t
Marasmus/kwashiorkor, 197t
Marfan's syndrome, 154t
Marginal perforation of tympanic membrane, 347t
Marijuana, 94, 101t
Mask, Standard Precautions and, 121t
Mask of pregnancy, 807
Mass
breast, 405-406t
fallopian tube, 759t
Masseter muscle, 252f
Mastalgia, 389
Mastitis, 408t
Mastoid fontanelle, 256f
Mastoid process, 252f, 324f
Maxilla, 252f
Maxillary sinus, 352, 353f
McMurray test, 592, 592f
Mean arterial pressure, 136
Mean corpuscular volume, 99
Measles, 242t
Measurement, 130f, 130-132, 131t, 132f
bedside assessment and, 788
sequence in health assessment, 764, 772, 777
Meatus
external auditory, 324f, 330-331
turbinate, 352, 352f
urethral, 725, 726f, 727f
Media of eye, 296
Medial canthus, 280f
Medial epicondyle, 570, 570f
Medial epicondylitis, 610t
Medial malleolus, 572, 573f
Medial meniscus, 572, 572f
Medial rectus muscle, 281f
Median sulcus of prostate, 711
Mediastinum, 414, 455
Medication history
in abdominal assessment, 533
in allergic skin eruption, 208
in anus, rectum, and prostate examination, 712
in health history
adult, 52
child, 61
older adult, 66
in nutritional assessment, 183
Medulla, 623, 623f
Meibomian gland, 280, 280f
Melanin, 204
Melanocyte, 204f
Melanoma, 245t
Melasma, 207
Melena, 712, 717
Memory
impairment of, 88t
mental status and, 72, 75
Menarche, 386, 386f, 727
malnutrition and, 185
Meniscal tear, 592, 592f
Meniscus, swelling of, 613t
Menopause, 728, 729, 749
breast changes in, 391
Menstrual history, 56, 729
pregnant woman and, 799
Mental disorder, 71
Mental health, 71
Mental illness during pregnancy, 825t
Mental status assessment, 71-92
abnormal findings in, 83-91
anxiety disorders in, 90-91
delirium, dementia, and amnestic disorders in, 88t
levels of consciousness and, 83t
mood and affect abnormalities in, 85t
mood disorders in, 89t
perception abnormalities in, 87t
schizophrenia in, 87t
speech disorders in, 84t
thought content abnormalities in, 87t
thought processes abnormalities in, 86t
of aging adult, 72
components of, 72-73
defining mental status and, 71
documentation and critical thinking in, 82
Mental status assessment (*Continued*)
of infants and children, 72
objective data in, 73-81
aging adult and, 80-81
appearance in, 73-74
behavior in, 74
cognitive functions in, 74-76
infants and children and, 79f, 79-80
Mini-Cog test and, 81, 81f
Mini-Mental State examination and, 78t, 78-79
thought processes and perceptions in, 76-78, 77f
Meperidine abuse, 101t
Metabolic syndrome, 200t
Metacarpophalangeal joint, 570, 571f
palpation of, 585, 585f
Metastatic malignant melanoma, 245t
Metatarsus adductus, 598
Meth mouth, 377t
Methamphetamine
appearance and behavior in abuse of, 101t
oral disease and, 377t
Methicillin-resistant *Staphylococcus aureus*, 120
Methylphenidate, 100
Mexican American heritage
bone mineral density and, 574
eating patterns and customs of, 177f, 177-178
female genitourinary development and, 727-728
lactose intolerance and, 531
male genital development and, 683
obesity and, 153, 532
Microaneurysm of retinal vessels, 321t
Microcephalic, term, 264
Microtia, 330
Mid-arm muscle area, 189
Mid-upper arm circumference, 189, 189f
Mid-upper arm muscle circumference, 189
Midaxillary line, 413, 414f, 529f
Midbrain, 623, 623f
Midcarpal joint, 570, 571f
Midclavicular line, 413, 413f
Middle ear, 324
Middle Eastern heritages, 177-178
Middle turbinate and meatus, 352, 352f, 361
Midposition uterus, 745f
Midsternal line, 412-413, 413f
Midsystolic click, 478, 489t
Midsystolic ejection murmur, 494t
Migraine, 257, 270t
Migratory glossitis, 379t
Migratory testes, 696
Milestones
developmental history of, 61
neurologic examination and, 632
Milia, 222, 222f
Mini-Cog test, 81, 81f, 835t
Mini-Mental State examination, 78t, 78-79, 835t
Mini Nutritional Assessment, 179, 179f
Miosis, 315t
Mirror pelvic examination, 734, 734f
Mitral area for heart auscultation, 475f
Mitral regurgitation, 495t
Mitral stenosis, 496t
Mitral valve, 457f, 458
prolapse of, 489t
prosthetic valve sounds of, 490t
Mixed hearing loss, 326
MMSE; *See* Mini-Mental State examination
Mobility
general survey and, 129
of skin, 215, 215f
in aging adult, 226
neonatal, 222
Modified Allen test, 509, 509f
Modified Caregiver Strain Index, 837, 838f
Modulation phase of pain, 161, 161f
Moisture of skin, 214
aging adult and, 225
neonatal, 222
Molding of neonatal cranial bones, 265
Mole, 207, 212, 213f, 538
Mongolian spot, 220, 220f
Moniliasis, 378t, 756t
Monocular blindness, 315t
Mons pubis, 725, 726f, 727f
Montgomery gland, 383, 384f
Mood, 72
abnormalities of, 85t
general survey and, 129
mental status and, 74
Mood disorders, 89t
Morgan's lines, 275t
Mormons, dietary practices of, 178t
Morning sickness, 531
Moro reflex, 656, 656f
Morphine abuse, 101t
Motor function assessment
facial nerve and, 635, 635f
glossopharyngeal and vagus nerves and, 635
in infant, 652f, 652-654, 653f
neurologic recheck of, 661, 661f
trigeminal nerve and, 634, 634f
Motor pathways, 624-625, 625f
Motor speech cortex, 84t
Motor system
aging related changes in, 629
cerebellar function and, 637-641, 638-641f
dysfunction of, 674t
inspection and palpation of muscles and, 636-637, 637f
of newborn, 652f, 652-654, 653f
Mouth, 352-354, 353-355f
buccal mucosa abnormalities and, 378-379t
health history of, 357-358
adult, 55
child, 62
older adult, 67
of infants and children, 368-369, 369f
lip abnormalities and, 375t
oropharynx abnormalities and, 381f
physical examination of, 362-366, 362-366f
of pregnant woman, 807
sequence in health assessment, 766, 774, 780
teeth and gums abnormalities and, 376-377t
tongue abnormalities and, 379-380t
MRSA; *See* Methicillin-resistant *Staphylococcus aureus*
Mucocele, 375t
Mucocutaneous junction, 709, 710f
Mucous plug, 728, 798
Multigravida, 796
Multipara, 796
Multiple fetuses, 823t
Multiple sclerosis, 674t
Murmur, 461, 494-497t
auscultation of heart and, 478-480, 478-480f
Murphy sign, 551, 551f
Muscle(s), 566, 567f
fibromyalgia and, 619t
movement abnormalities of, 670-671t
neck, 253, 253f
neurologic examination of, 636-637, 637f
pain or cramping in, 168, 575
Muscle testing, 578
elbow and, 584, 584f
knee and, 592, 592f
wrist and hand and, 587, 587f
Muscle tone
abnormalities of, 669t
of newborn, 652, 652f
testing of, 637, 637f
upper and lower motor neuron lesions and, 673t
Muscle weakness
facial nerve assessment and, 635, 635f
history of, 575, 630-631
in upper and lower motor neuron lesions, 673t
Muscular dystrophy, 674t
Musculoskeletal system, 565-620
abnormalities of, 608-619t
of ankle and foot, 615-616t
congenital, 618t
of elbow, 610t
of joints, 608t
of knee, 613-614t
of shoulder, 609t
of spine, 617t
of wrist and hand, 611-613t
of aging adult, 573-574
ankle and foot in, 572-573, 573f
changes from poorly controlled pain, 169t
cultural and racial variations in, 574
elbow in, 570, 570f
fibromyalgia and, 619t

Musculoskeletal system (*Continued*)
health history of, 574-577
adult, 56
aging adult and, 67
infants and children, 63
hip in, 571f, 571-572
of infants and children, 573
joints in, 565-566, 566f
knee in, 572, 572f
malnutrition and, 186t
muscles in, 566, 567f
osteoporosis and, 606
physical examination of, 577-607
of adolescent, 603, 603f
of aging adult, 604-605, 605f
ankle and foot and, 592-594, 593f, 594f
cervical spine and, 580, 580f
documentation and critical thinking in, 607
elbow and, 582-584, 583f, 584f
hip and, 588f, 588-589
of infant, 598-600, 599f, 600f
joint inspection in, 577
joint palpation in, 578
knee and, 589-592, 589-592f
muscle testing in, 578
patient preparation for, 577
of pregnant woman, 604, 604f
of preschool and school-age children, 601f, 601-603, 602f
range of motion assessment in, 578
shoulder and, 581f, 581-582, 582f
spine and, 594-598, 595-598f
temporomandibular joint and, 579f, 579-580
wrist and hand and, 584-587, 584-587f
of pregnant woman, 573
sequence in health assessment, 769, 770-771
shoulder in, 568-570, 569f, 570f
spine in, 568, 568f, 569f
temporomandibular joint in, 566, 567f
wrist and carpals in, 570, 571t
MyPyramid Dietary Guidelines, 181, 181f
Myalgia, 575
Mydriasis, 315t
Myelin, 621
Myocardium, 456, 457f
Myoclonus, 670t
Myoma, 758t, 824t
Myopia, 299f
Myxedema, 276t

N

NAAT; *See* Nucleic acid amplification test
Nabothian cyst, 740
N[um]agele's rule, 798
Nail(s), 205, 205f
abnormalities of, 248-250f
of aging adult, 226
health history of, 209
inspection and palpation of, 218f, 218-219, 219f
malnutrition and, 186t
Nail bed, 205, 205f
Nail matrix, 205, 205f
Nail plate, 205, 205f
Nares, 351, 351f
of newborn, 368
Nasal bone, 252f
Nasal cavity, 352, 352f, 360, 360f
Nasal discharge, 356, 360
Nasal furuncle, 374t
Nasal hair, 352, 355
Nasal mucosa, 352
Nasal polyp, 361, 374t
Nasal septum, 252f, 352, 360, 361f
perforated, 373t
Nasal vestibule, 351, 351f
Nasolabial fold, 252f, 253
Nasolacrimal duct, 280f
Nasopharynx, 352f, 354
National Center for Complementary and Alternative Medicine, 27
National Safety Council Home Safety checklist, 841t
National standards for cultural competence, 12f, 12-14, 13t
Naturalistic theory of illness, 21
Naturalization, 12
Nausea
in heart failure, 486t
history of, 533
during pregnancy, 531, 801
Near vision
accommodation and, 296, 296f
older adult and, 284
testing of, 288, 289f
Nearsighted, 299f
Neck, 251-278
brain injury prevention and, 267
dermatomes of, 628f
head size and contour abnormalities and, 271t
health history of, 256-259
adult, 55
child, 62
lymphatics of, 255f, 255-256
of older adult, 256
pediatric, 256, 256f
physical examination of, 259-269
aging adult and, 267
documentation and critical thinking in, 268-269
face and, 260
lymph nodes and, 260-262, 261f, 262f
pediatric, 264-267, 265f
pregnant woman and, 267
range of motion and, 260
skull and, 259-260
thyroid gland and, 263f, 263-264, 264f
trachea and, 262, 263f
of pregnant woman, 256, 807
sequence in health assessment, 766, 775, 779
swelling of, 272-273t
Neck vessels, 462-463, 463f
palpation of, 470-471, 471f
sequence in health assessment, 768
Neecham Confusion Scale, 835t
Neglect, 103
child, 108
elder, 107, 107t
intimate partner, 105-107, 106f, 107f
Neologism, 86t
Nerve, 626
Neuroanatomic pathway of pain, 159-160, 160f
Neurologic recheck, 632, 660-663, 661-663f
Neurologic system, 621-678
abnormal gaits and, 672-673t
abnormal postures and, 676t
of aging adult, 629
Alzheimer disease and, 667t
bedside assessment of, 789
central nervous system in, 621-626
motor pathways of, 624-625, 625f
sensory pathways of, 623-624, 624f
structures in, 621-623, 622f, 623f
upper and lower motor neurons of, 626, 626f
changes from poorly controlled pain, 169t
cranial nerve abnormalities and, 668-669t
frontal release signs and, 677t
health history of, 630-632
adult, 56
older adult, 67
pediatric, 63
of infant, 629
malnutrition and, 186t
motor system dysfunction and, 674t
muscle movement abnormalities and, 670-671t
muscle tone abnormalities and, 669t
pathologic reflexes and, 677t
peripheral nervous system in, 626-629, 626-629f
physical examination of, 632-666
cerebellar function assessment in, 637-639, 638f, 639f
coordination and skilled movements in, 640f, 640-641, 641f
cranial nerve testing in, 633-636, 634-636f
deep tendon reflexes testing in, 645-649, 646-649f
documentation and critical thinking in, 665-666
infant and, 651t, 651-657, 652-657f
muscle inspection and palpation in, 636-637, 637f
neurologic recheck and, 660-663, 661-663f
patient preparation for, 632-633
preschool and school-age children and, 657-660, 658f
sensory system assessment in, 641-645, 642-644f
superficial reflexes testing in, 650, 650f, 651f
Neurologic system (*Continued*)
of pregnant woman, 809
sensory loss and, 675-676t
sequence in health assessment, 769-770, 776
stroke and, 629
upper and lower motor neuron lesions and, 673t
Neuropathic pain, 162, 162f, 172t
Neurotransmitter, 161
Nevus, 212, 213f, 538
Nevus flammeus, 238t
New learning
aging adult and, 80
Four Unrelated Words Test and, 75
Newborn
abdomen of, 531
chest of, 435
CRIES Neonatal Postoperative Pain Measurement Score and, 169, 170f
eye of, 284, 304, 304f
female genitourinary examination in, 748, 748f
head circumference of, 145, 145f
hearing acuity of, 337
heart murmur in, 481
jaundice in, 214
lung of, 416-418, 417f
neurologic examination of, 651t, 651-657, 652-657f
neurologic system of, 629
normal respiratory rate of, 135t
nose of, 368
physiologic jaundice in, 222
pigmentation in, 220f, 220-221, 221f
sequence of health assessment of, 772-776
skin of, 205-206, 223, 223f
skull of, 256, 256f, 264-266, 265f
stool of, 553, 711
Nicking, 320t
Nicotine
appearance and behavior in abuse of, 101t
disease risk and, 370
fetal brain and, 417
Night blindness, 285
Nipple, 383, 384f
deviation in pointing of, 404t
discharge from, 389, 407t
inspection of, 393, 393f
retraction of, 404t
Nociceptive pain, 160-161, 161f, 172t
Nociceptor, 159-160
Nocturia, 684
aging male and, 688
cardiovascular assessment and, 468
Nocturnal emission, 687
Nocturnal enuresis, 686
Nodule, 232t
on ear, 342t
mucocele, 375t
subcutaneous, 583, 610t
thyroid gland, 272t
Noise-induced hearing loss, 338
Non-immigrant, 12
Non-stress test, 819
Nonmalignant persistent pain, 163
Nonsynovial joint, 565-566
Nonverbal behaviors of pain, 168-169
Nonverbal communication, 30, 36-37, 37t
child interview and, 38
cross-cultural, 47-48
Norbeck Social Support Questionnaire, 837
Normocephalic, term, 259
Nose, 351-352, 351-353f
abnormalities of, 373-374t
of child, 62, 368
health history of, 55, 356-357
physical examination of, 359-361, 359-361f
sequence in health assessment, 766, 774, 780
Nosebleed, 357, 373t
Nosocomial infection, 120
Note-taking during interview, 31, 31f
Nuclear cataract, 319t
Nucleic acid amplification test, 757t
Nucleus pulposus, 568, 569f
herniated, 617t
Numeric pain rating scales, 166-167, 167f
Nursing caries, 376t
Nursing diagnoses, 5
Nursing facility, functional assessment of older adult and, 839

Nursing process, 2-6, 3f, 5t
Nutrition
adult and, 57
general survey and, 128
older adult and, 68
Nutrition screening, 178t, 178-182, 179f, 180t
Nutritional assessment, 175-202
in abdominal examination, 534
adolescent and, 176
adult and, 176
aging adult and, 176-177
classification of malnutrition and, 196-197t
cultural considerations in, 177f, 177-178
documentation and critical thinking in, 195
guidelines for two thousand calories per day, 181t, 181-182
health history in, 182-185
health promotion and, 193-194
infants and children and, 176
Malnutrition Screening Tool in, 178t, 179
metabolic syndrome and, 200t
Mini Nutritional Assessment in, 179, 179f
MyPyramid Dietary Guidelines and, 181, 181f
nutritional consequences of bariatric surgery and, 200t
nutritional deficiencies and, 198-199t
nutritional status and, 175
physical examination in, 186-193
anthropometric measures in, 187-190f, 187-191
clinical signs of malnutrition and, 186t
infants and children and, 191, 193
laboratory studies and, 191-192
serial assessment in malnourished individual and, 193
pregnancy and lactation and, 176
religious dietary practices and, 178t
Subjective Global Assessment in, 180t, 180-181
Nutritional deficiencies, 198-199t
Nutritional history
of child, 61-62
of pregnant woman, 805
Nutritional status, 175
Nystagmus, 633

O

Obesity
abdominal distention in, 557t
anthropometric measures in, 195t
cardiovascular heart disease and, 466
cultural considerations in, 153, 532
in Cushing syndrome, 155t
epidemic of, 194
Objective data, 2, 49
Objective vertigo, 329
Oblique fissure, 414, 414f
Oblique muscles of eye, 281, 281f
Obsession, 87t
Obsessive-compulsive disorder, 90-91t
Obstetric history, 52, 729, 800-801
Obtunded level of consciousness, 83t
Occipital bone, 252f
neonatal, 256f
Occipital lobe, 622, 622f
Occipital lymph node, 255, 255f, 261f
Occlusion, 524t
Occult blood in stool, 717
Occupational hazards, 631
Occupational health
adult and, 59
older adult and, 68
pregnant woman and, 806
skin lesions and, 209
Ocular fundus
of child, 306
of older adult, 307-308, 308f
Oculomotor nerve, 627f
abnormalities of, 668t
damage to, 315t
infant reflexes and, 651t
pupillary responses in neurologic recheck, 662, 662f
testing of, 633
Older adult
abdomen of, 531
health history of, 535
physical examination of, 554
Older adult (*Continued*)
abuse and neglect of, 103-114, 104t
assessing for, 107, 107t
documentation of, 110f, 110-111, 111f
health effects of, 105
physical examination in, 108-109, 109t
anus, rectum, and prostate of, 717
breast of, 386-388
health history of, 391
physical examination of, 401
clinical setting for physical examination and, 125-126
ear of, 326-327, 337
eye of, 284-285
health history of, 67, 287
physical examination of, 306-308, 306-308f
female genitourinary system of, 728
health history of, 732
physical examination of, 749-750
functional assessment of, 67-69, 829-847
activities of daily living and, 830-832, 831f
acute care setting and, 837-838
advanced activities of daily living and, 832
altered cognition and, 844
assistive living and, 839
caregiver assessment and, 837, 838f
cognitive evaluation in, 835, 835t
community-based services and, 838
continuing care retirement communities and, 839
cultural considerations in, 843-844
depression and, 835-836, 836f
driving and, 840-841, 841t
exercise and, 839-840
health care maintenance and, 840
home care and, 839
instrumental activities of daily living and, 832, 833f
measuring physical performance in, 832-834
nursing facilities and, 839
pain and, 844
risk for functional decline during hospitalization in, 834f, 834-835
sleep and, 841t, 841-842, 842t
social domain and, 836-837, 837t
spiritual assessment and, 842-843
general survey of, 148-149
head and neck of, 256
health history of, 259
physical examination of, 267
health history of, 66f, 66-67
heart of, 465, 465f
health history of, 470
physical examination of, 483
height of, 191
interview of, 40, 40f
lungs of, 418
health history of, 421
physical examination of, 437
male genitourinary system of, 683
health history of, 687-688
physical examination of, 697
mental status assessment of, 72, 80-81
musculoskeletal system of, 573-574
health history of, 576-577
physical examination of, 604-605, 605f
neurologic system of, 629, 632
nose, mouth, and throat of, 355-356
health history of, 358-359
physical examination of, 370, 370f
nutritional assessment and, 176-177
health history in, 185-186
laboratory tests in, 193
physical examination in, 191
pain and, 163, 170-171, 171f
peripheral vascular system of, 504-505
health history of, 67
physical examination of, 517
positioning for physical examination, 125-126
preparation for physical examination, 126
sequence of health assessment of, 126, 780
skin of, 206
health history of, 210
physical examination of, 224-226, 224-226f
substance use assessment and, 96, 98
vital signs of, 149-150
Older Americans Resources and Service Multidimensional Functional Assessment Questionnaire, 832
Olecranon bursitis, 610t
Olecranon process, 570, 570f
Olfactory nerve, 352f, 627f
abnormalities of, 668t
testing of, 633
Olfactory receptor, 352
Oligohydramnios, 824t
Omohyoid muscle, 254f
Onycholysis, 249t
Opacities in lens, 319t
Open-angle glaucoma, 308
Open-ended questions, 32-33, 33t
Opening snap, 490t
Ophthalmoscope, 120, 120f, 296-297, 297f, 299f, 300f
Ophthalmoscopic examination, 296-302
macula and, 301-302
optic disc and, 300f, 300-301, 301f
retinal vessels and, 301
Opiates abuse, 101t
Opisthotonos, 652, 676t
Oppenheim reflex, 677t
Opthalmia neonatorum, 305
Optic atrophy, 320t
Optic chiasm lesion, 316t
Optic disc, 282, 282f, 283f
abnormalities of, 320t
ophthalmoscopic inspection of, 300, 300f
Optic fundus, 296-302
macula and, 301-302
ophthalmoscopic examination of, 296-297, 297f, 299f, 300f
optic disc and, 300f, 300-301, 301f
retinal vessels and, 301
Optic nerve, 281f, 282f, 627f
abnormalities of, 668t
infant reflexes and, 651t
lesion in, 316t
testing of, 633
Optimal nutritional status, 175
Oral cancer, 356, 370
Oral candidiasis, 378t
Oral cavity, 352-354, 353-355f
buccal mucosa abnormalities and, 378-379t
health history of
adult, 55
child, 62
older adult, 67
lip abnormalities and, 375t
oropharynx abnormalities and, 381f
physical examination of, 362-366, 362-366f
teeth and gums abnormalities and, 376-377t
tongue abnormalities and, 379-380t
Oral Kaposi sarcoma, 381t
Oral temperature measurement, 133
in infants and children, 147
Orbicularis oculi muscle, 252f, 280f
Orbicularis oris muscle, 252f
Orchitis, 706t
Organ of Corti, 325
Organic disorders, 71
Organs, enlarged, 562-563t
Orientation, 72
mental status and, 74-75
Oropharynx, 352f, 354
abnormalities of, 381f
Orthopnea, 419, 467, 486t
Orthostatic hypotension, 142, 483
Orthostatic vital signs, 141-142
Ortolani maneuver, 599, 599f
Oscillometry, 148
Osgood-Schlatter disease, 614t
Osteitis deformans, 271t
Osteoarthritis, 608t, 612t
Osteoma, 345t
Osteoporosis, 573, 574, 606, 608t
Otalgia, 327
Otitis externa, 341t, 344t
Otitis media, 327
Otitis media with effusion, 346t
Otomycosis, 348t
Otorrhea, 328
Otosclerosis, 326
Otoscope, 119, 119f

Otoscopy, 331f, 331-332
  abnormal findings in, 346t
  child and, 334-335, 335f
Oucher Scale, 167
Oval window, 324, 324f
Ovarian cancer, 760t
Ovarian cyst, 557t, 759t
Ovary, 529f, 726, 727f
Over-the-counter medications, 26
Overall pain assessment tools, 165
Overnutrition, 175-176
Overweight child, 534
Oxygen saturation, 150, 150f, 434
  bedside assessment of, 788

P

P wave, 461, 461f
Paget's disease of bone, 271t
Paget's disease of breast, 407t
Pain, 159-174
  abdominal, 168
    costovertebral angle tenderness and, 543, 543f
    history of, 532-533
    in infants and children, 534
    during pregnancy, 802
    rebound tenderness and, 551, 551f
    referred, 559, 559t
  aging adult and, 163, 170-171, 171f, 844
  assessment tools for, 164-167, 165-167f
  bone, 575
  breast, 389
  calf, 511
  chest, 420, 467
  child and, 167, 167f
  cultural considerations in, 163
  documentation and critical thinking in, 171
  earache, 327
  eye, 286
  in fibromyalgia, 619t
  gender differences in, 163
  headache, 256-257
  infant and, 163, 167, 167f, 169, 170f
  initial assessment of, 164
  joint, 574-575
  leg, 505
  muscle, 575
  neck, 258
  neuroanatomic pathway of, 159-160, 160f
  neuropathic, 162, 162f
  nociceptive, 160-161, 161f
  nonverbal behaviors of, 168-169, 169f
  penile, 685
  perception of, 624, 642, 642f
  in peripheral vascular disease, 521t
  physical examination in, 168
  poorly controlled, 169t
  in Raynaud's phenomenon, 520t
  in reflexive sympathetic dystrophy, 173t
  sinus, 357
  skin, 168, 210
  sources of, 162
  transcultural expression of, 25
  types of, 162-163, 172t
Pain assessment tools, 164-167, 165-167f
Pain rating scales, 166-167, 167f
PAINAD scale, 169, 170f
Palate
  cleft, 375t, 381t
  high-arched, 369
  physical examination of, 365f, 365-366, 366f
Palatine tonsil, 352f, 504, 504f
Pallor, 213, 229t
  arterial insufficiency and, 515
  cardiovascular assessment and, 468
  modified Allen test and, 509
  of optic disc, 320t
  in Raynaud's phenomenon, 520t
Palmar grasp, 654, 655f
Palpable friction rub, 443t
Palpation, 115-116
  of abdomen, 545-551
    aorta and, 550, 550f
    of child, 553, 553f
    enlarged organs and, 562-563t
    of infant, 552, 552f
    kidneys and, 550, 550f
    light and deep, 545f, 545-547, 546f
Palpation (*Continued*)
    liver and, 548, 548f
    normally palpable structures in, 547f
    of pregnant woman, 809f, 809-810, 810f
    spleen and, 549, 549f
  across precordium, 474, 474f
  of ankle and foot, 593, 593f7
  of anterior chest, 431f, 431-432, 432f
  of anus and rectum, 714f, 714-715, 715f
  of apical impulse, 474, 474f
  of breast, 395-398, 395-398f
  of carotid artery, 470-471, 471f
  of cervical spine, 580
  of elbow, 583, 583f
  of external ear, 330, 330f
  of female axillae, 395, 395f
  of female external genitalia, 736f, 736-737
  of hair, 217
  for inguinal hernia, 692, 692f
  of inguinal lymph nodes, 693, 693f
  of joint, 578
  of knee, 589-591, 589-591f
  of nails, 218f, 218-219, 219f
  of neck, 260-262, 261f, 262f
  of neonatal chest, 436
  of nose, 359-361, 359-361f
  of penis, 689f, 689-690, 690f
  of peripheral vascular system and lymphatics
    of arm, 506-509, 507-509f
    of leg, 509-516, 510-516f
  of posterior chest, 422-424, 423f
  of radial artery
    for blood pressure measurement, 138, 138f
    for pulse, 134, 134f
  rectovaginal, 747, 747f
  of scrotum, 690f, 690-692, 691f
  of shoulder, 581
  of sinuses, 361, 361f
  of skin, 212-217, 212-217f
  of skull, 259
  of spinous processes, 595
  of temporomandibular joint, 260
  of thyroid gland, 263f, 263-264, 264f
  of wrist and hand, 584f, 584-585, 585f
Palpebral conjunctiva, 280, 280f
Palpebral fissure, 252f, 279, 280f
Pancreas, 529f, 530
Pancreatitis, 559t
Panic attack, 90t
Panic disorder, 90t
Pansystolic regurgitant murmur, 478, 495t
Papanicolaou test, 740
  adolescent and, 748-749
  cultural considerations in, 728
Papillary muscle, 457f
Papilledema, 306, 320t
Papule, 232t
Paradoxical split of second heart sound, 478, 488t
Paralysis, 631, 670t, 673t
Paranasal sinus, 352, 353f
Paraphimosis, 702t
Paraplegia, 670t, 674t
Paraurethral gland, 725, 726f
Parent, interview of, 37-38, 38f
Parental bonding, 143
Paresis, 630, 670t
Paresthesia, 631
Parietal bone, 252f
  neonatal, 256f
Parietal lobe, 622, 622f
Parietal pleura, 415, 415f
Parkinsonian gait, 672t
Parkinsonism, 674t
Parkinson syndrome, 275t
Parolee, 12
Paronychia, 248t
Parotid gland, 253, 253f, 354, 354f
  enlargement of, 273t
Paroxysmal nocturnal dyspnea, 419
Pars flaccida, 324, 325f
Pars tensa, 324, 325f
Passive range of motion, 578
Past health
  in adult health history, 51-52
  in child health history, 60
  in older adult health history, 66
Past-pointing, 640
Patch, 232t
Patella, 572, 572f
  ballottement of, 590, 590f
Patent ductus arteriosus, 492t
Pathologic fourth heart sound, 491t
Pathologic reflexes, 626, 677t
Pathologic third heart sound, 490t
Patient-centered expected outcomes, 6
Patient positioning
  for anus, rectum, and prostate examination, 713, 713f
  for cardiovascular assessment, 470
  for eye examination, 287
  for female genitourinary examination, 733f, 733-735, 734f
  infant and, 122-123, 123f
  for nose, mouth, and throat examination, 359
  for pediatric otoscopic examination, 335, 335f
  toddler and, 123
Patient preparation
  for abdominal examination, 536
  for anus, rectum, and prostate examination, 713
  for breast examination, 392
  for cardiovascular assessment, 470
  for chest examination, 421
  for ear examination, 330
  for examination of pregnant woman, 806
  for eye examination, 287
  for female genitourinary examination, 732-733, 733f
  infant and, 123
  for male genitourinary examination, 688-689
  for musculoskeletal examination, 577
  for neurologic examination, 632-633
  for nose, mouth, and throat examination, 359
  for peripheral vascular and lymphatic examination, 506
  for skin examination, 211
  toddler and, 123-124
Pattern injury, 109t, 237t
Pattern of injuries, forensic term, 109t
PDA; *See* Patent ductus arteriosus
Peau d'orange skin, 215, 392, 404t
Pectinate line, 709, 710f
Pectoral lymph node, 385, 385f, 503f
Pectus carinatum, 440t
Pectus excavation, 440t
Pediculosis capitis, 247t
Pediculosis pubis, 752t
Pedigree, 52, 53f
Pedunculated rectal polyp, 722t
Pellagra, 198t
Pelvic examination, 732-751
  of adolescent, 748-749
  of aging adult, 749-750
  bimanual, 742-746, 743-746f
  documentation and critical thinking in, 750-751
  of infants and children, 747-748
  inspection of cervix and os in, 739f, 739-740
  inspection of external genitalia in, 735f, 735-737, 736f
  obtaining cervical smears and cultures in, 740f, 740-742, 741f
  patient preparation and equipment for, 732-733, 733f
  positioning for, 733f, 733-735, 734f
  of pregnant woman, 749, 814-819
    bimanual examination in, 815, 815f
    genitalia inspection in, 814
    pelvimetry in, 816f, 816-819, 817t, 818f
    speculum examination in, 814, 814f
  rectovaginal examination and, 746-747, 747f
  speculum examination in, 737f, 737-738, 738f
  vaginal wall inspection in, 742
Pelvic inflammatory disease, 757t, 759t
Pelvic musculature abnormalities, 754t
Pelvimetry, 816f, 816-819, 817t, 818f
Penis, 679, 680f
  abnormalities of, 702-703t
  circumcision and, 683
  health history of, 685
  of infant, 695f, 695-697, 696f
  lesions of, 701-702t
  physical examination of, 689f, 689-690, 690f
  Tanner's sexual maturity ratings and, 682t
Peptic ulcer, 559t

Perception, 72
abnormalities of, 87t
of health, 59
mental status assessment of, 76-78, 77f
of pain, 161, 161f
proprioception and, 624
Percussion, 116f, 116-117, 117f, 117t
of anterior chest, 432f, 432-433
in cardiovascular assessment, 475
of general abdominal tympany, 540, 540f
of infant abdomen, 552
of infant head, 267
of liver, 541f, 541-542
of lung fields, 424-426, 425f
of neonatal chest, 436
of posterior chest, 424-426, 425f
Perforation
of nasal septum, 373t
of tympanic membrane, 347t
Perforators, 501
Performance Activities of Daily Living, 832-834
Perianal area inspection, 714
Pericardial fluid, 456
Pericardial friction rub, 491t
Pericardium, 456, 457f
Perineum, 726f
Periorbital edema, 260, 312t
Peripheral arterial disease, 524t
Peripheral nervous system, 626-629, 626-629f
Peripheral neuropathy, 643, 675t
Peripheral vascular disease
in arm, 520t
arterial, venous, or diabetic leg ulcers in, 522t
in leg, 523t
pain profiles in, 521t
peripheral arterial disease in, 524t
Peripheral vascular pressure, 137, 137f
Peripheral vascular system, 499-525
of aging adult, 504-505
arteries in, 499-500, 500f
changes during pregnancy, 504, 808-809
health history of, 505-506
adult and, 55
older adult and, 67
of infants and children, 504, 504f
lymphatics and, 502-504, 503f, 504f
peripheral vascular disease and
in arms, 520t
arterial, venous, or diabetic leg ulcers in, 522t
in legs, 523t
pain profiles in, 521t
peripheral arterial disease in, 524t
physical examination of, 506-518
of aging adult, 517
arm inspection and palpation in, 506-509, 507-509f
documentation and critical thinking in, 518
of infants and children, 516-517
leg inspection and palpation in, 509-516, 510-516f
of pregnant woman, 517
variations in pulse contour and, 519t
veins in, 501, 501f
venous flow and, 501-502, 502f
Peritoneal friction rub, 562t
Peritoneal reflection, 710, 710f
Peritoneum, 529f, 710, 710f
Perl[ac]eche, 375t
Permanent resident alien, 12
Permanent teeth, 354, 355f
PERRLA mnemonic, 296
Perseveration, 86t
Persistent pain, 163, 169
Personal distance, 44t
Personal habits
adult and, 58
as cardiac risk factors, 468-469
child and, 64
Personal hygiene
general survey and, 129
mental status assessment and, 74
Personal questions in interview, 41
Perspiration, 214
Pes planus, 601
Petechiae, 109t, 240t
Peyer's patch, 504f
Peyronie disease, 703t
Phalen test, 587, 587f
Pharyngeal cancer, 356
Pharyngeal tonsil, 352f, 504, 504f
Pharyngitis, 381t
Pharynx, 354
abnormalities of, 381f
health history of, 357-358
adult, 55
child, 62
physical examination of, 366f, 366-367
Phimosis, 702t
Phobia, 87t
Phoria, 290
Photographic documentation in domestic violence, 110, 110f, 111f
Photophobia, 286
Physical abuse, 103, 104t
Physical appearance
of aging adult, 148
general survey and, 127
of infants and children, 142
nonverbal communication and, 36
Physical environment
of examination room, 120-121, 121t
functional assessment of older adult and, 840f, 840-842, 841t
interview and, 31, 31f
Physical examination
of abdomen, 536-556
of aging adult, 554
aorta palpation in, 550, 550f
auscultation of bowel and vascular sounds in, 539f, 539-540, 540f
of child, 553, 553f
contour and, 536, 536f
costovertebral angle tenderness and, 543, 543f
demeanor and, 539
documentation and critical thinking in, 555-556
fluid wave and, 543f, 543-544
hair distribution and, 538
iliopsoas muscle test in, 551, 551f
of infant, 552f, 552-553
inspiratory arrest in, 551
kidney palpation in, 550, 550f
light and deep palpation in, 545-547, 545-547f
liver palpation in, 548, 548f
liver span percussion in, 541f, 541-542
percussion of general tympany in, 540, 540f
pulsation or movement and, 538
rebound tenderness and, 551, 551f
shifting dullness and, 544f, 544-545
skin and, 537f, 537-538, 538f
spleen palpation in, 549, 549f
splenic dullness and, 542, 542f
symmetry and, 537, 537f
umbilicus and, 537
assessment techniques in, 115-126
auscultation in, 118, 118f
inspection in, 115
palpation in, 115-116
percussion in, 116f, 116-117, 117f, 117t
of breast, 392-401
adolescent and, 401
aging woman and, 401
breast self-examination education and, 398-399, 399f
documentation and critical thinking in, 402-403
infants and children and, 400-401
inspection and palpation of axillae in, 395, 395f
inspection of breast in, 392-394, 392-394f
lactating woman and, 401
male breast and, 400, 400f
palpation of breast in, 395-398, 395-398f
pregnant woman and, 401
in cardiovascular assessment, 470-485
aging adult and, 483
anterior chest inspection in, 473
apical impulse palpation in, 474, 474f
auscultation of heart in, 474-480f, 475-480
carotid artery auscultation in, 471, 471f
carotid artery palpation in, 470-471, 471f
documentation and critical thinking in, 484-485
estimation of jugular venous pressure in, 473, 473f
in infants and children, 480-482, 481f, 482f
jugular venous pulse and, 472, 472t
palpation across precordium in, 474, 474f
Physical examination (*Continued*)
patient preparation for, 470
percussion in, 475
pregnant woman and, 483
of chest and lungs, 421-439, 473
of acutely ill person, 437
adventitious lung sounds and, 429-430, 444-445t
of aging adult, 437
auscultation of anterior chest in, 433
breath sounds and, 427t, 427-429, 428t, 429f
diaphragmatic excursion and, 426, 426f
documentation and critical thinking in, 438-439
of infants and children, 434-437, 435f, 435t, 436f
inspection of anterior chest in, 430-431
inspection of thoracic cage in, 422
measurement of pulmonary function status in, 433-434
palpation of anterior chest in, 431f, 431-432, 432f
percussion of anterior chest in, 432f, 432-433
percussion of lung fields in, 424-426, 425f
of pregnant woman, 437
symmetric chest expansion and, 422f, 422-423
tactile fremitus and, 423f, 423-424
voice sounds and, 430, 446t
clinical setting for, 118-119, 119f
safety of, 120-121, 121t
in domestic violence assessment, 108-110, 109t
of ear, 330-340
aging adult and, 337
documentation and critical thinking in, 338-340
external canal and, 332
external ear and, 330f, 330-331
hearing acuity test and, 333
infants and children and, 334-336f, 334-337
otoscopic inspection in, 331f, 331-332
tympanic membrane and, 332f, 332-333
vestibular apparatus and, 334
of eye, 287-310
of aging adult, 306-308, 306-308f
anterior eyeball structures inspection in, 295-296, 296f
confrontation test in, 289f, 289-290, 290f
cover test in, 290, 291f
diagnostic positions test in, 291f, 291-292
documentation and critical thinking in, 309-310
external ocular structures inspection in, 292-294, 292-295f
Hirschberg test in, 290
of infants and children, 302-305f, 302-306
near vision test in, 288, 289f
ophthalmoscopy in, 296-302, 297-301f
Snellen Eye Chart and, 287-288, 288f
of female genitourinary system, 732-751
of adolescent, 748-749
of aging adult, 749-750
bimanual examination in, 742-746, 743-746f
documentation and critical thinking in, 750-751
of infants and children, 747-748
inspection of cervix and os in, 739f, 739-740
inspection of external genitalia in, 735f, 735-737, 736f
obtaining cervical smears and cultures in, 740f, 740-742, 741f
patient preparation and equipment for, 732-733, 733f
positioning for, 733f, 733-735, 734f
of pregnant woman, 749
rectovaginal examination in, 746-747, 747f
speculum examination in, 737f, 737-738, 738f
vaginal wall inspection in, 742
of head and neck, 259-269
aging adult and, 267
documentation and critical thinking in, 268-269
face and, 260
lymph nodes and, 260-262, 261f, 262f
pediatric, 264-267, 265f
pregnant woman and, 267
range of motion and, 260
skull and, 259-260
thyroid gland and, 263f, 263-264, 264f
trachea and, 262, 263f
of male genitourinary system, 688-698
of adolescent, 697
of aging adult, 697
documentation and critical thinking in, 698
of infant, 695f, 695-697, 696f
inguinal lymph nodes and, 693, 693f

Physical examination (*Continued*)
palpation for inguinal hernia in, 692, 692f
patient preparation for, 688-689
penis and, 689f, 689-690, 690f
scrotum and, 690f, 690-692, 691f
testicular self-examination education and, 693-694, 694f
urinary function assessment in, 694
of mouth, 362-366, 362-366f
musculoskeletal, 577-607
of adolescent, 603, 603f
of aging adult, 604-605, 605f
ankle and foot and, 592-594, 593f, 594f
cervical spine and, 580, 580f
documentation and critical thinking in, 607
elbow and, 582-584, 583f, 584f
hip and, 588f, 588-589
of infant, 598-600, 599f, 600f
inspection in, 577
joint palpation in, 578
knee and, 589-592, 589-592f
muscle testing in, 578
patient preparation for, 577
of pregnant woman, 604, 604f
of preschool and school-age children, 601f, 601-603, 602f
range of motion assessment in, 578
shoulder and, 581f, 581-582, 582f
spine and, 594-598, 595-598f
temporomandibular joint and, 579f, 579-580
wrist and hand and, 584-587, 584-587f
of neurologic system, 632-666
cerebellar function assessment in, 637-639, 638f, 639f
coordination and skilled movements in, 640f, 640-641, 641f
cranial nerve testing in, 633-636, 634-636f
deep tendon reflexes testing in, 645-649, 646-649f
documentation and critical thinking in, 665-666
infant and, 651t, 651-657, 652-657f
muscle inspection and palpation in, 636-637, 637f
neurologic recheck and, 660-663, 661-663f
patient preparation for, 632-633
preschool and school-age children and, 657-660, 658f
sensory system assessment in, 641-645, 642-644f
superficial reflexes testing in, 650, 650f, 651f
of nose, 359-361, 359-361f
in nutritional assessment, 186-193
anthropometric measures in, 187-190f, 187-191
clinical signs of malnutrition and, 186t
infants and children and, 191, 193
laboratory studies and, 191-192
serial assessment in malnourished individual and, 193
in pain assessment, 168
of peripheral vascular system and lymphatics, 506-518
of aging adult, 517
arm inspection and palpation in, 506-509, 507-509f
documentation and critical thinking in, 518
of infants and children, 516-517
leg inspection and palpation in, 509-516, 510-516f
of pregnant woman, 517
of pregnant woman, 806-821
abdominal inspection and palpation in, 809f, 809-810, 810f
auscultation of fetal heart tones in, 813, 813f
bimanual examination in, 815, 815f
blood pressure measurement in, 819
breasts in, 808, 808f
documentation and critical thinking in, 820-821
general survey in, 806-807
heart in, 808
Leopold's maneuvers in, 810-813, 811-813f
lungs in, 808
mouth in, 807
neck in, 807
neurologic system in, 809
patient preparation in, 806
pelvimetry in, 816f, 816-819, 817t, 818f
peripheral vasculature in, 808-809

Physical examination (*Continued*)
routine laboratory and radiologic imaging studies in, 819
skin in, 224, 807, 807f
speculum examination in, 814, 814f
of sinuses, 361, 361f
of skin, 211-228
of adolescent, 223, 224f
of aging adult, 224-226, 224-226f
edema and, 215
of infants and children, 220-223, 220-223f
inspection and palpation of nails in, 218f, 218-219, 219f
inspection of hair in, 217
lesions and, 216-217, 217f
mobility and turgor of skin and, 215, 215f
moisture of skin and, 214
of pregnant woman, 224
skin color and, 211t, 212f, 212-214, 213f
teaching skin self-examination in, 219, 219f
temperature of skin and, 214
texture of skin and, 215
thickness of skin and, 215
vascularity and bruising and, 216, 216f
of throat, 366f, 366-367
Physical growth
developmental history of, 61
as index of child's general health, 145
Physical neglect, 104t
Physical performance measurement, 832-834
Physical Performance Test, 832
Physiologic cryptorchidism, 696
Physiologic cup, 283f
Physiologic fourth heart sound, 491t
Physiologic jaundice, 222
Physiologic third heart sound, 490t
Pica, 534
PID; *See* Pelvic inflammatory disease
Pigeon toes, 602
Pigment crescent, 300
Pigmentation, 212, 212f
aging adult and, 224, 224f
changes in, 207
newborn and, 220
Pigmented nevus, 538
Pilar cyst, 273t
Pilonidal cyst, 720t
Pinguecula, 306, 307f
Pink eye, 317t
Pinna, 323
Piskacek sign, 815
Pitting edema, 215, 513f, 513-514
in heart failure, 486t
Pitting of nails, 249t
Pituitary gland, 623f
Placenta, 795-796
Placing reflex, 657, 657f
Plantar grasp, 655, 655f
Plantar reflex, 650, 651f
Plantar wart, 616t
Plaque, 232t
Plasma glucose, 191
Platypelloid pelvis, 816, 817t
Pleura, 415, 415f
Pleural cavity, 414
Pleural effusion, 450t
Pleural friction rub, 424, 443t, 444t
Pleximeter, 116
Plexor, 116
Plugged milk duct, 408t
Pneumocystis jiroveci pneumonia, 451t
Pneumonia
lobar, 448t
Pneumocystis jiroveci, 451t
Pneumothorax, 451t
Point location test, 645
Point of maximal impulse, 474
Polio, 614t
Polycyclic skin lesion, 231t
Polydactyly, 600, 613t
Polyhydramnios, 823t
Polyp
cervical, 755t
of ear, 345t
nasal, 361, 374t
rectal, 722t
Pons, 623, 623f

Poorly controlled pain, 169t
Popliteal aneurysm, 524t
Popliteal artery, 500, 500f
Popliteal pulse, 511f, 511-512, 512f
Popliteal vein, 501, 501f
Port-wine stain, 238t
Position testing, 643, 643f
Positional deformity of infant leg, 598
Positioning
for anus, rectum, and prostate examination, 713, 713f
for cardiovascular assessment, 470
of examination table, 119, 119f
for female genitourinary examination, 733f, 733-735, 734f
infant and, 122-123, 123f
for nose, mouth, and throat examination, 359
for pediatric otoscopic examination, 335, 335f
toddler and, 123
Positive signs of pregnancy, 796
Positive spleen percussion, 542
Post polio knee abnormality, 614t
Postcentral gyrus, 622f
Posterior auricular lymph node, 255, 255f, 261f
Posterior axillary lien, 413, 414f
Posterior cervical lymph node, 255, 255f, 261f
Posterior chamber, 280f, 282, 282f
Posterior column tract, 624, 624f, 642, 642f
Posterior fontanel, 256, 256f
Posterior nail fold, 205, 205f
Posterior palpation of thyroid gland, 263, 263f
Posterior spinothalamic tract, 624, 624f
Posterior thorax
auscultation of, 427f, 427-430, 428t, 429f
landmarks of, 412, 413f
lobes of lung and, 414, 414f
percussion of, 424-426, 425f
sequence in health assessment, 767
Posterior tibial artery, 500, 500f
Posterior tibial pulse, 512, 512f
Posterior triangle, 253-254, 254f
Postnatal status in child health history, 60
Posttraumatic stress disorder, 91t
Postural vital signs, 141-142
Posture
abnormal, 676t
of aging adult, 149, 573
general survey and, 128
heart murmur and, 479
mental status assessment and, 73
nonverbal communication and, 36
Poupart ligament, 681, 681f
PQRSTU mnemonic, 51
PR interval, 461
Prealbumin, 192
Preauricular lymph node, 255, 255f, 261f
Precentral gyrus, 622f
Precocious development, 401
Precordial bulge, 482
Precordium, 455, 456f
abnormal pulsations on, 492t
palpation across, 474, 474f
physical examination of, 473-480
auscultation of heart in, 474-480f, 475-480
inspection of anterior chest in, 473
palpation across precordium in, 474, 474f
palpation of apical impulse in, 474, 474f
percussion in, 475
Prediabetes, 191
Preeclampsia, 802, 822t
Pregnancy gingivitis, 369, 369f
Pregnancy-induced hypertension, 483
Pregnant woman, 795-828
abdomen of, 531, 558t
breasts of, 386
chloasma and, 267
culture and genetics and, 799
determining weeks of gestation, 798, 798f
developmental competence and, 798-799
disorders of pregnancy and, 825t
fetal size inconsistent with dates and, 823-824t
first trimester and, 796f, 796-797
genitourinary system of, 728
health history of, 799-806
breasts and, 391
heart and, 470
nutritional assessment and, 185

Pregnant woman (*Continued*)
heart of, 464-465
lungs of, 418
malpresentations and, 826t
mouth of, 355, 369, 369f
musculoskeletal system of, 573
nose and throat of, 355
nutritional assessment and, 176, 193
peripheral vascular system and lymphatics of, 504
physical examination of, 806-821
abdominal inspection and palpation in, 809f, 809-810, 810f
auscultation of fetal heart tones in, 813, 813f
bimanual examination in, 815, 815f
blood pressure measurement in, 819
breasts in, 401, 808, 808f
documentation and critical thinking in, 820-821
general survey in, 806-807
genitourinary system in, 749
heart in, 483, 808
Leopold's maneuvers in, 810-813, 811-813f
lungs in, 437, 808
mouth in, 807
musculoskeletal system in, 604, 604f
neck in, 807
neurologic system in, 809
nutritional assessment and, 191
patient preparation in, 806
pelvimetry in, 816f, 816-819, 817t, 818f
peripheral vascular system and lymphatics in, 517, 808-809
routine laboratory and radiologic imaging studies in, 819
skin in, 224, 807, 807f
speculum examination in, 814, 814f
placenta and, 795-796
preeclampsia and, 822t
second trimester and, 797
skin of, 206
substance use assessment and, 96
third trimester and, 797-798
thyroid of, 256
uterine enlargement in, 757t
weight gain and, 798
Prehypertension, 156t
Preload, 462, 462f
Premature beat, 476
Premature thelarche, 401
Prenatal status in child health history, 60
Prepatellar bursae, 572, 572f
Prepatellar bursitis, 614t
Prepuce, 679, 680f
abnormalities of, 702t
Presbycusis, 327, 328
Presbyopia, 284, 288
Preschool child
developmental history of, 61
female genitourinary examination in, 747
interview of, 38-39
musculoskeletal system of, 601f, 601-603, 602f
neurologic examination of, 657-659, 657-660, 658f
positioning for physical examination, 124, 124f
preparation for physical examination, 124f, 124-125
sequence of health assessment, 125, 777-780
weight measurement in, 143, 143f
Prescription medication abuse, 94, 100
Present health or history of present illness
adult, 50-51
pediatric, 60
Presentation of fetus, 810
Pressure overload, 492t
Pressure ulcer, 236t
Presumptive signs of pregnancy, 796
Presystole, 458, 459t
Preterm infant, 823t
Preterm labor, 825t
Pretibial edema, 513, 513f
Prevention
of brain injury, 267
of hypertension, 156t
of osteoporosis, 606
of stroke, 664
Priapism, 703t
Primary contact dermatitis, 243t
Primary hypertension, 156t
Primary open-angle glaucoma, 285
Primary skin lesion, 216, 232-233t
Primigravida, 796
Primipara, 796
Priority setting, 5, 5t
Privacy, interview and, 30
Probable signs of pregnancy, 796
Problem-centered database, 7-8
Professional interactions, 43
Professional jargon, 35-36
Profile sign, 506
Progesterone, pregnancy and, 796
Projectile vomiting, 561t
Prolapse
rectal, 721t
uterine, 754t
Pronation, 566, 567f
Pronator drift, 660
Proprioception, 624
Prostate, 680f, 709-724
abnormalities of, 723t
of infants and children, 711
palpation of, 715-716, 716f
structure and function of, 710f, 711
Prostate cancer, 723t
genetic factors in, 711
screening for, 697
Prostate-specific antigen, 697, 711
Prostatitis, 723t
Prosthetic valve sounds
aortic valve, 489t
mitral valve, 490t
Protein-calorie malnutrition, 197t
Protein malnutrition, 197t
Proteinuria in preeclampsia, 822t
Protodiastolic filling, 458, 459f
Protraction, 566, 567f
Protruding eyes, 312t
Protuberant abdomen, 536f
Pruritus, 207-208
Pruritus ani, 721t
PSA; *See* Prostate-specific antigen
Pseudofolliculitis, 207
Pseudoptosis, 306, 306f
Pseudostrabismus, 304, 304f, 311t
Psoriasis, 245t
Psychiatric mental illness, 71
Psychological abuse, 104t
Psychological neglect, 104t
Pterygium, 306, 318t
Ptosis, 313t, 633
Puberty
breast development during, 388
estrogen and, 726
male sexual development and, 681-683, 682t
prostate gland and, 711
Pubic hair, 538, 682t
Pubic lice, 217
Pubic symphysis, 529f
Public distance, 44t
Pulmonary artery, 456, 457f
Pulmonary changes from poorly controlled pain, 169t
Pulmonary circulation, 455, 456f
Pulmonary embolism, 452t
Pulmonary function status, 433-434
Pulmonary veins, 456, 457f
Pulmonic area for heart auscultation, 475f
Pulmonic regurgitation, 497t
Pulmonic stenosis, 494t
Pulmonic valve, 457f, 458
Pulsation in abdomen, 538
Pulse, 500
carotid artery, 462, 463f
in heart failure, 486t
jugular venous, 462, 463f
measurement of, 134f, 134-135
aging adult and, 149
infants and children and, 147
sites in arm and leg for, 500f
of pregnant woman, 483
variations in, 519t
Pulse deficit, 476
Pulse oximeter, 150, 150f, 434
Pulse pressure, 136, 136t
Pulsus alternans, 519t
Pulsus bigeminus, 519t
Pulsus bisferiens, 519t
Pulsus paradoxus, 519t
Puncta, 280, 280f
Puncture, forensic term, 109t
Pupil, 280f, 282, 282f
abnormalities of, 315t
inspection of, 295-296, 296f
of newborn, 305-306
responses in neurologic recheck, 662, 662f
Pupillary light reflex, 283, 284f, 295
Pure tone audiometer, 333
Purpura, 240t
Purpuric lesion, 240t
Purulent otitis media, 347t
Pustule, 233t
Pyloric stenosis, 561t
Pyramidal tract, 624-625, 625f
Pyrosis, 532

Q

QRS complex, 461
Quadrants
of abdomen, 530, 530f
of breast, 385, 385f
Quadriceps muscle, 572, 572f
Quadriceps reflex, 648, 648f
Quadriplegia, 670t
flaccid, 676t

R

Race
blood pressure and, 136
colorectal cancer and, 711
differences in eyes, 285
prostate cancer and, 711
stroke and, 629
Radial artery, 500, 500f
palpation of
for blood pressure measurement, 138, 138f
for pulse, 134, 134f
Radial pulse, 507, 507f
Radiocarpal joint, 570, 571f
Radiologic studies during pregnancy, 819
Radius, 570, 570f
fracture of, 611t
Rage, 85t
Range of motion, 578
of ankle and foot, 594, 594f
of cervical spine, 580, 580f
of elbow, 583f, 583-584, 584f
general survey and, 129
of hip, 588f, 588-589
infant and, 600, 600f
of knee, 591, 591f
of neck, 260
of shoulder, 581f, 581-582, 582f
of spine, 596f, 596-598, 597f
of temporomandibular joint, 579, 579f
of wrist and hand, 586, 586f
Rapid alternating movements, 640, 640f
Rapid Disability Rating Scale-2, 831-832
Rash
axillary, 391
of breast, 390
diaper, 209, 241t
female external genitalia, 752t
health history of, 208
in infants and children, 241-242t
in Lyme disease, 244t
neonatal, 221, 221f
Raynaud's phenomenon, 520t
Reactive airway disease, 449t
Reason for seeking care
in adult health history, 50
in child health history, 59
in older adult health history, 66
Rebound tenderness, 551, 551f
Recent memory, mental status and, 75
Receptive aphasia, 84t, 622
Rectal ampulla, 709, 710f
Rectal bleeding, 712
Rectal lesion, 559t
Rectal prolapse, 721t
Rectal temperature measurement, 133, 147
Rectocele, 754t
Rectosigmoid junction, 710f
Rectouterine pouch, 710, 710f, 726, 727f
Rectovaginal examination, 746-747, 747f
Rectovesical pouch, 710, 710f

Rectum, 529f
abnormalities of, 722t
colorectal cancer screening and, 718
female, 727f
health history of, 712-713
of infants and children, 711
physical examination of, 713-719
documentation and critical thinking in, 718-719
in infants and children, 717
inspection of perianal area in, 713
palpation in, 714f, 714-715, 715f
patient positioning for, 713, 713f
stool examination in, 716-717
sequence in health assessment, 771, 776
structure and function of, 709-710, 710f
Rectus abdominis, 527
Red eye, 286
Red reflex, 298
Reference lines of chest, 412-413, 413f, 414f
Referred pain, 162
abdominal, 559, 559t
Reflection in interview, 33-34
Reflex arc, 626f, 626-627
Reflexes
deep tendon, 645-649, 646-649f
of newborn, 654-657, 654-657f
pathologic, 677t
pediatric health history of, 631
superficial, 650, 650f, 651f
upper and lower motor neuron lesions and, 673t
visual, 283-284, 284f
Reflexive sympathetic dystrophy, 173t
Refugee, 12
Reinforcement test, 646, 646f
Religion, 15, 16, 17f
Religious dietary practices, 178t
Remodeling of bone, 573
Remote memory, mental status and, 75
Renal artery stenosis, 562t
Renal calculi, 700t
Renal colic, 559t
Renal system; *See* Genitourinary system
Residual volume, 418
Resonance, 425
Resonant percussion sound, 117t
RESPECT mnemonic, 27t
Respectful care, 12
Respiration
effect on heart sounds, 460
measurement of, 135, 135t
in aging adult, 150
in infants and children, 148, 148f
mechanics of, 416, 417f
patterns of, 441-442t
Respiratory center in brain, 416
Respiratory hygiene, Standard Precautions and, 121t
Respiratory infection, 420
Respiratory rate of newborn, 436
Respiratory system
bedside assessment of, 789
changes from poorly controlled pain, 169t
health history of
adult, 55
child, 62
older adult, 67
Rest
adult and, 57
child and, 64
older adult and, 68
Rest tremor, 671t
Retention cyst, 375t
epididymal, 705t
Retina, 281, 282, 282f
visual field loss and, 316t
visual pathway and, 282-283, 283f
Retinal detachment, 316t
Retinal vessels, 282, 283f
abnormalities of, 320-321t
ophthalmoscopic inspection of, 301, 301f
Retracted drum, 346t
Retraction, 566, 567f
Retraction of breast, 393f, 393-394, 394f, 404t
Retroflexed uterus, 745f
Retroverted uterus, 745f
Review of systems
in adult health history, 54-57
in child health history, 62-63
in older adult health history, 67
pregnant woman and, 804-805
Rheumatoid arthritis, 574-575, 608t, 612t
Rhinitis, 360, 374t
Rhinorrhea, 356
Rhonchal fremitus, 424, 443t
Rhythm of pulse, 135
Rib, 411
Rickets, 199t
Right atrium, 457, 457f
Right lymphatic duct, 502, 503t
Right subclavian vein, 503f
Right ventricle, 457, 457f
Rigidity, 669t
Ringworm, 243t, 246t
Rinne tuning fork test, 333
Risk diagnoses, 5
Ritalin; *See* Methylphenidate
ROM; *See* Range of motion
Romberg test, 334, 638-639, 639f
Rooting reflex, 654, 654f
Rotation, 566, 567f
Rotator cuff, 568
Rotator cuff tear, 609t
Rotter's lymph node, 385f
Round window, 324f
Rounded abdomen, 536f
Rubella, 242t, 803
Rubeola, 242t
Rugae
scrotal, 680, 680f
vaginal, 726, 727f

S

Sacral promontory, 529f
Sacral spinal nerves, 628f
Sacral vertebrae, 628f
Safety
adolescent psychosocial interview and, 65f
brain injury prevention and, 267
older adult driver and, 840-841, 841t
setting for physical examination and, 120-121, 121t
Sagittal suture, 251, 252f, 256f
Saline mount, 742
Saliva, 354
Salivary gland, 253, 253f, 354, 354f
Salmon patch, 222, 223f
SBAR framework, 793
Scabies, 248t
Scale, 233t
Scalp
lesion of, 217
ringworm of, 246t
Scaphoid abdomen, 536f
Scapula, 412, 413f
Scapular line, 413, 413f
Scar, 235t
surgical, 538, 538f
Scarred drum, 348t
Schizophrenia, 87t
School-age child
developmental history of, 61
female genitourinary examination in, 747
interview of, 39
musculoskeletal system of, 601f, 601-603, 602f
neurologic examination of, 657-660, 658f
positioning for physical examination, 125, 125f
preparation for physical examination, 125
respiratory rate of, 135t
sequence of health assessment, 125, 780
weight measurement in, 143, 143f
Scientific theory of illness, 21
Scissors gait, 672t
Sclera, 280f, 281, 282f
inspection of, 293, 293f
of newborn, 305
subconjunctival hemorrhage and, 317t
Scleral crescent, 300
Scleral icterus, 293
Scleroderma, 215, 277t
Scoliosis, 441t, 617t
screening for, 603, 603f
Scorbutic gums, 198t
Scotoma, 285, 316t
Scratch test, 542
Screening
for alcohol problems, 98
for anxiety disorders, 77, 77f
for breast cancer, 402
for cervical cancer, 729, 750
for child sexual abuse, during male genitourinary examination, 686
for colorectal cancer, 718
for cystic fibrosis, 799
Denver II, 79
for depression, 77
for elder abuse and neglect, 107, 107t
for glaucoma, 308
for hearing deficit, 333
for human immunodeficiency virus, 803
for intimate partner violence, 105-107, 106f, 107f
musculoskeletal, 577
for prostate cancer, 697, 711
for scoliosis, 603, 603f
for suicidal thoughts, 77
Scrotal tongue, 380t
Scrotum, 680-681
abnormalities of, 704-706t
health history of, 685
of infant, 695f, 695-697, 696f
physical examination of, 690f, 690-692, 691f
Tanner's sexual maturity ratings and, 682t
Seasonal rhinitis, 357
Sebaceous cyst, 342t
Sebaceous gland, 204f, 205
Sebaceous hyperplasia, 226, 226f
Seborrheic dermatitis, 247t
Seborrheic keratosis, 225, 225f
Second heart sound, 460, 460f, 476f, 476-477, 477f, 488t
Second-level priority problems, 5-6
Second trimester, 797
Secondary skin lesion, 216, 233-235t
Secondhand smoke, 438
Sedatives abuse, 101t
Seizure, 670t
child and, 631
history of, 630
pregnant woman and, 805
Self-care
in breast care, 390
in dental health, 358
in ear health, 329
in eye health, 286
in female genitourinary health, 729
in foot care, 517
high-fiber foods and, 713
in musculoskeletal health, 576
nutritional assessment and, 183
in respiratory care, 420
in skin care, 209, 219, 219f
testicular self-examination and, 693-694, 694f
Self-concept
adult and, 57
older adult and, 68
Self-esteem
adult and, 57
older adult and, 68
Self-examination
breast, 398-399, 399f
skin, 219, 219f
testicular, 693-694, 694f
Semi-coma, 83t
Semicircular canal, 324f, 325
Semilunar valve, 458
Seminal vesicle, 680f, 710f, 711
Senile angioma, 216, 216f
Senile cataracts, 319t
Senile keratosis, 225, 225f
Senile lentigines, 224, 224f
Senile purpura, 206
Senile tremor, 267, 659
Sensorineural hearing loss, 326
Sensory cortex, 624
Sensory function assessment, 641-645, 642-644f
facial nerve and, 635, 635f
glossopharyngeal and vagus nerves and, 635
newborn and, 654
trigeminal nerve and, 634, 634f
Sensory loss, 675-676t
Sensory pathways, 623-624, 624f

Index

Sensory perception, age-related changes in, 72
Sentinel tag, 720t
Septum, nasal, 360, 361f
Sequence of health assessment, 763-785
  abdomen and, 768
  chest and, 767
  documentation and critical thinking in, 781-785
  ears and, 765
  eyes and, 765
  female breasts and, 767
  female genitalia and, 772
  general appearance and, 764
  head and face and, 765
  health history and, 764
  heart and, 767, 768
  inguinal area and, 768
  lower extremities and, 769, 770
  male breasts and, 768
  male genitalia and, 771
  male rectum and, 771
  measurement and, 764
  mouth and throat and, 766
  musculoskeletal system and, 769, 770-771
  neck and, 766
  neck vessels and, 768
  neurologic system and, 769-770
  newborn and infant and, 123, 772-776
  nose and, 766
  school-age child, adolescent, and aging adult and, 780
  skin and, 765
  toddler and preschool child and, 124, 777-780
  upper extremities and, 767
  vital signs and, 765
Serous otitis media, 346t
Serum albumin, 192
Serum cholesterol, 466
Serum proteins, 192
Serum transferrin, 192
Serum triglycerides, 192
Sessile rectal polyp, 722t
Setting for physical examination, 118-119, 119f
  safety of, 120-121, 121t
Setting-sun sign, 304
Seventh-Day Adventists, dietary practices of, 178t
Sex
  blood pressure and, 136
  differences in pain behavior, 163
  general survey and, 127
Sex maturity ratings
  female, 727, 727t
  male, 681-682, 682t
Sexual abuse, 103
  screening for, 731
Sexual activity
  adolescent and, 65f, 687, 731-732
  aging male and, 683
  female and, 730-731
  male history of, 685-686
Sexual health
  adult health history of, 56
  child health history of, 63
  older adult health history of, 67
Sexual orientation, 45
Sexually aggressive person, interview of, 41-42
Sexually transmitted infection
  female history of, 731
  genital herpes in, 701t
  genital warts in, 701t, 742, 753t
  gonorrhea in, 742, 757t
  male history of, 686
Shaken baby syndrome, 105
Shallow anterior chamber, 318t
Shifting abdominal dullness, 544f, 544-545
Shingles, 244t
Short-form McGill Pain Questionnaire, 166
Short leg gait, 673t
Short Michigan Alcoholism Screening Test, 98-99, 99t
Short Portable Mental Status Questionnaire, 835t
Short process of malleus, 324, 325f
Shortness of breath, 467
  in heart failure, 486t
  history of, 419
Shoulder, 568-570, 569f, 570f
  abnormalities of, 609t
  physical examination of, 581f, 581-582, 582f
Sigmoid colon, f, 528f, 710f
Sign, 50, 441t
Silence
  cultural variations in, 47
  during interview, 33
Simian crease, 600
Sinoatrial node, 461, 461f
Sinus, 352, 352f, 353f
  adult health history of, 55
  child health history of, 62
  physical examination of, 361, 361f
Sinus arrhythmia, 135, 476
Sinus pain, 357
Sinusitis, 374t
Six-minute distance walk, 434
Skeletal muscle, 566, 567f
Skeleton, 565, 573
Skene's gland, 725, 726f
Skilled movements testing, 640f, 640-641, 641f
Skin, 203-250
  of abdomen, 537f, 537-538, 538f
  of aging adult, 206
  of arms and legs, 505
  artificial tanning and, 227
  biocultural differences in, 206-207
  of breast, 392
  cutaneous reflexes and, 648, 648f
  of ear, 330
  hair abnormalities and, 246-248t
  health history of, 207-211
    adult, 55
    child, 62
  of infants and children, 205-206
  lesions of, 230-245t
    in children, 241-242t
    common, 243-245t
    malignant, 245t
    pressure ulcer in, 236t
    primary, 232-233t
    secondary, 233-235t
    shapes and configurations of, 230-231t
    trauma or abuse-related, 237t
    vascular, 238-240t
  malnutrition and, 186t
  nail abnormalities and, 248-250f
  pain in, 168
  physical examination of, 211-228
    of adolescent, 223, 224f
    of aging adult, 224-226, 224-226f
    documentation and critical thinking in, 227-228
    edema and, 215
    of infants and children, 220-223, 220-223f
    inspection and palpation of nails in, 218f, 218-219, 219f
    inspection of hair in, 217
    lesions and, 216-217, 217f
    mobility and turgor of skin and, 215, 215f
    moisture of skin and, 214
    of pregnant woman, 224
    skin color and, 211t, 212f, 212-214, 213f
    teaching skin self-examination in, 219, 219f
    temperature of skin and, 214
    texture of skin and, 215
    thickness of skin and, 215
    vascularity and bruising and, 216, 216f
  of posterior chest, 422
  of pregnant woman, 206, 807, 807f
  scleroderma and, 277t
  sensory assessment and, 641
  sequence in health assessment, 765
  structure and function of, 203-205, 204f
Skin cancer, 245t
  artificial tanning and, 227
Skin color, 212f, 212-214, 213f
  of aging adult, 224, 224f
  changes in legs and feet, 514-515, 515f
  detecting changes in, 229-230t
  determination of, 204
  of ear, 330
  external variables influencing, 211t
  general survey and, 128
  of infant, 220
  of posterior chest, 422
Skin self-examination, 219, 219f
Skin tag
  aging adult and, 225, 225f
  on ear, 327t
Skinfold thickness, 188f, 188-189, 191
Skull, 251
  infant, 264-266, 265f
  neonatal, 256, 256f
  physical examination of, 259-260
  pilar cyst and, 266
Sleep
  adult and, 57
  older adult and, 68, 841-842, 842t
Small intestine, 528f, 529, 529f
  referred abdominal pain and, 559t
Small saphenous vein, 501, 501f
SMAST-G questionnaire, 98-99, 99t
Smear, cervical, 740f, 740-742, 741f
Smell, altered, 357
Smokeless tobacco, 370
Smoking
  appearance and behavior in, 101t
  cardiovascular heart disease and, 466
  fetal brain and, 417
  oral cavity health history and, 358
  pregnant woman and, 803
  secondhand smoke exposure and, 438
Smoking history, 420
Smooth, glossy tongue, 379t
Snellen E chart, 303, 303f
Snellen Eye Chart, 287-288, 288f
Snout reflex, 677t
Snuff, 370
Social distance, 44t
Social domain in functional assessment of older adult, 836-837, 837t
Social phobia, 90t
Socialization, 16
Soft palate, 353f, 354
Solar keratosis, 225, 225f
Solid viscera, 527
Solitary thyroid nodule, 272t
Somatic pain, 162, 172f
Somatotopic organization, 625
Somnolent level of consciousness, 83t
Sore throat, 357, 381t
Sound production during percussion, 117, 117f, 117t
Source of history
  in adult health history, 50
  in child health history, 59
South American heritages
  culture-bound syndromes in, 26t
  health and illness beliefs and practices in, 25t
Space, cultural considerations in, 44, 44t
Spastic hemiparesis, 672t
Spasticity, 669t
  neurologic examination of newborn and, 652
Specific gravity, 694
Specific phobia, 90t
Speculum examination, 737f, 737-738, 738f
  of pregnant woman, 814, 814f
Speech
  general survey and, 129
  mental status assessment and, 74
Speech disorders, 84t
Sperm, 681
Spermatic cord, 680f, 680-681, 681f
Spermatocele, 705t
Sphenoid bone, 252f
Sphenoid fontanelle, 256f
Sphenoid sinus, 352, 352f, 353f
Sphincter, anal, 709, 710f
Sphygmomanometer, 137
Spider angioma, 239t
Spina bifida, 600, 618t
Spinal accessory nerve, 627f
  abnormalities of, 669t
  testing of, 636, 636f
Spinal cord, 623, 623f
  hemisection or transection of, 675t
  pain and, 160, 160f
Spinal nerves, 628, 628f
Spine, 568, 568f, 569f
  abnormalities of, 617t
  of aging adult, 604-605, 605f
  ankylosing spondylitis and, 608t
  of infant, 600, 600f, 776
  physical examination of, 580, 580f, 594-598, 595-598f
  of preschool and school-age children, 601

Spinothalamic tract, 624, 624f
testing of, 642, 642f
Spinous process, 412, 413f, 568, 569f
palpation of, 595
Spiritual assessment in older adult, 842-843
Spiritual resources, 57-58
Spirituality, 15-16
Spirometer, 434
Spleen, 504, 504f, 528f, 529, 529f
enlarged, 563t
palpation of, 549, 549f
peritoneal friction rub and, 562t
Splenic dullness, 542, 542f
Splenomegaly in heart failure, 486t
Splinter hemorrhage, 249t
Splitting of second heart sound, 460, 477f, 477-478, 483, 488t
Spontaneous pneumothorax, 451t
Sputum, 419
Squamocolumnar junction, 726
Squamous cell carcinoma, 245t
Stab wound, 109t
Standard drink, 94t
Standard Precautions, 121t
Stapes, 324, 324f
Star angioma, 239t
Stationary hand percussion, 116, 116f
Stature, 128
Steatorrhea, 712
Stensen's duct, 354, 354f, 365
Steppage gait, 672t
Stepping reflex, 657, 657f
Stereognosis, 624, 644, 644f
Sternal angle, 412, 412f
Sternomastoid muscle, 252f, 253, 253f, 254f
Sternum, 411, 412, 412f
Stethoscope, 118, 118f
STI; *See* Sexually transmitted infection
Stomach, 528f, 529
referred abdominal pain and, 559t
Stomatitis, 375t
Stool
blood in, 712
examination of, 716-717
impaction of, 722t
of newborn, 553, 711
Storkbite, 222, 223f
Strabismus, 286, 304, 311t
Straight leg raises, 597f, 597-598, 662, 662f
Strawberry mark, 238t
Stress, blood pressure and, 137
Stress management
adult and, 58
child and, 64
older adult and, 68
Stretch marks, 206, 224, 797, 807, 807f
Stretch reflexes, 645-649, 646-649f
Striae, 537, 537t
Striae gravidarum, 206, 224, 797, 807, 807f
Stridor, 437, 445t
Striking hand percussion, 116-117, 117f
Stroke, 629
abnormal facies in, 277t
mental status assessment in, 73
prevention of, 664
Stroke volume, 134, 462
Structural scoliosis, 617t
Stupor, 83t
Stye, 314t
Subacromial bursa, 568, 569f
Subacromial bursitis, 609t
Subconjunctival hemorrhage, 317t
Subcultural groups, 14
Subcutaneous nodule, 583, 610t
Subcutaneous tissue, 204, 204f
Subjective data, 2
health history and, 49
interview and, 29
Subjective Global Assessment, 180t, 180-181
Subjective vertigo, 329
Sublingual gland, 253, 253f, 354, 354f
Subluxation, 577
of elbow, 582
Submandibular gland, 253, 253f, 354, 354f
Submandibular lymph node, 255, 255f, 261f
Submental lymph node, 255, 255f, 261f
Subscapular lymph node, 385, 385f, 503f
Substance abuse
alcohol and, 93, 94t, 95t
clinical signs of, 100-101t
defining of, 94
diagnosis of, 95t, 95-96
functional assessment and, 58
interview and, 41
nutritional assessment and, 183
prescription medications and, 100
Substance dependence, 95t
Substance use assessment, 93-102
aging adult and, 96
alcohol use and abuse and, 93, 94t
clinical signs of substance use disorders and, 100-101t
diagnosis of substance abuse and, 95t, 95-96
health history in, 96-99, 97t, 99t
illicit drug use and, 94
normal range of findings in, 99-100
pregnant woman and, 96
prescription medication abuse and, 100
Substantia gelatinosa, 160, 160f
Succussion splash, 561t
Sucking reflex, 654, 677t
Sucking tubercle, 368
Suicide
adolescent psychosocial interview and, 65f
screening for suicidal thoughts and, 77
Sulcus, 622f
Summary translation, 47
Summation sound, 491t
Sunken eyes, 313t
Superficial central axillary lymph node, 503f
Superficial cervical lymph node, 255, 255f, 261f
Superficial palmar arch, 500, 500f
Superficial reflexes, 626, 650, 650f, 651f
Superficial submandibular lymph node, 503f
Superficial varicose veins, 523t
Superior oblique muscle, 281f
Superior rectus muscle, 281f, 282f
Superior turbinate and meatus, 352, 352f, 361
Superior vena cava, 456, 457f
Supernumerary nipple, 386, 386f, 393, 393f, 808
Supination, 566, 567f
Supine Achilles reflex, 647, 647f
Supine quadriceps test, 648, 648f
Supraclavicular lymph node, 255, 255f, 261f
Suprapatellar pouch, 572
Suprapubic area, 530, 530f
Suprasternal notch, 412, 412f
Surfactant, 416-417
Surgical history
of adult, 52
of child, 60
of older adult, 66
Surgical scar, 538, 538f
Suspensory ligaments of breast, 384f, 385
Sutures, 251
Swallowing difficulty, 258, 358, 532, 631
Swan-neck deformity, 612t
Sweat gland, 204f, 205
Sweating, 206-207, 214
Swelling
of arms or legs, 505
of breast, 390
of eye, 286
of head or neck, 258-259, 272-273t
of joint, 577, 609t
of knee, 613t
of temporomandibular joint, 579
Swimmer's ear, 341t
Symmetric chest expansion, 422f, 422-423, 431, 431f
Symmetric corneal light reflex, 311t
Symmetry
of abdomen, 537, 537f
of body, 128
Symphysis pubis, 528f, 680f
Symptom, 50
Synapse, 622
Syncope, 630
Syndactyly, 600, 613t
Synovial fluid, 566
Synovial joint, 565-566, 566f
Synovitis, 614t
Syphilitic chancre, 702t, 752t
Systemic circulation, 455, 456f
Systole, 458, 459f
Systolic extra heart sounds, 489t
Systolic murmur, 478
Systolic pressure, 136, 136t

T

T wave, 461, 461f
Tachycardia, 134
in heart failure, 486t
in infant, 481
Tachydysrhythmias, 466
Tachypnea, 442t
Tactile discrimination, 644
Tactile fremitus, 423f, 423-424, 432, 432f, 443t
Tail of Spence, 383, 384f, 385, 385f
Talipes equinovarus, 618t
Tandem walking, 638, 638f
Tangential lighting, 118
Tanner sexual maturity ratings
female, 727, 727t
male, 681-682, 682t
Tanner staging of breast development, 386, 387t
Tanning, skin cancer risk and, 227
Taping of interview, 31-32
Target lesion, 231t
Tarsal plate of eyelid, 280, 280f
Taste alteration, 358
Taste bud, 355
Tearing, 286
Tears, 280
Teeth
abnormalities of, 376-377t
baby bottle tooth decay and, 376t
deciduous, 355f
of older adult, 355-356, 370, 370f
permanent, 354, 355f
physical examination of, 362, 363f
Telangiectases, 239t
Telegraphic speech, 38
Temperature measurement, 132-134
in aging adult, 149
in infants and children, 146-147, 147f
Temperature of skin, 214
Temperature perception testing, 642
Temporal artery, 253, 253f, 500
Temporal bone, 252f
Temporal lobe, 622, 622f
Temporalis muscle, 252f
Temporomandibular joint, 252f, 566, 567f
inspection of, 260
physical examination of, 579f, 579-580
Tennis elbow, 610t
Tenosynovitis, Achilles, 615t
Tension headache, 257, 270t
Tension pneumothorax, 451t
Tenting of skin, 222
Terminal hair, 205, 217
Testicular self-examination, 693-694, 694f
Testicular torsion, 704t
Testis, 680f, 680-681
Testosterone, 683
Tetralogy of Fallot, 493t
Texture
of hair, 217
of skin, 215
aging adult and, 225, 225f
neonatal, 222
Thalamus, 622, 623f
lesion of, 676t
Thenar eminence, 584
atrophy of, 611t
Thickness of skin, 215
in aging adult, 226
neonatal, 222
Thigh pressure, 142, 142f
Third heart sound, 460-461, 490t
Third-level priority problems, 6
Third trimester, 797-798
Thoracic aneurysm, 524t
Thoracic aorta, 457f
Thoracic cage, 411, 422
Thoracic cavity, 414f, 414-416, 415f
Thoracic duct, 502, 503t
Thoracic spinal nerves, 628f
Thoracic vertebrae, 628f

Thorax, 411-454
abnormal tactile fremitus and, 443t
of aging adult, 418
biocultural differences in diseases of, 418
common respiratory conditions and, 447-453t
configurations of, 440-441t
dermatomes of, 628f
health history of, 418-421
of infants and children, 416-417, 417f
mechanics of respiration and, 416, 417f
physical examination of, 421-439
of acutely ill person, 437
adventitious lung sounds and, 429-430, 444-445t
of aging adult, 437
auscultation of anterior chest in, 433
breath sounds and, 427t, 427-429, 428t, 429f
diaphragmatic excursion and, 426, 426f
documentation and critical thinking in, 438-439
of infants and children, 434-437, 435f, 435t, 436f
inspection of anterior chest in, 430-431
inspection of thoracic cage in, 422
measurement of pulmonary function status in, 433-434
palpation of anterior chest in, 431f, 431-432, 432f
percussion of anterior chest in, 432f, 432-433
percussion of lung fields in, 424-426, 425f
of pregnant woman, 437
symmetric chest expansion and, 422f, 422-423
tactile fremitus and, 423f, 423-424
voice sounds and, 430, 446t
position and surface landmarks of, 411-413, 412f, 413f
of pregnant woman, 418
respiration patterns and, 441-442t
sequence in health assessment, 767
thoracic cavity and, 414f, 414-416, 415f
Thought content, 72
abnormalities of, 87t
mental status assessment of, 76
Thought processes, 72
abnormalities of, 86t
mental status assessment of, 76-78, 77f
Thready pulse, 135, 519t
Threat of violence during interview, 42
Thrill, 474, 492t
Throat, 354
abnormalities of, 381f
health history of, 357-358
adult, 55
child, 62
of infants and children, 368-369
physical examination of, 366f, 366-367
sequence in health assessment, 766, 774, 780
Thrush, 365, 378t
Thumb, dermatomes of, 628f
Thymus gland, 504, 504f
Thyroglossal duct cyst, 266
Thyroid cartilage, 254-255
Thyroid disease, pregnant woman and, 805
Thyroid gland, 254f, 254-255
congenital hypothyroidism and, 274t
hyperthyroidism and, 276t
hypothyroidism and, 276t
nodules of, 272t
physical examination of, 263f, 263-264, 264f
of pregnant woman, 256
Thyroid hormones, 254
Thyroid-stimulating hormone, 797
Thyroxine, 254
Thyroxine-binding prealbumin, 192
Tibial torsion, 599
Tibial tuberosity, 572, 572f
Tibiotalar joint, 572, 573f
Tic, 670t
Tinea capitis, 246t
Tinea corporis, 243t
Tinea cruris, 701t
Tinea pedis, 243t
Tinea versicolor, 244t
Tinel sign, 587, 587f
inetti Gait and Balance Evaluation, 834
innitus, 329
TMJ; *See* Temporomandibular joint
Tobacco smoke exposure, 438
Toddler
female genitourinary examination in, 747
normal respiratory rate of, 135t
Toddler (*Continued*)
positioning for physical examination, 123
preparation for physical examination, 123-124
sequence of health assessment, 124, 777-780
Toeing in, 602
Tolerance, term, 100t
Tongue, 353f, 354
abnormalities of, 379-380t
of child, 368, 368f
hypoglossal nerve testing and, 636
magenta, 198t
malnutrition and, 186t
mucocele of, 375t
physical examination of, 363f, 363-364, 364f
tremor of, 367
Tongue-tie, 379t
Tonic neck reflex, 266, 656, 656f
Tonsil, 352f, 353f, 354, 504, 504f
physical examination of, 366, 366f
Tonsillitis, 381t
Toothache, 357
Tophi, 342t, 615t
Torsion
testicular, 704t
tibial, 599
Torticollis, 272t
Torus palatinus, 356, 365, 365f
Total arm length, 190
Total health database, 7
Touch
cultural considerations in, 48
nonverbal communication and, 37, 37t
Toxic alopecia, 246t
Trachea, 262, 263f, 415f, 416
Tracheal shift, 263
Tracheobronchial tree, 415f, 416
Traction alopecia, 246t
Tragus, 324f
Transcultural expression of illness, 25-27, 26t
Transduction phase of pain, 160-161, 161f
Transection of spinal cord, 675t
Transillumination, 361
of scrotum, 692
Transmission phase of pain, 161, 161f
Transverse diameter of pelvic outlet, 818, 818f
Transverse lie and shoulder presentation, 826t
Transversus muscle, 528f
Trapezius muscle, 252f, 253, 254f
Trauma
of breast, 390
lesions caused by, 237t
Traumatic alopecia, 109t, 246t
Traumatic pneumothorax, 451t
Tremor, 671t
history of, 630, 632
of tongue, 367
Trendelenburg sign, 602, 602f
Triceps reflex, 647, 647f
Triceps skinfold thickness, 188f, 188-189
Trichomoniasis, 756t
Trichotillomania, 247t
Tricuspid area for heart auscultation, 475f
Tricuspid regurgitation, 495t
Tricuspid stenosis, 496t
Tricuspid valve, 457f, 458
Trigeminal nerve, 627f
abnormalities of, 668t
infant reflexes and, 651t
testing of, 634, 634f
Triglycerides
metabolic syndrome and, 200t
nutritional assessment and, 192
Triiodothyronine, 254
Trisomy 21, 274t
Trochlear nerve, 627f
abnormalities of, 668t
infant reflexes and, 651t
testing of, 633
Tropia, 290
Tuberculosis, 418, 452t
Tumor, 232t
abdominal, 558t
testicular, 705t
Tunica vaginalis, 680f
Tuning fork test, 333
Tunnel vision, 308
Turbinates, 352, 361
Turgor of skin, 215, 215f
in aging adult, 226, 226f
neonatal, 222
TWEAK questions, 98
Twenty-four hour recall, 180
Two-point discrimination, 645
Tympanic membrane, 323-324, 324f, 325f
abnormal otoscopic findings of, 346t
abnormalities of, 346-348t
physical examination of, 332f, 332-333
vibratility of, 336
Tympanic membrane temperature measurement, 133-134
in infants and children, 146-147, 147f
Tympanostomy tube, 347t
Tympany percussion sound, 117t
Type 2 diabetes mellitus
cardiovascular heart disease and, 466-467
obesity and, 532

U

Ulcer, 234t
aphthous, 378t
decubitus, 236t
leg, 522t
peptic, 559t
venous, 510
Ulna, 570, 570f
Ulnar artery, 500, 500f
Ulnar deviation or drift, 612t
Ulnar nerve, 570f
Ulnar pulse, 507, 507f
Umbilical area, 530, 530f
Umbilical hernia, 552, 560t
Umbilicus, 537
Umbo, 324, 325f
Unauthorized resident, 12
Undernutrition, 175
Upper extremity examination, 581-587
elbow and, 582-584, 583f, 584f
sequence in health assessment, 767, 775, 779
shoulder and, 581f, 581-582, 582f
wrist and hand and, 584-586, 584-586f
Upper motor neuron, 626, 626f
lesions of, 277t, 673t
Upper respiratory infection, 357
Upward palpebral slant, 313t
Ureter, 529f, 680f
Ureteral colic, 559t
Urethra, 679, 680f
Urethral caruncle, 753t
Urethral meatus, 725, 726f, 727f
Urethral stricture, 700t
Urethritis, 700t, 753t
Urgency, 684
Urinalysis
in male genitourinary examination, 694
during pregnancy, 819
Urinary frequency, 684
Urinary system; *See also* Genitourinary system
health history of
adult, 56
child, 63
older adult, 67
problems of
female, 730
male, 700t
Urinary tract infection during pregnancy, 802, 805
Urine
color of, 684-685, 685f
discolorations of, 699t
output in heart failure, 486t
Urticaria, 232t
Uterine fibroids, 758t, 824t
Uterus, 529f, 726, 727f
of aging woman, 728
bimanual examination of, 744-745, 745f
enlargement of, 757-758t
during pregnancy, 796, 796f, 809f, 809-810, 810f
prolapse of, 754t
Uvula, 353f, 366, 366f
bifid, 356, 381t

V

V wave of jugular venous pulse, 463
Vaccine, human papillomavirus, 732, 750

Vagina, 726, 727f
of aging woman, 728
pediatric vulvovaginitis and, 760t
vulvovaginal inflammations and, 756-757t
Vaginal bleeding during pregnancy, 801, 825t
Vaginal discharge
history of, 730
newborn and, 748
during pregnancy, 728, 814
Vaginal examination, 732-751
of adolescent, 748-749
of aging adult, 749-750
bimanual examination in, 742-746, 743-746f
documentation and critical thinking in, 750-751
of infants and children, 747-748
inspection of cervix and os in, 739f, 739-740
inspection of external genitalia in, 735f, 735-737, 736f
obtaining cervical smears and cultures in, 740f, 740-742, 741f
patient preparation and equipment for, 732-733, 733f
positioning for, 733f, 733-735, 734f
of pregnant woman, 749, 814, 814f
rectovaginal examination and, 746-747, 747f
speculum examination in, 737f, 737-738, 738f
vaginal wall inspection in, 742
Vaginal orifice, 725, 726f
Vaginal pool, 740, 740f
Vaginitis, 756t
Vagus nerve, 627f
abnormalities of, 669t
infant reflexes and, 651t
testing of, 635
Validation of data, 2, 4
Valves of heart, 456-458, 457t
Valves of Houston, 709, 710f
Valvular defect-related murmur, 494-497t
Vancomycin-resistant *Enterococcus*, 120
Varicella, 242t
Varicocele, 705t
Varicose veins, 514, 514f, 523t
during pregnancy, 797, 808
Variety of fetus, 810
Vas deferens, 680f, 681
Vascular disorders of external eye, 317t
Vascular lesion, 238-240t
Vascular resistance, 137, 137f
Vascular sounds, 539f, 539-540, 540f, 562t
Vascular spider, 224
Vascular system, 499-525
of aging adult, 504-505
arteries in, 499-500, 500f
health history of, 505-506
adult, 55
older adult, 67
of infants and children, 504, 504f
lymphatics and, 502-504, 503f, 504f
peripheral vascular disease and
in arms, 520t
arterial, venous, or diabetic leg ulcers in, 522t
in legs, 523t
pain profiles in, 521t
peripheral arterial disease in, 524t
physical examination of, 506-518
of aging adult, 517
documentation and critical thinking in, 518
of infants and children, 516-517
inspection and palpation of arms in, 506-509, 507-509f
inspection and palpation of legs in, 509-516, 510-516f
of pregnant woman, 517
of pregnant woman, 504
variations in pulse contour and, 519t
veins in, 501, 501f
venous flow and, 501-502, 502f
Vascularity of skin, 216, 216f
neonatal, 222, 223f
Veins, 501, 501f
varicose, 514, 514f, 523t
Vellus hair, 204-205, 217
Venous flow, 501-502, 502f
Venous hum, 482, 562t
Venous lake, 239t
Venous leg ulcer, 522t
Venous stasis, 510, 522t
Venous ulcer, 510, 522t
Ventricle, 457
Ventricular gallop, 478, 490t
Ventricular septal defect, 493t
Verbal communication, 30
Vernix caseosa, 205, 222
Vertebra prominens, 251, 412, 413f
Vertebrae, 411, 568, 569f
Vertebral canal, 623
Vertebral foramen, 569f
Vertebral line, 413, 413f
Vertex presentation, 826t
Vertigo, 258, 326, 329, 630
Vesicle, 232t
Vesicular sounds, 428, 428t
Vestibular apparatus, 334
Vestibular gland, 726
Vestibule
of ear, 324f, 325
female urethral, 725, 726f
nasal, 351, 351f, 352f
Vestibulocochlear nerve, 324f, 627f
infant reflexes and, 651t
Vibratility of tympanic membrane, 336
Vibration perception testing, 643, 643f
Vibrissae, 352
Video recording of interview, 31-32
Violence
domestic violence assessment, 103-114
assessment for risk of homicide in, 112, 112f
child abuse and neglect and, 108
cultural considerations in, 113
definitions in, 103-104, 104t
denial in, 113
documentation in, 110f, 110-111, 111f
elder abuse and neglect and, 107, 107t
health effects of violence and, 104-105
history in, 108
intimate partner violence and, 105-107, 106f, 107f
physical examination in, 108-110, 109t
threat during interview, 42
Viscera, 527-529
Visceral pain, 162, 172f
Visceral pleura, 415, 415f
Visceral reflexes, 626
Viscosity of blood, 137, 137f
Vision difficulty, 285
Vision loss, 286
glaucoma and, 308
Visual acuity
infants and children and, 302f, 302-303
older adult and, 284, 306
testing of, 287-289, 288f
Visual fields, 282-283, 283f
infants and children and, 303
loss of, 316t
testing of, 289f, 289-290, 290f
Visual pathways, 282-283, 283f
Visual reflexes, 283-284, 284f
Vital capacity, 418
Vital signs, 132-150
of aging adult, 149-150
in bedside assessment, 788-789
blood pressure in, 136f, 136-142
common errors in, 141t
factors affecting, 136-137, 137f
Korotkoff sounds and, 139t
measurement in arm for, 138f, 138-140
measurement in thigh for, 142, 142f
documentation of, 153
of infants and children, 146-148, 147f, 148f
in neurologic recheck, 663
orthostatic or postural, 141-142
of pregnant woman, 483
pulse in, 134f, 134-135
respirations in, 135, 135t
sequence in health assessment, 765, 772
temperature in, 132-134
Vitamin D, pregnant woman and, 803
Vitiligo, 212, 212f
Vocal fremitus, 423f, 423-424, 432, 432f
Vocal resonance, 430
Vocal sounds, 430, 446t
Voice, nonverbal communication and, 37
Volume overload, 492t
Voluntary guarding, 546
Voluntary muscle, 566, 567f
Vomiting
in heart failure, 486t
history of, 533
during pregnancy, 531, 801, 825t
projectile, 561t
VRE; *See* Vancomycin-resistant *Enterococcus*
VSD; *See* Ventricular septal defect
Vulvovaginal inflammations, 756-757t
Vulvovaginitis, 760t

W

Waddling gait, 673t
Waist circumference, 132, 132f, 187
in metabolic syndrome, 200t
Waist-to-hip ratio, 187
Wart, plantar, 616t
Water-hammer pulse, 519t
Watering of eye, 286
Weak, thready pulse, 519t
Weakness
facial nerve assessment and, 635, 635f
history of, 575, 630-631
in upper and lower motor neuron lesions, 673t
Weber tuning fork test, 333
Weight
adolescent and, 535
after bariatric surgery, 200t
blood pressure and, 136
loss of, 193
measurement of, 130, 130f
in aging adult, 149, 149f
in infants and children, 143, 143f
in nutritional assessment, 182, 191
overweight child and, 534
during pregnancy, 191, 798
Wellness diagnoses, 5
Wen, 273t
Wernicke's aphasia, 84t
Wernicke's area, 84t, 622, 622f
Wet dream, 687
Wet prep, 742
Wheal, 232t
Wheeze, 430, 445t
in heart failure, 486t
Whispered voice test, 333, 446t
White head, 223, 224f
Why questions, 36
Withdrawal, 100t
Withdrawal delirium, 101t
Woman; *See* Female
Women's Experience with Battering Scale, 113
Wood's light examination, 217, 217f
Word comprehension, 75
Word salad, 86t
Working phase of interview, 32-34, 33t, 34f
Wound, forensic term, 109t
Wrist, 570, 571t
abnormalities of, 611-613t
physical examination of, 584-587, 584-587f
Wryneck, 272t

X

X descent of jugular venous pulse, 463
Xanthelasma, 307, 307f
Xerosis, 210, 225
Xerostomia, 358
Xiphoid process, 412f, 528f

Y

Yeast infection, 728
Yin/yang theory, 21

Z

Zosteriform skin lesion, 231t
Zygomatic bone, 252f
Zygomaticus muscle, 252f

Index

Assessment Terms: English and Spanish			
English	Spanish	English	Spanish
HISTORY TAKING			
How do you feel?	¿Cómo se siente?	Nausea	Náusea
Good	Bien	Does eating make you vomit?	¿El comer le hace vomitar?
Bad	Mal	How are your stools?	¿Cómo son sus heces?
Let me see …	Déjeme ver …	Are they regular?	¿Son regulares?
Let me feel your pulse.	Déjeme tomarle el pulso.	Have you noticed their color?	¿Se ha fijado en el color?
Is your memory good?	¿Es buena su memoria?	Are you constipated?	¿Está estreñido?
Do you have any pain in your head?	¿Le duele la cabeza?	Do you have diarrhea?	¿Tiene diarrea?
Did you fall? How did you fall?	¿Se cayó? ¿Cómo se cayó?	Have you any difficulty urinating?	¿Tiene dificultad en orinar?
Did you faint?	¿Se desmayó?	Do you urinate involuntarily?	¿Orina sin querer?
Have you ever had fainting spells?	¿Ha tenido desmayos alguna vez?	Are any of your limbs swollen?	¿Están hinchados algunos de sus miembros?
Have you slept well?	¿Ha dormido bien?	How long have they been swollen like this?	¿Desde cuándo están hinchados así?
Have you any difficulty in breathing?	¿Tiene dificultad al respirar?	Have you ever had:	¿Alguna vez usted ha padecido:
How long have you been coughing for?	¿Desde cuándo tose Ud?	cancer	del cáncer
Do you cough a little?	¿Tose poco?	diabetes	de la diabetes
Do you expectorate much?	¿Escupe mucho?	heart disease	de una enfermedad cardíaca
What is the color of your expectorations?	¿De qué color es el esputo?	respiratory disease	de una enfermedad respiratoria
Is your hearing affected?	¿Está afectado el oído?	cirrhosis	de la cirrosis
Do you have ringing in the ears?	¿Le zumban los oídos?	depression	de la depresión
When did your eyesight begin to fail you?	¿Desde cuándo ha disminuido su visión?	Do you smoke?	¿Fuma usted?
Do you sometimes see double?	¿Ve las cosas doble algunas veces?	How much do you smoke each day?	¿Cuánto fuma a diario?
Tell me what number this is.	Dígame qué número es éste.	When did you stop smoking?	¿Cuándo dejó de fumar?
Tell me what letter this is.	Dígame qué letra es ésta.	Do you drink?	¿Toma bebidas alcohólicas?
Do things look cloudy to you?	¿Ve las cosas nubladas?	How often do you drink?	¿Cuántos tragos habitualmente?
Can you see clearly?	¿Puede ver claramente?		
Better at a distance?	¿Mejor a cierta distancia?		